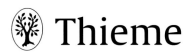
Thieme

Differential Diagnosis in Conventional Radiology

Francis A. Burgener, MD
Professor of Radiology
University of Rochester
Medical Center
Rochester, NY
USA

Martti Kormano, MD
Formerly Professor and Chairman
Department of Radiology
University of Turku
Turku
Finland

Tomi Pudas, MD
Department of Radiology
University of Turku
Turku
Finland

3rd edition

2190 illustrations

Thieme
Stuttgart · New York

© 2008 Georg Thieme Verlag,
Rüdigerstraße 14, 70469 Stuttgart, Germany
http://www.thieme.de

Thieme New York, 333 Seventh Avenue,
New York, NY 10001, USA
http://www.thieme.com

Typesetting by primustype Hurler GmbH,
D-73274 Notzingen
Printed in Germany by Grammlich, Pliezhausen

ISBN 978-3-13-656103-4 (TPS, Rest of World)
ISBN 978-1-58890-275-7 (TPN, The Americas)   1 2 3 4 5 6

Preface

Conventional radiography remains the backbone of our specialty despite the advent of newer and possibly more exciting imaging techniques such as computed tomography, magnetic resonance imaging, and, most recently, positron emission tomography. In contrast to many of these newer methods, conventional radiography is practiced not only by radiologists but also by a large number of clinicians and surgeons. With each examination, one is confronted with radiologic findings that require interpretation in order to arrive at a general diagnostic impression and a reasonable differential diagnosis. To assist the film interpreter in attaining this goal, this book is based upon radiographic findings, unlike most other textbooks in radiology that are disease oriented. Since many diseases present radiographically in a variety of manifestations, some overlap in the text is unavoidable. To minimize repetition, the differential diagnosis of a radiographic finding is presented in tabular form whenever feasible. Most tables list not only the various diseases that may present radiologically in a specific pattern, but also describe in succinct form other characteristically associated radiographic findings and pertinent clinical data. Radiographic illlustrations and drawings are included to demonstrate visually the radiographic features under discussion.

The transition from film to digital radiography has had a great impact on conventional radiology since the publication of the last edition. This change, however, did not affect the way radiologic diagnoses are ascertained. Since the publication of the last edition the names of a few disorders have changed (e. g., histiocytosis X is now known as Langerhans cell histiocytosis) and a few new diseases have been recognized (e. g., femoroacetabular impingement and severe acute respiratory distress syndrome or SARS). These facts were taken into consideration in this new edition. The chapters "Localized Bone Lesions" and "Joint Diseases" have been completely rewritten and newly illustrated since I took them over from Dr. Kormano. The chapter "Trauma and Fractures" has also undergone a major overhaul with the inclusion of specific fracture sites. Several chapters in the abdominal section considered to be of lesser importance in the age of computed tomography have been eliminated to comply with the publisher's request not to alter the overall volume of text. The chapter on mammography has been deleted because the subject could no longer be covered with the required depth to be useful in the framework of this text. In the remaining chapters, text has been updated, many illustrations replaced, and a large number of new illustrations added.

A "changing of the guard" has also taken place. Since Dr. Martti Kormano's professional endeavors no longer include clinical radiology, he was not able to take on the task of updating his original contributions to the text. Fortunately for all concerned, he was able to find in Dr. Tomi Pudas a very talented young radiologist to take over the revision of his original chapters.

I hope this new revised third edition will be as well received as the previous editions. The concept of an imaging pattern approach in tabular form rather than a disease-oriented text was introduced in 1985 with the first edition of *Differential Diagnosis in Conventional Radiology* and has since been adopted by many authors. I take this as a compliment; after all, imitation is the sincerest form of flattery.

This book is meant for physicians with some experience in conventional radiology who wish to strengthen their diagnostic acumen. It is a comprehensive outline of radiographic findings and will be particularly useful to radiology residents preparing for their specialist examination, especially since the exposure to conventional radiography during their training continuously decreased in the past in favor of newer imaging modalities. Any physician involved in the interpretation of conventional radiographs should find this book helpful in direct proportion to his or her curiosity.

It is my hope that the third edition of *Differential Diagnosis in Conventional Radiology* will prove as interesting as its predecessors to medical students, residents, radiologists, and physicians involved in the interpretation of conventional radiographs.

Francis A. Burgener, MD

Acknowledgements

It is impossible to thank individually all those who helped to prepare the third edition of this textbook. I wish to acknowledge the staff of our publisher Thieme, in particular Dr. Clifford Bergman and Mr. Gert A. Krüger. I also appreciate the willingness of Ms. Annie Hollins and Ms. Stefanie Langner, both of whom were recently assigned by Thieme to this project to deal with my old-fashioned style relying mainly on paper, pencils, hard copy, and the telephone.

I am deeply indebted to Dr. Gertrud Gollman, Steinach am Attersee, Austria, who translated the last edition of this text into German and suggested many alterations and corrections which have been incorporated into this new edition.

My gratitude goes to all the radiologists whose cooperation made available illustrative cases to complement the original collection or to replace older illustrations. I am indebted to Drs. Steven P. Meyers, Johnny U.V. Monu, and Gwy Suk Seo, all staff members of the University of Rochester Radiology Department, and to the former residents Drs. John M. Fitzgerald and Wael E.A. Saad for providing selected cases.

I greatly appreciate the invaluable contributions to this project by two former faculty members of our department.

Dr. Jovitas Skucas, professor emeritus, has provided me with a substantial number of gastrointestinal cases from his exquisite collection to replace or complement the illustrations in this text. Following his retirement, Dr. Robert F. Spataro donated his entire urogenital teaching file to me, from which I have selected a few outstanding cases for this new edition.

I also wish to express many thanks to Jill Derby, Iona Mackey, and Marcella Maier for their assistance in preparing the references and to Shirley Cappiello for her general assistance. Last, but not least, I am most grateful to Alyce Norder who left the University and me after 30 years for the richness of the industry. She is the only person capable of deciphering my longhand and, as in the past, did a superb job in typing, editing, and proofreading the manuscript of the new edition of this text. Despite her heavy workload as executive assistant in her new endeavor, Alyce was kind enough to perform this task in her spare time, for which I am deeply grateful.

Finally I appreciate the support of my wife Therese, who has generously given her precious family time for the preparation of this book.

Francis A. Burgener, MD

I would like to express my deepest gratitude to honorary professor Martti Kormano who invited me to carry on his work in this new edition. I continue to admire the massive amount of work that he and Dr. Burgener originally put into the project in the early nineteen-eighties. The hundreds of hours which Dr. Kormano and I have spent together editing this edition have been a great pleasure. It was a fascinating time in my life.

I especially want to thank Drs. Kimmo Mattila and Seppo Koskinen for introducing me to musculoskeletal radiology, and for their extraordinary teaching and support. Many thanks also belong to Drs. Erkki Svedström, Risto Elo, and Peter B. Dean for encouraging me on my way in the field of radiology. The many fascinating discussions I have had with Drs. Seppo Kortelainen and Teemu Paavilainen brought me much delight, on non-radiological topics as much as on professional subjects.

I also express sincere thanks to the staff of the publishers, Thieme, especially to Dr. Clifford Bergman and Mr. Gert Krüger. Finally, much gratitude is due to Mr. Markku Livanaien for his valuable assistance with technical questions, and to Ms. Pirjo Helanko for all her help with general matters. Many other individuals helped in various ways with this project, and though I cannot name them all, I am grateful for their contributions.

Tomi Pudas, MD

Contents

Abbreviations

ABC	aneurysmal bone cyst	IP	interphalangeal (joint)
AC	acromioclavicular (joint)	IV	intravenous
ACTH	adrenocorticotropic hormone	IVC	inferior vena cava
AIDS	acquired immune deficiency syndrome	L	left
ALL	acute lymphoblastic leukemia	LA	left atrium
AML	acute myeloblastic leukemia	LCH	Langerhans cell histiocytosis
ANCA	antineutrophil cytoplasmotic autoantibodies	LE	lupus erythematosus
ANT	anterior	LIP	lymphoid interstitial pneumonitis
AP	anteroposterior	LL	lower lobe
APVR	anomalous pulmonary venous return	LLL	left lower lobe
ARDS	acute respiratory distress syndrome	LLQ	left lower quadrant
ATN	acute tubular necrosis	LUL	left upper lobe
AV	arteriovenous	LUQ	left upper quadrant
AVF	arteriovenous fistula	LV	left ventricle
AVM	arteriovenous malformation	M	male
AVN	avascular necrosis	MAI	*Mycobacterium avium intracellulare*
BOOP	bronchiolitis obliterans organizing pneumonia	MCP	metacarpophalangeal (joint)
BPOP	bizarre parosteal osteochondromatous proliferation	MFH	malignant fibrous histiocytoma
		ML	middle lobe
Bx	biopsy	MPS	mucopolysaccharidosis
Ca	calcium	MR	magnetic resonance
CAD	coronary artery disease	MRI	magnetic resonance imaging
CAM	cystic adenomatoid malformation	MS	multiple sclerosis
CHF	congestive heart failure	MTP	metatarsophalangeal (joint)
CID	cytomegalic inclusion disease	NHL	non-Hodgkin lymphoma
CLL	chronic lymphatic leukemia	NUC	nuclear medicine
CMV	cytomegalovirus	PA	posteroanterior
CNS	central nervous system	PAPVR	partial anomalous pulmonary venous return
COP	cryptogenic organizing pneumonia	PATH	pathology
COPD	chronic obstructive pulmonary disease	PAVM	pulmonary arteriovenous malformation
CPP	calcium pyrophosphate dihydrate crystals	PCP	*Pneumocystis carinii pneumonia*
CPPD	calcium pyrophosphate dihydrate deposition disease	PDA	patent ductus arteriosus
		PE	pulmonary embolism
CRMO	chronic recurrent multifocal osteomyelitis	PET	positron emission tomography
CT	computed tomography	PFFD	proximal femoral focal deficiency
D	disease	PIP	proximal interphalangeal (joint)
DD	differential diagnosis	PNET	primitive neuroectodermal tumor
DDH	development dysplasia of the hip	PO	per oral
DIC	dissemination intravascular coagulation	PTLD	post-transplantation lymphoproliferative disorder
DIP	desquamative interstitial pneumonitis		
DIP	distal interphalangeal (joint)	PVNS	pigmented villonodular synovitis
DISH	diffuse idiopathic skeletal hyperostosis	RA	right atrium
DISI	dorsal intercalated segmental instability	RA	rheumatoid arthritis
EAC	external auditory canal	RBC	red blood cell
EG	eosinophilic granuloma	RDS	respiratory distress syndrome
F	female	RES	reticuloendothelial system
FAI	femoroacetabular impingement	RLL	right lower lobe
GE	gastroesophageal	RSD	reflex sympathetic dystrophy
GI	gastrointestinal	RUL	right upper lobe
GIP	giant cell interstitial pneumonitis	RV	right ventricle
GIST	gastrointestinal stromal tumor	SARS	severe acute respiratory distress syndrome
HAD	calcium hydroxyapatite crystals	SC	sternoclavicular (joint)
HADD	calcium hydroxyapatite crystal deposition disease	SI	sacroiliac (joint)
		SLAC	scapholunate advanced collapse
Hb	hemoglobin	SLE	systemic lupus erythematosus
HD	Hodgkin disease	STT	scaphotrapeziotrapezoidal
HIV	human immunodeficiency virus	TAPVR	total anomalous pulmonary venous return
HRCT	high-resolution CT	TB	tuberculosis
Hx	history	TFC	triangular fibrocartilage
IAC	internal auditory canal	TFCC	triangular fibrocartilage complex
IM	intramuscular		

TMJ	temporomandibular joint	US	ultrasound
TNM	tumor-node-metastasis	UVJ	ureterovesical junction
UIP	usual interstitial pneumonitis	VCUG	voiding cystourethrogram
UPJ	ureteropelvic junction	VISI	volar intercalated segmental instability

Bone

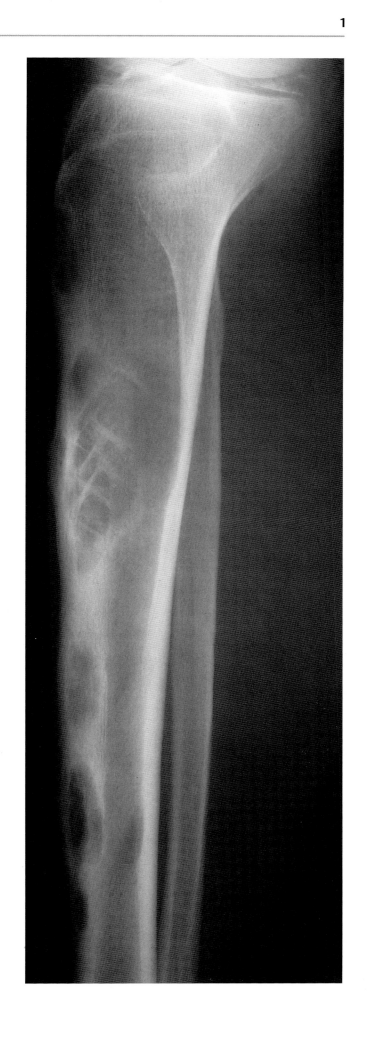

1 Osteopenia

Osteopenia is defined as a decrease in bone density caused by reduced bone formation and/or increased bone resorption. Reduction in bone formation may result from either inadequate matrix formation (e.g., disuse osteoporosis and protein deficiency of any etiology) or inadequate matrix calcification (e. g., osteomalacia). Primary hyperparathyroidism is an example of too much resorption of both bone matrix and mineral. A combination of these causes results in the undermineralization present in the majority of osteopenic disorders. Furthermore replacement of bone matrix by benign or malignant bone proliferation (e.g. thalassemia, multiple myeloma and leukemia) or bone marrow disease (e.g. metastases, infections and storage diseases) may also result in osteopenia.

Approximately 30% of the bone mineral must be lost before a difference in the bone density can be detected by conventional radiography. More sensitive techniques useful for earlier detection and quantification of osteopenia include axial computed tomography and photon or x-ray absorptiometry. It should also be borne in mind that the normal bone density changes with age, increasing from infancy to age 35–40 and then progressively decreasing at the rate of 8% per decade in women and 3% in men.

The radiographic findings of osteopenia are loss of bone density and cortical thinning. Osteopenia may either be generalized or localized, and its differential diagnosis is discussed separately in Tables 1.1 and 1.2.

In *osteoporosis,* a combination of loss of bone density and cortical thinning may result in an apparent increase in density of the cortex and vertebral endplates, that appear as thin, sharp lines (Figs. 1.1 and 1.2). Bone resorption occurs preferentially in the transverse trabeculae, while the trabeculae along stress lines are accentuated. Resorption of all trabeculae in a vertebral body produces the "empty box" sign. As a result of compression fractures the vertebral body may depict a depressed endplate or become wedge-shaped, biconcave (fish vertebra) or uniformly compressed (pancake vertebral body). Cartilaginous (Schmorl's) nodes are caused by displacement of a portion of the intervertebral disc into the vertebral body. With the exception of osteogenesis imperfecta, bones do not bend in osteoporosis. A predisposition towards fractures, however, exists in the brittle bones, especially in the vertebral bodies, ribs, hips and wrists. Fracture healing is delayed and the callus formation poor. Abundant callus formation in osteopenic bones may occur, however, with exogenous (iatrogenic) or endogenous (Cushing's syndrome) hypercortisolism and osteogenesis imperfecta. In osteoporosis, serum calcium, phosphorus and alkaline phosphatase are normal.

In *osteomalacia,* a nonspecific loss of bone density is often the only radiographic sign. Blurring of both cortical margins and trabeculae results in a "ground glass" appearance of the involved bone and is more characteristic. This is often most obvious in the vertebral bodies. In the skull, a blurred mottled appearance similar to hyperparathyroidism is characteristic. Bones are softened and have a tendency to bend resulting in deformities commonly found in the thorax, vertebral column, pelvis and extremities. Pseudofractures (Looser's zones or Milkman's syndrome) occur frequently and represent infractions with incomplete healing. They are found in

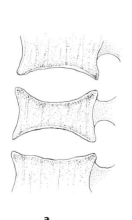
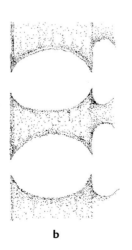
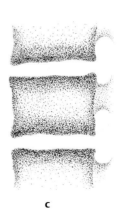

a   b   c

Fig. 1.1 **Osteopenia. a** *Osteoporosis*: Deossified, biconcave vertebral bodies (fish vertebrae) with thin but dense-appearing endplates and prominent vertical trabeculae. The superior endplates typically are affected more severely. **b** *Osteomalacia*: Uniform deossification with loss of trabecular detail ("ground-glass appearance") and compression fractures. Fish vertebrae tend to be smoother than in osteoporosis and involve superior and inferior endplates with equal severity. **c** *Hyperparathyroidism*: A "rugger jersey spine" is usually only found in secondary hyperparathyroidism (renal osteodystrophy), whereas primary hyperparathyroidism depicts a bony texture similar to osteomalacia.

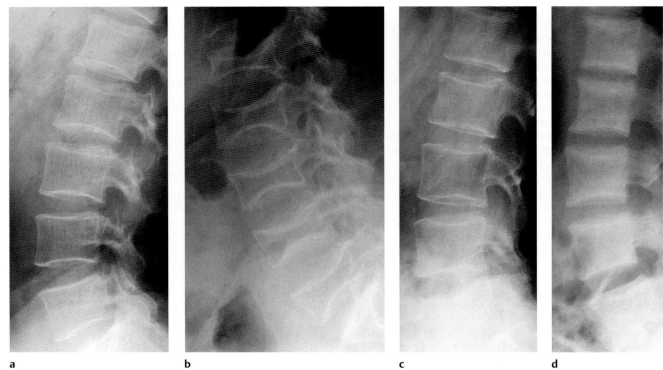

a   b   c   d

Fig. 1.**2   Osteoporosis (a), osteomalacia (b) and hyperparathy-roidism (c and d).** Osteoporosis (**a**): Thin sharply defined end-plates with accentuation of the vertical trabeculae are seen. Osteomalacia (**b**): Uniformly biconcave vertebral bodies with poorly defined endplates and blurred trabeculae are seen. *Primary hyperparathyroidism* (**c**): Thin poorly defined endplates with blurring of the trabecular pattern in the vertebral bodies are seen. *Secondary hyperparathyroidism* (**d**): Blurring of the trabecular pattern in the vertebral bodies is associated with thickening and sclerosis of the superior and inferior endplates ("rugger jersey spine").

the scapula (lateral margin), ribs, clavicle, ischial and pubic rami, femur (especially medial aspect of the neck), and other long bones. Characteristic laboratory findings in osteomalacia include a slightly low to normal serum calcium, a low serum phosphorus and an elevated alkaline phosphatase.

Bony lesions are found in less than half of the patients with *hyperparathyroidism*. Subperiosteal resorption along the radial margin of the phalanges is virtually pathogno-monic. These erosions occur most often in the proximal and middle phalanges of the index and middle finger (Fig. 1.**3**). Absorption of the terminal tufts and cortical striations ("tun-neling of the cortex") are commonly associated with this condition. Endosteal resorption occurs in long bones. Re-sorption may also be evident in the acromial ends of the

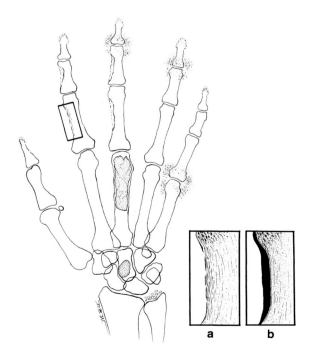

a   b

Fig. 1.**3   Hyperparathyroidism** of the hand. Subperiosteal re-sorption and cortical striations, usually best seen on the radial mar-gins of proximal and middle phalanges of second and third finger. A magnified view of these findings is demonstrated in insert a, whereas insert b shows a normal cortex for comparison. Additional findings include resorption of the tufts, periarticular soft-tissue calcifications, brown tumors (third metacarpal and capitatum), and joint cartilage calcification (often in the triangular fibrocar-tilage between ulna and corresponding part of the proximal carpal row).

clavicles, the sacroiliac joints, the symphysis, in the calcaneus at the insertion of the plantar fascia and in the ribs (usually in their upper borders). The bone is softened resulting in secondary deformities such as basilar impression in the skull and kyphoscoliosis. Cyst-like lesions and so-called brown tumors occur in tubular and flat bones. While brown tumors heal after removal of the parathyroid adenoma and may eventually even become sclerotic, cysts remain unchanged after treatment. Granular deossification of the skull results in a "salt and pepper" appearance. Resorption of the lamina dura around the teeth is commonly present. Soft tissue calcifications (especially arterial and para-articular), joint cartilage calcifications (especially menisci and the triangular fibrocartilage in the wrist), nephrocalcinosis, and nephroureterolithiasis are common features of hyperparathyroidism. Pancreatitis, peptic ulcer disease and gallstones may also be associated. Classic laboratory findings in primary hyperparathyroidism include a high serum calcium, a low serum phosphorus, and an elevated alkaline phosphatase in the presence of bone disease.

An increased bone density is often associated with secondary hyperparathyroidism (renal osteodystrophy). In these cases thickening of the superior and inferior endplates of the vertebral bodies can result in a "rugger jersey spine".

The skeletal changes in different forms of hyperparathyroidism are identical, although brown tumors are more common in primary hyperparathyroidism, whereas osteosclerosis and extensive soft-tissue calcifications are more often found in secondary hyperparathyroidism.

Table 1.1 Differential Diagnosis of Generalized Osteopenia

Etiology	Comments
Osteoporosis	Laboratory findings: serum calcium, phosphorus and alkaline phosphatase all normal.
Senile or postmenopausal	Most common form of osteoporosis. Females affected more often and more severely than males. Compression fractures typically spare the less weight-bearing cervical and upper thoracic spine.
Disuse atrophy	Prolonged immobilization from any cause (e.g., neuromuscular disorders, cast).
Protein deficiency (e.g., malnutrition, nephrosis) (Fig. 1.4)	Pure dietary protein deficiency is rare. In underdeveloped countries, extensive osteopenia is associated with *kwashiorkor*, a marasmic protein-calorie malnutrition affecting mostly children. Protein deficiency secondary to malabsorption is more common (see under osteomalacia). Abnormal protein metabolism is the underlying cause of osteoporosis in *scurvy* (vitamin C deficiency) and different *endocrinologic disorders*.
Juvenile (idiopathic)	Between ages 8 and 14, characterized by abrupt onset of bone pain. Rare, self-limiting disorder with commonly spontaneous healing.
Osteogenesis imperfecta (Fig. 1.5)	Osteogenesis imperfecta congenita (fractures present at birth) and tarda (fractures absent at birth). Deformities resulting from recurrent fractures in later life and bone bending characteristic. Both disorders inherited.
Homocystinuria	Inherited disorder that presents radiographically as combination of osteoporosis, Marfan-like changes (e.g., arachnodactyly), and metaphyseal and epiphyseal widening.
Anemia (Fig. 1.6)	Bone marrow hyperplasia causes widening of the medullary space, cortical thinning, and trabecular resorption by pressure atrophy. Occurs in severe *iron deficiency* and *sickle cell anemia*, but is more pronounced in *thalassemia*, where a generalized cystic appearance, particularly of the flat bones, is characteristic.
Bone marrow infiltration (e.g. multiple myeloma, carcinomatosis) (Fig. 1.7)	Deossification is caused by diffuse infiltration and proliferation of tumor cells in the bone marrow resulting in endosteal erosions, cortical thinning and trabecular resorption by both pressure atrophy and destruction. While osteopenia might be the only radiologic manifestation in multiple myeloma and diffuse skeletal bony metastases, patchy osteolytic areas are often present in these conditions. Bone marrow infiltration associated with cortical thinning and trabecular resorption can also be found in reticuloses (e.g. *Gaucher's* and *Nieman-Pick disease*), *histiocytoses* and *hyperlipoproteinemias*. In children, leukemia frequently causes osteopenia.
Connective tissue disease (especially rheumatoid arthritis)	Other more characteristic radiographic findings are often associated with the disease suggesting the correct diagnosis (see Chapter 6).

(continues on page 8)

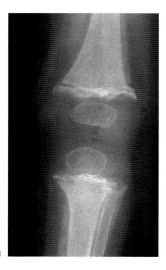

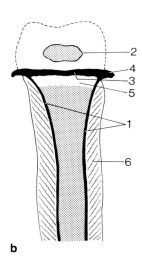

a

b

Fig. 1.**4 a, b Scurvy.** Characteristic findings include: (1) Osteopenia with markedly thinned cortex, (2) thin, dense, ring-like calcification around the epiphysis (Wimberger's line), (3) dense, linear calcifications in the distal metaphysis ("white line of Frankel"), (4) a small bone spur immediately adjoining the "white line of Frankel" (Pelkan's spur), (5) a radiolucent band proximal to the "white line of Frankel" (Trummerfeld zone), and (6) subperiosteal hemorrhage (calcifies only after therapy is instituted). Epiphyseal separation and/or fragmentation in the region of the metaphysis may also be associated.

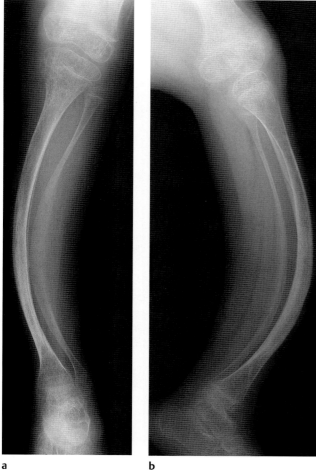

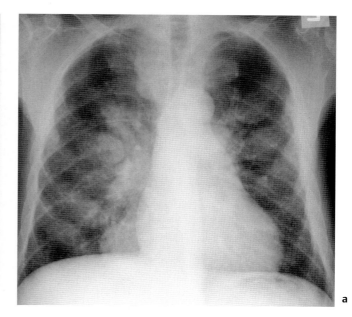

a

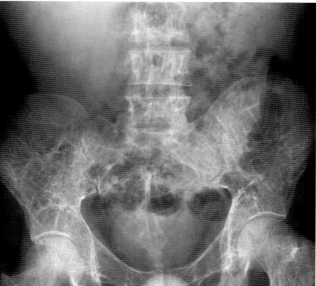

b

a   b

Fig. 1.**5 a**, **b**   **Osteogenesis imperfecta.** Diffuse osteopenia with bowing deformities of the narrowed (overconstricted) tibia and fibula shafts with flaring of the metaphyses is seen in anteroposterior (**a**) and lateral (**b**) projections.

Fig. 1.**6**   **Thalassemia major.** Chest (**a**) and pelvis (**b**). Generalized, cystic-appearing osteopenia caused by red bone marrow hyperplasia, with main involvement of the central or flat bones characteristic. Note also the bulbous widening of the anterior ends of the ribs.

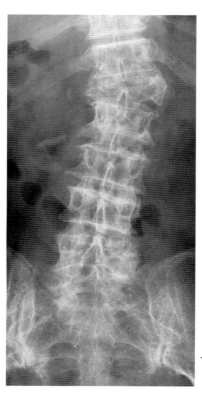

◁ Fig. 1.**7**   **Multiple myeloma** presenting as generalized osteopenia in the spine. In this case, however, extensive destruction of L1 and the destroyed left pedicle of L5 suggest the malignant process.

Table 1.1 (Cont.) Differential Diagnosis of Generalized Osteopenia

Etiology	Comments
Endocrine disorders	*Hypogonadism*: osteoporosis associated with delayed epiphyseal fusion (e.g., *Turner's syndrome, eunuchoidism*). *Cushing's syndrome*: chronic excess of glucocorticoids. *Addison's disease*: insufficiency of the adrenal cortex. *Diabetes mellitus*: osteopenia present in about 50% of patients. *Hyperthyroidism*: often associated with cortical striations best seen in metacarpal bones. See also under hyperparathyroidism in this table.
Drug-induced (e.g., steroids, heparin) (Fig. 1.8)	Steroids: large dosages over several months. Heparin: 15,000 to 30,000 units for six months or longer.
Osteomalacia **(Fig. 1.9)**	Laboratory findings in osteomalacia: serum calcium slightly low to normal; serum phosphorus low; alkaline phosphatase elevated.
Deficient absorption of calcium and/or phosphorus;	
1. vitamin D deficiency	Dietary causes, or lack of sunshine Adult: *osteomalacia*. Loss of bone density with blurring of both cortical margins and trabeculae characteristic. Bowing deformities and pseudofractures occur frequently. Children: *rickets* (Fig. 1.**10**). Most commonly found in premature infants. Develops most commonly between 6 and 12 months of age. Radiographic features include: indistinct, frayed and concave metaphyses ("cupping") with perpendicular trabeculae extending towards the epiphyseal areas. Delayed appearance of epiphyseal ossification centers with blurred margins (DD: Scurvy: sharply outlined epiphyses). Bulky growth plates in long bones result in swelling around the joints and a "rachitic rosary" at the costochondral junctions of the middle ribs.
2. Malabsorption	Diseases of the gastrointestinal tract, hepatobiliary system and pancreas associated with malabsorption are the most common cause of Vitamin D deficiency in developed countries. Rickets and osteomalacia is commonly associated with *sprue, celiac disease, Crohn's disease, scleroderma, small bowel fistulas, blind loop syndromes, small intestinal bypass surgery*, and *gastric* or *small bowel resection*.
3. Dietary calcium deficiency	Extremely rare.
Defects in renal tubular or intestinal calcium phosphate transport system:	
1. Vitamin D-resistant rickets (x-linked hypophosphatemia) and pseudo-vitamin D deficiency rickets (Figs. 1.11 and 1.12)	Proximal tubular resorption of phosphorus decreased. Inherited (X-linked dominant and autosomal recessive) disorders with similar clinical features (short stature, multiple fractures, varus or valgus deformities of the knees, bowing deformities of the long bones in the lower extremities and muscular weakness), but only the latter condition is commonly associated with convulsions. Enthesopathy in the spine may resemble ankylosing spondylitis but without erosions in the sacroiliac joints.

(continues on page 10)

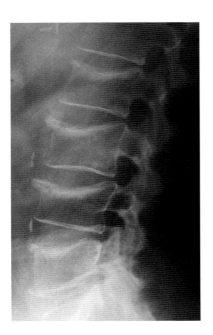

Fig. 1.8 Steroid-induced osteoporosis. Osteoporosis with thickening and sclerosis of the compressed end-plates is characteristic of exogenous or endogenous hypercortisolism.

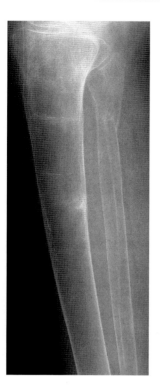

Fig. 1.**9** **Osteomalacia.** Marked demineralization with blurring of the inner cortical margins and loss of trabeculations are characteristic. Several pseudofractures are seen, presenting as sclerotic transverse lines in the tibia.

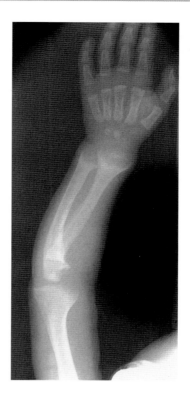

Fig. 1.**10** **Rickets.** Characteristic changes include: (1) osteopenia, (2) poorly calcified and defined epiphyses, (3) widening of the epiphyseal cartilage plate, (4) widening, cupping, and fraying of the metaphyses, (5) periosteal reactions, and (6) bowing deformities. Greenstick fractures are also commonly associated, but not present in this case.

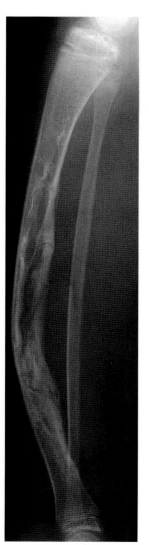

Fig. 1.**11** **Vitamin D-resistent rickets (x-linked hypophosphatemia).** Osteopenia with multiple fractures/pseudofractures and anterior bowing deformity of the tibia is seen.

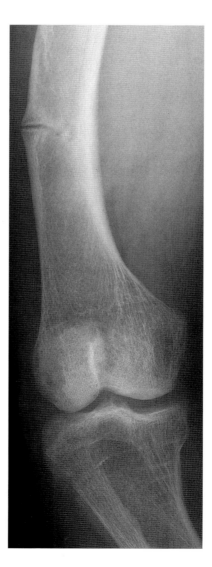

Fig. 1.**12** **Vitamin D-resistent rickets (x-lilnked hypophosphatemia).** Mild osteopnia with bowing deformity and pseudofracture in the distal femur and genu varum is seen.

Table 1.1   (Cont.) Differential Diagnosis of Generalized Osteopenia

Etiology	Comments
2. Renal tubular acidosis (Fig. 1.13)	Metabolic acidosis attributed to renal loss of alkali. Pathogenesis of osteomalacia in this condition is unclear. Commonly associated with nephrocalcinosis and nephrourolithiasis.
3. Fanconi's syndrome (De Toni-Debré-Fanconi syndrome)	Idiopathic or acquired disorder characterized by hypophosphatemia, glucosuria and amino-aciduria. The idiopathic form is often associated with *cystinosis* (widespread tissue deposition of cystine crystals). The acquired form may be secondary to *Wilson's disease* (rare familial disorder with impaired hepatic excretion of copper and characteristic pigmentation of the cornea [Kayser-Fleischer ring], *multiple myeloma* and *lead* or *cadmium poisoning*.
Chronic anticonvulsant drug therapy	Anticonvulsants (e.g. Phenytoin) and many tranquilizers induce hepatic enzymes that accelerate degradation of biologically active vitamin D metabolites.
Fibrogenesis imperfecta ossium and axial osteomalacia	Fibrogenesis imperfecta ossium (axial and appendicular bone involved) and axial osteomalacia (only axial skeleton involved) are rare disorders found in middle-aged males. Loss of bone density with a few coarse trabeculae may produce a "fishnet appearance." Occasionally, the bone density may increase.
Hypophosphatasia (Fig. 1.14)	Autosomal recessive disorder with a wide spectrum of clinical severity. Generalized deficient bony mineralization is found radiographically. The most severe skeletal involvement is observed in neonates, in whom the disease is often fatal. In childhood the disorder resembles rickets, but associated irregular lucent extensions into the metaphyses representing uncalcified bone matrix are characteristic. The adult form is characterized by radiolucent bones, pseudofractures, and fractures occurring after minor trauma that show delayed healing with minimal callus formation. Biochemical hallmark; low alkaline phosphatase.
Hyperparathyroidism (Figs. 1.15 and 1.16)	Laboratory findings of primary hyperparathyroidism: serum calcium high; serum phosphorus low; alkaline phosphatase elevated in the presence of bone disease.
Primary hyperparathyroidism	Found with parathyroid adenoma, primary chief cell or clear cell hyperplasia of all parathyroid glands, and parathyroid carcinoma.
Secondary hyperparathyroidism	Compensatory mechanism in any state of true hypocalcemia. Usually due to chronic renal failure, but may also be caused by hypovitaminosis D and malabsorption of calcium. In chronic renal disease, the skeletal changes are usually a combination of hyperparathyroidism, osteomalacia and osteosclerosis. This complex is best referred to as "*renal osteodystrophy*."
Tertiary hyperparathyroidism	Development of an autonomous parathyroid adenoma in chronically overstimulated hyperplastic parathyroid glands (e.g., following renal transplantation).

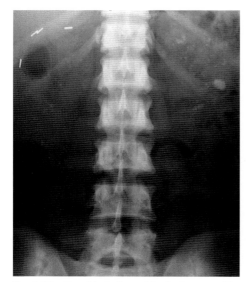

Fig. 1.**13   Renal tubular acidosis.** Increased bone density secondary to renal osteodystrophy is seen. Note also the extensive bilateral nephrocalcinosis.

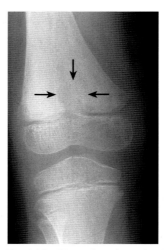

Fig. 1.**14   Hypophosphatasia.** Osteopenia and a radiolucent lesion (arrows) extending from the growth plate into the distal femur metaphysis representing uncalcified bone matrix are seen.

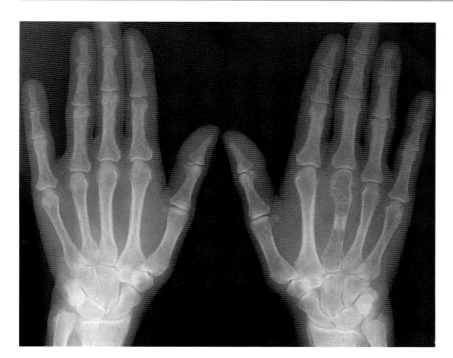

Fig. 1.**15** **Hyperparathyroidism.** Subperiosteal resorption best seen along the radial margin of the proximal phalanges of both index fingers. Brown tumors involving the distal phalanx of the left index finger and the entire right third metacarpal bone. Resorption of the tufts, especially in the thumbs. The cortex in the metacarpals and phalanges depicts fine striations.

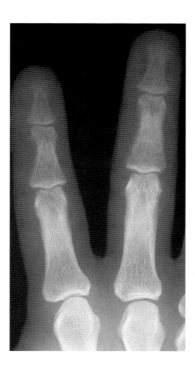

Fig. 1.**16** **Hyperparathyroidism.** Subperiosteal resorptions seen along the radial margins of the proximal and middle phalanges of the second finger and the middle phalanx of the third finger are virtually diagnostic. Cortical striations are also evident.

Table 1.2 Differential Diagnosis of Localized Osteopenia

Etiology	Comments
Disuse atrophy (local immobilization): 1. **fracture (more pronounced distal to the fracture site)** 2. **cast** 3. **neural paralysis** 4. **muscular paralysis**	Besides identical radiographic features as in generalized osteopenia, the localized form may also have a patchy appearance due to spotty cortical thinning (e. g., reflex sympathetic dystrophy).
Reflex sympathetic dystrophy (RSD, Sudeck's atrophy) (Fig. 1.17)	Rapid development of often patchy osteoporosis associated with painful soft-tissue swelling following trivial trauma. Cerebrovascular disorders, cervical spondylosis, discal herniation, postinfectious states, calcific tendinitis, vasculitis, and neoplasm are other implicated conditions. Probably of neurovascular origin.
Regional transitory osteoporosis	A painful self-limited osteoporosis in middle-aged or elderly patients. Most often found in the hip ("transitory demineralization of the femoral head") , but may also involve any other major joint. Associated with disability lasting 2 to 4 months.
Shoulder-hand syndrome (Fig. 1.18)	Pain and stiffness in the shoulder combined with pain, swelling and vasomotor phenomena in the hand following an acute illness (e.g. myocardial infarction, in which condition it is usually located on the left side). Radiographically, it resembles reflex sympathetic dystrophy.
Burns and frostbites	Radiographic findings consist of osteoporosis, bone resorption, osteonecrosis, and dystrophic soft tissue calcifications (burns).
Inflammatory: 1. **rheumatoid arthritis** 2. **osteomyelitis** 3. **tuberculosis**	Localized osteoporosis is usually the first, although nonspecific, radiographic manifestation of any inflammatory disease.
Bone infarct and hemorrhage	In their early stages, both bone infarcts and hemorrhages produce localized demineralization. With healing, lesions become calcified and eventually osteosclerotic.
Radiation osteonecrosis (Fig. 1.19)	Radiation changes are dose-related, with a threshold level of 30 Gy and cell death occurring at 50 Gy. Radiographic changes occur one year after radiotherapy at the earliest. They are initially often predominantly lytic, and progress with time to a mixed lytic and sclerotic stage.
Tumor (Fig. 1.20)	Osteolytic metastases and multiple myeloma must primarily be considered. Primary bone tumors (benign or malignant) may present as localized deossification, but only rarely.

(continues on page 14)

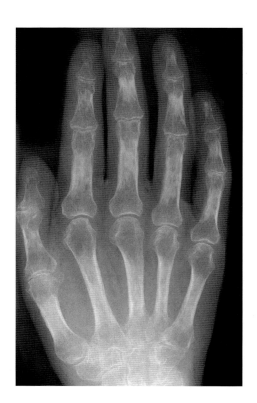

Fig. 1.**17** **Reflex sympathetic dystrophy.** Patchy demineralization most severe near the joints is quite characteristic.

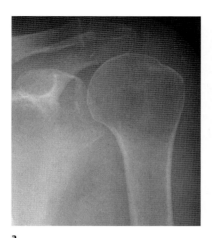

a

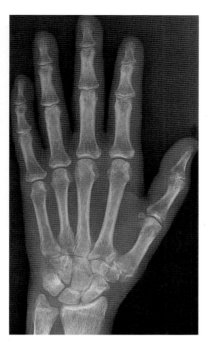

b

Fig. 1.**18 a, b** Shoulder-hand syndrome. Deossification limited to the left shoulder (**a**) and hand (**b**) several weeks following myocardial infarction is characteristic.

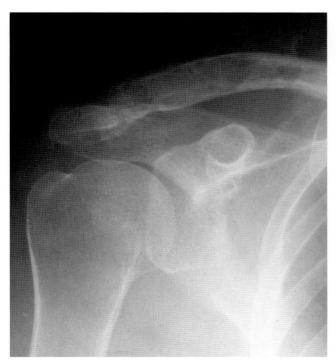

Fig. 1.**19** **Radiation osteonecrosis.** Deossification of the distal end of the clavicle with endosteal bone resorption is seen 4 years after irradiation for breast carcinoma.

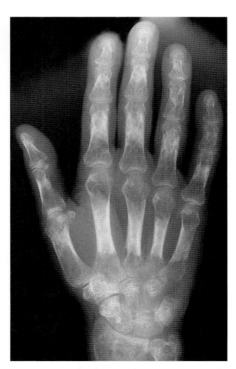

Fig. 1.**20** **Multiple myeloma.** Demineralization is most pronounced near the joints, as in reflex sympathetic dystrophy in Fig. 1.**17**.

Table 1.2   (Cont.) Differential Diagnosis of Localized Osteopenia

Etiology	Comments
Paget's disease (lytic phase) (Fig. 1.21)	Skull: osteoporosis circumscripta. Long bones: usually a well-defined and V- or wedge-shaped area of deossification originating in the subchondral bone of an epiphysis.
Fibrous dysplasia (Fig. 1.22)	Both purely lytic lesions and a homogeneous, "ground glass" appearance occur, besides predominantly sclerotic manifestations. Cortical thinning and bony expansion is commonly associated with lytic lesions in tubular bones.

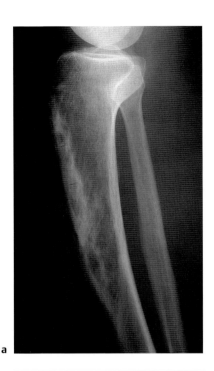

a

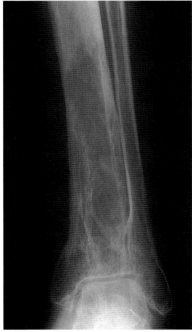

b

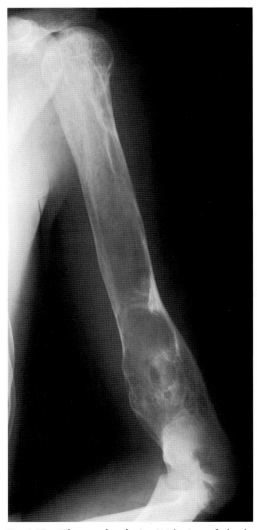

Fig. 1.**21 a, b**   **Paget's disease.** The lytic phase in two different patients. Relatively well-defined V-or flame-shaped areas of deossification containing strands of increased bony densities in a slightly expanded shaft are characteristic (a: proximal tibia, b: distal tibia and fibula).

Fig. 1.**22**   **Fibrous dysplasia.** Widening of the humerus, with a "ground glass" appearance and a few scattered patchy sclerotic areas, is evident.

2 Osteosclerosis

Osteosclerosis is defined as an increase in bone density caused by increased activity of osteoblasts or by osteogenic or chondrogenic tumor cells forming bone-like tissue. Calcification of tissue other than osteoid within bone is usually dystrophic in nature and may also increase the bone density radiographically.

Ossifications within the medullary cavity commonly present as homogeneous, fluffy, cotton-like or cloud-like densities. They most often are caused by bone islands or osteoblastic metastases (Figs. 2.1 and 2.2). Calcifications within the medullary cavity typically present as punctate, annular, comma-shaped or shell-like densities and are commonly associated with chondroid matrix tumors and bone infarcts (Figs. 2.3 and 2.4).

The increase in bone density may be scattered or diffuse. This distinction appears useful in the differential diagnosis of osteoblastic reactions, since certain diseases may exclusively present as scattered (solitary or multiple) sclerosis. Accordingly, the differential diagnosis of these entities will be discussed separately in Tables 2.1 and 2.2. Table 2.3 lists sites and commonly used eponyms for idiopathic avascular necrosis.

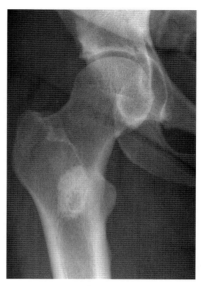

Fig. 2.1 **Bone island**. A sclerotic focus is seen in the intertrochanteric area. The lesion depicts both tiny radiating bone spicules in its periphery and a central radiolucency, both radiographic features that help to differentiate it from an osteoblastic metastasis.

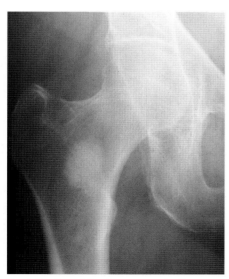

Fig. 2.2 **Osteoblastic metastasis (breast carcinoma)**. An osteoblastic lesion is seen in the intertrochanteric area.

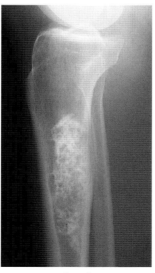

Fig. 2.3 **Enchondroma**. An oblong lesion consisting of multiple irregular, often punctate calcifications is seen in the proximal tibia shaft.

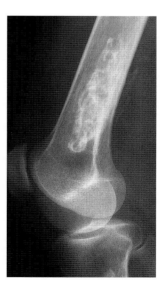

Fig. 2.4 **Bone infarct**. An oblong radiodense lesion with shell-like calcifications is seen in the distal femur shaft.

Table 2.1   Solitary or Multiple Scattered Osteosclerotic Lesions

Disease	Radiographic Findings	Comments
Bone island (enostosis) (Fig. 2.5)	Well-circumscribed isolated area of increased density rarely exceeding 1 cm in diameter. A very slow growth in size is occasionally observed. Margins demonstrate characteristically tiny spiculations or a "brush" border. A central radiolucency is occasionally observed. Occur at any location but pelvis and upper femora appear to be most common locations.	Radionuclide bone imaging is normal. (DD: Osteoblastic metastases are invariably associated with a markedly increased radionuclide uptake.) A large, very dense and structureless bone island within the medullary cavity is often called *enostoma* (Fig. 2.6). Without proper clinical history such a lesion is often indistinguishable from a surgically excised and *methylmethacrylate cemented bone lesion* (Fig. 2.7).
Osteopoikilosis (Fig. 2.8)	Multiple round or ovoid bone densities ranging in size from 2 mm to 2 cm. May demonstrate a radiolucent center. Can be found in all bones, but skull, mandible, ribs, sternum, and vertebrae are only rarely involved. In long bones they are characteristically located in metaphyses and epiphyses, whereas in the scapula and pelvis they are typically found around the glenoid fossa and acetabulum, respectively.	Rare familial disorder not associated with clinical symptoms and therefore incidentally discovered at any age. No increased radionuclide uptake is found in bone scans.
Osteopathia striata (Fig. 2.9)	Dense longitudinal striations that involve the metaphyses and may extend into the epiphyses and diaphyses. In the ilium, the linear densities radiate from the acetabulum. Vertebral bodies and skull may also be involved.	Rare and usually asymptomatic bone disorder. Occasionally associated with focal dermal hypoplasia *(Goltz's syndrome)*
Chondrodysplasia punctata (congenital stippled epiphyses) (Fig. 2.10)	Multiple punctate calcifications occurring in the epiphyses before the normal time of appearance of the epiphyseal ossification centers. DD: *Zellweger's cerebrohepatorenal syndrome*, where the stippling is limited to the patella.	Rare genetically heterogeneous epiphyseal dysplasia associated with a broad spectrum of clinical symptoms. Affected bones may be shortened, or the disorder may regress and leave no deformities. The epiphyseal calcifications may disappear by the age of 3, or may gradually increase in size and coalesce to form a normal-appearing single ossification center.
Multiple epiphyseal dysplasia (Fairbank's disease)	Irregular mottled calcifications of the epiphyses diagnosed in children and adolescents. Sequelae in the adult consist of epiphyseal irregularities, degenerative joint changes, and rarely, asymmetrical shortening of tubular bones.	Can be considered to be the tarda form of chondrodysplasia punctata. *Cretinism* with delayed appearance of stippled and fragmented epiphyseal ossification centers and sclerotic metaphyseal bands must be differentiated.

(continues on page 18)

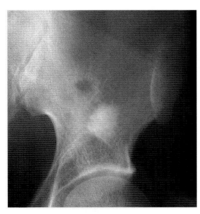

Fig. 2.**5**   **Bone island**. Well-circumscribed focus of increased density with tiny spiculations in its periphery ("brush" border) is seen in the ilium.

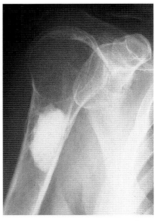

Fig. 2.**6**   **Large bone island (enostoma)**. A large, very dense and structureless lesion is seen in the proximal humerus.

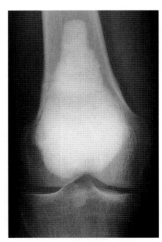

Fig. 2.**7**   **Methylmethacrylate bone cement**. Sequelae of excision with subsequent cementing of a giant cell tumor are seen in the distal femur.

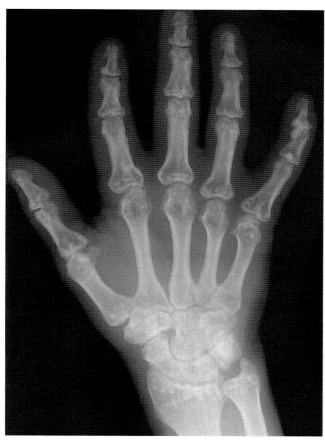

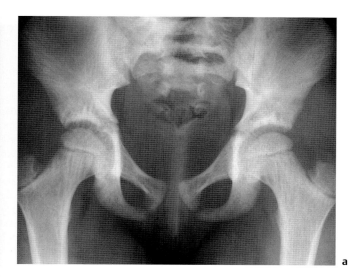

a

Fig. 2.**8** **Osteopoikilosis**. Multiple round to ovoid sclerotic lesions measuring a few millimeters in diameter are seen. In the tubular bones they are characteristically located in the metaphyses and epiphyses

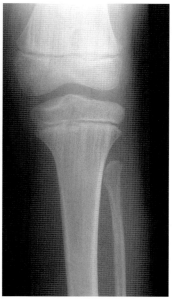

b

Fig. 2.**9** **Osteopathia striata**. Longitudinal striations involving the pelvis (**a**) and mainly the metaphyses of the femur and tibia (**b**) are seen.

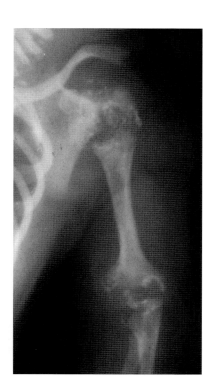

Fig. 2.**10** **Chondrodysplasia punctata**. Punctate calcifications are seen in the epiphyses. Note also the widened and irregular metaphyses

Table 2.1 (Cont.) Solitary or Multiple Scattered Osteosclerotic Lesions

Disease	Radiographic Findings	Comments
Melorheostosis (Fig. 2.11)	Presents in early stage as linear hyperostosis beginning at one end of a tubular bone, progresses with time towards the diaphyses, and results finally in cortical thickening involving either one side or the entire cortex. The lesion may simulate wax flowing down the side of a candle. Osteoma-like protrusions and soft tissue ossifications may be associated.	Often limited to a single limb, in which one or more bones may be affected. At an advanced stage it is part of the differential diagnosis of diffuse osteosclerosis and will be discussed in Table 2.2.
Osteoma (Fig. 2.12)	Protruding mass lesion composed of abnormally dense bone with structureless appearance. It rarely exceeds 2 cm in diameter, and is usually confined to bone that is produced by the periosteal membrane. It arises from the outer or inner table of the skull, the paranasal sinuses (especially frontal and ethmoid), from the mandible, maxilla, and rarely from the tubular bones of the extremities.	Benign hamartomatous lesion consisting exclusively of osseous tissue. *Gardner's syndrome*: Multiple osteomas associated with soft tissue tumors and pre-malignant polyposis, mainly of the colon.
Benign and malignant bone tumors (Figs. 2.13, 2.14 and 2.15)	Predominantly sclerotic lesions, either as a solitary focus (enchondroma, osteochondroma, chondrosarcoma, osteoid osteoma, osteoblastoma, osteosarcoma, and Ewing's sarcoma) or as multiple foci (enchondromatosis or Ollier's disease, hereditary multiple exostoses or diaphyseal aclasis, and osteosarcomatosis).	Differential diagnosis of bone tumors is discussed in detail in Chapter 5.

(continues on page 20)

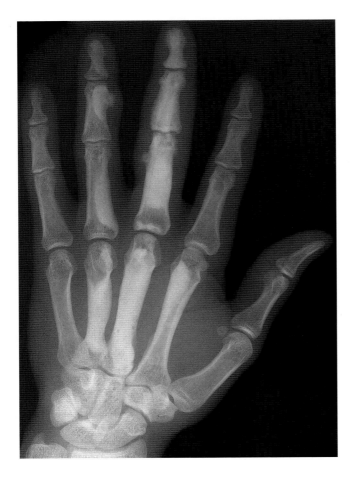

Fig. 2.**11** **Melorheostosis**. Sclerosis of several metacarpals and phalanges caused by cortical thickening, often with involvement of only one side of a bone. The presentation of the disorder has been compared with the "flowing of wax down a burning candle." Note also the involvement of the small osteoma-like protrusions from the proximal phalanx of the third finger (ulnar side) and the middle phalanx of the fourth finger (radial side).

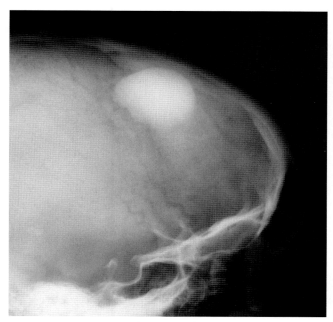

Fig. 2.**12** **Osteoma**. An abnormally dense lesion with structure-less appearance is characteristic. In this case, the osteoma originated from the outer table and could easily be palpated.

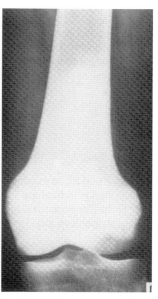

Fig. 2.**13 Osteosarcoma.** A rather homogeneous sclerosis of the distal femur sparing only a small portion of the subchondral bone in the lateral femur condyle is seen.

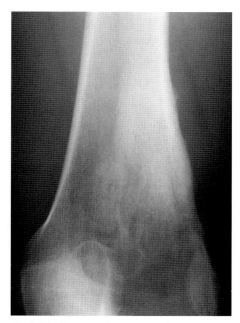

Fig. 2.**14** **Parosteal sarcoma**. This posterior cortical tumor of the distal femur diaphysis presents as an irregularly defined sclerotic lesion in this anteroposterior projection (viewed face-on). The lateral projection of this sarcoma is shown in Fig. 4.**49**.

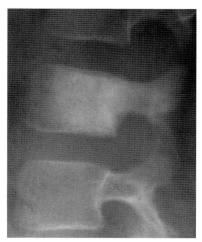

Fig. 2.**15** **Ewing's sarcoma**. A relatively poorly defined sclerotic lesion is seen in L3 involving the posterior two-thirds of the vertebral body and pedicles.

Table 2.1 (Cont.) Solitary or Multiple Scattered Osteosclerotic Lesions

Disease	Radiographic Findings	Comments
Osteoblastic metastases (Fig. 2.16)	Poorly defined areas of increased density with indistinct or lost trabecular structure. With increase in size, adjacent metastases may coalesce, resulting finally in most diffuse sclerosis. With the exception of renal and most thyroid carcinomas which produce invariably lytic and often expansile metastases, osteoblastic metastases may originate from virtually every carcinoma, but *carcinoma of the prostate* and *breast* are the most common sources. Other primary tumors include osteosarcomas, carcinoids, and carcinomas originating in the lung, nasopharynx, gastrointestinal tract and urinary bladder. Of the lymphomas, *Hodgkin's disease* and *histiocytic lymphoma* (reticulum cell sarcoma) are most likely to produce osteoblastic bone lesions.	In *children*, leukemia, neuroblastoma, and Ewing's sarcoma metastases must be considered, although these lesions are more commonly lytic before treatment is instituted.
Multiple myeloma	Focal sclerotic lesions are a rare initial manifestation.	Characteristic lytic lesions may become sclerotic with proper therapy.
Plasma cell granuloma (Fig, 2.17)	Solitary or scattered osteoblastic foci that are only slowly growing.	Consists histologically of a dense infiltrate of normal plasma cells. In contrast to multiple myeloma and plasmacytoma, all laboratory findings are normal. Nowadays considered to be a variant of *chronic recurrent multifocal osteomyelitis* (CRMO) or SAPHO (synovitis, acne, pustulosis, hyperostosis, osteitis), respectively
POEMS syndrome	Solitary or multiple osteosclerotic lesions and fluffy spiculated hyperostotic areas preferentially at sites of ligamentous attachment in axial and para-axial locations.	POEMS is the acronym for *polyneuropathy*, *organomegaly*, *endocrinopathy*, *M protein*, and *skin changes*.
Chronic or healed osteomyelitis (Fig. 2.18)	May present as localized, thickened sclerotic bone usually containing radiolucent areas.	Bacterial, tuberculous, and fungal organisms may all cause a chronic sclerosing-type osteomyelitis. *Sclerosing osteomyelitis of Garré* is a low-grade chronic infection not associated with bone destruction or sequestration.
Brodie's abscess (Fig. 2.19)	Central lucency surrounded by a slight to extensive reactive sclerosis. Located typically in the metaphysis and, less commonly in the epiphysis or diaphysis of tubular bones. Cortical thickening, periosteal new bone and sequestrum formation may be found with Brodie's abscess, but are not typical.	Chronic, often painful lesion.
Tropical ulcer	Often expansile lesion involving preferentially the lower half of the tibia. Associated with periostitis, resulting in localized fusiform periosteal and cortical thickening or even broad-based excrescences resembling osteomas.	In patients of all ages in Central and East Africa.
Callus formation (Fig. 2.20)	Healed fractures result in a localized increase in bone density.	Commonly in ribs or metatarsals following a fatigue fracture.
Stress fracture (Fig. 2.21)	Findings dependent on both location and time. A fracture line (cortical or complete) is not always evident. In the shaft of tubular bones, localized cortical thickening and periosteal reaction are characteristic. At the end of tubular bones (e.g. femoral neck, tibia plateau) and in cancellous bone, a band-like focal sclerosis without appreciable periosteal reaction is usually found.	Presents clinically with activity-related pain that is relieved by rest. Radionuclide examination and magnetic resonance imaging are both much more sensitive for early detection and diagnosis. A stress fracture occurring in normal bone under abnormal (increased) stress is referred to as a *fatigue fracture*, whereas a stress fracture occurring in abnormal (osteopenic) bone with normal stress is referred to as an *insufficiency fracture*.
Healed bone lesion (Fig. 2.22)	Spontaneously or under appropriate treatment, healed lytic lesion may become sclerotic.	Benign bone lesions such as fibrous cortical defects and nonossifying fibromas may spontaneously regress and persist as sclerotic foci. Lytic metastases (e.g., from bronchogenic carcinoma, breast carcinoma, lymphoma) and multiple myeloma manifestations may respond to local irradiation, chemotherapy, and/or hormone therapy by becoming osteosclerotic. Brown tumors in primary hyperparathyroidism become sclerotic after removal of the parathyroid adenoma.

(continues on page 23)

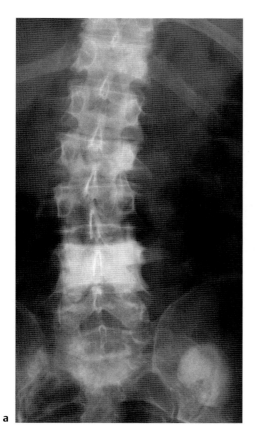

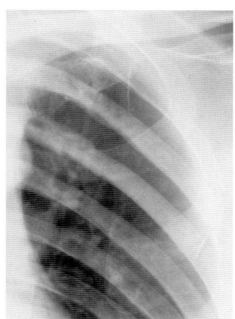

a

b

Fig. 2.**16　Osteoblastic metastases** from prostatic carcinoma (**a**) involving the spine and pelvis and from Hodgkin's disease (**b**) involving only the left fourth and fifth rib. The involvement of different vertebral bodies varies from barely visible, poorly defined areas of increased densities in some vertebrae to almost complete sclerosis ("ivory vertebra") in L4.

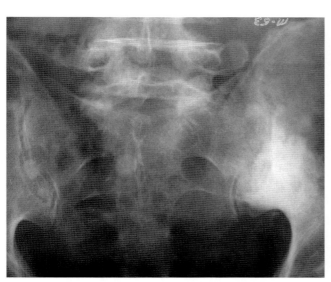

Fig. 2.**17　Plasma cell granuloma**. Scattered osteoblastic lesions and a larger osteoblastic area in the left ilium adjacent to the sacroiliac joint are seen.

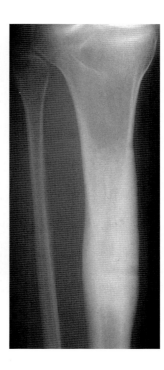

Fig. 2.**18　Sclerosing osteomyelitis of Garré**. A homogeneous sclerosis of the proximal spindle-shaped tibia shaft is seen.

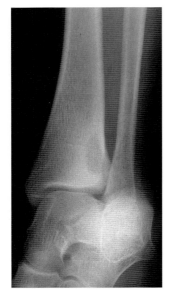

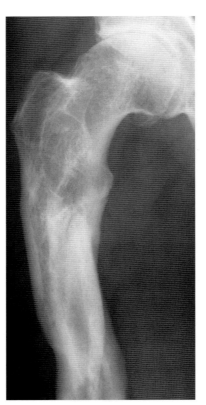

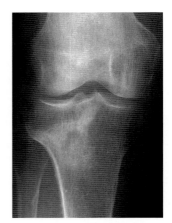

Fig. 2.**19**   **Brodie's abscess**. Radiolucent lesion with surrounding reactive sclerosis in the distal tibia metaphysis is characteristic

Fig. 2.**20**   **Healed fracture**. Irregular widening of the shaft, cortical thickening and sclerosis is seen in this healed comminuted fracture of the proximal femur.

Fig. 2.**21**   **Insufficiency fracture**. A poorly defined osteosclerotic zone is seen in the lateral aspect of the proximal tibia.

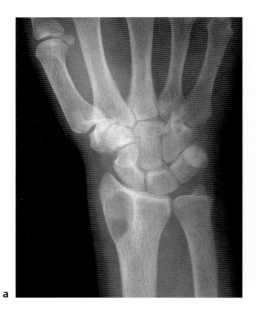

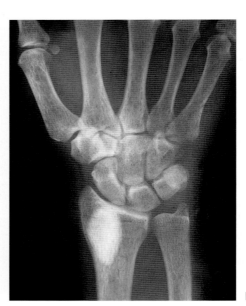

a

b

Fig. 2.**22**   **Brown tumor** in primary hyperparathyroidism, **a** before and **b** five years after removal of a parathyroid adenoma, Healing of the brown tumor resulted in a persistent sclerotic focus.

Table 2.1   (Cont.) Solitary or Multiple Scattered Osteosclerotic Lesions

Disease	Radiographic Findings	Comments
Bone infarcts (old) (Figs. 2.23 and 2.24)	Most often found in the proximal or distal ends of long tubular bones. Healed infarcts present as irregularly calcified areas in the medullary cavity, demarcated from the normal bone by a dense serpiginous contour or irregular streaks. The calcifications may eventually progress to ossification.	Infarcts are often associated with other diseases such as occlusive vascular disease, sickle cell anemia, pancreatitis, connective tissue disease, caisson disease, Gaucher's disease, and radiation therapy. A similar calcification in the medulla of long bones can occasionally be seen after *removal* of an *intramedullary rod*. Enchondromas can simulate bone infarcts (Fig. 2.**25**).

(continues on page 24)

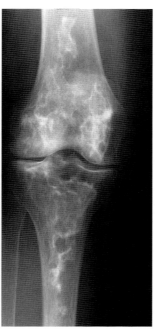

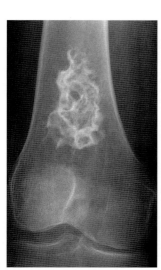

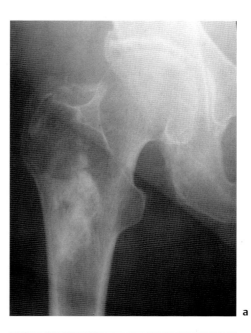

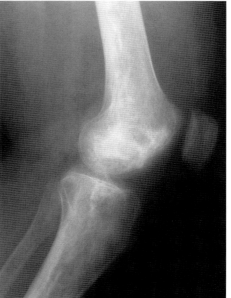

a   b

Fig. 2.**23 a, b   Bone infarcts**. Irregular peripheral rim calcifications are seen in the distal femur (**a**) and more extensive in both the distal femur and proximal tibia (**b**) in these patients with sickle cell anemia.

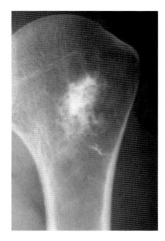

Fig. 2.**25   Enchondroma**. An irregular calcification is seen that is most dense in its center.

a

b

Fig. 2.**24 a, b   Bone infarcts**. In an attempt to heal the originally calcified infarct becomes ossified from its periphery towards the center and eventually presents as an irregular sclerotic lesion as seen in the proximal femur shaft in **a** and about the knee in **b**.

Table 2.1   (Cont.) Solitary or Multiple Scattered Osteosclerotic Lesions

Disease	Radiographic Findings	Comments
Radiation osteonecrosis (Fig. 2.26)	May present years after therapy as a mixture of sclerotic and lytic lesions even when no infarcts have occurred.	This condition can be differentiated from a local tumor recurrence with bone involvement by a normal or even depressed uptake on a bone scan.
Avascular (epiphyseal) necrosis (AVN) (Fig. 2.27)	Sequelae of avascular necrosis in epiphyses consist of sclerotic and cystic areas of flattened and irregular joint surfaces, which lead to early secondary degenerative changes, particularly in the weight-bearing joints. Most idiopathic avascular necroses occur during childhood and adolescence. Idiopathic avascular necroses occurring in adulthood are found in the medial femur condyle (*Ahlbäck's disease*, also reffered to as *spontaneous osteonecrosis about the knee* or *SONC*) and in the lunate (*Kienböck's disease*). Ahlbäck's disease typically occurs in the elderly with female predominance and occasionally affect the lateral femoral ar the tibial condyles. New evidence suggest it represents a stress (insufficiency) fracture rather than a spontaneous osteonecrosis. Kienböck's disease is usually found in young adults. In an advanced stage, the lunate shows increased bone density, fragmentation, and compression.	May be found in any disorder associated with medullary bone infarcts. Avascular necrosis is caused by interruption of the blood supply to the epiphyses with subsequent death of the hematopoetic cells in 6–12 hours, osteocytes in 12–48 hours, and lipocytes in 2–5 days. The etiology may be traumatic (e. g., femoral neck fracture), thromboembolic (e. g., sickle cell disease), vasculitic (e. g., systemic lupus erythematosus), stereoidal, marrow-infiltrative (e. g., Gaucher's disease) or idiopathic (e. g., Legg-Calvé-Perthes disease). An idiopathic genesis of this abnormality is commonly associated with an eponym (see Table 2.**3**).
Paget's disease (Fig. 2.28)	Can cause uniform areas of increased bone density in the sclerotic phase. In the reparative (mixed lytic and sclerotic) stage, the disease is characteristically associated with cortical thickening resulting in enlargement of the affected bone. Any bone can be affected; "cotton wool" appearance of the skull and "ivory vertebral body" are representative examples of the sclerotic phase of the disease.	Purely sclerotic phase is less common than the combined destructive and reparative stage virtually pathognomonic for the disease.
Fibrous dysplasia	Besides having a cyst-like or "ground glass" appearance, it can also present as purely sclerotic lesions. Manifestations are usually associated with bone expansion, particularly in tubular bones. With more extensive involvement, bone deformities almost invariably occur.	Occurs in monostotic and polyostotic forms. An *ossifying fibroma* of the skull, face and mandible cannot be histologically differentiated from fibrous dysplasia, and can be considered radiographically as a localized manifestation of this disease. Ossifying fibromas occuring in long bones, especially in the tibia and to a lesser extend fibula are referred to as *osteofibrous dysplasia* (Fig. 2.29)
Mastocytosis (Fig. 2.30)	Can present with focal or diffuse bone involvement. Focal form is characterized by scattered, well-defined sclerotic foci often alternating with areas of bone rarefaction. Skull, spine, ribs, pelvis, humerus, and femur are preferred sites of involvement.	Majority of patients develop skin lesions containing mast cells during the first year of life. Hepatosplenomegaly, lymphadenopathy, and pancytopenia may be associated.

(continues on page 26)

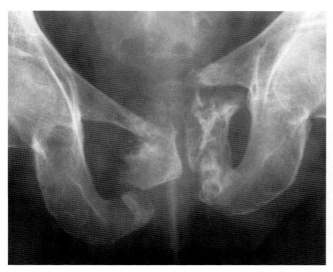

Fig. 2.**26** **Radiation osteonecrosis**. Mixed osteolytic and osteoblastic lesions are seen in both pubic bones with several pathologic fractures 7 years after irradiation for bladder carcinoma.

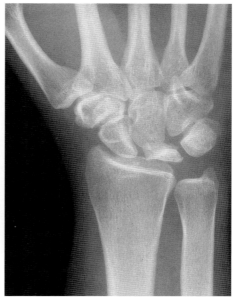

Fig. 2.**27** **Avascular necrosis of the lunate** (Kienbock's disease). Increased sclerosis of the lunate, which is compressed and shows early fragmentation. A shortening of the ulna (negative ulnar variance) as present in this case has been implicated as predisposing to Kienbock's disease through increased pressure on the lunate from the medial corner of the distal radius.

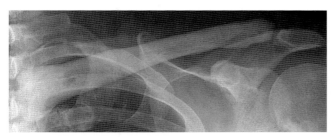

Fig. 2.**28** **Paget's disease**. A slightly thickened and uniformly sclerotic clavicle is seen.

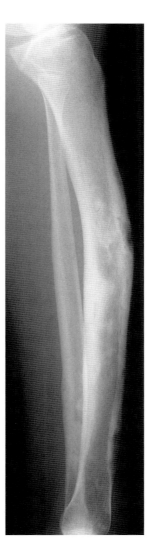

Fig. 2.**29** **Osteo fibrous dysplasia**. Anterior bowing of the sclerotic and slightly widened tibia shaft with a thickened irregular posterior cortex and several lytic lesions in the anterior cortex are seen. Similar but less severe changes are also present in the fibula.

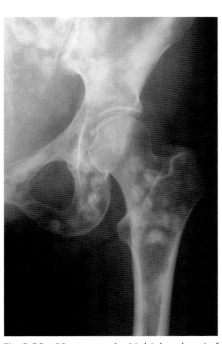

Fig. 2.**30** **Mastocytosis**. Multiple sclerotic foci are evident.

Table 2.1   (Cont.) Solitary or Multiple Scattered Osteosclerotic Lesions

Disease	Radiographic Findings	Comments
Tuberous sclerosis (Fig. 2.31)	Often presenting with scattered intracerebral calcifications, renal hamartomas, and bone lesions. Characteristic skeletal changes are patches of osteosclerosis ranging from a few millimeters to several centimeters in diameter. The lesions are not associated with any bone enlargement, and are most commonly found in skull, lumbar spine (especially pedicles), and pelvis, although all bones may be involved. Cyst like lesions may be seen in the hands and feet.	Rare familial disorder with defect in developing ectodermal structures. Present clinically with adenoma sebaceum of the face, with epilepsy, and with mental deficiency.
Sarcoidosis (Fig. 2.32)	Focal or generalized osteosclerosis is a rare manifestation involving spine, pelvis, skull, ribs, proximal long bones and terminal phalanges (acro-osteosclerosis).	A more characteristic presentation that is found especially in the bones of the hand consists of osteopenia with a coarsened, reticulated or lace-work trabecular pattern and localized cystic ("punched-out") lesions.

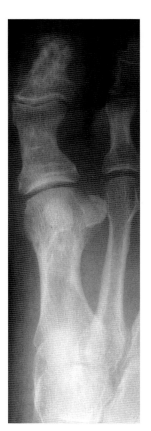

Fig. 2.**31** **Tuberous sclerosis**. Irregular sclerotic areas are interspersed with small cyst-like lesions.

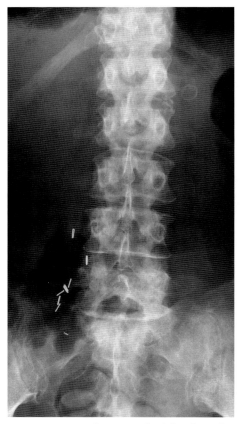

Fig. 2.**32** **Sarcoidosis**. Poorly defined patchy sclerotic areas are noted throughout the spine.

Table 2.2   Generalized Diffuse Osteosclerosis

Disease	Radiographic Findings	Comments
Physiologic osteosclerosis of newborn	Cortical thickening and abundant spongiosa formation can result in considerable osteosclerosis, mainly affecting the long tubular bones.	Sclerotic changes disappear gradually during the first weeks of life and have no pathologic significance. Can be found in more than half of all premature infants.
Congenital syphilis (Fig. 2.33)	Symmetrical involvement of metaphyses and diaphyses, with the epiphyseal ossification centers being spared. Metaphyseal involvement varies from transverse striping to destructive lesions originating in the corners adjacent to the cartilage plate and a frayed appearance of the metaphyseal ends similar to rickets. Particularly characteristic is a destructive lesion adjacent to the medial metaphyseal growth plate of the proximal tibia (Wimberger's sign). In the diaphyses, subperiosteal cortical thickening and periosteal reactions may be associated with focal destructive lesions.	Changes in congenital syphilis caused by a combination of luetic osteomyelitis and nonspecific trophic disturbances in enchondral bone formation. Radiographic changes may be present at birth or develop subsequently.
Rubella embryopathy (Fig. 2.34)	Predilection for distal femoral and proximal tibial metaphyses and adjacent diaphyses where irregular longitudinal lytic and sclerotic densities are found, giving a "celery-stick" appearance. Metaphyseal ends are irregular but not cupped.	Caused by maternal rubella infection in the first trimester of pregnancy. Associated clinical findings may include congenital heart disease, hepatosplenomegaly, cataracts, chorioretinitis, and thrombocytopenic purpura. *Toxoplasmosis* and *cytomegalic inclusion disease* may result in similar bony changes.
Erythroblastosis fetalis	Transverse metaphyseal bands and diffuse sclerosis of the diaphyses may be present.	Congenital hemolytic anemia caused by Rh factor incompatibility. Clinically, severe prolonged jaundice (icterus gravis neonatorum) and generalized edema (hydrops fetalis) are associated.

(continues on page 28)

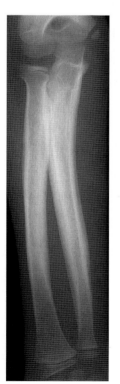

Fig. 2.**33   Congenital syphilis**. Sclerosis of the diaphysis is caused by cortical thickening and periosteal reactions. Destructive lesions are no longer recognizable in this healing phase.

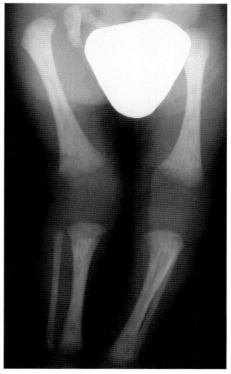

Fig. 2.**34   Rubella embryopathy**. Irregular longitudinal lytic and sclerotic densities in the distal femur and proximal tibia ("celery-stick" appearance) are characteristic. Metaphyses are slightly irregular, but not cupped.

Table 2.2 (Cont.) Generalized Diffuse Osteosclerosis

Disease	Radiographic Findings	Comments
Infantile cortical hyperostosis (Caffey's disease) (Fig. 2.35)	Cortical thickening, sometimes with asymmetrical distribution. Mandible clavicles, long bones (especially ulnae), ribs, skull, scapula and pelvis are involved, in that order of frequency. Tubular bones may have a spindle-shape appearance since only the diaphyses are involved. A laminated periosteal reaction is only associated in the healing phase.	Uncommon disease of unknown etiology with onset in the first 5 months. Clinically, the affected bones are associated with tender soft tissue swellings and fever. Recovery occurs over a period of a few weeks to several months. Roentgen changes regress within a year.
Ribbing's disease	Solitary or multiple, often asymmetric involvement of the diaphyses of long bones (especially femur and tibia) with sclerosis and hyperostosis.	Usually asymptomatic and often considered as forme fruste of Engelmann-Camurati disease. When a solitary bone is involved the differential diagnosis includes chronic *sclerosing osteomyelitis of Garré*.
Progressive diaphyseal dysplasia (Engelmann-Camurati disease) (Fig. 2.36)	Cortical thickening of the long bones beginning in the midshaft and progressing peripherally, resulting in a spindle-shape appearance with relatively abrupt transition to normal bone. Involvement of other bones with sclerosis is less common.	This autosomal dominant transmitted neuromuscular disease is usually diagnosed between 4 and 12 years of age. Characteristic clinical features include a peculiar wide-based, waddling gait, muscular weakness, and malnutrition.
Generalized cortical hyperostosis (van Buchem's disease) (Fig. 2.37)	Diffuse symmetrical sclerosis and cortical thickening, predominantly of the diaphyses of all tubular bones. Sclerosis and thickening occurs also in the vault and base of the skull, mandible, clavicles, ribs and spine (particularly affecting the spinous processes).	Rare autosomal recessive disorder occurring in adulthood with male predominance. *Worth's syndrome*: Autosomal dominant form, with similar but less severe radiographic findings, is often detected incidentally on radiographs obtained for unrelated reasons.
Hereditary hyperphosphatasia (Juvenile Paget's disease)	Marked cortical thickening can be found in all bones. In the long tubular bones the process involves the entire bone rather than only the diaphyses and bowing deformities occur, especially in the femora. Pseudofractures and "splitting" of the cortex may also be seen.	Rare autosomal recessive disease developing usually in the second or third year of life with striking, predilection for those of Puerto Rican descent. Radiographic features resemble Paget's disease. Alkaline phosphatase is elevated. Pseudoxanthoma elasticum may be associated.
Craniometaphyseal dysplasia	Osteosclerosis of the diaphyses of the tubular bones is only found in infancy, and is subsequently replaced by widened diaphyses with cortical thinning and metaphyseal expansion (Erlenmeyer flask deformity). Sclerosis of the skull (calvarium and base) occurs. Lack of aeration of the paranasal sinuses and mastoids is present. The mandible can be markedly thickened and sclerotic, with defective dentition.	Rare autosomal dominant or recessive disorders characterized by failure of normal tubulation of bone and skull abnormalities. Clinically, hypertelorism and a broad flat nose are characteristic, and cranial nerve deficits (progressive hearing and vision loss and facial paralysis) occur. In *craniodiaphyseal dysplasia* (autosomal recessive) massive and progressive hyperostosis of the skull and facial bones are associated with cortical thickening and lack of normal modeling of the long and short tubular bones (Fig. 2.37 A).
Hypoparathyroidism	Osteosclerosis, particularly of the axial skeleton, is the most common bony abnormality, but may be subtle and defy detection. Transverse sclerotic bands in the metaphyses of the long bones, increased density of the iliac crest, and marginal sclerosis of vertebral bodies can also be found. Ossification of muscle insertion and ligaments and subcutaneous calcifications occur. Enthesopathy in the spine resembles diffuse idiopathic skeletal hyperostosis (DISH). In the skull calvarial thickening, basal ganglion calcification and defective dentition are characteristic.	Hypocalcemia induces neuromuscular excitability, resulting eventually in tetany in both primary and the more common secondary hypoparathyroidism. The latter is most often caused by accidental removal of the parathyroid glands during thyroid surgery. *Pseudohypoparathyroidism* differs from the primary form by the presence of short metacarpal and metatarsal bones and the lack of response to parathyroid hormone substitution therapy. *Pseudopseudohypoparathyroidism* has similar radiographic features, but no blood chemical changes.

(continues on page 30)

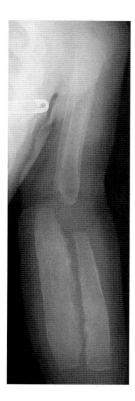

Fig. 2.**35 Infantile cortical hyperostosis (Caffey's disease)**. Periosteal reactions with subsequent cortical thickening result in widened and relatively dense diaphyses of the long bones in the upper extremity.

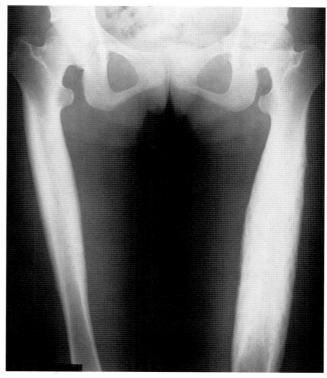

Fig. 2.**36 Progressive diaphyseal dysplasia (Engelmann-Camurati disease)**. Cortical thickening of different severity in both femurs of the same patient produced spindle-shaped, sclerotic diaphyses with a relatively abrupt transition to normal bone.

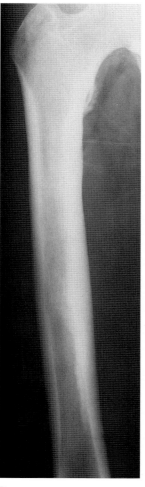 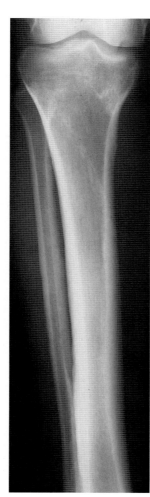

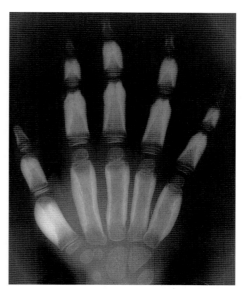

Fig. 2.**37 A Craniodiaphyseal dysplasia.** Marked cortical thickening of the short tubular bones of the hand in seen.

◁ Fig. 2.**37 Generalized cortical hyperostosis (van Buchem's disease)**. Symmetrical sclerosis and cortical thickening predominantly of the diaphyses of the femur (**a**) and the tibia and fibula (**b**), is seen.

a   b

Table 2.2 (Cont.) Generalized Diffuse Osteosclerosis

Disease	Radiographic Findings	Comments
Osteopetrosis (marble bones, Albers-Schönberg disease) (Fig. 2.38)	Symmetrical increase in bone density ranging from minimal to extreme may be found. All bones may be involved with no predilection for a specific location within one bone. Tubular bones lack modeling, often causing flaring of the ends (Erlenmeyer flask deformity). Longitudinal and transverse striations as well as "bone-within-bone" appearance occur.	Rare hereditary bone disorder with usually normal serum calcium, phosphorus, and alkaline phosphatase levels. At least four different types are differentiated, one of which is associated with tubular acidosis.
Pyknodysostosis	Diffuse Osteosclerosis occurs but differs from osteopetrosis by the absence of both Erlenmeyer flask deformities and "bone-within-bone" appearance. Hypoplasia of the mandible and short bones of the hands and feet with osteolysis of the distal phalanges are characteristic.	Rare autosomal recessive disorder consisting of osteosclerosis, short stature, frontal and occipital bossing, small face with receding chin, short broad hands, and hypoplasia of the nails.
Dysosteosclerosis	Sclerosis of skull, ribs, clavicles and tubular bones similar to osteopetrosis. However, platyspondylia and lucent areas in the expanded diametaphyses allow differentiation.	Autosomal recessive disorder manifested in early childhood with small stature, dental anomalies, abnormal bone fragility, and occasionally neurologic symptoms.
Melorheostosis (Fig. 2.39)	Causes asymmetrical or uniform cortical thickening. Usually limited to one extremity, with a predilection for tubular bones where it presents as continuous or interrupted streaks of sclerotic areas.	When features of melorheostosis are present together with findings of osteopoikilosis and osteopathia striata, then the disorder is often referred to as *mixed sclerosing bone dystrophy* (Fig. 2.**40**).

(continues on page 32)

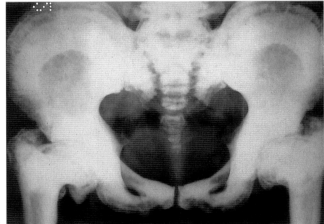

a

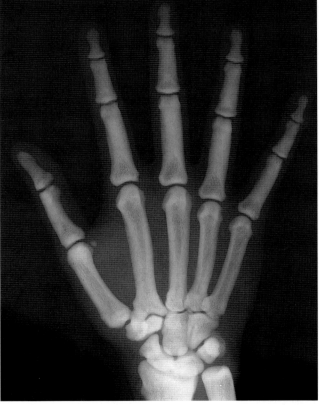

b

Fig. 2.**38** **Osteopetrosis**. Diffuse and symmetrical osteosclerotic involvement of the entire skeleton is characteristic. Note "bone-within-bone" appearance in the pelvis and tarsal bones (**a**) pelvis; (**b**) hand; (**c**) foot.

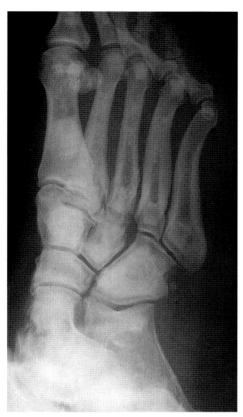

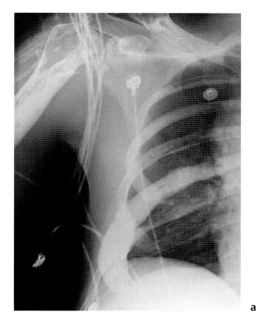

a

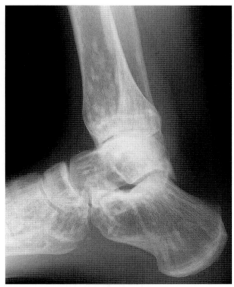

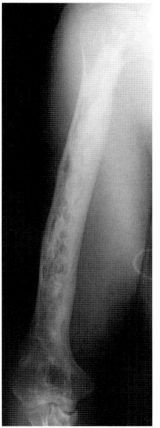

b

Fig. 2.**38 c**

Fig. 2.**40 Mixed sclerosing bone dystrophy**. Features of osteopoikilosis, osteopathia striata and melorheostosis are seen.

Fig. 2.**39 a, b Melorheostosis**. Extensive predominantly band-like ossificatins were seen in many bones of the right side of the patient shown here in the right hemithorax (**a**) and right humerus (**b**). The left side was normal.

Table 2.2   (Cont.) Generalized Diffuse Osteosclerosis

Disease	Radiographic Findings	Comments
Metastatic disease (extensive) (Fig. 2.41)	Generalized diffuse osteosclerosis.	Most commonly from carcinoma of prostate and breast.
Myelofibrosis (myelosclerosis, myeloid metaplasia) (Fig. 2.42)	Approximately half of the patients develop a diffuse (rarely patchy) osteosclerosis. Ribs, spine, pelvis, humeri, and femur are most often involved. Massive splenomegaly is usually apparent radiographically. Extramedullary hematopoiesis, evident as a paraspinal mass, may be present. Both findings may help to differentiate myelofibrosis from osteoblastic metastases, fluorosis, osteopetrosis, and renal osteodystrophy.	Clinically characterized by hepatosplenomegaly, anemia, thrombocytopenia.
Anemias and leukemias (Figs. 2.43 and 2.44)	Present radiographically more commonly with a loss of bone density and coarsening of the trabecular pattern. Generalized sclerosis may occur, particularly in *sickle cell anemia*.	Extramedullary hematopoiesis can be associated with all blood disorders. Splenomegaly is usually present except in the adult sickle cell patient (presumably because of multiple splenic infarctions).
Multiple myeloma	Uniform sclerosis is a very rare manifestation.	Characteristic bone marrow and laboratory findings.
Gaucher's disease (Fig. 2.45)	May present in the reparative stage with diffuse osteosclerosis. Characteristic for Gaucher's disease in the femur is the combination of avascular necrosis of the femoral head, Erlenmeyer's flask deformity of the distal end, and multiple osteolytic and/or sclerotic lesions in the shaft.	The radiographic findings described are seen in the chronic form of Gaucher's disease, whereas the acute infantile form is characterized by pathology in the respiratory and central nervous system and is usually fatal in the first year of life.

(continues on page 34)

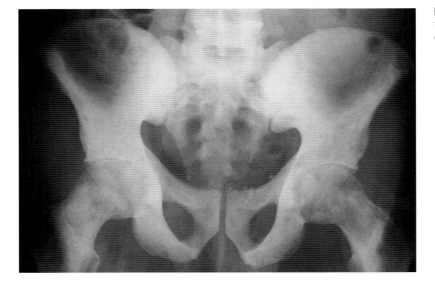

Fig. 2.**41** **Osteoblastic metastases** from prostatic carcinoma. Generalized diffuse osteosclerosis is seen.

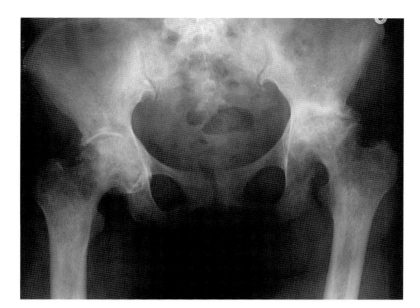

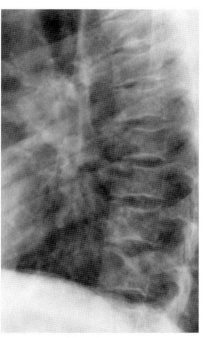

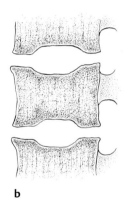

b

a

Fig. 2.**43** **Sickle cell anemia**. A nonuniform cuplike depression of only the central portions of the upper and lower endplates of several contiguous vertebral bodies is characteristic and assumed to be caused by local ischemia inhibiting central bone growth. The bone density may be decreased or increased and the trabecular pattern is often coarsened. **a**: thoracic spine; **b**: drawing.

Fig. 2.**42** **Myelofibrosis**. Diffuse symmetric and somewhat patchy osteopenia is seen involving the lumbosacral area, pelvis and proximal femora.

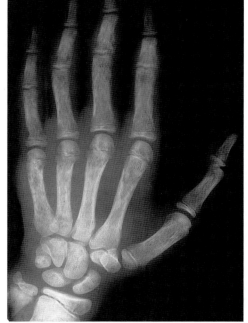

Fig. 2.**44** **Leukemia**. A coarsened trabecular pattern and "cortical tunneling" (longitudinal striations in the cortex) with an overall increased bone density are seen in this child with acute leukemia.

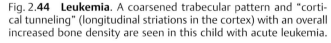

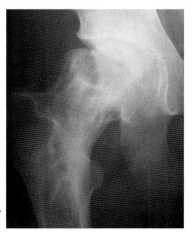

Fig. 2.**45** **Gaucher's disease**. Avascular necrosis of the femoral ▷ head and sclerotic changes in the proximal femur are evident.

Table 2.2 (Cont.) Generalized Diffuse Osteosclerosis

Disease	Radiographic Findings	Comments
Erdheim-Chester disease (lipid granulomatosis) (Fig. 2.46)	Symmetric patchy or diffuse osteosclerosis and cortical thickening of the diaphyses and metaphyses of the major long bones, with relative sparing of the epiphyses and axial skeleton, are characteristic.	Affects men and women in the fifth through seventh decade. Xanthomatous patches in the eyelids and mild skeletal pain can be present, but patients may also be asymptomatic.
Paget's disease (Fig. 2.47)	The advanced stage of the polyostotic form may eventually result in a deformed and diffusely sclerotic skeleton. Enlargement of all involved bones by cortical thickening is a radiographic hallmark of the disease.	Common cause of osteosclerosis observed in an asymptomatic patient aged over 40. The radiographic diagnosis is supported by markedly elevated serum alkaline phosphatase and normal serum calcium and phosphorus levels.
Fibrous dysplasia (polyostotic form) (Fig. 2.48)	Similar to Paget's disease. Can present as diffuse sclerosis of the involved bone associated with widening and cortical thickening. The manifestations are predominantly unilateral, and bone deformities are common.	Clinically, "cafe-au-lait" pigmentations with irregular outline ("coast of Maine" appearance) are found in approximately one third of patients with the polyostotic form. Alkaline phosphatase is normal or only mildly elevated.
Mastocytosis	Can present throughout the skeleton as diffuse sclerosis that is not sharply demarcated from normal bone and often intermingled with osteolytic areas.	See also Table 2.1
Tuberous sclerosis	Can present as diffuse osteosclerosis similar to mastocytosis.	See also Table 2.1
Sarcoidosis	Diffuse osteosclerosis is a rare manifestation.	See also Table 2.1
Renal osteodystrophy (Fig. 2.49)	Features of osteomalacia, hyperparathyroidism, and sclerosis. The latter might be the dominant finding and is often combined with soft tissue calcifications. A "rugger jersey" spine (dense endplates with relatively lucent centers resulting in a striped appearance of the spine) is most characteristic.	Represents the skeletal response to chronic renal disease of any origin. In *primary hyperparathyroidism*, sclerosis is virtually limited to cases that are healing.
Oxalosis (Fig. 2.50)	Sclerotic, metaphyseal bands and "woolly" or "Paget-like" sclerosis are combined with features of renal osteodystrophy, including a more generalized form of osteosclerosis.	Deposition of calcium oxalate crystals as a primary hereditary (autosomal-recessive) disorder, or more commonly associated with chronic renal disease. Extensive nephrocalcinosis, nephrolithiasis, and extrarenal soft-tissue deposition of calcium oxalate occur.
Hypervitaminosis D, idiopathic hypercalcemia of infancy (Williams syndrome), intoxication with lead, bismuth, or phosphorus (Fig. 2.51)	Present with dense transverse metaphyseal bands and generalized sclerosis.	In children.
Fluorosis (Fig. 2.52)	Fluorosis progresses from coarsening of the trabecular structures to a dense uniform sclerosis. Characteristically, the findings are most pronounced in the axial skeleton, although all bones may be involved. Periosteal reaction may be present. Extensive ligamentous calcifications are characteristic, particularly in the sacrospinous and sacrotuberous ligaments.	Can be found at any age. Clinically, the most characteristic feature is mottling of the enamel of the teeth. Chronic fluorine intoxication occurs, when the drinking water contains excessive fluoride concentrations (endemic in certain regions of India) or with chronic fluoride therapy in too high dosages (e.g., for osteoporosis).

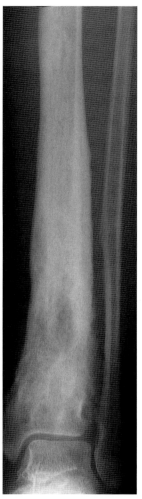

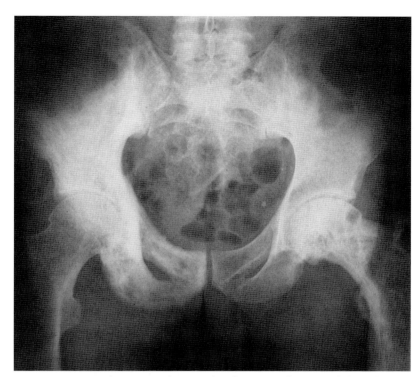

Fig. 2.**47** **Paget's disease**. Predominantly sclerotic involvement of the right hemipelvis, left ilium (inferior half) and left proximal femur is seen.

Fig. 2.**46** **Erdheim-Chester disease**. Inhomogeneous sclerosis with cortical thickening and relative sparing of the epiphysis is seen in the distal tibia.

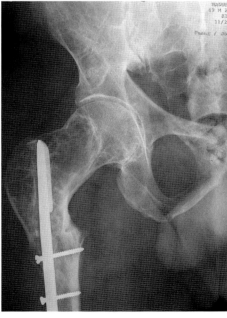

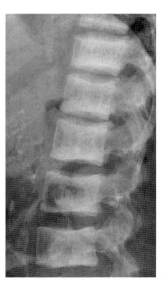

Fig. 2.**48** **Fibrous dysplasia (polyostotic form)**. Mixed osteolytic (some with ground glass appearance) and osteosclerotic involvement of the right hemipelvis and proximal femur is seen.

Fig. 2.**49** **Renal osteodystrophy**. Sclerosis is particularly dense at the endplates of the vertebral bodies, resulting in a characteristic "rugger jersey" spine appearance.

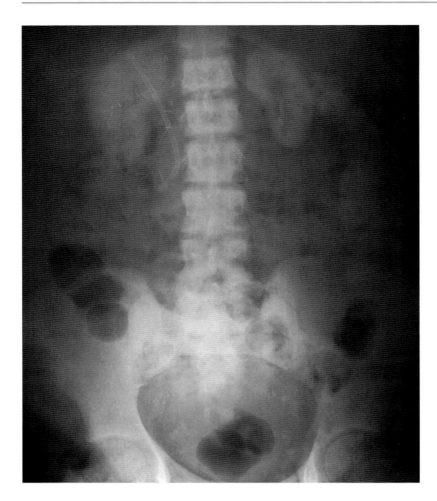

Fig. 2.**50** **Oxalosis**. Diffuse "woolly" sclerosis of the axial skeleton and proximal femora is associated with bilateral dense and small kidneys.

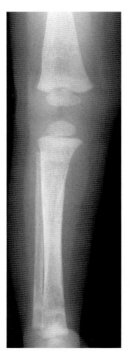

Fig. 2.**51** **Hypervitaminosis D**. Generalized sclerosis and transverse bands in slightly widened metaphyses are seen.

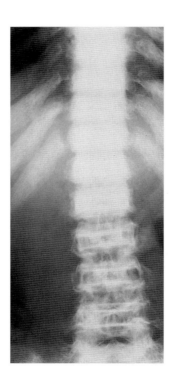

Fig. 2.**52** **Fluorosis**. Increased bone density varying from a markedly thickened and coarsened trabecular pattern to uniform sclerosis.

Table 2.3 Avascular Necrosis of the Bone

Location	Eponym or Name of Disease	Etiology	Time of Occurrence
Spine			
Vertebral body (vertebra plana)	Calvé-Kümmel-Verneuil	Idiopathic, posttraumatic, eosinophilic granuloma	Childhood
Vertebral epiphysis	Scheuermann	Idiopathic	Adolescence
Pelvis			
Iliac crest	Buchman	Idiopathic	Adolescence
Ischial apophysis	Milch	Idiopathic	Adolescence
Ischiopubic synchondrosis	Van Neck	Idiopathic	Childhood
Symphysis pubis	Pierson	Idiopathic	Adolescence
Upper extremity			
Clavicle (lower half of sternal end)	Friedrich	Idiopathic	Adulthood
Head of humerus	Hass	Idiopathic	Childhood
Head of humerus (Fig. 2.53)	Avascular necrosis	Post fracture and other causes similar to avascular necrosis of femoral head (see under this subject in this table)	Adulthood
Head of humerus	Osteochondritis dissecans	Idiopathic, posttraumatic	Adolescence, adulthood
Capitulum of humerus (Fig. 2.54)	Panner	Idiopathic, posttraumatic	Childhood, adolescence
Capitulum of humerus	Osteochondritis dissecans	Idiopathic, posttraumatic	Adolescence, adulthood
Head of radius	Brailsford	Idiopathic	Childhood
Distal ulna (epiphysis)	Burns	Idiopathic	Childhood
Hand			
Scaphoid	Preiser	Idiopathic	Childhood, adolescence
Scaphoid (proximal part)	Avascular necrosis	Posttraumatic	Adulthood
Lunate	Kienböck	Idiopathic, posttraumatic	Adulthood
Entire carpus	Caffey	Idiopathic (bilateral), posttraumatic	Childhood, adolescence
Heads of metacarpals	Dietrich	Idiopathic	Adolescence
Bases of phalanges	Thiemann	Idiopathic, posttraumatic	Adolescence

(continues on page 38)

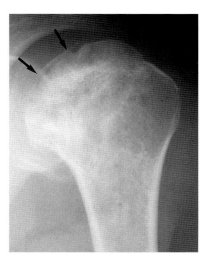

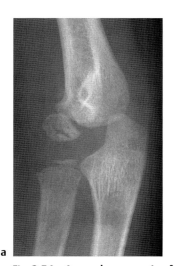

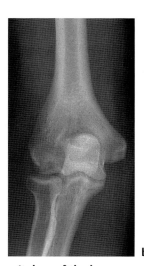

a

b

Fig. 2.**53** **Avascular necrosis of the humeral head.** Sclerotic and lytic changes in the humeral head with fragmentation of the joint surface (arrows) are seen.

Fig. 2.**54** **Avascular necrosis of the capitulum of the humerus (Panner)** (2 cases). **a:** Fragmentation of the slightly sclerotic capitulum humeri is seen (arrow). **b:** Sclerotic lesion in the capitulum humeri is seen with healing.

Table 2.3   (Cont.) Avascular Necrosis of the Bone

Location	Eponym or Name of Disease	Etiology	Time of Occurrence
Lower extremity			
Femoral head epiphysis (Fig. 2.55)	Legg-Calvé-Perthes	Idiopathic	Childhood
Femoral head epiphysis	Slipped capital femoral epiphysis	Idiopathic, posttraumatic	Adolescence
Femoral head	Osteochondritis dissecans	Idiopathic, posttraumatic	Adolescence, adulthood
Femoral head	Avascular necrosis	Idiopathic, degenerative and associated with a variety of diseases (e.g., congenital disorders, hematologic and reticuloendothelial diseases, posttraumatic (especially subcapital hip fracture), post-inflammatory diseases, endocrinologic and metabolic disorders, collagen diseases, pancreatic diseases, alcoholism, steroid therapy, post-irradiation, and caisson disease.	Adolescence, adulthood
Greater trochanter	Mandl	Idiopathic	Adolescence
Medial femur condyle (less commonly lateral femur condyle)	Osteochondritis dissecans	Idiopathic, posttraumatic	Adolescence, adulthood
Medial femur condyle (less commonly lateral femur condyle, rarely tibial condyles) (Fig. 2.55 a)	Ahlbäck (Spontenous osteonecrosis about the knee or SONC)	Idiopathic, stress (insufficiency) fractures	Adulthood (usually after age 60 with female predominance)
Medial or lateral femur condyle	Avascular necrosis	Posttraumatic and other causes similar to avascular necrosis of femoral head.	
Patella	Köhler	Idiopathic	Childhood
Patella (secondary ossification center at inferior aspect of patella)	Sinding-Larsen-Johansson	Idiopathic, posttraumatic	Adolescence
Patella	Osteochondritis dissecans	Idiopathic, posttraumatic	Adolescence, adulthood
Intercondylar spines of tibia	Caffey	Posttraumatic	Adolescence
Medial tibia condyle	Blount	Idiopathic, posttraumatic	Infancy, childhood, adolescence
Tibial tuberosity	Osgood-Schlatter	Idiopathic, posttraumatic	Childhood, Adolescence
Distal tibia (epiphysis)	Liffert-Arkin	Idiopathic, posttraumatic	Childhood
Foot			
Talus (Trochlea)	Diaz	Idiopathic	Childhood
Talus (Trochlea) (Fig. 2.56)	Osteochondritis dissecans	Idiopathic, posttraumatic	Adolescence, adulthood
Talus (Trochlea)	Avascular necrosis	Posttraumatic and other causes similar to avascular necrosis of femoral head (see under this subject in this table)	Adulthood
Epiphysis of calcaneus	Sever	Idiopathic	Adolescence
Navicular	Köhler	Idiopathic	Childhood
Navicular (Fig. 2.57)	Mueller-Weiss	Idiopathic, posttraumatic	Adulthood
Os tibiale externum	Haglund	Idiopathic, posttraumatic	Childhood, adolescence, adulthood
Base of fifth metatarsal	Iselin	Idiopathic	Adolescence
Head of metatarsals (most commonly first)	Osteochondritis dissecans	Idiopathic, posttraumatic	Adolescence, adulthood
Head of metatarsals (most commonly second) (Fig. 2.58)	Freiberg	Idiopathic, posttraumatic	Adolescence, adulthood
Base of phalanges	Thiemann	Idiopathic	Adolescence, adulthood

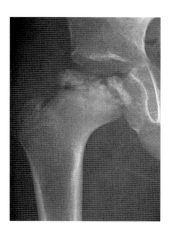

Fig. 2.**55** **Legg-Calvé-Perthes disease**. A flattened, fragmented and laterally displaced capital epiphysis is associated with a widened and shortened femoral neck.

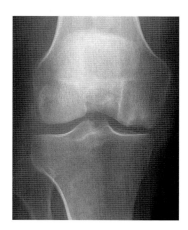

Fig. 2.**55 a** **Ahlbäck's disease (spontaneous osteonecrosis about the knee or SONC)**. An osteochondral defect with mild surrounding sclerosis is seen in the weight-bearing portion of the medial femur condyle.

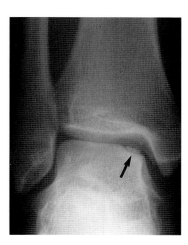

Fig. 2.**56** **Osteochondritis dissecans of the talus**. A small, oval-shaped bony fragment is seen in an articular defect located in the medial aspect of the talar dome (arrow).

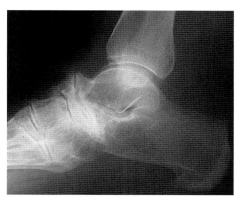

Fig. 2.**57** **Avascular necrosis of the navicular bone (Mueller-Weiss)**. A collapsed sclerotic navicular bone with secondary degenerative changes in the talonavicular joint is seen.

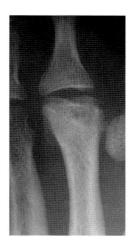

Fig. 2.**58** **Avascular necrosis of the head of the second metatarsal (Freiberg)**. Sclerosis and flattening of the head of the second metatarsal is seen.

BMA Library

BMA House, Tavistock Square, London WC1H 9JP

British Medical Association
BMA House
Tavistock Square
London
WC1H 9JP

BMA

CERTIFICATE OF POSTAGE RECEIPT to be obtained and retained. You are liable for any lost items.

3 Periosteal Reactions

A periosteal reaction is a common response to a variety of insults to the bone. Important differential diagnostic clues may be obtained from both patterns and locations of periosteal reactions. After an acute incidence, it usually takes three weeks before a periosteal reaction can be diagnosed radiographically. Periosteal reactions should be classified as either *solid* or *interrupted*. Each of these two basic forms of periosteal reaction consist of several subtypes. Furthermore, it appears useful for the differential diagnosis to discriminate between conditions with localized or generalized periosteal reactions.

Solid periosteal reactions can be *thin* (1 mm or less in thickness) or *thick* (2 mm or more). A thin periosteal reaction might represent an early stage of a highly aggressive bone lesion or a chronic, benign process (Fig. 3.1). On the other hand, a thick periosteal reaction usually suggests a benign condition. Thick periosteal reactions may be further subdivided into *straight*, *elliptical*, and *undulating*, each subtype suggesting somewhat different diagnostic possibilities (Fig. 3.2).

An *interrupted periosteal reaction*, in general, signals an acute and rapidly progressing process requiring immediate attention. These periosteal reactions can be *laminated ("onion skin"), perpendicular ("sunburst")*, or *amorphous* (Fig. 3.3). A destructive bone lesion associated with any interrupted periosteal reaction suggests acute osteomyelitis or a malignancy.

A local elevation of the periosteum that is calcified at the site of its bone insertion is known as *"Codman's triangle"* (Fig. 3.3b). Originally considered as a sign of a malignant bone neoplasm, it has been recognized that it can also occur with benign processes such as osteomyelitis, subperiosteal hemorrhage, and fracture. When the periosteal reaction eventually blends with the adjacent cortex, cortical thickening occurs. However, cortical thickening may also develop by excessive endosteal or periosteal new bone formation without stripping the periosteum away from the cortex. The differential diagnoses of various bone lesions with periosteal reactions are discussed in Table 3.1.

Under a variety of degenerative, traumatic and inflammatory conditions, a periostitis is found at the insertions of many tendons and ligaments causing the appearance of *"whiskering"* (Fig. 3.4). The most common location is the pel-

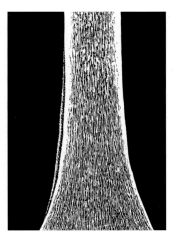

Fig. 3.**1** **Thin (1 mm or smaller) periosteal reaction.** This is an indeterminate finding, since it may indicate a chronic benign process that progresses slowly, if ever, to a solid thick periosteal reaction; or it may represent the earliest stage of an aggressive bone lesion that progresses rapidly to an interrupted periosteal reaction.

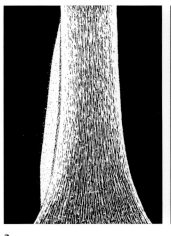
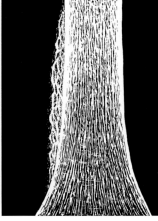

a   b

Fig. 3.**2** **Solid periosteal reactions** indicating a benign bone le- ▷ sion. **a** Thick (2 mm or larger) periosteal reaction. **b** Undulating periosteal reaction. **c** Periosteal cloaking. **d** Elliptical periosteal reaction.

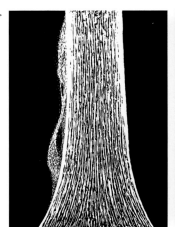
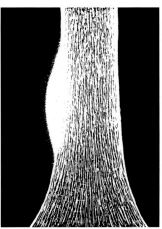

c   d

vis, where the iliac crests, the ischial tuberosities and the ischiopubic rami are affected. Other sites of extrapelvic involvement include the femoral trochanters, the patella, the calcaneus, the dorsum of the foot, the inferior clavicular margin at the attachment of the coracoclavicular ligament, the humeral tuberosities, and the olecranon. As the periostitis progresses the "whiskers" become more prominent, and may transform into spurs or other bony excrescences referred to as *enthesophytes*. They tend to remain relatively ill-defined or fluffy in *ankylosing spondylitis* (Fig. 3.5), *Reiter's syndrome* and *psoriasis*. In these inflammatory conditions, erosions or sclerosis of the adjacent bone may be associated.

The enthesophytes in *diffuse idiopathic skeletal hyperostosis (DISH)* (Fig. 3.6) are bilateral and symmetrical, but without adjacent erosions or reactive bone sclerosis. These spurs are well demarcated and often irregular in outline, especially in the calcaneus. Degenerative disease of tendons and ligaments in the elderly may produce similar enthesophytes, but they tend to be less prominent and less symmetric.

Localized spurring at the insertions of tendons and ligaments occurs in conjunction with *chronic stress* or as *sequelae of an old injury*. Spur formations are commonly found in the calcaneus, patella and trochanters with *acromegaly*. Ligamentous and tendinous calcifications resembling DISH and predominantly involving the axial skeleton are encountered in *fluorosis, hypoparathyroidism*, and *vitamin D-resistant rickets* (adults), but may be associated in these conditions with osteosclerosis, which is particularly striking in fluorosis.

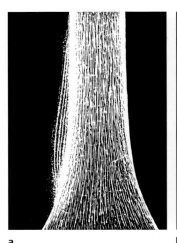 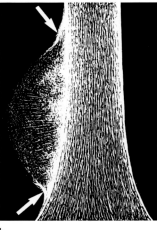 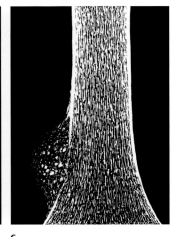

a b c

Fig. 3.**3 Interrupted periosteal reactions** indicating an aggressive or malignant bone lesion. **a** Laminated ("onion skin") periosteal reaction. **b** Perpendicular ("sunburst") periosteal reaction and Codman's triangles at both ends (arrows). **c** Amorphous periosteal reaction.

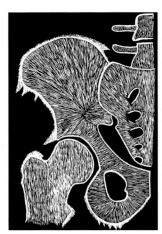

Fig. 3.**4 Whiskering**. Periostitis at the insertion of tendons and ligaments found with a variety of degenerative, traumatic and inflammatory conditions. Progression to formation of spurs or bony excrescences (enthesophytes) possible.

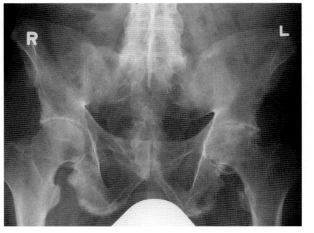

Fig. 3.**5 Ankylosing spondylitis**. Fluffy enthesopathy along the iliac crests and ischia with sclerosis of the adjacent bones is associated with fusion of the sacroiliac joints and the visualized part of the lumbar spine. Note the delicate bridging syndesmophytes in the lumbar spine. Arthritic changes with circumferential (axial) joint space narrowing and early erosions are also seen in both hips.

Fig. 3.**6 DISH**. Well defined enthesopathy with bony excrescences that can be differentiated in cortical and cancellous bone are associated with normal sacroiliac joints and fused lower lumbar spine by huge paravertebral ossifications.

Table 3.1   Diseases with Periosteal Reactions

Disease	Preferred Locations	Distribution	Periosteal Reactions	Comments
Physiologic periostitis in infants (Fig. 3.7)	Long bones	Generalized and symmetrical	Solid thin or thick	Develops in second or third month of life, especially in prematures.
Congenital syphilis (Fig. 3.8)	Long bones	Generalized and symmetrical	Solid thick or laminated	Associated with transverse striping of metaphyses and destructive lesions, initially involving the corners of the metaphyses adjacent to the cartilage plate.
Infantile cortical hyperostosis (Caffey's disease) (Fig. 3.9)	Mandible, clavicle, scapula, ribs, tubular bones (limited to diaphyses)	Solitary or multiple	Solid thick or laminated	Clinically tender soft-tissue swellings are associated with the affected bone. Onset occurs in the first five months of life.
Hypervitaminosis A	Tubular bones (especially ulna), metatarsals, clavicle, tibia, fibula (limited to diaphyses)	Generalized	Solid, undulating or occasionally laminated	Associated with tender soft masses in children usually between 1 and 3 years old. *Prostaglandin* infusions in neonates (to maintain patency of the ductus-dependent congenital heart disease) may result in similar bony changes. In older children and adolescents, periosteal reactions and hyperostosis in the axial and appendicular skeleton similar to DISH may bay be found with chronic administration of *retinoid drugs*.

(continues on page 44)

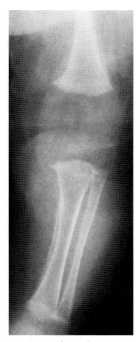

Fig. 3.7 Physiologic periostitis in infants. A solid, thin periosteal reaction is found along the medial aspect of the tibia and lateral aspect of the distal femur.

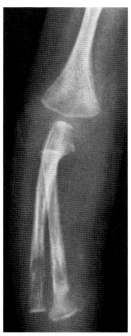

Fig. 3.8 Congenital syphilis. Solid, thick periosteal reactions are associated with destructive lesions in the radius and ulna and with irregular metaphyses.

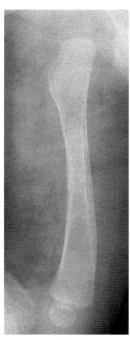

Fig. 3.9 Infantile cortical hyperostosis (Caffey's disease). A laminated periosteal reaction is seen along the femur diaphysis.

Table 3.1 (Cont.) Diseases with Periosteal Reactions

Disease	Preferred Locations	Distribution	Periosteal Reactions	Comments
Scurvy (healing) (Fig. 3.10)	Long bones	Generalized	Solid thick	Caused by calcification of the subperiosteal hemorrhage.
Rickets (healing) (Fig. 3.11)	Long bones	Generalized	Solid thin, thicker laminated	Caused by calcification of the subperiosteal osteoid. Associated with mineralization of the zone of provisional calcification that appears as an irregular dense area in the epiphyseal cartilage, separated by a thin radiolucent line from the metaphysis.
Dysproteinemia	Tubular bones, mandible	Generalized and symmetrical	Solid thin or thick, or laminated	In children with bone pain and often with fever. Hyperphosphatemia may also be present.
Pachydermoperiostosis (primary hypertrophic osteoarthropathy) (Fig. 3.12)	Long tubular bones, especially radius, ulna, tibia and fibula. Less common in metacarpals, metatarsals, and phalanges, pelvis, ribs and clavicles.	Generalized and symmetrical. May extend from the diaphyses into the metaphyses and epiphyses (DD: Secondary hypertrophic osteoarthropathy, where it does not extend into the epiphyses).	Solid thick, often with shaggy, irregular excrescences	Familial condition with skin thickening and cortical thickening. Periosteal new bone formation tends to blend with thickened cortex. Almost exclusively found in males with predilection for blacks. Onset in adolescence.
Secondary hypertrophic osteoarthropathy (Fig. 3.13)	Diaphyses of tubular bones	Generalized and symmetrical	Solid thin or thick (often undulating and cloaking) or laminated	In patients with bronchogenic carcinoma, and occasionally with chronic diseases of lung, gastrointestinal tract, or cardiovascular system.
Osteosarcoma (Figs. 3.14 and 3.15)	Femur, tibia, humerus, and mandible	Localized	Solid thin, laminated, perpendicular (thin spicules) or amorphous. Codman's triangle occurs	*Periosteal sarcoma*: Limited to the cortex of long bone diaphyses (especially femur and tibia). Perpendicular periosteal reaction and Codman's triangle are characteristic.
				Parosteal sarcoma: a large radiodense lesion with smooth lobulated or irregular margins is attached to the external cortex (Fig. 3.16).

(continues on page 46)

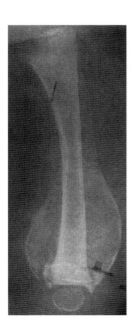

Fig. 3.**10** **Scurvy** (healing). This characteristic periosteal reaction is caused by calcification of the subperiosteal hemorrhage.

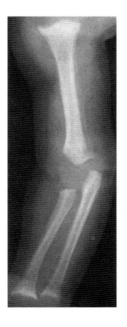

Fig. 3.**11** **Rickets** (healing). This periosteal reaction is caused by calcification of the subperiosteal osteoid.

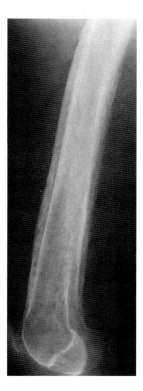

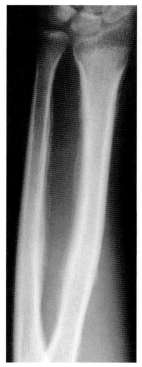

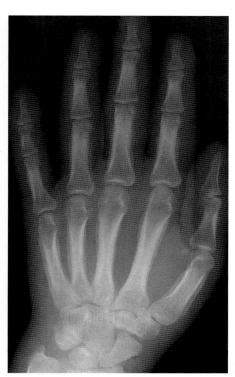

Fig. 3.**12 Pachydermoperiostosis (primary hypertrophic osteoarthropathy.** A solid, thick, and shaggy periosteal reaction is seen

Fig. 3.**13a**, **b Secondary hypertrophic osteoarthropathy.** Solid thin and laminated, occasionally undulating periosteal reactions are seen in the radius and ulna (**a**) and tubular bones of the hand (**b**).

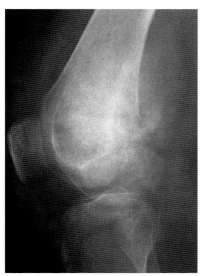

Fig. 3.**14 Osteosarcoma (osteolytic).** A poorly defined osteolytic lesion is seen in the distal femur associated with a large amorphous periosteal reaction posteriorly.

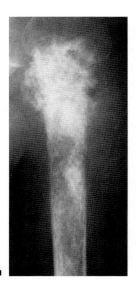

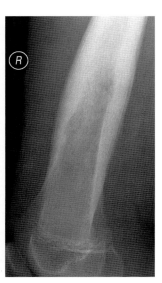

◁ Fig. 3.**15a**, **b Osteosarcoma (2 cases).** A permeative destructive lesion with osteoblastic areas and amorphous periosteal reaction, interspersed with thin perpendicular spicules, is seen in **a**. Cortical thickening with laminated periosteal reaction is seen in **b**.

Fig. 3.**16 Parosteal osteosarcoma.** A large, radiodense lesion with irregular margins is attached posteriorly to the distal femur in characteristic location. ▷

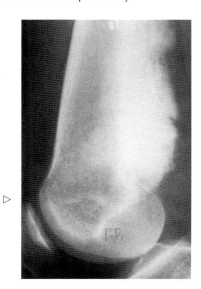

Table 3.1   (Cont.) Diseases with Periosteal Reactions

Disease	Preferred Locations	Distribution	Periosteal Reactions	Comments
Ewing's sarcoma (Figs. 3.17 and 3.18)	Under 20 yr: tubular bones Over 20 yr: flat bones	Localized	Solid thin, laminated or perpendicular (thin spicules). Codman's triangle occurs.	
Other sarcomas (e.g. chondrosarcoma, fibrosarcoma) and primary bone lymphoma (including reticulum cell sarcoma)	Long bones, flat bones	Localized	Solid thin, thick or amorphous. Rarely solid thick, laminated, perpendicular or amorphous. Codman's triangle is unusual.	Periosteal reactions are rare in these conditions. Cortical thickening in a chondroid matrix tumor suggests low-grade chondrosarcoma rather than enchondroma.
Leukemia and metastases (Figs. 3.19 and 3.20)	Long bones, ribs	Multiple	Solid thin or laminated. Perpendicular in skull. Rarely solid thick.	Interrupted periosteal reactions are common in children (e.g., leukemia and metastases from *neuroblastomas*). Solid periosteal reaction or localized cortical thickening is associated with metastases from *prostatic* and *breast carcinomas*.
Osteoid osteoma (Fig. 3.21)	Femur, tibia, fibula, humerus, vertebral arch	Localized	Elliptical and dense. Rarely solid thin.	Radiolucent intracortical nidus with or without central calcification is classical, but not always demonstrated.
Other benign tumors and cysts		Localized	Solid thin or thick.	Periosteal reactions usually associated with bone expansions and/or pathologic fractures.
Acute hematogenous osteomyelitis (Fig. 3.22)		Solitary, rarely multiple	Solid thin or thick, laminated or perpendicular (short and squat spicules). Codman's triangle occurs.	Earliest radiographic findings: bone destruction after 1 week, periosteal reactions after 2 weeks, and sequestrum formation after 3 weeks. Organisms: staphylococci, streptococci, salmonella (especially in sickle cell anemia), pseudomonas, klebsiella (often with intravenous drug abuse), less common: pneumococci, meningococci, brucella, fungi, viruses, and parasites.

(continues on page 48)

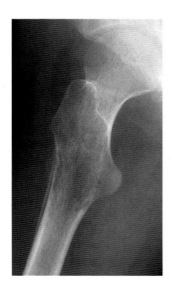

Fig. 3.**17   Ewing's sarcoma**. A poorly defined permeative osteolytic lesion is seen in the proximal femur with beginning laminated periosteal reaction on its outer cortex.

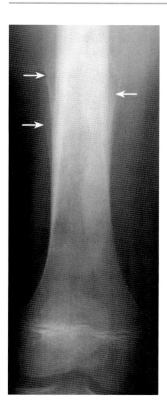

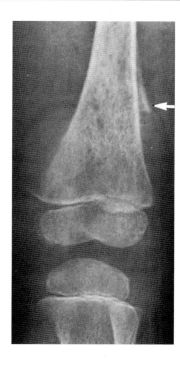

Fig. 3.**18** **Ewing's sarcoma**. A barely perceptive permeative osteolytic lesion in the femur shaft is associated with laminated periosteal reactions including three Codman's triangles (arrows).

Fig. 3.**19** **Neuroblastoma metastasis**. A permeative lesion with a Codman's triangle (arrow) and a faint perpendicular periosteal reaction is seen. A solitary neuroblastoma metastasis is radiographically often indistinguishable from a Ewing's sarcoma.

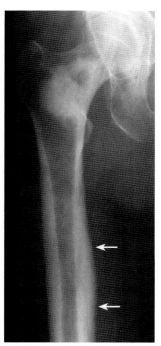

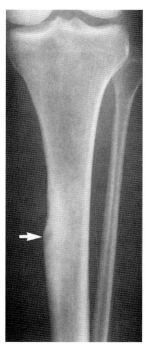

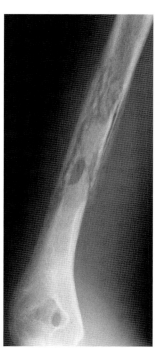

Fig. 3.**20** **Osteoblastic metastases (breast carcinoma)**. Besides a large osteoblastic metastases in the femoral neck and intertrochanteric area localized thickening of the cortex in the femur shaft is also evident (arrows).

Fig. 3.**21** **Osteoid osteoma**. A dense, elliptical periosteal reaction with a nidus (arrow) is diagnostic.

Fig. 3.**22** **Acute osteomyelitis**. A destructive bone lesion surrounded by a laminated periosteal reaction is seen.

Table 3.1   (Cont.) Diseases with Periosteal Reactions

Disease	Preferred Locations	Distribution	Periosteal Reactions	Comments
Chronic osteomyelitis (Fig. 3.23)		Solitary, rarely multiple	Solid thick, often undulating and cloaking.	Thick periosteal reaction associated with sclerosis, and scattered radiolucent areas which may contain a dense bone sequestrum.
Osteomyelitis from contiguous infective source (Fig. 3.24)	Hands, feet or adjacent to decubitus ulcers	Localized	Solid thin or thick.	Periosteal reaction associated with bone destruction and sclerosis. Commonly found in diabetes mellitus, quadriplegia and vascular insufficiency.
Tuberculous osteomyelitis (Fig. 3.25)		Solitary, rarely multiple	Solid thin or thick.	Similar to hematogenous osteomyelitis, but osteopenia is more pronounced, whereas periosteal reactions and osteosclerosis are less. Similar findings as in tuberculosis are seen in *atypical tuberculosis bacilli* and *BCG osteomyelitis*.
Syphilis	Long bones, skull	Localized or generalized	Solid thin or thick, often undulating and with squat spicules, or laminated.	In early acquired syphilis, an extensive generalized periosteal reaction and cortical thickening is the most common osseous manifestation. The radiologic hallmark of the tertiary stage of the disease consists of dense bony sclerosis with areas of destruction (gumma formation).
Yaws	Long and short tubular bones, skull	Localized or generalized	Solid thin or thick, often undulating and with squat spicules, or laminated.	Occurs in tropical climates, and is usually acquired before puberty. Radiographic features similar to syphilis and *bejel* (prevalent in the Middle East). The causative organisms of these three spirochetal diseases are morphologically indistinguishable.
Tropical ulcer	Tibia (anterior aspect of middle and distal third)	Localized	Solid thick, elliptical or undulating.	Common in Central and East Africa.
Leprosy	Hands, feet	Solitary or multiple	Solid thin or thick, or laminated.	May be associated with bone destruction. Neuropathic bone manifestations are, however, much more common and characteristic.
Rheumatoid arthritis (juvenile)	Peripheral and axial skeleton: periarticular and at tendon and ligament insertions	Localized or generalized	Solid thin or thick or laminated.	Common in juvenile rheumatoid arthritis; very rare in adults, and never a dominant feature.
Psoriatic arthritis (Fig. 3.26)	As above, preferentially in hands	Localized or Generalized	Solid thin or thick or laminated.	Periosteal reactions not uncommon. Irregular bony excrescences characteristic.
Reiter's syndrome (Fig. 3.27)	Calcaneus, short tubular bones of foot, tibia, and fibula	Localized, seldom generalized	Solid thin or thick (often "fluffy") or laminated.	Periosteal reactions common.
Polyarteritis nodosa	Long tubular bones (preferentially lower limbs) and metatarsals	Generalized and symmetrical	Solid thin or thick, characteristically undulating.	Radiographically similar to hypertrophic osteoarthropathy. Pain and swelling of the lower extremity may be associated.

(continues on page 50)

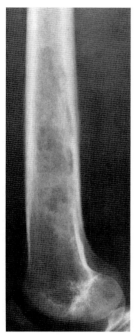

Fig. 3.**23** **Chronic osteomyelitis**. A poorly defined, mixed lytic and sclerotic lesion is associated with a solid periosteal reaction (serratia marcescens osteomyelitis in an intravenous drug abuser).

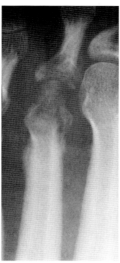

Fig. 3.**24** **Osteomyelitis in diabetes mellitus**. A destructive lesion around the third metatarsophalangeal joint with periosteal reaction is seen.

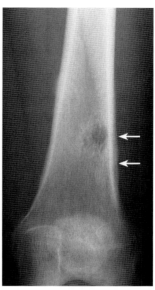

Fig. 3.**25** **Tuberculous osteomyelitis**. A poorly defined lytic lesion is associated with a thin solid periosteal reaction (arrows).

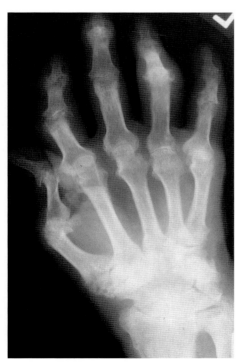

Fig. 3.**26** **Psoriatic arthritis**. Besides erosive arthritic changes extensive periostitis and sclerosis is seen producing an "ivory hand".

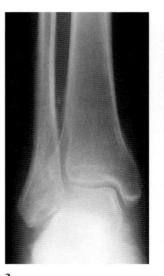
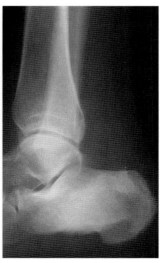

a   b

Fig. 3.**27** **Reiter's syndrome**. **a** Ill-defined periosteal reactions around the ankle and **b** fluffy "whiskering" in the posterior and inferior aspect of the calcaneus are quite characteristic.

Table 3.1 (Cont.) Diseases with Periosteal Reactions

Disease	Preferred Locations	Distribution	Periosteal Reactions	Comments
Fractures and stress fractures (Fig. 3.28)		Solitary or multiple	Solid thin or thick or laminated. Codman's triangle occurs.	Periosteal reactions are similar in traumatic and pathologic fractures.
Subperiosteal hemorrhages	Long tubular bones	Solitary or multiple	Solid thin or thick or laminated. Codman's triangle occurs.	Traumatic (including *battered child syndrome*) and *hemophilia*.
Electrical and thermal injuries	Upper extremity	Localized	Solid thin.	Osteolysis, osteosclerosis, periarticular calcifications and heterotopic bone formation are frequently associated.
Vascular and lymphatic disease (Fig. 3.29)	Lower extremity	Localized or generalized	Solid thin or thick, often undulating.	Any disease associated with venous and/or lymphatic stasis. Vascular calcifications and phleboliths may be associated.
Bone infarct	Long tubular bones	Solitary or multiple	Solid thin or thick.	Especially in sickle cell disease, where the periosteal reaction may also be caused by osteomyelitis. *Hand-foot syndrome:* infarctions of the short tubular bones causing periosteal reactions that are indistinguishable from osteomyelitis. Occurs in young children (average age 18 months) with sickle-cell disease.
Eosinophilic granuloma (Langerhans cell histiocytosis)		Solitary or multiple	Solid thin or thick. Rarely laminated.	Destructive bone lesions may contain bone sequestrum.
Gaucher's and other storage diseases	Long tubular bones, spine, and pelvis	Localized or generalized	Solid thin or thick, often undulating and cloaking.	Combination of avascular necrosis of the femoral head, Erlenmeyer flask deformity of the distal femur, circumscribed osteolytic lesions, and bone infarcts are characteristic for Gaucher's disease.
Thyroid acropachy (Fig. 3.30)	Tubular bones, particularly hands and feet	Bilateral and relatively symmetrical	Solid thin or thick, occasionally with short and squat spicules.	Usually one year and later after treatment with thyroidectomy or radioactive iodine.
Renal osteodystrophy (Fig. 3.31)	Long tubular bones, metatarsal, pubic rami	Generalized and symmetrical	Solid thin or thick, occasionally laminated.	Associated with findings of hyperpalathyroidism and osteosclerosis. Very rare in *primary hyperparathyroidism*.
Tuberous sclerosis	Tubular bones	Solitary or multiple	Solid thin or thick, often undulating.	
Neurofibromatosis	Long bones of lower extremity	Solitary or multiple	Solid thick, often undulating.	Pathogenesis of this manifestation is not clear.
Fluorosis	Tubular bones	Generalized and symmetrical	Solid thick, often undulating and cloaking.	Osteosclerosis and ossification of ligaments and tendons at their insertion.
Gardner's syndrome	Tubular bones	Multiple	Solid thin or thick, often undulating.	Osteomas and intestinal polyposis are associated.
DISH (diffuse idiopathic skeletal hyperostosis) (Fig. 3.32)	Spine, pelvis, lower extremity (commonly patella and calcaneus)	Multiple and often symmetrical	Solid thick.	Particularly at tendon and ligament insertions into bone ("whiskering").

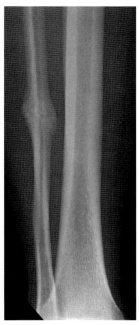

Fig. 3.**28** **Stress fracture**. A healing stress fracture is seen in the fibula shaft with exuberant callus formation.

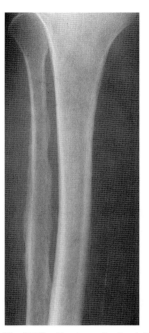

Fig. 3.**29** **Venous stasis**. A thick, undulating periosteal reaction in the proximal tibia, and particularly fibula is associated with extensive varicosis.

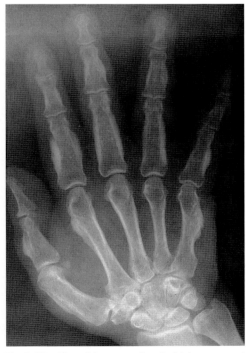

Fig. 3.**30** **Thyroid acropachy**. A thick, asymmetric, shaggy periostitis is seen in the fingers with predilection for the metacarpals and proximal phalanges.

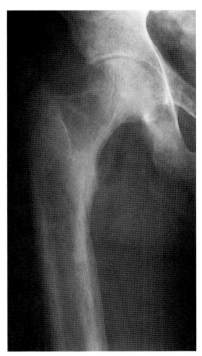

Fig. 3.**31** **Renal osteodystrophy**. Diffuse sclerosis is associated with a solid thick periosteal reaction in the lateral femur cortex and laminated in the medial femur cortex.

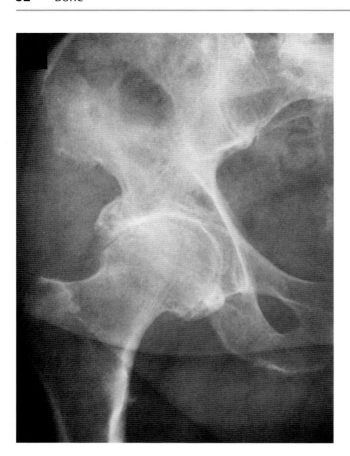

Fig. 3.**32** **DISH.** "Whiskering" along the iliac crest, ischiopubic ramus, and femoral trochanters associated with hypertrophic spurs at the superior and inferior margins of the acetabulum.

4 Trauma and Fractures

The radiologic diagnosis and differential diagnosis of an acute fracture is usually not associated with any problems. A sharply demarcated fracture line is the hallmark of an acute fracture. Depending on their radiographic appearances, fractures are classified into different types (Fig. 4.1). Occasionally, however, a frank fracture line cannot be demonstrated in undisplaced fractures immediately after injury even when films in several projections are taken. Demonstration of either a cortical break that has to be differentiated from a nutrient artery or disruption of the normal spongiosa pattern may be the only clue in these instances to diagnose a fracture. Magnetic resonance imaging or a nuclear medicine scan is otherwise required to arrive at the correct diagnosis.

In the presence of clinical evidence of a fracture, a zone of increased bone density or an abnormal angulation may suggest radiographically an acute fracture, although these findings can also be encountered in healing fractures and other bone diseases. At least some degree of soft-tissue swelling can be seen radiographically in virtually all acute fractures, but this finding is of little use to differentiate a fracture from a distortion or other soft-tissue injuries.

Fracture healing begins with an acute inflammatory response resulting in the organization of the fracture hematoma by invasion of fibrovascular tissue. At this stage, bone resorption along the fracture margins becomes evident and in undisplaced fractures may allow at this stage (several days after the injury incidence) an unequivocal radiographic diagnosis. Periosteal and endosteal callus formation usually becomes visible two to three weeks after injury and is first evident as a thin periosteal reaction and irregular mottled calcifications about the fracture, increasing with time in density, and finally developing bone texture. The healing process of a noncomplicated fracture from injury to consolidation takes one to several months. Fracture healing progresses more rapidly in oblique or spiral fractures, in a single fracture, and in younger patients. The healing process is slower in larger bones, in transverse fractures, in the presence of multiple fractures, and with increasing age of the patient.

A *delayed union* is found with poor reduction, incomplete immobilization, in the presence of infection, in vitamin C and/or D deficiencies, and in areas of preexisting bone disease (pathologic fractures). Infections are particularly common in *compound fractures*, where extensive soft-tissue damage is caused by either a fracture fragment piercing through the skin or by an object (e.g., a projectile) penetrating from the outside.

Malunion refers to a fracture that is healed with significant fracture fragment displacement and/or angulation. A *nonun-*

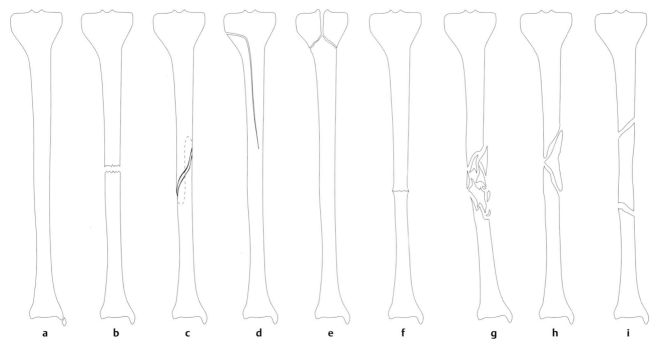

Fig. 4.1 Classification of fracture according to their radiographic appearance. a Avulsion fracture (secondary to forcible tearing of ligament or tendon attachment). A chip fracture has the same radiographic appearance, but is caused by direct impact. **b** Transverse fracture (secondary to shearing force to opposite sides of a bone or to impact force along transverse axis). An oblique fracture (not shown) occurs secondary to impact along an oblique axis. **c** Spiral fracture (secondary to rotary-type injury).

d Longitudinal fracture (secondary to impact force along longitudinal axis). **e** T-, V-, or Y-shaped fracture in proximity of joints (secondary to impact force along longitudinal axis). **f** Impacted fracture or compression fracture (secondary to impact force along longitudinal axis). **g** Comminuted fracture (secondary to severe external trauma or shattering effect of a projectile). **h** Fracture with butterfly fragment. **i** Segmental fracture.

ion is characterized by failure of fracture healing 6 to 9 months after injury. The fracture margins are well delineated and often sclerotic and a frank area of intervening translucency is present. Nonunion may result from the same complications associated with delayed union or by interposition of soft tissue between the fracture fragments. *Hypertrophic nonunion* is commonly caused by continued motion at the fracture site. In these cases the fracture line persists or exces-

sive and prolonged bone resorption at the fracture margins occurs. Eventually the bone ends become sclerotic, and there is a varying degree of non-bridging external callus formation. *Atrophic nonunion* is thought to result from extensive bone death. The radiographic appearance is that of a persistent fracture line without demonstrable callus formation (Figs. 4.2 and 4.3). Nonunion may eventually progress to *pseudarthrosis* formation (Fig. 4.4).

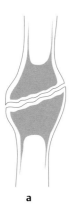 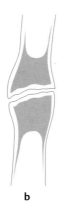  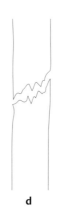

a b c d

Fig. 4.**2**   **Nonunion. a** Hypertrophic (elephant foot). **b** Hypertrophic (horse foot). **c** Oligotrophic. **d** Atrophic.

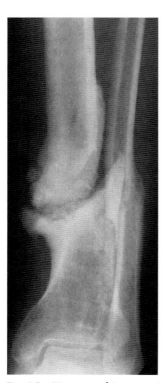

Fig. 4.**3**   **Hypertrophic nonunion.** The distal tibia shaft fracture shows relatively smooth, sclerotic borders without endosteal or periosteal bony bridging of the fracture line, A healed fibula fracture is also evident.

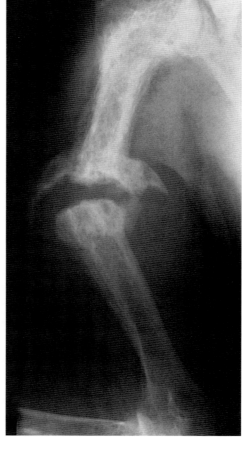

Fig. 4.**4**   **Pseudarthrosis** had developed 2 years after a fracture of ▷ the humerus that shows classical changes of Paget's disease.

Fracture healing in *osteogenesis imperfecta* is complicated by pseudarthrosis formation with a higher incidence than in normal bone. Pseudarthrosis is also a common feature in *neurofibromatosis*, where it is most often found in the lower two-thirds of the tibia (Fig. 4.5). Pseudarthrosis occurs also in *fibrous dysplasia*, which often demonstrates bone changes radiographically similar to neurofibromatosis. The two disorders can, however, often be differentiated by their skin manifestations. The cafe-au-lait spots in fibrous dysplasia are irregularly outlined ("coast of Maine" appearance), whereas they are smoothly outlined in neurofibromatosis ("coast of California" appearance). Furthermore, the presence of cutaneous fibromas is characteristic for the latter condition. *"Congenital pseudarthrosis"* is a rare condition that may or may not be related to neurofibromatosis or fibrous dysplasia (forme fruste?).

Fractures of the *proximal humerus* occur between one or all four major segments, which include the articular segment (anatomic neck fracture), the proximal humerus shaft (surgical neck fracture), the greater tuberosity and the lesser tuberosity. The modified *Neer four-segment classification* is based on the number of displaced segments. Any fracture that is not or only minimally (less than 1 cm) displaced and not or only minimally angulated (less than 45°) is disregarded. A one-part fracture may involve any or all four anatomic segments but there is no displacement or angulation between fracture fragments. A two-part fracture indicates that only one segment is displaced in relation to the three that remain undisplaced or are intact. A three-part fracture commonly consists of a displaced greater *or* lesser tuberosity fracture combined with a surgical neck fracture. A four-part fracture typically involves both greater and lesser tuberosity in addition to the surgical neck with displacement of all four segments. Two-part, three-part, and four-part fractures may be associated with either anterior or posterior dislocation. The involvement of the articular surface in an anterior fracture-dislocation is referred to as "head splitting" and in a posterior fracture-dislocation as "impression".

Fractures of the *elbow* may involve the distal humerus, and proximal radius and ulna. Extra-articular fractures of the distal humerus involve the epicondyles and supracondylar area. Intra-articular fractures of the distal humerus may involve either the trochlea or the capitellum alone (transcondylar fractures) or both (bicondylar or intercondylar fractures with or without supracondylar comminution). Fractures of the radial head are common in adults, but when nondisplaced or minimally displaced may be difficult to demonstrate with routine radiographic projections. An *Essex-Lopresti fracture* consists of a comminuted displaced fracture of the radial head associated with posterior subluxation of the distal ulna. Fractures of the proximal ulna may involve the coronoid process or the olecranon, but the former rarely occurs as an isolated injury.

A *Monteggia fracture* is the association of a proximal ulnar shaft fracture with dislocation of the radial head. Both the apex of angulation of the ulnar fracture and the dislocation of the radial head are anterior in type 1 (60%), posterior in type 2 (15%), lateral in type 3 (20%) and similar to type 1 but associated with a radius shaft fracture at the level of the ulnar fracture in type 4 (5%) (Fig. 4.6). A *Galeazzi fracture* consists of a fracture of the distal third of the radius with angulation apex dorsal and medial (ulnar) associated with dorsal and medial dislocation of the ulna in the distal radioulnar joint (Fig. 4.7).

Fractures of the *distal radius* include 1. *Colles fracture* (extra-articular, usually occurring about 2 to 3 cm from the articular surface with typically radial and dorsal displacement and angulation apex volar of the distal radius fracture fragment and frequent association of an ulnar styloid fracture). 2. *Smith fracture* (extra- or intra-articular fracture with volar displacement of the distal fragment). 3. *Barton fracture* (intra-articular oblique fracture of the dorsal distal radius) and 4. *Hutchinson or chauffeur's fracture* (fracture of the radial styloid process) (Fig. 4.8). The scaphoid is the most commonly fractured carpal bone. The fracture may be located in the distal pole (5%), tubercle (5%), waist (75%) or proximal pole (15%) (Fig. 4.9). Common complications of a

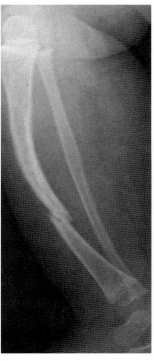

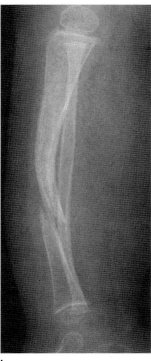

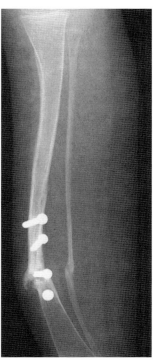

Fig. 4.5 Nonunion and pseudarthrosis formation in neurofibromatosis. a A fracture is seen in the tibia that shows anterior bowing.
b Six months after **a**. Periosteal callus formation and bone resorption occurred around the fracture fragments, but the fracture has not healed (nonunion). **c** Five years after **a**. Despite various conservative and surgical treatment attempts, the fracture has not healed, and a pseudarthrosis has formed. Note also the bowing and narrowing (overconstriction) of the fibula (characteristic of neurofibromatosis) in which a healed fracture is now seen.

a   b   c

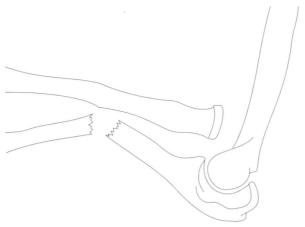

Fig. 4.**6** **Monteggia fracture** (type 1). Fracture of the proximal ulnar shaft with anterior angulation at the apex and anterior dislocation of the radial head is seen.

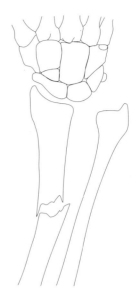

Fig. 4.**7** **Galleazzi fracture**. Fracture of the distal radius with angulation apex medial and dorsal and posteromedial dislocation of the ulna in the distal radioulnar joint is diagnostic. The radius fracture fragments may also overlap.

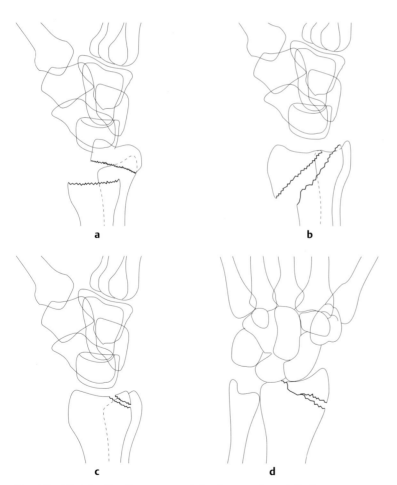

Fig. 4.**8** **Distal radius fractures**. **a** *Colles fracture*: Dorsal displacement and angulation apex volar of distal fragment. **b** *Smith fracture*: Volar displacement of distal fragment. **c** *Barton fracture*: Intra-articular fracture of the dorsal distal radius. **d** *Hutchinson* or *chauffeur's fracture*: Fracture of the radial styloid process.

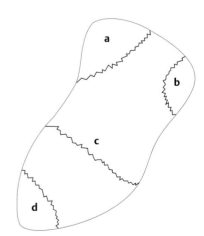

Fig. 4.**9** **Scaphoid fractures** may involve distal pole (**a**), tubercle (**b**), waist (**c**) or proximal pole (**d**).

scaphoid waist fracture include nonunion and avascular necrosis of the proximal fracture fragment.

The most frequent ligamentous injuries of the carpal bones are centered around the lunate and include scapholunate dissociation, perilunate dislocation, midcarpal dislocation and lunate dislocation. *Scapholunate dissociation (rotary subluxation of the scaphoid)* (Fig. 4.**10**) is associated with an injury to the scapholunate ligament. The condition is diagnosed on the dorsovolar view of the wrist by either widening of the space between the scaphoid and lunate measuring more than 2 mm in the midline between these to carpal bones or more than 4 mm at their proximal border, respectively, (*Terry Thomas sign*) and/or a volar tilt of scaphoid producing a foreshortened scaphoid with characteristic ring shadow (*signet ring sign*). In *perilunate dislocation* the lunate is volarly rotated, but remains in articulation with the radius and the capitate is dorsally dislocated with regard to the lunate. In *lunate dislocation* the volarly rotated lunate is also completely volarly dislocated with regard to both the radius and capitate which remain aligned (Fig. 4.**11**). *Pericarpal dislocation* can be considered a stage between perilunate and lunate dislocation with anterior subluxation of the volarly tilted lunate with regard to the radius and complete dorsal dislocation in the lunocapitate joint. Perilunate dislocations may be associated with carpal bone fractures. The prefix "trans-" indicates which carpal bone(s) is/are fractured (e.g., trans-scaphoid perilunate dislocation).

Intra-articular fractures of the base of the first metacarpal may be simple (*Bennett fracture*) (Fig. 4.**12**) or comminuted (*Rolando fracture*). In these conditions the first metacarpal is frequently dorsally and radially dislocated or displaced, respectively, caused by the pull of the abductor pollicis longus. A *boxer's fracture* involves the neck of a metacarpal (most commonly the fifth) with characteristic dorsal angulation at the apex. A *gamekeeper's thumb* (*skier's thumb*) (Fig. 4.**13**) results from rupture of the ulnar collateral ligament of the first

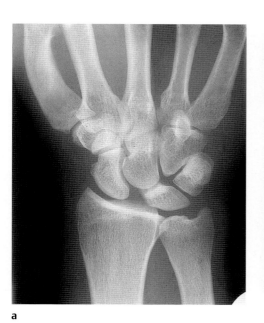

a

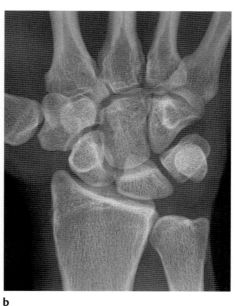

b

Fig. 4.**10 a, b Scapholunate dissociation** and rotary subluxation of the scaphoid. An injury to the scapholunate ligament is diagnosed by either widening of the distance between scaphoid and lunate (Terry Thomas sign) (**a**) or by rotary subluxation of the scaphoid producing the signet ring sign (**b**).

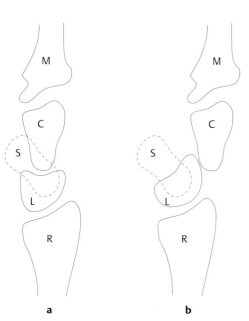

a

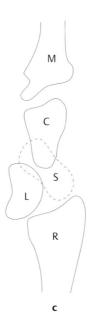

b   c

Fig. 4.**11 Perilunate and lunate dislocation.**
a Normal lateral wrist, **b** perilunate dislocation, **c** lunate dislocation. C: capitate. L: lunate. M: 3rd metacarpal. R: radius. S: scaphoid.

metacarpophalangeal joint that may be accompanied by the fracture of the base of the proximal phalanx.

In the *pelvis* stable and unstable fractures must be differentiated (Figs. 4.**14** and 4.**15**). In unstable fractures the pelvic ring formed by the sacrum and pelvis is totally disrupted in two or more places. Stable pelvic fractures include avulsion injuries (anterosuperior and anteroinferior iliac spines and ischial tuberosity) and/or complete disruption of the pelvic ring limited to a single location. Pelvic fractures may extend into the acetabulum where involvement of the dome (acetabular roof), anterior (iliopubic) wall or column and posterior (ilioischial) wall or column must be differentiated.

Fractures of the *proximal femur* may be classified as capital, subcapital, midcervical, basicervical, intertrochanteric and subtrochanteric (Fig. 4.**16**). Capital fractures are uncommon and usually associated with posterior hip dislocation.

After healing they may be impossible to differentiate from avascular necrosis of the femoral head. Frequent complications of displaced femoral neck fractures are avascular necrosis of the femoral head and nonunion.

Fractures about the *knee* may involve the distal femur or the proximal tibia. Distal femur fractures may be extra-articular (supracondylar) or intra-articular (condylar or intercondylar). Fractures of the proximal tibia may involve, besides the intercondylar eminence, the lateral or, less frequently, the medial tibia plateau or both. The articular surface of the tibia plateau may be split, depressed or both. Cruciate ligament injuries are frequently associated with fractures extending into the intercondylar eminence of the tibia. A *Segond fracture* is an avulsion fracture of the lateral proximal tibia just distal to the joint line at the insertion of the reinforced capsule. This fracture has to be differentiated from an avulsion of *Gerdy's*

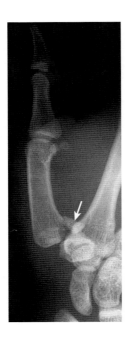

Fig. 4.**12** **Bennett fracture**. A simple intra-articular fracture (arrow) of the base of the first metacarpal with radial subluxation of the latter is seen.

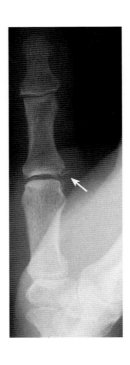

Fig. 4.**13** **Gamekeeper's (skier's) thumb**. A tiny avulsion fracture (arrow) of the ulnar aspect of the proximal phalanx of the thumb is seen.

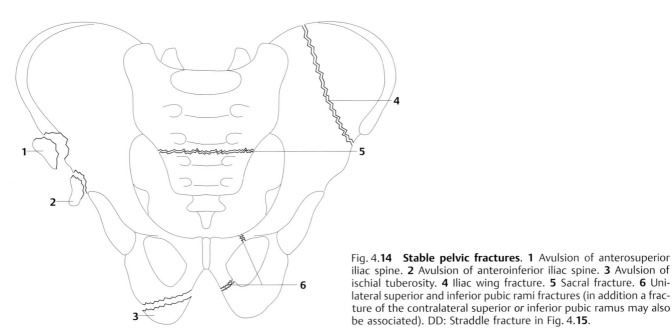

Fig. 4.**14** **Stable pelvic fractures**. **1** Avulsion of anterosuperior iliac spine. **2** Avulsion of anteroinferior iliac spine. **3** Avulsion of ischial tuberosity. **4** Iliac wing fracture. **5** Sacral fracture. **6** Unilateral superior and inferior pubic rami fractures (in addition a fracture of the contralateral superior *or* inferior pubic ramus may also be associated). DD: Straddle fracture in Fig. 4.**15**.

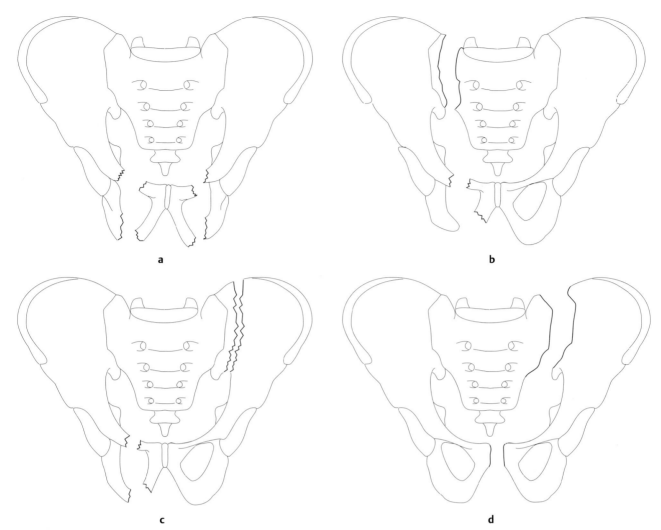

Fig. 4.15   Unstable pelvic fractures. a Straddle fracture (both superior and inferior pubic rami (or ischial rami) are fractured. **b** Malgaigne fracture (instead of the sacral wing fracture the ipsilateral sacroiliac joint may be disrupted or the ilium along the ispilateral sacroiliac joint may be fractured). **c** Bucket handle fracture. **d** Pelvic "dislocation" (pubic diastasis associated with unilateral or bilateral sacroiliac joint disruption).

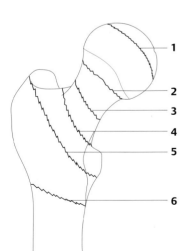

Fig. 4.16   Proximal femur fractures: **1**: capital, **2**: subcapital, **3**: midcervical, **4**: basicervical, **5**: intertrochanteric, **6**: subtrochanteric. Fractures **1–4** are intracapsular, **5** and **6** extracapsular. Fractures **2**, **3**, and **4** are femur neck fractures.

tubercle (insertion of the iliotibial tract) that is located anterior to the Segond fracture and usually only visualized on an external oblique but not on a frontal radiograph.

Fractures of the *ankle* can be classified as unimalleolar, bimalleolar, trimalleolar or complex (comminuted fracture of the distal tibia and fibula). A fracture of the distal tibia caused by axial load is called *pilon fracture* when the fracture line extends into the articular surface of the distal tibia, the tibia plafond. Injuries of the ankle are commonly caused by inversion (supination, adduction) or eversion (pronation, abduction) of the foot and may be associated with external (lateral) rotation of the foot. These injuries may be ligamentous, osseous, or both. Depending on their radiographic presentation (Fig. 4.17) both mechanism and severity of the injury can be assessed. Osteochondral fractures of the lateral or less commonly the medial talar dome may be associated

resulting from impingement of the talus on the fibula or tibia, respectively.

Fibular shaft fractures may be associated with ankle injuries. A *Dupuytren fracture* consists of a distal fibular fracture 2 to 7 cm above the ankle joint line associated with disruption of the distal tibiofibular syndesmosis and the medial collateral (deltoid) ligament. The same injury without disruption of the distal tibiofibular syndesmosis is termed *Pott fracture*. A *Maisonneuve fracture* (Fig. 4.18) is an eversion-lateral rotation type injury similar to the DuPuytren fracture and consists of a proximal fibula fracture, disruption of the tibiofibular syndesmosis and a medial malleolar fracture or torn medial collateral (deltoid) ligament.

Fractures of the talus tend to be vertical, typically involving the neck of the talus, or comminuted and occur most often from forced dorsiflexion of the foot. Osteochondral fractures

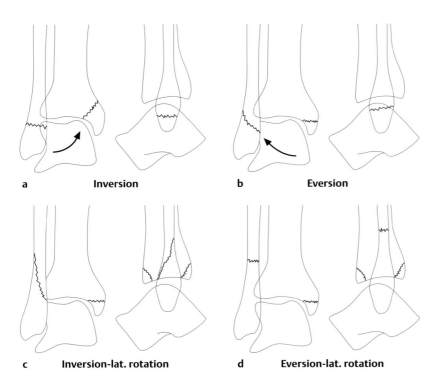

a   **Inversion**   b   **Eversion**

c   **Inversion-lat. rotation**   d   **Eversion-lat. rotation**

Fig. 4.**17** **Ankle fractures. a** Inversion injury (20%). Horizontal (avulsion) fracture of the lateral malleolus and oblique (talar impaction) fracture of the medial malleolus, both originating at or below the joint line. **b** Eversion injury (10%). Horizontal (avulsion) fracture of the medial malleolus and oblique (talar impaction) fracture of the lateral malleolus, both originating at or below the joint line. **c** Inversion-lateral rotation injury (60%). Oblique (spiral) fracture of the distal fibula originating anteromedial at or up to 1.5 cm above the joint line and extending in dorsal and proximal direction. Fractures of the medial and posterior malleolus and anterior tibial tubercle may be associated. **D** Eversion-lateral rotation injury. Fracture of the medial malleolus associated with a horizontal supramalleolar (2 cm or higher above the joint line) fracture of the distal fibula. Fractures of the posterior malleolus and anterior tibial tubercle may be associated. Note that instead of a malleolar fracture the corresponding ligament may be torn. Widening of the mortise (injury to the tibiofibular syndesmosis consisting of the anterior and posterior tibiofibular ligaments, inferior transverse ligament [immediately distal the latter] and interosseous membrane) can be diagnosed when the distal tibia and fibula no longer overlap on the mortise view. Avulsion fractures of the anterior tibial tubercle and posterior malleolus indicate injuries of the anterior and posterior tibiofibular ligaments respectively, and are only found with rotational injuries (modified Lange-Hansen classification).

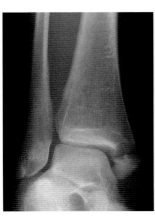
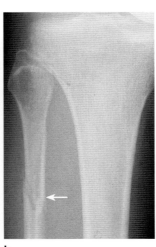

a   b

Fig. 4.**18 a, b** **Maisonneuve fracture.** A fracture of the medial malleolus with slightly widened mortise evident by the loss of the normal tibiofibular overlap is seen in (**a**). Fracture of the proximal fibula (arrow) is associated indicating disruption fo the tibiofibular syndesmosis (**b**).

of the medial or lateral talar dome may be associated with inversion or eversion injuries of the ankle. Talar dislocations may be peritalar involving the talocalcaneal and talonavicular joints or total involving besides the aforementioned joints also the tibiotalar joint ("floating talus").

Seventy-five percent of *calcaneal fractures* extend into the subtalar (talocalcaneal) joint. Depression of the subtalar joint is diagnosed by the Böhler's angle (angle between lines drawn on lateral radiograph from the highest point of the subtalar joint to the anterior process of the calcaneus and posterosuperior aspect of the calcaneus respectively) measuring less than 28 degrees.

Chopart fracture-dislocation involves both the talonavicular and calcaneocuboidal joints and abutting bones. *Lisfranc fracture-dislocation* (Fig. 4.19) involves the tarsometatarsal joints. In the homolateral form all metatarsals are dislocated laterally, whereas in the divergent form the first metatarsal is dislocated dorso-medially and remaining metatarsal laterally. Associated fractures most often occur at the base of the second metatarsal, followed by the base of the third metatarsal and the first and second cuneiforms. A first ray separation is diagnosed when the joint space between the medial and intermediate cuneiform is widened.

An *intra-articular avulsion fracture of the base of the fifth metatarsal* has to be differentiated from a *Jones fracture* referring to an extra-articular transverse fracture of the proximal fifth metatarsal shaft. Jones fractures have a high incidence of non-union.

Cervical spine injuries are caused by hyperflexion (e.g. anterior wedge fracture, anterior subluxation, and bilateral locked facets with anterior subluxation of the superior vertebra), hyperextension (e.g. avulsion of anteroinferior corner of a vertebral body, typically at C2), hyperrotation (e.g. rotary atlanto-axial dislocation), hyperflexion and rotation (e.g. unilateral locked facet), lateral hyperflexion (e.g. unilateral uncinate process or pillar fracture) and vertical compression (e.g. burst fracture). A *Jefferson fracture* is a burst fracture of C1 presenting classically with bilateral disruption of both anterior and posterior arches and with lateral displacement of both lateral masses.

Dens (odontoid) fractures (Fig. 4.20) are classified based on their location: Type I fractures occur cephalad to the base of the dens, and are usually obliquely oriented. They are stable and must be differentiated from an ossiculum terminale (ossicle of Bergmann) at the tip of the dens. Type II fractures are unstable transverse fractures at the base of the dens and must be differentiated from an os odontoideum. Type III fractures extend from the base of the dens into the body of C2 and are usually stable injuries. They can be differentiated from type II fractures on the lateral radiograph by disruption of the normal "ring shadow" of the axis caused by the pedicles.

A *hangman's fracture* (Fig. 4.21) is a hyperextension injury of the axis presenting with bilateral pedicle fractures and varying degrees of anterior subluxation or frank dislocation of the body of C2. This fracture can be considered as trau-

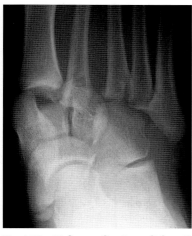

Fig. 4.**19 Lisfranc fracture-dislocation (homolateral form).** Lateral dislocation of all metatarsals is seen. Fractures of the bases of the second and third metatarsals are associated.

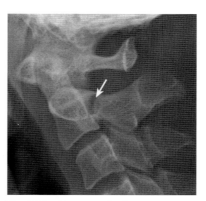

Fig. 4.**21 Hangman's fracture.** Fracture of the pedicles of C2 (arrow) with only minimal anterior subluxation of the body of C2 is seen.

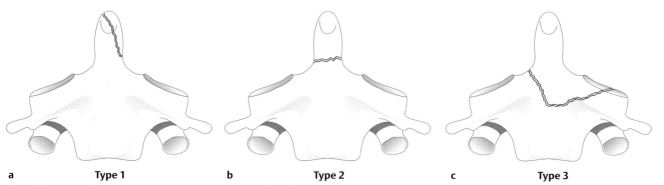

| a Type 1 | b Type 2 | c Type 3 |

Fig. 4.**20 Dens fractures. a** Type 1: Fracture (usually oblique) cephalad to the base of the dens. **b** Type 2: Transverse fracture at the base of the dens. **c** Type 3: Fracture extending from the base of the dens into the body of C2.

matic spondylolisthesis of C2 and is nowadays most commonly found in automobile accidents when the face strikes the windshield. A *clay-shoveler's fracture* (Fig. 4.22) is an oblique or vertical avulsion fracture of the spinous process of C6 or C7 (occasionally T1 to T3) caused by a sudden load on the flexed spine.

Teardrop fractures (Fig. 4.23) in the cervical spine may be associated with both hyperextension and hyperflexion injuries. In the extension teardrop fracture the avulsion arises from the anteroinferior corner of a vertebral body usually at the level of C2 or C3. This injury is in contrast to the flexion teardrop fracture stable and the triangular fracture fragment produced by hyperextension is small and does not exceed in size one quarter of the sagittal diameter of the vertebral body. However it has to be emphasized that many hyperextension injuries in the lower cervical region with few or no radiographic abnormalities may be unstable or result in severe neurologic damage. The flexion teardrop fracture is a highly unstable injury typically involving the lower cervical spine with C5 being most often affected. The vertebral body is divided into a smaller anteroinferior teardrop fragment and a larger posterior fragment. The teardrop fragment is frequently large but at most is only minimally anteriorly and inferiorly displaced whereas the remaining vertebral body is posteriorly displaced into the spinal canal.

Acute *thoracolumbar spine fractures* are best classified by mechanism of injury and location. For the latter the concept of the three-column spine is most useful. The anterior column comprises the anterior two-thirds of the vertebral body, the middle column the posterior third of the vertebral body and pedicles, and the posterior column the facet joints, lamina and spinous process. A column is also considered affected when the corresponding spinous ligaments are injured. Anterior and posterior one-column fractures are stable, whereas two- and three-column fractures and all fractures involving the middle column must be considered unstable.

Four types of major injuries can be discerned in the thoracolumbar spine (Fig. 4.24): 1. *Compression fractures* are flexion injuries resulting in compression of the anterior column. They present with anterior or less commonly lateral cortical buckling or wedging of a vertebral body. In severe compression fractures posterior ligamentous distraction injuries may be associated. 2. *Burst fractures* are the result of axial loading resulting in compression of both the anterior and middle columns with centropetal disruption. Characteristic radio-

graphic findings include increased sagittal diameter of the vertebral body, increased interpediculate distance, retropulsion of the posterosuperior portion of the vertebral body and moderate to marked anterior wedging. 3. *Seat-belt injuries (Chance fractures)* are caused by hyperflexion of the spine resulting in distraction injuries of both the middle and posterior columns associated at times with anterior compression of the vertebral body. The radiographic findings depend on whether the injury is predominantly osseous or ligamentous. A horizontal splitting of the vertebra beginning in the spinous process or lamina and extending through the pedicles into the vertebral body without anteroposterior subluxation is characteristic. Ligamentous injuries can be diagnosed by widening of the interspinous distance, increased height of the intervertebral foramina, and perching or locking of the facet joints. 4. *Fracture-dislocation injuries* refer to the complete disruption of all three spinal columns. The hallmark of these severe, usually mixed osseous-ligamentous injuries is the presence of intervertebral subluxation or dislocation, while the loss of height of the involved vertebral bodies characteristically is commonly relatively small.

Traumatic fractures of the spine have to be differentiated from subacute or chronic compression fractures associated with osteopenia. These fractures are frequently located in the mid thoracic spine, whereas traumatic fractures are preferentially located in the thoracolumbar region. A narrow zone of increased density below the fractured endplate, produced by impacted trabeculae and/or attempted fracture healing, is commonly present in compression fractures associated with osteoporosis.

Fractures in children may present with special features. *Greenstick fractures* (Fig. 4.25) are incomplete fractures of the relatively soft growing bone perforating only one cortex and ramifying within the medullary cavity. *Bowing fractures* (Fig. 4.26) present as antero-posterior or lateral bending of the radius, ulnar or fibula without evidence of a bony break. Comparison radiographs of the opposite side are often required for correct diagnosis. *Torus (buckling) fractures* (Fig. 4.27) produce a buckling of the metaphyseal cortex in children and osteopenic adults.

Trauma to the bone in children and adolescents often involves the cartilage (growth) plate, as long as the epiphyses are not closed. These injuries can be classified into different types using the Salter-Harris method (Fig. 4.28). A Salter-Harris type III fracture in the lateral distal tibia epiphysis is referred to as *juvenile Tillaux fracture* (Fig. 4.29). A *triplane*

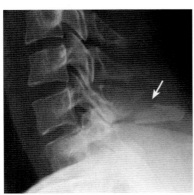

Fig. 4.22 Clay-shoveler's fracture. Oblique fracture of the spinous process (arrow) of C7 is seen.

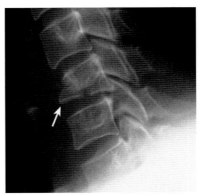

Fig. 4.23 Flexion teardrop fracture. A fracture at C5 is seen consisting of the smaller anteroinferior teardrop fragment (arrow) and a larger posterior fragment that is posteriorly displaced into the spinal canal.

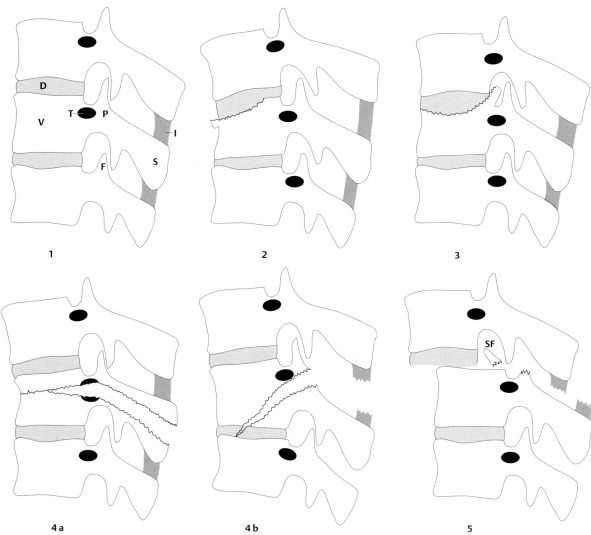

1   2   3

4 a   4 b   5

Fig. 4.**24 Thoracolumbar spine fractures**. **1** Normal. **2** Compression fracture. **3** Burst fracture. **4** Chance fracture (4**a**: one-level, 4**b**: two-level). **5** Fracture-dislocation. D: Intervertebral disc. I: Interspinous ligament. F: Facet (apophyseal) joint. P: Pedicle.

S: Spinous process. T: Transverse process. V: Vertebral body. SF in 5: Superior facet of the middle vertebra. Note that a torn interspinous ligament may also imply tears in the anterior and posterior longitudinal ligaments and ligamentum flavum.

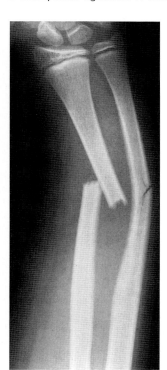

Fig. 4.**25 Greenstick fracture.** An incomplete ulnar fracture with bowing of its shaft and intact cortex on its radial side is seen in addition to the transverse overriding radius fracture.

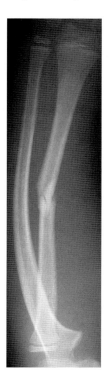

Fig. 4.**26 Bowing fracture.** A fracture of the radius shaft is associated with a marked bending deformity (bowing fracture) of the ulna without evidence of a cortical break.

fracture of the distal tibia in adolescents represents a variation of a Harris-Salter type IV injury (Fig. 4.**30**). Two, three or four fragments (parts) may result with two fragments being most common.

A *traumatic epiphysiolysis of the femur head* is particularly common in boys between 10 and 15 years of age, although a history of acute trauma is often not available. In these cases of *slipped capital femoral epiphyses (SCFE)*, repeated low-grade trauma is believed to be the triggering mechanism. The displacement of the femoral head in relation to the metaphysis is almost always in a posterior, inferior and medial direction (Fig. 4.**31**).

Multiple fractures and dislocations in an infant should raise the suspicion of an "*abused child syndrome.*" More subtle find-

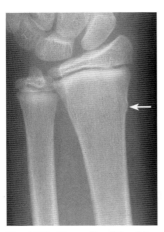

Fig. 4.**27   Torus (buckling) fracture**. Buckling of the metaphyseal cortex of the distal radius (arrow) is seen.

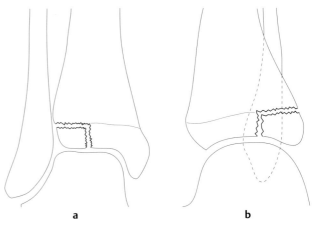

Fig. 4.**29   Juvenile Tillaux fracture** is a Harris-Salter type III fracture involving the posteriolateral (shown here) or anterolateral aspect of the distal tibia epiphysis (**a**: anteroposterior, **b**: lateral).

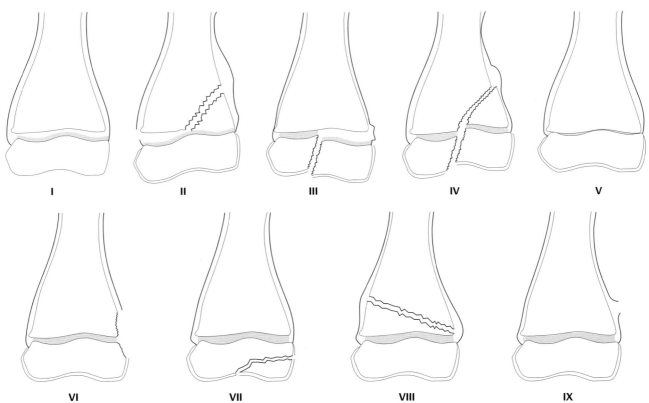

Fig. 4.**28   Salter-Harris classification** of growth plate injuries (types I-V) with **Rang and Ogden's** additions (types VI-IX). Type **I**: Injury limited to the cartilage plate, which shows complete transverse laceration. The bone itself is intact. Prognosis is good. Type **II**: Incomplete transverse laceration of the cartilage plate associated with oblique fracture of the metaphysis. Triangular fracture fragment remains attached to the epiphysis. Prognosis is good. Type **III**: Incomplete transverse laceration of the cartilage plate associated with longitudinal fracture through the epiphysis.

Prognosis is bad if the fracture is not reduced with smooth joint surface. Type **IV**: Oblique longitudinal fracture through epiphysis, cartilage plate, and metaphysis. Prognosis is bad if the fracture is not perfectly reduced. Type **V**: Crushing of the cartilage plate with intact bone. Premature closure of the plate and stoppage of growth is relatively common. Type **VI**: Trauma to the perichondrium with tethering of growth plate. Type **VII**: Fracture of the epiphysis. Type **VIII**: Fracture of the metaphysis. Type **IX**: Avulsion injury of the periosteum.

ings in this condition include injuries to the cartilage plate, metaphyseal fragmentation and avulsions, the latter producing a characteristic "bucket-handle" deformity, posttraumatic metaphyseal cupping and cortical thickening (Fig. 4.32).

The evaluation of *dislocations* requires radiologic examinations in at least two projections (Fig. 4.33). With a single projection, a dislocation as well as a potentially associated avulsion or compression fracture is easily missed. Traumatic, habitual, pathologic (secondary to joint disease), paralytic, and congenital dislocations are differentiated. There is no longer any contact between the two joint surfaces in a complete dislocation (luxation), whereas in subluxations (incomplete dislocations), a partial contact between the joint surfaces is still maintained.

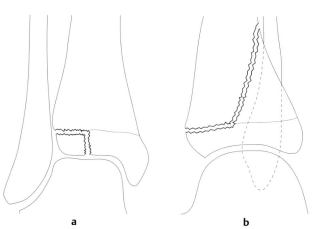

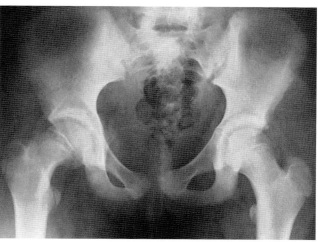

Fig. 4.**30 Triplanar (triplane) fracture** (two-part) of the distal tibia in children consists of a vertical fracture of the epiphysis in the sagittal plane, a horizontal fracture in the axial plane through the lateral and anterior aspect of the growth plate and an oblique fracture of the metaphysis in the coronal plane extending from the growth plate to the posterior cortex of the tibia (**a**: anteroposterior, **b**: lateral).

Fig. 4.**31 Traumatic epiphysiolysis (slipped capital femoral epiphysis).** The right femoral head is displaced medially, downward and backward. Note also the widening of the physis, the irregularities of the metaphysis, and the blurring of the junction between the metaphysis and the epiphyseal cartilage plate, all of which are early signs of an imminent slip. These findings are best appreciated when compared with the normal left hip.

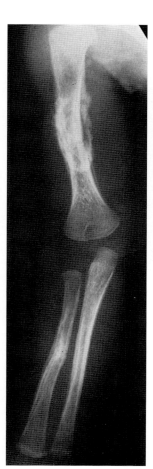

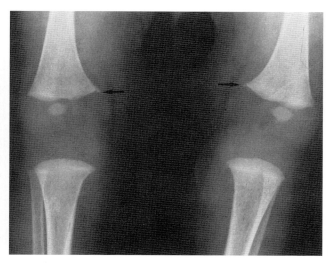

Fig. 4.**32 a, b Abused child syndrome. a** Healing fractures are seen in the humerus, radius, and ulna. **b** More recent avulsions of the metaphyseal corners (arrows) produce the characteristic "bucket-handle" deformity in infants.

Osteochondritis dissecans appears to be caused in a great majority, if not all cases, by stress, usually of chronic nature. The medial femur condyle is the most common site of involvement, but the disease has also been observed in the lateral femur condyle, the distal tibia, the talar dome, the capitulum of humerus (Fig. 4.34), the patella, and the heads of the femur, humerus, and metatarsals, especially the first. The bony fragment may still be located in the corresponding defect of the articular surface or may have become completely separated from the latter and form a loose intra-articular body. The differential diagnosis of loose intra-articular bodies is shown in Table 4.1.

Table 4.1 Differential Diagnosis of Loose Intra-Articular Bodies

Disease	Preferred Location	Number of Loose Bodies	Other Radiographic Findings	Comments
Osteochondritis dissecans	Knee	One	Defect (pit) in articular surface at the site of origin.	Preponderant in young males.
Osteochondromatosis (synovial) (Fig. 4.35)	Large joints, bursae	Multiple (often more than 10), relatively uniform in size, one-third not calcified	Joint effusion common.	Preponderant in young to middle-aged males. Hypertrophic cartilaginous synovial growths that may become detached, calcified and eventually ossified.
Trauma (chondral and osteochondral fractures)	None	One or more, not always calcified	Evidence of old trauma.	Secondary to avulsion of bone and/or cartilage (articular surface, meniscus).
Septic or tuberculous arthritis	None	One or more	Evidence of joint destruction and deformity.	Rare. Characteristic clinical history.
Degenerative joint disease	Weight-bearing joints	One or more detached spurs	Osteophytosis, sclerosis, subchondral cysts, and joint space narrowing.	Usually in elderly patients. *Synovial chondrometaplasia* may also occur simulating osteochondromatosis.
CPPD arthropathy (Fig. 4.36)	Large joints of upper and lower extremities	One or more	Similar to degenerative joint disease, but more destructive and progressive. Chondrocalcinosis and subchondral cyst formation are common and often prominent.	Elderly patients.
Avascular necrosis	Hip, knee, shoulder	One or more	Advanced stage with flattened or collapsed articular surface	Bone infarcts may also be present. May simulate osteochondritis dissecans in the knee, but is often bicondylar or bilateral.
Neuropathic arthropathy (hypertrophic form) (Fig. 4.37)	Weight-bearing joints	Multiple, varying size	Marked sclerosis, disintegration of articular surfaces and subluxation.	Loss of pain sensation (diabetes, syphilis [Charcot joint] and other neurologic disorders).

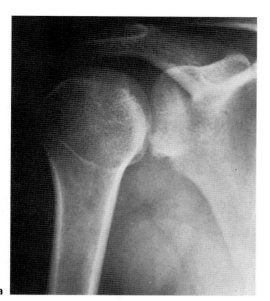

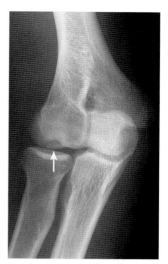

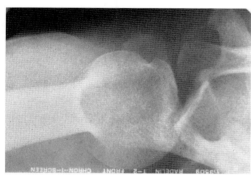

Fig. 4.**33 a, b** **Posterior dislocation of the shoulder with impaction fracture of the humeral head. a** In the oblique anteroposterior projection, the posterior dislocation is difficult to appreciate (normally there is a slight overlap between humeral head and glenoid fossa in this projection). **b** The axillary projection identifies clearly the posterior dislocation. Furthermore, an impaction fracture on the humeral head caused by the impingement of posterior ridge of the glenoid fossa is now evident.

Fig. 4.**34** **Osteochondritis dissecans.** A small bony fragment (arrow) is located in a subchondral defect of the capitulum of the humerus.

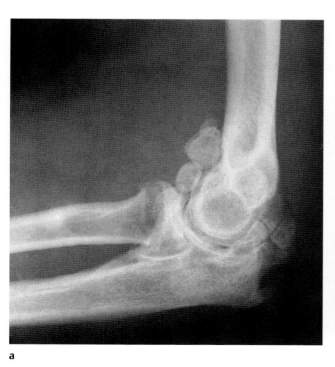

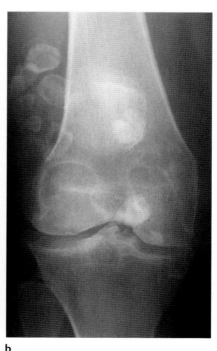

Fig. 4.**35 a, b** **Osteochondromatosis** (2 patients). **a** Elbow, **b** knee. Multiple loose bodies are seen in both joints.

Stress fractures can be subdivided into fatigue fractures and insufficiency fractures. *Fatigue fractures* occur in normal bones with the application of an abnormal stress or torque caused by a new strenuous or repeated activity. *Insufficiency fractures* occur when normal stress is placed on an abnormal (osteopenic) bone. Stress fractures are usually symptomatic. They begin as small cortical cracks, and may progress to subcortical infraction and eventually a fracture running transversely across the bone (Fig. 4.38). If the fracture line cannot be demonstrated radiographically, magnetic resonance imaging (MRI) or a radionuclide examination are always posi-

tive and may provide an early diagnosis. MRI, however, has comparable sensitivity and superior specificity to bone scintigraphy in the assessment of stress fractures. Osteomyelitis and bone tumors such as osteosarcoma and osteoid osteoma can be differentiated from a stress fracture on the basis of both characteristic location and the typical history of stress fractures (Table 4.2 and Fig. 4.39). At a later stage, periosteal reactions with subsequent localized callus formation and cortical thickening obscuring the fracture line, are found in the diaphyses of tubular bones (Fig. 4.40). In an epiphyseal and metaphyseal location (e.g., tibia plateau) and cancellous

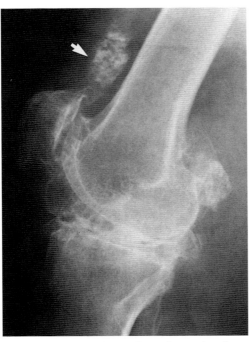

Fig. 4.**36 CPPD arthropathy.** Advanced arthritic changes with numerous calcific and osseous bodies in the joint space and suprapatellar bursa (arrow) are seen.

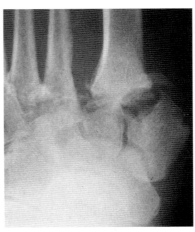

Fig. 4.**37 Neuropathic arthropathy.** Fragmentation of the joint surfaces with several irregular loose bodies, sclerosis and subluxations are seen in the metatarsophalangeal joints.

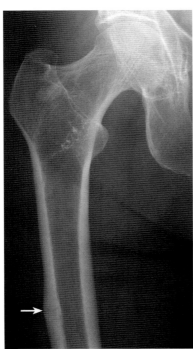

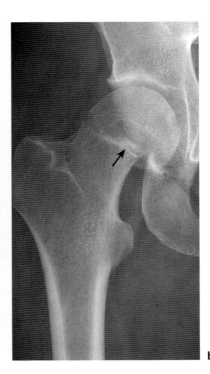

Fig. 4.**38 a, b Stress fractures** (2 patients). (**a**) A transverse linear radiolucency (arrow) is associated with mild localized cortical thickening in the femur shaft. (**b**) The stress fracture presenting initially as poorly defined sclerotic band (arrow) in the medial aspect of the femoral neck progressed to a complete subcapital fracture.

a

b

Table 4.2 Stress Fractures (Fig. 4.39)

Location	Activity
1. Lower cervical or upper thoracic spinous process	Shoveling
2. Clavicle	Postoperative (radical neck dissection)
3. Coracoid process of scapula	Trap shooting
4. Ribs	Carrying heavy pack (first rib), golf, coughing
5. Humerus: distal shaft	Throwing a ball
6. Ulna: coronoid process shaft	Pitching a ball, throwing a javelin, pitchfork work, propelling wheelchair
7. Hook of hamate	Holding golf club, tennis racket, baseball bat
8. Lumbar vertebra: pars interarticularis (spondylolysis)	Ballet, lifting heavy objects, scrubbing floors
9. Femur: neck shaft	Ballet, running Ballet, marching, running, gymnastics
10. Pelvis: obturator ring	Stooping, bowling, gymnastics
11. Patella	Hurdling
12. Tibia	Running (proximal shaft in children, mid- and distal shaft in adults)
13. Fibula: proximal or distal shaft	Jumping, parachuting running
14. Calcaneus	Jumping, parachuting, prolonged standing, recent immobilization
15. Navicular	Stamping on ground, marching, running
16. Metatarsals	Marching, stamping on ground, prolonged standing, ballet, postoperative bunionectomy
17. Sesamoids of great toe	Prolonged standing

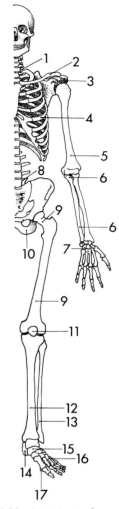

Fig. 4.**39 Locations of stress fractures.** The numbers in the Fig. correspond to the numbers in Table 4.**2**.

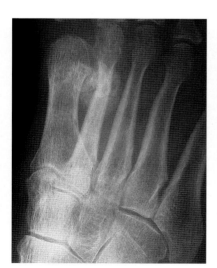

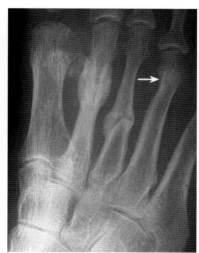

a   b

Fig. 4.**40 a, b Stress fractures. (a)** A healing stress fracture with extensive periosteal callus formation is seen in the second metatarsal. No other stress fracture was diagnosed at this time. Sequelae of arthroplasty including resection of the base of the proximal phalanx of the great toe are incidentally also evident. **(b)** Three months later the stress fracture in the second metatarsal has progressed in healing. A second healing stress fracture is now seen in the third metatarsal shaft and a new stress fracture with only minimal sclerosis in the neck of the fourth metatarsal (arrow).

bone, a band-like focal sclerosis usually without appreciable periosteal reaction is more characteristic (Fig. 4.41).

Osteoporosis and rheumatoid arthritis are the two most common conditions in which insufficiency fractures are encountered. *Reinforcement lines (bone bars)* presenting as well-defined, usually thin sclerotic lines extending partially or completely across the marrow cavity in patients with osteopenia have to be differentiated from poorly defined, band-like insufficiency fractures (Fig. 4.42). Reinforcement lines can be considered as unmasking of growth arrest lines occurring in childhood, although their pathogenesis is unclear. They are incidental findings without clinical relevance.

Pathologic fractures occur at sites of pre-existing abnormalities and are often caused by a minor trauma that would not fracture healthy bone (Figs. 4.43 and 4.44). The radiographic differential diagnosis between pathologic and nonpathologic fracture can at times be difficult, particularly when the injury occurred days to weeks prior to the first radiologic examination. In these cases, bone resorption oc-

curring at the site of a nonpathologic fracture may simulate an underlying pathologic lesion. On the other hand, a smaller underlying lytic or sclerotic bone lesion can be missed radiographically, particularly in the presence of displacement at the fracture site. In these cases, the demonstration of other lytic or sclerotic lesions as well as the absence of a history of trauma or the lack of fracture pain should suggest the possibility of a pathologic fracture. Pathologic fractures can also occur as early as five months after radiation therapy: that is, at a time when the bone does not reveal any radiation-induced changes.

Avulsion fractures (Fig. 4.45) at the site of ligament and tendon attachments can be differentiated from accessory ossicles by the lack of a clearly defined cortical margin characteristic of the latter condition (Figs. 4.46 and 4.47). The diagnosis can be further supported by the demonstration of a cortical defect or irregularity in the adjacent bone. Avulsion injuries are caused by either a single violent traumatic event or repetitive injuries. They are particularly common in child-

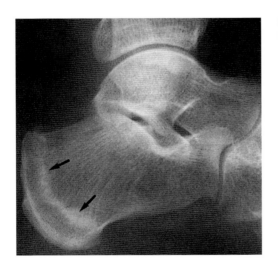

Fig. 4.**41** **Stress fracture.** An irregular sclerotic band is seen paralleling the posterior border of the calcaneus (arrows).

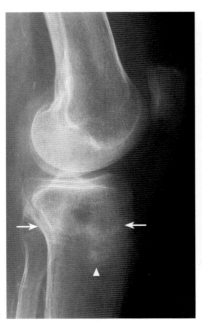

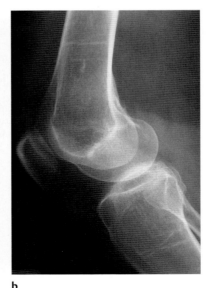

Fig. 4.**42 a, b** **Insufficiency fractures versus einforcement lines (bone bars).** (**a**) Osteopenia and a poorly defined sclerotic band (arrows) associated with a small sclerotic focus (arrowhead) are characteristic manifestations of insufficiency fractures. (**b**) Thin, well-defined sclerotic lines extending partially or completely across the distal femur and proximal tibia in osteopenia are virtually diagnostic for reinforcement lines (bone bars). In contrast to insufficiency fractures they have no clinical implications.

a

b

ren, since the physeal cartilage of an apophysis is considerably weaker than tendinous or ligamentous tissue. Several avulsion injuries about the pelvis and hips occur in young athletes including the anterior superior or inferior iliac spine, iliac crest, ischial tuberosity, pubic symphysis (adductor muscle insertion sites), and greater or lesser trochanter.

Calcifications and ossifications developing in a ligament after acute or repeated low-grade trauma can be impossible to differentiate from an ossicle, since both may be well corticated. A characteristic location (e. g., *Pellegrini-Stieda lesion* [Fig. 4.48] in the medial collateral ligament of knee) or the patient's history (e. g., *"rider's bone"* in the adductor muscles of the thigh) may, however, suggest the correct diagnosis.

Heterotopic bone formation in soft tissues following trauma is often termed myositis ossificans, since it occurs most commonly in muscle but is also found in tendons, ligaments, periosteum, and other connective tissues. It frequently develops after insertion of a joint prosthesis, particularly in the hip, and in paraplegic patients. Occasionally, myositis ossificans can mimic a parosteal sarcoma (Fig. 4.49). It can be distinguished from the latter by the fact that the periphery is both more dense and smoothly outlined ("eggshell calcification") and by the demonstration of a fine radiolucent line separating the lesion in its entire length from the adjacent bone (Fig. 4.50). A central amorphous calcification associated with a soft tissue mass is not found in myositis ossificans and suggests rather a synovial or extraosseous osteogenic sarcoma, where it is present in 30% and 50% of the cases, respectively.

Excessive callus formation following a fracture may occasionally have a tumor-like appearance. It is found in fractures that have not been properly immobilized. These fractures may not have been diagnosed because of a decreased sensitivity to pain secondary to a neurologic disorder. Since fractures are not immobilized in the battered child syndrome, excessive callus formation is common in that condition too. It is also associated with elevated steroid blood concentrations (e. g., Cushing's syndrome and steroid therapy).

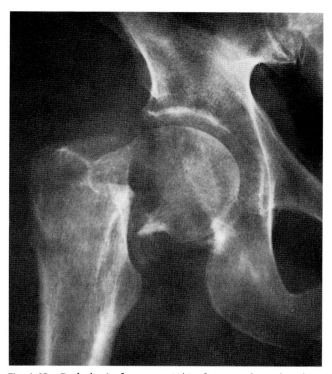

Fig. 4.**43 Pathologic fracture.** A hip fracture through a large osteolytic metastasis from a renal cell carcinoma involving the femur neck is seen.

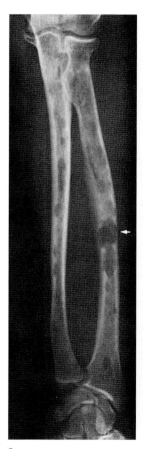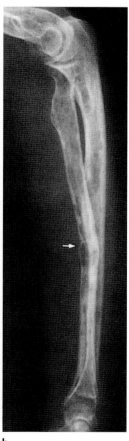

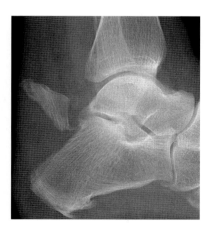

Fig. 4.**45 Avulsion fracture.** A fracture of the posterosuperior aspect of the calcaneus at the Achilles tendon insertion with superior displacement of the avulsed fracture fragment is seen.

a   b

Fig. 4.**44 a, b Pathologic fracture. a** The cortical break (arrow) is barely visible in the radius shaft of this patient with multiple myeloma in the anteroposterior projection. **b** In the lateral projection, the pathologic fracture (arrow) can be better appreciated because of some angulation of the radius at the fracture site.

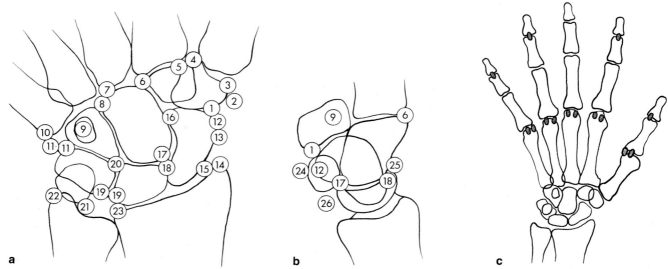

a   b   c

Fig. 4.**46 Characteristic locations of accessory bones (numbered) and sesamoids (shaded) in the wrist and hand. a** Anteroposterior projection of the wrist. **b** Lateral projection of the wrist. **c** Anteroposterior projection of the hand:

1. epitrapezium
2. calcification (bursa, flexor carpi radialis)
3. paratrapezium
4. trapezium secundarium
5. trapezoides secundarium
6. os styloideum (carpal bone or carpe bossu)
7. ossiculum Gruberi
8. capitatum secundarium
9. os hamuli proprium
10. os vesalianum
11. os ulnare externum (calcifications in bursa or tendon)

12. os radiale externum
13. avulsion of the scaphoid, not an accessory bone
14. persisting center of ossification of the radial styloid process
15. accessory bone belween scaphoid and radius (paranaviculare)
16. os centrale carpi
17. hypolunatum
18. epilunatum
19. accessory bone belween lunatum and triquetrum
20. epipyramis
21. avulsion of the styloid process of the ulna ("triangulare")
22. persistent nucleus of the styloid process of the ulna
23. small osseous element in the radioulnar joint
24. calcification on the pisiform
25. avulsion of the triquetrum, not an accessory bone
26. tendon or bursal calcification.

Fig. 4.**47 Characteristic locations of accessory bones (numbered) and sesamoids (shaded) in the ankle and foot. a** Anteroposterior projection of the ankle. **b** Lateral projection of the ankle. **c** Anteroposterior projection of the foot.

1. accessory bone (or sesamoid) between the medial malleolus and the talus
2. os subtibiale
3. talus accessorius
4. os sustentaculi
5. os tibiale externum
6. os retinaculi
7. accessory ossicle (or sesamoid) between the lateral malleolus and the talus
8. os subfibulare
9. talus secundarius
10. os trochleare calcanei
11. os trigonum
12. os talotibiale
13. os supratalare
14. os supranaviculare
15. os infranaviculare
16. os intercuneiforme
17. os cuneometatarsale
18. os intermetatarsale
19. os unci
20. secondary cuboid
21. calcaneus secundarius
22. os accessorium supracalcaneum
23. os subcalcis
24. os peronaeum (peroneal ossicle)
25. os vesalianum
26. os cuneonaviculare mediale
27. sesamum tibiale anterius
28. os cuneometatarsale 1 plantare
29. os intercuneiforme.

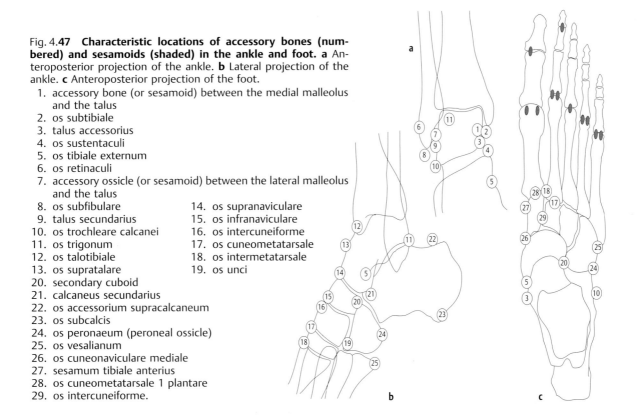

a

b   c

Finally, fractures occurring in osteogenesis imperfecta may to heal with excessive callus formation.

Fractures extending to the articular surface result in a *joint effusion (hemarthrosis)*. In fractures of the radial head, a joint effusion displacing the anterior and/or posterior fat pad may be the only radiographic finding (Fig. 4.51). The demonstration of a *fat-fluid level* in the shoulder or knee is presumptive evidence of an intra-articular fracture but can only be demonstrated when the exposure is made with a horizontal beam (Fig. 4.52). *Pseudofractures (Looser's zones, Milkman's syndrome)* are assumed to be incomplete stress (insufficiency) fractures, presenting radiographically as narrow (2 to 3 mm) radiolucent bands lying perpendicularly to the cortex (Fig. 4.53). At a later stage, sclerosis develops around these lesions, making them more readily detectable. Pseudofractures are present in vitamin D deficiency (osteomalacia,

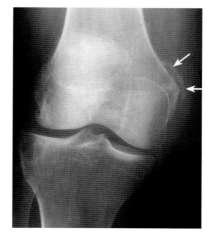

Fig. 4.**48 Pellegrini-Stieda lesion**. A shell-like ossification (arrows) along the medial femur condyle developed within one month after an acute injury to the medial collateral ligament of the knee.

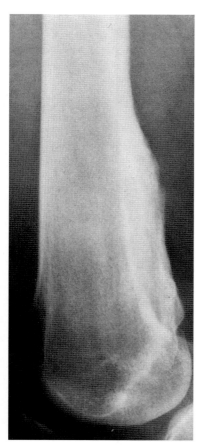

Fig. 4.**49 Parosteal osteosarcoma.** The densely sclerotic lesion is solidly attached to the posterior cortex of the distal femur.

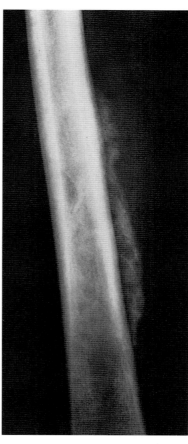

Fig. 4.**50 Myositis ossificans (post-traumatic).** The ossification along the medial femur shaft is separated in its entire length from the adjacent bone.

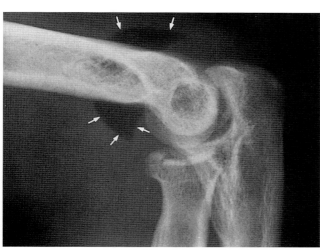

Fig. 4.**51 Joint effusion (hemarthrosis) secondary to radial head fracture.** The joint effusion is evident from the positive posterior and anterior fat pad sign, evident as sail-like radiolucencies along the distal humerus (arrows). Demonstration of any radiolucent area posteriorly always indicates a joint effusion (positive posterior fat pad sign), whereas a small oblong radiolucent area along the anterior aspect of the distal humerus can be normal. The anterior fat pad sign is only indicative of a joint effusion when it assumes a triangular or sail-like shape, as in this case. Note also the fracture in the radial head, which not uncommonly escapes radiographic detection even when radiographs in multiple projection are taken.

rickets), renal osteodystrophy, Paget's disease, fibrous dysplasia, and hereditary hyperphosphatasia ("juvenile Paget's disease") or are rarely idiopathic. They are located in the femur (neck and shaft), pubic and ischial ramus, scapula, clavicle, ribs, ulna (proximal shaft), radius (distal shaft), metacarpals, metatarsals, and phalanges.

Nutrient arteries pierce the diaphyses of tubular bones obliquely. Their site of entry and angulation are fairly constant and, characteristically, the vessels point away from the dominant growing end of the bone (the end with the epiphyseal center in short tubular bones, or the end with the later fusing epiphysis in long bones). In the long tubular bones of the upper extremity they run towards the elbow, whereas in the lower extremity they run away from the knee ("to the elbow/ go, from the knee/flee"). Nutrient arteries may be evident radiographically as oblique radiolucent cortical channels that should not be confused with fracture lines (Fig. 4.54).

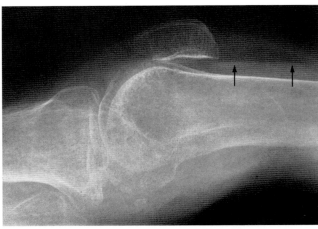

Fig. 4.**52** **Fat-fluid blood level secondary to tibia plateau fracture.** A fat-fluid level, pathognomonic of an intra-articular fracture, is seen in the suprapatellar bursa. It is caused by the lighter and more radiolucent fat (arrows) layering on top of the heavier blood in the joint (lipohemarthrosis). This finding can only be seen when the radiograph is taken with horizontal beam.

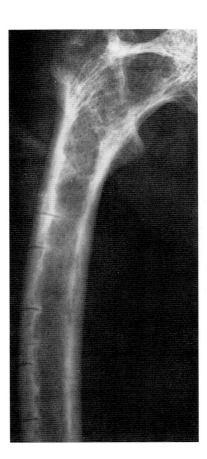

Fig. 4.**53** **Pseudofractures (Looser's zones) in Paget's disease.** Multiple pseudofractures are seen presenting as small radiolucent lines with adjacent sclerosis lying perpendicularly to the outer cortex of the femur shaft. Note also the bowing deformity, thickened cortices, and coarsened trabecular pattern of the femur characteristic of Paget's disease.

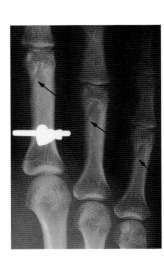

Fig. 4.**54** **Nutrient arteries.** Oblique radiolucent cortical channels are seen in characteristic location (arrows).

5 Localized Bone Lesions

Conventional radiography remains the primary imaging modality for the evaluation of skeletal lesions. The combination of conventional radiography, which has a high specificity but only an intermediate sensitivity, with radionuclide bone scanning, which has a high sensitivity but only a low specificity is still the most effective method for detecting and diagnosing bone lesions and differentiating between benign and malignant conditions. Conventional radiography, is, however, limited in delineating the intramedullary extent of a bone lesion and even more so in demonstrating soft-tissue involvement. Although magnetic resonance imaging frequently contributes to the characterization of a bone lesion, its greatest value lies in the ability to accurately assess the intramedullary and extraosseous extent of a skeletal lesion.

A solitary bone lesion is often a tumor or a tumor-like abnormality, but congenital, infectious, ischemic and traumatic disorders can present in similar fashion. Differentiation between a benign or malignant bone lesion is not always possible. Signs of an aggressive or malignant osseous lesion include rapid growth, large size, poor demarcation, cortical violation, interrupted periosteal reaction and soft tissue extension. Signs of a nonaggressive or benign osseous lesion include slow growth, small size, sharp margination, cortical expansion without cortical violation, solid periosteal reaction and no soft tissue extension. However these radiologic features are not infallible and many exceptions occur indicating the need for histologic confirmation in the appropriate setting.

In osteolytic lesions a **geographic, moth-eaten and permeative pattern of bone destruction** are commonly discerned. A *geographic lesion* (Figs. 5.1 and 5.2) has a well-defined margin separating it clearly from the surrounding normal bone. The zone of transition of normal to abnormal bone is short and a sclerotic border of various thickness may surround the lesion. Geographic lesions are usually benign, especially when they are marginated by a sclerotic rim. Multiple myeloma and metastases, however, frequently present as geographic lesions without sclerotic borders (Table 5.1).

A *moth-eaten lesion* (Fig. 5.3) is a poorly demarcated focus of bone destruction with a long zone of transition from normal to abnormal bone indicating its aggressive nature and rapid growth potential. Malignant bone tumors, osteomyelitis and eosinophilic granulomas frequently present with this pattern of bone destruction (Table 5.2).

A *permeative lesion* (Fig. 5.4) represents the most aggressive bone destruction pattern with rapid growth. The lesion merges imperceptibly with the normal bone. Highly malignant tumors infiltrating the bone marrow such as round cell sarcomas (e.g. Ewing's sarcomas and lymphomas) typically are associated with this pattern of bone destruction. It is, however, also found in acute osteomyelitis and rapidly developing osteoporosis such as reflex sympathetic dystrophy. Infiltration of the cortex may also be associated with these conditions, presenting as cortical striation or tunneling.

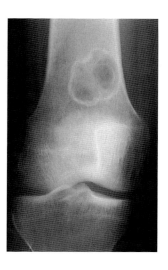

Fig. 5.**1** **Geographic lesion**. A well-demarcated lesion with sclerotic border is seen in the distal femur (nonossifying fibroma).

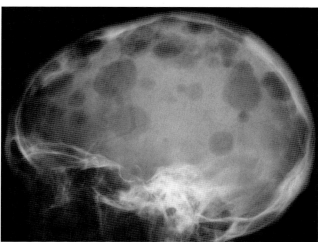

Fig. 5.**2** **Geographic lesions**. Multiple well-demarcated (punched-out) purely lytic lesions are seen in the vault of the cranium (multiple myeloma).

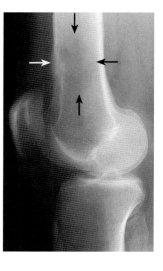

Fig. 5.**3** **Moth-eaten lesion**. A poorly demarcated osteolytic lesion (arrows) is seen in the distal femur (non-Hodgkin lymphoma).

Table 5.1 Solitary well defined osteolytic lesion

Subchondral cyst (associated with arthritis, osteonecrosis, or trauma)

Gout (intraosseous tophus)

Amyloidosis

Intraosseous ganglion

Simple (unicameral) bone cyst

Aneurysmal bone cyst

Epidermoid inclusion cyst

Glomus tumor

Intraosseous lipoma

Enchondroma

Chondroblastoma

Chondromyxoid fibroma

Nonossifying fibroma

Desmoplastic fibroma

Osteoblastoma

Giant cell tumor

Fibrosarcoma

Clear cell chondrosarcoma

Angiosarcoma

Plasmacytoma/multiple myeloma

Metastasis

Eosinophilic granuloma

Brown tumor (hyperparathyroidism)

Hemophilic pseudotumor

Osteonecrosis (bone infarct)

Brodie's abscess/cystic osteomyelitis

Fibrous dysplasia

Sarcoidosis

The cortex represents a barrier to nonaggressive lesions. Benign medullary processes may leave the endosteal surface intact or produce *endosteal scalloping* (Fig. 5.5). The latter finding is, however, also frequently seen with multiple myeloma and metastases. Progressive endosteal erosion associated with solid new periosteal bone deposition creates an expanded osseous contour indicative of a nonaggressive benign skeletal lesion. Aggressive skeletal lesions may penetrate the entire thickness of the cortex (Fig. 5.6) and sometimes induce a variety of interrupted periosteal reactions including onion-peel, sunburst and hair-on-end patterns or a

Table 5.2 Solitary poorly defined osteolytic lesion

Hemangioma

Chondroblastoma

Osteoblastoma

Giant cell tumor

Fibrosarcoma

Malignant fibrous histiocytoma

Chondrosarcoma

Osteosarcoma

Ewing's sarcoma

Angiosarcoma

Multiple myeloma

Metastasis

Lymphoma

Langerhans cell histiocytosis (eosinophilic granuloma)

Hemophilic pseudotumor

Osteonecrosis (bone infarct)

Osteomyelitis

Brodie's abscess

Sarcoidosis

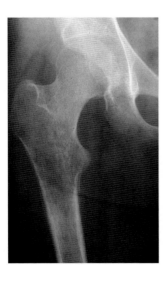

Fig. 5.4 Permeative lesion. A poorly defined osteolytic lesion merging imperceptibly with the normal bone is seen in the proximal femur. Note also the beginning laminated periosteal reaction in the subtrochanteric area (Ewing sarcoma).

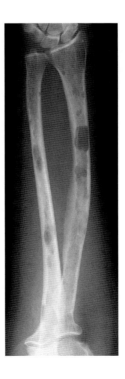

Fig. 5.5 Endosteal scalloping. Sharply demarcated erosions of the inner cortex of the radius and ulna caused by multiple osteolytic lesions is seen (multiple myeloma).

Codman's triangle. They are most commonly associated with osteosarcoma, Ewing's sarcoma, and osteomyelitis and are discussed in greater detail in chapter **3**.

The matrix of a skeletal lesion may be inhomogeneous because it contains areas of *calcification* or *ossification*. Calcifications appear as ring-like, flocculent or fleck-like radiodense areas (Figs. 5.**7** and 5.**8**). Intramedullary matrix calcification is primarily associated with cartilaginous tumors and bone infarcts (Table 5.3). Foci of intramedullary ossifications are more homogeneous and often ivory-like and are most often caused by bone islands, osteoblastic metastases and primary bone forming neoplasms (Fig. 5.**9**). They are discussed in detail in chapter **2**.

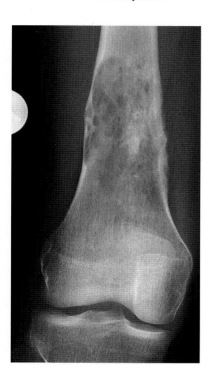

Fig. 5.**6** **Cortical penetration**. A poorly defined, mixed osteolytic and osteoblastic lesion is seen in the distal femur penetrating through the medial cortex. The lateral cortex is expanded and thinned but still intact (osteosarcoma).

Table 5.3 Bone lesions with calcification
Intraosseous lipoma
Osteochondroma
Enchondroma
Periosteal (juxtacortical) chondroma
Bizarre parosteal osteochondromatous proliferation (BPOP)
Chondroblastoma
Dysplasia epiphysealis hemimelica (Trevor's disease)
Fibrocartilagenous mesenchymoma
Chondromyxoid fibroma
Osteoid osteoma (nidus)
Osteoblastoma (nidus)
Ossifying fibroma
Gnathic tumors (see chapter 11)
Chordoma
Chondrosarcoma (all variants)
Metastasis (especially thyroid carcinoma)
Gout (intraosseous tophus)
Osteonecrosis (bone infarct)
Intraosseous hematoma
Osteogenesis imperfecta (popcorn calcifications in enlarged epimetaphyses)

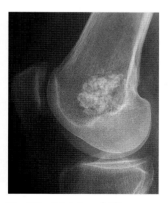

Fig. 5.**7** **Matrix calcification**. A flocculent, ring-like cluster of calcification is seen in the distal femur (enchondroma).

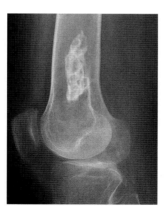

Fig. 5.**8** **Matrix calcification**. An irregular, shell-like calcification is seen in the distal femur (bone infarct).

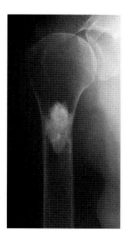

Fig. 5.**9** **Intramedullary ossification**. An irregular, ivory-like area of sclerosis is seen in the proximal humerus (enostosis or giant bone island).

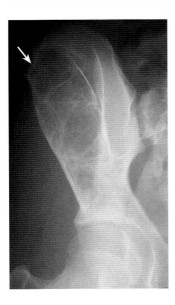

Fig. 5.**10** **Septation.** A lytic lesion with extensive delicate trabeculation induced by the tumor is seen in the iliac wing. Note also the localized cortical violation (arrow) in the superolateral aspect of the lesion (aneurysmal bone cyst).

Septation of the matrix represents another mechanism of new bone formation evoked by a neoplasm (Fig. 5.10). In other instances intratumoral septations represent the remnants of the original bone matrix largely destroyed by the neoplasm (Fig. 5.11). Septation is associated with both benign and malignant lesions. Delicate thin trabeculae typically are found in giant cell tumors and aneurysmal bone cysts, lobulated trabeculae in nonossifying fibromas, spiculated or radiating trabeculae in hemangiomas and irregular coarse trabecula in a variety of benign and malignant lesions, often of fibrous connective tissue origin (Table 5.4). A uniform hazy increase in radiodensity in an osteolytic lesion is termed *ground glass appearance*. It is most characteristic for fibrous dysplasia (Fig. 5.12), but is occasionally also found in simple (unicameral) bone cysts in the adult. The demonstration of a *sequestrum* (Fig. 5.13) representing a segment of

Table 5.4 Osteolytic lesions with trabeculation/ septation

Simple (unicameral) bone cyst
Aneurysmal bone cyst
Intraosseous lipoma
Hemangioma
Chondromyxoid fibroma
Nonossifying fibroma
Ossifying fibroma
Giant cell tumor
Gnathic tumors (see chapter 11)
Adamantinoma
Ameloblastoma
Fibrosarcoma
Malignant fibrous histiocytoma
Osteosarcoma, teleangiectatic
Plasmacytoma/multiple myeloma
Metastasis (e.g. blowout-metastases from kidney, thyroid or lung)
Brown tumor (hyperparathyroidism)
Hemophilic pseudotumor
Fibrous dysplasia
Sarcoidosis

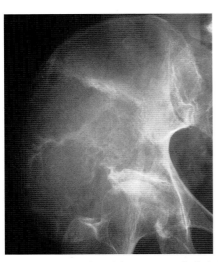

Fig. 5.**11** **Septation**. A large expansile lytic lesion with remaining remnants of the original bone matrix producing a septated appearance, is seen in the ilium (plasmacytoma).

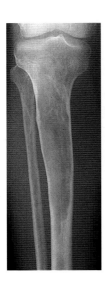

Fig. 5.**12** **Ground glass appearance** . A slightly expansile osteolytic lesion with a hazy increase in density is seen in the proximal tibia (fibrous dysplasia).

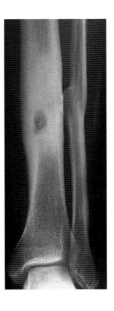

Fig. 5.**13** **Bone sequestrum**. A lytic lesion containing a small sclerotic sequestrum in its center is surrounded by dense sclerosis and cortical thickening in the tibia (chronic osteomyelitis). A healed fibula fracture is incidentally also seen.

dense necrotic bone is indicative of chronic osteomyelitis (Table 5.**5**).

  Bone expansion can be associated with both benign and malignant lesions. In a slowly growing tumor the bone erosion on the inner cortex is compensated by bone apposition on the outer cortex (Fig. 5.**14**). In this instance the cortex remains intact at all times, but the thickness of this new cortical shell may be different when compared to the original cortex. The interface between normal and expanded cortex may be filled in with dense bone and often is referred to as *buttressing* (Fig. 5.**15**). It is found, among others, with eosinophilic granulomas, aneurysmal bone cysts and osteoblastomas. In rapidly growing tumors the new bone formation cannot keep up with the bone breakdown resulting in *cortical violation* or *frank destruction* (Fig. 5.**16**) (Tables 5.**6** and 5.**7**).

Table 5.5 Osteolytic lesions containing a sequestrum or bone fragment

Simple (unicameral) bone cyst with pathologic fracture (fallen fragment sign)

Fibrosarcoma (sequestered bone fragment)

Metastasis (sequestered bone fragment)

Bone lesion with pathologic fracture (fracture fragment)

Eosinophilic granuloma (sequestrum)

Comminuted fracture (intramedullary displaced cortical fragment)

Osteomyelitis (sequestrum)

Brodie's abscess (sequestrum)

Infected pin tract (ring sequestrum)

Button sequestrum in skull (eosinophilic granuloma, metastases, epidermoid, osteoblastoma, osteomyelitis, radiation necrosis, bone flap undergoing avascular necrosis, burr hole and normal variants)

Table 5.6 Expansile osteolytic lesion with intact cortex

Simple (unicameral) bone cyst

Aneurysmal bone cyst (eccentric)

Enchondroma

Chondromyxoid fibroma (eccentric)

Nonossifying fibroma (eccentric)

Desmoplastic fibroma

Osteoblastoma

Giant cell tumor (eccentric)

Fibrosarcoma

Chondrosarcoma

Eosinophilic granuloma

Brown tumor (hyperparathyroidism)

Hemophilic pseudotumor

Healing/healed fracture

Osteomyelitis (e.g. spina ventosa [phalanges or metacarpals] in tuberculosis)

Fibrous dysplasia

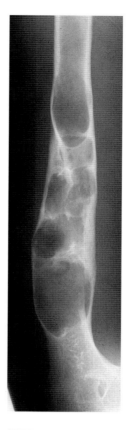

Fig. 5.**14** **Expansile lesion with intact cortex.** An expansile, multiloculated lesion with intact, thinned or thickened cortex is seen in the distal humerus (simple [unicameral] bone cyst).

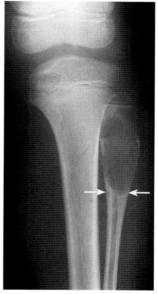

Fig. 5.**15** **Buttressing.** Localized cortical thickening (arrows) is seen in the proximal fibula at the interface between normal cortex and expanded cortex of the osteolytic lesion (aneurysmal bone cyst).

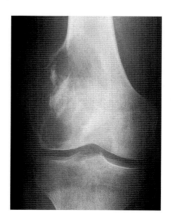

Fig. 5.**16** **Cortical destruction.** An eccentric, expansile, osteolytic lesion in the distal femur metaphysis and epiphyses broke through the cortex with only a few cortical remnants remaining (giant cell tumor).

The *location* of a solitary lesion within a bone provides an important clue to the correct diagnosis. In tubular bones the epiphysis is a common location for chondroblastomas, clear cell chondrosarcomas, metastases, lipomas, subchondral cysts, intraosseous ganglia and Brodie's abscesses. Giant cell tumors originate in the metaphysis, but quickly penetrate the closed growth plate and extend into the subchondral bone. Osteoid osteomas (intra-articular presentation), enchondromas and eosinophilic granulomas occasionally are also found in the epiphyses, but the diametaphysis is a more characteristic location for these tumors (Table 5.8). Lesions commonly located in the epiphyses are also found about the joints of flat bones, patella and carpal and tarsal bones.

Typical *metaphyseal lesions* include nonossifying fibroma which characteristically develops a short distance from the growth plate, chondromyxoid fibroma which abuts the growth plate, simple (unicameral) bone cyst, aneurysmal bone cyst, osteochondroma, Brodie's abscess, mesenchymal sarcomas such as osteosarcoma and chondrosarcoma and metastases. Common *diaphyseal lesions* include round cell tumors (e.g. Ewing's sarcoma and lymphoma), metastases, nonossifying fibromas, simple (unicameral) bone cysts in adults, enchondromas, osteoid osteomas, osteoblastomas, and fibrous dysplasia.

The diagnosis of a tubular bone lesion is also facilitated by the identification of its center with regard to the medullary canal and cortex. Typical *central lesions* include simple (unicameral) bone cysts, enchondromas, fibrous dysplasia and bone infarcts. *Eccentric lesions* include aneurysmal bone cysts, giant cell tumors and chondromyxoid fibromas. Typical *cortical lesions* are nonossifying fibromas and osteoid osteomas (Fig. 5.17). *Surface lesions* arise from the outer surface of the cortex (e.g. surface high-grade osteosarcoma). *Juxtacortical lesions* (Figs. 5.18 and 5.19) can be divided into those originating from the deep layer of the periosteum (periosteal lesions) and those derived from the outer layer of the periosteum and growing in an exophytic pattern (parosteal lesions). Typical examples of juxtacortical lesions include the periosteal osteosarcoma and parosteal osteosarcoma (Table 5.9).

Table 5.7   Expansile osteolytic lesion with cortical violation

Aneurysmal bone cyst (eccentric)

Epidermoid inclusion cyst

Glomus tumor

Hemangioma (skull)

Chondromyxoid fibroma (eccentric)

Desmoplastic fibroma

Osteoblastoma

Giant cell tumor (eccentric)

Fibrosarcoma

Malignant fibrous histiocytoma

Chondrosarcoma

Osteosarcoma

Angiosarcoma

Plasmacytoma/multiple myeloma

Metastases (from kidney, thyroid, lung)

Hemophilic pseudotumor

Table 5.8   Common location of tubular bone lesions

Epiphyses

Subchondral cyst (associated with arthritis, osteonecrosis or trauma)

Gout (intraosseous tophus)

Amyloidosis

Intraosseous ganglion

Intraosseous lipoma

Chondroblastoma

Dysplasia epiphysealis hemimelica (Trevor's disease)

Giant cell tumor (originates in metaphysis)

Clear cell chondrosarcoma

Metastasis

Brodie's abscess

Metaphyses

Simple (unicameral) bone cyst

Aneurysmal bone cyst

Osteochondroma

Chondromyxoid fibroma

Periosteal desmoid

Nonossifying fibroma

Desmoplastic fibroma

Fibrosarcoma

Malignant fibrous histiocytoma

Chondrosarcoma

Osteosarcoma

Metastasis

Osteomyelitis

Brodie's abscess

Fibrous dysplasia

Diametaphysis

Simple (unicameral) bone cyst (in adults)

Intraosseous lipoma

Enchondroma

Periosteal chondroma

Nonossifying fibroma

Bone island

Osteoid osteoma

Osteoblastoma

Adamantinoma (especially anterior tibia)

Fibrosarcoma

Malignant fibrous histiocytoma

Ewing's sarcoma

Angiosarcoma

Multiple myeloma

Metastasis

Lymphoma

Langerhans cell histiocytosis (eosinophilic granuloma)

Brown tumor (hyperparathyroidism)

Hemophilic pseudotumor

Osteonecrosis (bone infarct)

Osteomyelitis

Fibrous dysplasia

Osteofibrous dysplasia (especially anterior tibia)

The knowledge of the *age of a patient* is fundamental to the correct interpretation of any bone lesion. Most benign symptomatic bone tumors are diagnosed in patients below the age of 30 years. Asymptomatic benign bone lesions are however a frequent incidental finding at any age. Primary malignant bone tumors in children and adolescents usually consist of osteosarcomas and Ewing's sarcomas. Neoplasms typically diagnosed between the age of 20 and 40 years include giant cell tumors, parosteal sarcomas and adamantimomas. Symptomatic bone tumors diagnosed at the age of 40 years and older must be considered malignant until proven otherwise with the vast majority being either metastases, lymphoma or multiple myeloma.

The differential diagnosis of localized bone lesions is discussed in Table 5.**10**.

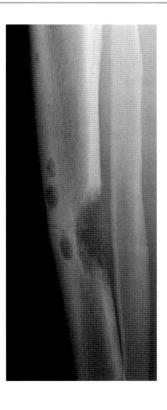

Fig. 5.**17** **Cortical lesions.** Multiple osteolytic lesions are seen within the cortex of the tibia. The largest lesion has extended from the cortex into the medullary space and adjacent soft tissue (metastases from bronchogenic carcinoma).

Table 5.9 Cortical lesions

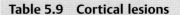

Localized elliptical cortical thickening

Osteoid osteoma

Osteomyelitis (chronic)

Stress fracture

Localized defect of external cortex

Periosteal desmoid (posteromedial aspect of distal femur)

Fibromatosis

Adamantinoma (especially anterior tibia)

Osteofibrous dysplasia (especially anterior tibia)

Ewing's sarcoma

Metastasis (especially from bronchogenic carcinoma)

Hyperparathyroidism including brown tumor

Gouty tophus

Adjacent soft tissue neoplasm or abscess

Subperiosteal osteomyelitis

Subperiosteal hematoma

Avulsion fracture/injury (chronic)

Juxtacortical tumors and tumor-like lesions

Parosteal lipoma (may induce cortical thickening or hyperostosis

Parosteal hemangioma (may induce cortical thickening or hyperostosis

Osteoma

Osteochondroma

Periosteal (juxtacortical) chondroma

Bizarre parosteal osteochondromatous proliferation (BPOP)

Periosteal (juxtacortical) desmoid

Peripheral chondrosarcoma

Periosteal chondrosarcoma

Periosteal osteosarcoma

Parosteal osteosarcoma

Parosteal myositis ossificans

Spurs (congenital, post-traumatic)

Enthesopathy

Osteophytosis

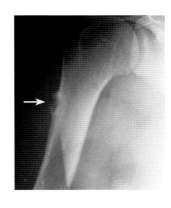

Fig. 5.**18** **Juxtacortical lesion.** A defect (arrow) with minimal punctate matrix calcifications is seen in the outer cortex of the proximal humerus surrounded by periosteal new bone formation (periosteal [juxtacortical] chondroma).

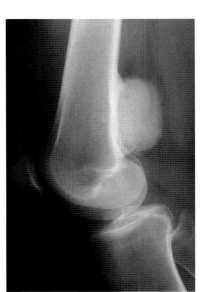

Fig. 5.**19** **Juxtacortical lesion.** An ossified mass with adjacent cortical thickening is seen in the posterior aspect of the distal femur (parosteal osteosarcoma).

Table 5.10   Localized bone lesions

Disease	Radiographic Findings	Comments
Subchondral cyst (Fig. 5.20)	Solitary or multiple defects measuring up to 3 cm in diameter with sclerotic border located in the subchondral bone (pressure segment) of a joint. Communication with joint may be present occasionally allowing gas to pass into the cyst (pneumatocyst).	Associated with osteoarthritis, calcium pyrophosphate dihydrate crystal deposition disease (CPPD), osteonecrosis (avascular necrosis) and rheumatoid arthritis. *Traumatic* cysts are the sequela of a bone injury, but may be larger and not necessarily associated with an arthritic process.
Intraosseous ganglion (Fig. 5.21)	Unilocular or multilocular, well-defined lytic epiphyseal lesion, often with sclerotic margin. The lesion does not communicate with the adjacent joint. Preferred locations are the medial malleolus of the tibia, femoral head, acetabulum and carpal bones.	A *herniation pit* (Fig. 5.22) is a well-circumscribed radiolucent defect usually measuring less than 1 cm in diameter with a thin sclerotic border in the superolateral aspect of the femoral neck caused by herniated synovium.
Simple (unicameral) bone cyst (Figs. 5.23, 5.24 and 5.25)	Centrally located, well-demarcated and often slightly expansile osteolytic lesion with cortical thinning is characteristic. The lesion may be septated or depict a scalloped inner margin. Most often located in long tubular bones (especially humerus and femur), initially in the metaphysis abutting the growth plate and with time migrating into the diaphysis. Pathologic fracture is relatively common with a fracture fragment occasionally located at the bottom of the cyst (fallen fragment sign).	Asymptomatic unless fractured. Usually diagnosed before the age of 20 years with a 3:1 male predominance. After that age bone cysts tend to appear more often in flat bones such as pelvis or calcaneus. *Echinococcal (hydatid) cysts* are found in 1% of infected patients presenting with single or multiple expansile cystic lesions ("bunch of grapes") preferentially located in the pelvis and sacrum.
Aneurysmal bone cyst (Figs. 5.26 and 5.27)	Presents most commonly as an eccentric, expansile osteolytic lesion with intact or disrupted cortex in the metaphysis of a long tubular bone. Extensive sclerosis at the interface between normal and expanded cortex ("buttressing") may be present. Delicate thin trabeculation is characteristic and an expansile ballooning lesion may produce a "soap-bubble" appearance. Other common locations include the posterior elements of the spine and the pelvis, where a large soft tissue component may simulate a malignancy.	Primary lesions are usually diagnosed in the first, second or less frequently third decades of life with slight female predominance. Secondary aneurysmal bone cysts (20%) are found in giant cell tumors and less frequently in osteoblastomas, simple bone cysts, nonossifying fibromas, teleangiectatic osteosarcomas, metastases, fibrous dysplasia, Paget's disease, and others.

(continues on page 84)

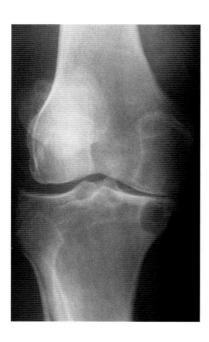

Fig. 5.**20 Subchondral cyst**. Degenerative changes with a large subchondral cystic lesion with sclerotic margin is seen in the medial tibia plateau.

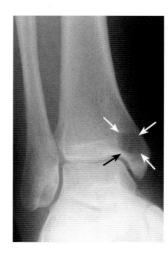

Fig. 5.**21 Intraosseous ganglion**. A small cystic lesion (arrows) with slightly sclerotic margin is seen in the medial malleolus in the absence of arthritis in the ankle.

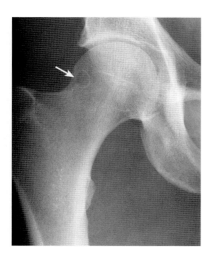

Fig. 5.**22** **Herniation pit**. A cystic lesion (arrow) with sclerotic margin is seen in the anterolateral aspect of the femoral neck.

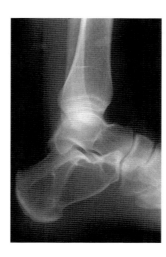

Fig. 5.**23** **Simple (unicameral) bone cyst**. A septated osteolytic lesion with cortical thinning is seen in the calcaneus.

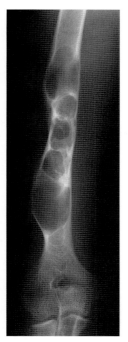

Fig. 5.**24** **Simple (unicameral) bone cyst**. A multiloculated cystic lesion with expanded cortex is seen in the humerus.

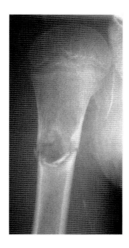

Fig. 5.**25** **Simple (unicameral) bone cyst with fallen fragment sign**. A cystic lesion with pathologic fracture and a linear dense fragment at the bottom of the cyst is seen in the proximal humerus.

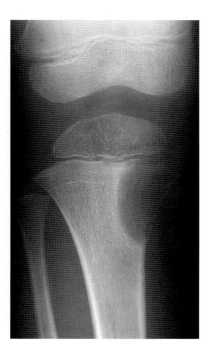

Fig. 5.**26** **Aneurysmal bone cyst**. An eccentric osteolytic lesion is seen in the proximal tibia abutting the open physis.

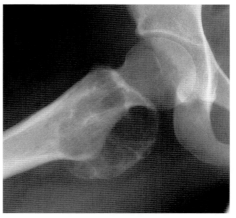

Fig. 5.**27** **Aneurysmal bone cyst**. An expansile trabeculated osteolytic lesion with "soap-bubble" appearance is seen originating from the greater trochanter.

Table 5.10 (Cont.) Localized bone lesions

Disease	Radiographic Findings	Comments
Epidermoid (inclusion cyst) Figs. 5.28 and 5.29)	Intraosseous lesion presents as well-defined osteolytic defect, often with sclerotic margin, occurring in the terminal phalanx of the hand or in the skull. The lesion may be expansile with thinning or destruction of the cortex. Skull lesions usually measure 1 to 5 cm in diameter and may be limited to the diploic space or extend through one or both tables. An irregularly shaped button sequestrum is usually present in larger skull lesions.	Usually diagnosed in the second to fourth decades of life with slight male predominance. A history of trauma is often present suggesting intraosseous implantation of ectodermal tissue with subsequent development of an epidermoid. The lesion is lined with a stratified squamous epithelium shedding keratin debris that breaks down and forms cholesterol.
Glomus tumor	Intraosseous glomus tumor presents as a well-defined osteolytic lesion in the terminal phalanges of the hand indistinguishable from an epidermoid on plain film radiography. Differentiation is however possible with MR imaging, where the glomus tumor depicts marked contrast enhancement, often with characteristic "salt and pepper" appearance.	Glomus tumors occur in patients of any age, typically are neither palpable nor visible and present in fingertips with aching pain and point tenderness. Secondary bone involvement from a soft tissue glomus tumor is much more common (e.g. temporal bone). In the hand such a lesion presents as shallow, well-marginated erosion in the adjacent bone, usually in the tuft of a terminal phalanx.
Lipoma (Fig. 5.30)	Well-circumscribed osteolytic lesion, often surrounded by a sclerotic border. Irregular thick bony ridges are frequently found in larger lesions. May contain a central calcified nidus (especially in the calcaneus). Demonstration of fatty tissue within the lesion by either CT or MR imaging is virtually diagnostic.	Besides the calcaneus intraosseous lipoma occur most commonly in the metaphyses of long tubular bones, especially the femur, tibia and fibula. A relatively typical location of larger lipomas is the femoral neck abutting the intertrochanteric line. In this location they resemble fibrous dysplasia. *Liposarcomas* rarely arise in bone.
Liposclerosing myxofibroma (Liposclerosing myxofibrous tumor, LSFMT) (Fig. 5.31)	Well defined lytic or "ground glass" lesion, often with markedly sclerotic-border occurring typically (80%) in the pretrochanteric and intertrochanteric region of the proximal femur. Fat is not always demonstrated with either CT or MRI.	Rare benign lesion commonly diagnosed as incidental finding or presenting with pain in patients between 20 and 70 years of age. Malignant transformation occurs in less than 10% of cases. May be a variant of fibrous dysplasia or represent a burned-out or infarcted intraosseous lipoma.

(continues on page 86)

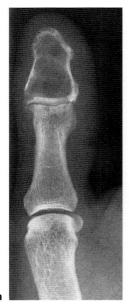
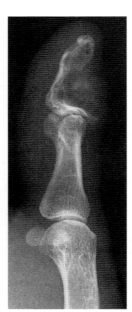
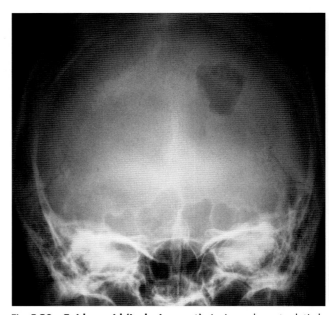

a b

Fig. 5.28 a, b **Epidermoid (inclusion cyst)**. An expansile osteolytic lesion is seen in the distal phalanx of the thumb.

Fig. 5.29 **Epidermoid (inclusion cyst)**. An irregular osteolytic lesion with slightly beveled margin is seen in the vault of the skull.

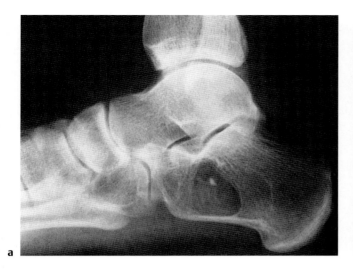

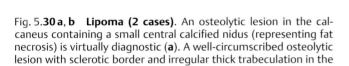

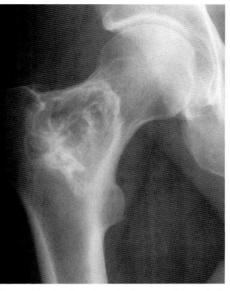

Fig. 5.**30 a, b   Lipoma (2 cases)**. An osteolytic lesion in the calcaneus containing a small central calcified nidus (representing fat
necrosis) is virtually diagnostic (**a**). A well-circumscribed osteolytic
lesion with sclerotic border and irregular thick trabeculation in the
femoral neck abutting the intertrochanteric line is quite characteristic (**b**). The demonstration of fatty content by either CT or MRI
differentiates this lesion from fibrous dysplasia.

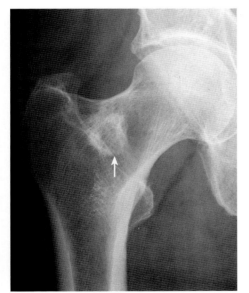

Fig. 5.**31   Liposclerosing myxofribroma**. A round lesion with sclerotic margin is
seen in the pretrochanteric region of the proximal femur (arrow).

Table 5.10   (Cont.) Localized bone lesions

Disease	Radiographic Findings	Comments
Hemangioma (Figs. 5.32, 5.33 and 5.34)	*Spine*: Coarse, vertical trabecular pattern ("corduroy" appearance) in the vertebral bodies is characteristic. Diameter of thickened vertical trabeculae is rather uniform (DD: Multiple myeloma, metastases and Paget's disease, which may present with irregular coarse trabecular thickening). Extension into the posterior elements, paraspinal tissues, and spinal canal is rare. *Skull*: Slightly expansile osteolytic lesion with radiating ("sunburst") pattern. *Tubular bones*: Poorly defined osteolytic lesion with lattice-like trabecular pattern.	Usually found in patients over 40 years of age with female predominance. Occasionally non-Hodgkin's lymphoma (especially the histiocytic type) and metastases (e.g. breast carcinoma) may simulate a hemangioma in the spine. *Cystic angiomatosis* (Fig. 5.35) is characterized by widespread cystic lesions often surrounded by a rim of sclerosis. They may progress to osteosclerotic lesions simulating metastases. The condition is frequently associated with widespread visceral involvement. *Cystic lymphangiomatosis* presents in a similar fashion. Accumulation of contrast material in lesions during lymphography is diagnostic.
Osteochondroma (Figs. 5.36 and 5.37)	Bony protuberance demonstrating cortical and medullary continuity with parent bone is diagnostic in the tubular bones. The lesion may be pedunculated (with narrow stalk and bulbous tip) or sessile (with a broad, flat base). Osteochondromas characteristically originate from the metaphyses and point away from the nearby articulation. The tip of the osteochondroma is covered by a hyaline cartilage cap that may contain regular stippled calcifications. A large cartilaginous cap containing irregular calcifications is suspicious of malignant transformation. Osteochondromas in the pelvis frequently are large and difficult to differentiate from lesions that have undergone malignant transformation. In the ribs osteochondromas frequently occur at the costochondral junction. Malignant transformation may be best assessed with MR imaging. A cartilage cap of 1 cm or less in thickness indicates a benign lesion, whereas a cap thicker then 2 cm is suspicious for malignant transformation.	Osteochondromas occur in children and adolescents as a slowly growing painless mass. They are intimately related to the physis and cease to enlarge with fusion of the adjacent growth plates. Rarely osteochondromas may develop in the adult after trauma. DD: 1. *Subungual exostosis* (Fig. 5.38) projects from the dorsomedial aspect of the tuft, usually of the great toe (80%) or other distal phalanges of the foot or hand. 2. *Reactive bony excrescence* in medial portion of base of distal phalanx of great toe (normal variant). 3. *Turret exostosis* arises on dorsal surface of proximal or middle phalanx in a finger (post-traumatic). 4. *Supracondylar process of humerus* (Fig. 5.39): Spur originating from the anteromedial aspect of the distal humerus pointing towards the elbow (phylogenetic vestige). 5. *Pes anserinus spur* may mimic a small osteochondroma in the medial aspect of the proximal tibia (enthesophyte, occasionally associated with anserinus bursitis). 6. *Post-traumatic spurs* secondary to healed avulsion fractures. 7. *"Tug" lesions* at tendinous attachment sites in the lower extremity. *Hereditary multiple exostoses* (Fig. 5.40) present with multiple, usually bilateral and symmetric osteochondromas in the axial and appendicular skeleton associated with bone modeling deformities. In *metachondromatosis* (Fig. 5.41) multiple osteochondromas and enchondromas coexist, especially in the hands and feet.

(continues on page 88)

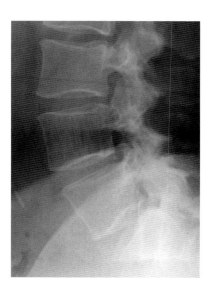

Fig. 5.**32** **Hemangioma**. A rather uniform coarse vertical striation pattern ("corduroy" appearance) seen in the vertebral body of L4 is virtually diagnostic.

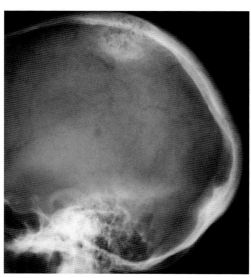

Fig. 5.**33** **Hemangioma**. A slightly expansile lesion with marginal sclerosis and characteristic radiating bony spicules within the lesion is seen in the vault of the skull.

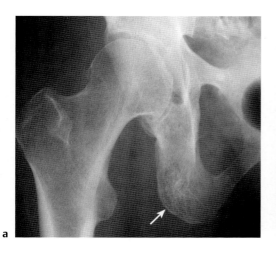

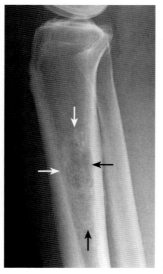

Fig. 5.**34 a, b** **Hemangioma** (2 cases). A poorly defined osteolytic lesion (arrows) with lattice-like trabecular pattern is seen in the ischiatic ramus (**a**) and proximal tibia (**b**).

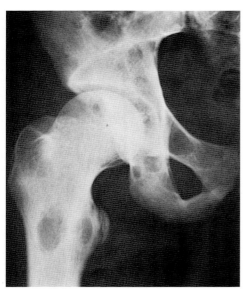

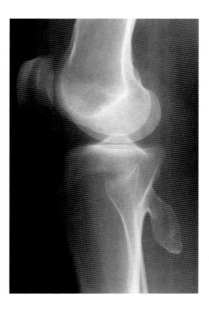

Fig. 5.**36** **Osteochondroma (pedunculated).** A bony protuberance demonstrating cortical and medullary continuity with the tibia and pointing away from the knee is characteristic.

Fig. 5.**35** **Cystic angiomatosis**. Multiple well-demarcated osteolytic lesions surrounded by sclerosis are seen in the pelvis and upper femur.

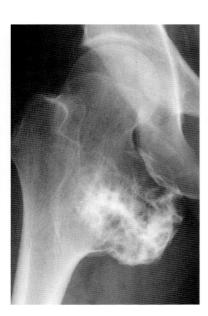

Fig. 5.**37** **Osteochondroma (sessile).** A broad-based bony outgrowth from the lesser trochanter with calcified cartilage cap is seen. This lesion cannot be differentiated from a low-grade peripheral chondrosarcoma.

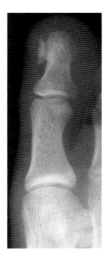

Fig. 5.**38** **Subungual exostosis.** An irregular bone protuberance originates from the dorsomedial aspect of the tuft of the great toe.

Table 5.10 (Cont.) Localized bone lesions

Disease	Radiographic Findings	Comments
Dysplasia epiphysealis hemimelica (Trevor's disease) (Fig. 5.42)	Lobulated osseous mass (articular chondroma) protruding from an epiphysis, carpal or tarsal bone. Presents initially in infants as irregular ossifications adjacent to the involved bone. Preferential involvement of the medial side of a lower extremity (e.g. distal femur, proximal and distal tibia and talus). Multiple bones in a single extremity are affected in two-thirds of cases.	Presents in children and young adults with swelling, pain and deformity localized to one side of the body.
Enchondroma (Figs. 5.43 and 5.44)	Well-circumscribed, often lobulated, osteolytic lesion with endosteal scalloping composed of hyaline-type cartilage with varying degrees of calcifications. Preferred locations are the metaphyses of the long tubular bones and the diaphyses in the short tubular bones of the hands and feet. Cortical expansion and pathologic fractures are frequent findings in the hands and feet, but malignant transformation is very rare in these locations. Transformation to chondrosarcoma in the long tubular and flat bones should be suspected with an enlarging radiolucent area, the disappearance of pre-existing calcifications or pathologic fracture.	Enchondromas are usually discovered in the third and fourth decades of life as incidental findings. The presence of pain should arouse suspicion of malignant transformation. Low-grade chondrosarcomas in the long tubular bones and axial skeleton are difficult if not impossible to differentiate from benign enchondromas. *Enchondromatosis (Ollier's disease)* (Figs. 5.**45** and 5.**46**) is characterized by multiple, asymmetrically distributed enchondromas, either exclusively or predominantly involving one side of the body. The affected bones often are shortened and deformed. After cessation of growth the lesion no longer increases in size unless malignant transformation has taken place, estimated to occur in 5 to 30% of patients. *Maffucci's syndrome* (Fig. 5.**47**) consists of multiple enchondromas and soft tissue hemangiomas containing multiple phleboliths.

(continues on page 90)

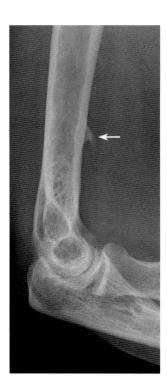

Fig. 5.**39** **Supracondylar process**. A spur is seen originating from the anteromedial aspect of the distal humerus and pointing towards the elbow.

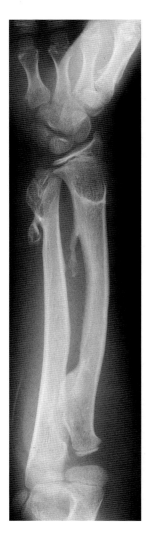

Fig. 5.**40** **Hereditary multiple exostoses**. Besides multiple osteochondromas modeling deformities in both the proximal and distal radius and ulna are also evident.

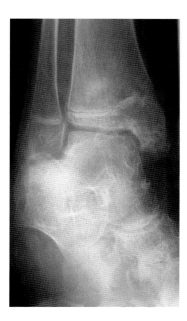

Fig. 5.**42** **Dysplasia epiphysealis hemimelica (Trevor's disease)**. An enlarged medial malleolus with an irregular, lobulated and partially calcified mass in its tip is seen. Calcified lesions are also present in the medial aspect of the talus and navicular bone.

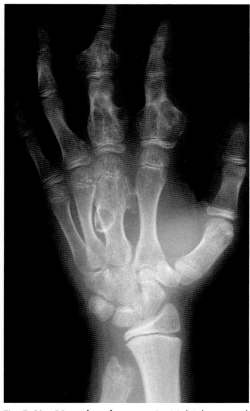

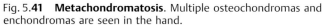

Fig. 5.**41** **Metachondromatosis**. Multiple osteochondromas and enchondromas are seen in the hand.

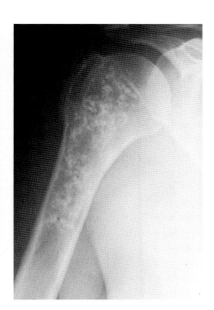

Fig. 5.**43** **Enchondroma**. A lesion containing flocculent, punctate and circular calcifications is seen in the proximal humerus. An old avulsion fracture of the greater tuberosity is incidentally also present.

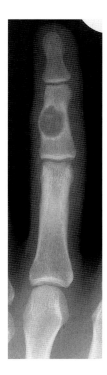

Fig. 5.**44** **Enchondroma**. An expansile osteolytic lesion with slightly sclerotic margin and faint matrix calcification is seen in the middle phalanx of the third finger.

Table 5.10 (Cont.) Localized bone lesions

Disease	Radiographic Findings	Comments
Periosteal (juxtacortical) chondroma (Figs. 5.48 and 5.49)	Calcified (50%) soft tissue mass with erosion of the adjacent cortex and varying degree of periostitis. Metaphyses of long bones and hands are most commonly affected.	All ages are affected but the tumor is usually diagnosed under age 30. Slight male predominance.
Bizarre parosteal osteochondromatous proliferation (BPOP) (Fig. 5.50)	Well-marginated sessile or pedunculated mass of heterotopic ossification arising from the cortical surface without medullary continuity between the lesion and the adjacent bone is characteristic.	Occurs usually in the hands and feet (occasionally in long tubular bones) without age and sex predilection. A history of trauma is evident in some patients.
Chondroblastoma (Figs. 5.51 and 5.52)	Well-defined, often lobulated lytic lesion involving the epiphysis or apophysis of a long tubular bone with or without thin sclerotic border and matrix calcification (> 50%) is characteristic. A solid periosteal reaction in the adjacent metaphyseal shaft can be induced by bone marrow edema surrounding the lesion. Approximately 10% of chondroblastomas occur in the hands and feet with predilection for the talus and calcaneus.	Benign cartilaginous lesion occurring between the ages of 5 and 25 years with slight male predominance.

(continues on page 92)

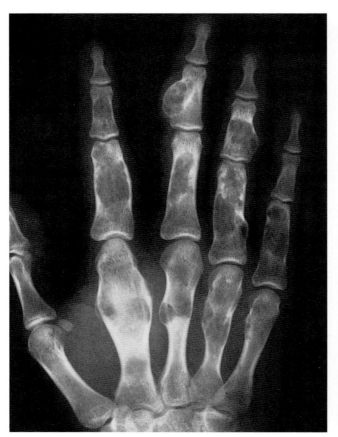

Fig. 5.**45 Enchondromatosis (Ollier's disease).** Multiple enchondromas are seen in the hand sparing the thumb and distal phalanges.

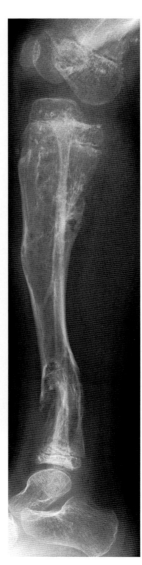

Fig. 5.**46 Enchondromatosis (Ollier's disease).** Multiple enchondromas are associated with severe modeling deformities in the distal femur, tibia and fibula.

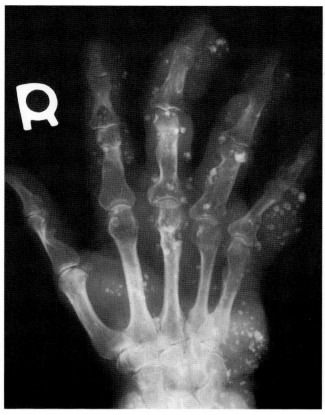

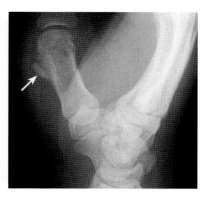

Fig. 5.**48** **Periosteal (juxtacortical) chondroma**. A cortical defect with surrounding sclerosis and adjacent soft tissue calcifications (arrow) is seen in the first metacarpal bone.

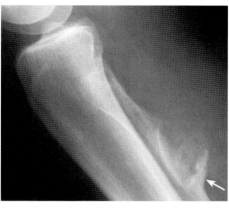

Fig. 5.**47** **Maffucci's syndrome**. Multiple enchondromas are associated with multiple soft tissue hemangiomas containing numerous phleboliths.

Fig. 5.**49** **Periosteal (juxtacortical) chondroma**. An eccentric osteolytic lesion with sclerotic margin, buttressing (arrow), and faint matrix calcifications is seen in the proximal fibula.

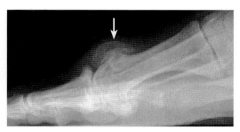

Fig. 5.**50** **Bizarre parosteal osteochondromatous proliferation (BPOP)**. A "mushroom cap"-like ossified mass (arrow) arising from the distal aspect of the first metatarsal bone is seen.

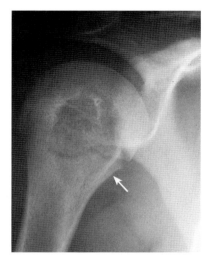

Fig. 5.**51** **Chondroblastoma**. A slightly lobulated osteolytic lesion with faint matrix calcification is seen in the humeral head. A solid periosteal reaction (arrow) and slight diffuse sclerosis of the metaphysis adjacent to the lesion is also evident.

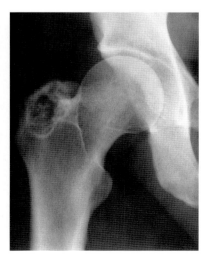

Fig. 5.**52** **Chondroblastoma**. A lytic lesion with sclerotic margin and matrix calcification is seen in the tip of the greater tuberosity.

Table 5.10   (Cont.) Localized bone lesions

Disease	Radiographic Findings	Comments
Chondromy-xoid fibroma (Fig. 5.53)	Eccentric metaphyseal osteolytic lesion with cortical expansion, coarse trabeculation, endosteal scalloping and scalloped sclerotic medullary border is commonly seen. Destruction of the cortex resulting in a hemispherical osseous defect or "bite" without periosteal reaction is characteristic of larger lesions. Predilection for the long tubular bones of the lower extremity, but occasionally also found in pelvis and foot.	Uncommon benign cartilaginous lesion occurring between the ages of 5 and 25 years with slight male predominance and presenting with slowly progressive pain, tenderness, swelling and restriction of motion is typical. *Fibrocartilagenous mesenchymoma* is a very rare solitary expansile osteolytic lesion with spotty or ring-like calcifications, cortical destruction and soft tissue invasion originating most often in the metaphysis of long tubular bones. Age distribution is similar to chondromyxoid fibroma.
Periosteal (juxtacortical) desmoid (Fig. 5.54)	Saucer-like defect in the posteromedial cortex of the distal femur often associated with adjacent sclerosis, periostitis and soft-tissue swelling.	Occurs between the age of 10 and 20 as sequelae of acute or chronic trauma at the adductor magnus tendon insertion in the linea aspera.
Nonossifying fibroma (Figs. 5.55, 5.56 and 5.57)	Small lesions present as round or oblong, well delineated, radiolucent areas in the cortex with normal or sclerotic adjacent bone. They typically arise in the metaphysis at a short distance from the physis. Larger lesions present as a well delineated, eccentric, ovoid osteolytic area in the diametaphyses. They frequently have a multiloculated appearance and both cortical expansion and thinning may be evident. The long tubular bones, especially the tibia and femur, are most frequently affected. With time the lesions may spontaneously disappear or become sclerotic.	Usually diagnosed in patients under the age of 20. Smaller lesions are referred to as *benign fibrous cortical defects*. They are asymptomatic and diagnosed as incidental finding on routine radiography and occasionally are multifocal. They usually regress spontaneously or less commonly enlarge and migrate with growth into the diaphyses eventually being referred to as nonossifying fibromas. Pathologic fractures in larger lesions are not uncommon. *Jaffe-Campanacci syndrome* consists of multiple nonossifying fibromas associated with café-au-lait spots, mental retardation and hypogonadism. *Benign fibrous histiocytomas* (Fig. 5.58) are histologically identical to nonossifying fibromas, but present as slightly more aggressive lesions in patients over age 20 without site predilection.
Desmoplastic fibroma (Fig. 5.59)	Central osteolytic lesion with trabeculated, soap bubble or honeycomb pattern in the metaphyses of long tubular bones, mandible or pelvis. Slight bony expansion with endosteal erosion and limited periosteal bone formation may be associated.	Rare benign neoplasm occurring in the second or third decades of life. Pain and swelling are the leading clinical symptoms or a pathologic fracture may be the presenting feature.

(continues on page 94)

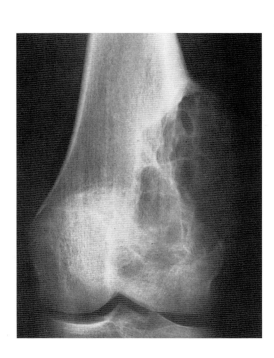

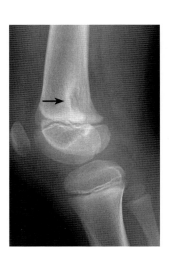

Fig. 5.**54   Periosteal (juxtacortical) desmoid**. A saucer-like defect in the posteromedial cortex of the distal femur with adjacent sclerosis in a child with unfused physis is virtually diagnostic.

Fig. 5.**53   Chondromyxoid fibroma**. An expansile eccentric osteolytic lesion with irregular trabeculation, dissolved cortex, and scalloped sclerotic medullary border is seen in the distal femur metaphysis.

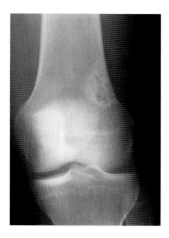

Fig. 5.**55 Nonossifying fibroma**. A slightly oblong eccentric lesion with multiloculated appearance and sclerotic margin is seen in the distal femur metaphysis.

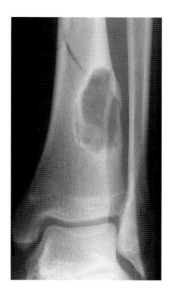

Fig. 5.**56 Nonossifying fibroma**. A large oblong eccentric osteolytic lesion with sclerotic margin and pathologic fracture is seen in the distal tibia.

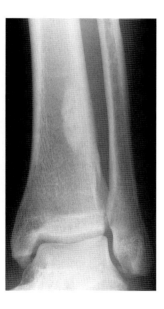

Fig. 5.**57 Nonossifying fibroma (healed)**. An oblong eccentric sclerotic focus is seen in the distal tibia.

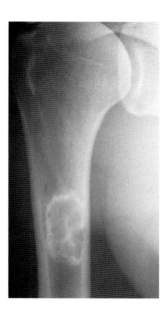

Fig. 5.**58 Benign fibrous histiocytoma**. A central intramedullary lesion with sclerotic margin and trabeculation is seen in the proximal humerus shaft.

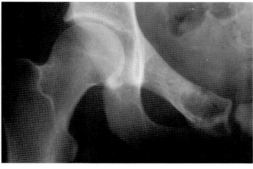
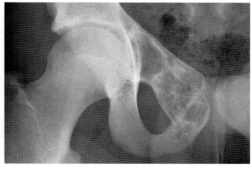

a   b

Fig. 5.**59 a, b Desmoplastic fibroma (2 cases)**. A central, relatively poorly defined, slightly expansile osteolytic lesion with honeycombing and surrounding new bone formation is seen in the superior pubic ramus and body of both patients.

Table 5.10   (Cont.) Localized bone lesions

Disease	Radiographic Findings	Comments
Bone island (enostosis) (Figs. 5.60 and 5.61)	Single or multiple intraosseous foci of homogeneously dense bone most often found in the pelvis, proximal femurs and spine. They may be round, ovoid or oblong and are aligned with the long axis of the trabecular architecture. Tiny bone spicules radiating from the periphery of the lesion are quite characteristic. A somewhat radiolucent center may occasionally be encountered. Range in size from a few millimeters to a few centimeters.	Incidental finding in all age groups. Lesions may slowly increase or decrease in size over years. Bone scintography is usually negative. (DD: osteoblastic metastases). A *curettaged* and *methylmethacrylate cemented bone lesion* may resemble a large enostosis. *Osteopoikilosis:* Numerous small sclerotic foci with symmetric distribution in periarticular locations.
Osteoma (Fig. 5.62)	Mass of either uniformly dense compact bone or less dense cancellous bone protruding from the skull and facial bones (especially the paranasal sinuses). Rarely osteomas arise from the cortical surface of the clavicle, pelvis and tubular bones.	*Gardner's syndrome:* Autosomal dominant disease consisting of multiple osteomas, colonic polyposis and soft tissue tumors (especially desmoids). *Tuberous sclerosis:* Multiple osteoma-like lesions may be associated, especially in the metacarpals and metatarsals.
Osteoid osteoma (Figs. 5.63, 5.64, 5.65, 5.66 and 5.67)	*Diaphysis of long tubular bones*: Cortical radiolucent lesion (nidus) measuring less than 1 cm in diameter surrounded by a zone of uniform bone sclerosis (elliptical thickening of the cortex) is virtually diagnostic. The nidus is not always identified with plain film radiography and occasionally has a calcified center. *Intra-articular location*: A nonconspicuous small radiolucent focus often without significant reactive sclerosis may be present inducing a synovial inflammatory response that may result in secondary arthritic changes. *Carpal and tarsal bones*: A partially or completely calcified lesion without or only mild reactive sclerosis is characteristic. *Spine*: An osteosclerotic focus in the posterior elements is the most common presentation. A scoliotic deformity is usually associated with the lesion and is located near its apex on the concave side of the curve.	Occurs in patients between 7 and 25 years of age with a male predominance of 3 to 1. Pain is the hallmark of the disease, usually more dramatic at night and ameliorated by aspirin. Bone scintigraphy shows an unusual intense uptake in the center of the lesion (nidus) differentiating it from chronic cortical osteomyelitis with small abscess formation. Localized cortical thickening caused by a stress fracture typically is associated with a transverse linear radiolucency. In the lumbar spine a unilateral osteosclerotic focus about a pedicle is frequently caused by a hypertrophied intra-articular pars caused by *unilateral spondylysis* of the contralateral side.

(continues on page 96)

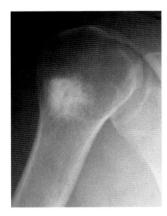

Fig. 5.**60**   **Enostosis (large bone island).** An osteoblastic lesion with tiny bone spicules radiating from its periphery is seen in the proximal humerus metaphysis.

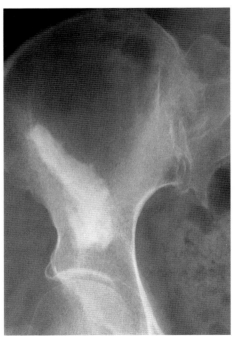

Fig. 5.**61**   **Enostosis (large bone island).** An irregular shaped large osteoblastic lesion with minimally spiculated border is seen in the ilium.

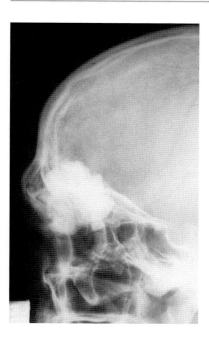

Fig. 5.**62** **Osteoma**. A slightly lobulated dense bone mass is seen protruding into the frontal sinus.

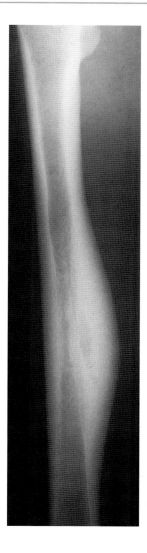

Fig. 5.**63** **Osteoid osteoma**. Elliptical cortical thickening is seen in the femur shaft. The nidus is not identified in this case with conventional film radiography.

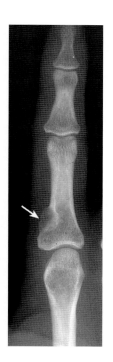

Fig. 5.**64** **Osteoid osteoma**. An expansile cortical lesion (arrow) with only minimal surrounding sclerosis is seen in the proximal phalanx of the index finger.

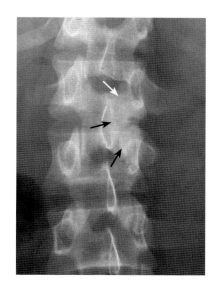

Fig. 5.**66** **Osteoid osteoma**. An osteosclerotic focus (arrows) is seen in the left posterior elements of L1 located at the apex on the concave side of the associated mild scoliosis.

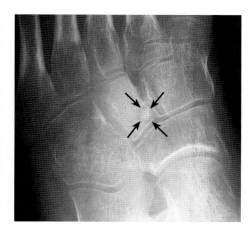

Fig. 5.**65** **Osteoid osteoma**. An osteolytic lesion (arrows) with calcified center (target lesion) is seen in the lateral cuneiform that depicts an overall slight increase in density with the exception of its lateral and distal aspect.

Table 5.10 (Cont.) Localized bone lesions

Disease	Radiographic Findings	Comments
Osteoblastoma Figs. 5.68 and 5.69)	*Long tubular bones*: Osteoblastomas typically originate in either the medullary or cortical bone of the diaphysis and present as expansile osteolytic lesions, often with areas of calcification or ossification, surrounding bone sclerosis and frequently exuberant solid periosteal reaction. *Spine*: A well-defined expansile osteolytic lesion that is partially or extensively calcified and surrounded by mild sclerosis at best, is commonly found in the posterior elements. *Hands, feet and pelvis*: Slightly expansile lytic lesions with varying degrees of matrix calcification/ossification and surrounding reactive sclerosis are the most common presentation	Usually diagnosed in the second and third decades of life with a male predominance of 2 to 1 and similar clinical presentation as in osteoid osteomas. The size of the nidus (actual size of the osteolytic lesion) may be used to differentiate between osteoblastomas (>2 cm) and osteoid osteomas (<2 cm). *Aggressive (malignant) osteoblastomas* are differentiated from the typical (conventional) osteoblastomas by a more aggressive pattern of tumor behavior including a much greater likelihood to recur. The radiologic features of both types are similar, but cortical violation with tumor extension into the neighboring soft tissues is suggestive of aggressive osteoblastomas.
Giant cell tumor (Figs. 5.70 and 5.71)	In the long tubular bones (85%) a giant cell tumor presents as an eccentric expansile osteolytic lesion, often with a delicate trabecular pattern ("soap bubble" appearance) extending from the metaphysis into the subchondral bone. The margins of the lesion may be well or poorly defined, but sclerosis and periosteal reactions are typically absent. Cortical breakthrough with spread into the adjacent soft tissues occurs. Occasionally the tumor is found in pelvis, sacrum, ribs, vertebral bodies, hands and feet.	Occurs usually in the third and fourth decades of life with equal sex distribution. Tumor recurrence is about 50% in excised and grafted lesions, but markedly reduced when cemented with methylmethacrylate instead of bone grafts. *Malignant giant cell tumors* (including malignant transformation of a benign giant cell tumor) account for about 5%. The *giant cell (reparative) granuloma* (Fig. 5.**72**) has a more benign course and similar histologic and radiologic features as the giant cell tumor, although cortical violation with spread into neighboring soft tissues does not occur and a predilection for facial bones and short tubular bones of the hands and feet exists.

(continues on page 98)

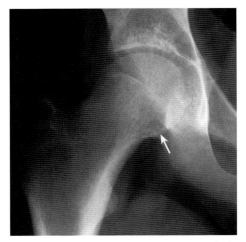

Fig. 5.**67** **Osteoid osteoma (intra-articular).** A nonconspicuous radiolucent focus (arrow) without periosteal reaction is seen medially at the junction between femoral head and neck.

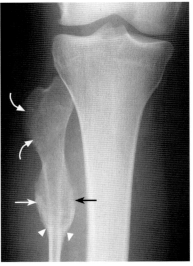

Fig. 5.**68** **Osteoblastoma.** An osteolytic lesion with exuberant solid periosteal reactions (arrows) and buttressing (arrowheads) is seen in the proximal fibular diaphysis. A second cortical lesion (curved arrows) with faint matrix calcification near the fibular head was caused by a **periosteal (juxtacortical) chondroma.**

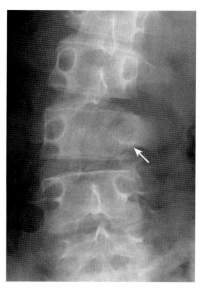

Fig. 5.**69** **Osteoblastoma**. An expansile osteolytic lesion with enlargement of the pedicle (arrow) and faint surrounding sclerosis is seen in the left posterior elements of L3 at the apex on the concave side of the associated scoliosis.

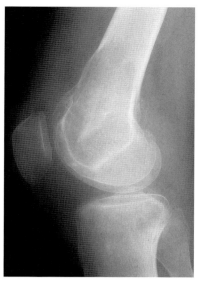

Fig. 5.**70** **Giant cell tumor**. A poorly demarcated osteolytic lesion with faint trabeculation and cortical violation is seen in the distal femur.

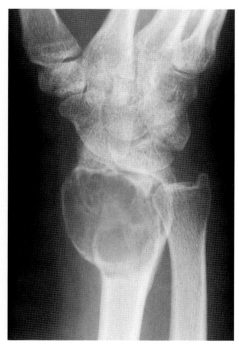

Fig. 5.**71** **Giant cell tumor**. An expansile, well-demarcated osteolytic lesion with "soap bubble" appearance is seen in the distal radius.

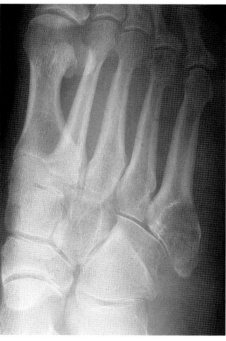

Fig. 5.**72** **Giant cell reparative granuloma**. A slightly expansile osteolytic lesion is seen in the base of the fifth metatarsal.

Table 5.10 (Cont.) Localized bone lesions

Disease	Radiographic Findings	Comments
Chordoma (Figs. 5.73 and 5.74)	Destructive expansile osteolytic lesion with large soft tissue mass and intratumoral calcifications in about half the cases is characteristic. Originates from the sacrum and coccyx (60 %), clivus (30 %) and spine, especially C2 (10 %). Sacral lesions characteristically grow anteriorly. In the spine vertebral collapse, sclerosis (ivory vertebra) and enlarged neural foramina are additional manifestations.	Saccrococcygeal chordomas occur in 40- to 60-year-old patients with male predominance. Spheno-occipital chordomas are usually diagnosed in 20- to 40-year-old patients without sex predilection. The *chondroid chordoma* is a variant comprising one-third of all clivus chordomas with better prognosis and particularly prominent calcifications. Hematogeneous metastases may eventually develop in about one-third of all chordomas.
Adamantinoma (angioblastoma) (Fig. 5.75)	Single or multiple, central or eccentric, multilocular, slightly expansile, sharply or poorly delineated osteolytic lesions with or without reactive sclerosis in the diaphysis of the tibia (85 %) with preferential involvement of its anterior cortex or other long tubular bones. Occasionally cortical destruction, exuberant periostitis and a soft tissue mass are associated.	Usually diagnosed in the third and fourth decades of life with slight male predominance. History of trauma is frequent. Local swelling is the major clinical finding. DD: *Osteofibrous dysplasia*. See under fibrous dysplasia at the end of this table.
Ameloblastoma (Fig. 5.76)	Presentation ranges from unilocular cyst to multilocular, often trabeculated lesion with cortical expansion or destruction and occasionally large soft tissue mass in the mandible or, much less commonly, the maxilla.	Usually diagnosed in the fourth and fifth decades of life without gender predilection. See chapter **11** for differentiation from other gnathic lesions.
Fibrosarcoma (Figs. 5.77, 5.78 and 5.79)	Well or poorly marginated osteolytic lesion with general lack of both periosteal reaction and osteosclerosis is typical. Irregular thin or thick intra-tumoral septation, cortical violation and soft tissue mass are frequently associated. Dystrophic calcifications and sequestered bone fragments are occasionally seen within the tumor. Preferential involvement of the metaphyses of the long tubular bones (70 %) with frequent extension into the diaphyses and epiphyses.	Rare malignant bone tumor occurring in the third to sixth decades of life without gender predilection. The histologic spectrum of fibrosarcomas ranging from well differentiated to poorly differentiated lesions is reflected in the greatly variable radiologic presentation. May complicate Paget's disease, bone infarcts, radiation necrosis and chronic osteomyelitis.

(continues on page 100)

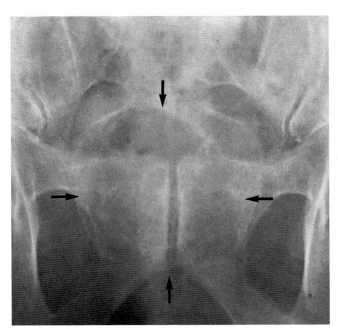

Fig. 5.**73** **Chordoma**. An osteolytic lesion (arrows) with slightly sclerotic margin and faint matrix calcification is seen in the sacrum.

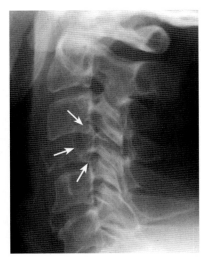

Fig. 5.**74** **Chordoma**. A hemispherical expansile osteolytic lesion (arrows) with slightly sclerotic margin originating in the posterior aspect of the vertebral body of C4 led to the infiltration of the remaining vertebral body with subsequent pathologic compression fracture.

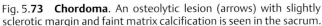

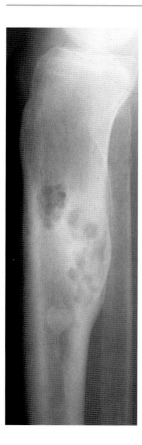

Fig. 5.**75 Adamantinoma**. A slightly expansile, well to poorly demarcated, multilocular lesion with reactive surrounding sclerosis is seen in the tibia.

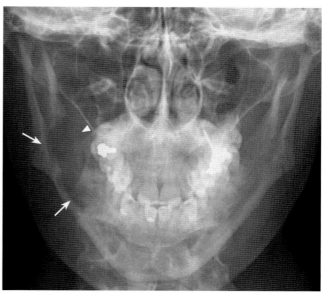

Fig. 5.**76 Ameloblastoma**. An expansile, multiloculated, osteolytic lesion with both endosteal scalloping (arrows) and cortical violation (arrowhead) is seen in the right mandible.

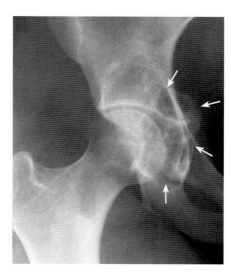

Fig. 5.**78 Fibrosarcoma**. An expansile trabeculated lesion is seen in the innominate bone of the acetabulum (arrows).

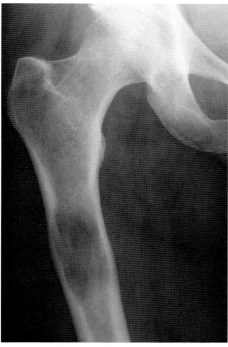

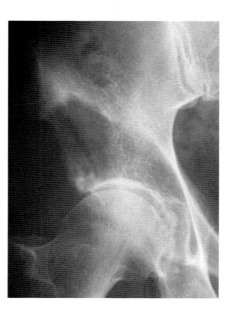

Fig. 5.**79 Fibrosarcoma**. A poorly defined osteolytic lesion is seen in the iliac bone above the acetabulum.

Fig. 5.**77 Fibrosarcoma**. A poorly demarcated lytic lesion with endosteal scalloping is seen in the femur diaphysis.

Table 5.10 (Cont.) Localized bone lesions

Disease	Radiographic Findings	Comments
Malignant fibrous histiocytoma (Figs. 5.80 and 5.81)	A poorly defined osteolytic lesion with cortical destruction, large soft tissue mass and absence of both periosteal reaction and new bone formation is the most common presentation. The ends of long tubular bones from diaphysis to epiphysis are affected in 75 percent of cases with strong predilection for the lower extremity. Osseous expansion is unusual but may be observed in flat bones such as pelvis, ribs, scapula, and sternum.	Occurs at any age, but the majority of cases are diagnosed in the fifth, sixth and seventh decades of life with slight male predominance. The lesion cannot be radiographically differentiated from a highly malignant fibrosarcoma. May develop in abnormal bone such as Paget's disease and bone infarcts or secondary to radiation therapy.
Chondrosarcoma, central (Figs. 5.82, 5.83 and 5.84)	A slightly expansile, multilobulated osteolytic lesion with cortical thickening, endosteal erosion and scattered stippled or irregular calcifications is characteristic. Matrix calcification representing the most specific finding is only present in about two-thirds of the cases. Lesions without matrix calcifications are virtually impossible to differentiate from fibrosarcomas. Demonstration of a poorly defined osteolysis, cortical violation and large soft tissue mass indicate a highly aggressive lesion, but an interrupted periosteal reaction typically is absent. However more often a geographic destruction pattern is present suggesting a less malignant process. The tumor has a predilection for the metaphyses of the long tubular bones (especially femur and humerus) and flat bones (especially pelvis) and the vertebrae.	Occurs usually between 30 and 60 years of age with male predominance. The tumor arises either de novo in the medullary cavity or is caused by malignant transformation of an enchondroma. Low-grade chondrosarcomas are extremely difficult to differentiate from enchondromas. Irregular matrix calcifications (as opposed to punctate, ring and arc-like calcifications), large areas of noncalcified tumor matrix, poorly defined osteolysis and cortical thickening (even solid) suggest all malignancy.
Chondrosarcoma, peripheral (Figs. 5.85 and 5.86)	Malignant transformation of a benign osteochondroma is suggested by demonstration of scattered and irregular calcifications in the cartilaginous cap of the tumor, associated soft tissue mass (non-calcified cartilage cap) and destruction or pressure erosion of the adjacent bone. Differentiation of an osteochondroma from a peripheral chondrosarcoma is not reliably possible on the basis of conventional radiography and supplementation with other imaging techniques such as bone scintigraphy and MRI is required.	Local pain and growth of an osteochondroma in adulthood suggests clinically malignant transformation. The risk of malignant transformation is much higher in patients with hereditary multiple exostoses (estimated to be up to 25 %) than in a solitary osteochondroma (about 1 %) Rarely a peripheral chondrosarcoma develops de novo from the periost (*periosteal* or *juxtacortical chondrosarcoma*).

(continues on page 102)

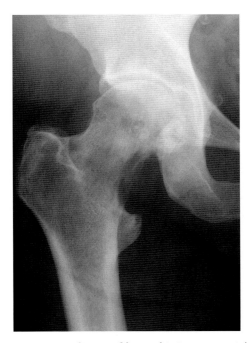

Fig. 5.**80 Malignant fibrous histiocytoma**. A highly aggressive permeative lesion involving the femoral head, neck, and intertrochanteric region without periosteal reaction is seen.

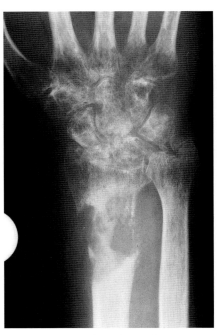

Fig. 5.**81 Malignant fibrous histiocytoma**. A highly destructive lesion originating in the distal radius and extending into the distal ulna and carpal bones is seen.

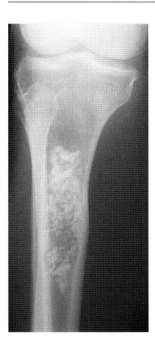

Fig. 5.**82** **Central chondrosarcoma (low grade)**. A slightly expansile lesion with extensive stippled calcifications, and endosteal scalloping is seen in the proximal tibia diaphysis. This lesion cannot be differentiated radiographically from an enchondroma.

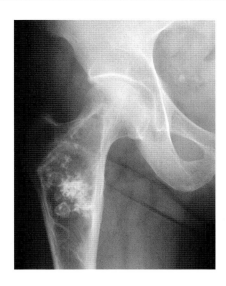

Fig. 5.**83** **Central chondrosarcoma**. A well to poorly demarcated osteolytic lesion with irregular matrix calcification and new cortical bone formation is seen in the proximal femur.

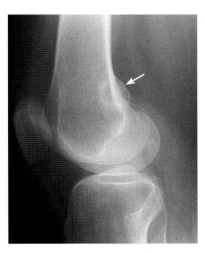

Fig. 5.**84** **Cortical chondrosarcoma (low grade)**. A small expansile cortical lesion (arrow) with faint matrix calcification and sclerotic margin originates from the posterior aspect of the distal femur metaphysis.

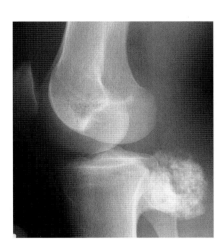

Fig. 5.**85** **Peripheral chondrosarcoma**. A broad-based bony protuberance with extensive irregular calcifications of the cartilaginous cap is seen originating from the posterior tibia metaphysis.

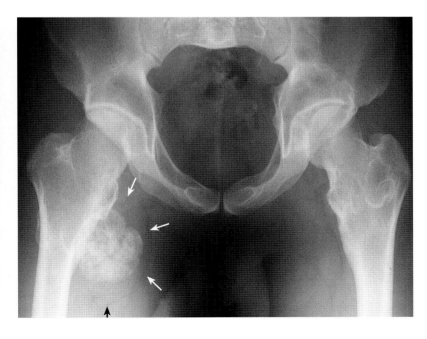

Fig. 5.**86** **Malignant transformation of osteochondroma in hereditary multiple exostoses.** Multiple exostoses with modeling deformities of the pelvis and both proximal femora is seen. The large exostosis originating beneath the right lesser trochanter with cartilage cap calcifications is associated with a soft mass (arrows) indicating malignant transformation.

Table 5.10 (Cont.) Localized bone lesions

Disease	Radiographic Findings	Comments
Clear cell chondrosarcoma (Fig. 5.87)	Poorly or well defined (sclerotic borders), slightly expansile epiphyseal lesion with central calcifications in about one-third of the cases is characteristic. Most frequent locations are the proximal ends of the femur, humerus and tibia.	Rare cartilaginous bone tumor occurring between 25 and 50 years of age with slight male predominance. Radiographic features are virtually identical to a chondroblastoma.
Dedifferentiated chondrosarcoma (Fig. 5.88 and 5.89)	Features of low-grade chondrosarcoma (nonexpansile osteolytic lesion with intact cortex and matrix calcifications) and of highly anaplastic sarcoma (expansile, poorly defined osteolytic lesion with cortical destruction and large soft tissue mass, but usually without calcification) are characteristic. The transition between these two tumor components is usually abrupt. Distribution of the tumor is similar to conventional chondrosarcoma with femur, humerus and pelvis being the most frequent sites of involvement.	Occurs in patients over 50 years of age without gender predilection. Presents with pain, soft tissue swelling or pathologic fracture (one-third of patients). The prognosis is very poor.
Mesenchymal chondrosarcoma (Fig. 5.90)	Features are indistinguishable from a high-grade conventional chondrosarcoma and include poorly defined osteolysis, matrix calcifications, cortical expansion and violation and soft tissue mass. Most frequent sites of involvement are femur, ribs and spine.	Occurs usually between 20 and 40 years of age and has a poor prognosis. Metastases to lymph nodes and other bones is not unusual. Approximately 50 percent of mesenchymal chondrosarcomas arise in the soft tissues.
Osteosarcoma (Figs. 5.91, 5.92, 5.93, and 5.94)	*Conventional osteosarcoma* presenting as a poorly defined intramedullary lesion most often originating in the metaphyses of long tubular bones with varying degrees of osteolysis and osteosclerosis is most characteristic. The tumor may however be purely osteolytic or osteoblastic. Cortical destruction associated with an interrupted periosteal reaction in the form of a Codman's triangle or with perpendicular ("hair-on-end" or "sunburst"), laminated ("onion skin") or amorphous appearance is most characteristic. Large soft tissue masses are commonly found in tumors with cortical violation. Most common sites of involvement are the long tubular bones (80%), especially the femur, tibia and humerus. Osteosarcomas are relatively infrequent in the pelvis, spine and facial bones, and rare in the remaining skeleton. *Teleangiectatic osteosarcomas* commonly present as large, often expansile and predominantly lytic lesions, often with cortical violation and tumor extension into the soft tissues, but without significant periosteal reaction and sclerosis. *Small cell osteosarcomas* commonly present as large predominantly osteolytic lesions, extending from the metaphysis to the diaphysis of a long tubular bone associated with interrupted periosteal reaction and large soft tissue masses. They resemble Ewing's sarcomas. *Intraosseous low grade osteosarcomas* present as purely osteosclerotic and mixed osteolytic/osteoblastic lesions often limited to the medullary portion of the diametaphyses of long tubular bones, especially of the tibia and femur. Irregular cortical thickening may however be associated. The tumor is frequently mistaken for a benign osteosclerotic process.	Osteosarcomas most commonly present in the second and third decades of life with pain, swelling, restriction of motion and pyrexia. Men are more frequently affected than women. In the elderly they may be a complication of Paget's disease or radiation therapy. *Gnathic osteosarcomas* present as purely osteoblastic, osteolytic or mixed lesions in the mandible or less frequently maxilla, occur in the middle-aged and elderly, and have a relatively benign course. *Intracortical osteosarcomas* are rare and originate in the cortices of the tibia and femur, presenting as slightly expansile osteolytic lesions with surrounding sclerosis. *Osteosarcomatosis* refers to simultaneous involvement of more than one skeletal site. It has to be differentiated from a unicentric lesion with distal skeletal metastases.

(continues on page 104)

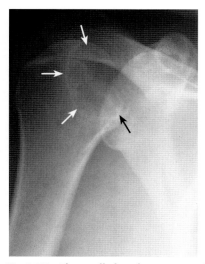

Fig. 5.**87** **Clear cell chondrosarcoma**. An ovoid osteolytic lesion (arrows) with slightly sclerotic border is seen in the humeral head.

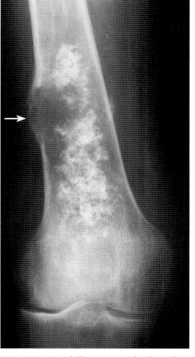

Fig. 5.**88** **Dedifferentiated chondrosarcoma**. A well-differentiated chondrosarcoma with extensive matrix calcification is seen in the distal femur associated with a poorly demarcated expansile osteolytic focus with cortical violation (arrow).

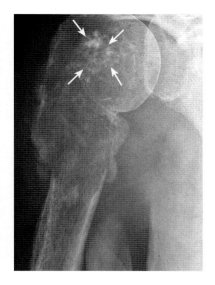

Fig. 5.**89** **Dedifferentiated chondrosarcoma**. A focus of punctate calcifications (arrows) in the humeral head is associated with a highly destructive permeative lesion with multiple pathologic fractures involving the proximal humerus shaft.

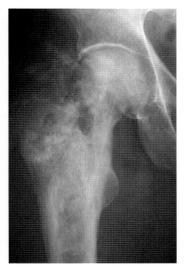

Fig. 5.**90** **Mesenchymal chondrosarcoma**. A highly destructive lesion with extensive irregular matrix calcification, cortical violation and large soft tissue mass is seen originating from the lateral aspect of the femoral neck and greater trochanter.

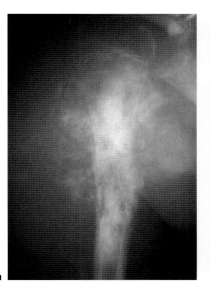

a

b

Fig. 5.**91 a, b** **Osteosarcoma (2 cases)**. A destructive osteoblastic lesion with extensive amorphous periosteal reaction and large soft tissue mass is seen in the proximal humerus shaft. A mixed, but predominantly osteolytic, relative poorly defined osteolytic lesion with cortical violation is seen in the distal femur.

Table 5.10 (Cont.) Localized bone lesions

Disease	Radiographic Findings	Comments
Periosteal osteosarcoma (Fig. 5.95)	Oblong dense lesion arising from the diaphyseal surface of a long tubular bone with irregular thickening and occasionally saucerization of the adjacent cortex is typical. A Codman's triangle and radiating or cloud-like osseous proliferation are frequently associated. Femur, tibia and humerus are the most common sites of involvement.	Usually diagnosed in the second and third decades of life with better prognosis than conventional osteosarcomas, but worse than parosteal osteosarcomas. Radiologic and histologic features of periosteal osteosarcomas and periosteal (juxtacortical) chondrosarcomas are similar if not identical. A *surface high-grade osteosarcoma* arises from the external surface of the cortex with clinical, histologic and radiologic features comparable to a conventional osteosarcoma.
Parosteal osteosarcoma (Fig. 5.96)	A large radiodense oval or round mass with smooth, lobulated, or irregular margins attached in sessile fashion to the external metaphyseal cortex of a long tubular bone is characteristic. A thin radiolucent line may separate the lesion outside its attachment (pedicle) from the cortex which itself may be thickened. With progressive enlargement the tumor tends to wrap around the bone. Ossification within the tumor proceeds from its base to the periphery and may be homogeneous or contain radiolucent areas. Tumor extension into the medullary bone is unusual. The most characteristic location is the posterior surface of the distal femur.	Most common type of osteosarcoma arising on the surface of a bone. Affected patients are adults most often in the third and fourth decades of life. Symptoms are typically insidious and include pain, swelling and a palpable mass. The prognosis is better than in both conventional and periosteal osteosarcomas. DD: *Post-traumatic myositis ossificans* (Figs. 5.97 and 5.98) can be differentiated from a parosteal osteosarcoma by the demonstration of a fine radiolucent line separating the lesion in its entire length from the adjacent bone. Furthermore the ossification in myositis ossificans is evenly radiodense throughout the lesion and its periphery is sharply delineated.

(continues on page 106)

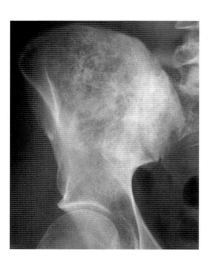

Fig. 5.**92 Osteosarcoma.** A poorly demarcated, mixed osteolytic and osteoblastic lesion is seen in the iliac wing.

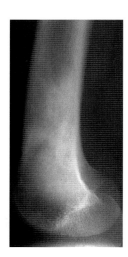

Fig. 5.**93 Osteosarcoma.** A purely osteosclerotic lesion is seen in the distal femur consistent with a low-grade intraosseous osteosarcoma.

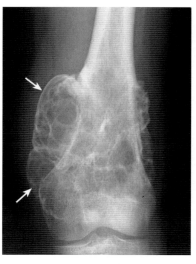

Fig. 5.**94 Teleangiectatic osteosarcoma with aneurysmal bone cyst.** A poorly defined, slightly expansile, trabeculated, osteolytic lesion with cortical violation is associated with an aneurysmal bone cyst (arrows) presenting as better defined eccentric lesion with "soap-bubble" appearance.

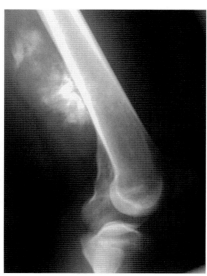

Fig. 5.**95 Periosteal osteosarcoma.** An oblong dense soft tissue lesion arising from the posterior femur diaphysis with cloud-like and radiating osseous proliferation is seen.

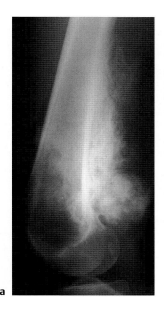
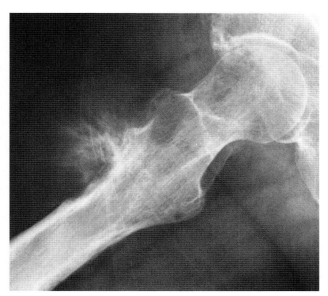

a

b

Fig. 5.**96 a, b Parosteal osteosarcoma (2 cases). a:** A large heterogeneous ossified mass containing radiolucent areas originates from the posterior surface of the distal femur and wraps around the shaft causing the inhomogeneous appearance of the latter. The tumor periphery is irregular and poorly defined. **b:** A partly ossified mass is attached by a sclerotic stalk to the irregular anterior cortex of the femur in the subtrochanteric area. The tumor ossification is concentrated around its stalk and gradually fades out towards the tumor periphery.

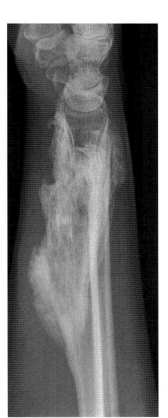

Fig. 5.**97 Posttraumatic myositis ossificans.** Following a complicated distal radius shaft fracture extensive heterotopic bone formation developed around the fracture site simulating a malignant osseous tumor.

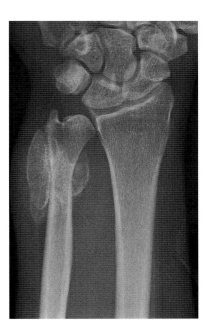

Fig. 5.**98 Posttraumatic myositis ossificans.** An ossified lesion with a complete rim of thin peripheral calcification ("eggshell calcification") is wrapping around the distal ulna. The lesion is separated in its entire length by a fine radiolucent line from the adjacent bone.

Table 5.10 (Cont.) Localized bone lesions

Disease	Radiographic Findings	Comments
Ewing sarcoma (Figs. 5.99, 5.100, 5.101, and 5.102)	A poorly defined osteolytic lesion with cortical violation and large soft tissue mass is characteristic. In tubular bones an interrupted periosteal reaction of the laminated ("onionskin") or less commonly perpendicular ("sunburst" or "hair-on-end") pattern is characteristically associated. Saucerization of the cortex is a rare but relatively characteristic manifestation of the disease. In flat and irregular bones osteosclerosis can be the dominant radiographic feature. The tumor can affect any bone, but has a predilection for the diametaphyses of long tubular bones and overall the lower half of the skeleton. The most common locations include femur, tibia, humerus, pelvis and sacrum.	Usually diagnosed between the ages of 5 and 30 years (peak 10 to 15 years) with slight male predominance. Involvement of the tubular bones occurs more often in children, whereas involvement of the flat bones is more commonly found in young adults. Patients present with localized pain and swelling occasionally combined with fever and leukocytosis. The tumor is rare in blacks. *Primitive neuroectodermal tumors (PNET)* (Fig. 5.**103**) have similar histologic and imaging features, but epiphyseal involvement, pathologic fractures, and distant metastases occur more frequently when compared to Ewing's sarcoma.
Angiosarcoma (Fig. 5.104)	Solitary or multiple, poorly or well demarcated lesions most commonly located in the medulla or cortex of long tubular bones, pelvis, spine and skull. Cortical thinning or violation and/or mild expansion without periostitis is occasionally associated.	Occurs in the fourth and fifth decades with male predominance. If multicentric it may simulate multiple myeloma, metastases, cystic angiomatosis, and cystic osteomyelitis (e.g. tuberculous or fungal). *Hemangioendothelioma* refers to a low-grade malignant angiosarcoma. *Hemangiopericytoma* is a borderline malignant tumor, with similar imaging features.
Plasmacytoma (Figs. 5.105 and 5.106)	Presents as an expansile trabeculated osteolytic lesion with cortical thinning and violation measuring up to several centimeters in diameter or as a well marginated purely osteolytic focus with endosteal scalloping. Rarely it may present as a sclerotic lesion (e.g. ivory vertebra). Most common locations are spine and pelvis. Complications in the spine include transdiscal tumor spread and pathologic fractures resulting sometimes in complete dissolution of a vertebral body.	Plasmacytoma may be considered a solitary manifestation of multiple myeloma with conversion to the latter occurring as late as 20 years after initial diagnosis. Plasmacytoma affects younger patients than multiple myeloma with about half the patients being 50 or younger at the time of diagnosis. It frequently presents with neurologic symptoms and radiographically may be mistaken for a giant cell tumor.

(continues on page 108)

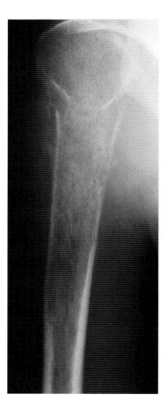

Fig. 5.**99** **Ewing sarcoma**. A permeative osteolytic lesion with cortical violation and beginning laminated ("onionskin") periosteal reaction is seen in the proximal humerus shaft.

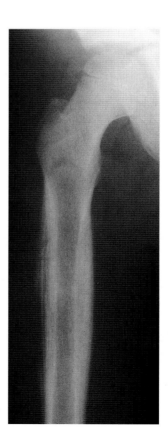

Fig. 5.**100** **Ewing sarcoma**. Extensive laminated ("onionskin") periosteal reaction and cortical tunneling is seen in the proximal femur shaft, while the permeative osteolytic lesion is barely perceptible.

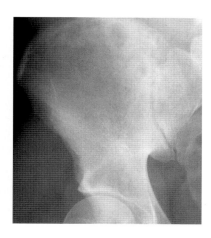

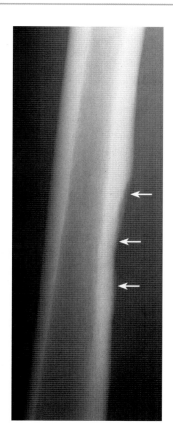

Fig. 5.**101 Ewing sarcoma**. A poorly demarcated mixed osteolytic and osteoblastic lesion involving the entire iliac wing is seen.

Fig. 5.**102 Ewing sarcoma**. Saucerization of the femoral cortex (arrows) is the only manifestation of the disease in this case.

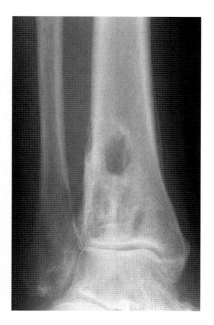

Fig. 5.**103 Primitive neuroectodermal tumor (PNET)**. A poorly defined, mixed osteolytic and osteoblastic lesion in the distal tibia with cortical violation and beginning amorphous periosteal reaction on its lateral side and early laminated periosteal reaction on its medial side is seen.

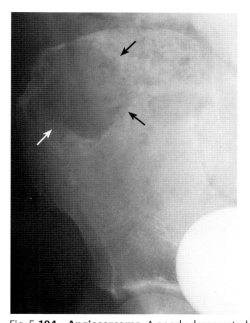

Fig. 5.**104 Angiosarcoma**. A poorly demarcated osteolytic lesion (arrows) with cortical violation is seen in the ilium.

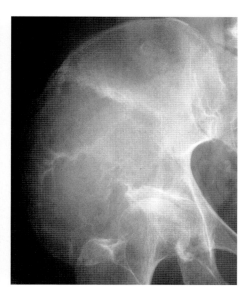

Fig. 5.**105 Plasmacytoma**. An expansile osteolytic lesion with trabeculation is seen in the ilium.

Table 5.10   (Cont.) Localized bone lesions

Disease	Radiographic Findings	Comments
Multiple myeloma (Figs. 5.107, 5.108, 5.109, 5.110 and 5.111)	Multiple well marginated ("punched out") or poorly delineated osteolytic lesions of relatively uniform size are characteristic. Endosteal scalloping is typically present with larger lesions in the long tubular bones. Diffuse osteopenia without well-defined areas of osteolysis is another common presentation. Periosteal new bone formation is exceedingly rare. Focal or multiple sclerotic lesions are an unusual initial presentation, but may develop after chemotherapy, irradiation or pathologic fracture. Preferred locations in order of decreasing frequency are spine, ribs, skull, pelvis, long tubular bones, and clavicles (distal end). Spine: Preferential osteolytic destruction of the vertebral bodies, sometimes associated with irregular thickening of the remaining vertebral trabeculae, relative sparing of the posterior elements, scalloping of the anterior margins of the vertebral bodies (pressure erosions from adjacent soft tissue lesions), and paraspinal or extradural tumor extension are common. Pathologic compression fractures are a frequent complication.	Occurs in patients over 40 years of age with male predominance, presenting with bone pain, anemia, hypercalcemia, proteinuria (including Bence-Jones proteins), and monoclonal gammopathy (high erythrocyte sedimentation rate, abnormal electrophoresis). *Waldenström's macroglobulinemia* presents with similar clinical and radiographic findings but the radiographic features are usually less conspicuous.

(continues on page 110)

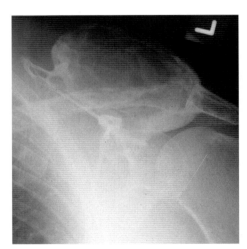

Fig. 5.**106   Plasmacytoma**. An expansile trabeculated osteolytic lesion ("soap bubble appearance") originating from the scapular spine is seen.

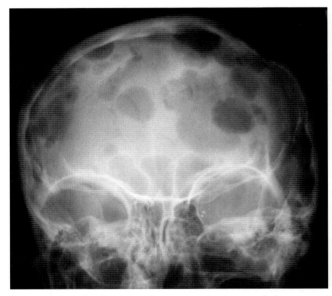

Fig. 5.**107   Multiple   myeloma**. Multiple   well-demarcated ("punched-out") osteolytic lesions are seen in the vault of the skull.

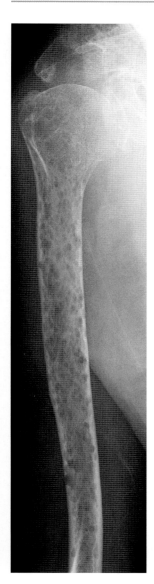

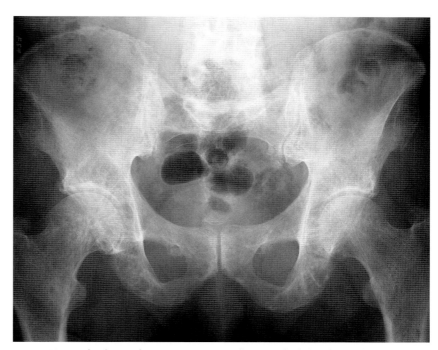

Fig. 5.**109** **Multiple myeloma**. Numerous well to poorly defined osteolytic lesions are scattered throughout the pelvis and proximal femora.

◁ Fig. 5.**108** **Multiple myeloma**. Innumerable well-defined osteolytic lesions of relatively uniform size are seen scattered throughout the humerus and the visualized part of the scapula.

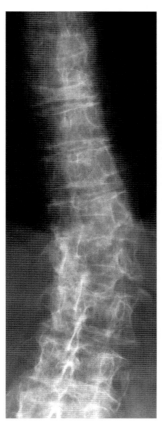

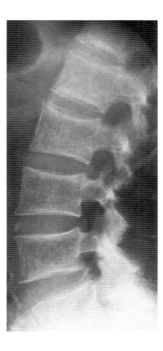

Fig. 5.**110** **Multiple myeloma**. Patchy osteopenia and tiny foci of increased bone density are evident throughout the thoraco-lumbar spine besides several compression fractures.

Fig. 5.**111** **Multiple myeloma**. Osteopenia with a prominent vertical trabecular pattern ("corduroy" appearance) is seen in all vertebral bodies of the lumbar spine.

Table 5.10   (Cont.) Localized bone lesions

Disease	Radiographic Findings	Comments
Metastases (Figs. 5.112, 5.113, 5.114, 5.115, and 5.116)	Solitary, or more commonly, multiple osteolytic, osteoblastic or mixed osteolytic-osteoblastic lesions with preferential involvement of the red marrow containing skeleton (spine, pelvis, ribs, skull, femora and humeri) is characteristic. Osteolytic metastases may be well or poorly marginated. Osteoblastic metastases may be focal or diffuse. In the spine, besides the vertebral bodies, the posterior elements including the pedicles are frequently also involved (DD multiple myeloma). Purely osteolytic metastases commonly arise from carcinomas of lung, kidney, thyroid and lymphoma. Purely osteoblastic metastases are most often associated with prostatic and breast carcinomas, but also with Hodgkin's lymphoma, carcinoids and medulloblastomas. Periosteal reactions are highly unusual in metastatic disease except in prostatic and breast carcinomas, gastrointestinal malignancies and neuroblastomas. Neither osseous expansion nor soft tissue masses are typically associated with bone metastases except in rib lesions, osteolytic metastases from carcinomas originating in the kidney, thyroid, lung and liver and osteoblastic metastases from prostatic and breast carcinomas. One or more sclerotic vertebral body (ivory vertebra) is most often caused by prostatic or breast carcinoma metastases, but also found with Hodgkin's lymphoma and Paget's disease. Pathologic fractures are a frequent complication, especially in the spine. Response of an osteolytic metastasis to treatment (e.g. chemotherapy or radiation therapy) is evident by progressive sclerosis proceeding from the periphery towards the center of the lesion with eventual reduction in size or disappearance of the osteolytic focus. The appearance of osteosclerotic foci during therapy is usually caused by progression of the disease, but may also indicate a healing response of pre-existing osteolytic metastases that could initially not be identified on radiographs. A positive treatment response of osteoblastic lesion is evident by decrease and eventual disappearance of the sclerotic focus.	Bone metastases are by far the most common skeletal malignancy occurring either by hematogenous spread or direct tumor extension. They most frequently originate from carcinomas of breast, prostate, lung, kidney, thyroid and gastrointestinal tract. Breast carcinoma metastases tend to be mixed, or, less commonly purely osteolytic or osteoblastic, often extensive and frequently associated with pathologic fractures. Prostate carcinoma metastases are characteristically osteoblastic, may be expansile (simulating Paget's disease) or associated with periostitis. Bronchogenic carcinoma metastases are typically osteolytic or mixed and occasionally expansile. An eccentric erosion of the external cortex of a long tubular bone ("cookie-bite" sign) is rare, but quite characteristic for a bronchogenic carcinoma metastasis manifestation. Kidney and thyroid carcinoma metastases are often solitary, purely osteolytic lesions that may be expansile and depict a septated (bubbly) appearance. Gastrointestinal tract metastases cover the whole spectrum from purely osteolytic to purely osteoblastic. Metastases from colon or rectum carcinoma may occasionally resemble an osteosarcoma and depict a sunburst periosteal reaction. Metastatic bone disease with unknown primary most often originates from prostate, lymphoma, breast, lung, kidney, thyroid or colon.

(continues on page 112)

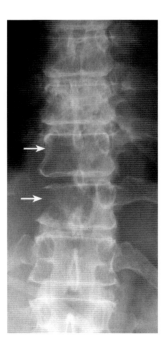

Fig. 5.**112 Metastases from bronchogenic carcinoma.** Scattered predominantly osteolytic metastases are seen in the thoracic spine with main involvement of the right pedicles and posterior elements of T10 and T11 (arrows) producing an "empty vertebral box" sign on that side.

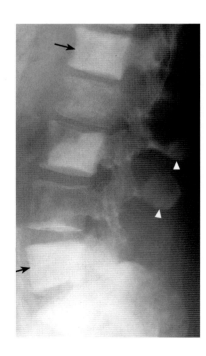

Fig. 5.**113 Metastases from breast carcinoma.** Predominantly osteoblastic metastases involving all vertebral bodies including the posterior elements of the lumbar spine. Ivory vertebrae are seen at L1 and L5 (arrows). Osteoblastic foci (arrowheads) are evident in the spinous processes of L2 and L3.

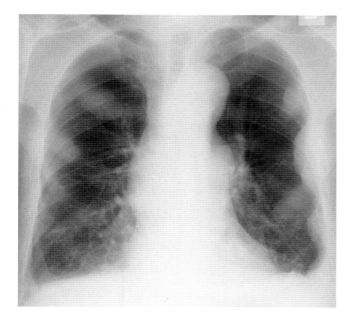

Fig. 5.**114** **Metastases from prostatic carcinoma**. Multiple bilateral expansile and purely osteoblastic metastases originating from the ribs are seen.

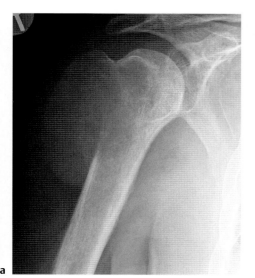
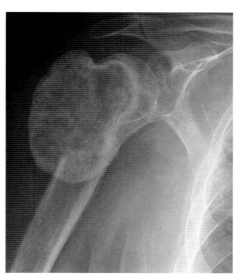

a   b

Fig. 5.**115 a, b** **Metastasis from renal cell carcinoma before (a) and after (b) radiation therapy**. A purely lytic, markedly expansile ("blow-out") lesion is seen originating from the dorsal aspect of the proximal humerus shaft (**a**). After radiation therapy the lesion became partially ossified depicting a trabeculated pattern and a well-demarcated sclerotic margin (**b**).

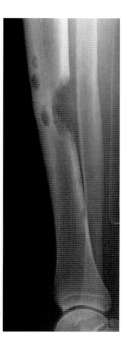

Fig. 5.**116** **Cortical metastases from bronchogenic carcinoma**. Multiple purely osteolytic lesions are seen in the cortex of the tibia. The largest lesion located posteriorly has broken through the cortex on both its inner and outer surface.

Table 5.10   (Cont.) Localized bone lesions

Disease	Radiographic Findings	Comments
Lymphoma (Figs. 5.117, 5.118, 5.119, 5.110 and 5.121)	Preferential sites of involvement include spine, pelvis, scapula and ribs. In long tubular bones involvement of the diametaphyses of the femur and tibia about the knee is most common. *Non-Hodgkin lymphoma* typically presents as solitary or, more often, multiple poorly defined osteolytic lesions. *Histiocytic lymphoma* (primary or secondary) frequently has a mixed osteolytic-osteoblastic appearance and may resemble Paget's disease without bony expansion. Purely osteoblastic lesions are uncommon in non-Hodgkin's lymphoma. *Hodgkin's disease* of the bone is always caused by secondary involvement. Its presentation ranges from purely osteolytic to purely osteoblastic lesions. Diffuse sclerosis of a vertebral body (ivory vertebra) is not an unusual manifestation. Osteolytic lesions tend to be poorly defined and are associated with periostitis in one-third of the cases.	Secondary involvement of bone caused by hematogenous spread or, less frequently, by direct invasion occurs in one-third of patients with non-Hodgkin's lymphoma and in 10% with Hodgkin's disease. Primary bone lymphoma is much less common, accounts for approximately 5% of all primary malignant bone tumors, is usually of the histiocytic-type (previously called reticulum cell sarcoma), and typically occurs in older patients with a 2:1 male predominance. *Burkitt's lymphoma* presents as expansile osteolytic lesions associated with a soft tissue mass. Involvement of the facial bones (especially the maxilla) is most characteristic in children of tropical Africa. Nonendemic Burkitt's lymphoma may be associated with immune dysfunction (e.g., organ transplantation and AIDS). *Mycosis fungoides* is a T-cell lymphoma with primary involvement of the skin. Discrete or poorly defined osteolytic lesions may be associated in the appendicular skeleton.
Leukemia (Figs. 5.122, 5.123 and 5.124)	Diffuse osteopenia with medullary widening and cortical thinning in tubular bones and vertebral compressions are the most common presentation. Moth-eaten or permeative osteolysis may be found in both tubular and flat bones. Radiolucent and/or radiodense metaphyseal bands, as well as periosteal new bone formation are particularly common in children. Complications may include intra-articular and subperiosteal hemorrhages, septic arthritis, osteomyelitis, osteonecrosis and secondary gout. *Granulocytic sarcomas (chloromas)* present as single or multiple, often expansile lytic lesions in the skull, spine, ribs, sternum and long tubular bones, usually in acute myelogenic leukemia.	Leukemias are classified based on cell maturity (acute with immature or blastic cells versus chronic with mature cells), cell morphology (myeloid versus lymphoid) or cell origin (thymus-derived T-cells versus blood marrow derived B-cells). Skeletal abnormalities are similar for all forms of leukemias, but are most common in acute childhood leukemias, where they occur in over 50% of cases, and least common in chronic leukemias.

(continues on page 114)

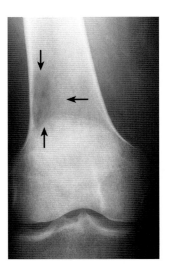

Fig. 5.**117   Non-Hodgkin lymphoma**. A poorly defined (moth-eaten) osteolytic lesion (arrows) is seen in the distal femur.

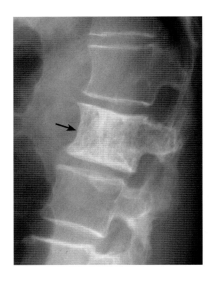

Fig. 5.**118   Non-Hodgkin lymphoma (histiocytic type)**. A mixed osteolytic and osteoblastic lesion with coarse irregular predominantly vertical trabeculation involving both the vertebral body and pedicles of L2 (arrow) is seen.

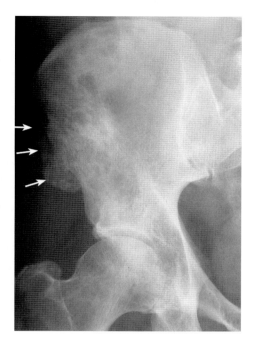

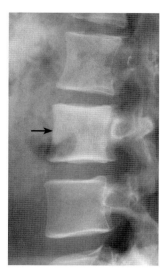

Fig. 5.**120** **Hodgkin's disease**. An ivory vertebral body is seen at L3 (arrow).

◁ Fig. 5.**119** **Non-Hodgkin lymphoma (histiocytic type)**. A mixed osteolytic and osteoblastic lesion is seen in the ilium. The lesion differs from Paget's disease by the absence of enlargement of the involved bone. Furthermore cortical violation (arrows) is also evident in this particular case.

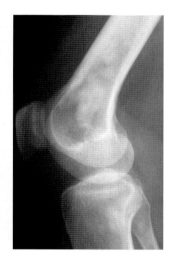

Fig. 5.**121** **Hodgkin's disease**. Several relatively poorly defined osteoblastic lesions are seen in the distal femur and the proximal tibia and fibula.

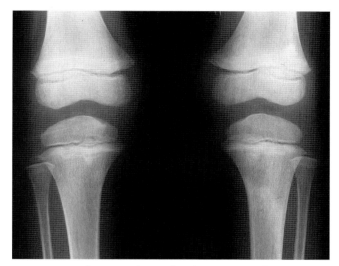

Fig. 5.**122** **Leukemia**. Sclerotic bands traversing all metaphyses about both knees are seen in this child.

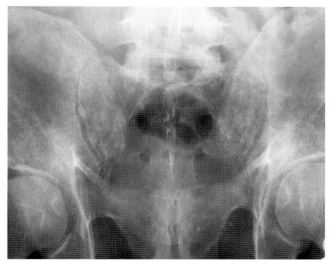

Fig. 5.**123** **Leukemia**. Innumerable tiny and poorly defined osteolytic and osteoblastic foci are scattered throughout the pelvis.

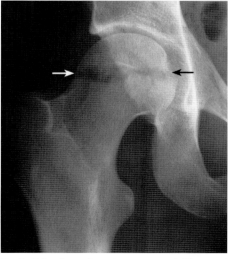

Fig. 5.**124** **Granulocytic sarcoma (chloroma)**. A barely perceptive permeative osteolytic lesion with pathologic fracture (arrows) is seen involving the femoral head and neck.

Table 5.10   (Cont.) Localized bone lesions

Disease	Radiographic Findings	Comments
Langerhans cell histiocytosis (Figs. 5.125, 5.126 and 5.127)	*Eosinophilic granuloma* presents as solitary or, less commonly, multiple lesions with preferential involvement of skull, mandible, spine, ribs and the diametaphyses (rarely epiphyses) of long tubular bones. Relatively well defined radiolucent areas with endosteal scalloping with or without slight bone expansion and periosteal new bone formation are typical in the long bones and may mimic osteomyelitis or even Ewing's sarcoma. Well-defined lytic lesions with or without sclerotic borders may be found in the skull and pelvis. A radiodense focus (button sequestrum) is frequently observed in skull lesions. Larger osteolytic areas in the skull typically depict beveled edges caused by the uneven destruction of the inner and outer tables. In the mandible radiolucent lesions about the teeth may lead to the "floating teeth" appearance. In the spine a collapsed vertebral body (vertebra plana) with intact intervertebral spaces or, less frequently, a lytic and occasionally slightly expansile lesion involving the vertebral body and/or the posterior elements may be found.	Langerhans cell histiocytosis comprises three major conditions. 1. *Eosinophilic granuloma* is both the most common and most benign variant representing approximately 70 % of cases. It is usually diagnosed between the age of 5 and 20. 2. *Hand-Schüller-Christian disease* is characterized by the triad of exophthalmos, diabetes insipidus and large lytic skull lesions ("geographic skull"). 3. *Letterer-Siwe disease* is the acute disseminated variant in children under age 2. Bone lesions are less common, but may include multiple widespread lytic lesions in the skull ("raindrop" pattern). Spontaneous healing of a solitary lesion occurs, typically progressing from the periphery towards its center and eventually resulting in its disappearance or transformation into a sclerotic focus.
Amyloidosis (Fig. 5.128)	Osteolytic lesions of variable size with endosteal scalloping simulating multiple myeloma preferentially located in the proximal humerus or proximal femur is the most common presentation. Subchondral amyloid deposition may result in avascular necrosis. Pathologic fractures are a relatively common complication. Subchondral cyst formation and erosions in the hand and wrist associated with periarticular or diffuse osteoporosis may simulate rheumatoid arthritis, although extensive nodular soft tissue masses, well-defined cystic lesions with or without surrounding sclerosis and preservation of the joint space are more characteristic for amyloidosis.	Musculoskeletal abnormalities are the result of amyloid deposition in bone, synovium and soft tissue. *Primary amyloidosis* occurs in patients above the age of 40 with male predominance. It may be associated with multiple myeloma. *Secondary amyloidosis* is associated with chronic renal disease, rheumatoid arthritis, lupus erythematosus, ulcerative colitis, chronic suppurative disease, and lymphoproliferative disorders.
Brown tumor in hyperparathyroidism (Fig. 5.129)	Single or multiple, occasionally expansile, well to poorly defined osteolytic lesions of the axial and appendicular skeleton. Eccentric or cortical location is not unusual. Common sites of involvement are facial bones, pelvis, ribs and femora. They may undergo necrosis and liquefaction producing cysts, or with proper treatment (removal of the parathyroid adenoma) become increasingly sclerotic.	Brown tumors are more commonly associated with primary than secondary hyperparathyroidism. Other manifestations of hyperparathyroidism are usually also apparent and include osteopenia, subperiosteal, endosteal and subchondral bone resorption, intracortical tunneling, chondrocalcinosis, and para-articular and vascular calcifications. Bone sclerosis is common in secondary hyperparathyroidism.

(continues on page 116)

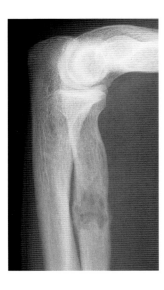

Fig. 5.125 Eosinophilic granuloma. An irregular, relatively well-defined osteolytic lesion with minimal endosteal scalloping, slight bone expansion and beginning periosteal reaction on its anterior margin is seen in the proximal radius shaft.

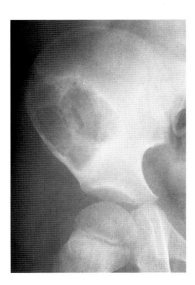

Fig. 5.126 Eosinophilic granuloma. A well defined, trabeculated osteolytic lesion with sclerotic margin and cortical violation is seen in the ilium.

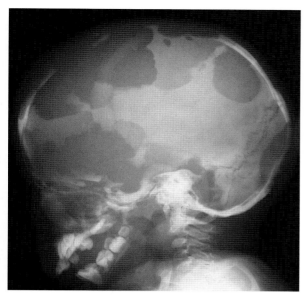

Fig. 5.**127** **Hand–Schüller–Christian disease**. Large, well-demarcated osteolytic lesions are seen in the vault of the cranium giving the appearance of a continental map ("geographic skull").

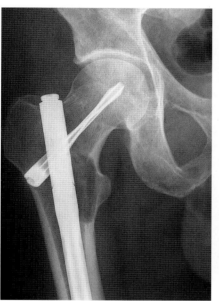

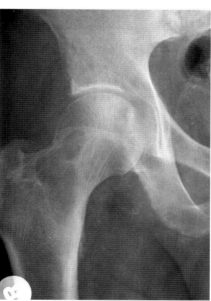

a   b

Fig. 5.**128 a, b** **Amyloidosis (2 cases)**. A large well-demarcated osteolytic lesion with endosteal scalloping is seen in the proximal femur shaft in this patient with multiple myeloma (**a**). A similar lesion is present in the second patient with chronic renal failure (**b**).

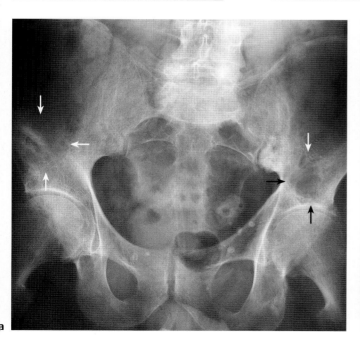

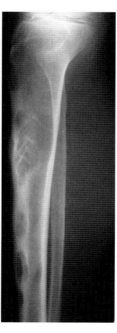

a   b

Fig. 5.**129 a, b** **Brown tumors in primary hyperparathyroidism**. Multiple poorly to well defined osteolytic lesions, some with trabeculation, are seen in the pelvis (arrows) and tibia. Most tibial lesions are cortical based (**a**: pelvis, **b**: tibia).

Table 5.10   (Cont.) Localized bone lesions

Disease	Radiographic Findings	Comments
Hemophilic pseudotumor (Figs. 5.130 and 5.131)	Central (intraosseous) or eccentric (subperiosteal), well-demarcated osteolytic lesion, are often associated with either solid or interrupted periosteal reaction and a large soft tissue mass. Minimal to massive calcification within the lesion is occasionally also encountered. Rarely, more than one bone contains a pseudotumor. Preferred locations are pelvis, femur, tibia and hand.	Lesions are late sequelae of intramedullary or periosteal hemorrhage occurring in fewer than 2% of hemophiliacs. Hemophilic arthropathy including dense joint effusions and joint contractures, avascular necrosis, especially of the femoral head and talus, spontaneous fractures and soft tissue hematomas may also be evident.
Intraosseous tophus in gout (Fig. 5.132)	One or more cystic lesions often with partial calcification may be found in the subchondral and deeper osseous areas simulating enchondromas. Larger intraosseous calcifications may mimic bone infarcts. These findings are most frequently seen is the hands and feet. Association with characteristic findings of gouty arthropathy is diagnostic.	Occurs in approximately 5% of patients with chronic gouty arthritis. Intraosseous urate deposition with subsequent calcifications usually originate from the adjacent joint, penetrate the cartilaginous surface and extend into the adjacent spongiosa.
Osteonecrosis (bone infarct and avascular necrosis) (Figs. 5.133, 5.134, 5.135 and 5.136)	Early signs are nonspecific and include mottled osteopenia, poorly defined osteolytic lesion(s), or patchy osteopenic and sclerotic areas. Findings are however more characteristic in an advanced late stage. In the diametaphyses they include a serpiginous peripheral rim of sclerosis surrounding an oblong area of bone rarefaction. Periostitis and matrix calcifications are frequently associated. Intramedullary calcifications are often the only finding and are typically shell-like whereas the calcifications in chondroid matrix tumors tend to be irregular and central and are surrounded by a rim of noncalcified, often slightly radiolucent tumor matrix. Solid periosteal reactions and cortical thickening may be associated with both conditions, but in the case of chondroid matrix tumor suggest a low-grade chondrosarcoma rather than enchondroma. Typical findings of osteonecrosis in the epiphyses include subchondral cyst(s) with sclerotic rim, arc-like subchondral radiolucency (crescent sign), subchondral fragmentation and eventually collapse of the articular surface, with considerable sclerosis and secondary degenerative changes in the affected joint.	Osteonecrosis can be divided in bone infarction, occurring more frequently in the metadiaphyseal regions of long bones (e.g. femur, humerus, and tibia) than in the axial skeleton and in avascular necrosis involving the subarticular bone. Solitary bone infarcts are frequently diagnosed as an incidental finding. Osteonecrosis may be idiopathic (25%) or associated with hematological and reticuloendothelial diseases (e.g. *sickle cell* and *Gaucher's disease*), collagen vascular diseases (e.g. *lupus erythematosus*), trauma (e.g. *subcapital hip fracture*), *renal transplantation, alcoholism, steroid use, pancreatitis, gout, irradiation* and *caisson disease.* *Radiation osteitis (osteonecrosis)* presents with a mixture of osteopenia, osteosclerosis and coarse trabeculation. Round to ovoid radiolucent lesions within the cortex of long tubular bones are quite characteristic as opposed to endosteal scalloping caused by tumor recurrence. Bony changes are dose-dependent with a minimal dose of 3000 cGy required and occur at the earliest one year after irradiation, at a time, when a nuclear medicine scan does longer depict an increased uptake. *Calcified intraosseous hematomas* may present radiographically similar to a calcified bone infarct.

(continues on page 118)

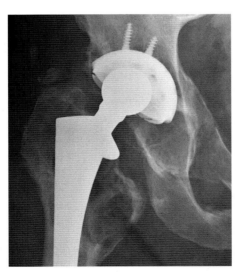

Fig. 5.**130** **Hemophilic pseudotumor**. Expansile osteolytic lesion with trabeculation developed in the greater and lesser trochanter as well as in the ischium and pubic bone adjacent to the components of the total hip prosthesis inserted 12 years earlier.

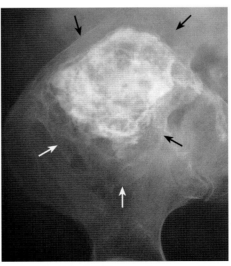

Fig. 5.**131** **Hemophilic pseudotumor**. A large expansile osteolytic lesion surrounded by a thin rim of solid new bone formation (arrows) and containing extensive central calcifications is seen in the ilium.

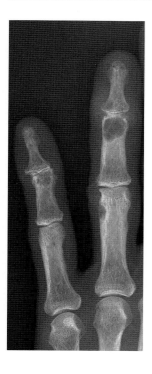

Fig. 5.**132 Intraosseous tophi in gout**. Well-demarcated osteolytic lesions with faint calcifications are seen in the fourth and fifth finger resembling enchondromas.

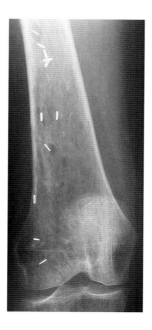

Fig. 5.**133 Osteonecrosis (bone infarct)**. Patchy demineralization and poorly defined osteolytic lesions seen in the distal femur are the earliest radiographic findings in osteonecrosis.

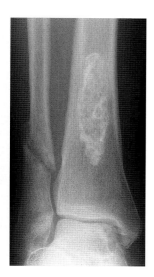

Fig. 5.**134 Osteonecrosis (bone infarct)**. An oblong shell-like calcification is seen in the distal tibia. A healing distal fibula fracture and a posttraumatic osteochondral defect in the medial talar dome are also present.

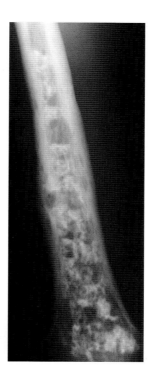

Fig. 5.**135 Radiation osteonecrosis**. Extensive bone infarction limited to the field of irradiation is diagnostic. Findings include widespread calcifications in the medulla and irregular cortical thickening with numerous round to oblong intracortical lucencies.

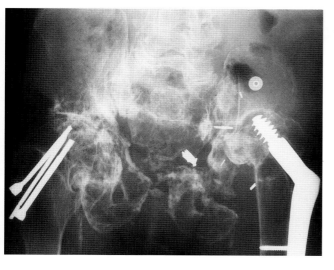

Fig. 5.**136 Radiation osteonecrosis**. A dysplastic osteopenic pelvis with extensive calcifications and numerous pathologic fractures and bilateral avascular necrosis of the femoral heads are the consequences of pelvic irradiation during childhood.

Table 5.10 (Cont.) Localized bone lesions

Disease	Radiographic Findings	Comments
Healing or healed fracture and stress fracture (Figs. 5.137 and 5.138)	Osteosclerosis and callus formation may simulate chronic osteomyelitis or an osteoid osteoma, respectively. Demonstration of a fracture line in an area of localized elliptical cortical thickening of a long tubular bone (as opposed to a round or ovoid intracortical abscess or nidus) is diagnostic.	In the absence of proper clinical information a healed fracture resulting in localized bony expansion and deformities can at times be difficult to differentiate from fibrous dysplasia.
Pigmented villonodular synovitis (PVNS) (Fig. 5.139)	Subchondral pressure erosions may be found at margins of "tight" joints such as hip, ankle, and wrist. They are caused by an often slightly dense appearing soft tissue mass due to hemosiderin deposition in both the effusion and synovial proliferation. Calcifications, osteoporosis and joint space narrowing are typically absent. Pressure erosions in the knee (most commonly involved joint) are uncommon.	Monoarticular proliferative synovial disorder presenting with insidious onset of swelling, pain of long duration and decreased range of motion occurring typically in young adults. A hemorrhagic (chocolate-brown) joint effusion in the absence of trauma is characteristic.
Osteomyelitis (acute) (Figs. 5.140, 5.141 and 5.142)	*Hematogenous osteomyelitis* presents initially in the medullary space with focal osteoporosis, endosteal scalloping, and osteolysis due to hyperemia, edema, abscess formation and trabecular destruction. Progression of the disease to the Haversian and Volkmann's canals results in cortical fissuring with subsequent destruction and subperiosteal abscess formation. A periosteal reaction (laminated or, less commonly, spiculated) is a characteristic finding at this stage. After one month, a sequestration (detached necrotic cortical bone presenting as radiodense bony spicule surrounded by granulation tissue and newly formed cortical bone (involucrum) may be evident. An opening in the involucrum is termed a cloaca. Sinus tracts leading to the skin surface are often evident. Occasionally intraosseous gas may be seen. In both infants and adults extension of the disease process into the adjacent joint is common whereas in childhood (1–16 years of age) the open growth plate represents an effective barrier to the spread of the infection from the metaphysis to the epiphysis and joint, respectively. *Osteomyelitis from a contiguous soft tissue infection* typically presents as focal osteoporosis due to edema with subsequent cortical erosion. Periostitis is another less frequent initial finding. Cortical destruction and bone marrow infection with abscess formation may ensue.	Affects all ages but is commonly found in children, diabetics, and intravenous drug abusers. Occurs by hematogenous route, spread from contiguous infection or direct implantation (punctures, penetrating injury and postoperative infection). Pyogenic osteomyelitis in children is most often caused by staphylococcus aureus, streptococci, escherichia coli, and hemophilus influenzae. Gram-negative organisms are not uncommon in adults and intravenous drug abusers. *Tuberculous osteomyelitis* (Figs. 5.**143** and 5.**144**) arises most commonly secondary to septic arthritis. Spinal involvement accounts for approximately 50 % of skeletal tuberculosis. Compared to pyogenic osteomyelitis osteoporosis is more pronounced, whereas new bone formation is less extensive. *Tuberculous dactylitis* ("spina ventosa") (Fig. 5.**145**) refers to cystic expansion of the short tubular bones of the hands and feet with varying degrees of periostitis. *Cystic tuberculosis* presents as one or multiple well-defined osteolytic foci without sclerosis preferentially in the peripheral skeleton. *Fungal osteomyelitis* (Fig. 5.**146**) resembles a tuberculous infection. Solitary or multiple osteolytic lesions with discrete margins, mild surrounding sclerosis and little or no periosteal reaction are a common presentation.

(continues on page 120)

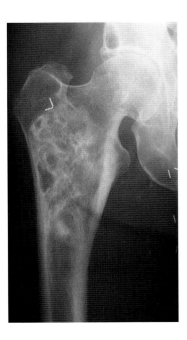

Fig. 5.**137 Healed fracture**. A widened proximal femur shaft with mixed osteolytic and osteoblastic texture is seen mimicking fibrous dysplasia. An ovoid subchondral cyst is incidentally seen in the lateral aspect of the acetabular roof.

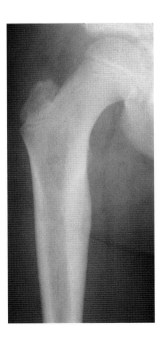

Fig. 5.**138 Healed stress fracture**. A localized elliptical cortical thickening is seen in the medial aspect of the proximal femur shaft.

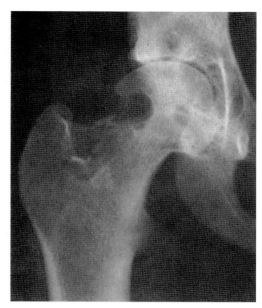

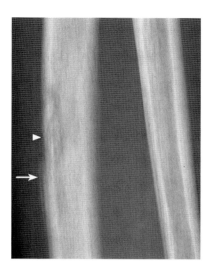

Fig. 5.**140** **Acute osteomyelitis**. Patchy demineralization, and beginning endosteal scalloping, cortical fissuring (arrowhead) and laminated periosteal reaction (arrow) are seen in the radius shaft representing the earliest radiographic manifestations of acute hematogenous osteomyelitis.

Fig. 5.**139** **Pigmented villonodular synovitis**. Several well-demarcated defects (pressure erosions) are seen in the lateral aspect of the femoral neck and head as well as in the acetabulum where they induced a reactive sclerosis.

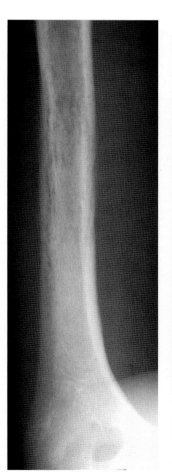

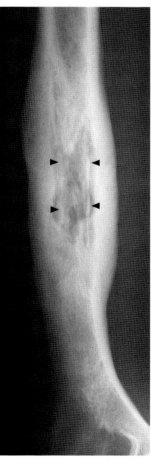

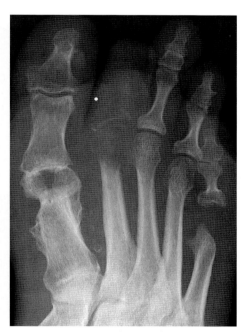

Fig. 5.**142** **Osteomyelitis in diabetic foot**. Besides neuropathic arthropathy manifestations in the first and fifth toe, osteolytic destruction of the second toe including the head of the second metatarsal is seen caused by osteomyelitis originating from an infected neuropathic skin ulcer in the second toe indicated by a metallic marker.

a   **b**

Fig. 5.**141 a, b** **Osteomyelitis**. A permeative osteolytic lesion with cortical fissuring and beginning sequestration of a large bone fragment in its center is seen in the humerus shaft (**a**). One year later an expansile lesion with extensive new cortical bone formation is found (**b**). The lesion depicts endosteal scalloping and contains the sequestered bone fragment (arrowheads).

Table 5.10 (Cont.) Localized bone lesions

Disease	Radiographic Findings	Comments
Brodie's abscess (Figs. 5.147 and 5.148)	Usually solitary, lytic and often elongated lesion with sclerotic border typically in the metaphyses of long bones. Epiphyses, diaphyses, flat and irregular bones (e.g. carpus and tarsus) are less common locations. In the epiphysis a circular well-defined osteolytic lesion is typical. In the diaphysis the abscesses may be found in central, subcortical or cortical locations. In the cortex the abscess is surrounded by periosteal new bone formation simulating an osteoid osteoma or a stress fracture.	Subacute pyogenic osteomyelitis (smoldering indolent infection), usually of staphylococcal origin is common in children, in whom the lesion is typically located in the proximal or distal tibia metaphysis and sometimes connected to the growth plate by a tortuous channel. Histologically a central purulent or mucoid fluid collection is surrounded by inflammatory granulation tissue and spongy bone eburnation. The lesion may occasionally contain a central sequestrum.
Osteomyelitis (chronic) (Fig. 5.149)	Thick irregular sclerotic bone with radiolucencies and extensive periosteal new bone formation is characteristic. Signs of remaining activity or reactivation include a change from the previous exam, poorly defined areas of osteolysis, thin laminated periosteal reaction, poorly defined bony excrescences, and demonstration of a sequestrum, sinus tract or soft tissue abscess. *Sclerosing osteomyelitis of Garré* (Fig. 5.151) is a low-grade infection without purulent exudate presenting as focal or circumferential cortical thickening and sclerosis in the mandible (most commonly) or diaphyses of long tubular bones. In the latter location osteoid osteoma, stress fracture and *Ribbing's disease* (hereditary multiple diaphyseal sclerosis with typically asymmetric distribution) must be considered in the differential diagnosis.	*Late acquired syphilis* resembles chronic osteomyelitis. Thickened sclerotic long bones caused by endosteal and periosteal new bone formation and ill-defined lytic lesions (gumma formation) are characteristic. *Chronic recurrent multifocal osteomyelitis (CRMO, chronic symmetric plasma cell osteomyelitis)* (Fig. 5.150) presents most commonly in children with a protracted clinical course and often symmetric involvement of the medial ends of the clavicles and metaphyses of long bones with a combination of osteolysis and osteosclerosis and extensive periosteal reaction and new bone formation. *SAPHO syndrome* (synovitis. acne, pustulosis, hyperostosis, osteitis) may be a related condition. *Epidermoid carcinoma* occurs in 1 % of osteomyelitis at the site of a chronically draining sinus and is evident as an enlarging soft tissue mass eroding the osteomyelitic bone.

(continues on page 122)

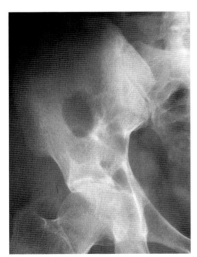

Fig. 5.143 Tuberculous osteomyelitis. A large multiloculated osteolytic lesion without significant reactive sclerosis is seen in the acetabular roof and adjacent ilium. The infection most likely originated from the hip where signs of tuberculous arthritis including joint space narrowing and early erosive changes in the femoral head are evident.

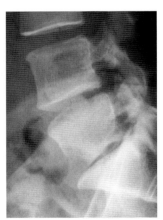

Fig. 5.144 Tuberculous spondylitis. An erosive lesion on the antero-inferior aspect of L5 is associated with marked disc space narrowing between L5 and S1.

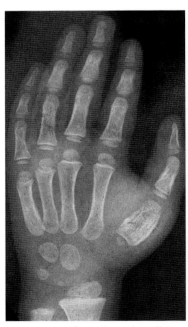

Fig. 5.145 Tuberculous dactylitis ("spina ventosa"). Expansile fusiform enlargement of the first metacarpal depicting a permeative osteolytic pattern is seen.

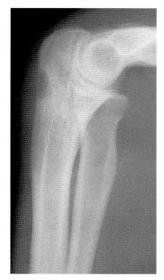

Fig. 5.**146** **Fungal osteomy-elitis (coccidioidomycosis)**. A solitary osteolytic lesion with discrete margin and mild surrounding sclerosis is seen in the olecranon.

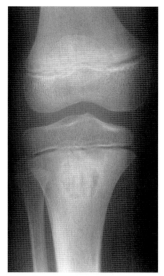

Fig. 5.**147** **Brodie's abscess**. An osteolytic lesion with sclerotic margin and multi-loculated appearance is seen in the proximal tibia meta-physis. The lesion is con-nected on its superomedial border by an osteolytic defect (channel) to the growth plate.

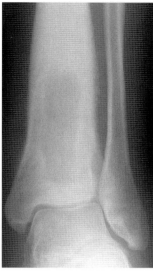

Fig. 5.**148** **Brodie's abscess**. An oblong osteolytic lesion with surrounding sclerosis and minimal periostitis is seen in the distal tibia.

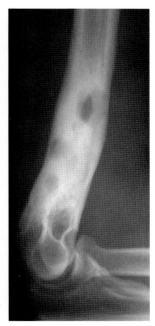

Fig. 5.**149** **Chronic osteo-myelitis**. A thick sclerotic dis-tal humerus shaft containing several radiolucencies is seen.

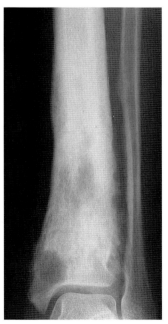

Fig. 5.**150** **Chronic recur-rent multifocal osteomyeli-tis**. A thickened sclerotic dis-tal tibia with several medul-lary and cortical osteolytic foci is seen.

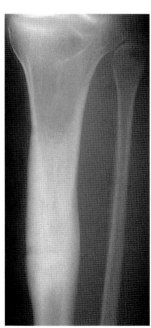

Fig. 5.**151** **Sclerosing osteo-myelitis of Garré**. Circumfer-ential cortical thickening and sclerosis is seen in the tibia diaphysis.

Table 5.10   (Cont.) Localized bone lesions

Disease	Radiographic Findings	Comments
Gorham's disease (vanishing bone disease) (Fig. 5.152)	Progressive, often massive osteolysis without attempt of repair (no periosteal or osteosclerotic reaction) spreading across joints or intervertebral spaces is characteristic. Preferential locations are the hip and shoulder regions, although any bone can be affected. Tapering or "pointing" of the long bones at the sites of osteolysis is typical. In the pelvis a rapidly destructive arthropathy of the hip presenting with destruction of primarily the femur head must be differentiated. This condition may be idiopathic, may represent unusual aggressive forms of osteoarthritis, osteonecrosis, CPPD or HADD, or may occur after intra-articular corticosteroid injections. *Proximal femoral focal deficiency (PFFD)* (Fig. 5.153) characterized by partial absence of the proximal femur is diagnosed in infancy.	Occurs sporadic at any age without sex predilection, but is usually diagnosed before the age of 40 years. Histologically a nonmalignant proliferation of angiomatous and fibrous tissue is evident. Other osteolysis syndromes diagnosed in infancy or childhood include acro-osteolysis of *Hajdu and Cheney, Joseph,* or *Shinz, carpal-tarsal osteolysis* (hereditary or associated with nephropathy), *Farber's disease* (elbows, wrists, knees and ankles) and *Winchester's syndrome* (carpal and tarsal areas and elbows).
Fibromatosis (Fig. 5.154)	Solitary or multiple soft tissue masses with erosions of the adjacent bone or osteolytic lesions. Cortical hyperostosis may be associated with bone involvement.	Variety of benign, but often aggressive fibrous proliferations presenting in both children and adults as tumor-like soft tissue lesions. Involvement of the adjacent bone is not uncommon in infantile forms of the disease.
Membranous lipodystrophy (polycystic lipomembranous osteodysplasia) (Fig. 5.155)	Symmetric and slowly progressive lytic lesions are found in the carpal and tarsal bones and the ends of long and short tubular bones. Bone deformities may eventually occur from pathologic fractures.	Rare hereditary disorder of adipose tissue affecting primarily the bones and brain. Presents commonly in the second or third decade of life with painful bones and joints and subsequently with presenile dementia.
Paget's disease (osteitis deformans) (Fig. 5.156, 5.157, 5.158, 5.159, 5.160, 5.161, and 5.162)	Monostotic or more commonly polyostotic asymmetric lesions with preferential involvement of the pelvis, femur, tibia, spine, skull, scapula, and humerus. The pattern of involvement ranges from purely osteolytic (e.g., osteoporosis circumscripta in the calvarium, and V- or flame-shaped defect in the diaphyses of long bones) to purely osteosclerotic (e.g., ivory vertebra). The mixed pattern (e.g., "picture frame vertebra" and "cotton wool" appearance of the skull) that is usually associated with bony enlargement, cortical thickening, and coarse trabeculation represents the most common manifestation. In long bones the disease characteristically progresses from an epiphysis to the diaphysis. Bone softening may result in bowing deformities of the long bones, acetabular protrusion, biconcave compression of vertebral end plates, and basilar invagination. Complications include cortical stress fractures (single or multiple horizontal radiolucent lines in the convex aspect of the deformed bone (lateral aspect of the femoral neck and shaft, anterior aspect of tibia), transverse pathologic fractures, and sarcomatous degeneration.	Common disorder of middle-aged and elderly patients that is often diagnosed as an incidental finding on radiographs obtained for unrelated purposes. The disease is present in 10% of patients over the age of 80 years and rare in patients under 40. Laboratory findings include elevated alkaline phosphatase and hydroxyproline levels in the serum and abnormally high hydroxyproline urine levels. Serum acid phosphatase values are normal. Neoplastic involvement in Paget's disease includes sarcomatous degeneration, giant cell tumor, aneurysmal bone cyst, and superimposition of metastases, multiple myeloma and lymphoma. Sarcomatous degeneration occurs in approximately 1% of patients usually over 55 years of age. Predominantly osteolytic osteosarcomas (60%), malignant fibrous histiocytoma/fibrosarcomas (25%) and chondrosarcomas (10%) are the most frequent tumors found in sarcomatous degeneration.

(continues on page 125)

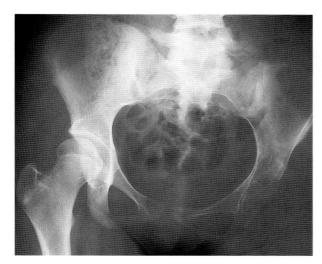

Fig. 5.152 Gorham's disease (vanishing bone disease). Complete osteolysis of the left proximal femur and beginning osteolysis of the left acetabulum and adjacent innominate bone without either periosteal reaction or reactive sclerosis is seen.

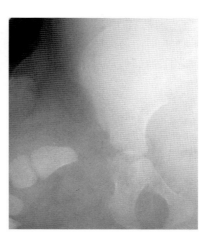

Fig. 5.153 Proximal femoral focal deficiency (PFFD). Dysplastic acetabulum and absent proximal femur are seen.

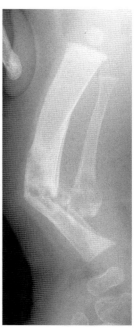

Fig. 5.154 Fibromatosis. Osteolytic lesions with pathologic fractures are seen in the distal tibia and fibula in this aggressive infantile form.

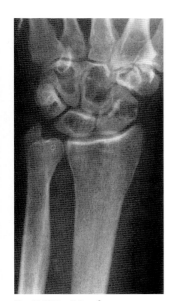

Fig. 5.155 Membranous lipodystrophy. Well-demarcated cystic lesions are seen in the carpal bones.

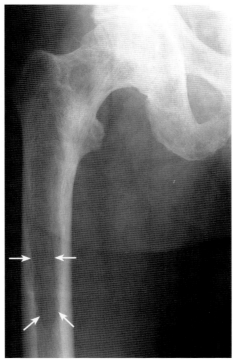

Fig. 5.156 Paget's disease. Mixed osteolytic and osteosclerotic form is seen in the proximal femur and pelvis and a predominantly osteolytic form with V- or flame-shaped osteolytic defect (arrows) in the femur shaft.

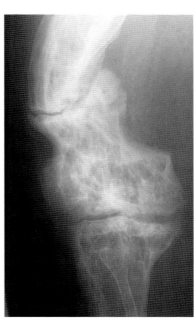

Fig. 5.157 Paget's disease. Mixed osteolytic and osteosclerotic form is seen in the distal femur and proximal tibia. Findings include bony expansion, coarse trabeculation, thickened cortices, bowing deformities and a pseudoarthrosis in the distal femur.

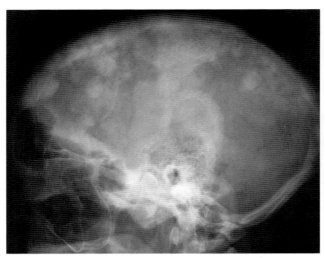

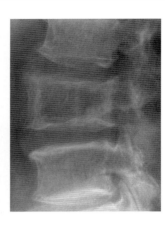

Fig. 5.**159**   **Paget's disease**. An enlarged vertebral body with coarse vertical striations and sclerotic margins ("picture frame vertebra") is seen in L3.

Fig. 5.**158**   **Paget's disease**. Sclerotic skull base, thickened vault (especially the inner table of the frontoparietal bone) and multiple sclerotic foci ("cotton wool" appearance) are diagnostic.

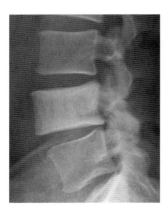

Fig. 5.**160**   **Paget's disease**. A slightly enlarged "ivory vertebra" is seen at L4.

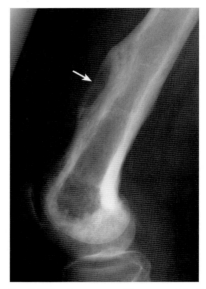

Fig. 5.**161**   **Aneurysmal bone cyst in Paget's disease**. A well-demarcated cortical lesion (arrow) with sclerotic border originates from the anterior cortex of the distal femur with characteristic findings of Paget's disease.

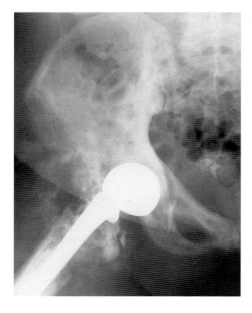

Fig. 5.**162**   **Osteosarcoma in Paget's disease**. A huge, partly ossified soft tissue mass is seen originating from the destructed proximal femur shaft around the hemiarthroplasty. Characteristic features of Paget's disease are present in the right hemipelvis and femur.

Table 5.10 (Cont.) Localized bone lesions

Disease	Radiographic Findings	Comments
Fibrous dysplasia (Figs. 5.163, 5.164, 5.165 and 5.166)	Solitary or multiple, often slightly expansile radiolucent lesions that may have a hazy quality ("ground glass" appearance). The matrix may also be uniformly dense, partially calcified or ossified, or thick dense bands may be present. A curvilinear sclerotic rim may outline lytic lesions. The monostotic form (75%) commonly involves a rib, femur, tibia, humerus, and mandible, whereas the polyostotic form (25%) frequently involves the skull and facial bones, pelvis, spine and shoulder girdle besides the long tubular bones. Polyostotic fibrous dysplasia may be unilateral or bilateral and may affect several bones of a single limb or both limbs. Solitary lesions in the long bones are located in the diaphyses or, less commonly, metaphyses. Bowing deformities are frequent in the polyostotic form.	Usually diagnosed before the age of 30. In the *McCune-Albright syndrome* precocious female sexual development and café-au-lait spots are associated with the polyostotic form. DD: *Neurofibromatosis*, where more irregularly contoured and darker café-au-lait spots are frequently associated with similar bone lesions. *Ossifying fibromas* are closely related to fibrous dysplasia and occur in the facial bones (especially mandible) and tubular bones (especially anterior aspect of tibia). In the latter location they are also referred to as *osteofibrous dysplasia* (Fig. 5.**167**).

(continues on page 127)

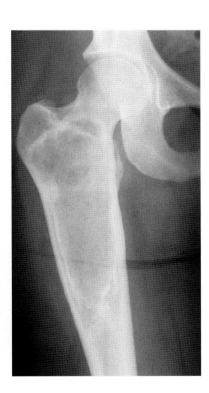

Fig. 5.**163 Fibrous dysplasia**. Slightly expansile, inhomogeneous lesion with "ground glass" appearance that is partially surrounded by a sclerotic margin is seen in the proximal femur.

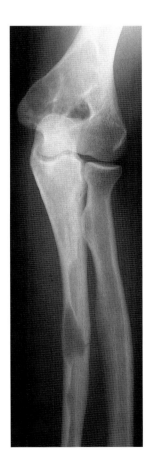

Fig. 5.**164 Fibrous dysplasia**. A slightly expansile, septated osteolytic lesion is seen in the distal humerus. Sclerotic expansion is evident in the proximal ulna. Osteolytic lesions with endosteal scalloping are present in the mid ulnar shaft.

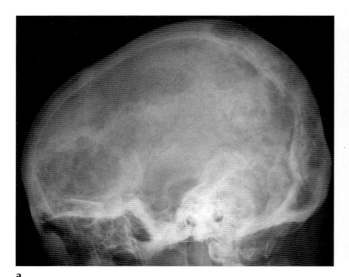

a

Fig. 5.**165 a**, **b** **Polyostotic fibrous dysplasia**. Extensive mixed osteolytic and osteoblastic lesions are seen. In the skull (**a**) the paranasal sinuses, base and vault are involved. Marked widening of the diploic space and expansion of primarily the outer table is best appreciated in the parieto-occipital area. Trabeculated osteolytic lesions with a hazy quality ("ground glass" appearance) are seen in the ilium and proximal femur (**b**). Slight bony expansion and beginning bowing deformity is also evident in the femoral neck and intertrochanteric area.

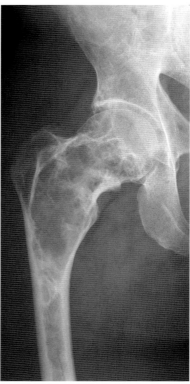

b

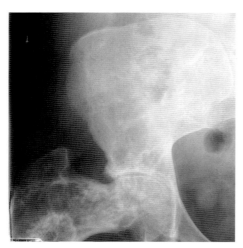

Fig. 5.**166** **Fibrous dysplasia**. Extensive mixed osteolytic and osteoblastic lesions with trabeculation and calcifications are seen in the ilium and hip. Coxa vara deformity ("shepherd's crook") is also evident.

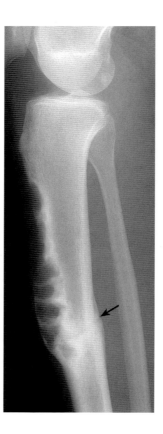

Fig. 5.**167** **Osteofibrous dysplasia**. An expansile multiloculated osteolytic lesion is seen originating from the anterior cortex of the tibia shaft that appears somewhat irregularly thickened. A healing pseudofracture (arrow) is also evident.

Table 5.10 (Cont.) Localized bone lesions

Disease	Radiographic Findings	Comments
Sarcoidosis (Fig. 5.168)	A solitary or multiple osteolytic lesions with a coarsened or lace-work trabecular pattern that may be associated with endosteal scalloping or cortical violation without periosteal reaction is the most common presentation. Purely osteolytic ("punched-out") cystic lesions or purely osteosclerotic foci are less common presentations. The hand is the predominant site of involvement, where acrosclerosis or acro-osteolysis may also be present.	Osseous sarcoidosis is usually associated with either skin lesions or pulmonary disease.
Particulate disease (Figs. 5.169, 5.170, and 5.171)	Presents typically as scalloped osteolytic lesion with or without sclerotic margins about a prosthetic component. Larger expansile lesions may become trabeculated and eventually break through cortex without inciting a periosteal reaction.	Foreign body reaction to wear debris of prosthetic components such as polymethylmethacrylate cement, polyethylene and silicone. Rarely an *intraosseous foreign body granuloma* is found that is not associated with joint replacement surgery or any other known cause of accidental foreign body implantation.

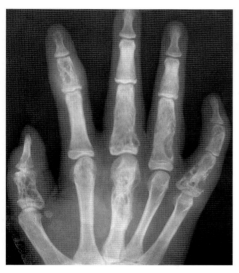

a

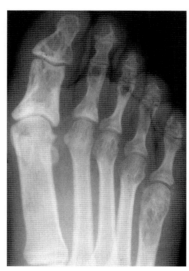

b

Fig. 5.**168 a, b Sarcoidosis**. Multiple osteolytic lesions with a honeycomb or lace-work trabecular pattern, some of which depict endosteal scalloping or cortical violation without periosteal reaction are seen in the hand (**a**) and foot (**b**).

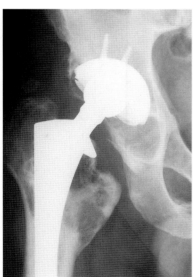

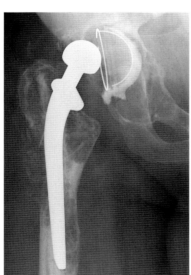

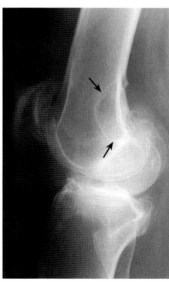

Fig. 5.**169 Foreign body granulomas.** An expansile trabeculated lesion with sclerotic margin is seen in the proximal femur shaft wrapping around the femoral component of the total hip prosthesis. A similar smaller second lesion is evident just below the acetabular component.

Fig. 5.**170 Particulate disease.** An aggressive osteolytic lesion with delicate trabeculation and cortical violation is surrounding the loose femoral component of the dislocated total hip prosthesis. A similar second lesion with bony expansion but without cortical violation is found around the loose acetabular component.

Fig. 5.**171 Foreign body granuloma.** An oblong eccentric lesion with sclerotic margin resembling a nonossifying fibroma is seen in the posterior aspect of the distal femur metaphysis (arrows). No history of accidental foreign body implantation was available in this case.

6 Joint Diseases

A multitude of radiologic changes occur in articular disorders. No single radiographic finding is however diagnostic for a specific arthropathy, since individual lesions in many conditions appear similar. The combinations of various radiologic parameters may lead to an accurate diagnosis, especially when pertinent clinical and laboratory findings are taken into consideration. The time and sequence of arthritic abnormalities observed with respect to the evolution of the disease may also offer important clues to the correct diagnosis. For example a rapidly progressing, destructive arthritic process involving a single joint is virtually diagnostic for septic (pyogenic) arthritis. Certain diseases such as rheumatoid arthritis show radiologic manifestations in a relatively early phase. Other arthritides such as gout depict radiographic abnormalities only late in their clinical course.

Proper radiographic analysis of any arthropathy must include the following criteria: 1. Number of joints involved (monoarticular versus polyarticular). 2. Distribution pattern of involved joints. 3. Joint space width. 4. Erosion. 5. Subchondral cysts. 6. Fragmentation of subchondral bone and loose intra-articular bodies. 7. Reactive (productive) bony changes (subchondral sclerosis, osteophytosis, enthesopathy, periostitis). 8. Osteoporosis (periarticular or generalized). 9. Joint deformities. 10. Chondrocalcinosis and periarticular soft tissue calcifications. 11. Joint effusions and para-articular soft tissue abnormalities.

Monoarticular arthritis (Table 6.1)

An arthritic process involving a single joint is commonly found in infectious arthritis, gout, secondary osteoarthritis and avascular necrosis. In pyogenic and tuberculous arthritis joint space narrowing, joint effusion and periarticular osteoporosis are characteristically present in the early stage followed by poorly defined bone destruction. Since periarticular osteoporosis and joint space narrowing are not present in gout, osteoarthritis and avascular necrosis, every monoarticular disease depicting these two radiographic abnormalities must be considered infectious in origin until proven otherwise. Osseous erosions and cysts in gout are sharply marginated as opposed to the poorly defined bone destruction in infectious arthritis. Osteoarthritis secondary to trauma may at times be difficult to differentiate from gout in small joints without proper clinical history and laboratory findings, since osseous erosions may simulate post-traumatic defects. Avascular necrosis in the early stage presents with normal radiographic findings. Subsequently patchy lucent and sclerotic areas may be seen in the subchondral bone on one side of a joint, followed by a diagnostic arc-like subchondral lucency (crescent sign) and eventually fragmentation and collapse of the involved bone.

Polyarticular arthritis (Table 6.2)

Rheumatoid arthritis, seronegative spondylarthropathy (psoriatic arthritis, Reiter's syndrome, ankylosing spondy-

litis and enteropathic arthropathy), gout, calcium pyrophosphate dihydrate crystal deposition disease (CPPD), osteoarthritis and neuropathic arthropathy are the most common polyarticular joint disorders. A symmetrically distributed articular disorder presenting with concentric joint space loss, erosions, osteoporosis, and fusiform soft tissue swelling is characteristic for rheumatoid arthritis. An erosive arthritis process involving both synovial and fibrocartilagenous joints (e.g. pubic symphysis and manubriosternal

Table 6.1 Monoarticular disease

Infectious arthritis:
  pyogenic
  tuberculous
  fungal
Gout
Hydroxyapatite deposition disease (HADD)
Traumatic arthritis
Secondary osteoarthritis
Avascular necrosis (osteonecrosis)
Pigmented villonodular synovitis
Synovial osteochondromatosis
Osteochondritis dissecans

Table 6.2 Polyarticular disease

Osteoarthritis
Erosive osteoarthritis
Rheumatoid arthritis
Psoriatic arthritis
Reiter's syndrome
Ankylosing spondylitis
Gout
Calcium pyrophosphate dihydrate crystal deposition disease (CPPD)
Hemochromatosis
Ochronosis
Multicentric reticulohistiocytosis
Hemophilia
Acromegaly
Jaccoud's arthritis
Systemic lupus erythematosus
Scleroderma
Multiple epiphyseal dysplasia

Table 6.3   Distribution patterns of polyarticular diseases

Involvement	Disease
Bilateral symmetric	Primary ostearthritis Erosive osteoarthritis Rheumatoid arthritis Ankylosing spondylitis CPPD Hemochromatosis Ochronosis Multicentric reticulohistiocytosis Neuropathic osteoarthropathy Hemophilia Acromegaly Jaccoud's arthritis Systemic lupus erythematosus Scleroderma Multiple epiphyseal dysplasia
Asymmetric	Secondary osteoarthritis Psoriatic arthritis Reiter's syndrome Gout
Distal interphalangeal joints (hand)	Osteoarthritis Erosive osteoarthritis Psoriatic arthritis Gout Multicentric reticulohistiocytosis Scleroderma
Proximal interphalangeal joints (hand)	Osteoarthritis Erosive osteoarthritis Rheumatoid arthritis Psoriatic arthritis Gout Multicentric reticulohistiocytosis Scleroderma
Metacarpophalangeal joints	Secondary osteoarthritis Rheumatoid arthritis Gout CPPD Hemochromatosis Jaccoud's arthritis Systemic lupus erythematosus
First carpometacarpal joint	Osteoarthritis Rheumatoid arthritis Gout Systemic lupus erythematosus
Common carpometacarpal joint Midcarpal joint	Rheumatoid arthritis Gout Osteoarthritis (scaphotrapeziotrapezoidal joint) Rheumatoid arthritis (including triquetropisiform joint) Gout CPPD (scaphotrapeziotrapezoidal joint)
Radiocarpal joint	Secondary osteoarthritis Rheumatoid arthritis Gout CPPD Hemochromatosis
Distal radioulnar joint	Rheumatoid arthritis Gout Scleroderma

joints) and the ligamentous attachments in the pelvis, femur and calcaneus in an often asymmetric fashion is characteristic for a seronegative spondylarthropathy. This diagnosis is further supported by the absence of osteoporosis, the presence of bony proliferation and intra-articular osseous fusion, and involvement of the spine and sacroiliac joints. Gouty arthropathy is characterized by asymmetric involvement of the appendicular skeleton, eccentric osseous erosions, bony proliferation, preservation of the joint space and absence of osteoporosis. In CPPD articular and periarticular calcifications are combined with joint space narrowing, eburnation, cyst formation, fragmentation and collapse. The presence of significant osteophytosis and the general absence of both intra-articular and extra-articular calcifications differentiates osteoarthritis from CPPD. Otherwise the radiographic findings in these two disorders are very similar, though fragmentation and bone collapse are less common in osteoarthritis. Neuropathic osteoarthropathy in an early stage may resemble osteoarthritis and CPPD, but extensive sclerosis associated with joint fragmentation, fractures and subluxations/dislocations is virtually diagnostic in a more advanced case.

Distribution patterns of articular diseases
(Table 6.3)

Symmetric joint involvement is typical of rheumatoid arthritis, primary osteoarthritis, CPPD and neuropathic arthropathy, whereas an asymmetric distribution of the affected joints favors the diagnosis of a seronegative spondylarthropathy, secondary osteoarthritis and gout.

In the hand nonerosive arthritic changes involving the distal interphalangeal joints suggests osteoarthritis, whereas erosive arthritic changes in the distal interphalangeal joints are common in psoriatic arthritis, erosive osteoarthritis and gout. Involvement of the proximal interphalangeal joints is common in rheumatoid arthritis and all aforementioned conditions affecting the distal interphalangeal joints. CPPD does not affect the interphalangeal joints, but has a predilection for the second and third metacarpophalangeal joints and the radiocarpal joint. Involvement of the metacarpophalangeal joints is common in both rheumatoid and psoriatic arthritis, but these joints are usually spared by both primary and erosive osteoarthritis.

In the wrist erosive arthritic changes without site predilection are very common in rheumatoid arthritis and gout and less frequent in psoriatic arthropathy. Both primary osteoarthritis and CPPD have a predilection for the first carpometacarpal joint and the joint between the scaphoid and trapezium-trapezoid.

In the foot primary osteoarthritis is typically located in both the first metatarsophalangeal joint (hallux rigidus), where it may be associated with hallux valgus deformity, and in the first tarsometatarsal joint. Rheumatoid arthritis commonly affects the interphalangeal joint of the great toe, both the metatarsal-phalangeal and tarsometatarsal joints, the talonavicular and the posterior subtalar joints. Seronegative arthropathies potentially affect any joint of the forefoot, but the most severe changes commonly occur in the metatarsophalangeal joints and the interphalangeal joint of the great toe. Gout shows a predilection for the first metatarsophalangeal joint and to a lesser degree the interphalangeal joint of the great toe, the metatarsophalangeal joints 2 to 5 and the tarsometatarsal joints, although any joint in the forefoot and midfoot can be affected. Neuropathic arthropathy in diabetes may involve the metatarsophalangeal joints and all joints of the midfoot and hindfoot.

Arthritic involvement of the calcaneus most commonly affects the sites of insertion of the Achilles tendon posteriorly and the plantar aponeurosis (fascia) inferiorly, as well as the posterosuperior aspect of the calcaneus that abuts the retrocalcaneal bursa. Retrocalcaneal bursitis leads to unilateral or bilateral erosions at this site in rheumatoid arthritis. Localized retrocalcaneal bursitis not related to a systemic arthritic process is termed *Haglund's syndrome* (Fig. 6.1). The condition is aggravaled by a prominent bony protuberance at the postero-superior aspect of the calcaneus (Haglund's deformity). The hallmark of the seronegative spondyloarthropathies are fluffy periostitis about the posterior and inferior aspect of the calcaneus and broadbased spurs (entesophytes) at the attachment of the Achilles tendon and plantar aponeurosis (Fig. 6.2). Erosions at these sites as well as near the retrocalcaneal bursa are not a dominant radiographic feature in these conditions. In osteoarthritis well-defined and typically narrow-based calcaneal spurs are found at the osseous tendon attachments. Similar bony excrescenses are associated with acromegaly, diffuse idiopathic skeletal hyperostosis (DISH) and CPPD (Fig. 6.3). In the latter condition linear calcific deposition in the Achilles tendon and plantar fascia may also be present. In gout tophaceous nodule in and about the Achilles tendon can lead to erosion near its calcaneal insertion.

In the knee bilateral and symmetric involvement of all three compartments (medial and lateral femorotibial space and patellofemoral joint) with marked joint space narrowing, osteoporosis and erosions is virtually diagnostic of rheumatoid arthritis. A tricompartmental distribution may also be found in seronegative spondylarthropathies, but the involvement is frequently asymmetric and less severe than in rheumatoid arthritis and periosteal new bone formation may be pronounced. In osteoarthritis the medial compartment is typically more severely affected than the lateral compartment resulting frequently in varus deformity. Significant degenerative changes in the patellofemoral joint may be associated. The compartmental distribution of CPPD in the knee is similar to osteoarthritis, but there is no preferential involvement of the medial compartment and both extensive chondrocalcinosis and rapid progression of the arthritic process including osseous destruction and fragmentation favor the former diagnosis. Isolated degenerative-like arthropathy of the patellofemoral joint should also raise the possibility of CPPD. Neuropathic arthropathy is characterized by disorganization of one or both knees including subluxation, fragmentation and extensive sclerosis.

In the hip the pattern of joint space loss may be useful to differentiate various articular diseases. Circumferential (axial or concentric) loss of joint space leads to migration of the femoral head in axial direction along the axis of the femoral neck (Fig. 6.4). Circumferential loss of joint space is associated with rheumatoid arthritis where both hips are affected in symmetric fashion. A unilateral (monoarticular) concentric loss of joint space suggests an infectious process but is also found with idiopathic chondrolysis of the hip. In ankylosing spondylitis a similar bilateral concentric joint space loss is found as in rheumatoid arthritis, but the presence of osteophytosis, commencing on the superolateral aspect of the femoral head and progressing to a collar about the femoral head-neck junction, is distinctive of the former disorder. Hip involvement in both psoriatic arthritis and Reiter's syndrome is similar to ankylosing spondylitis but un-

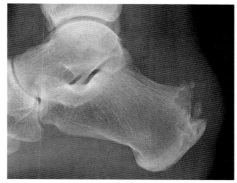

Fig. 6.**1 Haglund's syndrome**. Extensive erosive changes in the posterosuperior aspect of the calcaneus are associated with new bone formation and localized soft tissue mass secondary to retrocalcaneal bursitis.

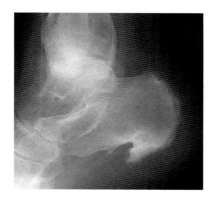

Fig. 6.**2 Inflammatory calcaneal spur (enthesophyte).** A broad-based plantar calcaneal spur is associated with fluffy periostitis about the posterior and inferior aspect of the calcaneus (Reiter's syndrome).

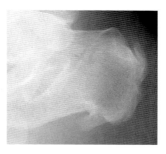

Fig. 6.**3 Degenerative calcaneal spurs (enthesophytes))**. Two well-defined calcaneal spurs depicting cancellous bone outlined by cortical margins are seen at the insertions of the Achilles tendon posteriorly and plantar aponeurosis inferiorly (acromegaly).

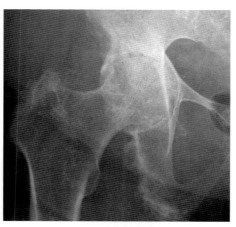

Fig. 6.**4 Circumferential loss of joint space**. Concentric (axial) narrowing of the joint space is associated with tiny articular erosions, extensive fluffy enthesopathy along the ischium and greater trochanter and fused sacroiliac joints. Mild protrusio acetabuli is also present (ankylosing spondylitis).

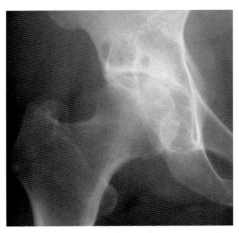

Fig. 6.5 Asymmetric loss of joint space. Narrowing of the joint space is limited to the superior (weight-bearing area of the hip and is associated with reactive sclerosis and subchondral cyst formation (osteoarthritis).

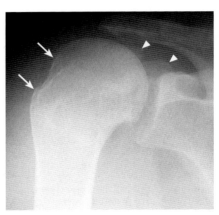

Fig. 6.6 Hatchet sign. An erosion limited to the lateral aspect of the humeral head (arrows) produces a deformity reminiscent of a hatchet. This finding is typically associated with ankylosing spondylitis or fungal arthritis as in this case. It should not be confused with a Hill-Sachs defect secondary to an anterior shoulder dislocation. Loose intra-articular bony fragments (arrowheads) and a decreased distance between humeral head and inferior aspect of the acromion indicating a chronic rotator cuff tear are also seen.

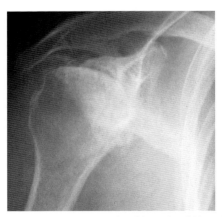

Fig. 6.7 Milwaukee shoulder. Cloud-like calcification in the rotator cuff and subacromial bursa projecting between the distal acromion and humeral head are associated with destructive shoulder arthritis and chronic rotator cuff tear evident by the decreased distance between humeral head and inferior aspect of the acromion.

common. In CPPD unilateral or bilateral concentric loss of joint space is associated with sclerosis, osteophytosis, cyst formation and eventually fragmentation of the femoral head. The demonstration of chondrocalcinosis in the acetabular labrum and pubic symphysis further supports the diagnosis of CPPD. Even in advanced cases of osteonecrosis (avascular necrosis) of the femoral head with bony collapse and fragmentation the joint space remains largely preserved. In osteoarthritis the loss of joint space narrowing is limited to the weight-bearing superior aspect of the joint or less frequently, to its medial aspect (Fig. 6.5). Besides the subchondral sclerosis, osteophytosis and cyst formation, cortical thickening or buttressing of the medial femoral neck cortex may also be apparent in this condition. *Protrusio acetabuli* (see Fig. 6.4) is associated with rheumatoid arthritis, ankylosing spondylitis, osteoarthritis (medial migration pattern), infection, acetabular trauma, Paget's disease and osteomalacia.

In the shoulder region bilateral symmetric loss of joint space in the glenohumeral joints combined with widened eroded acromioclavicular joints is characteristic for rheumatoid arthritis. Ankylosing spondylitis presents in similar fashion, but a large bony defect (erosion) on the superolateral aspect of the humeral head, the "hatchet" deformity (Fig. 6.6), the absence of osteoporosis and the presence of bony proliferation about the osseous erosions are clues to differentiate it from rheumatoid arthritis. Severe osteoarthritis in the glenohumeral joint is usually associated with previous trauma or overuse and is therefore most often unilateral. Acromioclavicular joint degeneration is frequent in middle-aged and elderly persons and may lead to shoulder impingement syndrome with the development of spurs protruding inferiorly from this joint and the adjacent undersurface of the acromion. In CPPD an advanced degenerative-like process in the glenohumeral joint may be associated with chondrocalcinosis. Calcium hydroxyapatite crystal deposition disease (HADD) presenting initially with cloud-like calcifications in the rotator cuff or subacromial bursa may progress to a destructive arthropathy of the glenohumeral joint with chronic rotator cuff tear, the so-called *Milwaukee shoulder syndrome* (Fig. 6.7).

Joint space width (Tables 6.4 and 6.5)

Analysis of the width of the joint space may provide important clues in the differential diagnosis of arthritic disorders. In these conditions the joint space may be narrowed, normal or widened. Furthermore joint space narrowing may be symmetric or asymmetric and occur early or late in the disease process. Symmetric joint space loss involving an entire joint early in the disease process is suggestive of an infectious or inflammatory arthritic disorder. An asymmetric joint space narrowing in the large joints of the lower extremity is indicative of osteoarthritis. In this condition subchondral sclerosis usually precedes a radiographically appreciable joint space loss. Advanced erosive or destructive joint disease with relatively well-maintained joint space and asymmetric joint involvement suggests gout and osteonecrosis, respectively. A widened joint space is typically associated with large joint effusions, especially in children, and hemathrosis secondary to trauma, hemophilia or other bleeding disorders. Joint laxity in neuromuscular disorders frequently presents with a widened joint space too. A *drooping shoulder* (Fig. 6.8) is an inferior "subluxation" of the humeral head caused by either a large hemarthrosis (e.g. in intra-articular proximal humerus fractures), any neurologic or muscular disorder affecting the supporting musculature or any direct injury of the capsule or rotator cuff itself. True subluxations and dislocations typically present also as joint space widening, but in certain projections these conditions may occasionally mimic a joint space narrowing. A considerable widening of the joint space in the fingers and toes can be found in psoriatic arthropathy when severe destruction of the subchondral bone is present. This condition has to be differentiated from sequelae of resection arthroplasties consisting of removal of one or both articular surfaces in an interphalangeal joint. A *widened acromioclavicular joint* (Fig. 6.**9**) is a frequent finding in rheumatoid arthritis and psoriatic arthropathy, but also encountered in infectious arthritis, traumatic separation, post-traumatic osteolysis (e.g. weight lifters), acromioplasty with resection of the distal clavicle, and hyperparathyroidism.

Erosions (Table 6.6)

Marginal articular erosions at osseous surfaces that do not possess protective cartilage are typical for early rheumatoid arthritis (Fig. 6.**10**). The erosions typically are poorly defined and without sclerotic margin. In the hand and wrist symmetric involvement with predilection for the proximal interphalangeal and metacarpophalangeal joints, trapezium, capitate, scaphoid, triquetrum and pisiform, and both the

Table 6.4 Narrowed joint space

Osteoarthritis (often asymmetric in weight-bearing joints)

Rheumatoid arthritis

Psoriatic arthritis

Reiter's syndrome

Ankylosing spondylitis

CPPD

Hemochromatosis

HADD

Ochronosis

Infectious arthritis

Hemophilia

Multiple epiphyseal dysplasia

Endstage of any arthritic process

Table 6.5 Widened joint space

Subluxation or dislocation (congenital, traumatic)

Hemarthrosis or large joint effusion

Joint laxity (neuromuscular, traumatic)

Psoriasis

Neuropathic osteoarthropathy

Acromegaly

Pigmented villonodular synovitis

Synovial osteochondromatosis

Synovial neoplasm

Resection arthroplasty

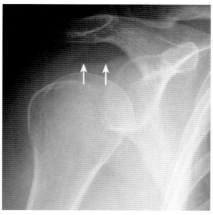

Fig. 6.**8 Drooping shoulder**. A large lipohemarthrosis with fat-blood level (arrows) secondary to a nondisplaced greater tuberosity fracture produces inferior subluxation of the humeral head evident by the increased distance between the latter and the inferior aspect of the acromion.

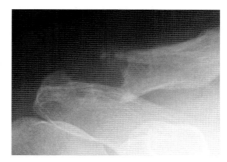

Fig. 6.**9 Widening of the acromioclavicular joint** is caused by erosion of the distal clavicle and to a lesser degree the distal acromion (secondary hyperparathyroidism).

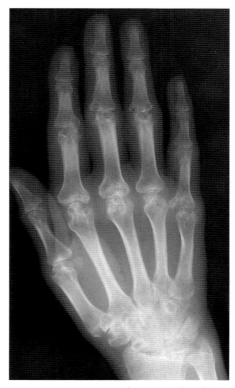

Fig. 6.**10 Erosions in rheumatoid arthritis**. Multiple preferentially marginal erosions with symmetric distribution and characteristic localization (sparring of the distal interphalangeal joints) are seen.

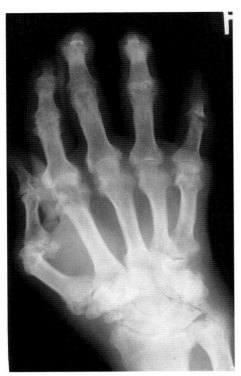

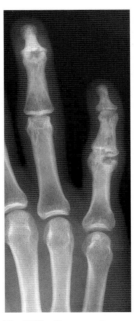

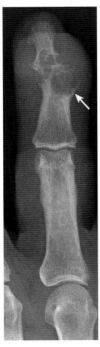

Table 6.6   Erosions

Erosive osteoarthritis

Rheumatoid arthritis

Psoriatic arthritis

Reiter's syndrome

Ankylosing spondylitis

Gout

HADD

Amyloidosis

Multicentric reticulohistiocytosis

Infectious arthritis

Scleroderma

PVNS (pressure erosions)

Synovial osteochondromatosis (pressure erosions)

Articular defects simulating erosions in CPPD, osteonecrosis, osteochondritis dissecans and osteochondral fractures

Fig. 6.11   Erosions in psoriatic arthritis. Multiple marginal erosions are associated with extensive bony proliferation evident as irregular excrescences with spiculated appearance. Note also the involvement of the distal interphalangeal joints and the partial resorption of the tufts on the third and fourth finger.

Fig. 6.12   Erosions in gout. Eccentric erosions with overhanging edge (arrow) and associated soft tissue mass is seen about the distal interphalangeal joint.

Fig. 6.13   Fragmentation of the articular surface in frostbite. Fragmentation of the distal articular surfaces of the proximal phalanx of the fifth finger and middle phalanx of the fourth finger secondary to osteonecrosis is seen. The remaining less exposed fingers were intact.

radial and ulnar styloid is characteristic. A poorly defined monoarticular erosive arthritic process suggests an infectious etiology. In psoriatic arthropathy (Fig. 6.11) marginal erosions characteristically are associated with adjacent bony proliferation evident as irregular excrescences with spiculated appearance. In gout (Fig. 6.12) one or more eccentric erosions with sclerotic margin and over-hanging edge may be evident. In erosive osteoarthritis the combination of osteophytosis and sharply marginated erosions in central location of the joint are characteristic. Fragmentation of an articular surface (e.g. in CPPD, osteonecrosis or secondary to trauma) may result in a defect that can mimic a true erosion (fig. 6.13).

Subchondral cysts (Table 6.7)

Single or multiple radiolucent lesions with sclerotic margins are commonly found with osteoarthritis, CPPD, and osteonecrosis (Fig. 6.14). In both osteoarthritis and osteonecrosis these cysts are typically located within the pressure segment of the joint, whereas in CPPD they are more widespread and frequently unusually large. A subchondral cyst occasionally is the sequela of a bone injury that becomes evident over a period of months after the traumatic episode (traumatic cyst). In rheumatoid arthritis the subchondral cysts frequently originate in the chondro-osseous junction and do not depict a surrounding sclerotic margin. An intraosseous ganglion presents as a solitary subchondral cystic lesion with sclerotic margin anywhere in the subchondral bone of a joint not affected by an arthritic process. Furthermore subchondral cysts can be mimicked by intraosseous gouty tophus, a Brodie's abscess and variety of neoplasms (e.g. chondroblastoma, giant cell tumor, intraosseous lipoma, clear cell chondrosarcoma, and skeletal metastases).

Fragmentation of subchondral bones and loose intra-articular bodies (Tables 6.8 and 6.9)

Fragmentation of the articular surface (Fig. 6.15) is commonly associated with CPPD, osteonecrosis, neuropathic arthropathy, far advanced osteoarthritis, and trauma (osteochondral fractures) resulting frequently in one or more loose intra-articular bodies. Detached osteophytes in osteoarthritis may also lead to loose intra-articular bodies. Joint destruction secondary to pyogenic or tuberculous arthritis may also be associated with loose intra-articular bony fragments. In osteochondritis dissecans the solitary osteochondral fracture fragment may be still located in the original articular defect (pit) or freely mobile in the joint. In synovial osteochondromatosis a large number of calcified/ossified loose bodies located within and around the involved joint and ranging in size from a few millimeters to several centimeters is characteristic.

Reactive (productive) bony changes

In osteoarthritis of weight-bearing joints sclerosis of the subchondral bone is frequently the first radiographic sign of the disease, since the causative joint cartilage degeneration

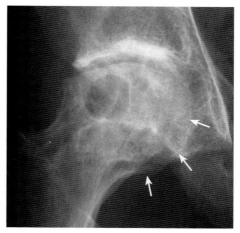

Fig. 6.**14** **Subchondral cyst in avascular necrosis (osteonecrosis)**. A cystic lesion with sclerotic margin is seen in the weight-bearing portion of the deformed and flattened femoral head. Secondary degenerative changes including remodeling and new bone formation (buttressing) along the medial aspect of the femoral head and neck (arrows) are also evident in this patient with sickle cell disease.

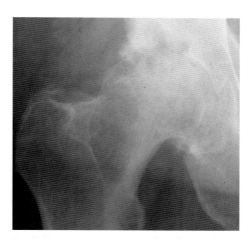

Fig. 6.**15** **Fragmentation of subchondral bone in osteoarthritis**. Degenerative changes in the weight-bearing portion of the hip are seen including subchondral cyst formation and beginning fragmentation of both acetabular dome and femoral head.

Table 6.7   Subchondral cystic lesions
Osteoarthritis
Rheumatoid arthritis
Gout
CPPD
Amyloidosis
Avascular necrosis (osteonecrosis)
Post-traumatic cyst without secondary osteoarthritis
Hemophilia
Infectious (Brodie's abscess)
Intraosseous ganglion
Intraosseous lipoma
Chondroblastoma
Giant cell tumor
Clear cell chondrosarcoma
Metastasis

Table 6.8   Fragmentation of articular surface
Intra-articular fracture
Osteoarthritis (advanced stage)
CPPD
HADD
Ochronosis
Infectious arthritis
Avascular necrosis (osteonecrosis)
Neuropathic osteoarthropathy
Osteochondritis dissecans

Table 6.9   Loose intra-articular bodies
Intra-articular fracture
Osteoarthritis (advanced stage)
CPPD
HADD
Ochronosis
Infectious arthritis
Avascular necrosis (osteonecrosis)
Neuropathic osteoarthropathy
Osteochondritis dissecans
Synovial osteochondromatosis

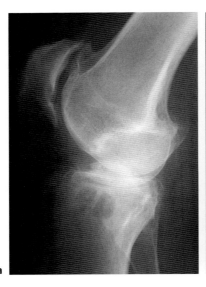 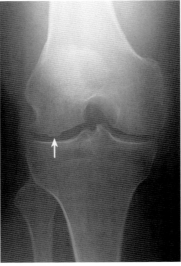

a   b

Fig. 6.**16 a, b   Osteophytosis in osteoarthritis**.
a: Marginal osteophytes are seen in the patellofemoral joint. **b**: A central (interior joint) osteophyte (arrow) presents as button-like excrescence originating from the subchondral bone largely denuded from its cartilage.

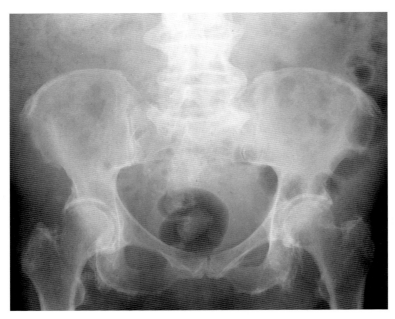

Fig. 6.**17   Enthesopathy in DISH**. Extensive well-defined bony proliferation is seen bilaterally along the iliac wings, ischiatic bones and greater and lesser trochanters. Note also the paravertebral ossifications in the lower lumbar spine and the normal sacroiliac joints.

can only be appreciated when a substantial loss of cartilage has occurred resulting in joint space narrowing. *Osteophytosis* (Fig. 6.**16**) is the hallmark of primary and secondary degenerative joint disease. *Marginal osteophytes* develop in the periphery of the articular surface of a joint and appear as lips of new bone. Less common are *central (interior joint) osteophytes* appearing as button-like or flat bony excrescences that may be demarcated at their bases by remnants of the original cartilage simulating occasionally loose intra-articular bodies.

Enthesopathy refers to bony proliferation at the site of osseous attachment of ligaments and tendons. Enthesophytes (Fig. 6.**17**) are commonly found with seronegative spondyloarthropathies and diffuse idiopathic skeletal hyperostosis (DISH). In the spine these conditions are characteristically associated with syndesmophytes (ossifications of the outer portion of the annulus fibrosus) or paravertebral ossification, respectively. The thin and vertically oriented, symmetric syndesmophytes in ankylosing spondylitis and enteropathic spondylarthropathy differ from the broader asymmetric syndesmophytes of psoriasis and Reiter's syndrome. Degenerative enthesophytes in osteoarthritis tend to be sharply marginated as opposed to the inflammatory enthesophytes associated with the seronegative spondylarthropathies that depict a more fluffy and often spiculated appearance.

Arthropathies commonly associated with periostitis (periosteal new bone formation) include psoriatic arthropathy, Reiter's syndrome, septic arthritis and juvenile rheumatoid arthritis. Intra-articular bone apposition on the medial aspect of the femoral neck is termed *buttressing*. It is most commonly observed with osteoarthritis and osteonecrosis, but occasionally is caused by a stress fracture or an adjacent osteoid osteoma.

Osteoporosis

In both the elderly patient and in advanced arthropathies of any etiology the presence of osteopenia is of little differential diagnostic value, since the finding may be either coincidental (e.g. senile osteoporosis) or caused by disuse. Periarticular or generalized osteoporosis are important radiographic features of rheumatoid, pyogenic, and tuberculous arthritis. These arthropathies have to be differentiated from reflex sympathetic dystrophy (Sudeck's osteodystrophy) and transient regional osteoporosis in which severe periarticular osteoporosis and articular pain are present in the absence of any radiographic joint abnormalities. Osteoporosis typically is not a feature of osteoarthritis, CPPD, gout and seronegative spondylarthropathies.

Joint deformities

Subluxations and dislocations are commonly caused by trauma, but are also associated with congenital and developmental diseases, neuromuscular disorders and most arthropathies. An erosive arthritic process associated with multiple joint deformities suggests the diagnosis of either rheumatoid arthritis or a seronegative spondylarthropathy such as psoriatic arthritis. The hand deformities associated with these diseases are depicted in Fig. 6.18. Similar hand and wrist deformities in the absence of erosions may be found with systemic lupus erythematosus or Jaccoud's arthritis secondary to rheumatic fever.

Common toe deformities include hallux valgus (valgus deformity in first metatarsophalangeal joint), hammer toe (hyperextended metatarsophalangeal, flexed proximal interphalangeal, hyperextended distal interphalangeal joints), claw toe (hyperextended metatarsophalangeal, flexed proximal interphalangeal and distal interphalangeal joints), curly toe (flexed proximal interphalangeal and distal interphalangeal joints), mallet toe (flexed distal interphalangeal joint), and cross-over toe (dorsal superimposition of a deviated toe over a neighboring toe). In rheumatoid arthritis spreading of the metatarsals, lateral deviation of the first to fourth toes in the metatarsophalangeal joints, and cock-up toe (hyperextended metatarsophalangeal joint with subluxation of the phalanx above the metatarsal head) are also frequently associated. Subluxation associated with articular fragmentations, osteophytosis and eburnation is most frequently found in neuropathic arthropathy.

Chondrocalcinosis and periarticular soft tissue calcifications (Tables 6.10, 6.11 and 6.12)

Calcification of articular cartilage is termed chondrocalcinosis (Fig. 6.19). It is the hallmark of calcium pyrophosphate dihydrate crystal deposition disease (CPPD). However chondrocalcinosis due to pyrophosphate and less frequently other crystals is also associated with many other conditions, most commonly with primary and post traumatic osteoarthritis and hyperparathyroidism. Periarticular soft tissue calcifications (Fig. 6.20) are frequently caused by calcium hydroxyapatite crystals, although other crystals such as calcium pyrophosphate dihydrate may be associated too. Extensive periarticular soft tissue calcifications are most commonly found with scleroderma (Fig. 6.21) and secondary hyperparathyroidism (renal osteodystrophy) whereas smaller and less conspicuous periarticular calcifications are typical for calcific tendinitis and bursitis, respectively.

Joint effusions

Joint effusions are commonly associated with synovial inflammation and trauma. In the absence of an injury a large monoarticular joint effusion suggests an infectious arthritic

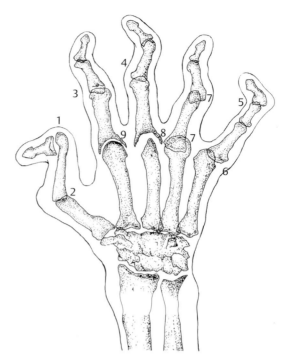

Fig. 6.**18**   **Hand deformities in inflammatory arthritis**. 1. Hyperextension and subluxation of the distal phalanx of the thumb. 2. Hyperextension at interphalangeal joint and flexion at the first metacarpophalangeal joint (Z-shaped deformity or hitchhiker's thumb). 3. Hyperextension distal interphalangeal and flexion proximal interphalangeal joint (boutonnière deformity). 4. Flexion distal interphalangeal and hyperextension proximal interphalangeal joint (swan-neck deformity). 5. Flexion distal interphalangeal joint (mallet finger). 6. Ulnar deviation at metacarpophalangeal joint. 7. Overriding dislocations at metacarpophalangeal and/or proximal interphalangeal joints ("telescoping" "opera-glass" deformity or "main en lorgnette"). 8. Whittled metacarpal head projecting in expanded base of proximal phalanx ("pencil-in-cup" deformity). 9. Erosion and compression of metacarpophalangeal joint ("ball-in-cup" or "cup-in-saucer" deformity). Boutonnière, and swan-neck deformities and ulnar deviation are more common in rheumatoid arthritis than psoriatic arthropathy, whereas "telescoping", "pencil-in-cup" and "ball-in-cup" deformities are more common in psoriatic arthropathy than rheumatoid arthritis.

Table 6.10   Chondrocalcinosis
Osteoarthritis (primary, secondary, post-traumatic)
Gout
CPPD
Hemochromatosis
Wilson's disease
HADD
Ochronosis
Acromegaly
Oxalosis

process. Joint effusions can only be differentiated from para-articular soft tissue swelling when the capsule of the affected joint is separated by a layer of fat from the surrounding tissues. This is the case in the elbow, knee and ankle where joint effusions can be reliably diagnosed by conven-

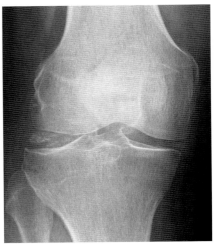

Fig. 6.**19** **Chondrocalcinosis in CPPD**. Extensive calcification is seen in the lateral and to a lesser degree medial meniscus.

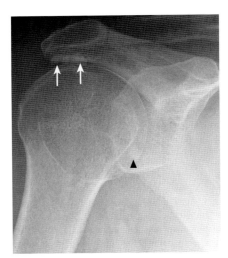

Fig. 6.**20** **Calcific tendinitis**. A localized calcification is seen in the supraspinatus tendon (arrows) of the rotator cuff. A smaller calcification is also present in the long biceps head tendon (arrowhead).

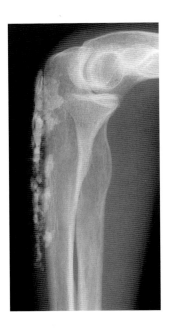

Fig. 6.**21** **Soft tissue calcification in scleroderma** is seen about the olecranon and dorsal aspect of the proximal ulna.

tional radiography (Fig. 6.22). Massive joint effusions may cause widening or pseudosubluxation of the involved joint such as inferior subluxation of the humeral head ("drooping shoulder") or widening of the distance between triquetrum and pisiform in a large radiocarpal joint effusion (Fig. 6.22d). After an intra-articular fracture a lipohemarthrosis can be diagnosed by the presence of a fat-blood level when the radiograph is obtained with horizontal beam technique. Occasionally intra-articular gas is also found in the absence of penetrating injury. Following a fracture or dislocation gas (mostly nitrogen) may accumulate in the joint, besides blood and bone marrow, in the form of one or more air bubbles as a result of negative intra-articular pressure. Such a pneumohemarthrosis or pneumolipohemarthrosis, respectively, is particularly common in the hip. A pyogenic arthritis caused by a gas-producing organism may also present with a large joint effusion containing gas. This condition has to be differ-

Table 6.11   Intervertebral disc calcification

Degenerative spine disease

Post-traumatic

CPPD

Hemochromatosis

Ochronosis

Acromegaly

Amyloidosis

Hyperparathyroidism

Paraplegia (e.g. poliomyelitis)

Spinal fusion of any etiology (e.g. congenital, surgical, traumatic, inflammatory, infectious, degenerative, DISH)

Table 6.12   Periarticular soft tissue calcification

Post-traumatic dystrophic calcification/myositis ossificans

Post-surgical dystrophic calcification/heterotopic bone formation

Paralysis

Thermal injury

Calcific tendinitis and bursitis

Gout

CPPD

HADD

Infectious arthritis (especially tuberculous)

Scleroderma and other connective tissue diseases

Hyperparathyroidism and renal osteodystrophy

Hypoparathyroidism

Hypervitaminosis D

Milk-alkali syndrome

Calcinosis circumscripta and tumoralis

Sarcoidosis

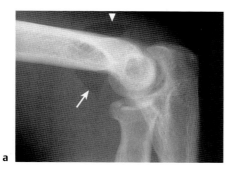

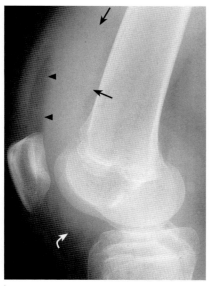

Fig. 6.**22 a, b, c, d   Joint effusions. a: Elbow**: Visualization of the posterior fat pad (arrowhead) is diagnostic. The anterior fat pad can normally be seen, but its elevation by the intra-articular fluid may produce a "sail" configuration (arrow) indicative of an effusion. A radial head fracture is also evident. **b: Knee**: Fluid accumulation in the suprapatellar bursa (arrows) that connects with the knee is diagnostic. The joint effusion (curved arrow) may also displace the inferior patellar fat pad anteriorly. A fat-fluid (blood) level (arrowheads) can be seen in the suprapatellar bursa in a post-traumatic lipohemarthrosis, when the examination is performed with horizontal beam technique. **c: Ankle**: A larger anterior (arrows) and smaller posterior (arrowhead) soft tissue bulge is characteristic. **d: Wrist**: Anterior subluxation of the pisiform is caused by the large hemarthrosis in the radiocarpal joint secondary to intra-articular fractures of the distal radius and ulna.

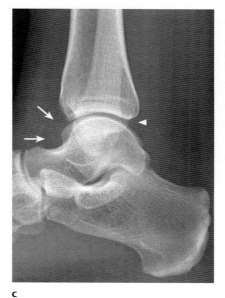

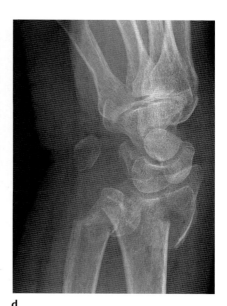

entiated from a transient, linear or crescent-shaped intra-articular vacuum phenomenon (gas in the intra-articular cavity) that is an occasional incidental finding (Fig. 6.**23**) indicating the absence of a significant joint effusion. Gas within a meniscus or disc is usually associated with degenerative disease.

Para-articular soft tissue abnormalities

(Table 6.**13**)

Fusiform para-articular soft tissue swelling commonly occurs with rheumatoid arthritis and psoriatic arthropathy, whereas sausage-like swelling of an entire digit is quite characteristic for the latter condition. Subcutaneous nodules are frequently associated with rheumatoid arthritis (Fig. 6.**24**) and are characteristically located in dorsal and lateral aspects of the fingers, about the olecranon, ischial tuberosities, femoral trochanters and the Achilles tendon region. Gouty tophi presenting as nodular soft tissue masses are commonly found in the knees, hands, ankles, elbows and may rarely calcify. In osteoarthritis of the hand Heberden's nodes about the distal interphalangeal joints and Bouchard's nodes about the proximal interphalangeal joints are posterolateral soft tissue nodules which in a more advanced stage may be associated with a bony outgrowth (osteophyte).

The differential diagnosis of articular disorders is discussed in Table 6.**14**.

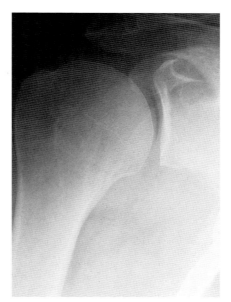

Fig. 6.**23   Vacuum phenomenon.** A crescent-shaped radiolucent line is seen in the glenohumeral joint indicating the absence of a joint effusion.

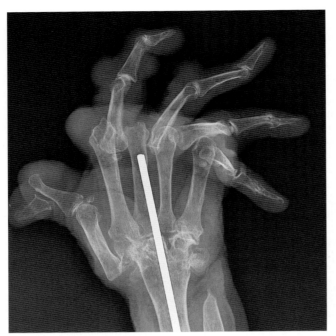

Fig. 6.24 **Subcutaneous soft tissue nodules in rheumatoid arthritis** are seen in the dorsal and lateral aspects of the fingers.

Table 6.13   Para-articular soft tissue nodules and swelling

Osteoarthritis (Heberden's nodes, Bouchard's nodes, bunion)

Rheumatoid arthritis (fusiform soft tissue swelling and rheumatoid nodules)

Rheumatic fever (similar to rheumatoid arthritis)

Psoriatic arthritis (fusiform soft tissue swelling and sausage finger)

Gout (tophi)

Multicentric reticulohistiocytosis (skin nodules and xanthomas)

Neuropathic osteoarthropathy

Infectious arthritis (fusiform soft tissue swelling and abscess formation)

Trauma (fusiform soft tissue swelling)

Foreign body granuloma (volar)

Hemophilia (hematomas)

Amyloidosis

Pigmented villonodular synovitis

Sarcoidosis (subcutaneous nodules)

Synovial cyst

Ganglion

Myositis ossificans (ossified)

Calcinosis circumscripta and tumoralis (calcified)

Xanthomatosis (subcutaneous nodules)

Weber-Christian disease (subcutaneous nodules)

Tumors (benign and malignant)

Aneurysm

Table 6.14 Differential Diagnosis of Articular Disorders

Disease	Characteristic Location	Radiographic Findings	Comments
Rheumatoid arthritis (RA) (Figs. 6.25, 6.26, 6.27, 6.28, 6.29, 6.30, and 6.31)	Symmetric polyarticular involvement of the synovial joints of the appendicular skeleton. Hands: Metacarpophalangeal and proximal interphalangeal joints including interphalangeal joints of the thumbs, with relative sparing of the distal interphalangeal joints. Wrists: Distal radioulnar joint including ulnar styloid, radiocarpal joint including radial styloid process and pisiform-triquetral joint. Feet: Medial aspects of the metatarsal heads, except in the fifth digit, where erosions on the lateral aspect may be the earliest manifestation. Interphalangeal joint of great toe (medial aspect) and calcaneus (erosions at insertions of Achilles tendon and plantar aponeurosis). Acromioclavicular joint (resorption of distal clavicles). Glenohumeral joints Elbows Hips (circumferential loss of joint space and protrusio acetabuli). Knees (symmetric involvement of the medial and lateral compartments). Ankles Cervical spine: Subluxations (anterior, lateral or vertical at C1-C2, less frequently at one or more subaxial levels). Vertical subluxation (telescoping) at the C1-C2 level may result in basilar invagination. Multilevel subluxations produce a "doorstep" or "stepladder" appearance.	Fusiform periarticular soft tissue swelling, regional osteoporosis and joint space narrowing associated with marginal and central erosions are the hallmark of the disease. The first erosions are frequently found in the metacarpophalangeal and proximal interphalangeal joints of the hands and the ulnar styloids. Besides marginal erosions originating typically in the bare bone areas of a joint without protective cartilage coverage, compressive erosions due to collapse of osteoporotic bone and surface erosions due to resorption of bone beneath inflamed tendons are also encountered. Synovitis resulting in fluid accumulation in joints, bursae and tendon sheaths is more difficult to appreciate with conventional radiographic technique. Progression of the disease leads to complete destruction of the involved joints and eventually to bony fusion, though the latter is rather uncommon. Subluxations and dislocation are frequent. In the hands flexion and extension contractures result in boutonnière or swan neck deformities of the fingers, hitchhiker deformity in the thumb and ulnar deviation in the metacarpophalangeal joints. In the wrist both volar (palmar) flexion instability (VISI) and dorsiflexion instability (DISI) occur besides dorsal subluxation of the distal ulna. Erosions may progress to extensive osteolysis in the distal clavicle, elbow and distal ulna. A chronic rotator cuff tear evident by progressive elevation of the humeral head (narrowing of the space between humerus and inferior surface of the acromion that typically becomes concave) is common in the advanced stage. In the spine diffuse narrowing of the disc spaces and facet joints without osteophytosis is characteristic.	Type III hypersensitivity connective soft tissue disorder with female predominance presenting clinically with morning stiffness, para-articular soft tissue swelling, especially of the wrist, hand and feet, and subcutaneous nodules at dorsal pressure points (e.g. olecranon). High sedimentation rate and positive rheumatoid factor in 90% are characteristic laboratory findings. Extra-articular manifestations (75%) are found in the lung (pulmonary fibrosis and rheumatoid nodules), pleura (unilateral or, less frequently, bilateral pleural effusions, usually not associated with parenchymal lung disease), cardiovascular system (pericarditis, myocarditis, aortitis and vasculitis), and lymphatic system (mild adenopathy and rarely splenomegaly). In *cystic rheumatoid arthritis* (Fig. 6.**32**) well-defined subcortical lesions often with sclerotic margins are the dominant radiographic feature, often in the absence of significant osteoporosis, joint space narrowing and erosions. In this condition 50% of patients are seronegative and there is no sex predilection. *Felty syndrome:* Rheumatoid arthritis associated with splenomegaly and neutropenia. *Sjögren's syndrome:* Connective tissue disorder with keratoconjunctivitis sicca, xerostomia and articular findings similar to rheumatoid arthritis.

(continues on page 144)

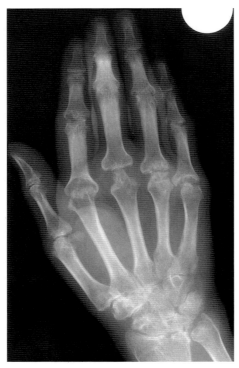

Fig. 6.**25** **Rheumatoid arthritis**. Osteopenia and erosive arthritic changes involving the hand and wrist with sparing of the distal interphalangeal joints are seen.

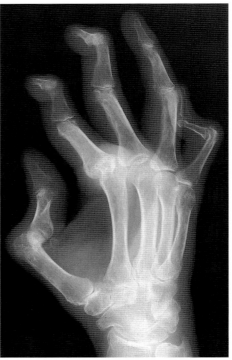

Fig. 6.**26** **Rheumatoid arthritis**. Osteopenia and erosive arthritic changes are associated with finger deformities including hitchhiker's thumb, swan neck deformities in digits 2 and 3, and boutonnière deformity in digit 5.

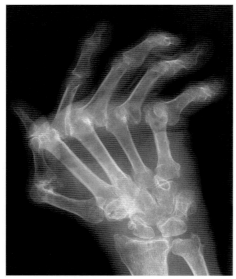

Fig. 6.**27** **Rheumatoid arthritis**. Severe osteopenia and erosive arthritic changes are associated with subluxations/dislocations and ulnar deviation in the metacarpophalangeal joints 2 to 5, ulnar subluxation in the radiocarpal joint and scapholunate dissociation.

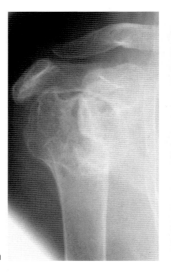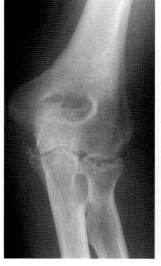

a

b

Fig. 6.**28 a, b** **Rheumatoid arthritis** (2 cases). **a** Shoulder: Extensive erosive changes in the glenohumeral joint and resorption of the distal clavicle are seen. **b** Elbow: Joint space narrowing and early erosions are evident.

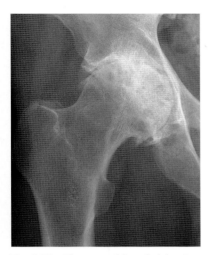

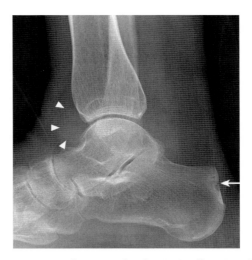

Fig. 6.**29** **Rheumatoid arthritis**. Concentric (axial) joint space narrowing is associated with osteopenia, erosions and small subchondral cysts. Beginning osteophytosis is indicative of early secondary degenerative changes.

Fig. 6.**30** **Rheumatoid arthritis**. Small erosions (arrow) with minimal surrounding sclerosis are seen in the posterosuperior aspect of the calcaneus. Generalized osteopenia and a large ankle joint effusion (arrowheads) are also evident.

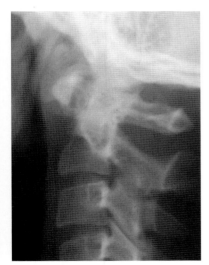

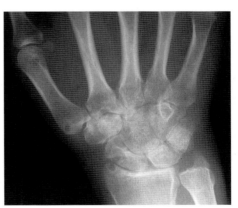

Fig. 6.**32** **Cystic rheumatoid arthritis**. Small well-defined subchondral cysts, some with sclerotic margins, are the dominant radiographic feature.

Fig. 6.**31** **Rheumatoid arthritis**. Early erosions about the dens associated with anterior atlanto-axial subluxation are seen.

Table 6.14   (Cont.) Differential Diagnosis of Articular Disorders

Disease	Characteristic Location	Radiographic Findings	Comments
Juvenile rheumatoid arthritis (JRA, chronic juvenile arthritis) (Figs. 6.33, 6.34, 6.35 and 6.36)	Symmetric, polyarticular. Hands (metacarpophalangeal and interphalangeal joints). Wrists, Feed (metatarsophalangeal, interphalangeal and intertarsal joints). Knees Hips Elbows Cervical spine Temporomandibular joint	Periarticular fusiform soft tissue swelling, osteoporosis and joint subluxations are common, similar to rheumatoid arthritis of the adult (RA). In contrast to the latter joint space narrowing and erosions are late manifestations in JRA, intra-articular bony ankylosis, periostitis and epiphyseal compression fractures are common and synovial cysts are rare. Growth disturbances including epiphyseal enlargement and either overgrowth or undergrowth of long bones with reduced diameters (overconstriction) are characteristic.	Rheumatoid arthritis in patients under 16 years of age with female predominance. Three types are differentiated: 1. Juvenile-onset adult type rheumatoid arthritis (15%) 2. Juvenile-onset ankylosing spondylitis (5%) 3. Still's disease (75%). Systemic and/or articular symptoms with negative rheumatoid factor. Three subtypes: a) Systemic disease. Acute febrile onset with skin rash, generalized lymphadenopathy, hepatosplenomegaly, pericarditis and myocarditis are usually associated with mild articular manifestations. b) Polyarticular disease. c) Para-articular or mono-articular disease: Usually confined to large joints. Associated iridocyclitis may lead to blindness.

(continues on page 145)

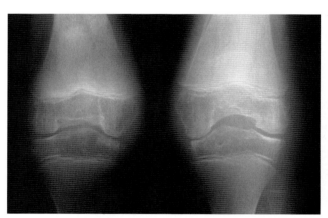

Fig. 6.**33**   **Juvenile rheumatoid arthritis**. Osteopenia, joint space narrowing and overgrowth of the epiphyses including widening of the intercondylar notch in the distal femora are seen.

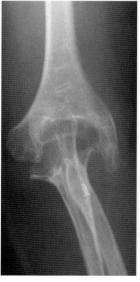

Fig. 6.**35**   **Juvenile rheumatoid arthritis**. Extensive erosive/destructive changes are seen in the elbow associated with overconstricted distal humerus and proximal radial and ulnar shafts.

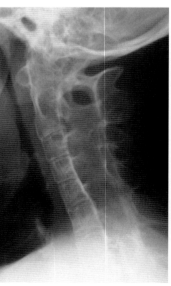

Fig. 6.**36**   **Juvenile rheumatoid arthritis**. A completely fused C-spine with uniformly marked disc space narrowing and severe osteopenia is seen.

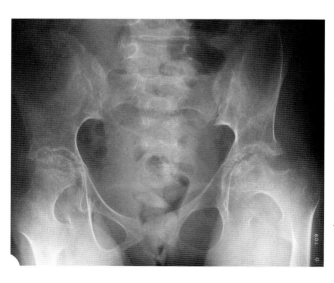

◁ Fig. 6.**34**   **Juvenile rheumatoid arthritis**. Severe generalized osteopenia and advanced erosive arthritis in both hips with right coxa valga and left coxa vara deformity are seen. Early erosive changes are evident in both sacroiliac joints.

Table 6.14 (Cont.) Differential Diagnosis of Articular Disorders

Disease	Characteristic Location	Radiographic Findings	Comments
Ankylosing spondylitis (Fig. 6.37, 6.38 and 6.39)	Symmetric involvement of synovial and fibrocartilagenous joints and sites of ligamentous and tendinous attachments (entheses). Sacroiliac joints Lumbar spine Thoracic spine Cervical spine (late) Tendinous insertion in pelvis ("whiskering") Pubic symphysis Hips Shoulders Sternoclavicular joints	Bilateral and symmetric involvement of the sacroiliac joints is the hallmark of the disease. Both synovial and ligamentous portions are affected, but involvement of the ilium is typically more severe. Erosive changes progress from loss of articular definition to superficial erosions, fraying of the subchondral bone and widening of the joint. Proliferative bony changes progress from focal sclerosis of the subchondral bone to irregular bony bridges and eventually complete ankylosis. In the spine syndesmophytes (thin vertical ossifications of the outer fibers of the annulus fibrosus) connecting the anterior and lateral corners resulting eventually in a bamboo spine formation and straightening (squaring) of the anterior vertebral margins are diagnostic. Other findings include increased sclerosis of the corners of the vertebral bodies ("shiny corner" sign), discal ballooning (biconvex shape of the disc secondary to osteoporosis), "dagger" sign (ossification of the interspinous ligament producing a central radiodense line on frontal radiographs) and "trolley-track" sign (three vertical lines on frontal radiographs related to the ossifications of the interspinous ligaments and apophyseal joints). The hip involvement is typically bilateral and symmetric with concentric joint space narrowing and osteophytosis. In the shoulder diffuse joint space narrowing and erosive changes predominantly in the superolateral aspect of the humeral head that may progress to complete destruction of that part ("hatchet" sign) are characteristic.	Chronic inflammatory disease primarily affecting the spine with male predominance of 4:1 to 10:1 and clinical onset with low back pain and stiffness at the age of 15–35 years. Histocompatibility antigen HLA-B27 is positive in 96%. Three times less common in blacks than Caucasians. Symmetric bilateral involvement of joints and sites of ligamentous attachment with subtle erosions and new bone formation (osteitis) with preferential involvement of the axial skeleton and large joints is characteristic. Erosive lesions in the spine at the discovertebral junction are termed Andersson lesions or, when located in the anterior margin, Romanus lesions. Complications of the ankylosed spine include fractures typically through a fused disc. Due to their instability these fractures are associated with significant morbidity and mortality, especially in the cervical region. Hand and wrist involvement occurs in 30% of patients, but is rarely a dominant feature of the disease. Radiographic findings in these locations are similar to psoriatic arthropathy.

(continues on page 147)

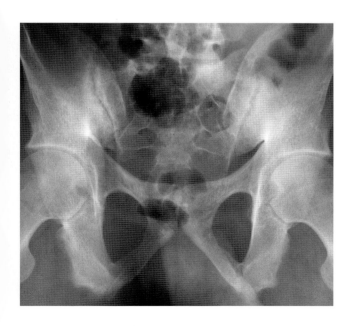

Fig. 6.**37** **Ankylosing spondylitis**. Symmetric bilateral sacroiliitis with erosions and joint space narrowing, mild concentric (axial) narrowing of both hips and extensive fluffy enthesopathy along the ischiatic bones are characteristic.

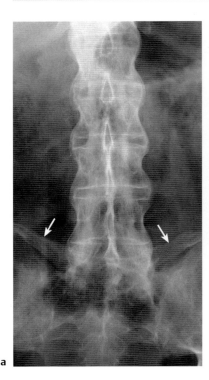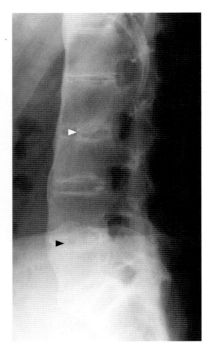

a

b

Fig. 6.**38 a, b** **Ankylosing spondylitis**. Fusion of the lumbar spine by delicate vertical syndesmophytes produces a "bamboo spine". Bilateral fused sacroiliac joints and ossification of both the interspinous ligament producing the "dagger" sign and the iliolumbar ligaments (arrows) are also evident in the anteroposterior projection (**a**). On the lateral film (**b**) straightening of the anterior vertebral margins, central disc calcifications (arrowheads) and either discal ballooning or discal narrowing are seen.

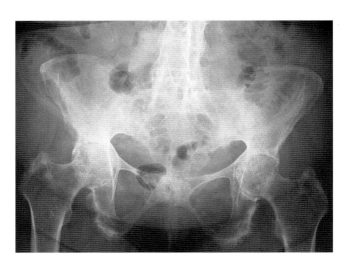

Fig. 6.**39** **Ankylosing spondylitis**. Generalized osteopenia, fusion of the lower lumbar spine and bilateral sacroiliac joints, marked concentric (axial) narrowing of the joint space in both hips with mild protrusio acetabuli on the right side, erosion and blurring of the subchondral bone with adjacent eburnation in the pubic symphysis, and extensive fluffy enthesopathy along the ischiatic bones and greater trochanters are seen.

Table 6.14 **(Cont.) Differential Diagnosis of Articular Disorders**

Disease	Characteristic Location	Radiographic Findings	Comments
Psoriatic arthritis (Figs. 6.40, 6.41, 6.42, 6.43, 6.44, 6.45 and 6.46)	Asymmetric polyarticular involvement of synovial and fibrocartilagenous joints and sites of tendinous and ligamentous attachments (entheses). Hands: Distal interphalangeal joints, proximal interphalangeal joints, metacarpophalangeal joints and tufts (tuftal resorption is almost always associated with nail involvement). Feet: Interphalangeal joints, metatarsophalangeal joints and tufts. Sacroiliac joints Sternoclavicular joints Acromioclavicular joints Spine Calcaneus Pubic symphysis	Fusiform soft tissue swelling about the involved joint or, less commonly, sausage-like swelling of entire digit is typical. Osteoporosis is not prominent or absent. Diffuse loss of joint space (similar to rheumatoid arthritis) is characteristic, but in the small joints of the fingers and toes considerable widening of articular space is not uncommon. Erosive/destructive changes tend to progress from the joint margins to the center. "Pencil-in-cup", or "ball-in-cup", "cup-and-saucer" appearance are quite characteristic in the digits. Bone proliferation is typically associated with erosive changes and may produce irregular excrescences with spiculated appearance. Exuberant periostitis and new bone formation in an entire phalanx may result in an ivory phalanx. Bony ankylosis is quite common in an advanced stage, especially in the hands and feet. Enthesopathy (bony proliferation at ligament and tendon attachment sites) occurs at the posterior and inferior surfaces of the calcaneus, femoral trochanters, the ischial tuberosities, medial and lateral malleoli, olecranon, radial tuberosity, and about the knees including the patella. Deformities in the hand and feet are less frequent than in rheumatoid arthritis. Sacroiliac joint involvement tends to be bilateral, but often somewhat asymmetric. Findings include erosions, sclerosis and widening or narrowing of the joint space, whereas complete ankylosis is relatively rare. In the spine thin and curvilinear to thick and fluffy paravertebral ossifications may be found with preferential involvement of the lower thoracic and upper lumbar spine. They may involve only one side of the spine, or when bilateral, may be asymmetric (DD: ankylosing spondylitis). In the cervical spine extensive proliferation along the anterior surface and both narrowing and sclerosis of the apophyseal joints are characteristic manifestations.	Arthritic changes are present in less than 5 % of patients with psoriasis. Skin disease is present in 85 % of patients with arthritic onset, but occasionally arthritis may antedate dermatological changes. HLA-B27 is positive in 80 % of patients whereas the rheumatoid factor is negative. Types: 1) True psoriatic arthritis (polyarthritis with distal interphalangeal joint involvement). 2) Seronegative polyarthritis simulating rheumatoid arthritis (DD: Psoriasis with coincidental rheumatoid arthritis). 3) Sacroiliitis and spondylitis. 4) Peripheral arthritis and sacroiliitis (combination of types 1 and 3) Radiographic features that differentiate psoriatic arthritis from rheumatoid arthritis in the hand include: 1) Lack of osteoporosis. 2) Tuftal resorption. 3) Asymmetric distribution of joint involvement 4) Involvement of the distal interphalangeal joints and relative sparing of the wrists. 5) Occasional widening of the articular space secondary to destruction of marginal and subchondral bone. 6) Bone proliferation including exuberant periosteal reaction, ankylosis and ivory phalanx formation 7) Sausage-finger.

(continues on page 150)

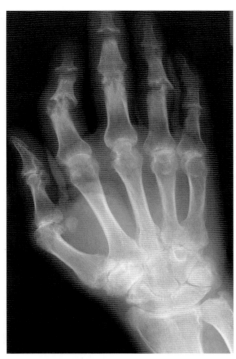

Fig. 6.**40** **Ankylosing spondylitis**. Erosive arthritic changes are seen in the hand and wrist that are indistinguishable from psoriatic arthritis.

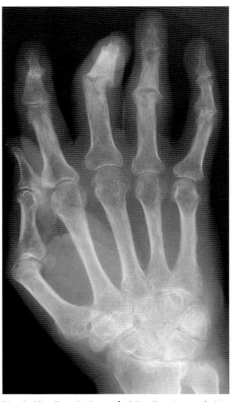

Fig. 6.**42** **Psoriatic arthritis**. Erosive arthritic changes involving primarily the proximal and distal interphalangeal joints and the wrist are seen. The margins of the erosions are frequently indistinct because of the associated new bone formation. Bony ankylosis of the distal interphalangeal joint of the index finger is also evident.

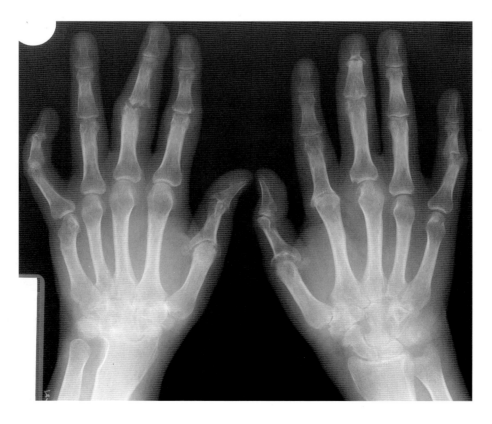

Fig. 6.**41** **Psoriatic arthritis**. Erosive arthritic changes with both asymmetric distribution and severity of joint involvement in both hands and wrists are seen.

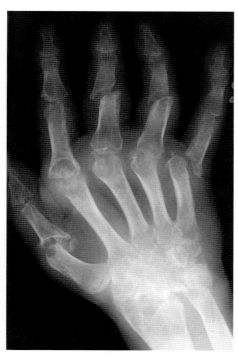

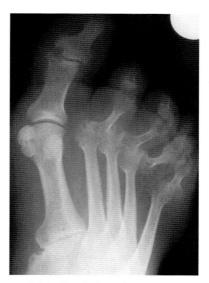

Fig. 6.**44** **Psoriatic arthritis**. Erosions associated with bone proliferation are seen in the interphalangeal joint of the great toe, the first tarsometatarsal joint and the dislocated metatarsophalangeal joints 2 to 5. Tuftal erosions are also evident in several toes.

Fig. 6.**43** **Psoriatic arthritis**. Severe destruction of the subchondral bone is seen in the hand and wrist leading to considerable widening of the articular space in several fingers.

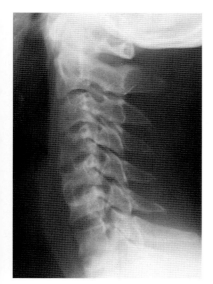

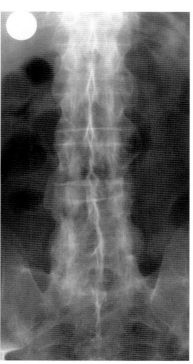

Fig. 6.**45** **Psoriatic arthritis**. Erosions of the bone adjacent to the intervertebral spaces of C4/5 and C5/6 with fluffy anterior syndesmophyte formation and beginning bony bridging.

Fig. 6.**46** **Psoriatic arthritis**. Fusion of the lumbar spine by large asymmetric syndesmophytes is seen. Narrowed bilateral sacroiliac joints with early erosions and mild reactive sclerosis on the right side are also present.

Table 6.14   (Cont.) Differential Diagnosis of Articular Disorders

Disease	Characteristic Location	Radiographic Findings	Comments
Reiter's syndrome (triad of arthritis, urethritis, and conjunctivitis) (Figs. 6.47, 6.48 and 6.49)	Usually asymmetric polyarticular involvement of synovial and fibrocartilagenous joints and entheses with preferential involvement of the lower extremity. Foot: Metatarsal phalangeal and interphalangeal joints including sesmoids. Calcaneus Ankle Knee Pubic symphysis Sacroiliac joints Spine Hand (especially proximal interphalangeal joints)	Periarticular osteoporosis may accompany acute episodes, but is not a prominent feature of the chronic stage. Loss of joint space and erosions are more frequently found in smaller than larger joints. Superficial bone resorption also occurs beneath inflamed bursae and tendon sheaths. Fluffy periosteal bone proliferation is characteristic, especially in the posterior and plantar aspect of the calcanei, ischial tuberosities and trochanters, but also in the metatarsal, metacarpal and phalangeal shafts, the malleoli and the knees. Sacroiliac joint involvement is common (in excess of 50% in advanced disease) and is usually bilateral symmetric or asymmetric. Osseous erosions associated with adjacent sclerosis varying from mild to severe predominate characteristically on the iliac site of the joint. In the lower thoracic and upper lumbar spine thin or thick vertical osseous bridges may extend across the intervertebral disc and initially are separated by a clear space from the lateral margin of the adjacent vertebral bodies. Spinal involvement is typically asymmetric.	Peak onset occurs between 15 and 35 years of age with male predominance. HLA-B27 is positive in 75% of patients. Transmission occurs in association with either epidemic dysentery or sexual intercourse. Urethritis is frequently the initial manifestation. Associated mucocutaneous lesions include balanitis circinata and keratosis blennorhagica in soles and palms. Conjunctivitis may progress to uveitis and keratitis. Seventy percent of patients develop radiographic bony alterations. Acute attacks may be associated with soft tissue swelling and osteoporosis. Radiographic features of Reiter's syndrome are virtually indistinguishable from psoriatic arthritis. Compared to the latter condition preferential involvement of the lower extremities, less frequent involvement of the spine and relatively rare bony ankylosis of the small joints of the hands and feet are favoring the diagnosis of Reiter's syndrome.
Enteropathic arthritis (Figs. 6.50, 6.51 and 6.52)	Monoarticular to bilateral symmetric Sacroiliac joints Spine Knees Ankles Feet Shoulder Elbows Wrists Hands	Central type: Symmetric involvement of the sacroiliac joints and spine indistinguishable from ankylosing spondylitis. Peripheral type: Monoarticular or pauciarticular acute synovitis presenting with soft tissue swelling and periarticular osteoporosis. A close temporal association between exacerbation of intestinal and arthritic findings is characteristic. Chronic changes are rare and include joint space narrowing, erosions and cyst formation mimicking rheumatoid arthritis. Clubbing of fingers and rarely periostitis of tubular bones simulating hypertrophic osteoarthropathy may also be found.	The incidence of arthritic changes: Ulcerative colitis 12% Crohn's disease 10% Whipple's disease 75% (predominantly peripheral type) Salmonella 2% Shigella 2% Yersinia 30% Intestinal bypass surgery 3% Hepatic disease (cirrhosis, hepatitis) 2% (exclusively peripheral type) Pancreatic disease 1% (exclusively peripheral type; associated osteonecrosis common). Intestinal infections caused by salmonella and yersinia may also cause septic arthritis and osteomyelitis by hematogenous spread.

(continues on page 152)

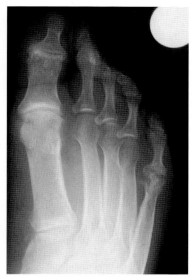
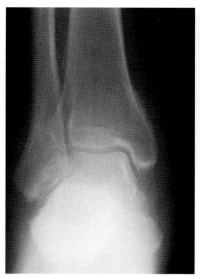
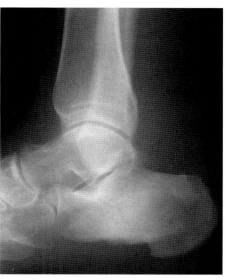

a

b

Fig. 6.47 Reiter's syndrome. Erosions with partial destruction of the metatarsal head and beginning fluffy bone proliferation are seen in the 5ᵗʰ metatarsal phalangeal joint. Joint space narrowing and beginning bony proliferation without erosions are evident in the interphalangeal joint and metatarsophalangeal of the great toe.

Fig. 6.48 a, b Reiter's syndrome. Extensive fluffy periostitis is seen in the medial aspect of the distal tibia metaphysis and about the lateral malleolus in **a**, and about the posterior and inferior aspect of the calcaneus in **b**.

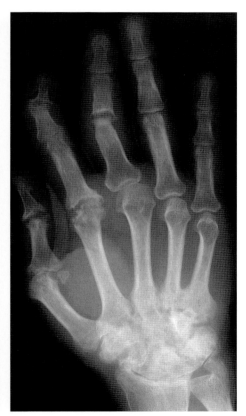

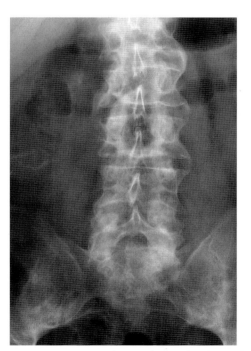

Fig. 6.49 Reiter's syndrome. Erosive arthritic changes with bone proliferation are seen in the several joints of the hand and the wrist. Note also the diffuse soft tissue thickening of digits 2 and 3 (sausage fingers).

Fig. 6.50 Enteropathic arthritis (Crohn's disease). Bilateral fused sacroiliac joints and delicate syndesmophyte formation in the lumbar spine are evident.

Table 6.14   (Cont.) Differential Diagnosis of Articular Disorders

Disease	Characteristic Location	Radiographic Findings	Comments
Jaccoud's arthritis (Fig. 6.53)	Bilateral symmetric Hands	Bilateral symmetric deforming non-erosive arthropathy. Ulnar deviation and flexion deformities of the metacarpophalangeal joints, especially in the fourth and fifth finger are characteristic. Hyperextension of the interphalangeal joints may be associated. Joint space narrowing and erosions are typically absent. Foot involvement with lateral deviation and subluxation of the metatarsophalangeal joints is less common.	Post-rheumatic fever arthropathy. Rheumatic fever is characterized by fever, carditis and polyarthritis following an episode of beta-hemolytic streptococcal infection. Reversible nature of the articular deformities is characteristic, but occasionally deformities may become fixed.
Systemic lupus erythematosus (Fig. 6.54)	Bilateral symmetric Hands Feet Hips Knees Ankles Shoulders	Bilateral symmetric deforming non-erosive arthropathy of the hands occurs in 25% of patients. Subluxation of the metacarpophalangeal joints with ulnar deviation, swan-neck and boutonnière deformities of the fingers and hyperextension of the interphalangeal joint of the thumb are characteristic. Joint space narrowing and erosions are rare. Occasionally hook erosions on the radial and volar aspects of the metacarpal heads are found, presumably produced by capsular pressure. Associated foot abnormalities may include hallux valgus deformity, metatarsophalangeal joint subluxations and splaying of the forefoot. Instability in knees, shoulders and atlanto-axial joint may also be present. Osteonecrosis is, besides deforming nonerosive arthropathy, the other classic feature of the disease occurring in up to 40% of patients. The femoral heads are most commonly affected site, but humeral heads, femoral condyles, tibial plateaus, talar domes, and the small bones of hands, wrists and feet are also frequently involved. Signs of avascular necrosis in these joints and cystic changes in the carpal bones are the corresponding radiographic features. Acrosclerosis and tuftal resorption complete the radiographic picture.	Relatively common connective tissue disorder with 10:1 female predominance and typical onset during child-bearing age. Three times more common in blacks. Laboratory findings include antinuclear DNA antibodies (87%), LE cell formation (78%), hypergammaglobulinemia (77%), anemia (78%) and leukopenia (77%). Nonspecific bilateral polyarthralgia involving hands, wrists, shoulders and knees is present in 90% of patients. Myositis and spontaneous tendon rupture are common and usually associated with systemic or local steroid therapy. Soft tissue calcifications occur, but are much less common than in either scleroderma or dermatomyositis. Osteomyelitis and septic arthritis (bacterial and mycotic) are relatively frequent complications. Both steroid administration and renal disease are major contributing factors to the susceptibility for infection. The deforming nonerosive lupus arthropathy differs from Jaccoud's arthropathy in the hand only by the site of involvement. In the former all metacarpophalangeal joints including the thumb are typically involved, whereas the latter has a preference for the fourth and fifth finger.

(continues on page 154)

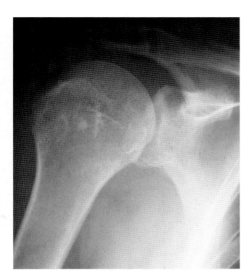

Fig. 6.**51** **Enteropathic arthritis (Crohn's disease)**. Erosions with fluffy spiculated bone proliferation are limited to the greater tuberosity.

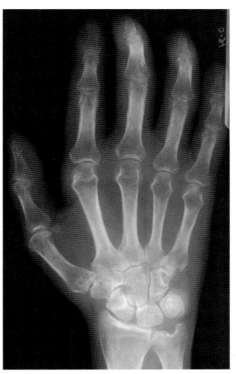

Fig. 6.**52** **Enteropathic arthritis (Crohn's disease)**. Juxta-articular osteoporosis and scattered early erosions are evident in the hand and wrist best appreciated in the volar aspect of the interphalangeal joint of the thumb and the ulnar aspect of the fifth carpometacarpal joint. Nonspecific arthritis with para-articular soft tissue swelling is seen in the distal interphalangeal joints of the third and fourth fingers.

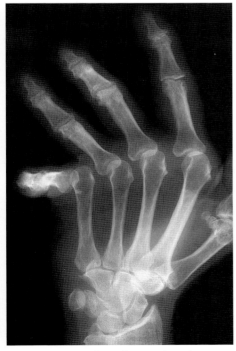

Fig. 6.**53** **Jaccoud's arthritis**. Ulnar deviation without erosions is seen in the metacarpophalangeal joints. It is most severe in the fifth digit where it progressed to complete dislocation.

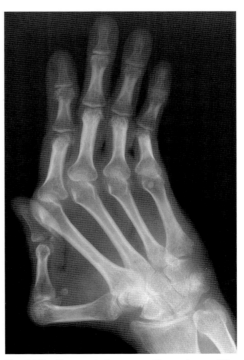

Fig. 6.**54** **Systemic lupus erythematosus**. Ulnar deviation in the metacarpophalangeal joints and hitchhiker's deformity of the thumb are seen.

Table 6.14   (Cont.) Differential Diagnosis of Articular Disorders

Disease	Characteristic Location	Radiographic Findings	Comments
Scleroderma (Fig. 6.55)	Monoarticular to bilateral symmetric. Hands (distal and proximal interphalangeal joints and metacarpophalangeal joints). Wrists (first carpometacarpal joint and distal radioulnar joint) Sternoclavicular joints Acromioclavicular joints Mandible (thickening of the periodontal membrane resulting in a widened periodontal gap between the tooth and the mandible is a characteristic finding).	Acro-osteolysis and soft tissue calcifications are the hallmark of the disease. Resorption of the tufts leads to "penciling" of the phalanx. Calcifications present as small punctate deposits at the phalangeal tip to more wide spread conglomerate deposits with periarticular distribution. Acrosclerosis (hyperostosis of the tuft) associated with soft tissue atrophy is another presentation. Nonspecific articular involvement of the hands and wrist may eventually progress to erosive destructive changes with or without intra-articular calcifications. Involvement ranges from monoarticular (e.g. first carpometacarpal joint) to bilateral symmetrical. Foot abnormalities are less frequent and usually limited to the metatarsophalangeal joints. Thinning of the 3rd to 6th ribs posteriorly, and resorption of both the proximal and distal ends of the clavicle and the distal acromion can also be found.	Autoimmune disease with 3:1 female predominance and peak age of 30 to 50 years. May be associated with CREST syndrome (Calcinosis of skin and subcutaneous tissue, Raynaud's phenomenon, Esophageal dysmotility, Sclerodactyly and Telangiectasia). Musculoskeletal abnormalities of scleroderma associated with other collagen vascular disease (e.g. rheumatoid arthritis or systemic lupus erythematosus) is referred to as mixed connective tissue disease or overlap syndrome, respectively. Soft tissue calcifications frequently occur also about large joints. (DD: Milk-alkali syndrome, hypervitaminosis D, renal osteodystrophy and tumoral calcinosis). *Dermatomyositis* (Fig. 5.56) presents with similar radiographic features as scleroderma, but both extensive linear subcutaneous and intermuscular fascial plane calcifications are typical for the former disorder.
Vasculitides	Hands Wrists Hips Knees Ankles	Nonspecific (periarticular soft tissue swelling, osteoporosis and joint effusions) or absent.	*Polyarteritis nodosa* (occasionally with periosteal new bone formation) *Giant cell (temporal) arteritis* *Polymyalgia rheumatica* *Henoch-Schönlein (anaphylactoid) purpura* *Cryoglobulinemia* (occasionally with small subchondral cysts) *Erythema nodosum*
Familial Mediterranean fever (Fig. 6.57)	Bilateral asymmetric Sacroiliac joints (unilateral or bilateral) Hips Knees	Osteoporosis Epiphyseal overgrowth in children. Articular erosions, sclerosis and fusion may eventually develop.	Rare genetic disorder predominantly in Sephardic Jews, Armenians and Arabs presenting with multiple episodes of fever associated with peritonitis, pleuritis and synovitis.
Relapsing polychondritis (Fig. 6.58)	Bilateral asymmetric Sacroiliac joints (unilateral or bilateral)	Bilateral sacroiliitis with joint space loss, erosion and eburnation without spinal alterations. Nonspecific findings in peripheral joints, sternoclavicular joints, manubriosternal and costochondral junctions ranging from usually mild nonerosive to occasionally multilating arthritis. Extra-articular findings include tracheal stenosis and calcifications of the auricular cartilage.	Episodic inflammation of cartilaginous tissue (e.g. external ear, nose, larynx, trachea, ribs and joints) and ocular structures (e.g. conjunctiva, sclera and urea) occurring in all age groups with peak in fourth decade.
Behçet's syndrome (Figs. 6.59 and 6.60)	Monoarticular or oligoarticular Knees Small peripheral joints Sacroiliac joints	Monoarticular or oligoarticular involvement with periarticular soft tissue swelling and osteoporosis and rarely joint space narrowing and small erosions	Triad of recurrent oral and genital ulcerations and ocular inflammation characteristic. Occurs at all ages (peak age 30 years) with male predominance.

(continues on page 156)

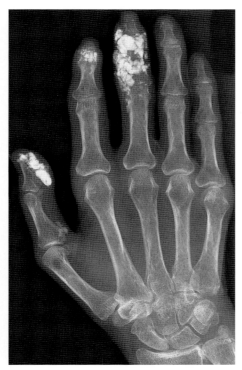

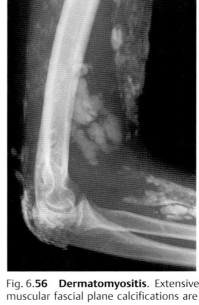

Fig. 6.**56** **Dermatomyositis**. Extensive subcutaneous and intermuscular fascial plane calcifications are evident.

Fig. 6.**55** **Scleroderma**. Osteopenia, soft tissue calcifications and resorption of the tufts in the thumb, index and middle finger are seen. The small cystic lesion in the distal aspect of the first metacarpal is an incidental finding most likely representing a small enchondroma.

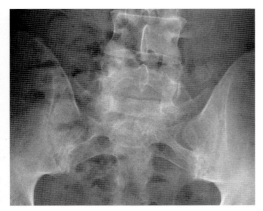

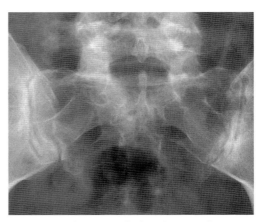

Fig. 6.**57** **Familial Mediterranean fever**. Osteopenia, joint space narrowing and early erosions are seen in both sacroiliac joints.

Fig. 6.**58** **Relapsing polychondritis**. Early erosions with reactive sclerosis are seen in both sacroiliac joints.

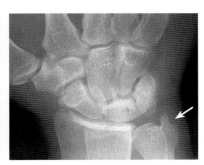

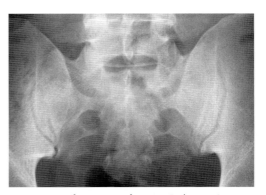

Fig. 6.**59** **Behçet's syndrome**. Minimal scattered erosive changes are seen in the wrist with the largest erosion being located in the ulnar styloid (arrow).

Fig. 6.**60** **Behçet's syndrome**. Early erosions are seen in both sacroiliac joints (same patients as in Fig. 6.**59**).

Table 6.14　(Cont.) Differential Diagnosis of Articular Disorders

Disease	Characteristic Location	Radiographic Findings	Comments
Hemophilia (Figs. 6.61 and 6.62)	Bilateral, not always symmetric Knees Ankles Elbows	Dense appearing (hemosiderin deposition) joint effusions and periarticular soft tissue swelling, osteoporosis, joint space narrowing, cartilaginous and osseous joint destruction with secondary sclerosis, osteophytosis and subchondral cyst formation and epiphyseal overgrowth (secondary to chronic hyperemia) are characteristic. Widening of the intercondylar femoral notch and squaring of the inferior pole of the patella, tibiotalar slanting in the ankle and widening of the trochlear and radial notches of the ulna in the elbow may be associated. Intraosseous hemorrhage may lead to osteonecrosis (especially in the femoral head and talar dome) and hemophilic pseudotumor formation simulating a variety of benign or malignant lesions and infections.	Occurs in approximately 1 in every 10,000 males due to X-linked deficiency of coagulation factor VIII (hemophilia A, 90% of patients) or factor IX (hemophilia B or Christmas disease, 10% of patients). Von Willebrand's disease (autosomal dominant with factor VIII and platelet deficiency) may occasionally present with similar features in both genders. Radiographic features of hemophilia and juvenile rheumatoid arthritis in large joints are virtually indistinguishable. Involvement of the spine and hands, bony ankylosis and growth inhibition are however findings only associated with juvenile rheumatoid arthritis.
Gout (Figs. 6.63, 6.64, 6.65, 6.66, 6.67, 6.68 and 6.69)	Monoarticular or asymmetric polyarticular involvement typical. Feet: Involvement of first metatarsophalangeal joint most characteristic with erosion frequently located on medial or dorsal aspect of first metatarsal head. Other metatarsophalangeal joints, interphalangeal joints, tarsometatarsal joints and intertarsal joints may also be affected. Hands: Distal and proximal interphalangeal joints are most commonly involved, but metacarpophalangeal joints and wrists may also be affected. Elbows: Bilateral olecranon bursitis with erosive and proliferative changes in the adjacent olecranon virtually pathognomonic. Knees Sacroiliac joints	Erosions caused by tophi may be intra-articular, para-articular or at a considerable distance from the joint and are typically surrounded by a sclerotic border producing a "punched out" appearance. An elevated bony spicule may form over the eroding tophus producing the "overhanging edge" sign that is found in almost half of the cases and quite characteristic. Bone proliferation may occasionally produce club-shaped metacarpal, metatarsal and phalangeal heads ("mushrooming"), enlarged ulnar styloids and thickened diaphyses. Tophi typically present as eccentric juxta-articular, lobulated soft tissue masses occasionally containing calcific deposits. Intra-osseous calcified tophi may mimic enchondromas in the hand. Calcium pyrophosphate deposition disease (CPPD) is occasionally associated presenting with chondrocalcinosis of the menisci of knee, pubic symphysis and triangular fibrocartilage of the wrist. Osteonecrosis is another associated complication.	Hyperuricemia is the hallmark of the disease. Deposition of urate crystals occurs in para-articular soft tissues, joints and bone causing inflammation and destruction. The disease is caused by either overproduction of uric acid or decrease in renal urate excretion. There is a 20:1 male predominance with the first attack occurring typically in the 5th decade of life, although any age is possible, in women the disease commences in the postmenopausal period. Stages: 1) Asymptomatic hyperuricemia 2) Acute gouty arthritis: Monoarticular or polyarticular attacks presenting with pain, tenderness and swelling, but usually without radiographic bony abnormality. 3) Chronic tophaceous gout: Develops eventually in fewer than half of the patients with recurrent acute attacks. *Secondary gout* rarely causes radiographically apparent arthropathy and is associated with myeloproliferative disorders and sequelae of their treatment and with chronic renal failure. *Lesch-Nyhan syndrome*: X-linked enzyme deficiency of uric acid metabolism presenting with mental retardation is associated with self-mutilation (amputation of fingertips), gouty erosions and retarded skeletal maturation. *Saturnine gout* is a complication of chronic lead poisoning caused by contamination of alcoholic beverages. *Type 1 glycogen storage disease* may also be associated with gouty arthritis

(continues on page 159)

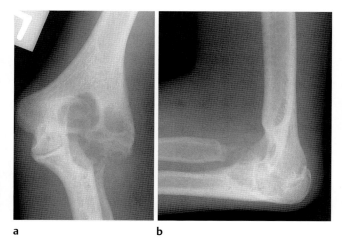

a   b

Fig. 6.**61 a, b** **Hemophilia**. Erosive/destructive changes with subchondral cyst formations are seen in the elbow in anteroposterior (**a**) and lateral (**b**) projections.

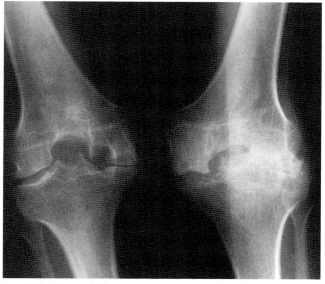

Fig. 6.**62** **Hemophilia**. Osteoporosis, widened intercondylic notch and joint space narrowing and destruction of the adjacent bone are seen bilaterally. Furthermore extensive reactive sclerosis with subchondral cyst formations is present in the lateral compartment of the left knee.

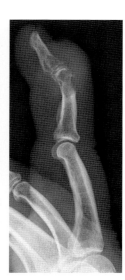

Fig. 6.**63** **Gout**. Well defined erosions with small bony spicules associated with a soft tissue mass are seen in the distal interphalangeal joint. Osteoporosis and joint space narrowing typically are absent.

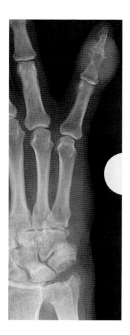

Fig. 6.**64** **Gout**. A large dense soft tissue mass surrounding the distal interphalangeal joint of the fifth finger where small subchondral and marginal erosions are seen, the latter with tiny overhanging bone spicules. Erosive and cystic changes with beginning bone proliferation are also seen in the wrist and distal radioulnar joint, most notably in the proximal aspect of the triquetrum.

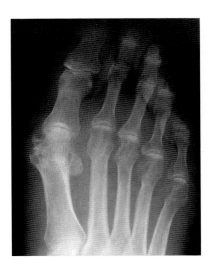

Fig. 6.**65** **Gout**. A large erosion with considerable amount of new bone formation is seen on the medial aspect of the first metatarsal head and neck without involvement of the articular surface of the adjacent joint. Only minimal erosive/cystic changes are seen in the other metatarsal heads and about the interphalangeal joint of the great toe.

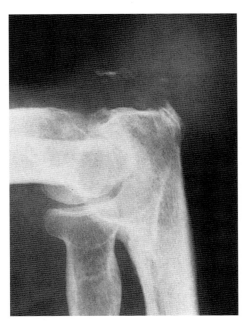

Fig. 6.**66** **Gout**. A large soft tissue mass with scattered calcifications is seen eroding the adjacent olecranon.

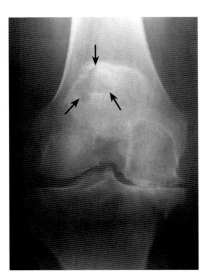

Fig. 6.**67** **Gout**. A large tophus (arrows) with sclerotic margin is seen in the patella. Joint space narrowing with small erosions and subchondral cysts and reactive sclerosis is seen in the medial compartment of the knee.

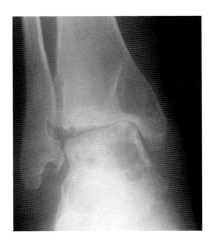

Fig. 6.**68** **Gout**. Well defined erosions of varying sizes and large cysts with or without sclerotic margins are seen in the distal tibia, lateral malleolus and talus.

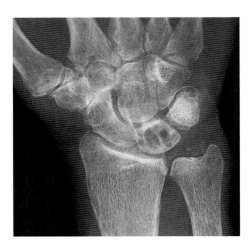

Fig. 6.**69** **Gout and CPPD**. A multiloculated cystic lesion in a slightly expanded lunate is associated with chondrocalcinosis in the triangular fibrocartilage. A smaller cyst with sclerotic margin is evident in the distal aspect of the triquetrum.

Table 6.14   (Cont.) Differential Diagnosis of Articular Disorders

Disease	Characteristic Location	Radiographic Findings	Comments
Calcium py-rophosphate dihydrate crystal deposition disease (CPPD) (Figs. 6.70, 6.71, 6.72 and 6.73)	Bilateral and symmetric distribution. Knees Wrists Metacarpophalangeal joints (especially 2nd and 3rd) Pubic symphysis Hips Intervertebral discs	Chondrocalcinosis is the hallmark of the disease and refers to linear or punctate calcifications of both the fibrocartilagenous cartilage (e.g. menisci of the knee, triangular fibrocartilage of the wrist, pubic symphysis, annulus fibrosus of the intervertebral disc, and acetabular and glenoid labra) and the hyaline cartilage (e.g. wrist, knee, elbow, hip and shoulder). The calcifications in the fibrous cartilage tend to be irregular, thick and shaggy and in the hyaline cartilage thin and linear. Synovial, capsular, tendinous, bursal and ligamentous calcifications are frequently associated. Arthritic changes of CPPD and osteoarthritis are very similar and include joint space narrowing and subchondral sclerosis. In CPPD, however, subchondral cysts tend to be larger and more numerous, and subchondral bone collapse and fragmentation with formation of intra-articular loose bodies are much more common, whereas osteophytosis is often less prevalent. CPPD also tends to affect joints that are not commonly involved in osteoarthritis, such as the metacarpophalangeal joints, midcarpal and radiocarpal compartments of the wrist, elbows and shoulders. In the knee the medial compartment is most frequently involved, similar to primary osteoarthritis, but isolated involvement of either the patellofemoral or lateral compartment is somewhat suggestive of either CPPD or post-traumatic osteoarthritis. In the wrist a predilection for the radiocarpal compartment results in "degenerative" changes between the distal radius and the proximal carpal row. The scaphoid moves proximally and appears compressed and deformed by the adjacent radius, whereas the lunate moves distally and hereby producing a "stepladder" appearance. This pattern is also referred to as scapholunate advanced collapse (SLAC) and, besides CPPD is also found a sequela of occupational or accidental trauma. Isolated "degenerative" changes in the second and third metacarpophalangeal joints including collapse of the metacarpal heads are another quite characteristic CPPD manifestation. Irregular, beak-like osteophytes on the radial aspects of the metacarpal heads may be associated. In the hip CPPD may be suggested when advanced degenerative changes are associated with concentric loss of joint space.	Most common crystalline deposition arthropathy affecting primarily the middle-aged and elderly population without sex predilection. Clinically CPPD may be asymptomatic or mimic osteoarthritis, rheumatoid arthritis, neuropathic arthropathy or gout, the latter beginning frequently referred to as *pseudogout*. CPPD is usually idiopathic, but a hereditary form is also recognized. A variety of diseases have been associated with CPPD including osteoarthritis, diabetes mellitus, gout, hyperparathyroidism, hemochromatosis, and Wilson's disease. Chondrocalcinosis may be found in both primary and post-traumatic osteoarthritis and thus the demonstration of cartilage calcification should not automatically lead to the diagnosis of CPPD arthropathy, particularly since the accumulation of other crystals than calcium pyrophosphate dihydrate (CPP) might be responsible for this finding. *Wilson's disease* (hepatolenticular degeneration) is a rare autosomal recessive disease with excessive copper retention caused by the inability of the liver to excrete it into the bile. It presents with degenerative changes in the brain, especially the basal ganglia, hepatic cirrhosis and diagnostic greenish-brown Kayser-Fleischer corneal rings. Articular changes in the metacarpophalangeal joints, wrist, hand, foot, hip, shoulder, elbow resemble CPPD or osteochondritis dissecans. Additional radiographic findings include osteoporosis and fluffy new bone formation at sites of capsular, ligamentous or tendinous attachments. In the spine wedged vertebral bodies with irregular plates and Schmorl's nodes simulate Scheuermann's disease.

(continues on page 161)

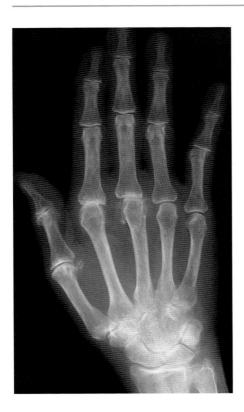

Fig. 6.**70** **CPPD**. Chondrocalcinosis of the triangular fibrocartilage associated with severe arthritic changes in the second and third metacarpophalangeal joint is a characteristic presentation. Other typical findings seen in this case include calcifications of the lunotriquetral ligament, joint space narrowing in the radiocarpal and scaphotrapeziotrapezoidal joints, tiny, beak-like osteophytes on the radial side of the second and third metacarpal heads and capsular calcifications about the third metacarpophalangeal joint.

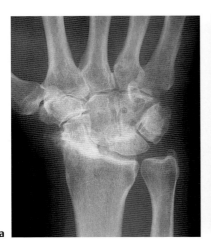

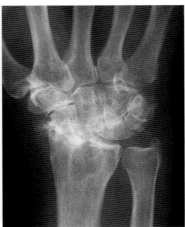

a   b

Fig. 6.**71 a, b** **CPPD**. Faint calcifications in the triangular fibrocartilage are associated with advanced arthritic changes in the radiocarpal joint including sclerosis and compression of the proximal scaphoid that appears embedded in the distal radius and increased scapholunate distance. This pattern is also referred to as scapholunate advanced collapse (SLAC). Multiple small cysts in other carpal bones and "degenerative" changes in the scaphotrapeziotrapezoidal joint without involvement of the first carpometacarpal joint are also seen in (**a**). One year later significant progression of the arthritic process including a new large subchondral cyst formation in the distal radius is seen in **b**.

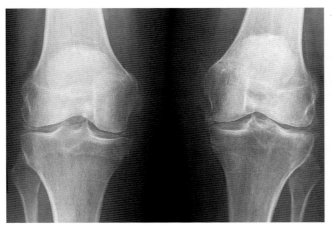

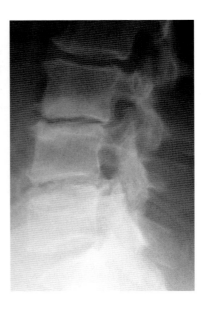

Fig. 6.**73** **CPPD**. Disc space narrowing with faint calcifications of the intervertebral discs, sclerosis of the adjacent plates and mild osteophytosis is seen.

Fig. 6.**72** **CPPD**. Chondrocalcinosis in the menisci and calcifications of the joint capsule and collateral ligaments, respectively, are seen in both knees.

Table 6.14 **(Cont.) Differential Diagnosis of Articular Disorders**

Disease	Characteristic Location	Radiographic Findings	Comments
Calcium hydroxyapatite crystal deposition disease (HADD) (Figs. 6.74, 6.75 and 6.76)	Tendons Bursae Joint capsule Shoulder	Periarticular hydroxyapatite (HA) crystal deposition is found in calcific tendonitis and bursitis. It is much more common than intra-articular HA deposition and almost always precedes the latter. Intra-articular HA crystal accumulation leads to joint space narrowing, destruction of subchrondral bone, subchondral sclerosis, intra-articular debris and joint disorganization. In the shoulder a chronic rotator cuff tear is invariably associated resulting in superior migration of the humeral head with possible erosion of the adjacent inferior aspect of the acromion and distal clavicle. The condition is *termed cuff tear arthropathy* or *Milwaukee shoulder syndrome.* HADD may also involve the knee (often limited to the lateral compartment), hip, elbow and the small joints of the hands and feet.	Periarticular HADD affects both men and women and is particularly common between 40 and 70 years of age. Symptoms include pain, tenderness, local edema and restricted motion. HA deposits are however also frequently found in asymptomatic patients. HADD arthropathy simulates CPPD, but does not produce the characteristic calcifications found in chondrocalcinosis. Cloud-like intra-articular opacities may however be evident in HADD. In *mixed calcium phosphate deposition disease* both HA and CPP crystals are found in the aspirated synovial fluid. This condition is not uncommon and should be expected when radiographically chondrocalcinosis and periarticular calcifications are present to a similar extend.

(continues on page 162)

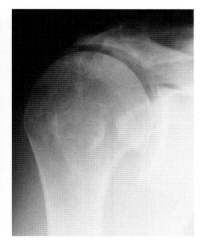

Fig. 6.**74** **HADD (Milwaukee shoulder)**. Rotator cuff calcifications are associated with a chronic rotator cuff tear evident by the superior migration of the humeral head with markedly decreased distance between the humeral head and distal acromion with eroded inferior margin and concave demarcation. Arthritic changes in the glenohumeral joint including a minimally deformed humeral head are also present.

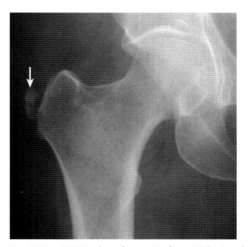

Fig. 6.**75** **HADD (trochanteric bursitis)**. A calcification (arrow) adjacent to the greater trochanter is seen.

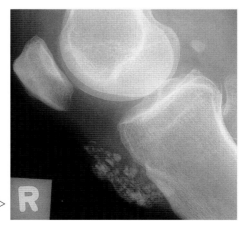

Fig. 6.**76** **HADD (housemaid's knee)**. Multiple calcifications are ▷ noted in an enlarged subcutaneous infrapatellar bursa.

Table 6.14   (Cont.) Differential Diagnosis of Articular Disorders

Disease	Characteristic Location	Radiographic Findings	Comments
Hemochromatosis (Fig. 6.77)	Metacarpophalangeal joints Wrists	Findings are almost identical to CPPD including chondrocalcinosis, but are commonly associated with a more uniform loss of joint space and osteoporosis. Characteristic involvement of the metacarpophalangeal joints (primarily 2nd and 3rd, less commonly 1st, 4th and 5th) include symmetric joint space loss, sclerosis, subchondral cysts, and fragmentation or flattening of the metacarpal heads. Compared to CPPD, the 4th and 5th metacarpophalangeal joints are more frequently involved, irregular beak-like osteophytes on the radial aspects of the metacarpal heads are more prevalent, the wrist involvement tends to be more widespread with diffuse affection of all midcarpal and common carpometacarpal joints, but with relative sparing of radiocarpal compartment.	*Primary hemochromatosis* is an inherited disorder with abnormal iron deposition resulting in cirrhosis, diabetes, skin pigmentation and heart failure. It has a 10:1 male predominance with symptoms occurring after the age of 40 years. *Secondary hemochromatosis* is associated with an increased intake of iron such as multiple blood transfusions in myeloproliferatory disorders and refractory anemias. An arthropathy is found in approximately one-third of patients commencing typically in the small joints of the hands and eventually progressing to the large joints.
Ochronosis (alkaptonuria) (Fig. 6.78)	Bilateral, not always symmetric Spine Hips Knees Shoulders Sacroiliac joints Pubic symphysis	In the spine widespread, often laminated disc space calcifications involving both nucleus pulposus and annulus fibrosis with predilection of the lumbar spine is most characteristic. Associated findings include marked uniform disc space narrowing at all levels, multiple vacuum phenomena and osteoporosis. Progressive discal ossification and bony bridging eventually results in a bamboo spine. Extraspinal manifestations in large joints resemble CPPD. Findings include asymmetric or symmetric joint space loss, severe subchondral sclerosis, and eventually collapse and fragmentation of the articular surface with intra-articular loose bodies. In contrast to CPPD subchondral cysts are absent or inconspicuous, whereas severe involvement of both the sacroiliac joints and pubic symphysis with eburnation and fragmentation is suggestive of ochronosis.	Rare hereditary metabolic disease with inability to metabolize homogentisic acid that is excreted by the kidneys. The urine is colorless when passed but darkens when exposed to light. Ochronotic pigmentation of the ears and sclera is usually first observed at the age of 20 to 30 years. Symptoms and signs of ochronotic arthropathy usually appear in the fourth decade of life.

(continues on page 164)

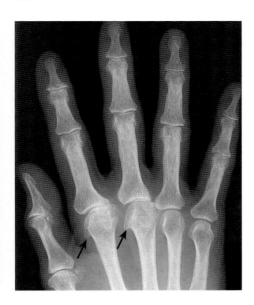

Fig. 6.**77**   **Hemochromatosis**. Symmetric joint space loss with mild subchondral sclerosis and large beak-like osteophytes (arrows) on the radial aspects of the metacarpal heads are seen in the second and third metacarpophalangeal joints.

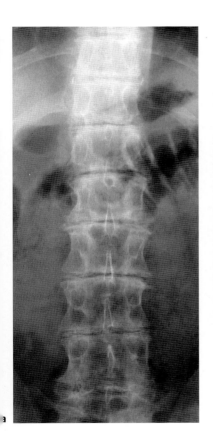
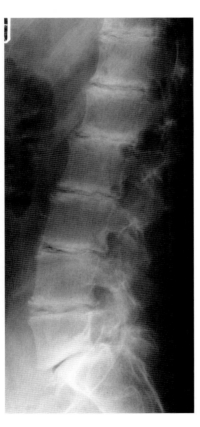

Fig. 6.**78 a, b   Ochronosis**. Marked uniform disc space narrowing with irregular and slightly sclerotic endplates, discal calcification and multiple vacuum phenomena is seen in anteroposterior (**a**) and lateral (**b**) projection throughout the lumbar and visualized lower thoracic spine. The syndesmophytosis in this case is rather minimal. Grade 1 anterolisthesis of L5 against S1 is also present secondary to spondylolysis at L5.

a

b

Table 6.14   (Cont.) Differential Diagnosis of Articular Disorders

Disease	Characteristic Location	Radiographic Findings	Comments
Acromegaly (Fig. 6.79)	Bilateral symmetric Hands Feet Mandible Spine Soft tissue thickening (heel, phalanges)	Hands and feet: Soft tissue thickening of the phalanges, joint space widening (especially metacarpophalangeal and metatarsophalangeal joints), thickening and squaring or overconstriction of phalanges, metacarpals and metatarsals, enlargement of the tufts and bases of the terminal phalanges, enlarged sesmoids and large enthesophyles at ligament and tendon attachment sites. Spine: Enlarged intervertebral disc, increased anteroposterior and lateral diameters of the vertebral bodies with exaggerated concavity of their posterior aspects. Premature osteoarthritis with prominent osteophytosis is seen at a later stage, especially in the weight-bearing joints and spine.	Hypersecretion of growth hormone due to eosinophilic adenoma or hyperplasia of the pituitary gland leads to gigantism in the immature skeleton and acromegaly in the mature skeleton. Stimulation of endochondral ossification results in enlargement of the costochondral junctions (acromegalic rosary). Stimulation of periosteal bone formation leads to enlargement of the mandible, phalanges, metacarpals, metatarsals and various tuberosities. Cartilage proliferation results in widened articular and intervertebral spaces.
Amyloidosis (Figs. 6.80 and 6.81)	Monoarticular to bilateral asymmetric Hand Wrists Shoulders Hips	Articular involvement includes asymmetric soft tissue masses, periarticular osteoporosis, erosions and cystic lesions with or without surrounding sclerosis and preservation of the joint space. Joint contractures and subluxations may also be present. Avascular necrosis may complicate amyloidosis in larger joints. Periarticular amyloid nodules or masses are frequently observed about the olecranon, shoulder, hand and wrist, where they can cause the carpal tunnel syndrome. Osteolytic lesions producing endosteal scalloping and, occasionally pathologic fractures and generalized osteoporosis are additional manifestations.	Primary amyloidosis occurs without coexistent disease or is associated with multiple myeloma. Secondary amyloidosis is associated with various chronic diseases including rheumatoid arthritis, sepsis, inflammatory disorders such as Crohn's disease, neoplasm and chronic hemodialysis. Primary amyloidosis is more frequent in men with an onset between 40 and 80 years. Amyloid joint disease shares many radiographic features with gout, xanthomatosis and pigmented villonodular synovitis.
Multicentric reticulohistiocytosis (lipoid dermatoarthritis) (Fig. 6.82)	Bilateral symmetric Hands Feet Wrists Shoulders Elbows Hips Knees Ankles Spine Sacroiliac joints	Predilection of the interphalangeal joints of the hands and feet with erosions originating at the joint margins and spreading centrally associated with soft tissue nodules is characteristic. The erosions are well circumscribed resembling defects seen in gout. The joint space is frequently preserved. Osteoporosis and new bone formation are absent. Progression to arthritis mutilans is seen in about one-third of cases. Severe erosive destructive changes in the cervical spine, especially the atlantoaxial joint is also a common manifestation. Erosions and bony ankylosis may be observed in the sacroiliac joints.	Uncommon systemic disease of unknown cause with female predominance and typical onset in middle age. In approximately two-thirds of patients polyarthritis is the first manifestation of the disease, followed after months to years by eruption of red to purple skin nodules measuring up to 1 cm in diameter. Patients may also reveal xanthomas preferentially involving the eyelids. Abnormal laboratory findings include anemia, hypercholesterolemia and elevated erythrocyte sedimentation rate.

(continues on page 166)

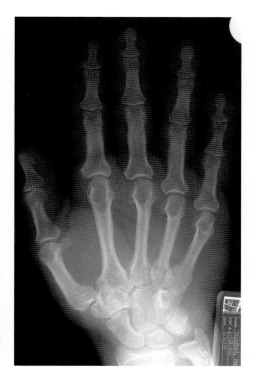

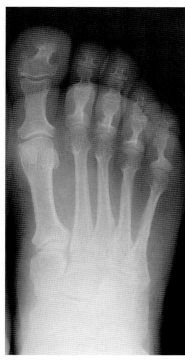

Fig. 6.**79 a, b** **Acromegaly**. Soft tissue thickening of the phalanges, joint space widening (especially metacarpophalangeal and metatarsophalangeal joints) enlarged tufts and bases of the terminal phalanges and prominent metacarpal and metatarsal heads are seen in the hand (**a**) and foot (**b**).

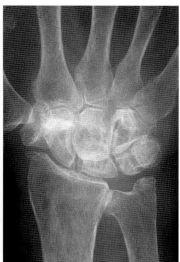

Fig. 6.**80** **Amyloidosis**. Osteopenia and multiple carpal cysts with relatively well preserved joint spaces are seen in the wrist.

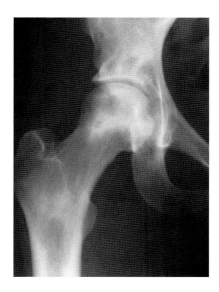

Fig. 6.**81** **Amyloidosis in chronic renal failure**. Poorly defined osteolytic lesions are seen in acetabular dome, femoral head and proximal femur shaft. In the former two locations the lesions are surrounded by an irregular and poorly demarcated sclerosis.

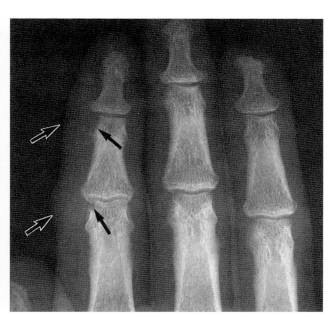

Fig. 6.**82** **Multicentric reticulohistiocytosis**. Soft tissue nodules (white arrows) are associated with marginal erosions (black arrows) in the proximal and distal interphalangeal joints of the index finger.

Table 6.14   (Cont.) Differential Diagnosis of Articular Disorders

Disease	Characteristic Location	Radiographic Findings	Comments
Osteoarthritis (degenerative joint disease (Figs. 6.83, 6.84, 6.85, 6.86, 6.87, 6.88, 6.89 and 6.90)	*Primary osteoarthritis:* Oligo-articular to polyarticular, often bilateral and relatively symmetric Hand (interphalangeal joints, rarely metacarpophalangeal joints). Wrist (first carpometacarpal joint, scaphotrapezio-trapezoidal joint) Hip Knee Foot (first metatarsophalangeal joint, tarsometatarsal joints and talonavicular joint) Acromioclavicular joint	Joint space loss, subchondral sclerosis, cyst formation and osteophytosis are the hallmark of osteoarthritis. The joint space loss in weight-bearing articulations typically is asymmetric and localized predominantly in the area that is subjective to excessive pressure (e.g. superior or weight-bearing portion of the hip, medial compartment of the knee). Subchondral sclerosis typically is confined to the area of joint space narrowing with progressive obliteration of this space. The sclerosis may extend both vertically and horizontally into the adjacent bone. Subchondral cysts (geodes) form within the pressure segment of the subchondral bone. The cysts commonly are multiple, and of variable size and depict sclerotic margins. They may or may not communicate with the joint. Osteophytosis: Marginal (peripheral) osteophytes are most common, developing as lips of new bone around the edges of the articular cartilage. Central osteophytes are button-like or flat excrescences within the articular surface denuded of cartilage. Thickening of the intra-articular cortex on the medial aspect of the femoral neck is termed buttressing and represents a periosteal osteophyte. Capsular osteophytes originating from the capsular attachment sites may be found in the interphalangeal joints producing the "seegull sign" as dorsal talar beak in the talonavicular joint. Degenerative enthesopathy may produce bony excrescences in the trochanters and ischial tuberosities and spurs in the calcaneus, patella and olecranon. Bony proliferation may be seen at syndesmotic insertion sites. Flattening and collapse of the articular surface may become apparent in a more advanced stage which is not always caused by the development of secondary avascular necrosis. Both joint effusions and synovial proliferation are not prominent features in osteoarthritis. Large effusions should suggest an inflammatory, infectious or traumatic arthritic process. Complications of osteoarthritis include malalignment (e.g. varus or, less commonly, valgus deformity and lateral subluxation in the knee, lateral displacement of the femoral head, radial subluxation in the first carpometacarpal joint, and radial or ulnar deviation in the interphalangeal joints) and the formation of loose intra-articular cartilagenous or osseous bodies.	Osteoarthritis is by far the most common joint disorder, one of the most common chronic diseases in the elderly and a leading cause of disability. There is a poor correlation between clinical symptoms and radiographic findings. The correlation between joint degeneration and advancing age is not linear. Rather, an age related predisposition to osteoarthritis appears to increase exponentially after the age of 50. Osteoarthritis refers to degenerative disease of synovial joints. Abnormalities, however, predominate in the cartilaginous and osseous tissues, whereas alterations in the synovium are generally mild. Primary (idiopathic) osteoarthritis occurs in the absence of any underlying abnormality. Secondary osteoarthritis refers to joint degeneration produced by a pre-existing condition. *Secondary osteoarthritis* (Figs. 6.**91**, 6.**92** and 6.**93**) is associated with pre-existing articular disease or deformity, trauma and chronic overuse and thus frequently involves articular sites that are not commonly affected in primary osteoarthritis. Secondary osteoarthritis may follow inflammatory or infectious arthritis, episodes of minor or major trauma, and congenital disorders. Chronic athletic and occupational overuse is associated with joint degeneration at specific locations: Workers using vibrating or pneumatic tools (e.g. miners or jackhammer operators) develop arthritic changes in the elbows, wrists and hands (especially carpal cysts), ballet dancers in the ankles and feet, football and soccer players in the ankles, feet, hips and knees, cyclists in the patellofemoral joints, boxers and wrestlers in the hands, wrists, elbows, and baseball players in the shoulder and elbows. *Sacroiliac joints* (Fig. 6.**94**): Besides focal or diffuse, well-defined subchondral sclerosis with or without loss of joint space, erosions are occasionally also seen in degenerative sacroiliac joint disease. An anterior bridging osteophyte is not uncommon and may mimic an osteoblastic metastasis centered over the sacroiliac joint. Subchondral cysts are relatively uncommon, but may contain gas (pneumatocyst) even in the absence of a vacuum phenomenon in the sacroiliac joint. *Rapidly destructive osteoarthritis of the hip* refers to an osteolytic destruction of the hip without osteophytosis within weeks. Besides osteoarthritis, CPPD, HADD and osteonecrosis have also been implicated (Fig. 6.**95**).

(continues on page 169)

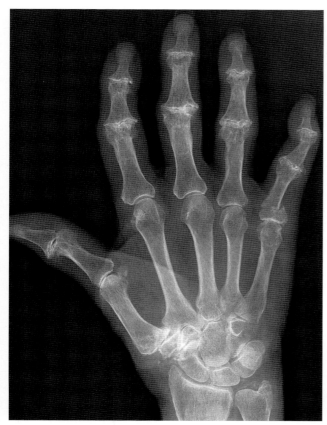

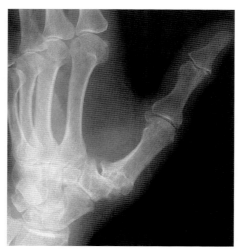

Fig. 6.**84** **Osteoarthritis**. Advanced degenerative changes including joint space narrowing, sclerosis, subchondral cyst formation and mild lateral subluxation are present in the first carpometacarpal joint.

Fig. 6.**83** **Osteoarthritis**. Arthritic changes including joint space narrowing and osteophytosis are seen in all interphalangeal joints,he first carpometacarpal joint and the scaphotrapeziotrapezoidal joint whereas the metacarpophalangeal joints are spared. Osteopenia and a fracture of the base of the proximal phalanx of the fifth finger are incidentally also present. Calcification of the triangular fibrocartilage is also evident.

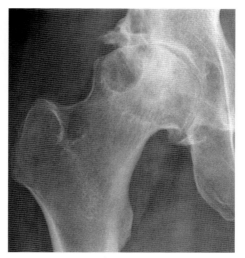

Fig. 6.**85** **Osteoarthritis**. Joint space narrowing in the superolateral aspect of the hip is associated with adjacent subchondral cyst formation in the acetabulum and femoral head. Considerable osteophytosis is also seen in the acetabulum.

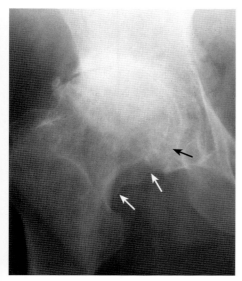

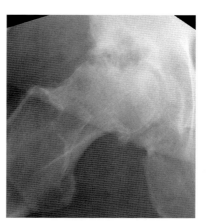

Fig. 6.**86** **Osteoarthritis**. Joint space narrowing limited to the weight-bearing portion of the hip associated with subchondral sclerosis is seen. New bone formation (buttressing) along the medial aspect of the femoral head and neck is also evident (arrows).

Fig. 6.**87** **Osteoarthritis**. Advanced degenerative changes with fragmentation of the subchondral bone of both the femoral head and acetabulum in the weight-bearing portion of the hip is evident.

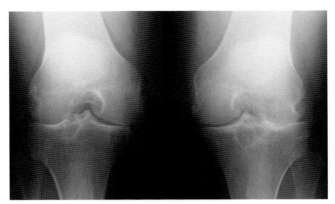

Fig. 6.**88** **Osteoarthritis**. Advanced degenerative changes with joint space narrowing, sclerosis, osteophytosis, subchondral cysts and loose bodies in the intercondylar notch are seen in both knees.

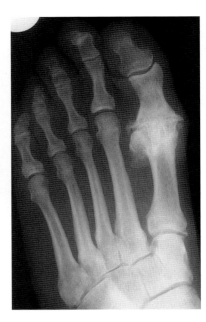

Fig. 6.**89** **Osteoarthritis (hallux rigidus)**. Advanced degenerative changes with joint space narrowing, extensive subchondral sclerosis and osteophytosis are seen in the first metatarsophalangeal joint.

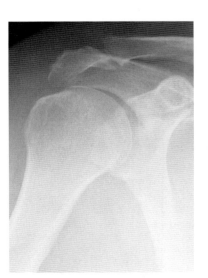

Fig. 6.**90** **Osteoarthritis**. Hypertrophic degenerative changes with inferior spurring are seen in the acromioclavicular joint causing impingement on the supraspinatus muscle and tendon (impingement syndrome).

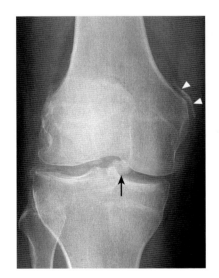

Fig. 6.**91** **Post-traumatic osteoarthritis**. Chondrocalcinosis in the lateral meniscus, a large intra-articular loose body (arrow) and a shell-like ossification (arrowheads) along the medial femoral condyle (Pelligrini-Stieda ossification) indicative of a chronic medial collateral ligament injury are seen.

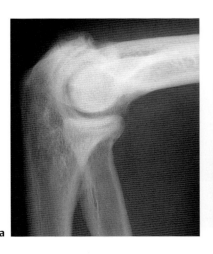

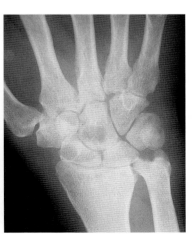

Fig. 6.**92 a, b** **Chronic overuse osteoarthritis.** **a Javelin thrower:** Degenerative changes including subchondral sclerosis, mild osteophytosis and healed fracture of the tip of the olecranon are seen in a javelin thrower. **b Jackhammer operator:** Multiple carpal cysts and early degenerative changes in the radiocarpal and distal radioulnar joints are seen in a patient with normal bone mineralization.

a   b

Table 6.14   (Cont.) Differential Diagnosis of Articular Disorders

Disease	Characteristic Location	Radiographic Findings	Comments
Erosive osteoarthritis (Fig. 6.96)	Bilateral symmetric Interphalangeal joints of the hand	Findings of advanced osteoarthritis (joint space narrowing, subchondral sclerosis and prominent marginal osteophytes) are associated with erosions. They commonly originate in the central portion of the joint as sharply marginated defects. Their central location differs from the marginal erosions seen in rheumatoid and psoriatic arthritis. Progression to bony ankylosis is not infrequent. In contrast to psoriatic arthritis the distribution pattern tends to be bilateral symmetric.	Presents clinically with acute inflammatory episodes including painful Heberden's and Bouchard's nodes (marginal osteophytes and soft tissue thickening about the distal and proximal interphalangeal joints, respectively) in women (male/female ratio is 1:10). May be associated with primary (noninflammatory) osteoarthritis in other joints of the hand and wrist.

(continues on page 170)

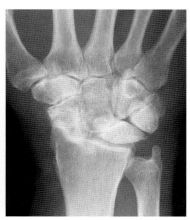

Fig. 6.**93   Post-traumatic scapholunate advanced collapse (SLAC).** Sclerosis and compression of the proximal scaphoid secondary to a healed fracture, scapholunate dissociation, and proximal migration of the scaphoid with obliteration of the radioscaphoid space are seen. Mild compression, rotation and sclerosis of the lunate with degenerative changes in the lunocapitate joint are also associated.

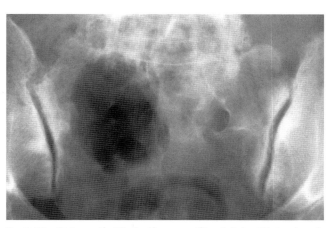

Fig. 6.**94   Osteoarthritis in the sacroiliac joints.** Bilateral well-defined subchondral sclerosis without erosions or joint space narrowing is seen.

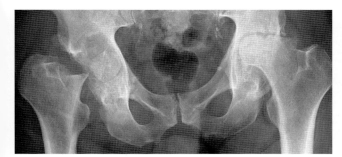

Fig. 6.**95   Rapidly destructive osteoarthritis of the hip.** Bilateral osteolytic destruction of both acetabula and femoral heads is seen. On the right side the process is further advanced and involves also the femoral neck.

Fig. 6.**96   Erosive osteoarthritis.** Joint space narrowing, sub- ▷ chondral sclerosis and osteophytosis are associated in several interphalangeal joints with central erosions. Degenerative changes with small subchondral cyst formation are also seen in both first carpometacarpal joints.

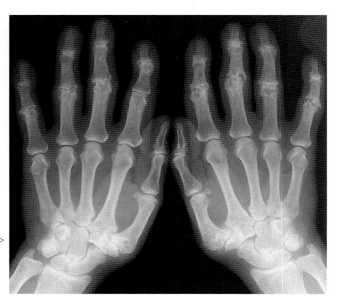

Table 6.14   (Cont.) Differential Diagnosis of Articular Disorders

Disease	Characteristic Location	Radiographic Findings	Comments
Degenerative disease of the spine (Figs. 6.97, 6.98, 6.99, 6.100, and 6.101)	Middle and lower cervical spine Lower lumbar spine	Degeneration of the intervertebral disc (*osteochondrosis*) may present with disc space narrowing, reactive sclerosis of the adjacent endplates, osteophytosis and vacuum phenomena (gas) within the disc. (DD: vacuum phenomenon within a vertebral body suggests ischemic necrosis). Degenerative disc calcification is uncommon. In children nucleus pulposus calcification occurs in the cervical spine as an isolated finding and may rupture into the adjacent vertebral body, intervertebral foramen or spinal canal. Large anterolateral osteophyte formations caused by disc displacement in that direction is referred to as *spondylosis deformans*. Superior and inferior disc displacement produces a cartilagenous (Schmorl's) node evident as a radiolucent lesion surrounded by a sclerotic rim. Posterior and posterolateral disc displacement is of greatest clinical significance because of its relationship with neurological structures, but cannot be assessed with plain film radiography. Degenerative changes in the apophyseal (facet) joints (*spondylarthrosis*) are also common and present with joint space narrowing, bony eburnation and osteophytosis. Ligamentous laxity may result in mild anterolisthesis (not associated with pars defect) or retrolisthesis. The neural foramina in the cervical spine below C2 may be encroached by osteophytes, frequently originating from the uncovertebral (Luschka's) joints.	Conditions associated with degenerative disease of the spine include costovertebral osteoarthritis, Baastrup's disease and Bertolotti's syndrome. *Costovertebral osteoarthritis*: The costovertebral joints are located between the head of the ribs and the vertebral bodies and between the necks and tubercles of the ribs and the transverse processes. Degenerative changes, predominant in the articulations of the 11th and 12th ribs, include joint space narrowing, bony eburnation and osteophytosis and may progress to complete bony ankylosis with pagetoid appearance of the posterior portion of the affected rib. *Baastrup's disease*: Extensive disc space loss or excessive lordosis of the lumbar spine leads to approximation and contact of the often unusually large spinous processes. Degenerative changes including reactive sclerosis and osteophytosis may develop between the "kissing spines" and may be associated with considerable pain. *Bertolotti's syndrome*: Degenerative changes may be found in the articulations between the transverse processes of a transitional vertebra in the lumbosacral junction and the adjacent sacral wing. The relationship of back pain to this finding is however debated.

(continues on page 172)

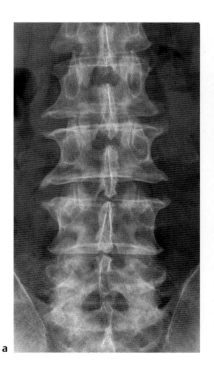
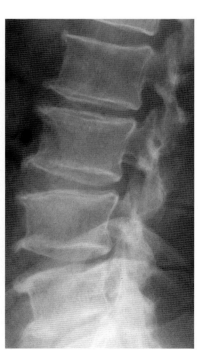

Fig. 6.97 a, b   Degenerative disease of the spine (spondylosis deformans). Anterolateral osteophytosis throughout the lumbar spine is the dominant radiographic manifestation seen in anterolateral (**a**) and lateral (**b**) projection.

a   b

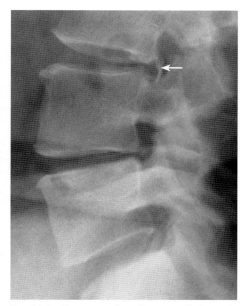

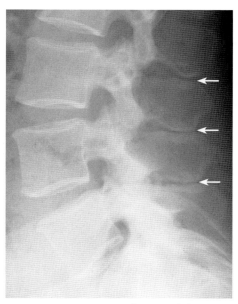

Fig. 6.98 Degenerative disease of the spine (osteochondrosis). Narrowing of the intervertebral space with relatively little osteophytosis is the dominant radiographic manifestation best seen at L4/5. Less severe disc space narrowing with calcification of the posterior longitudinal ligament (arrow) that is posteriorly displaced by the bulging disc and small anterior osteophyte formation is seen at L3/4.

Fig. 6.99 Degenerative disease of the spine (spondylarthrosis and Baastrup's disease). Spondylarthrosis: Degenerative changes in the apophyseal (facet) joints presenting with joint space narrowing, bony eburnation and osteophytosis are seen in all segments of the lumbar spine. Baastrup's disease: Degenerative changes including reactive sclerosis are also seen between the unusually large spinous processes (arrows) which appear in contact with each other ("kissing spines").

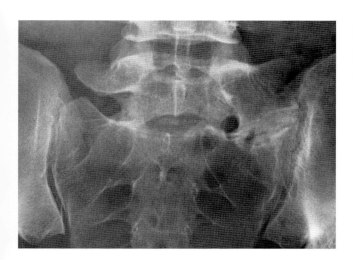

Fig. 6.100 Bertolotti's syndrome. Partial sacralization of L5 is seen. Degenerative changes between the enlarged left transverse process of this transitional vertebra and the adjacent sacral wing are evident by the extensive sclerosis at the contact site of these two parts.

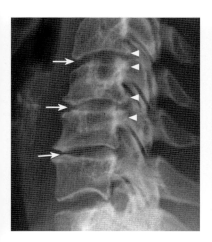

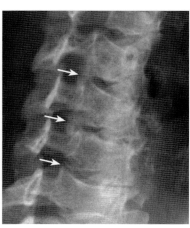

b

Fig. 6.101 a, b Degenerative cervical spine disease. Disc space narrowing with mild osteophytosis is seen between C4/5, C5/6, and C6/7 (arrows). Small osteophytes (arrowheads) protruding posteriorly into the spinal canal are seen in **a**. Encroachment of the right neural foramina by small osteophytes (arrows) originating from the uncovertebral (Luschka's) joints are evident in **b**.

Table 6.14   (Cont.) Differential Diagnosis of Articular Disorders

Disease	Characteristic Location	Radiographic Findings	Comments
Diffuse idiopathic skeletal hyperostosis (DISH, Forestier's disease) (Figs. 6.102 and 6.103)	Spine (especially lower thoracic and upper lumbar area) Pelvis Calcaneus Patella Olecranon	Diagnostic criteria in the spine include: 1. Flowing ossifications along the anterolateral aspect of at least 4 contiguous vertebral bodies. 2. Relative preservation of the disc space and absence of significant degenerative signs such as reactive sclerosis and vacuum phenomena in the involved segment. 3. Absence of bony ankylosis in the apophyseal joints and no evidence of sacroiliitis. Pelvis: Bony proliferation ("whiskering") in the iliac crests, ischial tuberosities and trochanters. Broad osteophytes at the lateral acetabular edges, inferior portions of the sacroiliac joints and superior aspect of pubic symphysis. Ossifications of iliolumbar, sacrotuberous and sacroiliac ligaments. Enthesophytes without adjacent reactive bone sclerosis or erosions at numerous sites, most commonly in the calcaneus, patella and olecranon.	Common ossifying diathesis characterized by bone proliferation at sites of tendinous and ligamentous attachment (entheses). Presents usually with mild symptoms of restricted spinal motion and tendinitis in patients over 50 years of age with 3:1 male predominance. The cause of DISH is unknown. It might be considered a hypertrophic variant of spondylosis deformans. Bony hyperostosis of the spine somewhat similar to DISH is associated with endocrine disorders such as acromegaly, hypoparathyroidism and diabetes mellitus. Hyperostosis of the spine and ligamentous calcifications are also found with fluorosis, but the latter condition is associated with diffuse osteosclerosis of the axial skeleton. Prolonged therapy for skin disorders with retinoid drugs (e.g. Acutane®), which are chemically similar to vitamin A, may also induce hyperostosis in both the axial and appendicular skeleton. Excessive heterotopic bone formation after prosthetic hip or knee replacement is frequently observed with DISH. *Ossification of the posterior longitudinal ligament (OPLL)* (Fig. 6.**104**) affects the cervical spine and is often associated with DISH.

(continues on page 174)

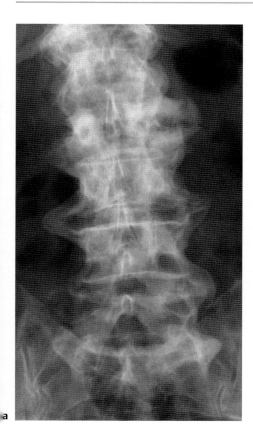

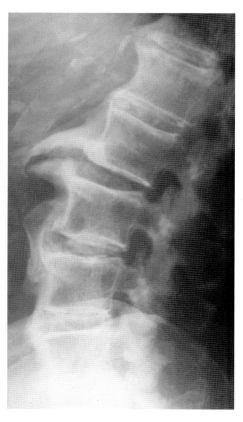

Fig. 6.**102 a, b**   **DISH**. Huge para-vertebral flowing ossifications with preservation of the disc spaces are noted throughout the lumbar spine in anteroposterior (**a**) and lateral (**b**) projection. Note also the absence of bony ankylosis in the apophyseal (facet) joints and the normal sacroiliac joints.

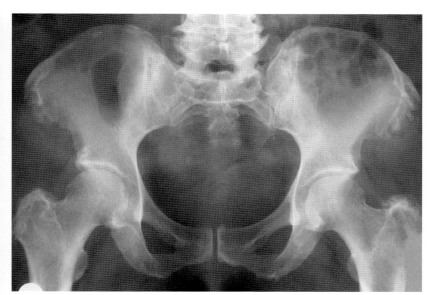

Fig. 6.**103**   **DISH**. Symmetrical bony proliferation ("whiskering") is seen in the iliac crests, greater trochanters and to a lesser degree in the ischial tuberosities.

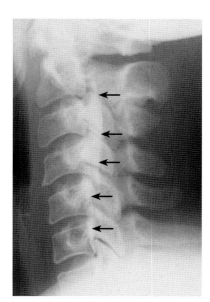

Fig. 6.**104**   **Ossification of the posterior longitudinal ligament (OPLL)** is seen in the cervical spine (arrows).

Table 6.14 (Cont.) Differential Diagnosis of Articular Disorders

Disease	Characteristic Location	Radiographic Findings	Comments

Neuropathic osteoarthropathy (Charcot joint) (Figs. 6.105, 6.106, 6.107, 6.108, 6.109 and 6.110)	Congenital indifference to pain and meningomyeloceles:
	  Knees
	  Ankles
	  Intertarsal joints
	Syringomyelia:
	  Shoulders
	  Elbows
	Tabes dorsalis:
	  Hips
	  Knees
	  Ankles
	  Spine
	Diabetes mellitus:
	  Midfoot
	  Forefoot
	Leprosy:
	  Hands
	  Feet
		Persistent joint effusion, often with cartilaginous and osseous debri (detritic synovitis) resulting from fragmentation of the articular surface are early findings. More advanced abnormalities include progressive rapid bone resorption or extensive joint destruction with marked sclerosis and osteophytosis, intra-articular osseous fragments, subluxations, massive effusions and fractures of neighboring bones. The end result is a completely disorganized joint with predominant features of bone resorption, new bone formation, or both.
		Diabetic foot: Fragmentation, sclerosis, subluxations or dislocations are characteristically found in the tarsometatarsal joints resembling a Lisfranc fracture/dislocation. Collapse of the plantar arch with talar malalignment and fragmentation of various tarsal bones is also a common manifestation. Flattening and fragmentation of the metatarsal heads resembling Freiberg's infarction or partial to complete resorption of the metatarsal heads and adjacent proximal phalanges with tapering of the remaining shafts are other presentations. Furthermore ischemic and infectious processes are frequently superimposed on the neuropathic changes in the diabetic foot.
			Hypertrophic bone changes are caused by repetitive trauma/microtrauma with attempted repair. Atrophic resorptive changes are caused by sympathetic dysfunction resulting in hyperemia and bone resorption. Congenital causes include myelomeningoceles and congenital indifference to pain. Acquired causes include brain and cord injuries or tumors, syringomyelia, tabes dorsalis, diabetes mellitus and leprosy.
			Axial neuropathic osteoarthropathy is usually productive and best described as greatly exaggerated degenerative changes in the spine with malalignment, profound reactive sclerosis and osteophytes reaching mammoth proportions. Osteolytic or destructive changes are less common and may result in rapid disintegration of vertebral bodies and/or apophyseal joints that can mimic infection or metastases. It is relatively common in *tabes dorsalis* with preferential involvement of the lumbar spine, but also seen in *syringomyelia* where it primarily affects the cervical spine.
			Congenital indifference to pain becomes manifest in infancy or childhood. Findings include amputation of fingers and toes caused by self-mutilation and fractures of the long bones with frequent epiphyseal separation.
			Leprosy: Skeletal abnormalities occurring on a neurological basis are much more frequent and severe than those produced by direct leprous infiltration. Acro-osteolysis and tapered resorption of the end of phalanges, metacarpals and metatarsals resulting in "licked candy stick" appearance are characteristic.

(continues on page 176)

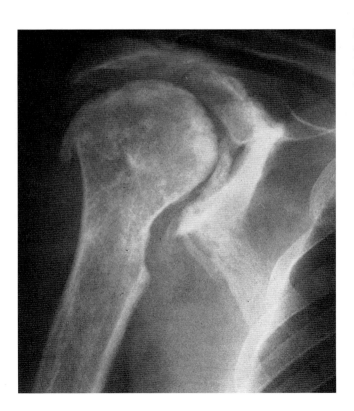

Fig. 6.**105 Neuropathic osteoarthropathy (syringomyelia).** Advanced arthritis with destruction of the glenoid, intra-articular fragments, sclerosis and osteophytosis is seen. Superior migration of the humeral head indicating a chronic rotator cuff tear is also evident.

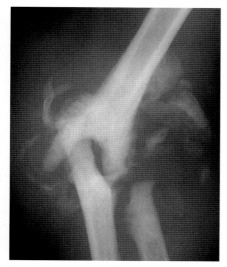

Fig. 6.**106** **Neuropathic osteoarthropathy (syringomyelia)**. A completely disorganized elbow with multiple fracture fragments and extensive sclerosis is seen.

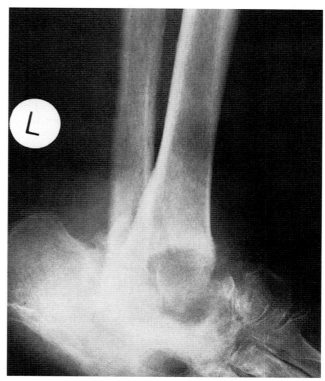

Fig. 6.**107** **Neuropathic osteoarthropathy (tabes dorsalis)**. Destruction of the ankle, subtalar and talonavicular joints with collapsed plantar arch and extensive sclerosis is seen.

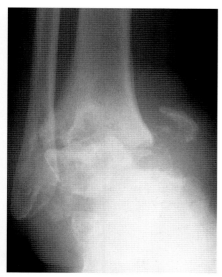

Fig. 6.**108** **Neuropathic osteoarthropathy (congenital indifference to pain)**. Extensive soft tissue swelling is associated with multiple fractures in the distal tibia and talus, angular deformity of the ankle, numerous loose fracture fragments, sclerosis and periostitis.

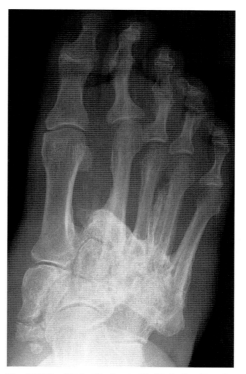

Fig. 6.**109** **Diabetic foot**. Multiple healing fractures with extensive callus formation in the mid and forefoot are associated with a collapsed and disrupted Lisfranc joint. Arteriosclerotic calcifications characteristically are also present.

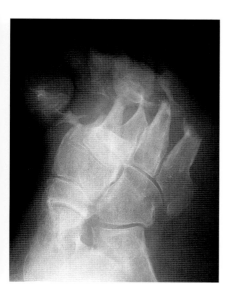

Fig. 6.**110** **Leprosy**. Multiple subluxations/dislocations and extensive osteolysis are seen in the forefoot resulting in a tapered appearance of many metatarsals and phalanges ("licked candy stick" appearance).

Table 6.14   (Cont.) Differential Diagnosis of Articular Disorders

Disease	Characteristic Location	Radiographic Findings	Comments
Pyogenic (septic) arthritis (Figs. 6.111, 6.112, 6.113 and 6.114)	Monoarticular Hip Knee Spine	Every monoarticular inflammatory arthritic process should be considered infectious until proven otherwise. Acute stage: Para-articular soft tissue swelling, joint effusion (frequently producing widening of the joint space in children) and juxta-articular osteoporosis followed by diffuse joint space narrowing due to rapid destruction of the articular cartilage and marginal and central bony erosions. Subacute/chronic stage: Subchondral bone destruction with reactive bone sclerosis, secondary degenerative changes and eventually bony ankylosis may be found. In the spine disc space narrowing and loss of normal definition of the adjacent endplates progressing rapidly to frank destruction of the subchondral bone plate or enlarging destructive foci is characteristic. After 2 to 3 months reparative changes become evident in the form of reactive sclerosis. In children a hematogenous infection of the intervertebral disc alone ("diskitis") without involvement of the neighboring vertebral bodies may occur as long as the blood supply to the discs remains intact. Diskitis may occur in adults by direct inoculation of the offending agent during diagnostic or surgical procedures. Sacroiliac joint infection typically is unilateral differentiating it from many other arthritic processes that are frequently bilateral.	A hematogenous infection-induced arthritis is either caused by direct infiltration and subsequent multiplication of the viable organism or without direct contamination of the joint. The latter is referred to as *reactive arthritis* and found with rheumatic fever and Lyme disease where it is caused by an antigen-mediated immune response to the offending organism. A sympathetic joint effusion adjacent to a site of inflammation may also mimic an acute infectious arthritic process. *Routes of infectious joint contamination* include *hematogenous spread, contiguous spread* (intra-articular extension of osteomyelitis or neighboring soft tissue abscess) and *direct implantation* (penetrating trauma or iatrogenic procedure). In infants and children monoarticular involvement of the knee or hip is the most common presentation. In the adult the lumbar spine and knee are the most common sites of involvement. Common organisms include staphylococcus aureus and streptococcus pyogenes at all ages, hemophilus influenza in children, and neisseria gonorrhoeae (often more than one joint involved) and brucella in adults. A prompt and definite diagnosis requires an arthrocentesis, blood cultures and possibly bone biopsy (spine).

(continues on page 178)

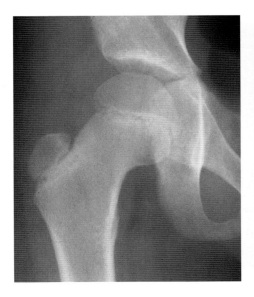 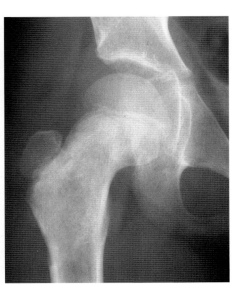

Fig. 6.**111 a, b   Pyogenic (septic) arthritis**. A joint effusion evident by the slight lateral subluxation of the femoral head is the only abnormality seen in **a**. Six weeks later narrowing of the joint space, especially medially, due to destruction of the articular cartilage and poorly defined mixed osteolytic and osteosclerotic areas in the femoral neck and adjacent shaft are seen in **b**.

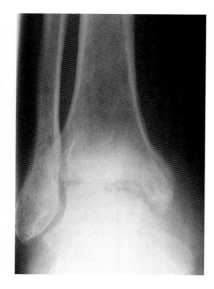

Fig. 6.**112**   **Pyogenic (septic) arthritis**. Joint space narrowing with destruction and fragmentation of the subchondral bone in the medial talar dome and adjacent tibia plafond is seen. Beginning periostitis in the distal tibia and fibula is also evident.

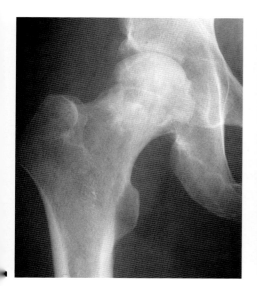 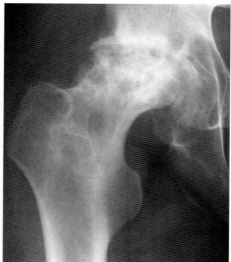

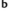

Fig. 6.**113 a, b**   **Pyogenic (septic) arthritis**. Joint space narrowing and poorly defined osteolytic and osteosclerotic lesions are seen in the femoral head and proximal neck in **a**. One year later marked disease progression with destruction and fragmentation of both the femoral head and acetabulum, osseous debris accumulation in the hip with lateral subluxation of the femoral head, extension of the osteomyelitic process into the intertrochanteric area and beginning repair (sclerosis of the acetabular roof with adjacent osteophyte formation) is seen in **b**.

b

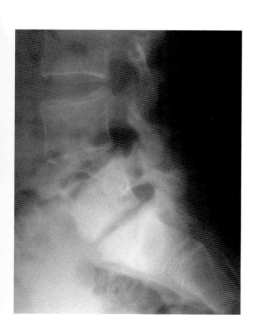

Fig. 6.**114**   **Diskitis**. Narrowing of the intervertebral space between L5 and S1 with slightly irregular adjacent endplates and marked sclerosis of the adjacent bone is seen.

Table 6.14   (Cont.) Differential Diagnosis of Articular Disorders

Disease	Characteristic Location	Radiographic Findings	Comments
Tuberculous arthritis (Figs. 6.115, 6.116 and 6.117)	Monoarticular Spine Hip Knee	Tuberculous spondylitis most commonly affects the thoracolumbar area. It may involve more than one intervertebral disc and has a predilection for the anterior aspect of the vertebral body. Extension into the adjacent ligaments and soft tissue is frequent allowing osseous or disc invasion at distant sites or leading to the formation of a psoas abscess that tends to calcify. A gibbus deformity in the thoracolumbar area may be the end result. In the appendicular joints Phemister's triad is characteristic consisting of juxta-articular osteoporosis, marginal erosions and gradual narrowing of the joint space. Compared to a pyogenic arthritis a delay in destruction of the articular cartilage or intervertebral disc, absence of reparative sclerosis, and calcification of the associated soft tissue abscesses are all suggestive of tuberculosis.	Skeletal tuberculosis can affect persons of all ages, but less than 1% of patients infected with tuberculosis have bone or joint manifestations. Tuberculous spondylitis is the most frequent skeletal manifestation presenting with an insidious onset of back pain, stiffness, local tenderness and possibly fever. Appendicular tuberculous arthritis may present with pain, swelling, weakness, muscle wasting and a draining sinus. Globally tuberculosis is the leading infectious cause of morbity and mortality. In industrialized nations the disease has retreated from the general population, affecting selected groups. In the United States an upsurge in tuberculosis has been noted since 1985 that is linked to the HIV epidemic.
Fungal arthritis (Fig. 6.118)	Monoarticular Large appendicular joints Spine	Joint involvement is usually caused by direct extension from an adjacent osseous focus and rarely by direct hematogenous implantation. Soft tissue swelling, effusion, joint space narrowing, erosions or bony destruction, with or without osteoporosis are observed in these cases.	Usually in patients with compromised immune system. Cryptococcosis, North American blastomycosis, coccidioidomycosis, histoplasmosis, sporotrichosis (especially hand and foot), and candidiasis are common organisms. *Madura foot*: Single or multiple osseous defects to extensive destruction with periostitis and sclerosis leading to extensive intra-articular osseous fusion ("melting snow" appearance).
Viral arthritis	Monoarticular to polyarticular Peripheral joints Often polyarticular	Nonspecific joint effusion without bony involvement. Chronic arthropathy following rubella vaccination/infection is occasionally seen resembling juvenile rheumatoid arthritis	Transient arthritis associated with rubella, mumps, mycoplasma infections, and hepatitis. Osteomyelitis and arthritis (suppurative and nonsuppurative) were in the past well-known complications of smallpox (variola).
HIV infection (AIDS) (Fig. 6.119)	Oligoarticular to polyarticular Knee Ankle Foot Hand	Reiter's-like asymmetric oligoarticular or polyarticular involvement of preferentially the lower extremity with considerable enthesopathy, especially in the foot (AIDS-foot). Peripheral arthropathy similar to psoriatic arthritis is also found. Involvement of the axial skeleton with the exception of the sacroiliac joint is uncommon.	HIV shares certain aspects of cellular immune deficiency elements with seronegative spondylarthropathies such as Reiter's syndrome and psoriasis. Septic, tuberculous and fungal arthritis are not uncommon in AIDS patients either (Figs. 6.**120** and 6.**121**). This infective arthritic process is monoarticular and, besides the knee and the sacroiliac joint, the larger joints of the upper extremity, and the acromioclavicular and sternoclavicular joints are frequently affected.

(continues on page 180)

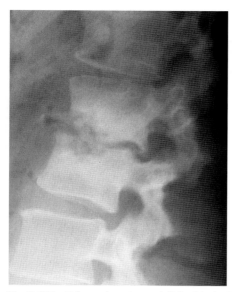

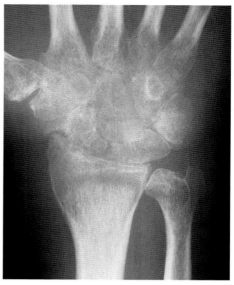

Fig. 6.**115** **Tuberculous spondylitis**. Marked disc space narrowing and a destructive lesion with fragmentation affecting the anterior aspect of the adjacent two vertebral bodies resulting in focal kyphosis (gibbus deformity) is seen at L1/2.

Fig. 6.**116** **Tuberculous arthritis**. Severe localized osteopenia associated with joint space narrowing and multiple small erosions is seen in the wrist involving the radiocarpal, intercarpal and carpometacarpal joints. The normal contralateral wrist in this patient differentiates this condition radiographically from rheumatoid arthritis.

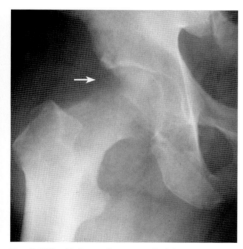

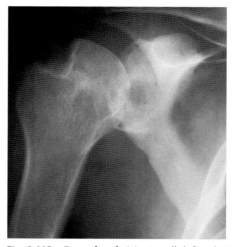

Fig. 6.**117** **Tuberculous arthritis**. Juxta-articular osteopenia, joint space narrowing and a poorly defined erosion (arrow) in the lateral aspect of the femoral head are seen.

Fig. 6.**118** **Fungal arthritis**. A well defined triangular osseous defect with sclerotic margin is seen in the greater tuberosity. Several poorly defined osteolytic lesions with surrounding sclerosis in the humeral head and glenoid are also seen in this patient with AIDS.

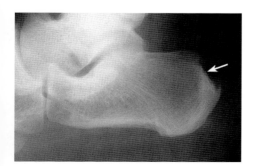

Fig. 6.**119** **HIV infection**. An erosive lesion (arrow) with minimal spiculated new bone formation is seen in the superolateral aspect of the calcaneus.

Table 6.14   (Cont.) Differential Diagnosis of Articular Disorders

Disease	Characteristic Location	Radiographic Findings	Comments
Pigmented villonodular synovitis (PVNS) (Figs. 6.122, 6.123 and 6.124)	Monoarticular Knee Hip Ankle Elbow Wrist	Dense appearing soft tissue swelling around the involved joint due to hemosiderin deposition in synovial proliferation and joint effusion. Pressure erosions and cysts are common in joints with tight capsule (e.g. hip, ankle, wrist). Osteoporosis and intra-articular calcifications/loose bodies are absent. Joint space is preserved until very late in the disease.	Highly vascularized, tumor-like synovial proliferation with multinucleated giant cells ingesting hemosiderin. Occurs typically in adults in the 3rd and 4th decade of life. Hemorrhagic (chocolate-brown) effusions in the absence of trauma are characteristic.
Synovial osteo-chondroma-tosis (Figs. 6.125, 6.126 and 6.127)	Usually monoarticular Occasionally bilateral Knee Hip Elbow Shoulder	Multiple calcified/ossified synovial nodules or loose bodies ranging in size from a few millimeters to several centimeters are characteristic. One-third of chondromas are not calcified. Lesions may cause pressure erosions in the adjacent bone (e.g. hip) and widening of the joint space. No osteoporosis is evident. Secondary osteoarthritis occurs in advanced disease from chronic mechanical irritation by the loose bodies. Malignant transformation to chondrosarcoma is extremely rare.	Presents in the 3rd to 5th decades of life with chronic joint pain, limitation of motion and locking with 3:1 male predominance. *Synovial chondrometaplasia* occasionally occurs in the elderly patient with advanced primary osteoarthritis causing chronic synovial inflammation and subsequently secondary osteochondromatosis. Differential diagnosis includes *synovial hemangioma*, *lipoma arborescens* and pigmented villonodular synovitis.

(continues on page 182)

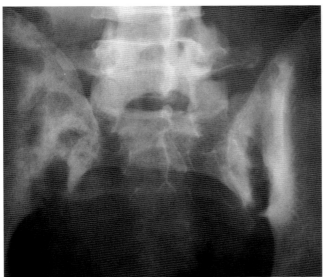

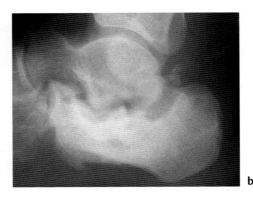

a

b

Fig. 6.**120 a, b   Septic arthritis in AIDS** (2 cases). **a** Widening of both sacroiliac joints caused by erosion and destruction of the adjacent bone with extensive sclerosis is seen. The bilateral involvement is unusual for septic arthritis. **b** Destruction of the subtalar joint is associated with extensive sclerosis primarily of the calcaneus.

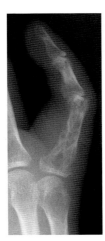

Fig. 6.**121   Tuberculous arthritis in AIDS**. Osteolysis of the proximal phalanx of the fifth finger with a coarsened, reticulated pattern reminiscent of sarcoidosis is seen extending into the proximal interphalangeal joint.

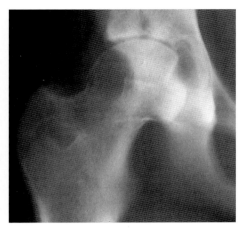

Fig. 6.**122**   **Pigmented villonodular synovitis**. Extrinsic pressure erosions present as scalloped extrinsic osteolytic lesions in the lateral aspect of the femoral neck and acetabulum.

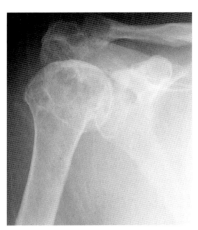

Fig. 6.**123**   **Pigmented villonodular synovitis**. Multiple lobulated cystic lesions often with minimally sclerotic margins are seen in the humeral head, acromion and distal clavicle.

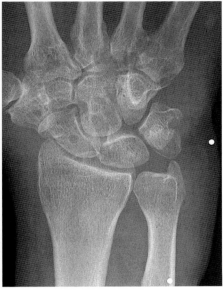

Fig. 6.**124**   **Pigmented villonodular synovitis**. A large soft mass along the distal ulna outlined by two metallic skin markers is associated with multiple erosions/cystic lesions in many carpal bones and the bases of metacarpals 3 to 5.

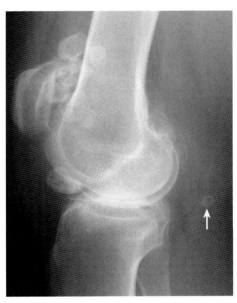

Fig. 6.**125**   **Synovial osteochondromatosis**. Multiple ossified loose bodies are seen in the knee joint, suprapatellar bursa and popliteal (Baker) cyst (arrow).

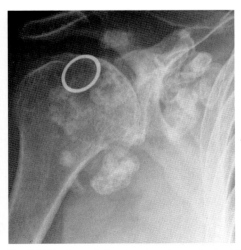

Fig. 6.**126**   **Synovial osteochondromatosis**. Multiple calcified or ossified loose bodies are seen in the glenohumeral joint including the axillary and subscapular recesses.

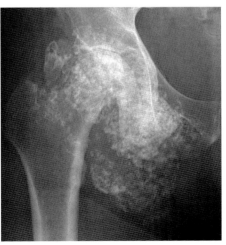

Fig. 6.**127**   **Synovial osteochondromatosis**. Innumerable small calcified loose bodies are seen in a hugely enlarged hip joint.

Table 6.14 (Cont.) Differential Diagnosis of Articular Disorders

Disease	Characteristic Location	Radiographic Findings	Comments
Osteochondritis dissecans (osteochondral fracture) (Figs. 6.128, 6.129, 6.130 and 6.131)	Knee: Medial femoral condyle. Less commonly lateral femoral condyle, tibia, and patella. Talus: Lateral and medial dome Elbow: Capitellum Shoulder: Humeral head and glenoid	Osteochondral fracture with characteristic location. The spectrum ranges from an in situ lesion with intact articular cartilage over a detached osteochondral body still located in the original pit (mouse bed) to a completely detached osteochondral fragment (mouse) away from the pit evident as a subchondral defect with sclerotic margin. Soft tissue swelling and joint effusions are frequently associated. Knee: The most common location is the nonweight-bearing portion of the medial femoral condyle at the intercondylar notch (70%). Other locations in the knee include the weight-bearing portions of either the medial or lateral femoral condyle and rarely the anterior aspect of the lateral femoral condyle and the medial facet of the patella	Presents most commonly in male adolescents and young adults with pain aggravated by motion, clicking and locking or maybe asymptomatic. It represents a subchondral fatigue fracture, but a single traumatic event is occasionally identified (especially in the talus). A purely cartilaginous lesion cannot be appreciated by plain film radiography and requires MR imaging or CT arthrography for accurate diagnosis. Avascular necrosis of the knee may also present with findings resembling osteochondritis dissecans, but in this condition frequently both knees or both condyles in the same knee are affected.

(continues on page 183)

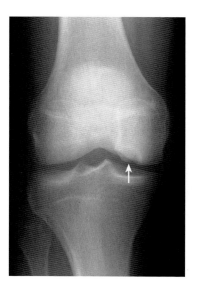

Fig. 6.**128 Osteochondritis dissecans.** A 1 cm oval shaped bony fragment (arrow) is seen in an osteochondral defect (pit), located classically along the lateral non-weight-bearing segment of the medial femur condyle. At a later stage, the bony fragment may become dislodged from the pit and found as a loose body anywhere in the knee joint.

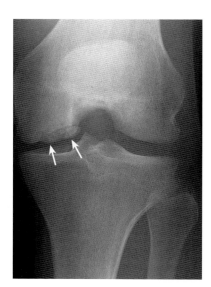

Fig. 6.**129 Osteochondritis dissecans.** An osteochondral defect extending from the intercondylar notch to the weight-bearing segment of the medial femur containing two osteochondral fracture fragments (arrows) is seen (extended classic variant).

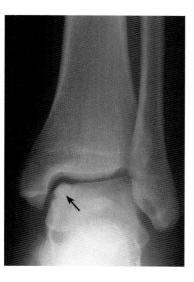

Fig. 6.**130 Osteochondritis dissecans.** A radiolucent line separates an oval shaped osseous body (arrow) from the medial talar dome. The lesion is referred to as in-situ when the articular cartilage covering the osseous fragment remains intact.

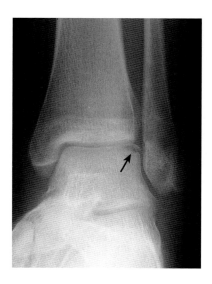

Fig. 6.**131 Osteochondral fracture.** An acute osteochondral fracture (arrow) is seen in the lateral talar dome. In the subacute/chronic stage this lesion may be impossible to differentiate from osteochondritis dissecans.

Table 6.14 (Cont.) Differential Diagnosis of Articular Disorders

Disease	Characteristic Location	Radiographic Findings	Comments
Avascular necrosis (osteonecrosis) (Figs. 6.132, 6.133, 6.134, 6.135, 6.136, 6.137 and 6.138)	Monoarticular, occasionallly bilateral Hip Knee Talus Scaphoid Shoulder	Articular involvement affecting only one site of the joint is characteristic. In an early stage plain film findings are absent or nonspecific and include mixed lytic and sclerotic changes producing a mottled appearance of the subchondral bone with preservation of the joint space. An arc-like subchondral lucent line (crescent sign in femoral head) is more specific. Progression of the disease results in subchondral cyst formation, fragmentation and eventually collapse of the affected epiphysis. At this stage loose intra-articular bony fragments are frequently present. The endstage is severe secondary osteoarthritis involving the entire joint. Post-traumatic avascular necrosis is most frequent in the femoral head (subcapital fracture, dislocation, or slipped capital femoral epiphysis), talar dome (talar neck fracture), humeral head (anatomic neck fracture, or severe fracture-dislocation), and proximal pole of scaphoid (scaphoid waist fracture).	For early diagnosis of avascular necrosis either radionuclide bone scintigraphy or magnetic resonance imaging is required. Primary avascular necrosis is uncommon in the adult except in the lunate (*Kienböck's disease*) and the knee (*Alhbäck's disease*). It is, however, common in children and adolescents (see Chapter 2). Secondary avascular necrosis is associated with trauma (fracture or dislocation), hemoglobinopathies (e.g. sickle cell anemia), exogeneous or endogeneous hypercortisolism, transplantation, alcoholism, pancreatitis, caisson disease, small vessel disease (e.g. systemic lupus erythematosus), Gaucher's disease, gout and radiation therapy. In many of these conditions more than one joint is involved and bone infarcts in the diametaphyses of the long bones may also be evident. *Ahlbäck's disease* or *spontaneous osteonecrosis of the knee (SONC)* usually occurs in patients over 60 years of age with female predominance. It presents with flattening of the weight-bearing portion of the medial femoral condyle. Involvement of the lateral condyle, tibial plateau or both knees are all uncommon. Progression of the disease results in further depression of the affected condyle with increased sclerosis and possible loose body formation. More recently a stress (insufficiency) fracture rather than osteonecrosis has been implicated as cansative factor for this condition.

(continues on page 185)

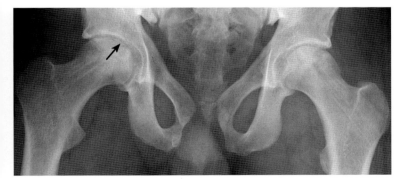

Fig. 6.**132 Avascular necrosis.** Early avascular necrosis presents with mixed lytic and sclerotic changes in both femoral heads without alteration of their shape. An arc-like subchondral lucent line (crescent sign) seen in the right femoral head (arrow) is a more specific finding and indicates progression of the disease. Sequelae from bilateral core decompression are evident by the oblique tracks extending from the greater trochanters to the femoral heads. Post-traumatic diastasis of the pubic symphysis is incidentally also present.

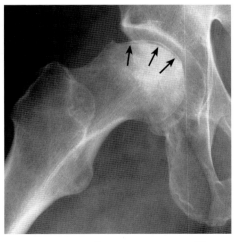

Fig. 6.**133 Avascular necrosis.** An arc-like subchondral lucent line (crescent sign) is seen (arrows).

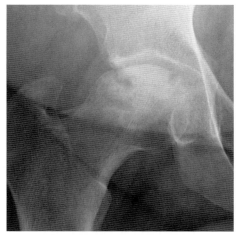

Fig. 6.**134** **Avascular necrosis**. Fragmentation of the femoral head in the weight-bearing segment results in flattening and collapse of the femoral head.

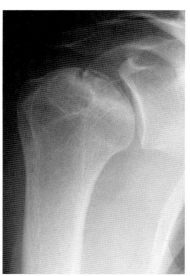

Fig. 6.**135** **Avascular necrosis**. Localized fragmentation of the humeral head in its superomedial aspect is seen. The osteochondral fracture fragment with crescent sign resides in an irregular pit with sclerotic margin. A large subchondral cyst infero-lateral to the pit is also evident.

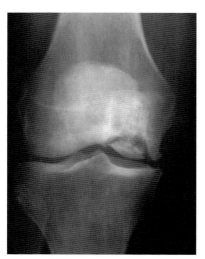

Fig. 6.**136** **Avascular necrosis**. A large detached osteochondral fragment is seen in the weight-bearing portion of the sclerotic medial femur condyle in this patient with systemic lupus erythematosus.

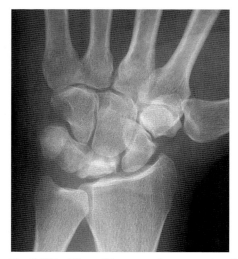

Fig. 6.**137** **Idiopathic avascular necrosis of the lunate (Kienböck's disease)**. A compressed, sclerotic lunate with several small cysts is seen.

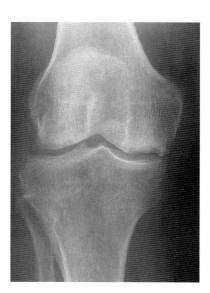

Fig. 6.**138** **Spontaneous osteonecrosis of the knee (Ahlbäck's disease)**. An irregular osteochondral defect with sclerotic border is seen in the weight-bearing portion of the medial femur condyle

Table 6.14 (Cont.) Differential Diagnosis of Articular Disorders

Disease	Characteristic Location	Radiographic Findings	Comments
Multiple epiphyseal or spondyloepiphyseal dysplasia (Figs. 6.139)	Polyarticular, bilateral, symmetric Hips Knees Ankles Shoulders Wrists	Epiphyseal centers of long bones are late in appearance and fragmented. After ossification they have a mulberry-like appearance and are commonly displaced. After puberty the affected articular surfaces of the long bones remain irregular and abnormal in shape and the joints may appear dysplastic. Femoral heads and condyles are flattened and often fragmented and deformities include coxa vara, genu valgum or varum, tibiotalar slant and V-shaped deformities of the wrist. Secondary osteoarthritis is present before the 3rd or 4th decade of life.	Heterogeneous group of dysplasias with minimal to advanced spinal changes (spinal beaking to platyspondyly). Radiographic differential diagnosis includes *cretinism, avascular necrosis, mucopolysaccharidosis, juvenile rheumatoid arthritis* and in the hip *Legg-Calvé-Perthes disease* and *Meyer's dysplasia* (delayed and fragmented epiphyseal ossification resulting eventually in normal hip, bilateral in 50% of cases).

(continues on page 186)

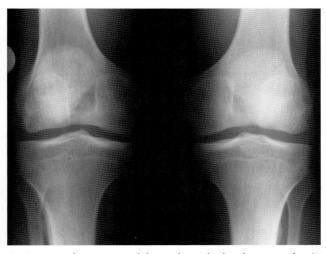

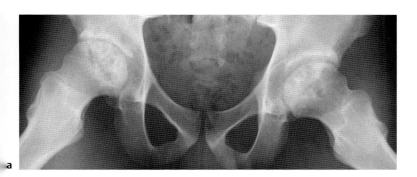

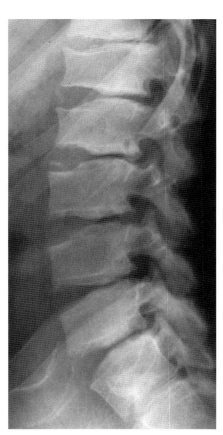

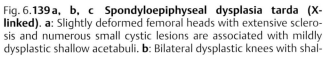

Fig. 6.**139 a, b, c Spondyloepiphyseal dysplasia tarda (X-linked). a**: Slightly deformed femoral heads with extensive sclerosis and numerous small cystic lesions are associated with mildly dysplastic shallow acetabuli. **b**: Bilateral dysplastic knees with shallow intercondylar notches and hypoplastic tibial spines are seen. **c**: Dysplastic vertebral bodies with characteristic osseous humps in their central and posterior portions causing narrowing of the disc spaces posteriorly and widening anteriorly are seen.

Table 6.14   (Cont.) Differential Diagnosis of Articular Disorders

Disease	Characteristic Location	Radiographic Findings	Comments
Hyper-parathyroid-ism (Figs. 6.140 and 6.141)	Bilateral, symmetric sacroiliac joints Sternoclavicular joints Acromioclavicular joints Pubic symphysis	Subchondral bone resorption in the axial or less commonly appendicular skeleton may mimic an erosive arthritic disease.	Other radiographic findings include osteopenia, acro-osteolysis, subperiosteal bone resorption, chondrocalcinosis, soft tissue calcifications and brown tumors. Osteosclerosis is a feature of secondary hyperparathyroidism (renal osteodystrophy).
Sarcoidosis (Fig. 6.142)	Monoarticular to polyarticular Hands Feet	Articular involvement in the chronic form is usually an extension of the osseous disease causing destruction and collapse of the joint	In the acute form radiographic findings are nonspecific and include soft tissue swelling, effusions and occasionally osteopenia affecting small and medium-sized joints.
Particulate synovitis (Figs. 6.143 and 6.144)	Associated with prosthetic joint implants	A joint effusion is the initial presentation. Tiny radiopaque particles may be evident in the joint fluid and synovial lining when the synovitis is induced by radiopaque bone cement. Subsequently subchondral cysts and erosions, often with thin sclerotic margins may be found. Osteoporosis is not a prominent finding differentiating this condition from infection.	Caused by shed particles from a joint prosthesis secondary to normal wear or damaged prosthesis. May induce a foreign body synovitis and subsequent osseous involvement of the affected joint *(particulate disease)*. Particles of polymethylmethacrylate, silicone and polyethylene are the most common offending agents.

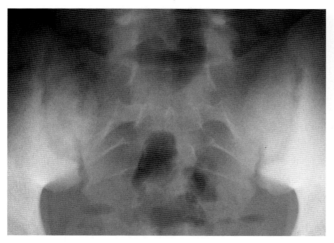

Fig. 6.**140** **Hyperparathyroidism (secondary)**. Bilateral widening of the sacroiliac joint with diffuse sclerosis, especially of the iliac bones is seen.

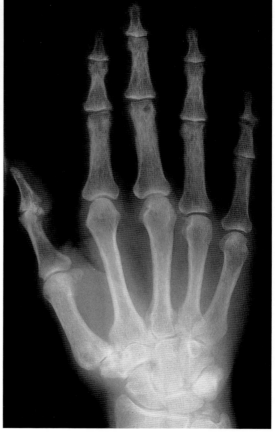

Fig. 6.**141** **Hyperparathyroidism**. Subchondral erosions imitating articular disease are seen in the distal interphalangeal joints of the second and fifth finger, the interphalangeal joint of the thumb and the first carpometacarpal joint. Other findings include heavy calcification of the triangular fibrocartilage, subperiosteal resorption along the radial margin of several phalanges, acro-osteolysis and a small brown tumor in the distal aspect of the proximal phalanx of the third finger.

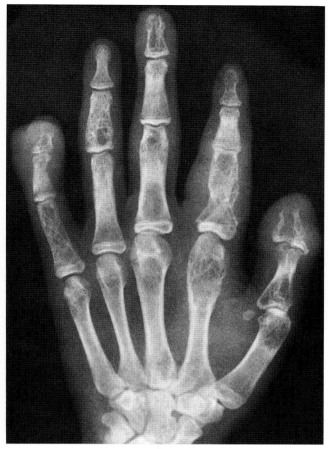

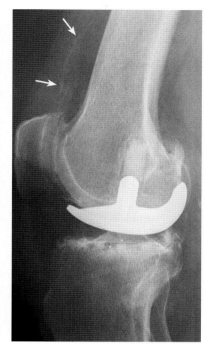

Fig. 6.**143** **Cement synovitis**. A unicompartmental (Repicci) prosthesis is seen in the medial compartment of the knee with signs of loosening of the femoral component and wear of the tibial component. Osteoarthritis is evident in the lateral knee compartment and patello-femoral joint. A small joint effusion with slightly distended suprapatellar bursa outlined by tiny radiopaque cement particles is seen (arrows).

Fig. 6.**142** **Sarcoidosis**. Soft tissue lesions are associated with a coarsened lacework trabecular pattern or small cysts in many phalanges and distal metacarpals. Articular involvement of the interphalangeal joint of the thumb is an extension of the osseous involvement of the distal phalanx. Note also the acro-osteolysis in several fingers.

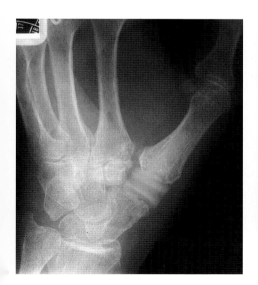

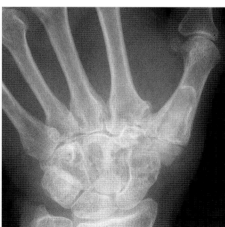

Fig. 6.**144 a, b** **Silicone-induced arthritis**. An intact silicone implant is seen in the first carpometacarpal joint following arthroplasty including trapezectomy for degenerative joint disease in **a**. Six years later partial collapse of the implant and osteolysis about its stem in the proximal first metacarpal is evident in **b**. In addition extensive erosive and cystic changes occurred in many carpal bones.

b

7 Joint and Soft-Tissue Calcification

Deposition of calcium in abnormal locations may take two forms: *calcification or ossification.* They can be roentgenologically differentiated from each other. Calcification is seen as structureless density; ossification shows organization into trabeculae and cortex (Figs. 7.**1** and 7.**2**).

Calcification of soft tissues is classified as *metastatic* (disturbance of calcium or phosphorus metabolism leading to ectopic calcification in primarily normal tissue), *calcinosis* (deposition of calcium in soft tissues in the presence of normal calcium metabolism), or *dystrophic* (calcium deposition in damaged tissues without generalized metabolic derangement). Ossification of soft tissues is usually due to *myositis ossificans* or *tumoral ossification* of soft tissues.

Tables 7.**1**–7.**6** present the differential diagnosis of calcification or ossification of joints and soft tissues of the extremities.

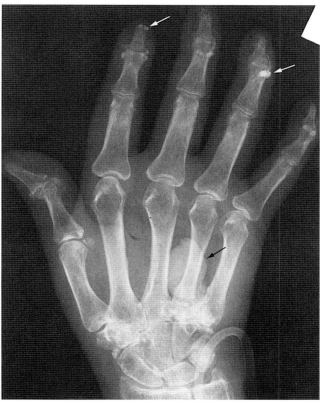

Fig. 7.**1 Structureless calcifications (arrows) in the soft tissues of the hand.** Chronic renal failure.

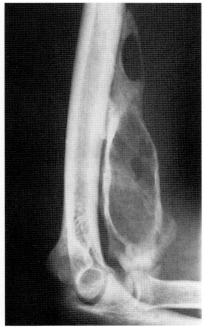

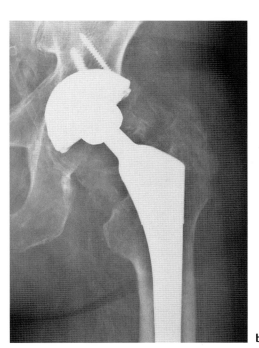

b

Fig. 7.**2 a, b Myositis ossificans. a** Bone formation in the soft tissues of the upper arm after trauma is seen. **b** Total hip prosthesis is the most common cause of myositis ossificans.

Table 7.1   Intra-articular calcified or ossified body (single or multiple)

Associated Disorders	Common Locations and Remark
Degenerative joint disease with detached spur.	Knee and other large joints. May resemble synovial osteochondromatosis, but usually contains one or few calcifications.
Fracture with avulsed fragment in joint (bone, articular cartilage meniscus).	Occurs especially in avulsed medial epicondyle of pediatric elbow. Cartilaginous fragments may or may not calcify.
Osteochondrosis dissecans (Fig. 7.5)	Knee, elbow, hip, shoulder, ankle; similar to synovial osteochondromatosis, but only one or few calcifications. A residual pit in the articular surface.
Synovial osteochondromatosis (Fig. 7.3)	Knee, hip, elbow, shoulder. Multiple small calcified or ossified densities within the joint capsule. Some of the synovial chondromas remain uncalcified and are not detected on plain films.
Neuropathic joint (Fig. 7.4)	Knee, hip, ankle, shoulder. Disintegration of joint surfaces, sclerosis and malalignment. May occur in diabetes, syringomyelia, syphilis and leprosy
Intra-articular tumor calcification (synovial sarcoma, intra-capsular chondroma).	Knee. Associated with a soft-tissue mass. A tumor may simulate a loose body.
Sequestrum from tuberculous or pyogenic arthritis.	Rare. Associated with arthritis or postarthritic deformity

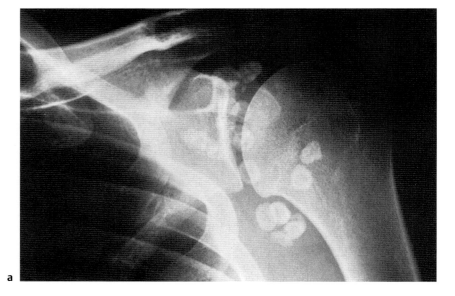

a

Fig. 7.**3**   **Synovial osteochondromatosis.**
a Shoulder joint. **b, c** Knee joint. There is
severe secondary osteoarthritis in the knee
joint.

Fig. 7.**3 b, c**   ▷

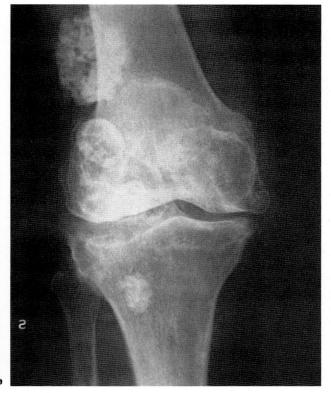

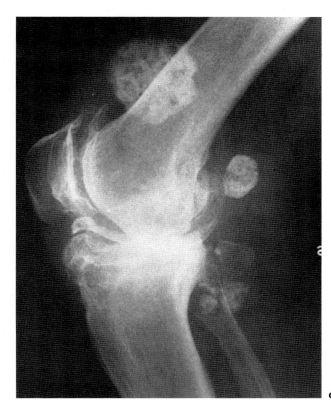

Fig. 7.**3 b, c**

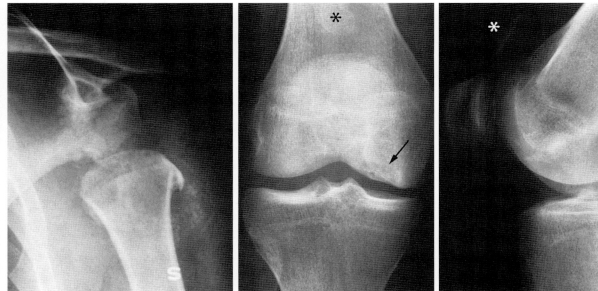

Fig. 7.**4 Syringomyelia.** Destruction of the glenoid fossa and humeral head, which is displaced inferiorly. The joint cavity contains calcific fragments.

Fig. 7.**5 a** Anteroposterior and **b** lateral views of the knee with **osteochondrosis dissecans**. A residual pit in the articular surface of the medial femoral condyle is demonstrated (arrow) and the calcified loose body is seen above the patella (asterisk).

Table 7.2   Calcification of articular cartilage or meniscus

Associated Disorders	Common Locations and Remark
Calcium pyrophosphate dihydrate deposition disease (CPPD) Pseudogout (Figs. 7.6 and 7.7).	Knees, wrists, hips. May be associated with various degrees of secondary osteoarthritis.
Idiopathic, primary osteoarthritis, trauma	Calcification of cartilage without crystal arthropathy.
Secondary osteoarthritis.	Premature osteoarthritis with chondrocalcinosis.
Hyperparathyroidism, renal osteodystrophy	Wrists, knees, hips, shoulders, elbows. Seen also in oxalosis with secondary renal failure.
Gout	Knee. Chondrocalcinosis is a secondary manifestation.
Ochronosis (alkaptonuria)	Menisci, intervertebral disks. Intervertebral disk calcification is also seen in *hypervitaminosis D, hypophosphatasia, ankylosing spondylitis, spondylosis* and *disk degeneration*
Acromegaly (Fig. 7.8)	Knee. Cartilage proliferation widens joint spaces. Calcification may happen.
Hemochromatosis	Autosomal recessive hereditary disorder in which iron accumulation causes the diseace. 20–60% of patients may have chondrocalcinosis. Calcification may be similar to CPPD.
Wilson's disease	Rare autosomal recessive disorder characterized by copper accumulation. Affects particularly basal ganglia and liver. In skeletal system it causes osteopenia, subchondral bone fragmentation and chondrocalcinosis.

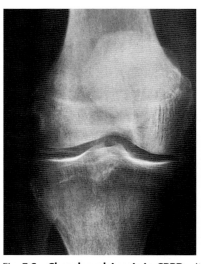

Fig. 7.**6**   **Chondrocalcinosis in CPPD** with calcification of menisci and articular cartilage of the knee.

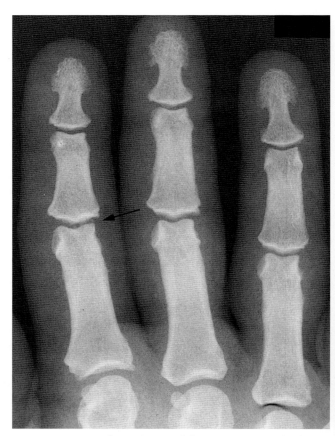

Fig. 7.**8**   **Acromegaly.** Widening of the joint spaces and calcification of the proximal interphalangeal joint cartilage of the index finger (arrow).

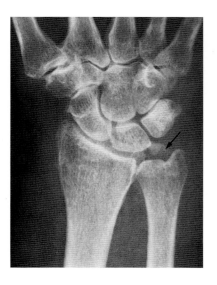

Fig. 7.**7**   **CPPD.** Calcification in the region of the triangular cartilage of the wrist (arrow). Osteoarthritic changes in the joint surfaces of the larger multangular bone.

Table 7.3 Periarticular soft tissue calcification or ossification

Associated Disorders	Common Locations and Remark
Hyperparathyroidism (Fig. 7.9) **Renal osteodystrophy**	Associated with other radiographic signs of hyperparathyroidism.
Other disorders of calcium and phosphate metabolism (hypoparathyroidism, chronic hemodialysis, widespread bone destruction, vitamin D intoxication, milk-alkali syndrome, etc.)	Ligamentous subcutaneous and intracranial calcifications sometimes occur. Not seen in postsurgical hypoparathyroidism.
Scleroderma (Fig. 7.10)	Most common in hands. Association of extensive calcinosis with scleroderma is called *Thibierge–Weissenbach syndrome*. The tetrad of skin calcification, Raynaud's phenomenon, sclerodactyly, and telangiectasia (*CRST syndrome*) is a variant of scleroderma.
Dermatomyositis (Fig. 7.11) **Polymyositis (Fig. 7.12)**	Associated with generalized or localized calcinosis of subcutaneous tissues.
Polyarteritis nodosa **Raynaud's syndrome** **Rheumatoid arthritis** **Systemic lupus erythematosus**	Periarticular calcifications in these connective tissue diseases are rare. May be reversible in systemic lupus erythematosus. Idiopathic soft tissue calcifications identical to the ones found in connective tissue diseases but without symptoms of the latter are termed *calcinosis universalis tumoralis and circumscripta*, respectively (Fig. 7.**13**).
Sarcoidosis	Large periarticular soft-tissue masses with or without calcifications are a rare manifestation.

(continues on page 194)

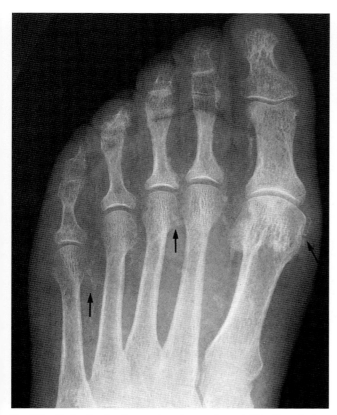

Fig. 7.**9** **Periarticular** (arrows) and **vascular calcifications in hyperparathyroidism**.

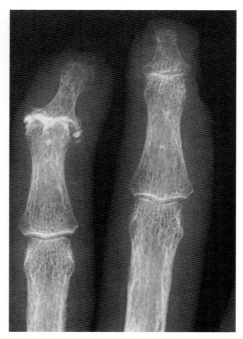

Fig. 7.**10** **Scleroderma.** Periarticular soft-tissue calcification in one finger and a soft-tissue defect in another.

Table 7.3   (Cont.) Periarticular soft tissue calcification or ossification

Associated Disorders	Common Locations and Remark
Gout	Periarticular calcified lump associated with chondrocalcinosis is diagnostic of gout. Most commonly occurs at the first metatarsophalangeal joint, the insertion of the Achilles tendon and the olecranon bursa.
Ochronosis (alkaptonuria)	Periarticular calcification occurs in spine and large joints.
Ehlers–Danlos syndrome	See subcutaneous calcifications, table 7.5.
Werner's syndrome (adult progeria)	Periarticular ligamentous calcifications, especially about the knees, may occur in this rare condition. Other radiographic findings include osteoporosis, premature atherosclerosis with calcification, and osteoarthritis.
Hydroxyapatite deposition disease (HADD) (Fig. 7.14)	Examples: shoulder (calcific tendinitis, periarthrosis). Hip (calcified trochanteric bursa).

(continues on page 195)

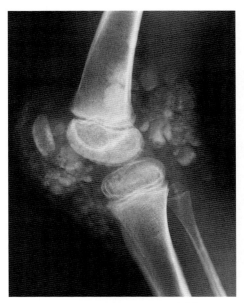

Fig. 7.11   Dermatomyositis in a child. Periarticular soft-tissue calcifications around the knee have some resemblance to synovial osteochondromatosis.

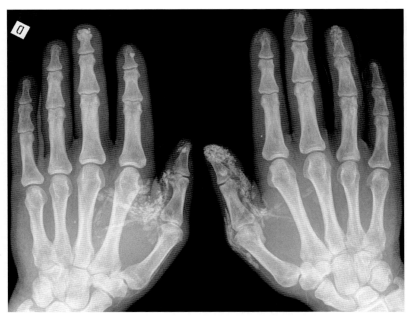

Fig. 7.12   Polymyositis and Raynaud's syndrome. Extensive soft tissue calcifications around thumb, fewer calcification at distal ends of other fingers.

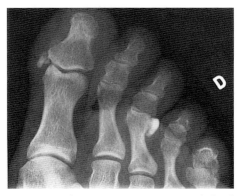

Fig. 7.13   Calcinosis circumscripta. Calcific deposits in the toes are as in scleroderma, but there are no other abnormalities.

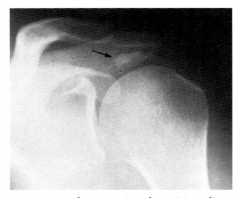

Fig. 7.14   Hydroxyapatite deposition disease. Calcification of the subacromial bursa of the shoulder.

Table 7.3 (Cont.) Periarticular soft tissue calcification or ossification

Associated Disorders	Common Locations and Remark
Myositis ossificans (localisata) (Fig. 7.15)	Calcification occurs about one month after trauma (hematoma, capsular or ligamentous damage), later it ossifies. Also common around joint replacement and in association with chronic neurological diseases (paraplegia). Ossification is always separated from bone by a radiolucent zone, unlike a malignant bone tumor.
Posttraumatic calcification (Fig. 7.16)	Pellegrini–Stieda calcification in the proximal attachment of the medial collateral ligament of the knee is a common presentation.
Synovial sarcoma (Fig. 7.17)	Most common in knee. Only small percentage of these tumors are intra-articular. The periarticular mass often contains calcific flecks, but not extensive calcification.
Pigmented villonodular synovitis	Most common in knee. A high-density lobulated mass may sometimes appear calcified due to hemosiderin deposits, although the tumor calcifies extremely rare.
Healed tuberculous arthritis (Fig. 7.18) (Caries sicca)	Large joints, spine. Fibrous ankylosis and extensive soft-tissue calcification often occurs.
Tumoral calcinosis (lipocalcinogranulomatosis)	Usually painless calcifications, most often of the bursae in the vicinity of joints (hip, elbow, shoulder) or near bony protuberances. If cystic, may show layering of calcific fluid. Small calcific nodules may progress to a large solid lobulated tumor. The joint is not involved.

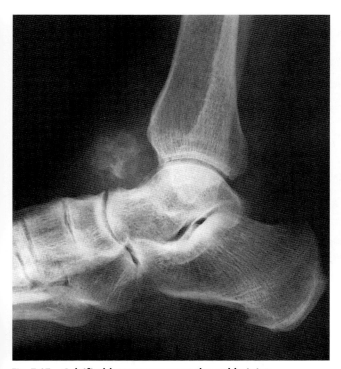

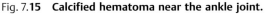

Fig. 7.**15** **Calcified hematoma near the ankle joint.**

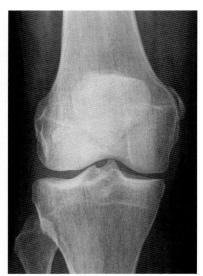

Fig. 7.**16** **Pellegrini–Stieda calcification.** Curvilinear soft tissue calcification at medial aspect of the femoral condyle.

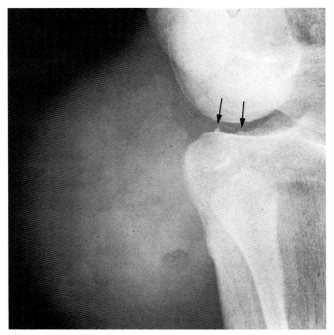

Fig. 7.**17**   **Synovial sarcoma of the knee joint.** A large soft-tissue mass and small calcifications near the joint space (arrows).

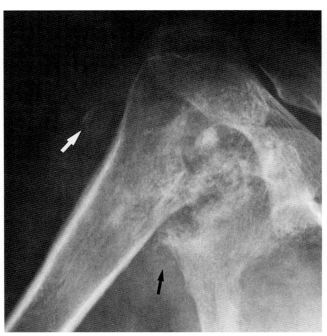

Fig. 7.**18**   **Healed tuberculous arthritis of the right shoulder.** Severe deformity and soft-tissue calcifications (arrows).

Table 7.4   Connective tissue and muscular calcification or ossification (Figs. 7.19–7.26)

Associated Disorders	Common Locations and Remark
Universal calcinosis (idiopathic) Scleroderma Dermatomyositis (Figs. 7.19–20) systemic lupus erythematosus (rare) Carbon monoxide poisoning (rare).	Variable: neck, thorax, limbs. Usually no ossification takes place.
Myositis ossificans progressiva (rare) (Fig. 7.21)	A rare hereditary connective tissue disorder. Ectopic ossification in early childhood. Neck, shoulders, proximal arms, pelvis. Associated with short first metacarpals and metatarsals and finger or toe anomalies.
Parasitic calcifications:	
– **Cysticercosis (Taenia solium) (Fig. 7.22)**	Multiple, ovoid (about 1 cm long and 3 mm thick) calcifications have their long axis along muscle planes.
– **Hydatid disease (Echinococcus)**	If calcifications occur in muscle, they tend to parallel the long axis of the limb.
– **Guinea worm disease (Dracunculus medinensis)**	Small irregular or linear serpinginous calcifications measuring up to several cm (calcified female worm) in legs, abdominal, or thoracic muscles.
– **Loiasis (Filaria loa loa)**	U- or V-shaped calcific dots in web spaces.
– **Schistosomiasis (Schistosoma haematobium)**	Fibrosis and granulomatous calcification, more commonly in the lower urinary tract.
– **Trichinosis (Trichinella spiralis)**	1 mm or less, rarely visible radiographically.
– **Armillifer armillatus.**	Multiple, comma-shaped peritoneal or pleural calcifications.

(continues on page 198)

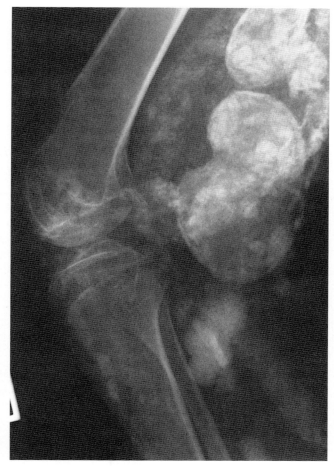

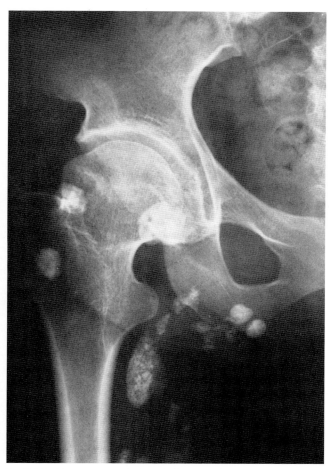

Fig. 7.**19** **Dermatomyositis.** Extensive connective tissue calcification in the leg.

Fig. 7.**20** **Dermatomyositis.** Calcification of connective tissues.

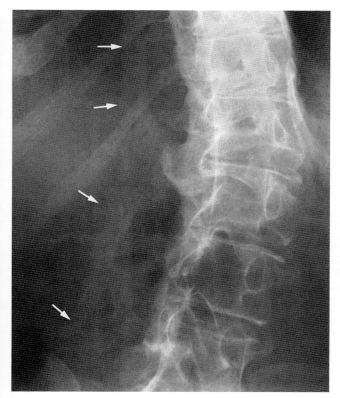

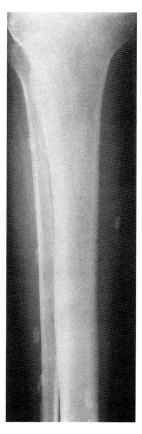

Fig. 7.**22** **Cysticercosis.** Multiple ovoid calcifications in the soft tissues of the leg.

Fig. 7.**21** **Myositis ossificans progressiva.** Paraspinal soft-tissue ossification (arrows) associated with myositis in this region.

Table 7.4   (Cont.) Connective tissue and muscular calcification or ossification (Figs. 7.19–7.26)

Associated Disorders	Common Locations and Remark
Idiopathic or degenerative (Fig. 7.23)	Ligaments of the shoulder girdle and pelvis often calcify in normal individuals.
Fluorosis	Paraspinal sacrotuberal and iliolumbal ligaments can calcify extensively in fluorosis. Sclerosis of the axial skeleton is more diagnostic.
Traumatic or postoperative	Common around total hip replacement.
Periosteal due to hematoma (Fig. 7.24)	In early phase may mimic periosteal sarcoma, but is denser at the periphery, whereas sarcoma is denser at the center.
Neurological causes, especially paraplegia	Myositis ossificans around hip joints is a common presentation.
Tumors:	
– Osteosarcoma	Rarely develops in the soft tissues, and may show fuzzy or spicular calcification.
– Chondrosarcoma	
– Fibroma	Small calcific flecks may be present in both benign and malignant tumors.
– Fibrosarcoma	
– Synovial sarcoma	Most tumors are extra-articular and commonly show calcific flecks.
– Lipoma (Fig. 7.25)	Both benign and malignant tumor may contain extensive ossification. Predilection in medial thigh and popliteal areas.
– Liposarcoma (Fig. 7.26)	
– Metastases	Bone-forming metastases occur in the carcinomas of the colon, breast, and urinary tract.
Leprosy	Nerve abscesses of tuberculous leprosy are seen as soft-tissue masses which may calcify.

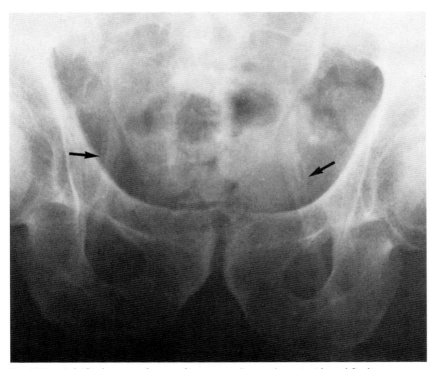

Fig. 7.**23**   **Calcified sacrotuberous ligaments** (arrows), an incidental finding.

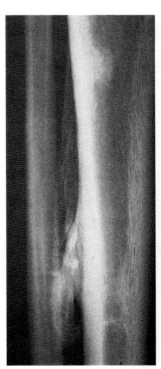

Fig. 7.**24**   **Calcification of periosteum and the interosseus ligament following hematoma.**

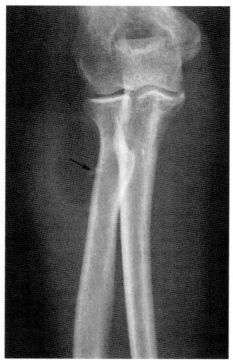

Fig. 7.**25** **Lipoma.** A low-density mass in the arm has a well-defined outline. It contains a calcified spot characteristic of fat necrosis (arrow).

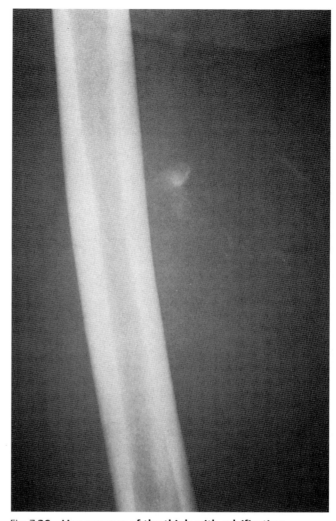

Fig. 7.**26** **Liposarcoma of the thigh with calcification.**

Table 7.5 Subcutaneous calcification or ossification

Associated Disorders	Common Locations and Remark
Dermatomyositis and other causes of generalized or circumscribed interstitial calcinosis. (Fig. 7.27)	Thighs, abdomen, thorax, shoulders, neck, hands, feet.
Ehlers–Danlos syndrome	Generalized inherited disorder of connective tissue and loose joints. Fatty nodules in the subcutaneous tissue of the extremities may calcify. They may mimic phleboliths, having central lucencies.
Pseudoxanthoma elasticum	Hereditary systemic disorder with widespread premature degeneration of elastic fibers. Middle and deep layers of the dermis may calcify, as well as tendons, ligaments, and large vessels.
Basal cell nevus syndrome	Soft-tissue calcification can be a feature of this inherited disorder characterized by multiple basal cell carcinomas, palmar pits, dentigerous cysts of the mandible, anomalies of the spine and ribs, and brachydactyly, as well as neurologic abnormalities.
Postinjection or traumatic fat necrosis (or heavy metals)	Irregular dense deposits in buttocks may contain heavy metals, but calcification of fat necrosis may follow injections of antibiotics etc.
Venous thrombosis Varicose veins	Lower extremities, subcutaneous ossification secondary to chronic venous stasis.

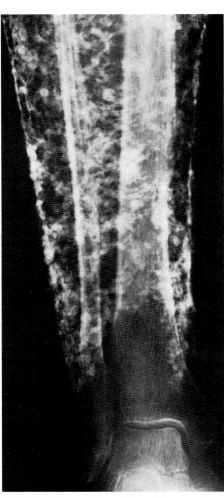

Fig. 7.**27** **Dermatomyositis** with extensive subcutaneous calcification.

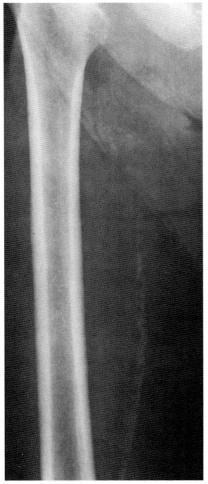

Fig. 7.**28** **Atheromatous calcifications** in the arteries of the thigh.

Table 7.6   Differential Diagnosis of Vascular calcifications

Findings	Associated Disorders	Common Locations and Remarks
Atheromatous calcifications (patchy) (Fig. 7.28)	*Arteriosclerosis* *Aneurysm* *Takayasu's arteritis*	Causes of premature atherosclerosis: familial hyperlipemia; secondary hyperlipemia (e.g., diabetes)
Mainly medial sclerosis of arteries evident as parallel lines (Monckeberg's medial sclerosis) (Fig. 7.29)	*Idiopathic hypercalcemia syndromes* *Nephropathies*	Hypercalcemia syndromes: hyperparathyroidism, hypervitaminosis D, immobilization, milk-alkali syndrome, sarcoidosis, idiopathic, paraneoplastic, or secondary to massive bone destruction.
Calcified thrombus (rare)	*Venous thrombosis, varicose veins*	Seen as an irregular calcification along the course at an artery or, more commonly, a vein.
Phlebolith (small rounded opacities, characteristically with central lucencies) (Fig. 7.30)	*Normal*	Common in pelvis, more rarely spleen, ankle, orbits.
	Angiomatous malformation, hemangioma	Usually a localized collection of phleboliths. Cavernous hemangioma associated with enchondromatosis is called *Mafucci's syndrome*.
	Varicose veins	Lower extremities.

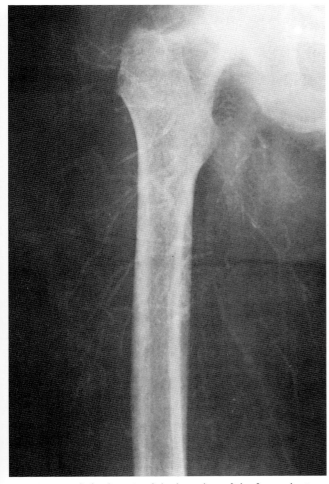

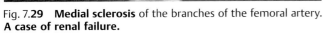

Fig. 7.**29** **Medial sclerosis** of the branches of the femoral artery. **A case of renal failure.**

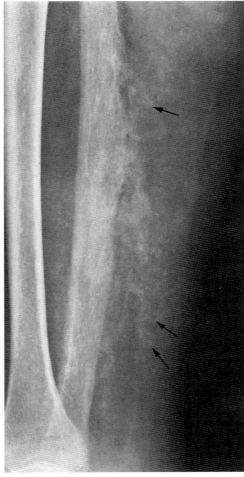

Fig. 7.**30** **Soft-tissue calcification associated with varicose veins.** Both ossifications (myositis ossificans) and calcified phleboliths (arrow) are seen.

8 Skull

Calcifications

Calcifications are a common finding on skull radiographs. With computed tomography, many more calcifications within the skull can be appreciated that escape detection with plain film radiography. Numerous artifacts on the scalp (e.g., dirt, fragments, ointments, and braids) may simulate intracranial calcifications and therefore must be taken into consideration (Fig. 8.1).

Physiologic Intracranial Calcifications

Physiologic and pathologic intracerebral calcifications occur, although the boundaries between the two can be blurred. Locations of characteristically physiologic calcifications are summarized in Table 8.1 and Fig. 8.2.

Table 8.1 Physiologic Intracranial Calcifications
Pineal
Habenula
Choroid plexus
Dura (falx, tentorium)
Ligaments (petroclinoid and interclinoid)
Pituitary
Internal carotid artery (cavernous portion)
Basal ganglia and dentate nucleus

A *calcified pineal* is found in 5% of children under the age of 10 and in almost two-thirds of the adult population (Fig. 8.3). With CT scanning, a considerably higher rate of pineal calcification is found. It appears amorphous or ring-like, and varies considerably in size but measures usually less than 1 cm. A pineal calcification exceeding 1 cm in diameter suggests neoplasm, either a pinealoma or even more commonly a teratoma. A calcified aneurysm of the vein of Galen may occasionally also simulate an abnormal pineal calcification.

The pineal lies midline in the anteroposterior projection. A displacement of a pineal more than 3 mm to one side of the midline suggests an intracranial mass lesion displacing the pineal away from the midline. On the lateral radiograph, the pineal projects approximately 3 cm above the highest posterior elevation of the pyramids. Numerous methods have been described to assess pineal displacement in this projection, but since their usefulness is rather limited, they will not be discussed in this context.

The *habenula* is located a few millimeters anterior to the pineal and calcifies in almost one-third of patients (Fig. 8.3). Habenular calcification characteristically assumes the shape of a "C" open posteriorly. Habenular displacement by intracranial lesions occurs in the same way as pineal displacement.

Although the *choroid plexus* can calcify in all ventricles, it most commonly occurs in the atrial portions of the lateral ventricles (junction of the body of the lateral ventricles with the posterior and temporal horns), projecting on the lateral view approximately 2 to 3 cm behind and slightly below the pineal (Fig. 8.3). In the anteroposterior projection, plexus

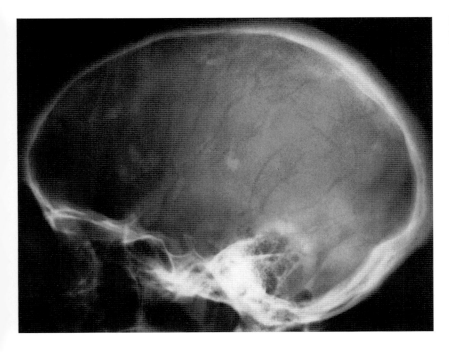

Fig. 8.**1** **Artifacts.** Corn rows (tight African-style braiding of the hair) simulate scattered intracranial calcifications

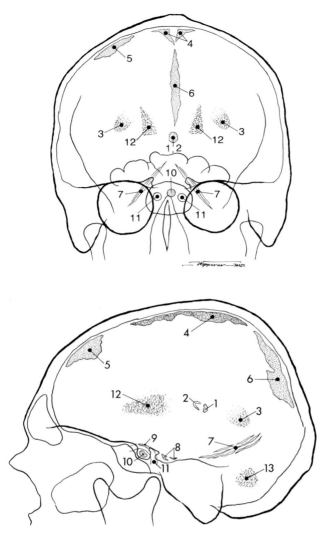

Fig. 8.**2a, b** **Physiologic intracranial calcifications** in **a** antero-posterior and **b** lateral projection. 1 pineal; 2 habenula; 3 choroid plexus; 4 falx around sagittal sinus; 5 dura; 6 falx (free edge); 7 tentorium; 8 petroclinoid ligament; 9 interclinoid ligament; 10 pituitary; 11 internal carotid artery (cavernous portion); 12 basal ganglia; 13 dentate nuclei.

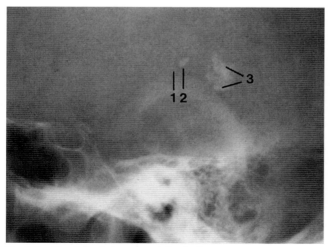

Fig. 8.**3** **Physiologic intracranial calcifications.** From anterior to posterior: 1 C-shaped habenula, 2 pineal gland, and 3 the two superimposed choroid plexuses are seen projecting just above the ear.

calcifications project approximately 3 cm from the midline and are usually symmetrical, although some disparity in size between the two sides occurs occasionally. The amount of calcification can vary greatly and is of no clinical significance. The calcifications have a characteristically fine to coarse granular appearance, occupying a circular area of 1 cm or more in diameter. Extensive plexus calcifications can be found in neurofibromatosis.

Calcification of dura, falx, and/or *tentorium* occurs in approximately 10% of cases, and each has quite a characteristic appearance (Fig. 8.4). Dural calcification around the sagittal sinus has a V-shaped appearance at the vertex in the anteroposterior projection. Calcifications in this area may occasionally be caused by calcified *Pacchionian (arachnoid) granulations* (diverticula-like outpouchings of the arachnoid space penetrating the dura mater and projecting into the lumen of the main sinuses and adjacent venous lakes). Falx calcifications are normally situated anteriorly, and are evident as linear streaks or lamellae in one or both leaves of the falx. Calcifications in the free edge of the tentorium have an inverted V-shape on the anteroposterior projection. The amount of calcification in the dura, falx, and tentorium usually has no clinical significance, particularly when the calcification is more or less diffuse. Falx and dura calcifications have been found in two thirds of patients with *basal cell nevus syndrome (Gorlin),* and extensive dura calcifications have been reported in *pseudoxanthoma elasticum.*

Calcifications of the petroclinoid and interclinoid (diaphragma sella) *ligaments* are common in the elderly. The former lies between the tip of the dorsum sella and the apex of the petrous bone, whereas the latter may result in interclinoid (sellar) bridging.

Pituitary calcifications are rarely recognizable on skull films, as opposed to histologic examinations. On skull films, they may represent calculi.

Arteriosclerotic calcifications of the internal carotid artery are commonly seen as it passes through the cavernous sinus. These calcifications can range from a small flake to complete visualization of the carotid syphon (8.5). On the lateral view, these calcifications are superimposed on the sella turcica, whereas ring-like calcifications may be seen on either side of the sella in anteroposterior projection.

Basal ganglia calcifications are found in a number of diseases (see "pathologic calcifications"), but are most often found incidentally in a healthy adult and have no clinical implications. The calcifications range from punctate to conglomerate densities in characteristic locations: on the anteroposterior examinations, the calcifications are symmetrical and parasagittal, whereas on the lateral view, they may assume a gentle curve, roughly paralleling the squamosal suture. However, sclerosis along the squamosal suture, presenting on the lateral view occasionally as a dense band (see Fig. 8.26b), should not be confused with basal ganglia calcifications.

Calcifications in the dentate nucleus of the cerebellum are less common than in the basal ganglia, but are found in the same conditions. On the lateral skull film, these calcifications are often obscured by the mastoid air cells, but are best seen in the occipital (Towne's) view as symmetrical crescent-shaped densities.

Pathologic Calcifications

Pathologic intracranial calcifications can be subdivided into localized or scattered. Localized calcifications are often suggestive of a specific disease process when both location and

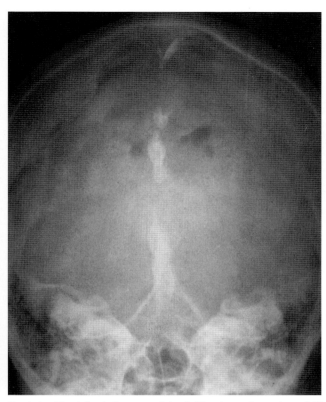

Fig. 8.**4** **Physiologic Intracranial calcifications.** Extensive calcifications of the falx (midline and V-shaped around the sagittal sinus) and tentorium (tent-like above the foramen magnum) are seen. Incidentally, small parasagittal radiolucencies are also noted, representing Pacchionian (arachnoid) granulations.

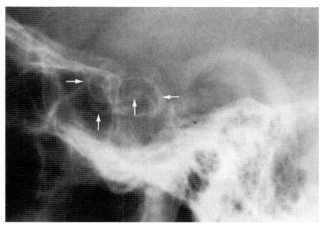

Fig. 8.**5** **Internal carotid artery calcifications.** Both completely calcified carotid syphons (arrows) are superimposed on the sella turcica.

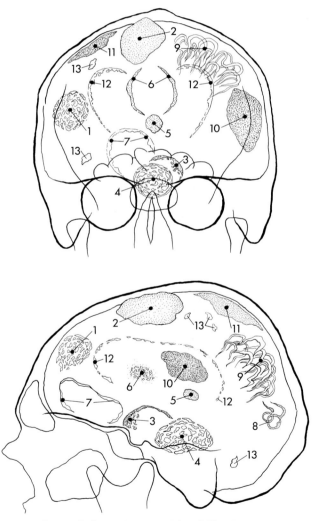

Fig. 8.**6 a, b** **Pathologic intracranial calcifications** in anteroposterior and lateral projection. 1 Glioma; 2 meningioma; 3 craniopharyngioma; 4 chordoma; 5 pinealoma or teratoma; 6 corpus callosum lipoma; 7 aneurysm; 8 arteriovenous malformation; 9 Sturge-Weber syndrome; 10 old intracerebral hemorrhage ("brain stone") or granuloma; 11 old subdural or epidural hematoma; 12 cytomegalic inclusion disease or congenital toxoplasmosis; 13 tuberous sclerosis.

shape of the calcification are taken into account. Scattered intracerebral calcifications are virtually limited to a variety of infectious processes, tuberous sclerosis and metastatic carcinomatosis (e.g., from breast carcinoma). Pathologic intracranial calcifications are summarized in Fig. 8.**6**.

Intracranial tumors represent the largest fraction of localized intracerebral calcifications. Their differential diagnosis is shown in Table 8.**2**.

Vascular lesions that calcify include (1) aneurysm, (2) arteriovenous malformations, and (3) old hemorrhages (intracerebral, subdural).

Arterial aneurysms occur most commonly in the region of the circle of Willis and calcify in less than 1%. Ring-like or arc-like calcifications are characteristic. Erosion of the adjacent bone may occur. A *calcified aneurysm of the vein of Galen* is rare, and is usually associated with obstructed hydrocephalus.

Calcifications in *arteriovenous malformations* are present on skull films in slightly less than 20%. Multiple small peripheral ring shadows combined with scattered flecks or streaks of calcification are almost always pathognomonic. Increased vascular markings in the skull are often an associated radiologic finding. A double-track ("tramline") calcification in the posterior parietal and/or occipital area is virtually diagnostic of the *Sturge-Weber syndrome* (meningofacial angiomatosis) (Fig. 8.**13**). In these cases, an ipsilateral port wine-colored nevus flammeus of the face in the distribution of the trigeminal nerve is almost invariably present. Mental retardation, seizure disorders, and contralateral hemiplegia may also be associated. The ipsilateral hemispheric brain atrophy may be evident radiographically

Table 8.2   Brain Tumors

Tumor	Preferred Location	Calcifications	Comments
Glioma: **Astrocytoma**	Adults: Central white matter of cerebrum Children: Cerebellum (40%), brainstem (20%), supratentorial (30%)	8% Grade 1 (well-differentiated): 25% Grade 2 (anaplastic): 6% Grade 3 (glioblastoma multiforme): 2%	50% of all brain tumors are gliomas of which four-fifths are astrocytomas and oligodendrogliomas. Gliomas are found in patients of all ages. Glioma calcification ranges from a few ill-defined dots and/or irregular linear streaks to a dense calcified nodule.
Oligodendroglioma (Fig. 8.7)	Frontal lobe	50%	
Ependymoma (Fig. 8.8)	Ventricles	15%	
Medulloblastoma	Infratentorial	Rare (<10%)	Highly malignant posterior fossa tumor usually diagnosed in infancy and childhood. It is a primitive neuroectodermal tumor (PNET).
Choroid plexus papilloma	Ventricles	25%	
Meningioma (Fig. 8.9)	Parasagittal, base of skull, falx, tentorium	5% to 15% (granular, curvilinear, or dense nodular ["ball of calcium"])	15% of all intracranial tumors. Predominantly in the middle-aged and elderly, rarely in children. M:F = 1:3. Associated and often diagnostic radiographic findings in 50%: 1 local hyperostosis; 2 increased meningeal vascular markings; and 3 enlarged foramen spinosum.
Craniopharyngioma (Fig. 8.10 a)	Suprasellar	75% (nodular and/or curvilinear)	Usually but not always associated with sellar abnormalities. Bimodal age distribution with peaks in 1st and 2nd decades (75%) and 5th decade.
Teratoma (Fig. 8.10 b)	Midline (half in pineal region)	75% (may contain teeth, etc.)	
Dermoid (cerebral)	Midline, most often posterior fossa	Almost always	Majority in children and adolescents. DD: epidermoid ("cholesteatoma") which is not necessarily midline, occurs at all ages and may be either extradural (rarely calcified) or intradural (commonly calcified).
Pinealoma	Pineal region	50% (pineal calcification exceeding 1 cm in diameter)	Majority in the first 2 decades of life, strong male predominance.
Pituitary adenoma	Pituitary fossa	Rare (4%)	Calcifications occur only in large, usually chromophobe or rarely eosinophil adenomas, which are always associated with an abnormal sella.

(continues on page 208)

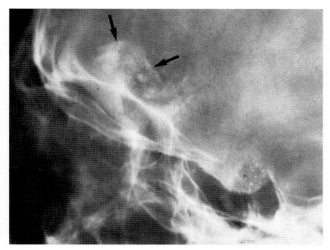

Fig. 8.**7** **Oligodendroglioma.** A tumor calcification is seen in the frontal lobe projecting just above the sphenoid wing (arrows).

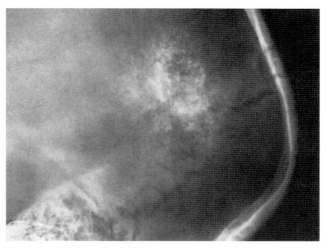

Fig. 8.**8** **Ependymoma.** A tumor calcification is seen projecting above the lambdoid suture.

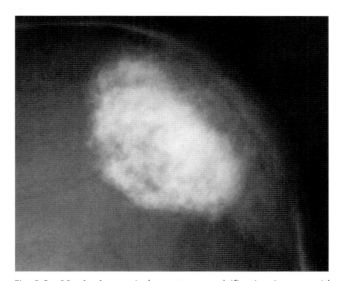

Fig. 8.**9** **Meningioma.** A dense tumor calcification is seen with thickening of the adjacent inner table of the skull.

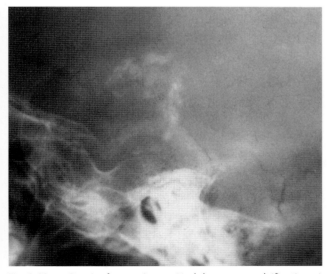

Fig. 8.**10 a** **Craniopharyngioma.** Nodular tumor calcifications in semicircular configuration are seen above a normal-sized sella. Although sellar abnormalities are commonly associated with this tumor, a normal-sized sella, as in this case, is not unusual in young children. Note the poor definition of the dorsum sellae secondary to increased intracranial pressure.

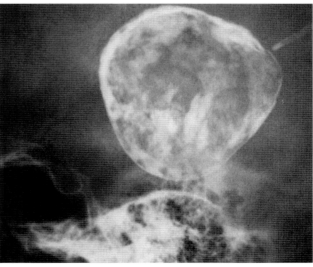

Fig. 8.**10 b** **Pineal teratoma.** A large calcified mass is seen midline.

Table 8.2   (Cont.) Brain Tumors

Tumor	Preferred Location	Calcifications	Comments
Chordoma (Fig. 8.11)	Skull base (clivus)	70% (retrosellar, parasellar or suprasellar)	Predominantly in 3rd and 4th decade. Usually associated with destruction of clivus. Extension to sella (destruction) and nasopharynx (soft-tissue mass) possible. Calcifications are particularly prominent in chondroid chordomas, a more benign variant.
Enchondroma, osteochondroma, chondrosarcoma	Dura, skull base	50%	Mimic meningiomas and chordomas.
Osteoma	Cranial vault, sinuses	Very dense, homogeneous ossification.	Protrudes from the outer or inner table of the cranial vault; in the latter case, it may mimic a meningioma.
Lipoma (Fig. 8.12)	Corpus callosum	2 curvilinear calcifications with concavity facing the midline around the area of the corpus callosum. Lipoma can sometimes be recognized as a radiolucent mass.	Corpus callosum lipoma usually diagnosed as incidental finding when calcified.
Von Hippel-Lindau disease	Orbits (retina) and cerebellum	Rare	Autosomal inherited disorder producing hemangioblastomas in both the cerebellar hemispheres and retina, associated with renal cysts and carcinomas. Pheochromocytomas and polycythemia may also be present.
Metastases	None	Rare	(e.g., from osteogenic sarcoma, mucinous adenocarcinoma of colon)
Other tumors	None	Extremely rare	(e.g., angioma, neurofibroma, hamartoma, etc.)

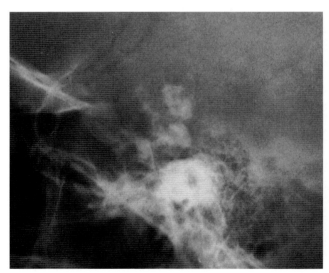

Fig. 8.**11**   **Chordoma.** Predominantly retrosellar tumor calcifications and destruction of clivus with sellar extension are seen.

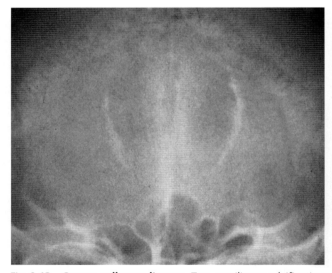

Fig. 8.**12**   **Corpus callosum lipoma.** Two curvilinear calcifications with the concavity, facing the midline, are diagnostic.

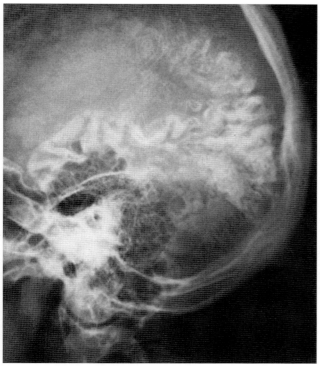

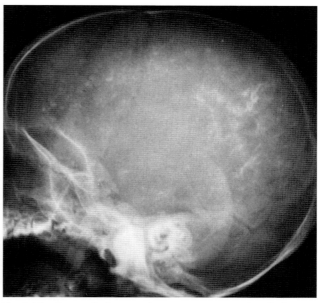

Fig. 8.**14 Congenital toxoplasmosis.** Scattered calcifications around the enlarged lateral ventricles, characteristically sparing the subtentorial area, are seen.

Fig. 8.**13 Sturge-Weber syndrome.** Extensive double-track ("tramline") calcifications in the posterior parietal and occipital area extending into the temporal lobes are seen. Ipsilateral large mastoid air cells are also present.

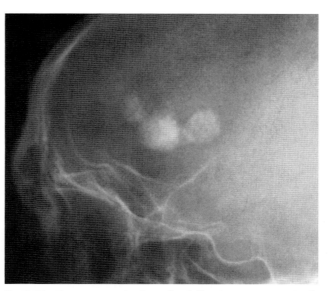

Fig. 8.**15 Cryptococcosis.** Round calcifications are seen in the frontal lobe area.

as elevated skull base and compensatory enlargement of the ipsilateral mastoid air cells with increased aeration.

Calcifications in *intracranial hemorrhages* occur. An *intracerebral hematoma* of either traumatic or spontaneous origin may ultimately result in a dense nodular and amorphous calcification ("brain stone"). *Cerebral infarcts* may rarely calcify also. *Subdural* and less frequently *epidural hematomas* can result on occasion in a thin calcified layer over the hemispheres. The extent of calcification may vary from a small focus to a huge deposit that envelops large portions of one or both hemispheres.

Numerous *inflammatory conditions* (infections and infestations) may result in intracranial calcifications. When they are located in the brain they are commonly scattered. *Congenital cytomegalic inclusion disease* is by far the most important diseases in this group, although other viral encephalitides (e.g., *polio, herpes,* and *rubella*) have been implicated as a cause of intracerebral calcifications. The incidence of calcification in cytomegalic disease is estimated at approximately 25%. The calcifications are found in the periphery of the often enlarged first and second ventricles.

Calcifications secondary to *congenital toxoplasmosis* occur in approximately half of the patients, and are virtually indistinguishable from cytomegalic inclusion disease (Fig. 8.**14**). Other parasitic infestations that can cause scattered intracerebral calcifications are *cysticercosis* (scattered nodular calcifications 1–3 mm in diameter) , *trichinosis* (punctate calcifications of 1 mm or less) and *paragonimiasis* (punctate to cystic, often in clusters and measuring up to 3–4 cm in diameter). Rarely, *echinococcal disease* may cause one or several larger intracranial calcifications.

Tuberculosis is for all practical purposes the only bacterial infection that has to be included in the differential diagnosis of intracranial calcifications. It may present as a single nodule, or less commonly as multiple calcified intracerebral nodules. A healed *brain abscess*, a *syphilitic gumma*, or a granuloma caused by a fungal infection (e.g., *cryptococcosis,* Fig. 8.**15**) are rare causes of similar localized intracerebral calcifications. Irregular calcifications resulting from tuberculous meningitis are found in the subarachnoid cisterns and project radiographically around and above the sella. Basal arachnoiditis produced by fungal diseases (e.g., *coccidioidomycosis*) can result in a similar radiographic picture.

Scattered intracerebral calcifications are found in 50% of patients with *tuberous sclerosis*. In contrast to toxoplasmosis and cytomegalic inclusion disease, the intracerebral calcifications in tuberous sclerosis are much more variable in size (lesions may exceed 1 cm in diameter), do not have a paraventricular distribution, and can also be found subtentorially (e.g., dentate nuclei). Calcifications occur also in the basal ganglia. Small areas of localized hyperostosis of the skull are often associated with tuberous sclerosis, and may actually be confused with intracerebral calcifications. In *neurofibromatosis* granular unilateral or bilateral temporal lobe calcifications may be found that appear to extend along the choroid plexus of the temporal horn. Scattered cerebral calcifications occur also with *metastatic carcinomatosis* (e.g., from breast neoplasms) or rarely develop after irradiation or a variety of other insults to the brain resulting in scarring and proliferation of neuroglial cells *(gliosis)*.

When the *basal ganglia* and *dentate nucleus calcifications* are not idiopathic, *primary hypoparathyroidism* appears to be the most frequent cause (Fig. 8.16), whereas these calcifications are rarely seen following surgical removal of the parathyroids. The calcifications in *pseudohypoparathyroidism* are radiographically indistinguishable. Calcifications of the basal ganglia and dentate nuclei may also be found in diseases associated with scattered intracerebral calcifications (e.g., tuberous sclerosis, or less commonly toxoplasmosis) and rarely in a few other conditions such as *Fahr's disease* (idiopathic familial cerebrovascular ferrocalcinosis), *lead* and *carbon monoxide intoxications, birth anoxia*, and certain congenital or acquired neurological disorders.

Vascular Markings, Sutures, and Fracture Lines

Vascular structures are responsible for a wide range of radiolucent markings in the normal skull (Fig. 8.17). With the exception of *emissary veins* that connect the venous systems inside and outside the skull and may produce bony channels, which are not wider than 2 mm, vascular structures cause indentations only on one table of the skull. Meningeal arteries and veins and dural sinuses produce indentations on the inner table that are fairly constant in position and thus relatively easily recognizable. *Pacchionian (arachnoid) granulations*, which are arachnoid extensions projecting into the lumen of the main sinuses and adjacent venous lakes, may erode through the inner table into the diploe. They most frequently produce irregular defects in the parasagittal area and the region around the torcula (see Fig. 8.4).

Diploic veins, on the other hand, are extremely variable in size, shape, and number. Besides diploic veins, there are *diploic lakes* that appear as irregular oval or round radiolucencies, rarely exceeding 2 cm in diameter. Occasionally larger and slightly expansile defects originating from the diploe can be found when a diploic vein forms a larger outpouching (Fig. 8.18). Diploic veins may resemble osteolytic lesions. The demonstration of an irregular and well-demarcated contour,

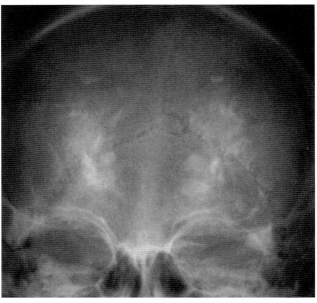

Fig. 8.16   Primary hypoparathyroidism. Extensive calcifications of the basal ganglia are seen. Calcifications of the dentate nuclei were also present, but cannot be recognized in this projection.

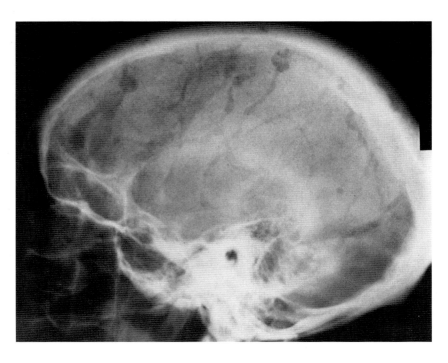

Fig. 8.**17   Normal vascular structures.** A wide range of radiolucent markings are seen in the skull.

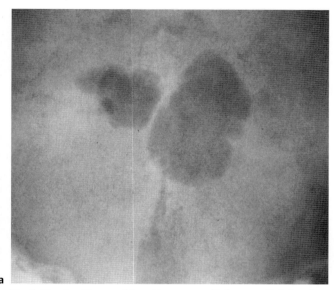

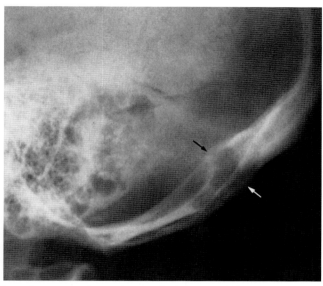

Fig. 8.**18 a, b** **Venous lakes.** Two unusually large well-defined, irregular radiolucencies are seen in the occiput. These large outpouchings of the diploic vein are slightly expansile as seen on the lateral projection (arrows). A single defect would be indistinguishable from an epidermoid originating from the diploe.

which is characteristic for venous lakes, may be helpful to differentiate them from osteolytic lesions.

The outer table may be indented by the *supraorbital artery* and the *middle branch of the superficial temporal artery*. The former is located in the frontal bone above the orbits, whereas the latter runs vertically across the temporal squama and fades out in the inferior part of the parietal bone (Fig. 8.**19**).

Vascular grooves have to be differentiated from *acute fractures*, which are usually more radiolucent, since they extend through both the inner and the outer table. Fracture lines also have very sharp and distinct margins (Fig. 8.**20**). Occasionally a fracture presents as an apparent dense line when the margins overlap in relation to the roentgen beam. This occurs most often with depressed fractures. *Sutures* may also be confused with acute fractures, when the suture in the outer table with the characteristic serrated appearance is obliterated and only the suture in the inner table remains visible as a relatively straight line. Sutures can, however, be differentiated from fractures by their constant anatomic location, their decreased radiolucency, and their less well-defined margins. Traumatic separation of a suture (diastasis) occurs occasionally in the adult. In children, traumatic suture diastasis has to be differentiated from raised intracranial pressure. In the latter condition, erosion of the dorsum sella, increased convolutional markings, and pineal displacement may also be found. A suture which is normally obliterated can occasionally persist (e.g., the metopic suture in the frontal bone or the mendosal and midsagittal sutures in the occipital bone) and should not be confused with a fracture line (Fig. 8.**21**).

Wormian bones are small bones occurring within a suture, most commonly within the lambdoidal suture (Fig. 8.**22**). They have no clinical significance and are found in healthy persons. However, a higher than normal incidence of multiple wormian bones has been found in a variety of congenital disorders such as *osteogenesis imperfecta, cretinism (hypothyroidism), cleidocranial dysostosis, progeria, hypophosphatasia, rickets*, and many others.

Compared with tubular bones, the osseous healing of skull fractures is slow and often incomplete, with only fibrous tissue formation. Such old fractures may persist as radiolu-

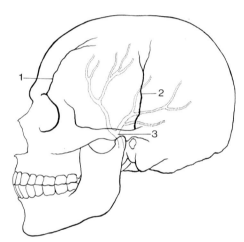

Fig. 8.**19** **Arterial grooves** on the outer and inner table. They have a constant anatomic location and should not be mistaken for fracture lines. 1 Supraorbital artery (outer table), 2 middle branch of the superficial temporal artery (outer table), and 3 middle meningeal artery (inner table). (Modified from Schunk H, Marayama Y Acta Radiol. 1960; 54: 186).

cent lines, which are often difficult to differentiate from vascular markings and sutures.

A *localized increase in vascular markings* can be a very important finding in the diagnosis of a *meningioma* when the increased vascular markings are associated with a calcified lesion or a local hyperostosis. It can be found relatively frequently in *arteriovenous malformations* which are calcified in almost 20% of cases.

Hypervascular primary or secondary tumors of the skull may also be associated with increased vascular markings. They may be observed in Paget's disease or fibrous dysplasia too, although the radiographic changes in these conditions are usually diagnostic by themselves. Because of a great variation in healthy persons, a generalized increase in the vascular markings is difficult to diagnose, but could indicate collateral circulation in cases with occlusion of major arteries or veins.

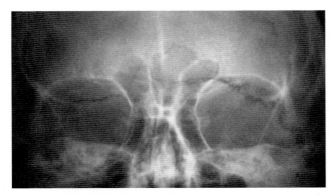

Fig. 8.20   Fracture and suture diastasis. Note the sharp and distinct margins of the fracture line projecting into the right orbit and the traumatic separation of the left lambdoid suture, whereas the normal lambdoid suture projecting into the frontal sinus has an indistinct margin and is barely visible.

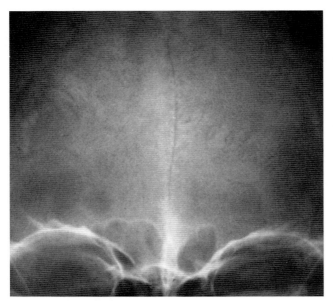

Fig. 8.21   Metopic suture. This suture is normally obliterated, but may occasionally persist and present as a poorly defined radiolucent line in the middle of the frontal bone, and should not be confused with a fracture.

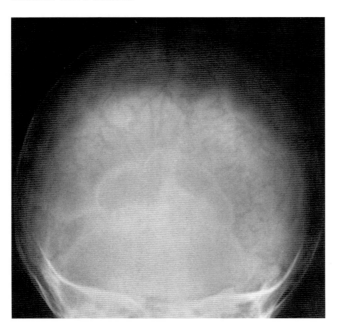

Fig. 8.22   Wormian bones. Numerous small bones are seen in the lambdoidal suture.

Osteosclerotic Lesions of the Vault of the Skull

For the differential diagnosis, sclerotic changes of the skull vault are best divided into localized and diffuse lesions.

Localized Sclerosis (Single or Multiple Osteoblastic Lesions) of the Skull Vault

As described in more detail in Chapter 2, the differential diagnosis of solitary or multiple localized sclerotic lesions includes benign tumors (e.g., *osteoma, osteochondroma*), malignant tumors (e.g., *osteosarcoma, metastases*) (Fig. 8.23), *chronic osteomyelitis* (Fig. 8.24), *ischemic necrosis* (especially in bone flaps), *radiation osteonecrosis* (Fig. 8.25), *fibrous dysplasia, neurofibromatosis, Paget's disease* ("cotton wool" appearance), *mastocytosis*, and *tuberous sclerosis* (often associated with scattered intracerebral calcifications). Formation of a band-like sclerosis along sutures is relatively common and without any clinical significance. Such a sclerosis along the squamosal suture should not be confused on the lateral view with calcifications in the basal ganglia (Fig. 8.26). *Hyperostosis frontalis interna* is an idiopathic irregular thickening of the inner table, mainly of the frontal bone (Fig. 8.26). The lesions are characteristically bilateral and symmetrical and spare the midline. They are most commonly found in women over 40 years of age, and progress at a very slow pace over the years. Thickening of the inner tables of other cranial bones or a more generalized thickening of the inner tables occur rarely. The latter condition is called *hyperostosis interna generalisata*.

An *ossified cephalhematoma* or *subdural hematoma* may also present as a localized area of increased density contiguous with either the outer or inner table, respectively (Fig. 8.27). *Meningiomas* invading the skull vault may present as localized thickening of the inner table (commonly in the parasagittal region or sphenoidal ridge) and may progress until they involve the whole thickness of the skull (Fig. 8.28). When the lesion is protruding outside the skull vault, sunburst spiculations may be present (Fig. 8.29).

Besides meningiomas, a localized *osteoblastic lesion with sunburst spiculations* can also be seen with *osteosarcomas, osteoblastic metastases* (e.g., from neuroblastomas), and hemangiomas (Fig. 8.30); *diffuse sunburst spiculations* of the vault with the exception of the occipital bone inferior to the internal occipital protuberance are encountered in severe anemias, particularly in *thalassemia* and to a lesser degree in *sickle cell anemia*.

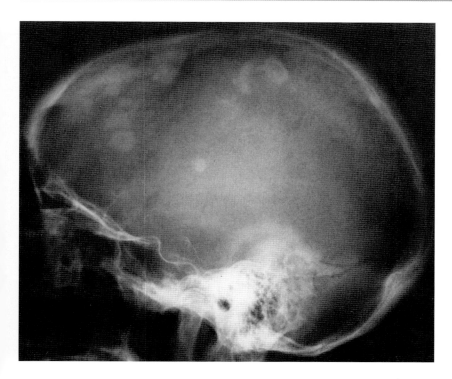

Fig. 8.**23 Osteoblastic metastases** from breast carcinoma. Round lesions of increased density are particularly well seen in the frontal area. Note also the normal thickness of the skull that helps to differentiate this condition from Paget's disease. Incidentally physiologic occipital thinning presenting as increased radiolucency of the squama occipitalis is also noted.

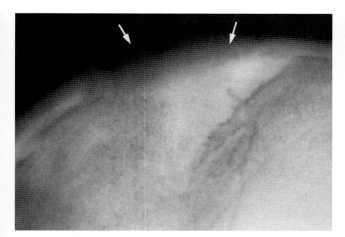

Fig. 8.**24 Chronic osteomyelitis.** A defect (arrows) seen in the frontal bone with adjacent sclerosis.

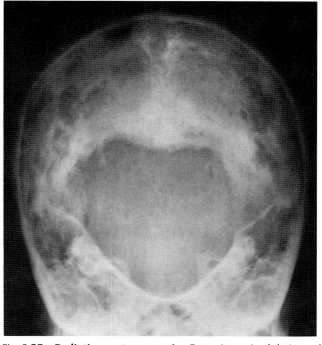

Fig. 8.**25 Radiation osteonecrosis.** Extensive mixed lytic and sclerotic bone involvement is found around a large surgical defect in the occiput.

Diffuse Sclerosis of the Skull Vault

A diffuse increase in bone density of the cranium may be caused by an abnormal osteoblastic response in the diploe triggered, for example, by osteoblastic metastases or myelofibrosis. Both sclerotic obliteration of the diploic space and thickening of the calvarium are the hallmark of *osteopetrosis* (Fig. 8.31) and many other constitutional diseases, such as *pyknodysostosis, van Buchem's disease* (generalized cortical

hyperostosis) (Fig. 8.32), *Engelmann–Camurati disease* (progressive diaphyseal dysplasia), *osteopathia striata* (Fig. 8.33), *melorheostosis* and *hyperphosphatasia*, which have already been discussed in Chapter 2. In these conditions, diffuse sclerosis of the calvarium is commonly associated with osteosclerosis in other bones too. Similar radiographic findings are found in children with *hypervitaminosis D, idiopathic hypercalcemia of infancy* (Williams syndrome), *hypoparathyroidism* and *pseudohypoparathyroidism*.

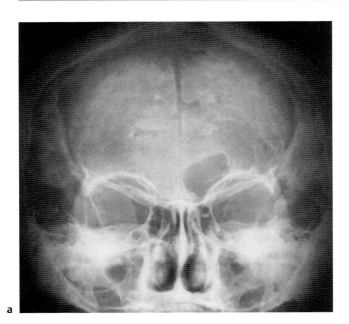

a

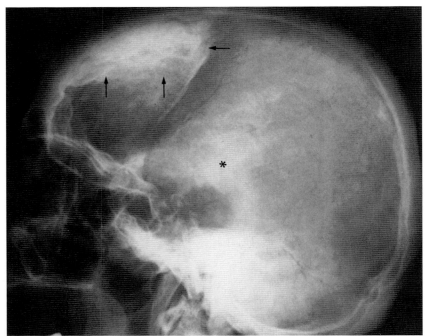

b

Fig. 8.**26 a, b   Hyperostosis frontalis interna.** Symmetrical thickening of the inner tables, mainly of the frontal bone, is seen (arrows). Incidentally, a wide sclerotic band in the area of the squamosal suture is also evident in the lateral projection (asterisk).

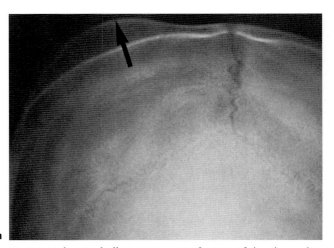

a

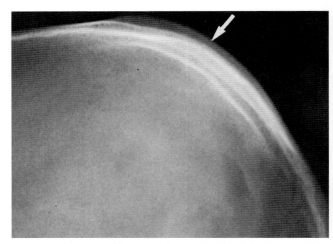

Fig. 8.**27 a, b   Cephalhematoma.** Ossification of the elevated periosteum over the parietal bone produces a localized thickening of the skull.

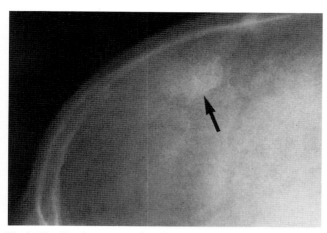

Fig. 8.**28** **Meningioma.** A localized thickening of the inner table is seen (arrows).

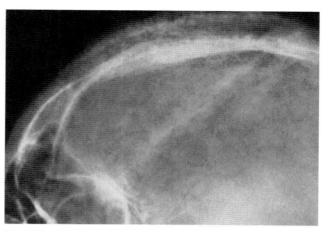

Fig. 8.**29** **Meningioma.** Localized thickening of both tables and the diploe as well as sunburst spiculations are seen.

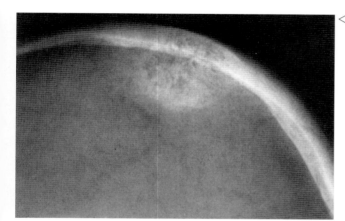

◁ Fig. 8.**30** **Hemangioma.** A slightly expansile lesion with marginal sclerosis and characteristic radiating bony spicules within the lesion is seen.

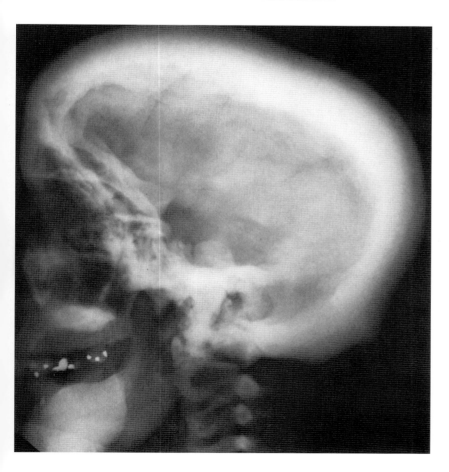

Fig. 8.**31** **Osteopetrosis.** Extensive sclerosis of the skull with complete obliteration of the diploic space and marked thickening of the calvarium is present. Note also the sclerosis and thickening of the facial bones and particularly of the mandible.

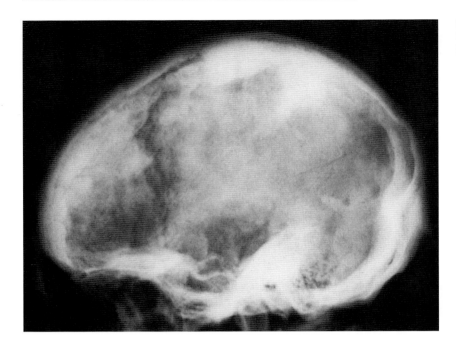

Fig. 8.**32** **Van Buchem's disease (general-ized cortical hyperostosis).** Extensive hy-perostosis of the entire skull is evident.

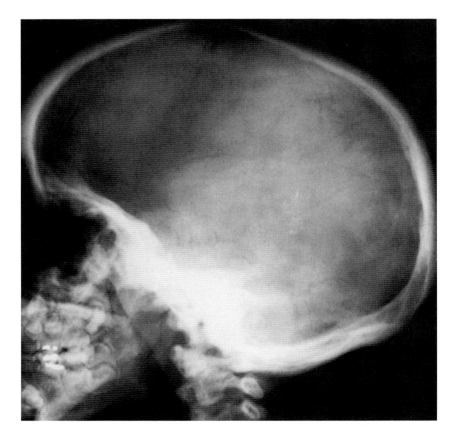

Fig. 8.**33** **Osteopathia striata.** Macro-cephaly and sclerosis of the skull are oc-casionally associated with the more charac-teristic bony changes of this disease in the tubular and flat bones, representing a dis-tinct autosomal dominant syndrome.

An increase in density of the skull vault may, however, also be the result of an abnormally thick calvarium. A great varia-tion in the normal range of the thickness of the calvarium ex-ists. A dense skull caused by an increased width of both outer and inner tables and the diploe, and observed as an isolated finding, has no clinical significance and may be called *id-iopathic.*

Thickening of the skull has been observed with *chronically increased intracranial pressure.* In childhood, both *cerebral atrophy* and *successful relief of increased intracranial pressure* (e.g. following surgery for hydrocephalus) may result in generalized calvarial thickening.

In *acromegaly,* thickening of the calvarium, particularly of the inner table, is associated with a large frontal sinus, exces-

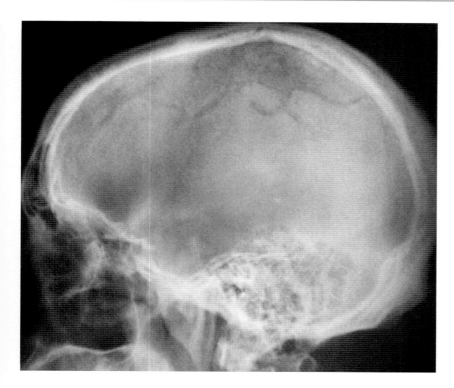

Fig. 8.**34** **Acromegaly.** Thickening of the skull, particularly of the inner table, prominent external occipital protuberance, excessive pneumatization of the mastoids, enlarged sella with straightening of the dorsum, and a large mandible (not shown) are characteristic. The frontal sinuses appear normal in this case, but are usually enlarged in this condition.

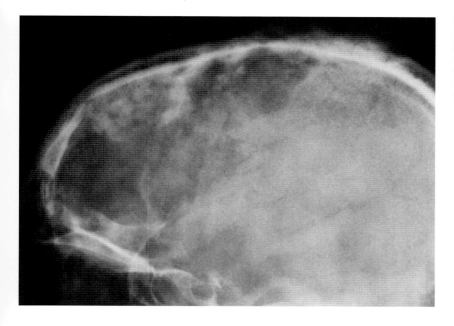

Fig. 8.**35** **Fibrous dysplasia.** Mixed lytic and sclerotic lesions are seen in the frontoparietal area. The disorder involves the outer table, that appears interrupted and expanded on the top of the vault, whereas the inner table remains intact in the entire skull.

sive pneumatization of the mastoids, prominent external occipital protuberance, and enlarged sella turcica (Fig. 8.**34**).

Sclerosis of the calvarium in *fibrous dysplasia* can be extensive but is usually not uniform. It is generally caused by expansion of the outer table while the inner table is usually not involved. Irregular radiolucencies can also be present (Fig. 8.**35**). Sclerosis of the skull base and/or paranasal sinuses by fibrous dysplasia is commonly associated with involvement of the vault of the skull.

In the combined destructive and sclerotic phase of *Paget's disease*, both inner and outer tables are thickened and the diploe is markedly widened and contains irregular areas of sclerosis ("cotton wool" appearance, Fig. 8.**36**). In the

sclerotic phase, a uniform thickening of the calvarium can be found with loss of differentiation between the tables and the diploe. Petrous pyramids and paranasal sinuses are often involved also.

The skull changes in *congenital hemolytic anemias* (e.g., thalassemia, sickle cell anemia) and less commonly in *acquired anemias* (e.g., iron deficiency) and *cyanotic congenital heart disease* result from erythroid hyperplasia of the marrow causing widening of the diploic space with external displacement and thinning of the outer table, which can assume a sunburst appearance (Fig. 8.**37**). The thickened diploe and outer table can often no longer be differentiated, whereas the inner table usually remains clearly defined.

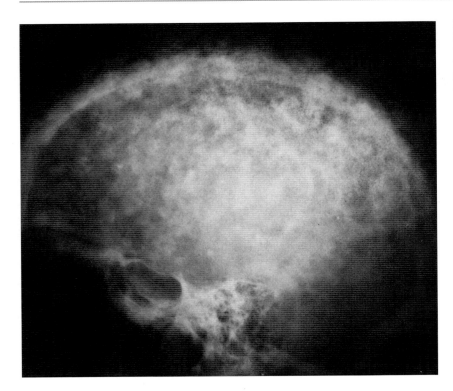

Fig. 8.**36** **Paget's disease.** Thickening of both the outer and inner table, widening of the diploë, loss of differentiation between tables and diploë, and irregular areas of sclerosis ("cotton wool" appearance) are diagnostic.

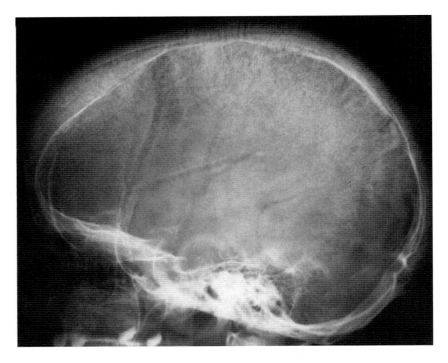

Fig. 8.**37** **Thalassemia.** Widening of the diploe and thinning of the outer table with sunburst appearance and sparing of the occipital bone below the internal occipital protuberance are characteristic. Poor pneumatization of the sinuses is also associated.

Characteristically, the occipital bone inferior to the internal occipital protuberance is not involved, because of the lack of bone marrow in this area. With the exception of thalassemia, where poor pneumatization of the sinuses can be found, there is no involvement of the paranasal sinuses. In *hyperparathyroidism,* granular deossification *("salt and pepper" skull)* with loss of the sharp definition of both the outer and inner table is typical. Small cyst-like lesions are also occasionally seen (Fig. 8.**38**). A "salt and pepper"-like skull can

occasionally be found as a normal variant; more commonly, it is associated with osteopenia of any etiology. However, in these conditions the outer and inner table remain sharply defined (Fig. 8.**39**).

Long-term *phenytoin therapy* may also be associated with diffuse calvarial thickening, besides radiographic evidence of rickets and osteomalacia, respectively. In *fluorosis* (secondary to chronic fluorine poisoning of the drinking water or in response to fluorine treatment of osteoporosis) calvarial

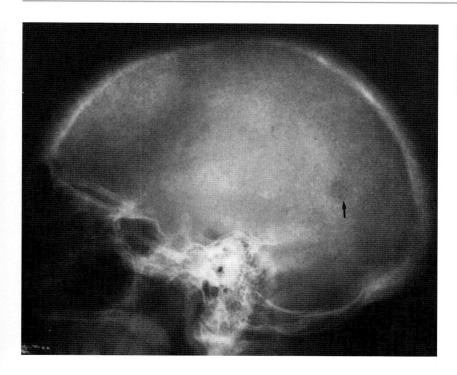

Fig. 8.**38** **Primary hyperparathyroidism.** Thickening of the calvarium with granular deossification ("salt and pepper" skull) and loss of definition of the tables are seen. A small cyst-like brown tumor is evident in the posterior parietal area (arrow),

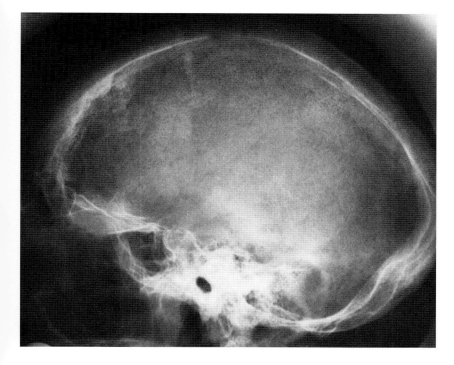

Fig. 8.**39** **Senile osteoporosis.** Granular deossification of the skull similar to the hyperparathyroidism in Fig. 8.**38** is seen. However, in contrast to the latter condition, both tables are still well defined and evident as distinct thin lines.

sclerosis occurs, but is less prominent than in the axial skeleton. Finally, *proper treatment of hyperparathyroidism* and *rickets* may also induce a generalized sclerosis of the skull. Similarly, *hypervitaminosis D* and *idiopathic hypercalcemia of infancy* (Williams syndrome) are further rare causes of diffuse osteosclerosis in children that may also affect the skull.

Solitary or Multiple Bone Defects in the Skull

When a bone defect is diagnosed in the skull, tangential views of the lesions are useful in determining whether the erosion is caused by an extracranial or intracranial mass, or originates within the bone. If the thinning of the skull is caused by pressure from an adjacent benign mass, then the bone defect has a curved and usually smooth appearance, and the thinning increases progressively from the periphery

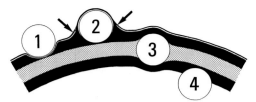

Fig. 8.40 Nondestructive expansile lesions originating from the vault of the skull or adjacent to it. (Solid black bands: outer and inner table, respectively; crosshatched area: diploë; black line: periosteum.) 1 Lesion originates from the scalp outside the periosteum. An extrinsic defect is produced in the outer table. 2 Lesion originates beneath the periosteum. An extrinsic defect in the outer table similar to 1 is produced, but in addition there is new bone formation by the elevated periosteum. This is usually most pronounced at both edges, where the new bone assumes a triangular shape (arrows). 3 Lesion originates form the diploë. Symmetrical erosion and expansion of both tables result. 4 Lesion originates from the meninges or brain. An extrinsic defect is produced on the inner table.

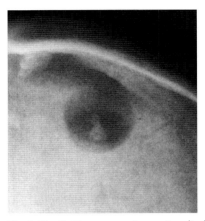

Fig. 8.41 Button sequestrum. A radiodense focus is seen within a lytic cranial lesion (eosinophilic granuloma).

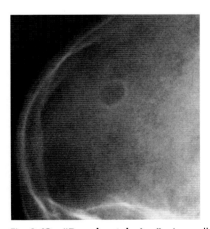

Fig. 8.42 "Doughnut lesion". A small round lytic defect surrounded by a sclerotic margin is evident.

to the center of the lesion. An erosion along the outer table indicates a scalp lesion, whereas an erosion on the inner table reflects an intracranial abnormality. Expansile lesions originating in the diploë erode and/or displace both inner and outer tables (Fig. 8.40).

Extracranial lesions eroding the vault or base of the skull are relatively rare and either of neoplastic or inflammatory origin. They are almost invariably associated with a soft-tissue mass or abnormality that can be diagnosed clinically. Carcinoma of the nasopharynx and sphenoid sinus, and glomus jugulare tumors, may invade the base of the skull, whereas skin carcinomas (rodent ulcers) may invade the skull vault. Pressure defects on the outer table of the skull may be produced by epidermoid cysts.

Lesions originating from the meninges and brain destroy the inner table first. Besides primary and secondary intracranial neoplasms, common causes for these are chronic subdural hematomas and abscesses, vascular structures and abnormalities (arteriovenous malformations and aneurysms), and cystic lesions (porencephalic cysts and meningoceles). Differential diagnosis of intracranial lesions causing bone destruction is rarely possible with conventional radiography unless other characteristic features (e.g., calcifications or location) are present.

Occasionally, a radiodense focus is found within a lytic cranial lesion and termed button sequestrum (Fig. 8.41). *Button sequestra* are found with eosinophilic granulomas, metastases (especially from breast carcinoma), epidermoids, osteomyelitis (including tuberculosis and syphilis), radiation necrosis, bone flaps undergoing avascular necrosis, and burr holes. A button sequestrum can also be mimicked by a radiolucent vascular channel forming a loop around a center of normal bone.

"Doughnut lesions" are small radiolucent areas in the skull surrounded by a sclerotic margin of variable thickness (Fig. 8.42). They often contain a central area of sclerosis simulating a button sequestrum. They are usually discovered incidentally on routine skull radiographs, and have no clinical significance.

A great variety of lesions originate from the skull itself, causing solitary or multiple bone defects. The differential diagnosis of lytic skull lesions is summarized in Table 8.3.

Abnormal Sella Turcica

There is a great variation in size and configuration of a normal sella turcica. On a lateral skull film, the greatest anteroposterior dimension of the normal sella ranges from 4 to 16 mm (average 10.5 mm), and its greatest depth (diaphragma sellae to floor) ranges from 4 to 12 mm (average 8.1 mm).

A *small sella* diagnosed as an incidental finding on a skull radiograph has no clinical significance and can be considered as a normal variant. A small sella has been described with hypopituitarism and several congenital syndromes and abnormalities,

The sella may demonstrate an abnormal shape without necessarily being enlarged. A *double-floor sella* on the lateral view suggests an intrasellar tumor with asymmetrical ex-

(continues on page 227)

Table 8.3 Solitary or Multiple Bone Defects in the Vault of the Skull

Disease	Radiographic Findings	Comments
Pacchionian (arachnoid) granulations (see Fig. 8.4)	Irregular smooth erosions in the inner table, located usually in the parasagittal area within 3 cm of the midline.	Pacchionian granulations are diverticula-like outpouchings of the subarachnoid space penetrating the dura mater and projecting into the lumen of the main sinuses and adjacent venous lakes. They may erode through the inner table into the diploic space.
Vascular markings (see Figs. 8.17 and 8.18)	Diploic veins and lakes may produce irregular, well demarcated oval or round radiolucencies, rarely exceeding 2 cm.	Other vascular structures may cause channel-like lucencies in the skull.
Parietal foramina (Fig. 8.43)	Smoothly marginated symmetric, parasagittal defects measuring up to 3 cm in diameter in the posterior parasagittal region.	Normal variant (nonossification of embryonal rests in parietal fissure) through which emissary veins pass.
Parietal thinning (Fig. 8.44)	Symmetric, crescent-shaped thinning of the superior portion of the parietal bones.	Normal variant in elderly males involving the outer tables.
Lacunar skull (craniolacunia, Lückenschädel) (Fig. 8.45)	Multiple radiolucent areas of calvarial thinning in newborns and infants, producing a pattern of exaggerated convolutional impressions.	Mesenchymal dysplasia of calvarial ossification. Usually associated with another malformation such as meningoceles of the skull or spine, hydrocephalus (e.g., in aqueductal stenosis) or Arnold-Chiari malformation. Spontaneous regression within first 6 months of life. DD: *Convolutional impressions* (normal variant visible between 2 and 8 years of age) and *"hammered silver" appearance* caused by increased intracranial pressure.
Meningocele, meningoencephalocele (Fig. 8.46)	Round to oval midline defect with smooth and often slightly sclerotic margins. Defect varies greatly in size and involves both inner and outer table. Frontal and occipital bone are the most common locations.	Congenital defect with herniation of meninges with or without brain. *Cranium bifidum* refers to a congenital midline defect without herniation.
Epidermoid (Fig. 8.47)	Solitary lytic and often expansile lesion measuring up to several cm in diameter. Its borders are always well-marginated and may be scalloped and sclerotic. Occasionally, a button sequestrum can be found.	Benign tumor caused by either posttraumatic implantation or congenital inclusion of epidermal elements. Appearance varies considerably with site of origin (e.g., scalp, diploë, or dura; see Fig. 8.**40**).
Dermoid	Small radiolucent defect without sclerotic margin, usually occurring in the midline.	Benign cystic lesion caused by congenital inclusion of elements from all dermal layers.
Arachnoid cyst	Smooth defect, often with a thin sclerotic rim.	Usually congenital, rarely traumatic or inflammatory in origin. Localized pressure causes thinning and outward bowing of the skull (see also posttraumatic [leptomeningeal] cyst in this table).
Primary bone tumors (benign and malignant)	Solitary, rare	Usually mixed lytic-sclerotic or predominantly sclerotic appearance.
Metastases (Fig. 8.48)	Usually multiple; irregular, ill-defined radiolucencies ("moth-eaten"); clear-cut defects occasionally with larger lesions. Button sequestrum (central nidus of intact bone in lytic defect) occurs, especially in breast carcinoma metastases.	Most frequent pathologic cause. All primaries that can produce lytic bone metastases, but breast carcinoma metastases are most common DD: vascular markings, Pacchionian (arachnoid) granulations.

(continues on page 224)

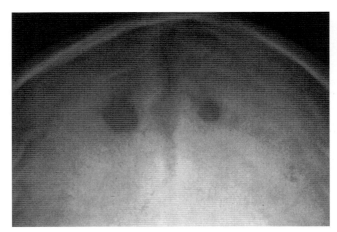

Fig. 8.**43**   **Parietal foramina.** Two symmetrical parasagittal defects are seen in characteristic location.

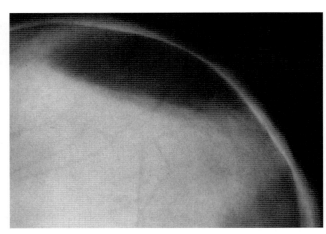

Fig. 8.**44**   **Parietal thinning.** An oblong radiolucent area is seen in the parietal bone, which is symmetrical and caused primarily by thinning of the outer tables.

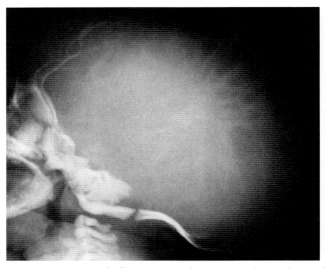

Fig. 8.**45**   **Lacunar skull.** A pattern of exaggerated convolutional impressions is caused by multiple areas of calvarial thinning

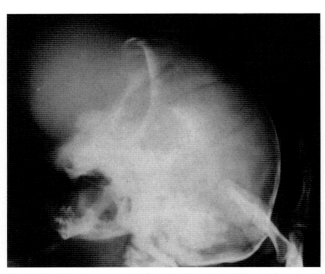

Fig. 8.**46**   **Meningoencephalocele.** Round, midline defect in the frontal bone with the meningoencephalocele evident as a soft-tissue mass.

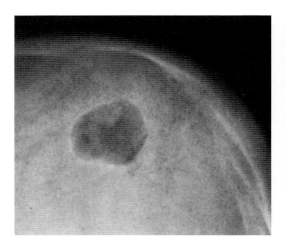

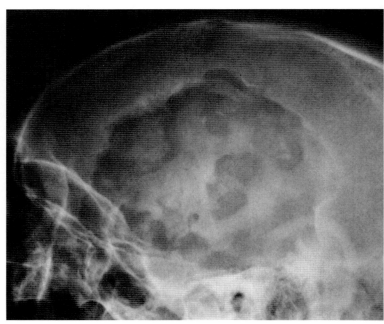

Fig. 8.**47**   **Epidermoids** (2 cases), **a** A relatively small lytic lesion with slightly sclerotic margins is seen. **b** A large defect with scalloped margins containing irregular bony fragments is evident.

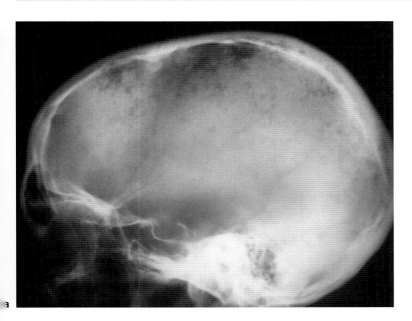

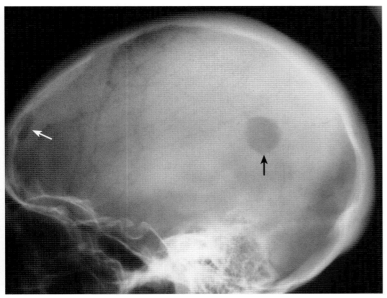

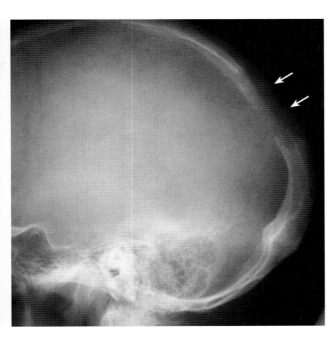

Fig. 8.**48** **Osteolytic metastases** (3 cases). **a** Multiple irregular, ill-defined and partially confluent radiolucencies ("moth-eaten" appearance) are seen (breast carcinoma). **b** Two well-defined ("punched-out") osteolytic lesions (arrows) are seen (thyroid carcinoma). **c** A large osteolytic lesion (arrows) extending along the diploic space with destruction of the outer table is seen in the parieto-occipital region (bronchogenic carcinoma).

Table 8.3   (Cont.) Solitary or Multiple Bone Defects in the Vault of the Skull

Disease	Radiographic Findings	Comments
Lymphoma, leukemia, malignant reticulosis	Multiple small erosions that can become confluent.	
Multiple myeloma (plasmacytoma) (Fig. 8.49)	Multiple (rarely solitary) sharply circumscribed ("punched-out") lesions are characteristic. May, however, also present similar to metastases.	Almost always in patients over 40 years of age.
Langerhans cell histiocytosis (eosinophilic granuloma, Hand–Schüller–Christian disease) (Figs. 8.50 and 8.51)	Solitary or multiple. Margins are usually well defined and often beveled and may become sclerotic. Button sequestra occur. Undulating margin when several lesions become confluent ("geographic skull").	Usually in patients under 40 years of age.
Hemangioma (see Fig. 8.30)	Solitary, Slightly expansile lesion with or without some marginal sclerosis. Virtually diagnostic when radiating bone spicules are present within the lesion.	
Neurofibromatosis (Fig. 8.52)	Lytic defects in occipital and temporal bone occur, but are rare. A round to oval calvarial defect involving the left lambdoid suture and extending toward the midline is considered to be most typical.	Neurofibromatosis more commonly involves the base of the skull (defects in sphenoid wing and posterior superior wall of the orbit are virtually diagnostic).
Fibrous dysplasia (Fig. 8.53)	Single or multiple but rarely purely lytic.	Usually mixed lytic and sclerotic pattern in the vault.
Paget's disease (Fig. 8.54)	Osteoporosis circumscripta: Destructive phase of Paget's disease in the vault . Area of destruction well demarcated, bilateral, and involving primarily the outer table of more than one bone in the calvarium.	In patients over 40 years of age. DD: Physiologic symmetrical *thinning of the squama occipitalis* is a common finding, best seen on lateral views.
Osteomyelitis (acute) (Fig. 8.55)	Irregular, poorly defined lytic areas, which may coalesce. Button sequestrum may be present.	Usually spread by continuity from infection adjacent to calvarium (e.g., paranasal sinus, middle ear, scalp) or secondary to fracture. Hematogenous spread to the skull is rare.
Tuberculosis	Solitary, round, sharply defined, purely lytic lesion, rarely containing a sequestrum.	
Syphilis	Multiple, poorly defined lytic lesions that may coalesce and contain one or more scattered sequestra.	
Fungal infections	Solitary or multiple, simulating either tuberculosis or metastases.	
Sarcoidosis	Solitary or multiple small purely lytic lesions.	
Burr holes, craniotomies	Edges of lesions initially beveled and smooth, but may become irregular with new bone formation.	Enlarged parietal foramina (symmetrical parasagittal defects in posterior parietal region) must be differentiated from burr holes (see Fig. 8.**40**).

(continues on page 226)

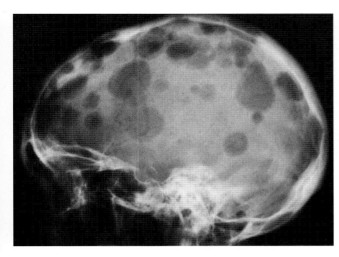

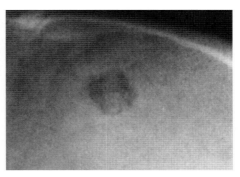

Fig. 8.**50 Langerhans cell histiocytosis** (eosinophilic granuloma). A solitary relatively well-defined lytic lesion with button sequestrum (central nidus of intact bone) is seen.

Fig. 8.**49 Multiple myeloma.** Multiple, sharply circumscribed ("punched-out") lytic lesions are characteristic.

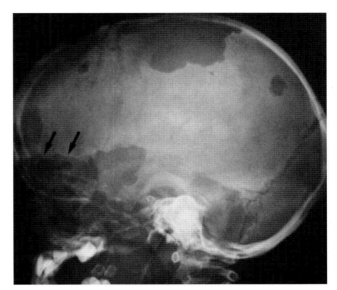

Fig. 8.**51 Langerhans cell histiocytosis** (Hand-Schüller- ▷ Christian disease). Destructive lesions with undulating and beveled margins are seen, resulting in the "geographic skull" appearance. The beveled margin (arrows) indicates that the outer and inner table are unevenly destroyed.

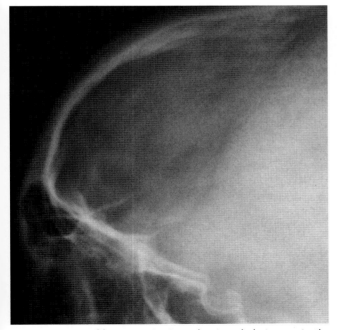

Fig. 8.**52 Neurofibromatosis.** A predominantly lytic area in the frontoparietal area is an unusual location in this disorder.

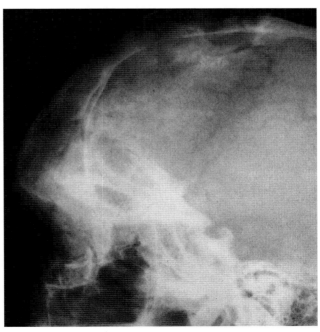

Fig. 8.**53 Fibrous dysplasia.** Extensive sclerosis of the skull base and paranasal sinuses is associated with expansile and predominantly lytic lesions originating from the outer table of the frontal bone, whereas the inner table appears intact.

Table 8.3   (Cont.) Solitary or Multiple Bone Defects in the Vault of the Skull

Disease	Radiographic Findings	Comments
Posttraumatic (lepto-meningeal) cyst (Fig. 8.56)	Solitary, often large defect with scalloped and beveled margin (inner table more eroded than outer table).	
Fibrosing osteitis	Solitary, poorly defined, lytic defect often with slightly sclerotic margin in outer table secondary to a fracture. Button sequestrum may be found.	Caused by transformation of fragmented bone into fibrous tissue.
Radiation osteonecrosis	Scattered small and irregular lytic defects occurring a year or more after irradiation. Button sequestrum occurs.	A mixed pattern of lytic and sclerotic lesions is more characteristic.
Brown tumors and hemorrhagic cysts in primary hyperparathyroidism (see Fig. 8.38)	Solitary or multiple poorly defined lesion(s) surrounded by granular demineralization ("salt and pepper" skull). After treatment (removal of parathyroid adenoma), cysts are often better demarcated because of the remineralization of the surrounding bone.	After treatment, brown tumors heal by filling in with bone and may eventually disappear or persist as sclerotic foci for many years.

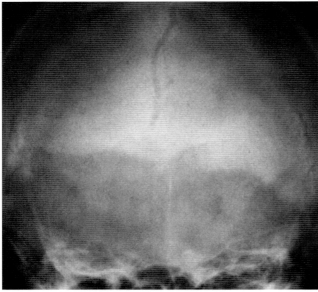

a

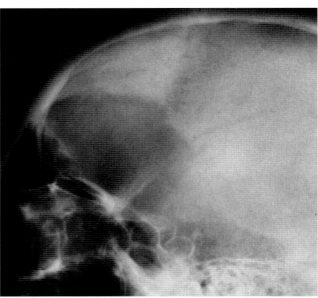

Fig. 8.**54 a, b Paget's disease.** A large, well-demarcated and somewhat asymmetric area of destruction in the frontal bone with extension into the temporal squama is seen (osteoporosis circum- scripta). Incidentally calcification of the carotid syphon that projects on the lateral view into the sella is also present.

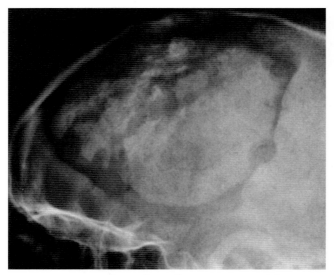

Fig. 8.**55   Osteomyelitis in bone flap.** Destruction of the antero- superior part of the bone flap is evident, while its posteroinferior portion is not affected.

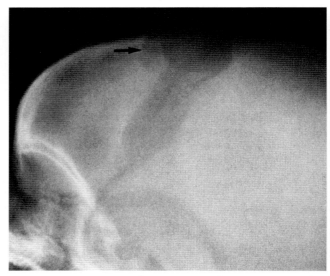

Fig. 8.**56   Posttraumatic (leptomeningeal) cyst.** A large defect with beveled margin (arrow) is seen six weeks after skull fracture during birth.

pansion (Fig. 8.57). Both a normally tilted sella and a super-imposed bony structure (e.g., from the sphenoid sinus or carotid sulcus) may simulate a pathologic double floor and must be differentiated from the latter.

The *J-shaped sella* refers to an elongated sella with a shallow anterior convexity caused by the sulcus chiasmaticus. It is more commonly seen in healthy children than adults. An enlarged sulcus chiasmaticus is a common finding in a *glioma of the optic chiasm* (Fig. 8.58). It is a rare finding in pituitary tumors extending anteriorly and in suprasellar tumors. In children, it can also be associated with *Hurler's syndrome* (mucopolysaccharidosis type 1) and with *chronic low-grade hydrocephalus*.

The *dorsum sella* shows a range of normal variations. On the lateral view, both the anterior and posterior margins consist of a well-defined cortex outlining a medulla of varying thickness and spongy texture. Pneumatization of the dorsum sella results occasionally from the extension of a large sphenoid sinus into the dorsum. In chronically elevated intracranial pressure or prolonged arterial hypertension, loss of definition of the entire dorsum sella occurs (see Fig. 8.10a), whereas the anterior cortex of the dorsum remains characteristically intact in osteopenia.

Enlargement of the sella turcica is caused by many intrasellar and parasellar mass lesions, which are summarized in Table 8.4

Table 8.4 Enlarged Sella Turcica

Disease	Radiographic Findings	Comments
Empty sella syndrome (Fig. 8.59)	Sella slightly enlarged and globular. No erosions, destructions, or posterior displacement of the dorsum.	Probably caused by a developmental defect in the diaphragma sellae allowing the prolapse of a small fluid-containing pocket of arachnoid into pituitary fossa. Enlargement of sella caused by fluid-transmitted pulsations. CT and MRI are diagnostic.
Increased intracranial pressure	Enlargement begins with erosion of the anterior cortex of the dorsum, proceeds to the floor of the sella, and may result in complete dissolution of the dorsum. Anterior and posterior clinoids can be thinned or eroded.	In chronically raised intracranial pressure caused by intracranial masses, cerebral edema, over-production of cerebrospinal fluid, obstruction of cerebrospinal fluid pathways or intracranial venous thrombosis.
Pituitary tumor (Fig. 8.60)	Ballooned sella with undercutting of the anterior clinoid processes, unequal downward displacement of the floor (double-floor appearance), and backward bowing to complete destruction of the dorsum.	Chromophobe adenomas virtually always produce considerable sellar enlargement. Eosinophil adenomas produce usually some enlargement of the sella and give rise to acromegaly. Basophil adenomas (causing Cushing's syndrome) and prolactin secreting microadenomas (causing amenorrhea and galactorrhea) do not generally cause any sellar abnormality. Adenocarcinomas are rare and cause an extremely rapid enlargement of the sella.
Craniopharyngioma (Fig. 8.61)	Elongated sella with short curved dorsum characteristic, but more often sellar changes indistinguishable from pituitary tumor.	Suprasellar tumor found predominantly in children and young adults. Calcified in 75% but incidence of calcification decreases with age. DD: Similar sellar changes in other juxtasellar or suprasellar tumors (meningiomas and, less commonly, other benign or malignant tumors originating in the adjacent structures, and metastases).

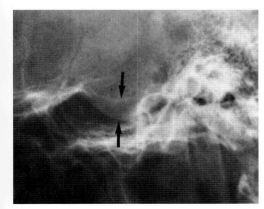

Fig. 8.**57 Double-floor sella.** Asymmetric growth of an eosinophil adenoma of the pituitary gland caused a double-floor sella (arrows).

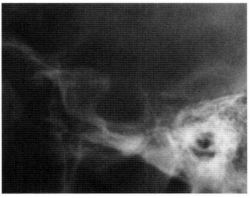

Fig. 8.**58 J-shaped sella.** A glioma of the optic chiasm undercutting the anterior clinoid processes caused this sellar configuration and enlargement. Note also the straightening and partial destruction of the dorsum.

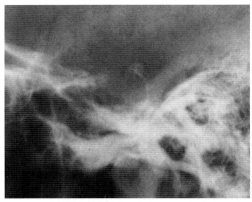

Fig. 8.59 Empty sella syndrome. A slightly enlarged and globular-appearing sella with an intact and normally configurated dorsum is characteristic. However, a relatively small pituitary adenoma can occasionally produce identical radiographic changes.

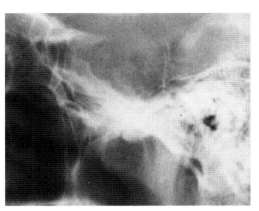

Fig. 8.60 Chromophobe pituitary adenoma. An enlarged sella with undercutting of the anterior clinoid processes and straightening and destruction of the dorsum is seen.

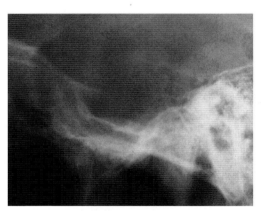

Fig. 8.61 Craniopharyngioma. An enlarged and elongated sella with completely destroyed dorsum is seen (see also Fig. 8.**10 a**).

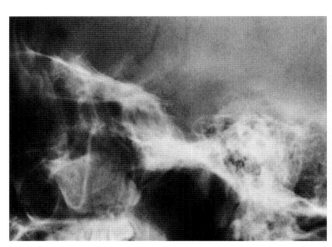

Fig. 8.62 Langerhans cell histiocytosis. Sellar destruction is associated with sclerotic lesions in the base of the skull and facial bones.

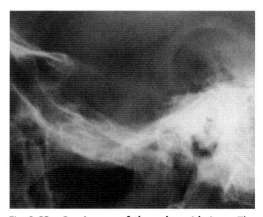

Fig. 8.63 Carcinoma of the sphenoid sinus. The sellar destruction is caused by direct invasion of the sphenoid sinus carcinoma that is often evident as a soft-tissue density in the sinus.

Basilar Invagination and Platybasia

Basilar invagination (impression) means elevation of the floor of the posterior fossa with invagination of the margins of the foramen magnum upward into the skull. This condition is readily diagnosed on radiographs taken either in anteroposterior or lateral projection (Fig. 8.**64**). Basilar invagination is often associated with platybasia (flattening of the base of the skull), in which an increased basal angle is found (Fig. 8.**65**). Basilar invagination and platybasia are found in a variety of congenital anomalies (e.g., *osteogenesis imperfecta, Klippel-Feil deformity, Arnold-Chiari malformation,* and *cleidocranial dysostosis*) and in acquired diseases producing bone softening. *Paget's disease* (Fig. 8.**65b**), *osteomalacia, hyperparathyroidism* and *rheumatoid arthritis* are the most common causes in the adult which produce these findings.

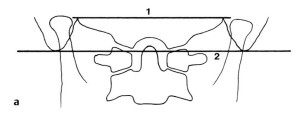

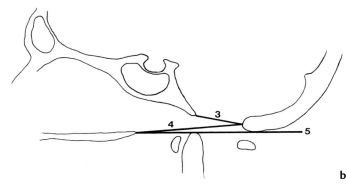

b

Fig. 8.**64 a, b Radiologic assessment of basilar invagination a** in anteroposterior and **b** lateral projection. 1 Digastric line. Tip of odontoid process is normally located below this line. 2 Bimastoid line. Tip of odontoid process projects normally not more than 10 mm above this line. 3 Foramen magnum or McRae line. Tip of odontoid process projects normally below this line. 4 Chamberlain line (hard palate to posterior margin of foramen magnum). Tip of odontoid process projects normally not more than 3 mm above this line. 5 McGregor line (hard palate to outer contour of occiput). Tip of odontoid process projects normally not more than 5 mm above this line

Sclerosis of the Base of the Skull

The following differential diagnosis is limited to those diseases that either frequently involve the base of the skull or are exclusively found in this area. Virtually all disorders presenting elsewhere in the skeleton with osteoblastic lesions or diffuse osteosclerosis may involve the base of the skull also. This is a particularly common finding in all constitutional diseases associated with osteosclerosis (Fig. 8.66). For a complete differential diagnosis, the reader is referred to Chapter 2.

Meningiomas may arise from various locations at the base of the skull such as cribriform plate, planum sphenoidale, tuberculum sellae, clinoid processes, and petrous bone. They cause a localized thickening and sclerosis of the involved bone (Fig. 8.67). Erosions of neighboring bony structures may also be associated. Differentiation from localized fibrous dysplasia can be difficult, but the presence of tumor calcification and the demonstration of trabeculae in the thickened sclerotic bone are only found with meningiomas and may help to distinguish these two entities.

Carcinomas originating in the ear, sphenoid sinus, and nasopharynx and invading the base of the skull are usually destructive, but may become sclerotic after radiotherapy. *Lymphoepitheliomas* (nonkeratinizing squamous cell carcinomas) of the nasopharynx or paranasal sinuses occasionally produce a localized sclerotic reaction in the adjacent bone before any treatment has been instituted.

Low-grade and chronic infections in the sphenoid sinus and mastoids produce localized sclerosis combined with poor pneumatization of the area. A localized sclerosis in the middle ear may be caused by chronic inflammation. Sclerotic changes in *otosclerosis* can only be appreciated with computed tomography, but not with conventional radiography.

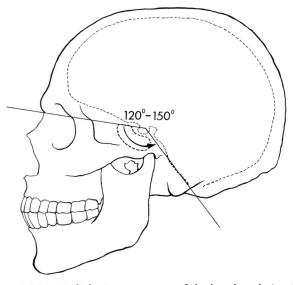

a

Fig. 8.**65 a Radiologic assessment of the basal angle** (angle between a line drawn through the nasion and the roof of the sphenoid sinus and a line paralleling the slope of the clivus or drawn through the tuberculum sella and the anterior margin of the foramen magnum). The normal basal angle ranges form 120 to 150 degrees (mean 135 degrees). An angle larger than 150 degrees indicates platybasia, whereas an angle smaller than 120 degrees indicates basal kyphosis. Platybasia is usually associated with basilar invagination, and basal kyphosis with prognathism.

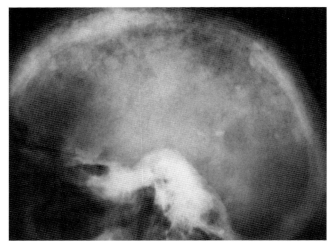

b

Fig. 8.**65 b Basilar invagination and platybasia in Paget's disease** evident as marked sclerosis of the base of skull. Note also the characteristic changes of Paget's disease in the vault of the skull.

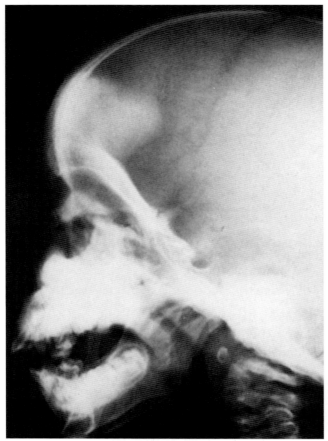

Fig. 8.**66** **Craniometaphyseal dysplasia.** Sclerosis of the base of the skull and facial bones with obliteration of all paranasal sinuses is seen. With the exception of a localized area of dense sclerosis in the frontal bone the vault of the skull is not affected, which is usually the case in this condition.

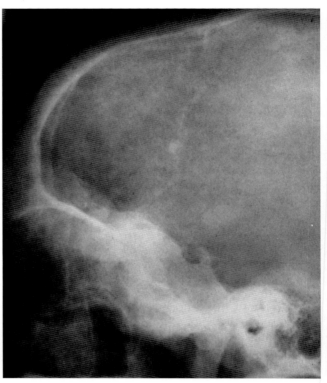

Fig. 8.**68** **Fibrous dysplasia.** Extensive sclerosis and thickening of the base of the skull with extension into the frontal bone is seen. The trabecular pattern in both the sclerotic and "ground glass" appearing areas is characteristically effaced.

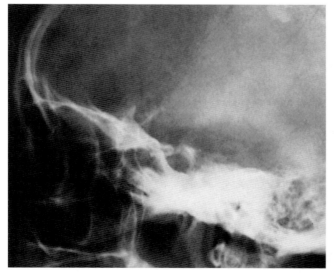

Fig. 8.**67** **Meningioma.** Sclerosis and thickening of the base of the skull was caused by a sphenoidal meningioma.

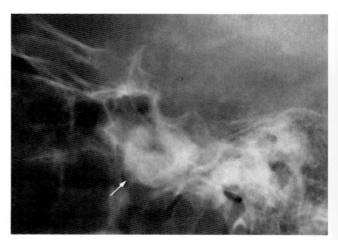

Fig. 8.**69** **Paget's disease.** Involvement of the base of the skull is seen, including a localized area of dense sclerosis (arrow).

Sclerotic changes caused by *fibrous dysplasia* in the base of the skull can be localized, but are often more widespread than in a meningioma, and manifestations of fibrous dysplasia may be found elsewhere in the skull. The bone changes may be purely sclerotic or a mixture of sclerosis and radiolucencies. The bone of fibrous dysplasia does not contain trabeculae and, for its thickness, does not appear very dense (Fig. 8.68).

Paget's disease can present as widespread sclerosis of the skull base usually associated with involvement of the vault and/or facial bones (Fig. 8.69). Encroachment of foramina and fissures occurs causing nerve compression symptoms.

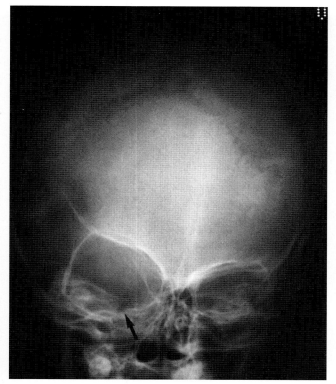

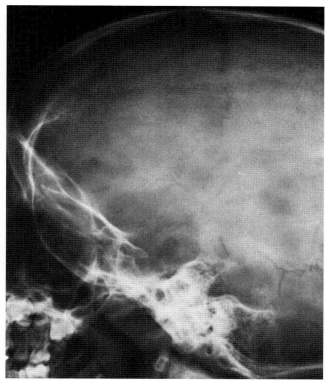

Fig. 8.**70 a, b** **Neurofibromatosis.** Asymmetry of the skull with enlarged right orbit, absent right superior orbital fissure, and erosion of the tip of the right petrous apex (arrow) are characteristic.

Basilar impression is a common finding with Paget's disease involving the base of the skull (see Fig. 8.**65b**).

In *Langerhans cell histiocytosis*, sclerotic involvement of the base of the skull is usually associated with destructive lesions, particularly in the sellar and parasellar region (see Fig. 8.**62**).

Erosion, Destruction or Lytic Defects in the Base of the Skull

Lytic lesions in the base of the skull may be caused by a variety of conditions that often can be differentiated from each other on the basis of location and radiographic appearance.

In *neurofibromatosis*, a unilateral defect in the sphenoid wings with absent superior orbital fissure and orbital enlargement can be found (Fig. 8.**70**). The disease may also be bilateral and erode the clinoid processes and the tip of the petrous apex.

Acoustic neuroma is the most common tumor of the inner ear, found usually in the middle-aged or elderly patient. The tumor presents radiographically as erosion and expansion of the internal auditory canal or erosion of the petrous apex (Fig. 8.**71**). Comparison with the normal contralateral side facilitates the diagnosis, but one has to keep in mind the fact that complete symmetry between the two sides is only seen in approximately 50% of healthy subjects. The length of the internal auditory canal varies greatly from individual to individual (3–16 mm; average 7–9 mm). Its diameter is more constant and should not exceed 5 mm. A diameter larger than 5 mm or a side difference in excess of 1 mm should raise the suspicion of a tumor.

A osteolytic defect projecting into the middle ear or the antrum mastoideum is most commonly caused by a *cholesteatoma* (Fig. 8.**72**). Primary cholesteatomas that are developmental in origin are rare. Secondary cholesteatomas

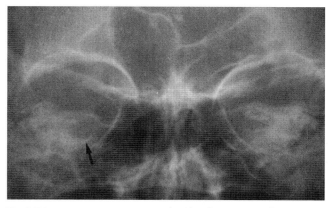

Fig. 8.**71** **Acoustic neuroma.** A localized erosion and expansion of the right internal auditory canal near the petrous apex is seen (arrow).

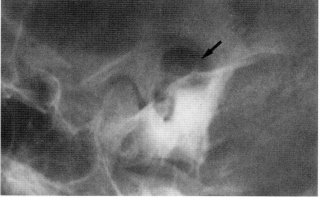

Fig. 8.**72** **Cholesteatoma.** A large round defect in the antrum mastoideum (arrow) is seen besides significant sclerosis of the mastoid indicating chronic mastoiditis (Schüller's view).

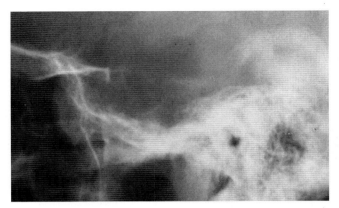

Fig. 8.**73** **Chordoma.** Destruction of the clivus, petrous pyramids and sella is seen (see also Fig. 8.**11**).

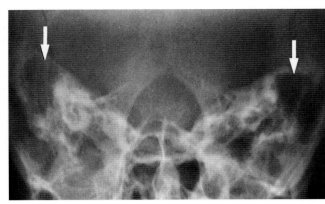

Fig. 8.**74** **Langerhans cell histiocytosis.** Two large areas of destruction simulating bilateral cholesteatomas are seen in the petrous bones (arrows). On the left side, the tumor had been removed one month earlier, with a surgical defect remaining that is impossible to differentiate from the original lesion.

Table 8.5　Destructive Lesions Affecting the Petrous Pyramid, Middle Ear and Antrum

A. Petrous pyramid
Neoplasm
  Acoustic neurinoma
  Meningioma
  Glioma
  Neuroma of the trigeminal and facial nerve
  Chordoma
  Glomus jugulare tumor
  Epidermoid (cerebellopontine angle cistern)
  Carcinoma of the nasopharynx
  Parotid tumors

Petrositis (Gradenigo's syndrome: diplopia, periorbital pain, and otorrhea)

Aneurysm (e.g., intrapetrous carotid artery)

Langerhans cell histiocytosis

B. Middle ear, antrum, and mastoids
Choleastoma (primary and secondary)

Neoplasm
  Carcinoma, primary or metastatic
  Sarcoma
  Glomus tumor

Abscess

Granuloma

Surgical defect

Langerhans cell histiocytosis

Glomus tumors are locally invasive chemodectomas arising in the chemoreceptor organs located in the jugular fossa or rarely in the hypotympanum of the middle ear. The glomus jugulare tumor erodes the jugular foramen and the interior aspect of the midpetrous pyramid in the early stage, whereas in a later stage, it may extend into the middle ear and the posterior fossa. Women are three times more frequently affected than men.

Chordomas originate from notochordal remnants found in the clivus and entire dorsal spine. The clivus is the second most common origin of this tumor, after the sacrococcygeal region. A destructive lesion of the clivus, dorsum sella, and petrous pyramid is virtually diagnostic when associated with a dense retrosellar calcification that is found in 70 % of patients (Fig. 8.73).

Meningiomas and *gliomas* may erode into the base of the skull causing a localized bone destruction, although an area of increased bone density is a more common manifestation in the former tumors.

Carcinomas of the nasopharynx, paranasal sinuses, and mastoids as well as a variety of *primary or metastatic bone tumors* have to be considered in the differential diagnosis when a destructive lesion is found in the base of the skull.

Surgical defects can simulate a neoplastic lesion and may be impossible to differentiate from a local tumor recurrence on a single examination. Proper patient history and/or follow-up examinations are usually required for a correct diagnosis (Fig. 8.74).

Langerhans cell histiocytosis (histiocytosis X) can mimic different diseases in the skull base and produce one or more lytic lesions. Sella turcica, sphenoid wings, petrous pyramids, and mastoid air cells are most often involved. Sellar destruction is not necessarily associated with diabetes insipidus, and vice versa. In the middle ear, the disease simulates unilateral or bilateral otitis media with or without cholesteatomas both clinically and radiographically (Fig. 8.74).

An *aneurysm of the internal carotid artery* may, depending on its location, cause erosion of the dorsum sella, petrous pyramid, carotid canal, and superior orbital fissure. The latter may also be eroded by a *carotid cavernous fistula* that is usually the consequence of a fracture involving the base of the skull.

are the result of ear infections and are quite common. A surgical defect following the excision of a cholesteatoma is usually impossible to differentiate from a cholesteatoma by conventional radiography. A large mastoid air cell can at times mimic a lytic defect in this area and must be differentiated. A summary of all destructive lesions involving the petrous pyramid, middle ear, and antrum is given in Table 8.**5**.

9 Orbits

Calcifications

Calcifications within the soft tissues of the orbits are uncommon, but their radiologic demonstration often has clinical significance and may be pathognomonic of a specific disease. Calcifications of the lens presenting as a circular density of approximately 7 mm on the posteroanterior projection and as an oval density on the lateral view occur in *cataracts*.

In *retrolental fibroplasia* (retinopathy developing in premature infants with oxygen being the primary offending agent), flecks of intravitreal calcifications are found that may be combined in a more advanced stage with lenticular calcifications (Fig. 9.1).

Finely stippled to conglomerate calcifications in children are seen with *retinoblastomas*, which are bilateral in approximately 20 %. Calcifications can also be found in intraorbital *meningiomas, gliomas, dermoids, angiomas, aneurysms, hematomas,* and *arteriovenous malformations*. These calcifications are similar in appearance to the previously described intracranial calcifications of the same lesions (Chapter 8). Multiple phleboliths have been reported in *venous malformations* and *cavernous hemangiomas* of the orbit. In *von Hippel–Lindau disease* (retinal, intracranial, and sometimes visceral angiomatosis) calcifications, though rare, may occur.

Bacterial and *parasitic infections* may rarely cause intraorbital calcifications. *Mucoceles* from the frontal or ethmoidal sinus may erode into the orbital cavity. Gross calcification of the cyst-like wall of a mucocele occurs in 5 % of these cases. *Phthysis bulbi* refers to shrinkage and wasting of the eye, usually the sequelae of severe, longstanding ophthalmic disease (e.g., trauma with intraocular foreign body, rupture of the globe, and chronic inflammatory disease). Calcification of the choroid, vitreous body and lens is common in this condition. In systemic conditions such as *hypercalcemia (e.g., hyperparathyroidism)* and *connective tissue disease*, intraorbital calcifications may occasionally be found. An intraorbital *foreign body* has to be differentiated from a pathologic calcification when the density of both is similar. The radiographic demonstration of even the smallest amount of intraorbital air *(orbital emphysema)* after a traumatic incident is virtually diagnostic of a fracture into an adjacent paranasal sinus, most commonly secondary to a fracture of the lamina papyracea of the ethmoid sinus (Fig. 9.2).

Erosions and Bony Defects in the Orbit

Dermoids and *epidermoids* occur most often in the superolateral portion of the orbit near its anterior margin. They grow slowly and produce a smoothly marginated defect often with slightly sclerotic margins.

Lacrimal gland tumors are benign mixed neoplasms that deepen the normal shallow fossa of the lacrimal gland in the superolateral quadrant of the orbit (Fig. 9.3). They do not produce a sharply marginated bony defect as observed with dermoid tumors in the same location. Rarely, lacrimal gland tumors undergo malignant transformation and cause irregu-

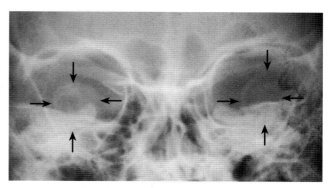

Fig. 9.**1** **Retrolental fibroplasia.** Lenticular calcifications (arrows) are seen in both orbits in this far advanced stage of the disease.

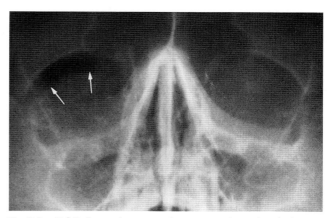

Fig. 9.**2** **Orbital emphysema.** A crescent-shaped radiolucency (arrows) is seen under the right orbital roof post fracture of the lamina papyracea of the ethmoid sinus, which cannot be appreciated on this examination,

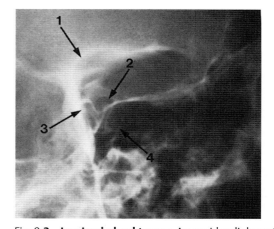

Fig. 9.**3** **Lacrimal gland tumor.** An ovoid radiolucent defect with a relatively poorly defined inferior margin is seen in the superolateral aspect of the orbit caused by deepening of the normally shallow fossa of the lacrimal gland in this location (arrow 1). Note also the oval-shaped optic canal (arrow 2), the pneumatized anterior clinoid projecting laterally to the optic canal (arrow 3), and the caroticoclinoid canal projecting inferiorly to it (arrow 4) on this standard optic canal projection.

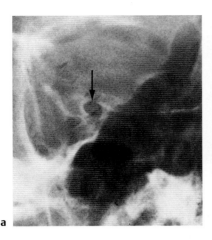
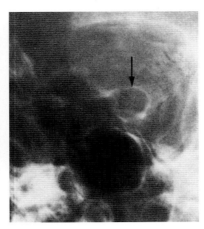

Fig. 9.**4 a, b   Optic nerve glioma.** A concentric enlargement of the left optic canal measuring 10 mm in diameter is seen in **b** (arrow). The normal right optic canal is shown for comparison in **a** (arrow).

a

b

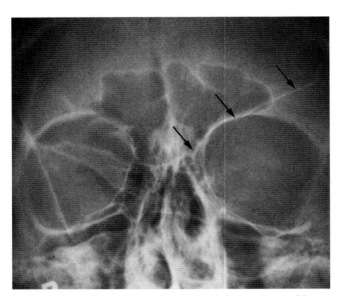

Fig. 9.**5   Neurofibromatosis.** Agenesis of the greater and lesser wings of the left sphenoid with absence of the superior orbital fissure and marked elevation of the sphenoid ridge (arrows) is seen in the enlarged left orbit ("empty orbit" sign). Hypoplasia of the left ethmoidal cells is also evident.

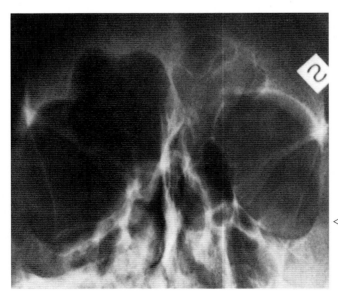

larly marginated lytic defects with or without a diffuse increase in density of the surrounding bone.

Hemangiomas and *retinoblastomas* in children, and *melanomas* in adults, are relatively common primary orbital tumors, but destruction of the orbital wall is unusual.

Carcinomas invading the orbit from the *nasopharynx* and *paranasal sinuses* can cause irregular bone destruction. *Gliomas* and *meningiomas* may also produce local areas of destruction, although a purely lytic involvement of the orbital wall by a meningioma is unusual. A *glioma* of the optic nerve produces localized enlargement of the optic canal (Fig. 9.**4**). This is the most common cause of a concentrically enlarged optic canal.

Orbital pseudotumors consist of a variety of chronic inflammatory conditions that rarely produce changes on conventional radiographic examinations. Enlargement of the superior orbital fissure or optic canal occurs exceptionally with lesions located posteriorly in the orbits.

Neurofibromatosis can be associated with unilateral orbital enlargement, large lytic defects in the orbital roof, walls, and floor, enlargement of the optic canal or superior orbital fissure and hypoplasia of the ipsilateral maxillary and ethmoid sinuses. Agenesis of the sphenoid wings produces the characteristic "empty orbit" sign (Fig. 9.**5**). Besides neurinomas and neurofibromas, gliomas and meningiomas are also found in this condition.

Metastases, lymphomas, multiple myeloma, and *primary bone* and *soft-tissue tumors* may involve the orbit, occasionally causing a destructive lesion. They must be considered in the differential diagnosis of an osteolytic or osteoblastic orbital bone lesion, but their presentation is not different from other locations.

Sinusitis may spread from the frontal sinus and less commonly from the ethmoid and maxillary sinuses into the soft tissue of the orbit. In such cases destruction of the intervening bone is common, but some increase in bone density along the margins is often present, suggesting the inflammatory etiology of the lesion. Similarly, a *mucocele* from an adjacent paranasal sinus may slowly erode into the orbit, causing a bony defect with smooth margins (Fig. 9.**6**).

◁ Fig. 9.**6   Mucocele of the frontal sinus** invading the right orbit and ethmoidal cells. A mucocele of the frontal sinus, which appears relatively radiolucent because of the considerable thinning of its walls that overcompensates the loss of aeration caused by the mucocele itself, has destroyed the right orbital roof and ethmoidal cells.

Table 9.1   Erosion and Enlargement of Optic Canal and Superior Orbital Fissure

Disease	Optic Canal	Superior Orbital Fissure
Increased intracranial pressure	Rare; concentric, bilateral	Rare; bilateral erosions of the margins of superior orbital fissures.
Glioma	Glioma of the optic nerve is the most common cause of concentric enlargement.	
Meningioma	Meningioma involving the optic nerve sheet. Rare. Enlargement concentric.	Rare. In meningiomas that originate from the middle fossa.
Pituitary tumor, craniopharyngioma or chordoma extending anteriorly	Unilateral or bilateral erosions beginning at the lateral wall.	Chromophobe adenomas are the second most common cause of superior orbital fissure widening.
Carcinoma of sphenoid sinus	Destruction of optic canal (particularly medial wall).	Rare
Intraorbital mass extending posteriorly	Rare (e.g., retinoblastoma)	Rare
Metastases	Rare	Rare
Inflammatory lesions	Rare. Concentric enlargement by granulomas (e.g., sarcoid, tuberculosis). Erosion of medial wall by mucocele of sphenoid sinus.	Rare (e.g., mucocele of sphenoid sinus).
Orbital pseudotumor	Rare	Rare
Aneurysm	Ophthalmic artery: concentric enlargement. Internal carotid artery (cavernous portion): lateral wall erosion.	Aneurysm of internal carotid artery (cavernous portion) most common cause of superior orbital fissure enlargement.
Arteriovenous malformation	Concentric enlargement with ophthalmic artery involvement.	Superior orbital fissure enlarged with ophthalmic vein involvement (e.g. , carotid-cavernous sinus fistula).
Orbital varix		Congenital dilatation of orbital veins that can occasionally cause an enlargement of the superior orbital fissure.
Langerhans cell histiocytosis (histiocytosis X)	Localized destruction of the optic canal is rare.	Limitation of destructive lesions to superior orbital fissure is uncommon.
Neurofibromatosis	Concentric enlargement of optic canal usually caused by associated optic nerve glioma.	Congenital enlargement of superior orbital fissure that is not associated with any mass lesion (orbital dysplasia) occurs. Neurofibromas and posterior orbital encephalocele can occasionally enlarge the superior orbital fissure but are not always associated with neurofibromatosis.

Langerhans cell histiocytosis produces irregularly marginated defects in the orbit. With healing, either spontaneously or after therapy, the margin of the lesion may become sclerotic. The lesions can vary considerably in size and seem to have a predilection for the roof and lateral wall of the orbit.

Conditions causing a more localized enlargement of the optic canal and superior orbital fissure are summarized in Table 9.1. The diameter of the *optic canal* ranges from 4 to 6 mm and its radiographic appearance varies considerably. In healthy subjects it is usually oval and rarely truly circular. Normal variants include "figure-of-eight" and "keyhole" ap-

pearances, the latter being essentially an incomplete "figure-of-eight." Pneumatization of the anterior clinoid may create the appearance of a second canal projecting laterally to the true optic canal. The caroticoclinoid canal is a developmental anomaly found in approximately 35% of skulls and projects inferiorly to the true optic canal (see Fig. 9.3).

The *superior orbital fissure* is the largest communication between middle fossa and orbit and has the shape of an inverted comma. Variations in size and shape are common, however, and an asymmetry between the two orbital fissures is found in 9% of cases.

Sclerosis of the Orbit

Sclerosis of the orbital walls must be differentiated from an intraorbital mass lesion causing an increased soft tissue density. Besides the orbital bones, an increased soft tissue density also obscures normal radiolucent areas such as the superior orbital fissure, whereas bony sclerosis outlines these areas more sharply and may even narrow the superior orbital fissure and the optic canal.

Meningiomas arising in the orbital walls are commonly associated with localized bone thickening and sclerosis. This is particularly true for meningiomas involving the greater and lesser sphenoid wings, where homogeneous sclerosis and thickening is quite characteristic ("meningioma en plaque"). When these sphenoid meningiomas are medially located, encroachment and narrowing of the superior orbital fissure and optic canal occur that can result in compression of the corresponding nerves (Fig. 9.**7**).

Chronic *frontal sinusitis* can cause a dense sclerosis of the orbital roof with irregular and poorly defined margins. Small osteolytic areas may be present within the sclerotic, thickened bone. *Sphenoid sinusitis* can also produce an osteitic reaction and reduce the lumen of the optic canal. Similarly, the superior orbital fissure can also be narrowed by a nonspecific sclerotic osteitis.

Fibrous dysplasia frequently involves the anterior portion of the base of the skull (Fig. 9.**8**). Thickening and sclerosis are often found in the roof and posterior wall of the orbit. The process is often bilateral and extensive. Differentiation from a meningioma can, however, be difficult when the process is unilateral and more localized. The age of the patient may be helpful in differentiating these two conditions, since fibrous dysplasia is usually discovered before the age of 20, whereas meningiomas occur usually in middle-aged and elderly persons. Symptoms of nerve compression are rare in fibrous dysplasia, even when the superior orbital fissure and optic canal appear encroached.

Paget's disease involves the orbits only in a late stage of the disease. As in other areas of the skull, coarse trabeculation and mottled sclerosis in a thickened bone are characteristic, and enchroachment of neural foramina can also occur.

Osteopetrosis affects the sphenoid wings including the superior orbital fissure and optic canal at an early stage. Symptoms related to nerve compression are a common initial complaint in these patients. At this stage, the degree of sclerosis is more impressive than the bone thickening. The radiographic changes are usually bilateral. A familial history is often helpful in establishing the diagnosis at this early stage. The involvement of the skeleton is usually already widespread in late childhood and adolescence.

Langerhans cell histiocytosis can present in the orbit a diffuse sclerosis often interspersed with some lytic lesions (Fig. 9.**9**). The disease may spread into adjacent bones but characteristically does not involve the sphenoid wings. Enlargement of the orbital fissure and optic canal is exceedingly rare.

In *craniometaphyseal dysplasia*, sclerosis of the orbits is often associated with narrowing of the optic canal (Fig. 9.**10**). "Erlenmeyer flask" deformities of the metaphyses of the long bones are characteristically also present in this condition.

Sclerosis of the orbital walls may be caused by many other lesions already discussed in Chapter **2**. The presence of these lesions in the orbit is, however, merely coincidental and their radiographic presentation does not differ from other locations in the skeleton. The orbital involvement may also be a manifestation of a more generalized disease process that is easily diagnosed when all findings are taken into consideration. For a complete differential diagnosis of sclerotic orbital lesions, the reader is therefore urged to consult Chapter **2**, which deals with osteosclerosis in general.

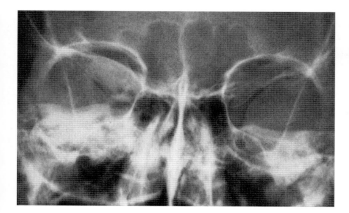

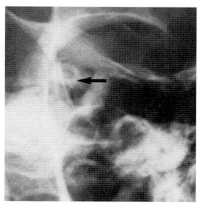

Fig. 9.**7 a, b**
Meningioma. Significant sclerosis of the lesser and greater right sphenoid wings with marked narrowing of the right superior orbital fissure and right optic canal (arrow in **b**) is seen.

Fig. 9.**8**   **Fibrous dysplasia.** Sclerosis and thickening of the right facial bones including roof and posterior wall of the orbit is seen.

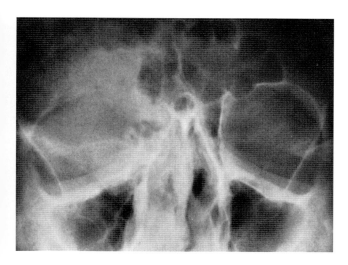

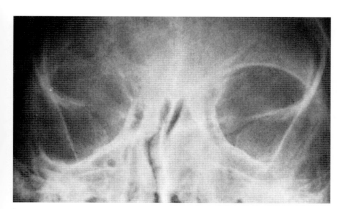

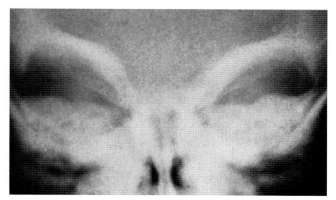

Fig. 9.**9**   **Langerhans cell histiocytosis.** Sclerosis and destruction of the superomedial wall of the right orbit with involvement of the adjacent frontal sinus and ethmoidal cells is evident.

Fig. 9.**10**   **Craniometaphyseal dysplasia.** Symmetrical sclerosis of both orbits is associated with sclerotic changes in the base of the skull and facial bones.

10 Nasal Fossa and Paranasal Sinuses

The paranasal sinuses consist of the frontal sinus, sphenoid sinus, maxillary antra, and ethmoidal air cells. They communicate with the nasal fossa and are lined with a mucous membrane contiguous with that of the nasal cavity. These are two important factors for the understanding of the development and spread of any pathologic process. Pneumatization and expansion of the sinuses occurs during the first and second decade of life, reaching its full extent only in early adulthood. The size of the sinuses varies greatly from individual to individual and even between the right and left side of the same individual. *Unilateral* or *bilateral hypoplasia* is not uncommon and has no clinical significance, except in some congenital syndromes where it might be a finding in a much wider spectrum of radiographic abnormalities (e.g., hypoplastic maxillary antra in *dysostosis cleidocranialis*). Enlarged paranasal sinuses are a constant feature of *acromegaly*, but as an isolated finding are best disregarded.

Since the paranasal sinuses are air-containing cavities, soft-tissue changes occurring in them can already be well demonstrated by conventional radiographic technique. Complete opacification of a sinus may at times be more difficult to appreciate than less severe mucosal thickening that is still contrasted by air. As a rule of thumb, the maxillary antra should normally have a similar transparency as the orbits in the Water's view. Fluid accumulation in a paranasal sinus can easily be demonstrated using a horizontal roentgen beam. In this case the fluid will accumulate in the deepest part of the sinus and form a sharp interface with the air topping it. It must, however, be remembered that when using a vertical beam, any fluid accumulation in a sinus produces a diffuse loss of translucency that is indistinguishable from mucosal thickening.

An *air–fluid level in a sinus* is caused by the accumulation of blood, pus, or exudate produced by the mucosa. An air–fluid level produced by blood is most commonly the result of a *fracture* (Fig. 10.1). Occasionally the only radiographic clue to a paranasal sinus fracture consists of a localized soft-tissue swelling caused by mucosal or submucosal bleeding. This is particularly common in *blow-out fractures of the orbit*, presenting as a small, soft-tissue bulge on the antral roof (Fig. 10.2). A more extensive hemorrhage can cause a complete loss of translucency of the involved paranasal sinus. In the maxillary antrum, a soft-tissue hematoma of the overlying cheek must be differentiated from a hemorrhage within the sinus, since both can cause a generalized loss of translucency. Clinical examination of the patient and radiographs in different projections allow differentiation between these two conditions.

Fractures of the paranasal sinus can sometimes only be diagnosed radiographically by demonstrating the leak of air from a sinus into a neighboring structure. *Orbital emphysema* is encountered with maxillary and ethmoidal sinus fractures (see Fig. 9.2). Air within the cranial cavity *(pneumocephalus)* may result from a fracture involving the frontal or ethmoid sinus.

Acute sinusitis is the most common cause of an air–fluid level in a paranasal sinus. Although air–fluid levels occur

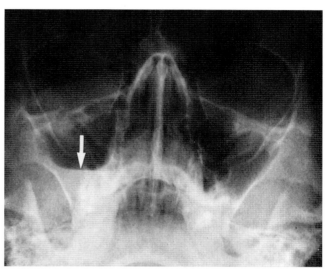

Fig. 10.**1 Air-fluid (blood) level secondary to trauma.** A fracture in the right antral roof with bleeding into the right maxillary antrum evident by the air-fluid level (arrow) is seen.

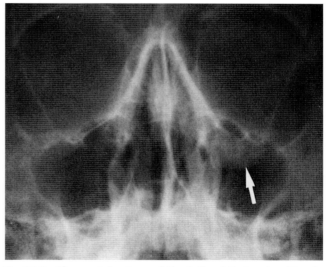

Fig. 10.**2 Blow-out fracture of the left orbit.** A polypoid soft-tissue mass (arrow) hanging from the left antral roof is the only radiographic evidence of this fracture.

with allergic sinusitis, they are more common with infectious sinusitis. The latter condition is often limited to one sinus, and mucosal thickening paralleling the bony walls is characteristically found. In allergic sinusitis a diffuse involvement of the nose (swelling of the turbinates) and all sinuses is usually present. In this condition, the mucosal thickening often produces a scalloped lining, and polyp formations are frequently encountered.

A soft-tissue thickening or mass with or without destruction of the adjacent bone can, however, be found in many other conditions, which will be discussed in Table 10.1. Asymmetry of the sinuses between the right and left side or localized osteosclerosis in a sinus wall can also produce a unilateral decrease in translucency that should not be confused with soft-tissue thickening within a sinus (Fig. 10.3).

Benign and malignant tumors of cartilagenous or osseous origin may occasionally develop in the facial bones. Their presentation, however, does not differ from any other location and their differential diagnosis has been covered in Chapter 5. A *rhinolith* in the nasal cavity should not be mistaken for such a lesion (Fig. 10.4).

Table 10.1   Soft-tissue Thickening or Mass in Paranasal Sinuses

Lesion	Radiographic Appearance	Comments
Benign tumors (see Fig. 10.18)	Variable, ranging from a localized soft-tissue mass to a dense bony lesion (osteoma).	Except for osteomas, these tumors are very rare and include *lipomas, hemangiomas , dermoids* and *chondromas*.
Carcinoma (Figs. 10.5 and 10.6)	Soft-tissue mass associated almost invariably with bone destruction. Sclerotic reaction of infiltrated bone occurs on rare occasions.	Usually found in patients over 50. Squamous cell carcinoma is by far the most common histologic type.
Sarcoma	Findings indistinguishable from carcinoma except when new bone is formed (e.g. , osteosarcoma).	Rare. All ages. *Benign mesenchymal neoplasms* are even less common.
Extrinsic neoplasm invading sinus (Fig. 10.7)	Usually malignant but also benign (e.g., chordoma, enchondroma, pituitary adenoma in sphenoid sinus, and juvenile angiofibroma.	*Juvenile angiofibroma*: Highly vascular tumor originating in nasopharynx of adolescent males. May bow the posterior wall of the maxillary antra anteriorly or invade the adjacent sinuses, orbits and even the cranium.
Odontogenic lesions (cysts, tumors)	Limited to the base of maxillary antra.	For differential diagnosis see Chapter 11.
Lymphoma (usually nonHodgkin) (Fig. 10.8)	Involvement often bilateral with soft-tissue thickening (occasionally polypoid) and frequently bone erosions.	Lymphadenopathy is usually the dominant clinical feature.
Wegener's granulomatosis (Fig. 10.9)	Unilateral or more commonly bilateral soft tissue thickening, often associated with erosion and/or sclerosis of the adjacent bone.	Usually associated with pulmonary, vascular, and renal disease. *Limited form of Wegener's granulomatosis*: Confined to respiratory tract including nasal cavity and paranasal sinuses and of relatively good prognosis.
Midline granuloma	Ulcerating granulomatous masses with progressive destruction of paranasal sinuses, nose, and hard and soft palate.	Destructive process may erode through the skin, resulting in mutilation of the face. Without proper treatment, the disease is fatal. Good response to high-dose local radiotherapy. The sinus involvement is radiographically indistinguishable from Wegener's granulomatosis, but there is neither pulmonary nor renal involvement.
Fibrous dysplasia (Fig 10.10)	Expansion and nonhomogeneous opacification of the involved sinuses. Associated with predominantly sclerotic involvement of the adjacent facial bones.	Similar findings in *ossifying fibromas* that can be regarded as localized form of fibrous dysplasia in facial bones. *"Leontiasis ossea"* (deformity and bilateral enlargement of the face) is caused by widespread involvement of the frontal and facial bones by fibrous dysplasia.

(continues on page 242)

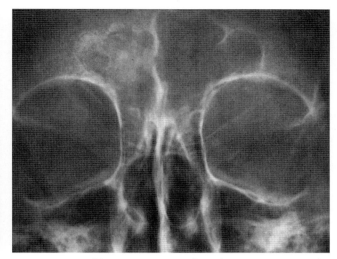

Fig. 10.**3** **Osteoblastic metastases** from breast carcinoma. The poorly defined increased density in the right frontal sinus is caused by osteoblastic bone metastases and should not be mistaken for soft-tissue thickening in this sinus.

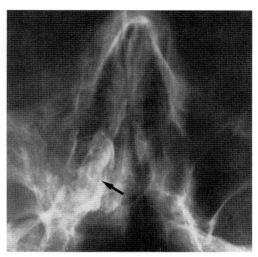

Fig. 10.**4** **Rhinolith.** An irregular sclerotic lesion is seen in the right nasal cavity (arrow).

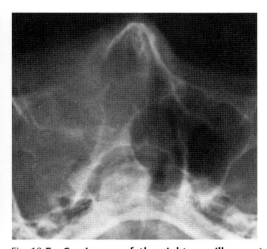

Fig. 10.**5** **Carcinoma of the right maxillary antrum.** A large soft-tissue mass originating from the right maxillary antrum with extensive destruction of the facial bones including the nose is seen.

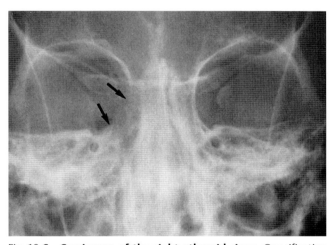

Fig. 10.**6** **Carcinoma of the right ethmoid sinus.** Opacification of the ethmoidal air cells with destruction of the adjacent medial wall (arrows) of the right orbit is seen.

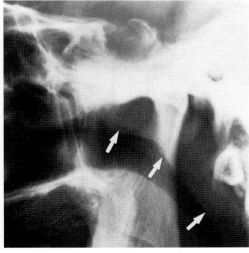

Fig. 10.**7** **Carcinoma of the nasopharynx** with invasion into the sphenoid sinus and pituitary fossa. The carcinoma, evident in the nasopharynx as increased soft-tissue density (arrows), has invaded into the sphenoid sinus, which is opacified, and destroyed the floor of the pituitary fossa.

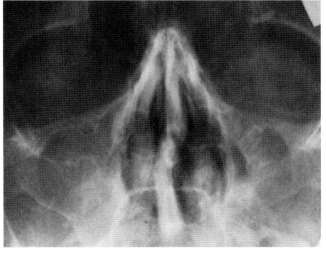

Fig. 10.**8** **Non-Hodgkin's lymphoma.** Complete obliteration of both maxillary antra by soft-tissue masses is seen. There is also a suggestion of bony erosions in both the left maxillary roof, where the infraorbital foramen can no longer be outlined, and the inferolateral wall of the left antrum, which can barely be recognized

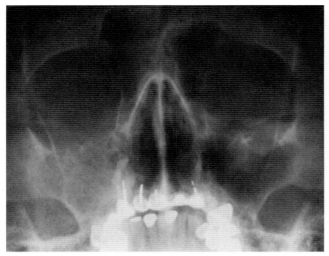

Fig. 10.**9   Wegener's granulomatosis.** Complete opacification of the right maxillary antrum with destruction of its superomedial wall and a soft-tissue mass protruding into the adjacent orbit is evident. Soft-tissue thickening including a round granulomatous mass is also present in the roof of the left maxillary antrum, but its wall appears to be intact.

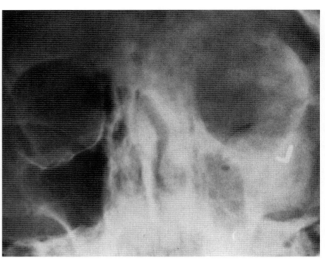

Fig. 10.**10   Fibrous dysplasia.** Enlargement of the left half of the face and left orbit by predominantly sclerotic lesions and nonhomogeneous opacification of the left maxillary antrum are seen. Involvement of the frontal bone is also evident.

Table 10.1   (Cont.) Soft-tissue Thickening or Mass in Paranasal Sinuses

Lesion	Radiographic Appearance	Comments
Neurofibromatosis (Fig. 10.11)	Deformed and enlarged facial bones and sinuses associated with large soft-tissue masses (neurofibromas) which may erode into the adjacent bones.	Changes in skull and orbit are more common and characteristic.
Paget's disease (Fig. 10.12)	Obliteration of sinuses occurs occasionally, but is solely caused by thickening and sclerosis of the bone without soft-tissue involvement.	Involvement of skull is much more common and characteristic.
Sinusitis – acute (Figs. 10.13 and 10.14)	Air-fluid levels, soft-tissue swelling, and polyps. Secondary osteomyelitis of adjacent bone is very rare.	Allergic or infectious. Infectious sinusitis is usually secondary to upper respiratory tract infections (e.g. , streptococci, staphylococci, or viral infections). Maxillary sinusitis can also be of dental origin.
Sinusitis, chronic granulomatous (Fig. 10.15)	Nasal and/or upper respiratory tract diseases are associated and usually prominent. Soft-tissue swelling, polypoid lesions, bone destruction, and sclerosis occur in sinuses.	*Bacterial*: tuberculosis, syphilis, leprosy, glanders (*Pseudomonas mallei*), listeriosis, yaws, actinomycosis, and *rhinoscleroma* (probably caused by *Klebsiella rhinoscleromatis*). *Fungal*: aspergillosis, blastomycosis, histoplasmosis, coccidioidomycosis, cryptococcosis, mucormycosis, sporotrichosis, rhinosporidiosis. *Idiopathic*: sarcoidosis, erythema nodosum.
Polyp and cyst (Fig. 10.16)	Smooth spherical or domeshaped opacities which may alter slightly their convex borders in different projections when the lesions are cystic and not under tension. Broadbased cystic lesions originating from the floor of the maxillary sinus may mimic occasionally an airfluid level. Sinus is uniformly opaque when completely occupied by lesion. The walls of the sinus are not affected.	"Polyp": Inflammatory hypertrophic swelling of mucosa. "Cyst": 1. Encapsulated exudate, pus, or blood. 2. Retention cyst containing mucus or serous material. 3. Surgical: Ciliated cyst developing in maxillary sinus post Caldwell-Luc operation (surgical production of window connecting the antrum with the inferior meatus of the nose).

(continues on page 244)

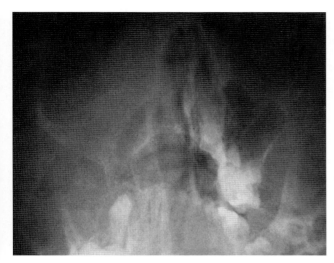

Fig. 10.**11** **Neurofibromatosis.** Enlarged right half of the face associated with huge soft-tissue masses (neurofibromas), that have eroded the adjacent bone is evident.

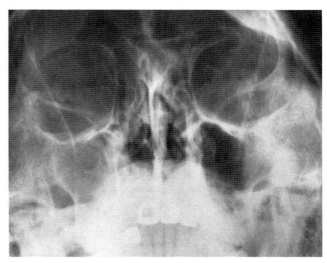

Fig. 10.**12** **Paget's disease.** Thickening and sclerosis of the facial bones bilaterally with complete obliteration of the right maxillary antrum is seen. Note also the sclerotic changes in the left skull vault.

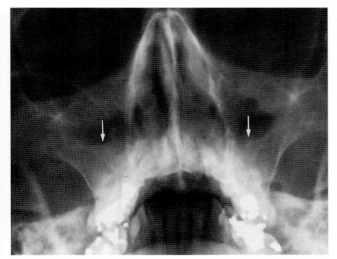

Fig. 10.**13** **Acute sinusitis.** Bilateral soft-tissue thickening and air-fluid levels (arrows) are seen in both maxillary antra. A viral upper respiratory tract infection preceded this examination.

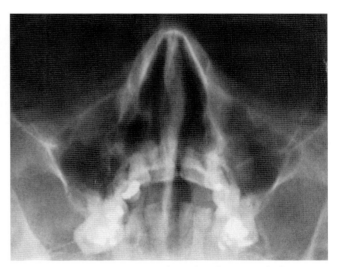

Fig. 10.**14** **Acute sinusitis.** Polypoid soft-tissue thickening in both maxillary antra is found in this patient with allergic history.

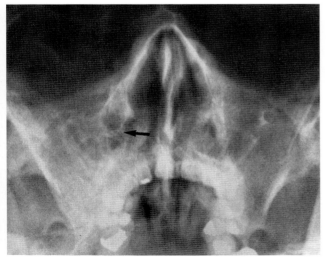

Fig. 10.**15** **Chronic granulomatous sinusitis.** Complete opacification of both maxillary antra with localized destruction of the medial wall on the right side (arrow) is caused by aspergillosis.

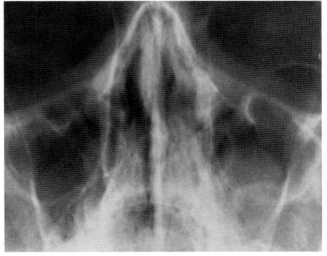

Fig. 10.**16** **Retention cyst.** A large polypoid soft-tissue density is seen in the base of the left maxillary antrum.

Table 10.1   (Cont.) Soft-tissue Thickening or Mass in Paranasal Sinuses

Lesion	Radiographic Appearance	Comments
Mucocele (Fig. 10.17)	Most common in frontal sinus, May occasionally produce an increased translucency of involved sinus when thinning of the adjacent bone outweighs the increased density from the fluid content. Erodes into neighboring structures (see also Fig. 9.**6**).	Develops when ostium of sinus remains closed after an infection has subsided. Retained aseptic fluid produces changes by pressure erosion. *Osteomas*, which are also most commonly found in the frontal sinus, have a much greater density than mucoceles and should not be confused with the latter (Fig. 10.**18**).
Fracture (see Fig. 10.1)	Localized submucosal hematoma may simulate polyp (e.g., blowout fracture: polypoid mass on antral roof). Air–fluid (blood) level may be present. Partial to complete sinus opacification may be found in an acute fracture or as sequela of an old fracture. Complex facial fractures include *blowout fractures of the orbit* (see Fig. 10.**2**), *tripod fracture* (Fig. 10.**19**), and *Lefort fractures* (Fig. 10.**20**).	In *barotrauma* (e.g., among divers and pilots of unpressurized aircraft) similar changes can be found. In this condition, polypoid mucosal swelling to complete opacification of a sinus is caused by submucosal hemorrhage, mucosal thickening, and/or outpouring of secretion.

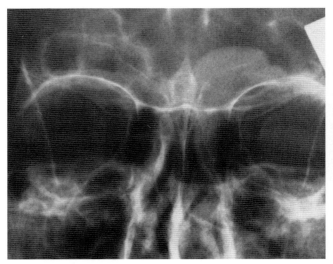

Fig. 10.**17**   **Mucocele.** A slightly lobulated soft-tissue mass is seen in the base of the left frontal sinus that is unusually large.

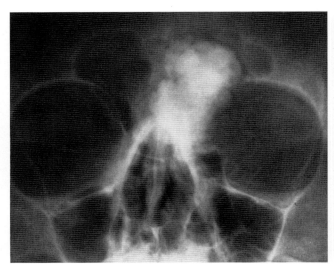

Fig. 10.**18**   **Osteoma.** A very dense, structureless, and lobulated lesion involving the left frontal and ethmoidal sinuses is seen.

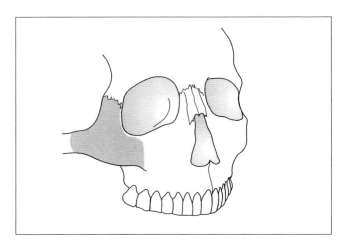

Fig. 10.**19**   **Tripod fracture.** Fracture sites include the frontozygomatic suture, zygomatic arch, and lateral wall of maxillary sinus with the anterior orbital rim.

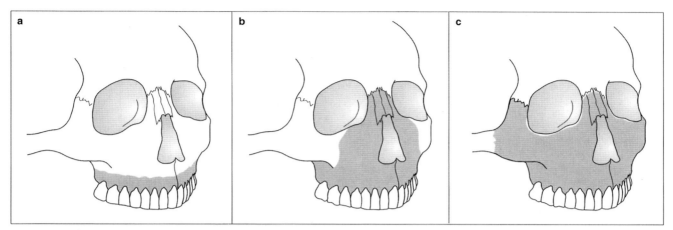

Fig. 10.**20**   **Lefort fractures. a** Lefort I: horizontal fracture line extending across the floor of the maxillary sinus above the dentition line ("floating palate"). **b** Lefort II: fracture runs vertically through the maxilla and across the nasal bridge and back to the pterygoid plates ("floating maxilla"). **c** Lefort III: fracture line passes across the bridge of the nose, orbits, and frontozygomatic sutures into the zygomatic arches and pterygoid plates ("floating face").

11   Jaws and Teeth

Calcifications in the soft tissues around the jaws may be caused by the same conditions as anywhere else in the body. They are commonly arteriosclerotic in origin or due to calcified lymph nodes secondary to granulomatous disease. These conditions must, however, be differentiated from *salivary gland calcifications*, which are usually caused by salivary calculi. They are radiopaque in approximately 80% because of their high calcium carbonate content and occur most often in the submandibular glands, less commonly in the parotid glands, and virtually never in the sublingual glands. A salivary stone tends to be oval in shape and usually has a relatively homogeneous density (Fig. 11.**1**).

Dysfunction of the temporomandibular joint may affect as many as 25% of the adult population and causes a variety of clinical symptoms ranging from headache to myofascial pain. This entity has gained increasing attention in recent years and is now referred to as temporomandibular joint syndrome. Unfortunately, plain film radiography is generally of little use in evaluating this condition, since in the vast majority of cases the disorder is related to an abnormality of the meniscus that divides this joint, and hence arthrography, computed tomography, or magnetic resonance imaging is required for proper diagnosis. In far-advanced cases, flattening or atrophy of the mandibular head, flattening of the articular tubercle, sclerosis, cysts, and spur formations around the joint may be seen with conventional radiographic technique (Fig. 11.**2**).

In the jaws, many pathologic conditions are related to the teeth. The emphasis in the remaining part of this chapter is on the differential diagnosis of these odontogenic lesions. The radiographic presentations of nonodontogenic lesions that may be confused with odontogenic lesions will be briefly discussed. For a more complete differential diagnosis of nonodontogenic lesions, the reader should refer to Chapters 1, 2, and 5.

Periodontal Abnormalities

The periodontium represents the supporting structure of the teeth comprising gingiva, periodontal ligament (membrane), alveolar bone, and cementum (Fig. 11.**3**). Radiographically, the cementum outlining the roots of the teeth cannot be differentiated from dentin. The periodontal membrane, evident radiographically as a radiolucent line of less than 1 mm in width, separates the root of a tooth in its socket from the alveolar bone of the jaw. A thin cortical line, the lamina dura, demarcates the latter from the periodontal membrane. From this observation, it becomes obvious that periodontal pathology can manifest itself radiographically as loss of lamina dura, widening of the periodontal membrane, or both. These subtle changes cannot, however, be appreciated with conventional x-ray technique, and require special dental films with high resolution for proper evaluation. Excessive bone resorption around the root of a tooth is commonly referred to as *"floating tooth."*

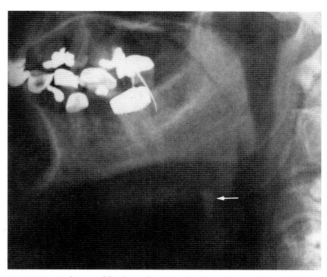

Fig. 11.**1** **Submandibular gland calculus.** An ovoid soft-tissue calcification (arrow) is seen below the right mandibular angle.

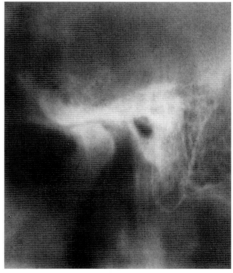

Fig. 11.**2** **Advanced degenerative changes in the temporomandibular joint** (tomography). Anterior spur and degenerative cyst are seen in the deformed and sclerotic head of the condylar process. There is also considerable flattening of the articular tubercle located anteriorly to the glenoid fossa, with significant sclerosis of both these structures.

Resorption of the lamina dura is common in primary and secondary *hyperparathyroidism*. In this condition, it is usually not associated with an appreciable widening of the periodontal membrane space. Reappearance of the lamina dura occurs after proper treatment. A generalized loss of the

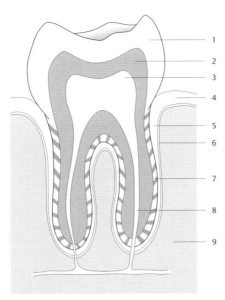

Fig. 11.**3** **Anatomy of a normal molar tooth.** 1 Enamel; 2 dentin; 3 pulp; 4 gum; 5 periodontal membrane; 6 lamina dura; 7 cement; 8 apical canal; 9 alveolar bone.

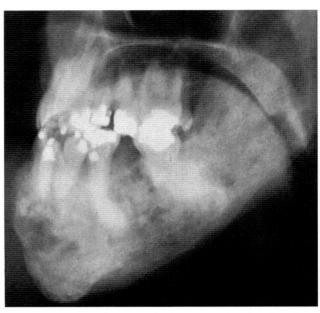

Fig. 11.**4** **Paget's disease.** Thickening and sclerosis of the mandible resulted in an apparent loss of the lamina dura around the teeth.

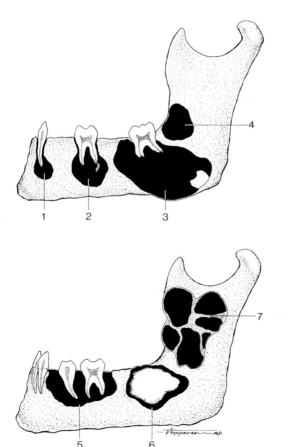

Fig. 11.**5 a, b** **Lytic mandibular lesions.** 1 Dental granuloma; 2 periodontal cyst (occasionally containing small root remnant); 3 dentigerous cyst; 4 primordial cyst; 5 "floating teeth" (e.g., eosinophilic granuloma); 6 odontoma; 7 ameloblastoma.

lamina dura can also be found with *osteoporosis* of any etiology (e.g., senile, steroid therapy, Cushing's syndrome), but in these cases remnants of the lamina can often still be recognized unless the osteoporosis has progressed so far that the correct diagnosis can easily be established by other radiographic findings. In both *periodontosis* (non-inflammatory, degenerative) and *periodontitis* (inflammatory), resorption of bone including the lamina dura occurs characteristically around the neck and proximal part of the root of a tooth while the lamina dura around the apex remains intact. If the process proceeds to a *periodontal abscess*, resorption of the entire lamina dura combined with widening of the periodontal membrane space may be found.

The radiographic absence of lamina dura is not only the result of its resorption but may also be caused by an increase in bone density of the adjacent cancellous bone as seen, for example, in *sclerosing osteomyelitis*. The radiographic loss of lamina dura observed in *Paget's disease* (Fig. 11.4), *fibrous dysplasia*, and *osteomalacia* is commonly the result of both bone resorption and sclerosis.

The width of a normal periodontal membrane space measures radiographically less than 1 mm. Generalized *widening of the periodontal membrane space* with intact lamina dura is characteristic for *scleroderma*, but may also be found in patients with the *habit of forcibly clenching the teeth*. The most common cause for a localized widening of the periodontal gap associated with resorption of the lamina dura is a severe inflammation such as *periodontal abscess*. More extensive bone resorption around one or several teeth produces radiographically the impression of *"floating teeth."* In addition to a periodontal abscess, this finding is common in *eosinophilic granuloma (Langerhans cell histiocytosis)*, but may also be encountered in any other condition producing a large lytic lesion such as *ameloblastoma, lymphoma, leukemia, multiple myeloma, metastases,* and *odontogenic lesions*.

Localized lytic lesions of odontogenic origin can represent an inflammatory, cystic, or neoplastic process or may be a developmental anomaly. The most common lytic lesions in the mandible are shown schematically in Fig. 11.5, while their more complete differential diagnosis is discussed in Table 11.1.

Only a few localized sclerotic lesions are unique for the jaw. *Odontomas* consist of an irregular opaque mass of different dental tissues such as enamel, dentin and cementum surrounded by a radiolucent line or band representing the fibrous capsule. Symmetric and bilateral sclerotic bony pro-

tuberances are occasionally found in the midline of the palate or along the lingual surface of the mandible (primarily in the canine-premolar region) and are termed *torus palatinus* and *mandibularis*, respectively. These are benign static growths without clinical significance. They must be differentiated from *osteomas*, which are protruding mass lesions composed of abnormally dense bone that is formed in the periosteum. They are most common in the skull and facial bones.

Table 11.1   Differential Diagnosis of Lytic Lesions in the Jaw

Lesion	Radiographic Appearance	Comments
Periodontal abscess	Localized poorly to well-defined defect in the periphery of a tooth.	*Periodontitis* is an extension of gingivitis to the underlying periodontal tissues. An abscess develops usually in a periodontal pocket that is partially or completely occluded, or is occasionally caused by a foreign body lodged in the periodontium.
Periapical abscess	Localized poorly to well-defined defect around the apex of a tooth.	Results from progression of pulpitis. In the acute stage, the tooth is extremely painful and tender to percussion. In the chronic stage, draining sinuses to the oral cavity, maxillary antra and even the surface of the skin may occasionally develop.
Periapical granuloma	Round or oval, fairly well-circumscribed radiolucency rarely exceeding 1 cm in diameter. May ultimately be transformed into periodontal cyst.	Forms as the reparative process following the resolution of a periapical abscess.
Periodontal cyst (dental, radicular or apical cyst) (Fig. 11.6)	Sharply defined radiolucent lesion with thin sclerotic margin, measuring from a few millimeters to several centimeters. Rarely remnants of the root of a primary tooth are found within the lesion. Bone expansion can be found with an enlarging cyst.	Most common cyst of jaw. Epithelium-lined sac, usually situated at the apex of the root. Acquired and probably of inflammatory origin (see periapical granuloma). A *residual cyst* (Fig. 11.7) is a cystic lesion remaining after tooth removal. Occasionally infected, particularly when root of tooth is retained (residual infection). *Multiple cysts* are rare and either developmental or associated with extensive caries.
Dentigerous cyst (follicular cyst) (Fig. 11.8)	Sharply defined, oval or round radiolucent lesion varying in size from 1 cm to a large expansile defect involving both the body and ramus of the mandible. The lesion characteristically contains the *crown of an unerupted tooth.*	Arises from the follicle of an unerupted tooth and is usually found in young persons. Cysts eventually destroyed by late tooth eruption have been referred to as "*eruptive cysts.*"

(continues on page 250)

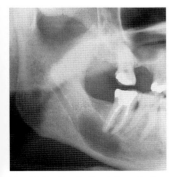

Fig. 11.6   Periodontal cyst. A well defined radiolucent lesion with very thin sclerotic margins involving the apex of the roots of the last molar is seen.

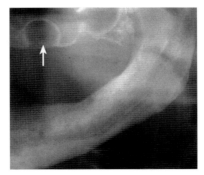

Fig. 11.7   Resdiual cyst. A cystic lesion with sclerotic border is seen in the maxilla (arrow). Irregular thickening and sclerosis of the left body and ramus of the mandible is also evident due to *sclerosing osteomyelitis of Garré.*

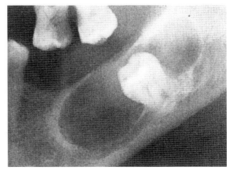

Fig. 11.8   Dentigerous cyst. A sharply defined, lytic lesion containing a molar crown is seen involving the left body of the mandible.

Table 11.1   (Cont.) Differential Diagnosis of Lytic Lesions in the Jaw

Lesion	Radiographic Appearance	Comments
Primordial cyst (Fig. 11.9)	Purely lytic, well-marginated, unilocular, round or oval lesion most commonly located posterior of the third molar in the angle or ramus of mandible.	Develops from embryonal tooth sac before any calcified structures have been formed.
Keratocyst (Fig. 11.10)	Radiolucent, often multiloculated lesion with smooth or scalloped border located in the body or ramus of the mandible. Occurs frequently in conjunction with impacted tooth. Differentiation from an ameloblastoma is often not possible.	Account for 5 to 10% of all jaw cysts and have a high recurrence rate. Multiple keratocysts can be found in *Gorlin's syndrome*, where they are associated with nevoid basal cell carcinomas and soft tissue calcifications. Other bony abnormalities include small flame-shaped cystic lesions and sclerotic foci, bifid ribs and anomalies of the spine and hands.
Fissural cyst	Most commonly located in midline of mandible or maxilla (e.g., incisive canal cyst or nasopalatine cyst), rarely lateral (e.g., globulomaxillary cyst between lateral incisor and canine tooth).	Arises from the epithelial remnant of an existing fissure or suture (sites of embryonic fusions).
Solitary bone cyst of the mandible (traumatic cyst) (Fig. 11.11)	In general relatively poorly defined and irregular radiolucency of varying size usually located in the body of the mandible. Larger lesions characteristically have a scalloped superior border that appears to undulate around the roots of teeth into the interdental bone. The teeth are neither splayed nor loosened.	Occurs most often in younger persons. History of trauma often present ("traumatic" or "hemorrhagic" cyst). May regress spontaneously.
Ameloblasioma (adamantinoma) (Fig. 11.12)	Unilocular or more commonly multilocular cystic (bubble-like) appearance often with coarse trabecular structures filling in part of the cystic cavities. Size varies from 1 cm to huge tumors causing cortical expansion or destruction with deformity of the face. Rarely, a small tumor mimics a simple cyst.	Most common tumor of the mandible that can occur at any age but is usually diagnosed after 30 years of age. Local invasion into surrounding structures and even distant metastases occur. *Adenoameloblastoma* (Fig. 11.13) and *ameloblastic fibroma* are rare tumors occurring both in the first two decades of life. They are clinically less aggressive than ameloblastomas. Clusters of calcifications and retained teeth may be found in these lesions.
Calcifying epithelial odontogenic tumor (Pindborg tumor) (Fig. 11.14)	Similar to ameloblastoma, but more dense when the characteristic honeycomb appearance is present within the lesion.	Clinical behavior similar to ameloblastoma: Locally invasive and tendency to recur.

(continues on page 252)

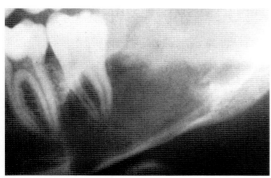

Fig. 11.**9** **Primordial cyst.** A well-defined cystic lesion is seen in the angle of the left mandible.

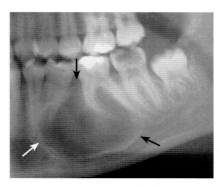

Fig. 11.**10** **Keratocyst**. A lytic lesion with partially sclerotic border (arrows) is seen in the body of the left mandible.

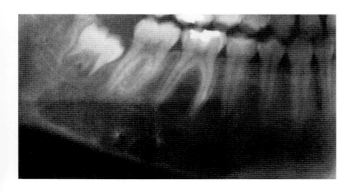

Fig. 11.**11** **Solitary (traumatic) cyst of the mandible.** A poorly-defined radiolucency with scalloped margins involving large portions of the right mandibular body extends superiorly between the roots of the teeth.

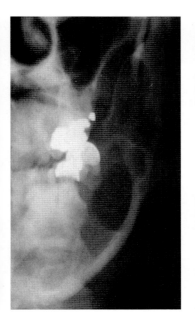

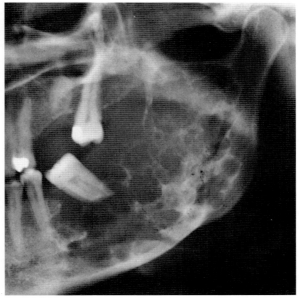

Fig. 11.**12 a, b** **Ameloblastoma** (2 cases). **a** A multilocular cystic and slightly expansile lesion with cortical thinning involves the left ramus and part of the adjacent body of the mandible. **b** A more aggressive lesion with soap-bubble appearance in similar location caused destruction of the cortex and resorption of the roots of an encroached molar.

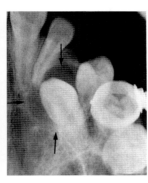

Fig. 11.**13** **Adenoameloblastoma.** A cystic lesion (arrows) associated with an unerupted tooth is characteristic.

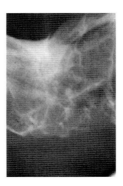

Fig. 11.**14** **Calcifying epithelial odontogenic tumor** (Pindborg). A lytic lesion with honeycomb appearance and small calcifications is seen.

Table 11.1 (Cont.) Differential Diagnosis of Lytic Lesions in the Jaw

Lesion	Radiographic Appearance	Comments
Odontoma (Figs. 11.15–21)	Well-circumscribed lesion containing varying amounts of different dental tissues evident usually as radiopaque material.	Odontomas represent abnormal developments of dental tissue and should be regarded rather as hamartomatous lesions than true neoplasms. Histologically ameloblastic (Fig. 11.15), complex (Fig. 11.16), and compound odontomas (Fig. 11.17), dentinoma (Fig. 11.18), odontogenic fibromyxoma (Fig. 11.19), and cementoma (Fig. 11.20) are distinguished. Hypercemtosis (Fig. 11.21) is excessive formation of cementum on the surface of the root of a tooth.

(continues on page 253)

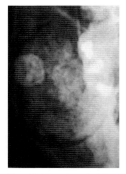

Fig. 11.**15 Ameloblastic odontoma.** A well-circumscribed cystic lesion containing a crown of a molar and amorphous opaque material is seen.

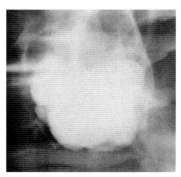

Fig. 11.**16 Complex odontoma.** A cystic lesion containing a very dense and homogeneous mass with a somewhat irregular outline is evident

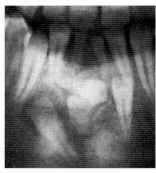

Fig. 11.**17 Compound odontoma.** A lesion containing several dwarfed and misshapen teeth is seen.

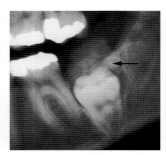

Fig. 11.**18 Dentinoma.** A radiopaque lesion (arrow) projects characteristically on top of the crown of an unerupted molar.

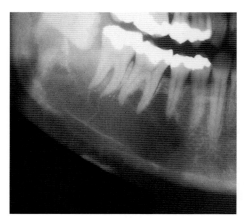

Fig. 11.**19 Fibromyxoma.** A poorly-defined radiolucent lesion extending superiorly between the roots of the teeth and eroding the inferior cortex is seen in the body of the mandible. The lesion is traversed by a few very delicate septa, some of which appear to extend beyond the eroded inferior cortex, giving it the appearance of a perpendicular periosteal reaction.

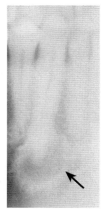

Fig. 11.**20 Cementoma.** A slightly radiopaque lesion with sclerotic border (arrow) is around the right lower canine.

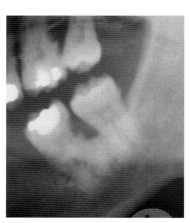

Fig. 11.**21 Hypercementosis.** Poorly defined radiopaque material (cement) is formed around the apex of the root of the left second mandibular molar.

Table 11.1   (Cont.) Differential Diagnosis of Lytic Lesions in the Jaw

Lesion	Radiographic Appearance	Comments
Stafne's mandibular defect (Fig. 11.22)	Round cyst-like lesion with dense sclerotic border located anterior to the mandibular angle. The continuity of the inferior border may be interrupted.	Developmental defect in the mandible caused by an accessory salivary gland. Sialography is diagnostic. Incidental finding in routine dental or mandibular radiography.
Nonodontogenic benign tumor	Similar to counterparts occurring elsewhere (see Chapter 5).	Rare. Aneurysmal bone cyst, giant cell tumor, hemangioma, neurofibroma, etc.
Gnathic osteosarcomas (Figs. 11.23 and 11.24)	Purely lytic, mixed or purely osteoblastic lesion originating in the mandible or less frequently in the maxilla.	Account for 8 % of all osteosarcomas. Differ from conventional osteosarcomas by the older age of onset (average age about 30 years) and decreased tendency for metastases.
Nonodontogenic primary malignant tumor (Fig. 11.25)	Similar to counterparts occurring elsewhere (see Chapter 5).	Rare. Fibrosarcoma, Ewing's sarcoma, chondrosarcoma, lymphoma and plasmacytoma occur.
Metastases (Fig. 11.26)	Similar to counterparts elsewhere (see Chapters 1, 2, and 5).	Hematogenous or per continuitatem from malignancy of oral or nasal cavity, salivary gland or skin.

(continues on page 254)

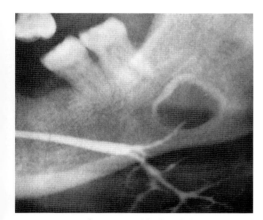

Fig. 11.**22** **Stafne's mandibular defect.** A round, cyst-like defect with a dense sclerotic border located anterior to the mandibular angle is caused by an accessory salivary gland . Sialography demonstrates the accessory duct draining this area.

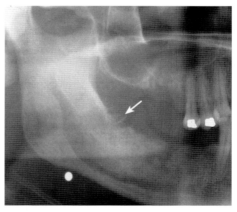

Fig. 11.**23** **Gnathic osteosarcoma**. A poorly defined, mixed osteolytic and osteoblastic lesion with violation of the superior cortex and small radiating spicule formation (arrow) is seen in the right body and angle of the mandible.

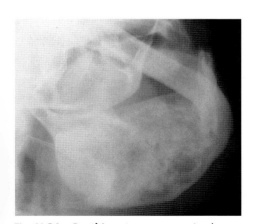

Fig. 11.**24** **Gnathic osteosarcoma**. A relatively well marginated and predominantly osteoblastic lesion with marked expansion but no definite cortical violation is seen in the body and ramus of the mandible.

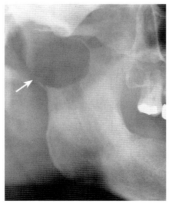

Fig. 11.**25** **Burkitt's lymphoma**. An expansile, well-defined, purely osteolytic lesion with minimal cortical violation (arrow) is seen in the ramus and condylar process of the right mandible.

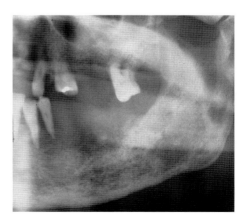

Fig. 11.**26** **Bronchogenic carcinoma metastasis.** A poorly defined, destructive osteolytic lesion is seen in the left mandible.

Table 11.1   (Cont.) Differential Diagnosis of Lytic Lesions in the Jaw

Lesion	Radiographic Appearance	Comments
Fibrous dysplasia (Fig. 11.27 and 11.28)	Expansile, lytic-to-sclerotic, fairly well circumscribed, unilateral lesion. Polyostotic form less common. The *ossifying fibroma* (/Fig. 11.**29**) of the jaw is a well-circumscribed slowly growing, expansile lesion measuring up to 5 cm in diameter with radiographic features similar to fibrous dysplasia.	"*Leontiasis ossea*" (deformity and bilateral enlargement of the face) is usually caused by widespread involvement with fibrous dysplasia. Similar changes, but usually without the sclerotic component, can be found in *neurofibromatosis* (Fig. 11.**30**).
Cherubism (hereditary fibrous dysplasia of the jaw)	Symmetrical enlargement of the mandible (especially in the region of the angles) by fibrous and cystic changes. Tooth anomalies (agenesis, noneruption, and displacement) are associated. Maxillary tuberosities are occasionally also involved.	Histologically indistinguishable from fibrous dysplasia, but autosomal dominant inherited and without manifestations outside the jaws. Develops as early as one year of age, and regresses after puberty.
Paget's disease (see Fig. 11.4)	Lytic, mixed, and sclerotic phase of the disease occurs. Loss of lamina dura in the involved bone. Gross enlargement of the mandible in the mixed and sclerotic phase is common.	Rarely in patients under 40 years of age.
Langerhans cell histiocytosis (eosinophilic granuloma) (Fig. 11.31)	Lytic lesion with "teeth floating in space" characteristic.	
Hyperparathyroidism	Generalized loss of lamina dura without widening of the periodontal membrane, Brown tumors (often multiple) may be evident as cystic lesions.	

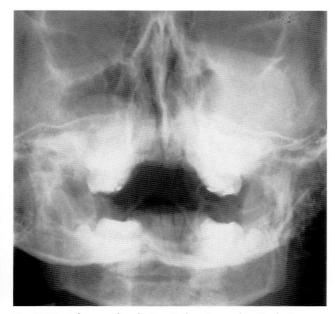

Fig. 11.**27** **Fibrous dysplasia.** Deforming sclerotic lesions are seen in the facial bones with main involvement of the left maxilla.

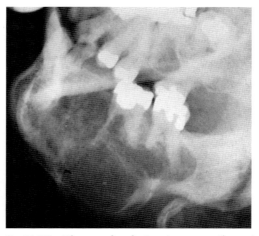

Fig. 11.**28** **Fibrous dysplasia.** An expansile, mixed lytic and sclerotic lesion is seen in the right mandibular body.

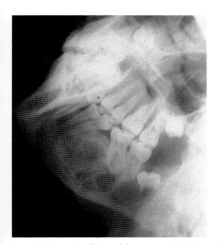

Fig. 11.**29** **Ossifying fibroma.** A lobulated, mixed osteolytic and osteoblastic lesion with slight bone expansion is seen in the body of the mandible.

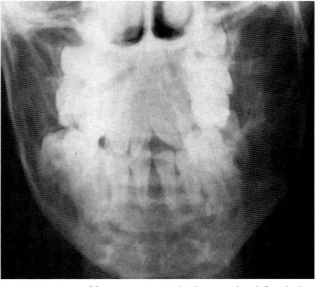

Fig. 11.**30** **Neurofibromatosis.** Multiple, poorly defined, lytic areas are seen in the grotesquely, but somewhat asymmetrically enlarged mandible.

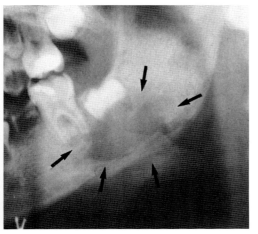

Fig. 11.**31** **Langerhans cell histiocytosis** (eosinophilic granuloma). A lytic lesion is seen in the left mandible around the last molar, that appears to float in space.

12 Spine and Pelvis

Spine

The development, structure, and function of the spine is complex. Consequently a great number of either primary or secondary abnormalities are encountered in various portions of the spinal column. Intraspinal lesions may not cause an abnormality on plain films despite serious clinical symptoms. In such cases MRI is advisable. In order to detect all available information from plain films, one should inspect them in a systematic fashion, paying attention to a number of different features.

The *alignment* of vertebrae in the normal spine includes a forward curvature (kyphosis) in the thoracic portion and a backward curvature (lordosis) in the cervical and lumbar portions. *Loss of normal curve* or straightening of the spine, often secondary to muscular spasm of variable etiology, may be difficult to evaluate in films taken on a Bucky table. The true extent of anteroposterior curves, as well as eventual lateral curvatures (*scoliosis*), is better evaluated in a weight-bearing (standing) position, if such positioning is not contraindicated by acute spinal trauma. Likewise, slippage of one vertebral body on the next either *forward* (*spondylolisthesis*) or *backward* may be better appreciated by taking flexion and extension views in a weight-bearing position.

A number of congenital or acquired diseases cause either general or local changes in the *size, shape, structure,* and/or *density* of the vertebral bodies and neighboring disk spaces. Such changes may or may not involve the neural arch. Plain films do not show intervertebral disks. For the evaluation of disk degeneration, protrusion or prolapse, MRI should be used. Facet joints are seen in plain films but for accurate evaluation of facet joint abnormalities and associated effects on root channels or spinal canal, a multislice CT examination or MRI is required.

Tables 12.1 and 12.2 are lists of some cardinal roentgen features of the spine and pelvis, respectively. They may serve as a reference point for differential diagnosis.

The *occipitovertebral junction* is developmentally a specialized area presenting a number of congenital anomalies. The latter as well as some acquired abnormalities of the upper cervical spine have radiographic features not seen elsewhere in the spinal column, and are presented in Table 12.3. Cervical spine fractures are caused by hyperflexion, hyperextension, hyperrotation, hyperflexion and rotation, lateral hyperflexion, and vertical compression. Fractures of spinal column are summarized in Table 12.4.

Table 12.5 presents a list of localized abnormalities involving the spine and their radiographic characteristics. Tumors involving the pelvis are presented together with tumors of the spine in Table 12.6. A more detailed discussion of bone tumors, including spine and pelvic bones, is found in Chapter 5.

Pelvis

Sacrum and coccyx are an integral part of the pelvis, although they essentially belong to the spine. Localized abnormalities of the sacrum, coccyx, and the rest of the pelvic girdle are therefore presented here together. Localized processes in the pelvic bones are not different radiographically from similar lesions in any flat bone. Abnormal *size and shape of the pelvis* may be typical of some congenital syndromes.

Involvement of *sacroiliac joints* may have great differential diagnostic significance. Early changes in the sacroiliac joints may be difficult to recognize, especially in young patients, whose sacroiliac joints are not completely ossified. CT and MRI cross-sectional images are helpful in demonstrating subtle changes. The involvement of sacroiliac joints in arthritides has been discussed already in Chapter 6, and is only briefly summarized in Table 12.2. Table 12.7 presents localized lesions usually involving the pelvis only.

Conditions Involving Both Spine and Pelvis

Abnormal size and shape of the pelvis may be typical of some congenital syndromes. Often they also present with spinal abnormalities. Many of the rare congenital syndromes are not included. The reader should consult texts of pediatric bone radiology in cases of rare congenital osteochondrodysplasias. Table 12.8 presents some congenital and acquired conditions with both pelvic and spinal radiographic findings.

Fractures of Spine

Fractures of the spine are summarized in Table 12.4. All seven cervical vertebral bodies must be visible on radiographs. In a case when good quality radiographs can not be obtained one has to consider CT imaging. Multiple fractures occur frequently. Multislice CT with reformats is nowadays highly recommended when serious spinal fracture is suspected. Multislice CT often reveals fractures not seen on radiographs.

Table 12.1   Some Radiographic Changes Characteristic of the Spine and Their Differential Diagnosis

Radiographic Finding	An Alphabetical List of Causes
Kyphosis, scoliosis or kyphoscoliosis 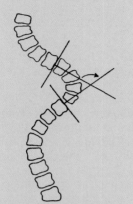	Chest wall abnormality (congenital or postoperative rib abnormality) Chronic unilateral lung disease Congenital spinal anomaly (e.g., fused vertebrae, vertebral hypoplasia or hemivertebra, dysraphism, rachischisis) Congenital syndromes (achondroplasia, cretinism, mucopolysaccharidosis, neurofibromatosis, osteogenesis imperfecta, etc.) Fracture, traumatic or pathologic, dislocation Idiopathic or postural Infection (spondylitis, tbc) Neoplastic (metastatic, multiple myeloma, primary tumor) Neuromuscular disorders Osteoid osteoma of the spine Osteoporosis (most often senile or postmenopausal) Paget's disease Rheumatoid or ankylosing spondylitis Scheuermann's disease (adolescent kyphosis) Neurotrophic spine (Charcot spine) Spasm due to an abdominal or retroperitoneal disease
Atlantoaxial subluxation (> 3 mm, children > 5 mm) 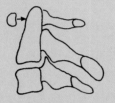	Ankylosing and psoriatic spondylitis Congenital cervicobasilar anomaly Down's syndrome Juvenile rheumatoid arthritis Morquio's syndrome Pseudogout Retropharyngeal abscess in a child Rheumatoid arthritis (common, see Chapter 6) Trauma (fracture or torn ligaments)
Increased diameter of one or more vertebrae 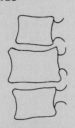	Acromegaly Benign bone tumor (hemangioma, giant cell tumor, aneurysmal bone cyst, osteoblastoma) Butterfly vertebra Compression fracture Fibrous dysplasia Paget's disease (sclerosis, framed) Hydatid disease (echinococcus) (uncommon) Scheuermann's disease (increased sagittal diameter) (common) (Degenerative ligamentous ossification)
Increased height of one or more vertebrae 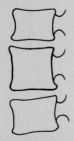	Arachnodactyly Compensatory growth (from non-weight bearing) Congenital or block vertebra
Biconcave vertebral bodies 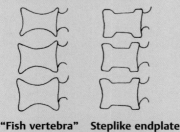 **"Fish vertebra" Steplike endplate depression**	Gaucher's disease (fish vertebra) Hereditary spherocytosis (fish vertebra) Homocystinuria (fish vertebra) Osteopenia (fish vertebra) (common) Renal osteodystrophy (fish vertebra) Sickle cell anemia (central steplike endplate depression or fish vertebra) Thalassemia major (rarely) (fish vertebra)

(continues on page 259)

Table 12.1   (Cont.) Some Radiographic Changes Characteristic of the Spine and Their Differential Diagnosis

Radiographic Finding	An Alphabetical List of Causes
Squared vertebral bodies	Ankylosing spondylitis (common)
	Paget's disease
	Psoriatic arthritis
	Reiter's syndrome
	Rheumatoid arthritis
Dense vertebra, solitary or multiple	Homogeneously dense or "ivory"
	Fluorosis
	Lymphoma (especially Hodgkin)
	Myelosclerosis
	Osteoblastic metastases
	Osteopetrosis
	Paget's disease
	Sclerotic or patchy, nonhomogeneous
	All the above, plus:
	Bone island
	Fracture (compression or healing)
	Hemangioma
	Idiopathic hypercalcemia
	Intervertebral disk disease
	Mastocytosis
	Nondiscogenic sclerosis (idiopathic)
	Osteoblastoma
	Osteomyelitis
	Renal osteodystrophy
	Radiation therapy
	Sarcoidosis
	Sarcoma (osteosarcoma, chondrosarcoma, Ewing's)
	Sickle-cell anemia
	Tuberous sclerosis
Collapse or flattening of one or more vertebrae	Aseptic necrosis (Kummel-Verneuil's syndrome)
	Congenital platyspondyly syndromes (e.g., achondroplasia, mucopolysaccharidosis, osteogenesis imperfecta)
	Eosinophilic granuloma
	Fracture (traumatic or pathologic) (common)
	Hemangioma
	Hyperparathyroidism
	Lymphoma
	Metastasis (pedicle involvement common)
	Myeloma, plasmocytoma (pedicle involvement rare)
	Osteomalacia
	Osteomyelitis
	Osteoporosis
	Paget's disease
	Scheuermann's disease
Anterior scalloping of one or more vertebral bodies	Aneurysm of aorta
	Inflammatory lymphadenopathy
	Lymphoma
	Metastatic lymph nodes
	Tuberculosis (spondylitis anterior)

(continues on page 260)

Table 12.1   (Cont.) Some Radiographic Changes Characteristic of the Spine and Their Differential Diagnosis

Radiographic Finding	An Alphabetical List of Causes
Posterior scalloping of one or more vertebral bodies 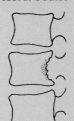	Achondroplasia Acromegaly Congenital syndromes (arachnodactyly, mucopolysaccharidosis, etc.) Increased intraspinal pressure Neurofibromatosis I (von Recklinghausen's disease) Syringomyelia Tumor of spinal canal
Enlarged intervertebral foramen 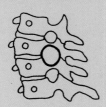	Congenital absence of pedicle Lateral meningocele Neurofibroma, neurinoma (common) Tumor (chordoma, dermoid, lipoma, lymphoma, meningioma, neuroblastoma) Vertebral artery aneurysm or tortuosity
Vertebral pedicle erosion or destruction 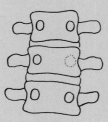	Benign bone tumor (aneurysmal bone cyst, giant cell tumor, hemangiopericytoma) Congenital absence Eosinophilic granuloma Granulomatous disease (tuberculosis, fungus) Intraspinal neoplasm or cyst (neurofibroma, meningioma) Metastasis (common) Multiple myeloma (rare) Syringomyelia
Localized widening of interpedicular distance 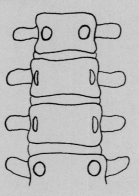	Diasthematomyelia Intrathecal tumors (e.g., ependymoma) Myelocele or meningomyelocele Rotation of vertebra in scoliosis (apparent widening) Hurler's syndrome Morquio's syndrome
Calcification of one or more intervertebral discs (either annulus fibrosus, nucleus pulposus, or both) 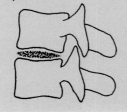	Acromegaly Ankylosing spondylitis Degenerative disk disease Hemochromatosis Hyperparathyroidism Hypervitaminosis D Idiopathic Ochronosis Poliomyelitis Pseudogout Spinal ankylosis for any reason (congenital, DISH, surgical) Transient calcification (in children)

(continues on page 261)

Table 12.1   (Cont.) Some Radiographic Changes Characteristic of the Spine and Their Differential Diagnosis

Radiographic Finding	An Alphabetical List of Causes
Syndesmophytes Ossification of the annulus fibrosus. Thin, vertical, and symmetrical. 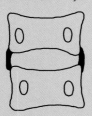	Ankylosing spondylitis Fluorosis Ochronosis (Alkaptonuria)
Paravertebral ossification Ossification of paravertebral connective tissue. Separated from the edge of the vertebral body and disk. 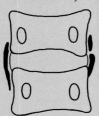	Fluorosis Hypoparatyroidism Psoriatic arthropathy Reiter's syndrome
Osteophytes Arising from the vertebral margin with no gap and having a claw appearance 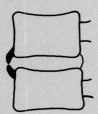	Acromegaly Stress response (spondylosis)
Traction spurs The tip not protruding beyond the horizontal plane of the vertebral endplate 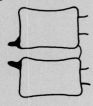	Shear stress across the disk
Anterior Ossification Undulating ossification of the anterior longitudinal ligament, intervertebral disk, and paravertebral connective tissue 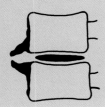	Diffuse Idiopathic Skeletal Hyperostosis (DISH)

Table 12.2 Some Radiographic Changes Characteristic of the Pelvis and Their Differential Diagnosis

Radiographic Finding	An Alphabetical List of Causes
Abnormal size or shape of pelvis	Acquired softening of bone (e.g., Paget's disease, osteomalacia) Congenital syndromes (e.g., achondroplasia, Down's syndrome, mucopolysaccharidosis, hereditary onycho-osteodysplasia) Posttraumatic Rheumatoid arthritis

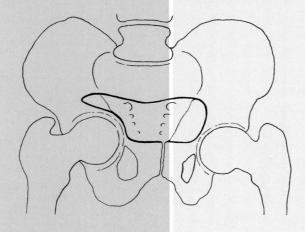

Protrusio acetabuli 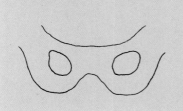	Acquired softening of bone (osteomalacia or rickets, hyperparathyroidism, Paget's disease, irradiation) Congenital or idiopathic (coxa vara with retroversion of the femoral neck, Otto pelvis) Degenerative joint disease, primary or secondary (including hemophilia, pseudogout, hemochromatosis, ochronosis) Femoroacetabular impingement (Pincer type) Infectious arthritis Osteogenesis imperfecta Traumatic (medial dislocation of the hip) Rheumatoid arthritis Rheumatoid variants (especially ankylosing spondylitis)
Widening of the pubic symphysis	Ankylosing spondylitis Congenital (bladder extrophy, epispadia, hypospadia, anal atresia, prune belly syndrome, cleidocranial dysplasia, pubic hypoplasia, spondyloepiphyseal dysplasia) Hyperparathyroidism Massive osteolysis Neurogenic osteolysis (paraplegia) Osteitis pubis and other infections (pyogenic, tuberculous, luetic) Pregnancy (common) Pubic osteonecrosis Rheumatoid arthritis Traumatic dislocation Tumor destruction
Bridging of the pubic symphysis	Ankylosing spondylitis Fluorosis Hyperparathyroidism (healed) idiopathic Healed infection Ochronosis Osteoarthritis Posttraumatic Postradiation therapy Rheumatoid arthritis Surgical fusion

(continues on page 263)

Table 12.2   (Cont.) Some Radiographic Changes Characteristic of the Pelvis and Their Differential Diagnosis

Radiographic Finding	An alphabetical List of Causes	Usual Appearance
Sacroiliac joint disease (erosion, widening, sclerosis and/or fusion) **a) Erosion, widening** **b) Fusion**	Agenesis (caudal dysplasia) Ankylosing spondylitis Crohn's disease Enteropathic arthritis Familial Mediterranean fever Gout Hyperparathyroidism Infection (pyogenic or tuberculous) Multicentric reticulo histiocytosis Neoplastic destruction (primary, metastatic) Osteitis condensans ilii Osteoarthritis Paraplegia Psoriatic arthritis Reiter's disease Relapsing polychondritis Rheumatoid arthritis Sacroiliitis circumscripta	Bilateral symmetric Bilateral symmetric Bilateral symmetric Bilateral symmetric Bilateral asymmetric Bilateral asymmetric Bilateral symmetric Unilateral Bilateral symmetric Unilateral Bilateral symmetric Bilateral asymmetric Unilateral Bilateral asymmetric Bilateral asymmetric Bilateral asymmetric Bilateral asymmetric

Table 12.3   Differential Diagnosis of Cervicobasilar Abnormalities (Occiput, C1, C2)

Disease	Radiographic Findings	Comments
Anomalies of the occipital bone:		
Manifestations of occipital vertebra	May appear in various forms and combinations: *Tertiary condyle* (1): A midline bony process at the anterior edge of foramen magnum. A joint between tertiary condyle and odontoid may be present. Seen in the lateral view.	Relatively uncommon (less than 1%). May limit the mobility of the atlanto-occipital joint.
	Basilary process: Bilateral, often asymmetric small protuberances at the anterior margin of the foramen magnum. Often too small to be appreciated.	Commonly present (12%). No clinical significance as such.
	Paracondylic (2) and *epitransversary processes* (3). Bony protuberances lateral to the occipital condyles. When connected to the occipital bone, they are called paracondylic. The name epitransversary refers to their connection with the transverse process of the atlas. Best seen in AP and Stenver's views.	Relatively uncommon (less than 1%). May cause a special form of atlantooccipital fusion.
	Posterior (4) or *lateral* (5) ponticles refer to bony rings in the arch and transverse process of the atlas, respectively. The posterior ponticle is seen in the lateral view, whereas the lateral ponticle may be visible in anteroposterior projection.	The posterior ponticle (Kimmerle's anomaly) is present in approximately 3%. They have no clinical significance.
Basilar impression	*Anterior* basilar impression results from platybasia and short clivus, evident on lateral skull film.	The frequency of primary basilar impression is approximately 1%. Platybasia: Angle between the clivus and a line connecting the nasion and the superior wall of the sphenoid sinus exceeds 150 degrees. For the measurement of basilar impression see Chapter 8.
	Medial basilar impression results from elevation of the hypoplastic occipital bone and associated condyles. It may be unilateral and associated with tilting of the head. The dens is used as a reference.	Anterior basilar impression can be measured from lateral skull films. Medial basilar impression can be reliably measured only from AP projection (digastric line).
Occipital condylar hypoplasia	Hypoplasia of the occipital condyle without basilar impression results in a relatively high position of the atlas and axis. The odontoid seldom extends into the foramen magnum. The digastric line is the key to detect this abnormality.	Usually asymptomatic, but can be symptomatic if associated with altered size of the foramen magnum. It may also limit the mobility of of the atlanto-occipital joint (functional atlanto-occipital fusion). Elevation of the odontoid may occur in severe rheumatoid arthritis.
Anomalies of the atlas and the axis:		
Atlanto-occipital fusion (atlasassimilation)	The atlas is either completely or partially fused into the occipital bone. If unilateral, may cause tilting of head.	Frequency approximately 0.25%. Often associated with other anomalies like Klippel-Feil syndrome, spina bifida of the atlas or basilar impression. Clinical significance usually depends on associated anomalies. May cause atlantoaxial subluxation (in 50% of cases).

(continues on page 265)

Table 12.3 (Cont.) Differential Diagnosis of Cervicobasilar Abnormalities (Occiput, C1, C2)

Disease	Radiographic Findings	Comments
Anomalies of the arch of the atlas 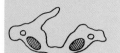	The dorsal arch may be totally absent or may have variable defects or clefts most commonly in the dorsal midline.	Dorsal cleft of the arch of the atlas is present in 4% of population. Arch defects are clinically asymptomatic.
Atlantoaxial fusion or malsegmentation	The lateral masses of the atlas and the body of the axis form a butterfly-looking complex in AP film. The dens and the anterior arch of the axis may be hypoplastic or totally missing. Various partial coalitions of the two bones may be present as a sign of abnormal segmentation.	These anomalies may be symptom-free or cause reduced mobility at the craniovertebral junction.
Odontoid bone (separate odontoid) (hypoplastic dens) (Figs. 12.1 and 12.2)	The dens of the axis is hypoplastic, seen as a protuberance at the site of the normal dens. The rounded odontoid bone is located either at the site of normal dens or higher up and anterior, maybe fused with clivus. The posterior arch of the axis is often absent. Atlas is usually ventrally subluxated.	In case of pseudoarthrosis of a fractured dens, the size and form of the odontoid process is normal. A small ossification center at the V-shaped tip of the dens is called ossiculum terminate Bergman. It has no clinical significance since it is not associated with atlantoaxial subluxation.

(continues on page 266)

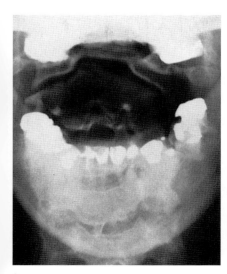

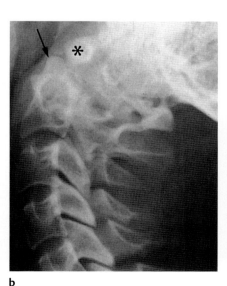

a
b

Fig. 12.**1 a, b** **Hypoplastic dens** (arrow) as seen **a** in AP and **b** lateral in projection. The atlas (asterisk) is posteriorly displaced.

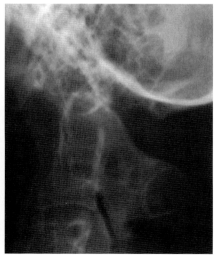

Fig. 12.**2** Hypoplastic dens, fusion of C2 and C3 and anterior displacement of the atlas. The posterior arch of the atlas is lacking **(Klippel-Feil anomaly, Type I).**

Table 12.3   (Cont.) Differential Diagnosis of Cervicobasilar Abnormalities (Occiput, C1, C2)

Disease	Radiographic Findings	Comments
Fractures: – **Jefferson fracture** – **Fracture of the arch of the atlas** – **Fractures of the dens** – **Hangman's fracture (fracture of the arch of the atlas)** 	See Table 12.4 and Chapter 4	See Table 12.4 and Chapter 4

Table 12.4   Differential Diagnosis of Fractures and Dislocations of the Spine

	Radiographic Findings	Comments
Cervical spine		
Occipitocervical (atlanto-occipital) dislocation	The only sign of occipitocervical dislocation on radiographs may be widened prevertebral soft tissues. The distance between occipital condyles and C1 is increased. Distance from basion to odontoid in normal adult is less than 4–5 mm (in children less than 10 mm). On odontoid view increased distance between occipital condyles and C1.	Usually due to motor vehicle accident. Often fatal and therefore rare in hospitals. All major structures crossing occipitocervical junction are ruptured. Mechanism of the injury is complex or unknown.
Occipital condyle fracture 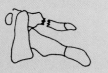	Usually conventional radiography fails demonstrate this fracture. Important to keep in mind when interpreting cervical radiographs (or CT).	Rare condition. CT is recommended method if occipital condyle fracture is suspected. Classification according to Anderson and Montesano: Type I: Occipital condyle impaction fracture caused by axial loading force like Jefferson fracture. Usually stable, if contralateral side intact. Type II: A component of basilar skull fracture. Usually stable. Type III: Avulsion of alar ligaments from occipital condyle. Potentially unstable.
Jefferson fracture (Fig 12.3)	Best seen on open-mouth AP view. Lateral dislocation of one or both lateral masses of the atlas in anteroposterior projection. A small fragment may be seen medial to the lateral mass, representing an avulsion of the attachment of the transverse ligament. Additional lower level fractures in 25–50 % of cases.	Caused by an axial force (e.g., diving). Fracture lines are located posterior or anterior to the lateral mass in the arch of the axis. May be unstable or stable.
Fracture of the arch of the atlas (Fig. 12.4)	Unilateral fracture is often seen only in the oblique view. Bilateral may be seen in lateral view. In hyperflexion fracture the posterior fragment of the arch of the atlas is angulated and/or displaced downwards. In hyperextension fractures the posterior fragment of the atlas projects upwards.	Some patients have a lateral cleft in the arch of the axis, which should be differentiated from a fracture. Fractures of the anterior arch are rare except for in the combined fractures of the occipitovertebral region. Usually due to hyperextension trauma. Considered as stable. Fracture of the dens may be associated and therefore may be unstable (see below).

(continues on page 268)

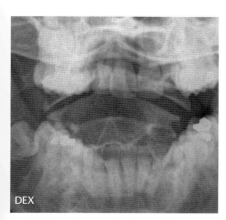

Fig. 12.**3** **Jefferson fracture.** The space between left atlanto-axial facets has increased on AP view.

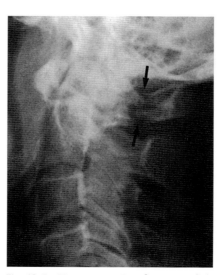

Fig. 12.**4** **Hyperextension fracture** of the arch of the atlas (arrows). The posterior fragment of the atlas projects characteristically upwards.

Table 12.4 (Cont.) Differential Diagnosis of Fractures and Dislocations of the Spine

	Radiographic Findings	Comments
Fractures of the dens (Fig. 12.5) **Type I**  **Type II** 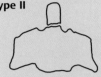 **Type III** 	Lucent linear defect through C2 which may take place mainly at three levels: Type I: Fracture (usually oblique) cephalad to the base of the dens. Usually obliquely oriented. Type II: Transverse fracture at the base of the dens. Type III: Fracture extending from the base of the dens into the body of C2. On lateral view the normal ring shadow of the axis is disrupted. Hyperflexion fractures of the dens are often combined with anterior subluxation of the atlas and fracture of the posterior arch of the atlas. In typical hyperextension fractures both the dens and atlas are posteriorly displaced and the fractured posterior arch of the axis is displaced.	Over 10% of fractures of the cervical spine involve dens. Isolated, nondisplaced fracture of the dens may not be detected until resorption of the fracture line. Type I: Usually stable Type II: Usually unstable Type III: Usually stable Unossified fracture or congenital nonunion of odontoid tip may result in odontoid bone (Figs. 12.**1**, **2**). May be difficult to detect in elderly people with osteoporosis and degenerative changes. Multislice CT with coranal and sagittal reformats is recommended.
Hangman's fracture (fracture of the arch of the axis) (Fig. 12.6) **Type I** **Type II** **Type III** 	Best seen on lateral view. Bilateral fractures close to the body in the pedicles of C2 can be seen. Variable degree of anterior subluxation of C2.	Hyperextension injury of the axis presenting with bilateral pedicle fractures and varying degrees of anterior subluxation or frank dislocation of the body of C2. Nowadays most commonly found in automobile accidents when face strikes the windshield. Hangman's fracture is considered as unstable fracture. Three types are recognized: Type I: Fracture line close to the body in the pedicle without anterior displacement of the body. Type II: Concomitant disruption of intervertebral disk C2–C3. Type III: This is type II fracture with associated C2–C3 facet dislocation.

(continues on page 269)

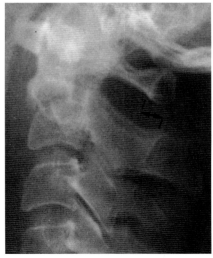

Fig. 12.**5** **Fracture of the dens** with anterior subluxation of the atlas and the dens.

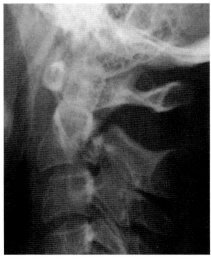

Fig. 12.**6** **Hangman's fracture** of the arch of the axis with anterior subluxation of the body of the axis.

Table 12.4   (Cont.) Differential Diagnosis of Fractures and Dislocations of the Spine

	Radiographic Findings	Comments
Burst fracture of C3–C7	On lateral view burst fracture is characterized by an anterior wedged deformity of vertebral body and retropulsion of a fragment from the posterior superior marging of vertebral body. On AP view widening of interpedicular distance may be seen.	Fracture mechanism is identical to Jefferson fracture, but fracture happens at the lower part of the cervical spine. Burst fracture is stable, if posterior ligaments are intact. Burst fracture becomes unstable if posterior ligaments disrupt. CT is recommended for evaluation of spinal canal.
Flexion tear drop fracture (see Fig. 4.23)	Radiological features of flexion tear drop fractures include backward displacement of fractured vertebral body, posterior displacement of upper column, widening of interspinous spaces, and kyphotic deformity of the cervical spine on the lateral view. On AP view widening of interlaminar spaces, a sagittal split fracture through the vertebral body and one or both laminae is often seen.	The flexion tear drop fracture is a specific form of burst fracture. Usually accompanied by spinal cord injury. Flexion tear drop fracture is highly unstable. About 15% of all cervical fractures are flexion tear drop fractures.
Extension tear drop fracture (Fig 12.7)	Lateral view of the spine demonstrates the tear drop fracture of anterior inferior corner of vertebral body and there is no subluxation.	Extension tear drop fracture is usually stable, but may be unstable at the lower part of the cervical spine. The most common location is at the level of C2–3. Defect in the ossification of the endplate may simulate fracture.
Endplate compression fracture (Fig. 12.8) Anterior Lateral Posterior	Endplate compression fractures are usually hyperflexion injuries that leave the posterior height of the vertebral body normal while the anterior vertebral height decreases. In thoracic and lumbar vertebrae, an increased density or diameter and irregularities of the anterior margin of the vertebral body may be associated. Widening of the facet joint space may be present in acute trauma.	If the anterior vertebral height in the cervical spine is 3 mm less than the posterior height, a compression fracture is suspected. In thoracic and lumbar spine, this measurement is not valid because many diseases cause wedge-shaped or collapsed vertebrae (e.g., Scheuermann's disease). Compression fractures are common in the lower cervical spine and in the lower thoracic spine. Compression of the posterior inferior margin of the vertebral body is likely due to an extension injury.
Fractures of the pedicle, neural arch (Fig. 12.9), or articular process	May resemble simple dislocation in the lateral view. Fracture of the pedicle may be better appreciated in the frontal view.	Neural arch is the most common site of a fracture in cervical spine. The articular pillar is particularly vulnerable in fractures.
Clay-shoveler's fracture (see Fig. 4.22)	Oblique or vertical avulsion fracture of the tip of the spinous process of C6 or C7 (occasionally T1–T3).	Caused by a repeated sudden load on the flexed spine. Must be differentiated from hyperflexion fracture, in which the fracture line is more horizontal.

(continues on page 270)

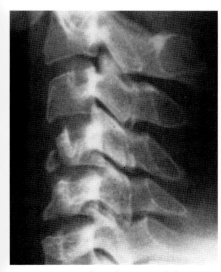

Fig. 12.**7   Tear drop fracture** of the anterior inferior margin of C4 resulting from extension injury. There is slight posterior dislocation of C4. Prevertebral soft tissue is thickened.

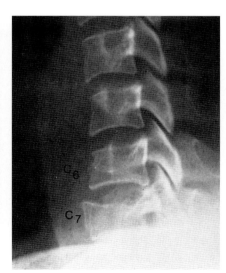

Fig. 12.**8   Compression fractures** of the anterior superior margins of C6 and C7. The height of the anterior C6 body is decreased, whereas C7 has a chip fracture. Prevertebral soft-tissue thickening is also observed.

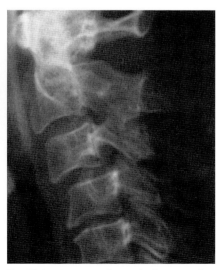

Fig. 12.**9   Fracture through the neural arch** of C3 anterior dislocation of the body of C3.

Table 12.4   (Cont.) Differential Diagnosis of Fractures and Dislocations of the Spine

	Radiographic Findings	Comments
Locked facets Unilateral (Fig. 12.10) **Bilateral (Fig. 12.11)**	Lateral and oblique views are sufficient to demonstrate facet joint locking. On the lateral view inferior and superior articular processes are in apposition. Facet joints have changed configuration so that laminar cortices intersect at one point. On AP view mild rotation may be seen especially in unilateral facet locking.	A locking can be unilateral or bilateral. Unilateral locking is relatively stable. Bilateral locking is result of extreme flexion and is unstable condition. Relatively often missed on plain films.
Anterior subluxation	Kyphosis at the affected level on lateral view. The space between the inferior articular process of the upper vertebra and the upper process of lower vertebra shows of abnormal extent. The degree of subluxation may show milder than needed to rupture ligamentous complex due to regressed distortion.	Hyperflexion trauma, in which disruption of posterior ligamentous complex happens. Unstable.

(continues on page 271)

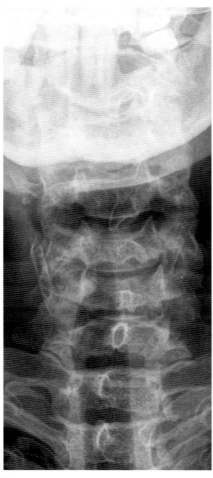

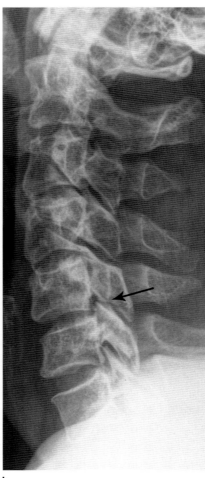

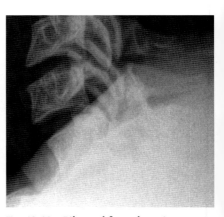

Fig. 12.**11   Bilateral facet luxation.**

◁ Fig. 12.**10   Unilateral locked facet.** On AP view the spinous processes of lower cervical spine curve to the left. On lateral view unilateral locking of the facets between C5 and C6 can be seen (arrow).

a   b

Table 12.4   (Cont.) Differential Diagnosis of Fractures and Dislocations of the Spine

	Radiographic Findings	Comments
Thoracolumbar spine		
Compression fractures: (Figs. 12.12a and 4.24) anterior lateral	Cortical bucking or wedging of anterior or less commonly lateral part of the vertebral body. Usually confined to the superior end plate. A zone of sclerosis is often present beneath the end plate. Note that posterior cortical line remains intact.	Flexion injury of the spine resulting in compression of the anterior column. In severe compression fractures posterior ligamentous distraction may be associated while middle column serves as the fulcrum. This is called as flexion-distraction fracture.
Flexion-distraction fracture	Cortical bucking or wedging of anterior part of the vertebral body. Posterior cortical line remains intact. Distinguished from a simple anterior compression fracture by horizontal fracture in the posterior elements e.g., pedicle. Widening of posterior bony elements of adjacent vertebrae.	This is a variant anterior compression fracture, in which middle column serves as a fulcrum and posterior column distracts leading to horizontal fractures of posterior bony elements or in the disruption of interspinosus ligaments.
Burst fractures (Fig. 12.12b)	On lateral view increased sagittal diameter and moderate to marked anterior wedged deformity of the vertebral body. Retropulsion of a fragment from the posterior superior marging of vertebral body. On AP view widening of interpedicular distance may be seen.	Most commonly at thoracolumbal region. Caused by hyperflexion and axial load. Intervertebral disc usually herniated into the vertebral body. Retropulsion of osseous material into spinal canal often causes neurological symptoms. Burst fracture is considered as unstable.
Chance fracture (seat-belt injuries) (Fig. 12.12 c)	The radiographic findings depend on whether the injury is predominantly osseous or ligamentous (see Fig. 4.**24**). Horizontal split of the vertebral body pedicles, lamina and spinous process in one level fracture. In two level chance fracture the fracture line passes through bone and ligaments.	Caused by hyperflexion of the spine resulting in distraction injuries of both the middle and posterior columns. Associated at times with anterior compression of the vertebral body. Most frequently at L1–L3. Change fracture is considered unstable.
Fracture dislocations (Fig. 12.12 d)	Intervertebral subluxation or dislocation. The loss of height of the vertebral body may be relatively small. Fragmentation of the injured vertebral bodies, dislocation of facet joints and fractures in the spinous processes and arches. Lateral plain films may show a wedge-formed vertebral body, kyphosis and distraction of the spinous processes. A small bony fragment arising from the anterior superior margin of the vertebrae below the dislocation. This may indicate an avulsion fracture created by the annulus.	Complete disruption of all three spinal columns. Usually mixed osseous–ligamentous injury.

(continues on page 273)

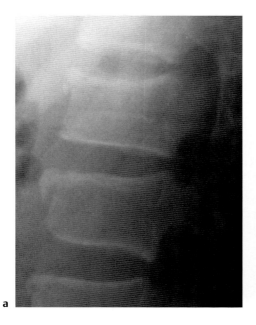

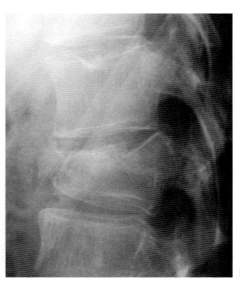

a

b

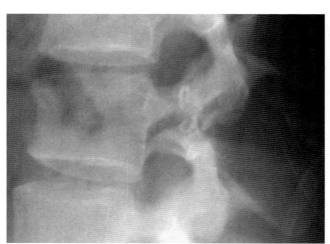

c

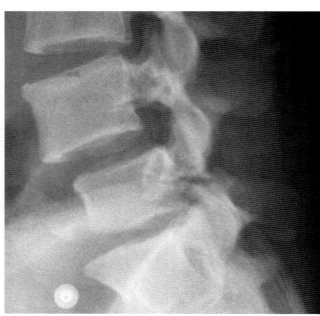

Fig. 12.**12   a Anterior compression fracture of upper end plate.** The fracture does not extent to posterior margin of the body. **b Burst fracture of L1.** A bony fragment is seen protruding into the spinal canal from superior posterior aspect of the body. **c Chance fracture.** Mild wedging of the body of L3. Fracture ex-tends through pedicles and transverse processes. **d Fracture dis-location between L4 and L5.** The space between processus spino-sus of L4 and L5 has increased and processus interticularis frac-ture of L5 is visible. L5 body is in mild retroposition. Anterior com-pression fracture on upper end plate of L4.

Table 12.4   (Cont.) Differential Diagnosis of Fractures and Dislocations of the Spine

	Radiographic Findings	Comments
Osteoporotic compression fractures (Figs. 12.13 a, b)	Wedge-shaped or biconcave vertebral body. Seen often on lateral view of chest X-ray. In acute fracture anterior wedge deformity usually involving the superior end plate with increase in bone density beneath the end plate. In old healed osteoporotic fracture a fine line of cortical bone is intact and there is no increased density of bone beneath the end plate. In an old fracture an anterior superior spur of an affected vertebra end plate is often present.	Determining whether the fracture is acute or not may be problematic. Previous images e.g., chest X-ray may be helpful.
Fractures of posterior spinal structures (spondylolysis)	See Table 12.5	Stress fractures, see spondylolysis in Table 12.5.
Pathologic fracture	See Table 12.5	

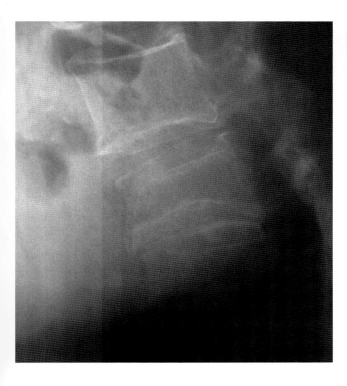

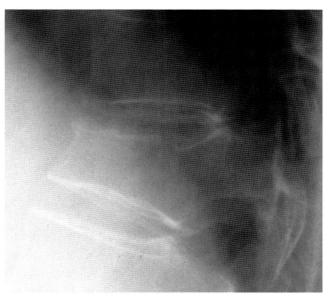

b

Fig. 12.**13   a Biconcave** (cod fish) **osteoporotic fracture. b** An old wedge-shaped osteoporotic fracture of T12.

Table 12.5   Differential Diagnosis of Anomalies of the Spine below the Axis

Disease	Radiographic Findings	Comments
Block vertebra (fusion of two or more vertebral bodies) (Figs. 12.14 and 12.15; see Figs. 12.16, 12.17, and 12.18 for comparison)	Variable grades of blocking from isolated hypoplasia of the intervertebral disk to complete fusion of bodies and even neural arches may be present. Decreased diameter of vertebrae at the site of segmentation defect, concavity of the anterior aspect of the block, and/or fusion of the neural arches are diagnostic of *congenital* block vertebra. Anterior blocking of several vertebral bodies is called *vertebral coalition*. It results in kyphosis due to asymmetric growth.	Most common at C2–3. Somewhat similar changes in the spine may be produced by vertebral infection, rheumatoid spondylitis, and operative fusion. Several other disorders may occasionally lead to spinal block, e.g., vertebral hemangioma, fibrous dysplasia, Paget's disease, fracture, chondrosarcoma, and other primary neoplasms, achondroplasia, spinal stenosis. Multiple anterior blocks may occur secondary to Scheuermann's disease and senile kyphosis.
	Klippel-Feil anomaly: Type I: Short neck with block vertebrae, vertebrobasilar anomalies (including basilar impression), scoliosis, Sprengel's deformity, etc. Type II: Segmentation anomalies of one or two pairs of cervical vertebrae only. Type III; Thoracic or lumbar anomalies together with Type I or II.	Clinically short neck, low-lying hairline, and limited cervical motion. Type I is most common, Type II is rare. In addition to spinal anomalies, also genitourinary abnormalities, deafness, and synkinesia are common. Several other skeletal, cardiovascular, and neurological abnormalities occur.

(continues on page 276)

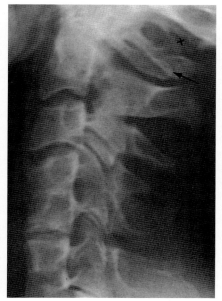

Fig. 12.**14   Congenital block vertebrae** C4–5, C6–7, T1–2 (not shown), associated with posterior ponticle (foramen arcuale) (*) and a defect in the posterior arch of the atlas (arrow) (Klippel-Feil type III).

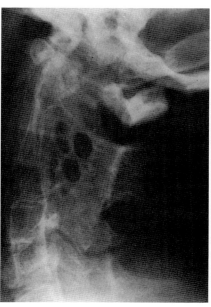

Fig. 12.**15   Severe segmentation anomalies** of the vertebrobasilar junction and blocking of the cervical spine (Klippel-Feil type I).

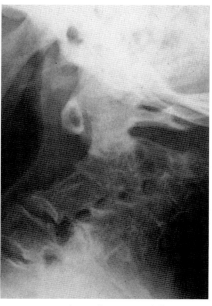

Fig. 12.**16   Tuberculous spondylitis** of the cervical spine resulted in multiple block vertebrae, which resemble Klippel-Feil anomaly.

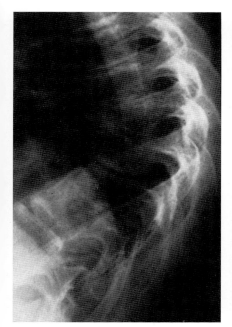

Fig. 12.**17   Tuberculous block vertebra** (T10 and T11) associated with a gibbus.

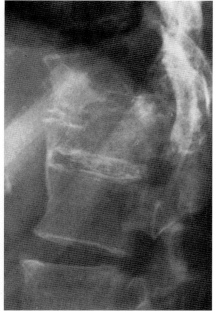

Fig. 12.**18   Posttraumatic block** T11, T12, and partially L1.

Table 12.5   (Cont.) Differential Diagnosis of Anomalies of the Spine below the Axis

Disease	Radiographic Findings	Comments
Spondylolysis (Fig. 12.19) 	Anterior slipping of one vertebral body on its subjacent neighbor while the posterior portions stay behind; is usually secondary to bilateral defects of pars interarticularis, called *spondylolysis*. Spondylolysis is best demonstrated in oblique films. Most common locations of spondylolysis are L5 and L4, rarely higher lumbar vertebrae or C6.	*Spondylolysis* may be a congenital failure of ossification or more likely traumatic, either an acute or a fatigue fracture. It is seen in 5% of the white population. When the facet joints are deformed or malpositioned, being more sagittal than coronal, the whole vertebra, including the posterior portion, slides forward. This results in dislocation, called *pseudospondylolisthesis* or degenerative spondylolisthesis with an intact neural arch. Hypertrophic osteoarthritis of the apophyseal joints is a basic finding. Spondylolisthesis should be differentiated from traumatic ventral luxation of vertebra without fracture. On perfectly positioned lateral films of the lumbar spine, an apparent defect of the pars interarticularis of L2 or L3 may resemble spondylolysis. This is a superimposition artifact (pseudospondylolysis), located slightly more superiorly on the pars than are true defects.
Spondylolisthesis (Figs. 12.20 and 12.21) **Pseudospondylolisthesis (Fig. 12.33)** 	Spondylolisthesis does occur secondary to congenital elongation of posterior elements without fracture (interarticular dysplasia). Spondylolysis is often present without spondylolisthesis. Rarely an arch cleft is retrosomatic (in the pedicle) or retroisthmic (in the lamina). Isolated lateral deviation and rotation of a spinous process seen in anteroposterior radiographs of the lumbar spine are associated with inequality in the length of pars interarticularis. The spinous process deviates toward the intact side or the side with the smaller spondylolytic defect. Unilateral spondylolysis may produce hypertrophy and sclerosis of the contralateral pedicle (Fig. 12.**44b**). A posteriorly wedged, slightly hypoplastic L5 is often present.	

(continues on page 278)

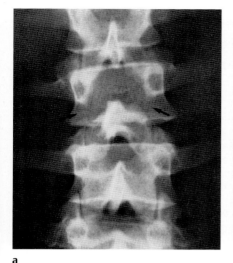

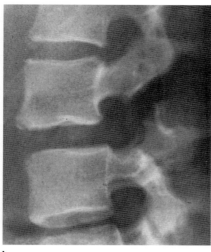

a

b

Fig. 12.**19 a, b   Spondylolysis** with minimal Spondylolisthesis of L3. Bilateral defect in the pars interarticularis is well seen in both AP (**a**) and lateral (**b**) views.

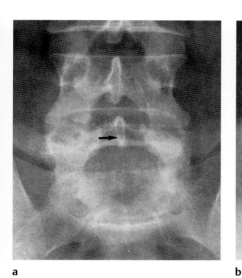

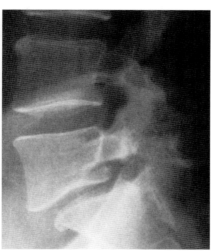

a

b

Fig. 12.**20 a, b   Spondylolisthesis. a** The spinous process deviates slightly to the left (arrow) indicating shorter left pars interarticularis. **b** Anterior displacement of the characteristically wedge-shaped L5 on the lateral film.

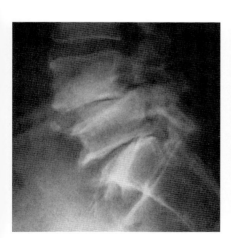

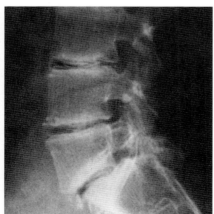

a

b

Fig. 12.**21 a, b   Spondylolisthesis.
a** Anterior slipping of L4 with disk degeneration and osteophytes both in spaces L4–L5 and L5–S1. **b** Spondylolisthesis of L5 in a patient with multiple calcified disk degenerations due to *ochronosis*.

Table 12.5 (Cont.) Differential Diagnosis of Anomalies of the Spine below the Axis

Disease	Radiographic Findings	Comments
Open dysraphisms *Myelomenigocele* *Myelocele* *Hemimyelomeningocele* *Hemimyeocele* **Closed spinal dysraphisms** *Lipomyelocele* *Lipomyelomeningocele* *Meningocele* **(Figs. 12.22–12.23)** *Myelocystocele* *Spina bifida* **(Fig. 12.24)** *Tight filum terminale*	Occasionally one of the posterior neural arches will remain permanently open. This is commonly seen at S1 or L5, but may occur in any area. The cleft may be only 1 to 2 mm wide and vertical or oblique in orientation. Such a defect, if unassociated with other deformity, is called occult spina bifida. If multiple or associated with widened spinal canal (broad interpedicular distance or posterior scalloping of the vertebral body), they are likely due to a significant abnormality.	In open dysraphisms the placode is exposed to the environment. In closed spinal dysraphisms skin or other cutaneus appendage covers spinal structures. Advanced imaging modalities are suggested. MRI shows the depth of defect. CT may be needed for evaluating bony structures. Subtle neurologic deficits such as gait disturbance, foot deformity, or impaired sphincter control may occur in diastematomyelia. Syringomyelia, meningomyelocele, or an intraspinal tumor may also cause broad interpedicular distance. Posterior scalloping may also occur in neurofibromatosis, achondroplasia, increased intraspinal pressure, and tumors of the spinal canal.
Vertebral hypoplasia and asymmetry **(Figs. 12.25–26)**	A wide spectrum of anomalies involving focal hypoplasia of part or all of a vertebral element occurs. Hypoplastic lesions may involve more than one level. Lateral hemivertebra results in scoliosis. Posterior hemivertebra in kyphosis or gibbus. Posterior hemivertebra is usually displaced approximately 3 mm posteriorly from the neighboring vertebral bodies. Hypoplasia or absence of a pedicle or lamina may also cause scoliosis.	A hemivertebra may cause encroachment of the neural canal. Unlike fractures, hemivertebrae are outlined by a cortical margin. Absent pedicle (usually cervical) may simulate an expanding mass in the intervertebral canal or metastatic destruction of the pedicle. Hemivertebra or "butterfly" vertebra of the thoracic or lower cervical region may be part of a neurenteric canal anomaly (fistula, sinus or enteric cyst) or more rarely associated with pulmonary or cardiac anomalies. Severe forms of sacral hypoplasia may be associated with major anomalies of the gastrointestinal and genitourinary tracts. Narrowing of the arch associated with enlargement of the neural foramen is usually due to a neurinoma (Fig. 12.**27**) or neurofibroma (Fig. 12.**28**).

(continues on page 280)

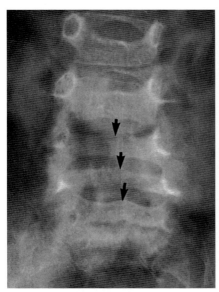

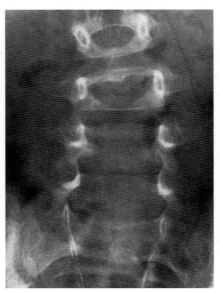

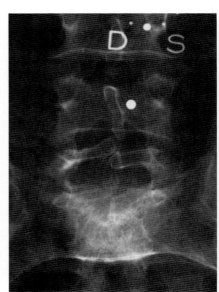

Fig. 12.**22** **Multiple clefts** in the posterior neural arches (arrows) and widening of the spinal canal due to meningocele.

Fig. 12.**23** **Meningocele.** Defects in the neural arches are wide and involve three lumbar and all sacral segments.

Fig. 12.**24** **Spina bifida** occulta of L5.

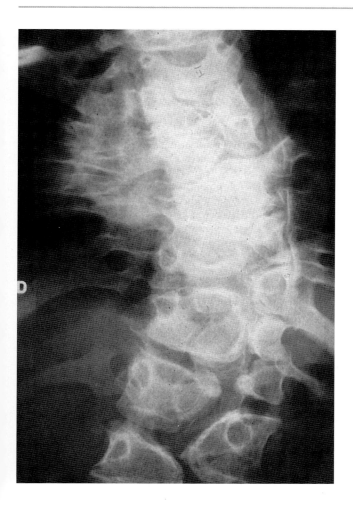

Fig. 12.**25** **Multiple segmentation anomalies** throughout the spinal column. Not a single normal vertebral body is present. Rib fusions are an associated finding.

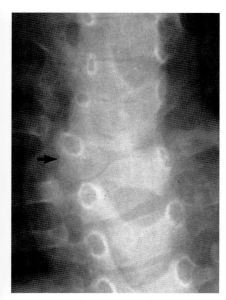

Fig. 12.**26** **Lateral hemivertebra** with scoliosis (arrow).

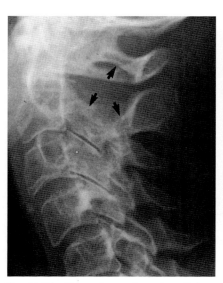

Fig. 12.**27**   Narrowing and erosion of the arch of the axis and atlas due to **neurinoma** (arrows).

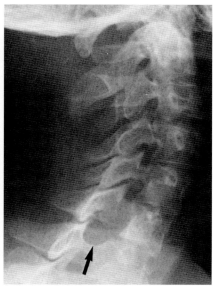

Fig. 12.**28** **Neurofibroma.** The neural foramen C6–C7 is enlarged (arrow). A dorsal cleft in the arch of the atlas is seen as an incidental finding.

Table 12.5 (Cont.) Differential Diagnosis of Anomalies of the Spine below the Axis

Disease	Radiographic Findings	Comments
Spinal stenosis (Figs. 12.29–30)	The decreased diameter of the spinal canal is due to short, heavy pedicles and enlarged apophyseal joints. (Stenosis at the level of Cl is due to craniovertebral anomalies, basilar impression, manifestations of occipital vertebrae, and atlantoaxial subluxation.) The normal sagittal diameter of the midcervical and lumbar canal is 15 mm or more; values below 13 mm may indicate stenosis. Congenital spinal stenosis may involve lumbar and, less frequently, cervical spine. Intervertebral foramina have a figure-of-eight configuration (Fig. 12.30 b) and lumbar lordosis is increased. In developmental lumbar and/or cervical spinal stenosis, the plain radiographic changes are less striking. The pedicles tend to be short and the lamina convergent, intervertebral foramina moderately narrowed in anteroposterior direction and elongated axially. Plain films may be deceptive in younger patients. In older patients the pattern is superimposed by spondylarthritic changes.	The most common cause of congenital spinal stenosis is achondroplasia. Abnormal enchondral bone formation and premature fusion of the cartilaginous synchondroses result in broad, squat vertebrae with concave dorsal surfaces and prominent intervertebral disks. Developmental stenosis is not associated with vertebral malformations and is asymptomatic until degenerative changes in the spine precipitate symptoms of neurogenic claudication or myelopathy. Except for high cervical stenosis, localized spinal stenosis is usually acquired, commonly involves midcervical or lower lumbar segments, and is associated with spondylotic and spondylarthritic changes. Lateral recess stenosis can occur in a canal with a normal sagittal diameter. Spinal stenosis is not adequately seen on plain films. CT or preferentially MRI should be available for assessment.

(continues on page 281)

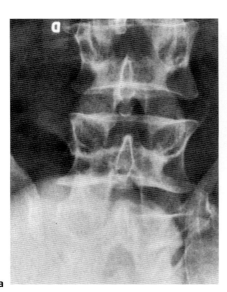
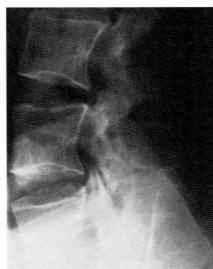

a b

Fig. 12.**29 a, b** **Spinal stenosis in achondroplasia. a** Anteroposterior film demonstrates lateral narrowing of the spinal canal in L4 and 5. Hypoplastic sacrum is also obvious. **b** Lateral film of another patient demonstrates narrow sagittal diameter of the spinal canal and posterior scalloping of the vertebral bodies.

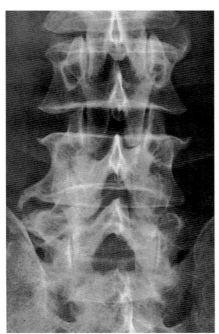
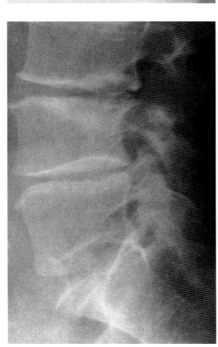

a b

Fig. 12.**30 a, b** **Acquired spinal stenosis. a** The lamina are convergent and the articular processes hypertrophic with superimposed spondylarthritis. **b** Short pedicles and decreased sagittal diameter of the spinal canal associated with narrowed disk spaces L3–L4 and L4–L5.

Table 12.5   (Cont.) Differential Diagnosis of Anomalies of the Spine below the Axis

Disease	Radiographic Findings	Comments
Inflammatory lesions Pyogenic vertebral spondylitis (Figs. 12.31 and 12.32)	The radiographic changes follow a certain pattern, but may take weeks or months to become apparent, depending on the aggressiveness of the process. 1 Disk space narrowing 2 Loss of the normally sharp adjacent subchondral plates 3 Areas of cortical demineralization 4 Destruction of the vertebral body, possibly collapse 5 Sclerotic new bone formation, sometimes spontaneous fusion. The process more commonly involves the anterior two-thirds of the vertebral body than the posterior part. Changes are usually seen in one disk space and two adjacent vertebral bodies. Destruction of only one end plate is very rare. Involvement of multiple levels and soft-tissue abscesses occur in approximately 20% each.	Pyogenic spondylitis refers to two distinct entities: 1. *Infectious diskitis*: occurs in children and adolescents, who have vascularized disks (Fig. 12.32). 2. *Blood-borne osteomyelitis* of the vertebral bodies in adults begins under the vertebral end plate and involves the disk secondarily, because the disk is avascular. In adults, primary infection of the disk is possible after surgery, needling, or trauma. Staphylococcus aureus is the infectious agent in approximately 90%. A history of recent primary infection, surgery, or urogenital instrumentation is common. Drug abusers have increased incidence of gram-negative infections and cervical involvement that is otherwise rare.

(continues on page 282)

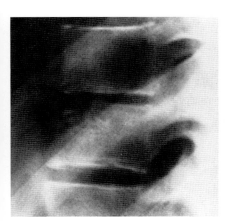
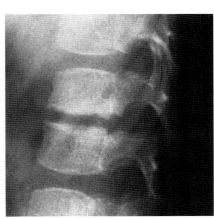

Fig. 12.**31 a, b   Pyogenic spondylitis.**
a There is disk space narrowing, destruction of the anterior portion of two adjacent vertebral bodies, more so in the inferior. **b** Three months later, sclerotic new bone formation is seen as a sign of healing.

b

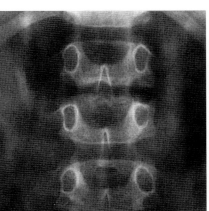
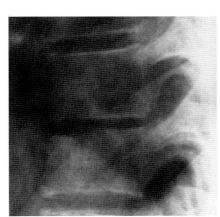

Fig. 12.**32 a, b   Infectious diskitis** in a child. Narrowing of the disk space with erosion and sclerosis of the adjacent end plates.

b

Table 12.5 (Cont.) Differential Diagnosis of Anomalies of the Spine below the Axis

Disease	Radiographic Findings	Comments
Spinal tuberculosis (Fig. 12.33)	Characteristic findings are: involvement of the thoracolumbar or midthoracic spine, osteoporosis, large paravertebral abscess relative to the amount of bone destruction, narrowing of one or more disk spaces after erosion of endplates, anterior compression of adjacent vertebra. Reactive sclerosis is not a rule. A pedicle may rarely be the primary focus. Roentgen findings that favor spinal tuberculosis are: involvement of three or more vertebral bodies, skip lesions in the spine, a large or calcified paraspinal mass, and the rare involvement of neural arches.	Secondary to hematogenous spread from primary pulmonary tuberculosis. Neurological symptoms are common due to extradural compression of the cord by paravertebral abscess, even before gibbus appears. Distinction of spinal tuberculosis from pyogenic vertebral osteomyelitis is often impossible. Subligamentous spread of spinal tuberculosis with anterior irregularities (anterior gouge defects) resembles lymphoma. If only one vertebra is involved it mimics metastasis. Spinal brucellosis is rare. Its roentgen appearance is distinguishable from spinal tuberculosis.
Fungal infections: **Actinomycosis** **Coccidioidomycosis** **Blastomycosis** **Cryptococcosis** **Aspergillosis**	All mimic spinal tuberculosis, and diagnosis depends on biopsy and culture of the organism. Involvement of the posterior arch and ribs is common in actinomycosis, coccidioidomycosis, blastomycosis, and cryptococcosis. Absence of vertebral collapse and sparing of the disk is typical of actinomycosis and coccidioidomycosis. Aspergillosis is virtually indistinguishable from spinal tuberculosis.	All are rare. Actinomycosis spreading from the retropharyngeal space affects the cervical spine. Presence of draining sinus tracts is common in actinomycosis, Coccidioidomycosis, and blastomycosis.
Fractures of the vertebral body	See Table 12.4	See Table 12.4
Fractures of the pedicle, neural arch, or articular process	See Table 12.4	See Table 12.4
Neuropathic spine (Fig. 12.34)	Neuropathic changes are usually limited to one to three contiguous vertebral bodies. Sclerosis or destruction together with fragmentation and altered alignment are typical.	The progression of roentgen changes is relatively rapid and osteophyte formation is florid, involving also the posterior elements, which is not a feature in infectious spondylitis. Unlike metastases, disk spaces are involved.

(continues on page 284)

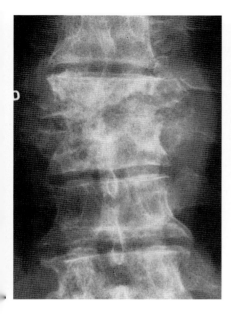
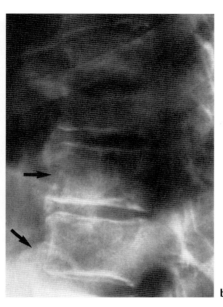

Fig. 12.**33 a, b   Tuberculous spondylitis.**
Paravertebral abscess is demonstrated in the AP view. Extensive destruction of two adjacent vertebral bodies with surrounding sclerosis. Anterior defects are seen in two lower vertebral bodies (arrows).

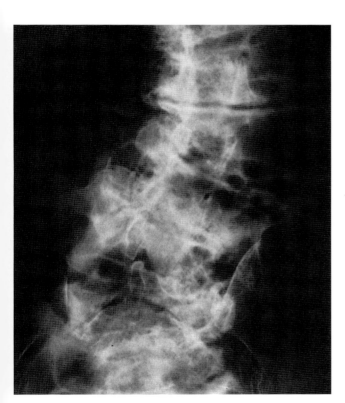

Fig. 12.**34   Neuropathic spine.** There is sclerosis, destruction, fragmentation and altered alignment, as well as spondylosis.

Table 12.5   (Cont.) Differential Diagnosis of Anomalies of the Spine below the Axis

Disease	Radiographic Findings	Comments
Scheuermann's disease (adolescent kyphosis) (Fig. 12.35)	Commonly involves thoracic vertebrae (T4–T12). The radiographic findings include: 1 slightly wedge-shaped vertebral bodies (kyphosis), with possibly narrowing of the anterior disk space 2 irregular but sharply demarcated endplates 3 increased sagittal diameter of involved bodies 4 Schmorl nodes 5 compensatory growth of a neighboring vertebra towards a Schmorl node 6 rarely fatigue fracture of the spinous process.	The most common disease of the spine in adolescents and young adults, considered as an aseptic necrosis of the vertebral endplate. May be painful or asymptomatic. At least three vertebral bodies should be involved to allow the diagnosis. Apophyseal separations may be incorrectly attributed to an acute injury.

(continues on page 285)

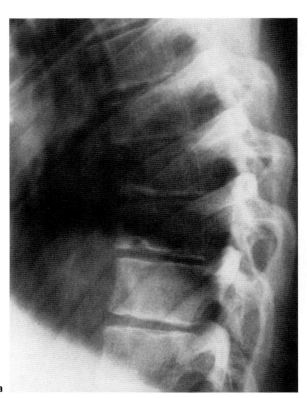

a

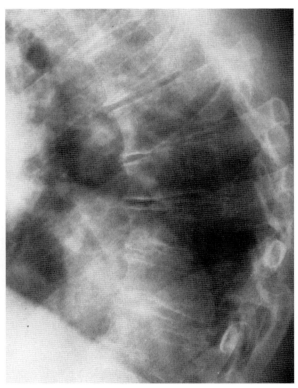

b

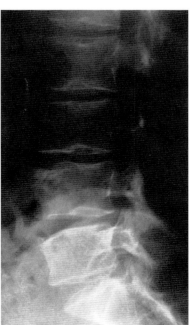

c

Fig. 12.35 a–c   **Scheuermann's disease.** Irregular endplates, increased sagittal diameter of the vertebral bodies, and Schmorl nodes are observed, **a** Age 18, **b** age 41. Increased kyphosis due to wedge-shaped thoracic vertebral bodies. **c** Changes in the lumbar spine. Several endplates contain Schmorl nodes. Apophyseal separations in the upper anterior corners of L4 and L5 simulate fractures.

Table 12.5 (Cont.) Differential Diagnosis of Anomalies of the Spine below the Axis

Disease	Radiographic Findings	Comments
Disk degeneration (Figs. 12.36–12.38)	The disk space is narrower than usual. Later the adjacent endplates may become sclerotic and osteophytes develop. A streak of gas within the disk space is indicative of disk degeneration. Degeneration may induce de- creased or increased motility of the neighboring vertebrae. A "sciatic hook" is a secondary osteophyte projecting posteriorly and indicates old disk herniation. Disk degeneration together with lumbar hyperlordosis predisposes to false joint formation between spinous processes (Baastrup syndrome (Fig. 12.**37b**).	Most common between L4/L5 and L5/S1. Osteophytes developing around a not narrowed disk space is called spondylosis anterior. Small osteophytes throughout the thoracic spine, associated with increased kyphosis and osteoporosis is typical of senile kyphosis. The anterior portions of the disks are narrowed. Occasionally the vertebral bodies may even fuse together. Calcification of disks is common in a thoracic spine with spondylosis. Multiple disk degenerations associated with disk calcifications are characteristic of ochronosis (alkaptonuria) (Fig. 12.38).

(continues on page 286)

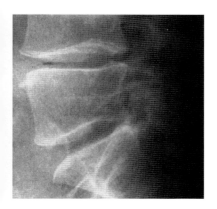

Fig. 12.**36 Disk degeneration** between L4/L5. The disk space is narrow and contains gas.

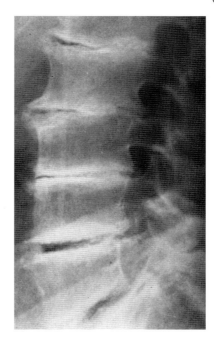

Fig. 12.**38 Multiple disk degenerations** and calcification of disk spaces secondary to **ochronosis**. There is anteposition of L5 relative to S1 (pseudolisthesis)

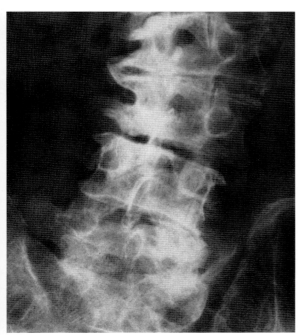

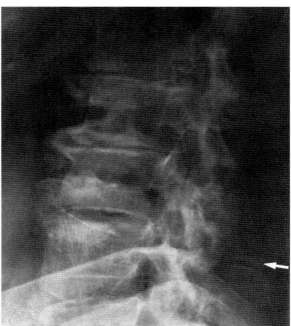

b

Fig. 12.**37 a, b Multiple disk degenerations** with scoliosis and extensive osteophytes. In the lateral view the osteophytes appear as sclerotic lines overlaying the vertebral bodies. Sclerosis in the adjacent spinous processes (arrow) indicates early Baastrup syndrome.

Table 12.5   (Cont.) Differential Diagnosis of Anomalies of the Spine below the Axis

Disease	Radiographic Findings	Comments
DISH **(Diffuse idiopathic skeletal hyperostosis, ankylosing hyperostosis, Forestier's disease)** **(Fig. 12.39)**	Flowing calcification and ossification along the anterolateral aspects of 4 or more contiguous vertebral bodies. The disk height in the involved segment is preserved, and apophyseal and sacroiliac joint manifestations are absent. Most commonly affects the thoracic and lumbar spine.	Additional findings include bony profile ration at sites of ligament and tendon attachments, calcification of iliolumbal and sacrotuberous and even other ligaments, and para-articular osteophytes. Etiology is unknown, but the condition often accompanies arthropathies, seronegative rheumatoid arthritis, diabetes, and other diseases. The only constant association is older age, generally over 50.
Paget's disease **(Osteitis deformans)** **(Figs. 12.40 and 12.41)**	Both vertebral body and arch are enlarged, having a rim of thickened cortex (a picture frame appearance), coarse trabeculae. Ivory appearance or squaring of the anterior margin are other presentations. Pathologic fractures may occur. May involve one or several vertebrae.	Involvement of the neural arch and spinous processes helps to differentiate Paget's disease from carcinoma metastases. Thickened cortex is not a feature of vertebral hemangioma. Squaring of the anterior margin helps to differentiate Paget's disease from osteoblastic metastases and Hodgkin's disease.
Nondiscogenic sclerosis (Fig. 12.42)	Homogeneously dense areas involving large segments of one or two vertebral bodies. They are usually continuous with the cortex or endplate and there is no narrowing of the disk space.	An asymptomatic localized, stable, benign, nonneoplastic form of vertebral body osteosclerosis of unknown etiology. It should be differentiated from bone island or sclerosis secondary to disk degeneration (discogenic sclerosis).

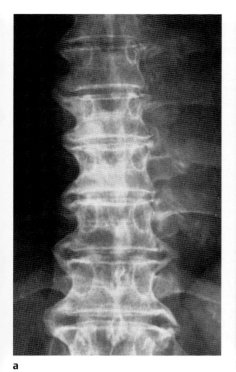
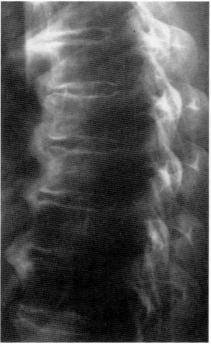
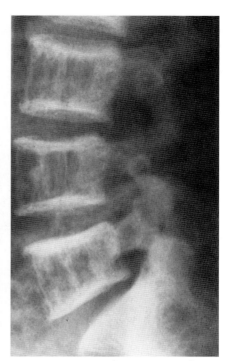

a

b

Fig. 12.**39 a, b   DISH.** Extensive ankylosing osteophytes and calcification of disks, but the disk spaces are not narrowed.

Fig. 12.**40   Paget's disease.** Squared vertebral bodies have a framed appearance and coarse trabeculae. The process also involves the neural arches.

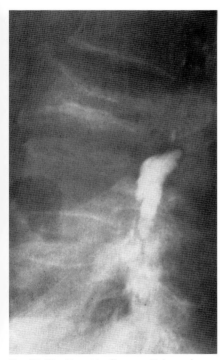
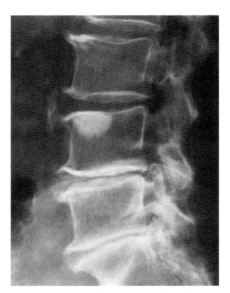

Fig. 12.**42   Non-discogenic sclerosis.** A homogeneous density associated with the upper endplate of L4 without other abnormalities. Two disk degenerations (L4 and L5) are also seen.

Fig. 12.**41   Paget's disease.** Enlarged diameter of a partially collapsed vertebral body. Dural sac contains oily myelograph contrast media.

Table 12.6   Differential Diagnosis of Bone Tumors in the Spine and Pelvis

Disease	Radiographic Findings	Comments
Benign bone tumors		
Aneurysmal bone cyst	Lytic expansile lesion covered by a thin shell of bone. Involves primarily the posterior elements and possibly the body of the vertebra. May cross a vertebral interspace and involve adjacent vertebrae, a feature not often seen in other tumors, with the exception of chordoma.	Approximately 20% of aneurysmal bone cysts appear in the spine and another 15–20% in the pelvis. Rare after 25 years of age. The second most common benign spinal tumor.
Hemangioma (Fig. 12.43)	Vertebral lesions in the thoracic and lumbar areas with prominent or thickened vertical trabeculae are generally called hemangiomas, but some may only represent telangiectasia or varicosity of osseous veins. A true hemangioma may also present as an expansile or lucent lesion in the vertebral body.	Approximately 15% of true hemangiomas appear in the spine. Small hemangiomas are very common in spine (incidence over 10%), but they cannot be seen in roentgenograms.
Osteoid osteoma (Fig. 12.44a) Osteoblastoma (Fig. 12.45)	Located almost always in the posterior elements and seen as a "dense pedicle." Lesions less than 1.5 cm in diameter are called osteoid osteomas and those greater than 1.5 cm are called osteoblastomas. Expansion of the bone is common in bigger lesions. Scoliosis is common and the tumor is usually at the apex of the concavity. Another presentation of osteoblastoma is a lytic lesion with occasionally sclerotic margin, which is useful in differentiating it from an aneurysmal bone cyst.	Approximately 40% of osteoblastomas and 5% of osteoid osteomas appear in the spine, rarely in pelvis. Over 15% of benign spinal tumors belong to this category. Unilateral spondylolysis or hypoplasia of the posterior elements may induce localized hypertrophy and sclerosis in the contralateral pedicle and pars interarticularis, mimicking an osteoid osteoma (Fig. 12.**44b**).
Giant cell tumor	A radiolucent lesion with well-defined margins without sclerosis of adjacent bone. Expansile in the sacrum and pelvis. Rarely crosses the sacroiliac joint.	Over 10% of giant cell tumors occur in the spinal column, mostly in the sacrum. The most common benign tumor of the spine. Pelvis is almost as commonly affected.
Other spinal lesions		
Eosinophilic granuloma (Fig. 12.46)	The destructive phase with spotty radiolucencies in the centrum of the vertebra is followed by vertebral collapse and a residual vertebra plana. The disk spaces are preserved.	The majority of eosinophilic granulomas occur in children under 10 years of age. More common in pelvis (above acetabulum) than in spine. Reactive sclerosis along the margin of a destructive pelvic lesion is typical.

(continues on page 290)

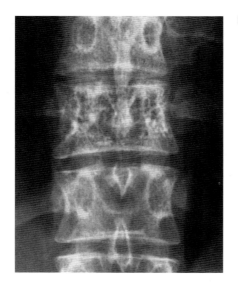

Fig. 12.**43**   **Hemangioma** of T11.

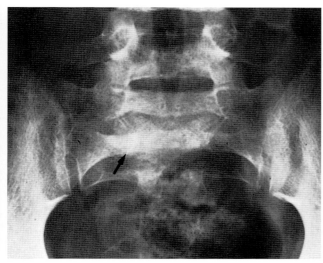

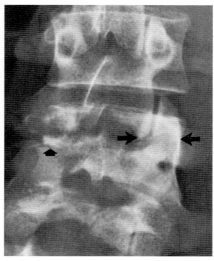

Fig. 12.**44 a**   **Osteoid osteoma** of sacrum seen as a sclerotic area (arrow).

Fig. 12.**44 b**   **Unilateral spondylolysis** with sclerosis of the contralateral pedicle mimicking osteoid osteoma. Spondylolysis of the right pars interarticularis (short arrow) of L4 is associated with a hypertrophic sclerotic left pedicle (arrows) in the same vertebra.

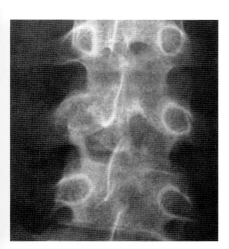

Fig. 12.**45**   **Osteoblastoma.** An expansile lytic lesion surrounded by some sclerosis, also involving the pedicle of L3.

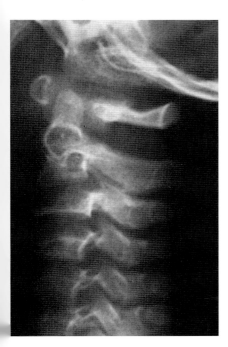

Fig. 12.**46**   **Eosinophilic granuloma.** Collapse of the body of C3.

Table 12.6   (Cont.) Differential Diagnosis of Bone Tumors in the Spine and Pelvis

Disease	Radiographic Findings	Comments
Malignant bone tumors		
Chordoma (Fig. 12.47)	A lytic, expanding lesion in the sacrum, coccyx or less commonly C2 or elsewhere in the cervical spine, with stippled calcifications in approximately 30% of cases. It may expand to adjacent vertebrae and soft tissues.	About 50% occur in the sacrococcygeal area, where it is characteristically associated with a presacral soft-tissue mass, 30% in the clivus, and the remaining 20% in cervical or lumbar areas.
Sacrococcygeal teratoma	A soft-tissue mass in the sacrococcygeal area with irregular calcification or ossification.	Teratomas are composed of mixed tissues, often containing bone and cartilage. Less than 40% are malignant, presenting as a large soft-tissue mass.
Fibrosarcoma (Fig. 12.48)	Medullary fibrosarcoma is more frequent and appears as a poorly marginated or even permeative osteolytic lesion. Periosteal fibrosarcoma causes cortical erosion and minimal periosteal reaction.	Fibrosarcoma appears relatively often in the pelvis and sacrum, rarely in the upper spinal columns. Malignant fibrous histiocytoma may have identical appearance.
Osteosarcoma	See Table 5.10.	Rare in the spine, relatively common in the pelvis.
Plasmocytoma	A lytic, often expansile lesion of the vertebral body or pelvic bone. Sclerotic margin is rare.	A precursor of multiple myeloma.
Ewing's sarcoma (Figs. 12.49 and 12.50)	The lesion in the spine is either sclerotic or lytic and may resemble osteosarcoma. A large paraspinal soft-tissue mass is frequently associated.	Primary Ewing's sarcoma of the spine is rare, but it is relatively common in sacrum. Pelvis is the second most common location. Metastatic involvement of the spine is frequent.

(continues on page 292)

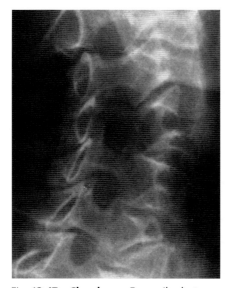

Fig. 12.**47   Chordoma.** Expansile destruction of C4, including enlargement of the neural foramen.

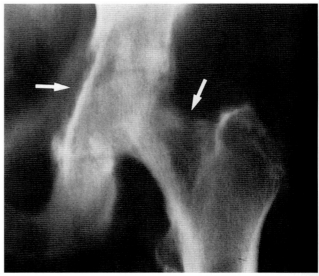

Fig. 12.**48   Fibrosarcoma.** Tomography reveals poorly marginated destruction of the acetabulum and the femoral neck (arrows).

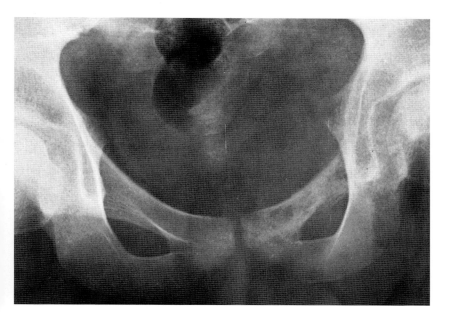

Fig. 12.**49** **Ewing's sarcoma.** Permeative destruction of the left acetabulum, ischium, and pubic bone. Lamellated periosteal reaction is seen in the pubic bone.

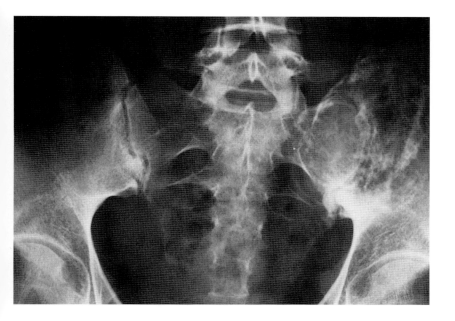

Fig. 12.**50** **Mixed lytic and sclerotic destruction** of the left ilium and sacrum by a tumor with histological characteristics of **Ewing's sarcoma**.

Table 12.6　(Cont.) Differential Diagnosis of Bone Tumors in the Spine and Pelvis

Disease	Radiographic Findings	Comments
Lymphomas (Figs. 12.51–12.53)	Spinal lymphoma is osteolytic in the majority of cases, but osteosclerosis and periosteal reaction occur. In Hodgkin's disease, marginal erosion of the vertebral bodies by lymph nodes is sometimes seen. The ivory type of sclerotic vertebra is more common in Hodgkin's than non-Hodgkin's lymphoma.	Extranodal disease including spinal and pelvic involvement is more common in non-Hodgkin's lymphomas than in Hodgkin's disease.
Chondrosarcoma (Figs. 12.54–12.55)	See Table 5.10	Pelvis is the most common location.
Hemangiopericytoma	Osteolytic, poorly marginated lesion. May affect either entire vertebra or a part of it.	A poorly understood, rare vascular neoplasm encountered in middle-aged patients, usually in the spine or pelvis. Differentiation from malignant fibrous tumors or metastasis is difficult.
Metastasis (Fig. 12.56)	Either lytic, mixed or sclerotic destruction of the vertebral body and pedicle is characteristic (see Chapter 5).	Primary malignancies are rare as compared with the high incidence of metastases. If several vertebrae are affected, metastases or multiple myeloma are likely.
Multiple myeloma (Fig. 12.57)	Loss of bone density and accentuation of trabecular pattern in spine and diffuse osteolytic lesions in pelvis are the most common patterns. (For other features, see Chapter 5)	Sparing of pedicles in the presence of osteolytic destruction of vertebral bodies differentiates multiple myeloma from typical osteolytic metastases.

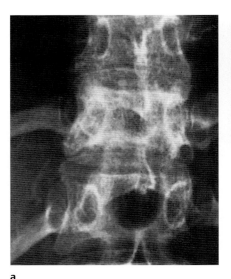

Fig. 12.**51**　**Mixed lytic and sclerotic destruction** of the left pubic area by a **non-Hodgkin's lymphoma** of bone.

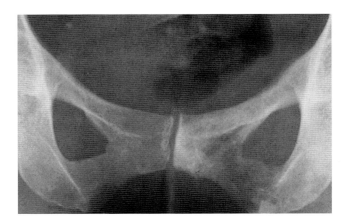

a　　　　　　　　　　　　　　　　　　b
Fig. 12.**52 a, b**　**Non-Hodgkin's lymphoma** of T11 causing mostly sclerotic destruction of the vertebral body and pedicle.

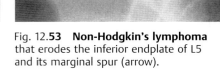

Fig. 12.**53**　**Non-Hodgkin's lymphoma** that erodes the inferior endplate of L5 and its marginal spur (arrow).

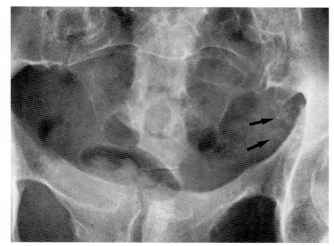

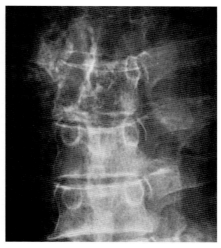

Fig. 12.**54**   **Chondrosarcoma** of pelvis that started from a preexisting exostosis in the inferior aspect of the iliac bone. Typical tumor calcification is seen near the apex of the exostosis (arrows).

Fig. 12.**55**   **Chondrosarcoma** of the thoracic spine involving two adjacent vertebrae as an osteolytic lesion with sclerotic margins and tumor calcification.

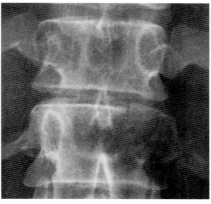

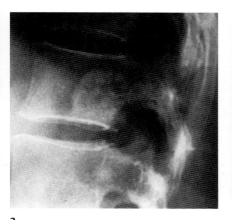

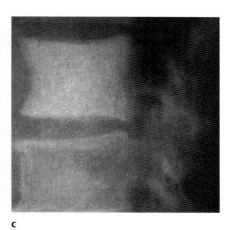

a   **b**   **c**

Fig. 12.**56 a–c**   **Metastatic lesions** of the spine.
a Osteosclerotic metastases from breast carcinoma involving both the body and pedicle, **b** Osteolytic metastasis from renal adeno-

carcinoma with destruction of the pedicle, **c** "Ivory" vertebra due to metastatic carcinoma of the prostate, uncharacteristically only involving the body.

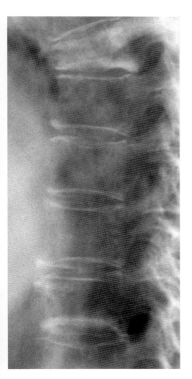

Fig. 12.**57**   **Multiple myeloma.** Patchy demineralization of spinal bodies. One vertebral body has collapsed superiorly.

Table 12.7   Differential Diagnosis of Localized Lesions of the Pelvis

Disease	Radiographic Findings	Comments
Caudal hypoplasia	Absence or hypoplasia of the sacral segments and sacroiliac joints. Hypoplasia and deformity of pelvic bones.	Often a baby of a diabetic mother. Associated with urogenital, gastrointestinal, and neural anomalies. Widening of pubic symphysis and other anomalies often are associated with urogenital anomalies.
Cleidocranial dysostosis	Most constant radiologic findings are in the skull, clavicles, and pelvis. There is separation of pubic symphysis, defective ossification of the ischia, pubis, hypoplasia of iliac wings, and hypoplastic sacrum.	A congenital dysostosis with faulty intramembranous bone formation which results in large head relative to small facial bones, narrow chest, and ragging shoulders. Hypoplastic changes are present in facial bones and clavicles. Spine may show fusion defects.
Hereditary onycho-osteodysplasia (Nail-patella syndrome)	Osteocartilagineous exostoses extending posteriorly from the iliac wings (iliac horns) are characteristic. The patella may show subluxation, hypoplasia, or aplasia. Radial head may also be hypoplastic.	An autosomal dominant disorder of ectodermal and mesodermal tissues, mainly manifesting dysplastic changes in nails, pelvis, knees and elbows. Iliac horns without associated abnormalities are called Fong's disease (Fig. 12.**58**).
Down's syndrome (Trisomy 21–22)	Flaring of the iliac wings, flattening of the roofs of the acetabula, and ischial tapering are characteristic radiological findings. Atlantoaxial subluxation is common.	Upward slanting eyes and characteristic face are detectable at birth. In trisomy 17–18 syndrome, the pelvis has an "antimongoloid" configuration.
Paget's disease (osteitis deformans) (Fig. 12.59)	Cortical thickening, particularly of the pelvic rim, enlargement of the pubis and ischium, and coarse trabecular pattern are characteristic.	Pelvis is commonly involved, showing usually mixed lytic and sclerotic changes,
Osteitis condensans ilii (hyperostosis triangularis ilii) (Fig. 12.60)	Bilateral sclerosis of the iliac bones with normal sacroiliac joints. Triangular sclerosis is limited to the anterior aspect of the lower two thirds of the height of the sacroiliac joint.	Common among women of childbearing age. The bilateral triangular pattern distinguishes this condition from unilateral sclerotic conditions like a bone island, blastic metastases, sacroilitis circumscripta, or Paget's disease.
Sacroiliitis circumscripta (Fig. 12.61)	A circular or polycyclic, well-delineated area of sclerosis involving both sacral and iliac sides of the sacroiliac joint, with minimal erosion of the joint surfaces.	A rare inflammation of unknown etiology. Should be differentiated from osteitis condensans ilii, in which sacrum is not involved. Capsular calcifications of the sacroiliac joint (joint surfaces unaffected).

(continues on page 296)

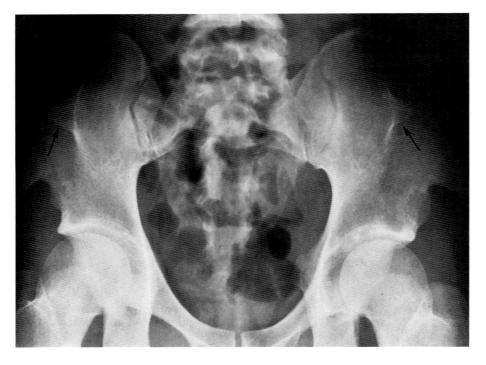

Fig. 12.**58**   **Iliac horns** (arrows), **Fong's disease**.

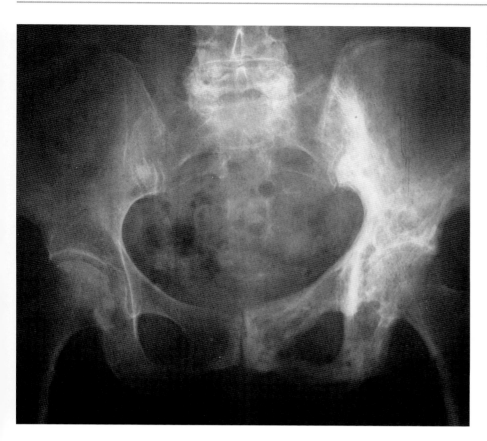

Fig. 12.**59** **Paget's disease** in the left pelvic bones. Enlargement of pubis and ischium and coarse trabecular pattern:

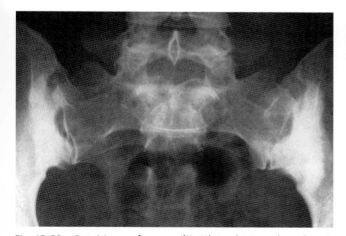

Fig. 12.**60** **Osteitis condensans ilii.** Bilateral triangular sclerosis of the iliac bones, normal sacroiliac joints.

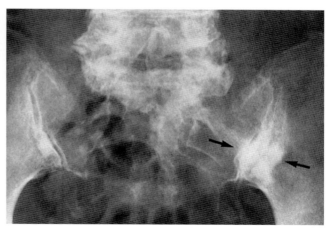

Fig. 12.**61** **Sacroiliitis circumscripta.** Polycyclic sclerosis on both sides of the sacroiliac joint. Tomography revealed minimal erosion.

Table 12.7 (Cont.) Differential Diagnosis of Localized Lesions of the Pelvis

Disease	Radiographic Findings	Comments
Pyogenic or tuberculous sacroiliitis (Fig. 12.62)	Usually unilateral destruction of sacroiliac joint. May be surrounded by sclerosis and soft tissue calcification. Old sacroiliitis may be seen as fusion of the joint.	Destruction of the sacroiliac joint cartilage is rare in relapsing polychondritis.
Osteochondrosis sacri	Sclerotic fragmentation of the lateral sacral apophyses with normal outline of the iliac joint contour.	A rare aseptic necrosis of the sacral apophyses. Occurs at the age of 16 to 20. Absence of erosions differentiates from juvenile ankylosing spondylitis and infection.
Osteolysis syndromes	Regional loss of bone around the sacroiliac joint (or elsewhere).	Very rare conditions, which may be associated with angiomatosis or lymphangiomatosis of bone in a child (massive osteolysis Gorham-Stout) or osteolysis secondary to paraplegia.
Osteonecrosis pubis	Erosion and/or sclerosis of the inferior and/or middle portion of the pubic symphysis (the attachment of the gracilis, adductor longus, and adductor brevis muscles).	A painful bone reaction similar to fatigue fractures. Usually occurs in young athletes, with pain in the pubic area.
Osteitis pubis (Fig. 12.63)	Demineralization, erosion, sclerosis of the pubic symphysis. Bridging of the pubic symphysis may result when healing,	Bacterial or aseptic inflammation of the pubic synchondrosis. Usually occurs 4 to 12 weeks after prostatectomy or other urogenital operation. Pregnancy, ankylosing spondylitis and other arthritides are more common causes of widening and/or erosion of the pubic symphysis.

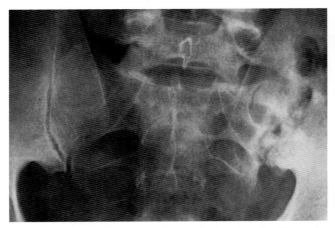

Fig. 12.**62** **Tuberculous sacroiliitis** with deep localized bone destruction, surrounding sclerosis, and calcification of soft tissue.

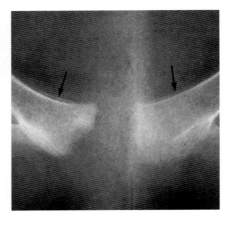

Fig. 12.**63** **Osteitis pubis** (aseptic). Widening of the symphysis, erosion of bone, and periosteal reaction at the pelvic rim (arrows).

Table 12.8 Differential Diagnosis of Disease with Generalized Involvement of Both Spine and Pelvis

Disease	Radiographic Findings	Comments
Achondroplasia (Fig. 12.64)	At birth, the spine shows flattened vertebral bodies and an increased height of the intervertebral spaces. The spinal canal is narrow, Hypoplasia of upper lumbar vertebra with kyphosis, partial beaking of lumbar vertebral bodies, and posterior scalloping may be present, The pelvis is smaller than normal due to short iliac bones and narrow sacrum. Milder forms exist. (See also spinal stenosis Fig. 12.**29**)	A hereditary bone dysplasia with a defect in enchondral bone formation.
Hurler's syndrome (mucopolysaccharidosis I) (gargoylism) (Figs. 12.65)	The vertebral bodies are oval with an anterior inferior beak. A hypoplastic "sail" vertebra may be present in the upper lumbar region causing angular kyphosis.	An autosomal recessive disease with dwarfism, retardation, and coarse facial features. The patients excrete heparan sulfate and dermatan sulfate in urine. Bone changes are seen after 2 years of age. The spinal changes may suggest an intraspinal mass.

(continues on page 298)

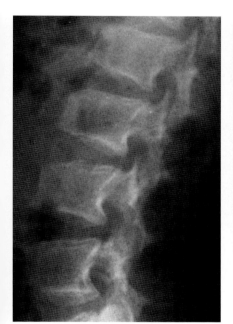
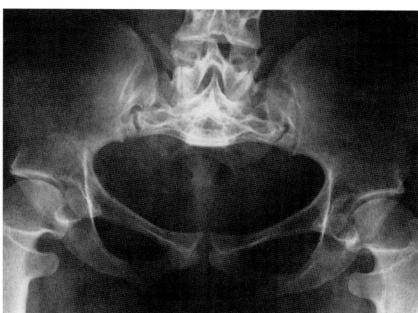

b

Fig. 12.**64 a, b** **Achondroplasia. a** Abnormal vertebral bodies with partial beaking and posterior scalloping of vertebral bodies, **b** Hypoplastic sacrum, abnormal shape of pelvis and hip joints.

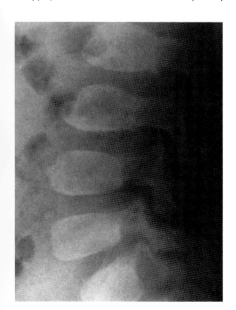

Fig. 12.**65** **Hurler's syndrome.** Oval vertebral bodies with an anterior inferior beak.

Table 12.8   (Cont.) Differential Diagnosis of Disease with Generalized Involvement of Both Spine and Pelvis

Disease	Radiographic Findings	Comments
Hunter's syndrome (mucopolysaccharidosis II) Fig. 12.66)	Hypoplasia of the pedicles and widening of the interpediculate spaces with posterior vertebral scalloping may be present.	The inferior beaking of ovoid bodies distinguish this condition from Morquio's syndrome. Hunter's syndrome is radiologically similar to Hurler's syndrome, but has a slower rate of progression.
Morquio's syndrome (mucopolysaccharidosis IV) (Fig. 12.67)	Universal vertebra plana show a central anterior beak in contrast to the inferior anterior beak seen in Hurler's syndrome. Other spinal findings include hypoplastic dens with atlantoaxial instability, dorsolumbar rotary kyphoscoliosis, and increased interpediculate distance as well as small sacrum with a narrow ovoid pelvic inlet and wide acetabula.	Manifests clinically during the second year of life. The patients excrete keratan sulfate in the urine. The trunk is short, whereas extremities are relatively normal. There is usually no mental retardation, but multiple deformities of the extremities and pigeon breast are present. Spondyloepiphyseal dysplasia congenita can be differentiated from Morquio's syndrome by absence of corneal clouding and mucopolysacchariduria and by manifestations present at birth, although spinal changes are similar in these two conditions.
Progeria	The vertebral bodies retain their infantile central notching. Bilateral coxa valga is constantly present.	A rare disease of unkown etiology characterized by dwarfism and premature aging. Beaked nose, receded chin, and baldness are typical.
Arachnodactyly (Marfan's syndrome)	Lumbar vertebrae may be abnormally tall, ilium may be vertical with wide pelvic cavity. Widening of the spinal canal and posterior scalloping of vertebral bodies are noted. Scoliosis is common.	An autosomal dominant growth disturbance caused by failure to produce normal collagen. Long slender metatarsals, metacarpals, and phalanges are characteristic.
Homocystinuria	Flattening and biconcavity of osteoporotic vertebral bodies are a distinctive difference to Marfan's syndrome.	A hereditary, somewhat heterogeneous condition, usually a lack of enzyme cystathionine beta synthetase. One third of patients show changes similar to those seen in Marfan's syndrome.
Neurofibromatosis I (von Recklinghausen's disease) (Fig. 12.68)	Radiographic findings in the spine are multiple. Kyphoscoliosis with dysplastic vertebral bodies, erosion of intervertebral foramina due to "dumbbell" neurofibromas and posterior scalloping of the vertebral bodies with or without meningoceles are commonly observed. Several other spinal or pelvic anomalies are encountered, but they are not diagnostic of this disease.	A hereditary disturbance of mesodermal and neuroectodermal tissues. Neurofibromas, smooth marginated cafe-au-lait spots on the skin, and bone deformities are characteristic findings.

(continues on page 300)

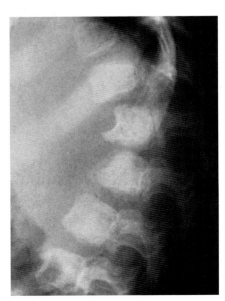

Fig. 12.**66   Hunter's syndrome.** A hypoplastic vertebra with characteristic inferior beak and kyfosis is seen.

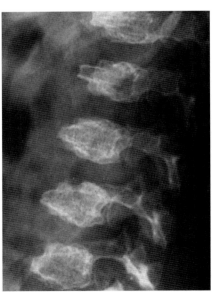

Fig. 12.**67   Morquio's syndrome.** Universally flat vertebrae have a central anterior beak.

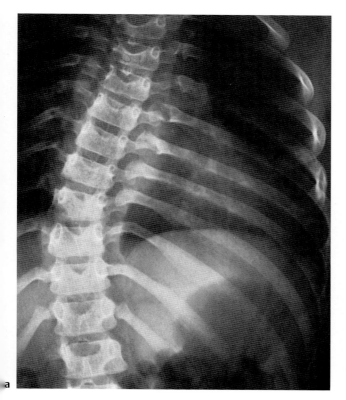

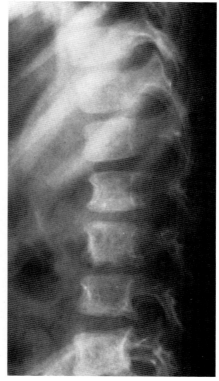

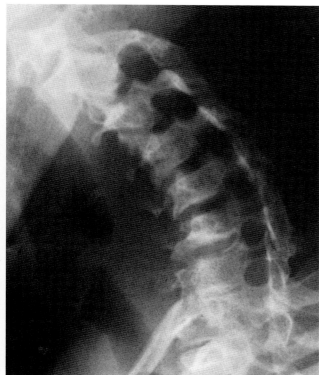

Fig. 12.**68 a, b, c   Neurofibromatosis. a** AP projection shows scoliosis and rib abnormalities (arrows), **b** Lateral projection demonstrates posterior scalloping of vertebral bodies. Slightly enlarged neural foramina at the thoracolumbar region. **c** Oblique view of the cervical spine demonstrates dysplastic cervical vertebrae with scoliosis and wide neural foramina.

Table 12.8   (Cont.) Differential Diagnosis of Disease with Generalized Involvement of Both Spine and Pelvis

Disease	Radiographic Findings	Comments
Osteogenesis imperfecta (Fig. 12.69)	The vertebral bodies are osteoporotic and have a nonuniform biconcave configuration. Scoliosis and protrusio acetabuli are common.	An inherited autosomal dominant connective tissue disorder. The congenital form is present at birth; the tarda form may manifest in puberty or adulthood. Osteoporosis, multiple fractures, bowing of the long bones and blue sclera are characteristic.
Sickle-cell anemia (Fig. 12.70)	The spine is radiolucent even in young adults. The trabecular pattern is coarse, producing areas of increased and decreased bone density. Vertebral bodies tend to be biconcave. A cuplike depression involving the central three-fifths of both upper and lower endplates of several vertebral bodies is typical. In children, the anterior vertebral notch may be exaggerated.	A condition in which the red blood cells assume a sickled configuration at reduced oxygen tension. An abnormal hemoglobin S is Genetically transmitted. The signs and symptoms of sickle-cell disease are due to anemia, e.g., rapid destruction of abnormal erythrocytes.
Thalassemia	Biconcavity of vertebral bodies is not a feature of thalassemia, but loss of density and coarse trabecular pattern may be seen in spine and pelvis.	A heterogeneous group of microcytic anemias based on a decreased rate of synthesis of one or more hemoglobin polypeptide chains. Heterozygotes are mildly affected. The radiographic changes in bones result from erythroid hyperplasia of the marrow.
Cretinism (congenital hypothyroidism)	Kyphosis, flattened vertebral bodies, and increased width of intervertebral spaces. An upper lumbar vertebra may have a wedge or hook configuration (sail vertebra).	The changes are not present at birth. Sail vertebrae occur also in achondroplasia, Hurler's syndrome and Morquio's syndrome.
Osteopetrosis (Albers-Schönberg disease) (Fig. 12.71)	All bones may be involved, with loss of distinction between cortex and medulla, The vertebrae and pelvis may be uniformly dense or there may be a "bone-within-a-bone" appearance of the vertebral bodies. Increased density of endplates may give rise to "sandwich vertebrae." Similar alternating. bands occur in pelvis, too.	Hereditary failure of absorption of primary spongiosa. The congenital form is inherited as an autosomal recessive and is manifest at birth. The tarda form is dominantly inherited, clinically benign and asymptomatic in 50 %. Anemia is a common clinical symptom. Somewhat similar, osteosclerosis, but without bone-within-a-bone and without anemia, is seen in a rare hereditary condition called pycnodysostosis. In osteopoikilosis, the sclerotic patches tend to occur around acetabula but not in the spine, whereas osteopathia striata may involve both pelvis and spine.

(continues on page 302)

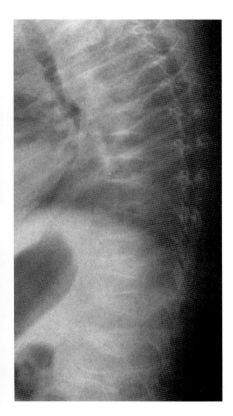

Fig. 12.**69 Osteogenesis Imperfecta** Radiolucent spine, biconcave lumbar vertebral bodies.

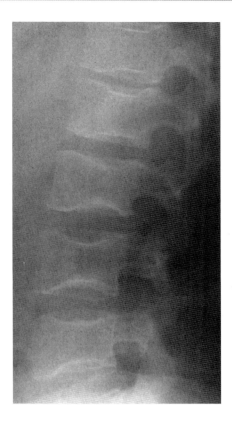

Fig. 12.**70 Sickle-cell anemia.** Cup-like depressions in the central endplates are clearest in the thoracolumbar region.

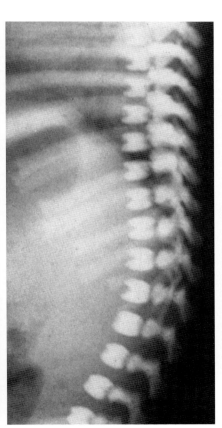

a

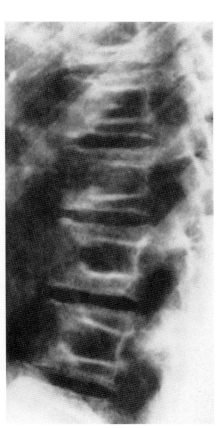

b

Fig. 12.**71 a, b Osteopetrosis. a** Uniformly dense vertebrae and ribs in a child, **b** "Sandwich vertebrae," increased density of the endplates.

Table 12.8   (Cont.) Differential Diagnosis of Disease with Generalized Involvement of Both Spine and Pelvis

Disease	Radiographic Findings	Comments
Myelofibrosis (myelosclerosis) (Fig. 12.72)	Variable degrees of osteosclerosis are seen in 50% of patients. The spine and pelvis are often involved. The increase of bone density may have either trabecular or "ground glass" pattern and it may be patchy.	Progressive fibrosis of the bone marrow with a leukemoid blood picture (splenomegaly) and osteosclerosis, usually in patients over 50. The condition is often preceded by polycytemia vera.
Mastocytosis (urticaria pigmentosa) (Fig. 12.73)	Spine and pelvis are commonly affected, showing a mixture of sclerosis (either diffuse or trabecular) and osteoporosis of the cancellous bone.	Abnormal number of mast cells in skin, resulting in umbilicated papules. Anemia is common. Bone marrow involvement results in sclerosis.
Tuberous sclerosis (Fig. 12.74)	Irregular patches of osteosclerosis without bone enlargement or coarsening of trabeculation. Lesions in the ilium are centrally located; pelvis and lumbar spine are involved in 40%.	A familial defect of ectodermal development. Adenoma sebaceum of the face, epilepsy, mental deficiency, hamartomas of the kidney, and small scattered intracranial calcifications are common.
Hypervitaminosis D	Vertebral bodies show dense endplates and a subcortical radiolucency.	Excessive intake of vitamin D. Metastatic calcifications are common (Chapter 7). Idiopathic hypercalcemia in a chronic form may also cause peripheral cortical sclerosis of vertebral bodies.
Fluorosis (Fig. 12.75)	Thickening of the trabecular pattern of the vertebral bodies and pelvis (also ribs and clavicles) is followed by dense, uniform, symmetrical sclerosis. Osteophytes are characteristically large and sclerotic. Bones may be widened. Calcification of the iliolumbar and sacral ligaments is common.	Excessive intake of fluoride, which inhibits normal bone resorption.

(continues on page 304)

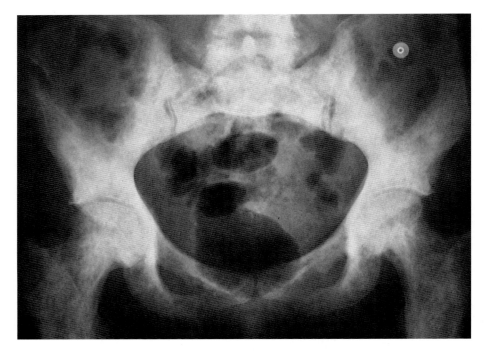

Fig. 12.**72   Myelofibrosis.** Patchy sclerosis of the pelvis, lower lumbar spine, and upper femora. The pattern mimics widespread osteosclerotic metastases (e.g., carcinoma of prostate).

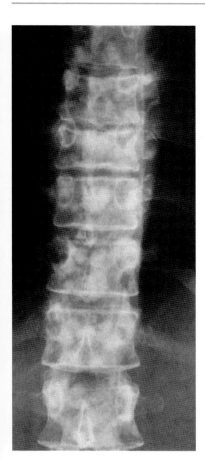

Fig. 12.**73** **Mastocytosis.** The vertebral bodies show patchy sclerosis

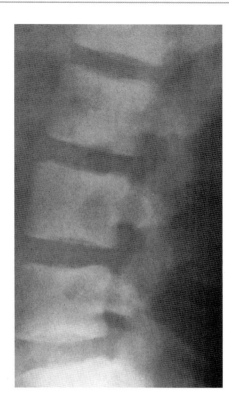

Fig. 12.**74** **Tuberous sclerosis.** Irregular patches of sclerosis are present around the pelvic rim, sacroiliac joints, and in the sacrum and lumbar spine. A scoliosis is an associated finding in this case.

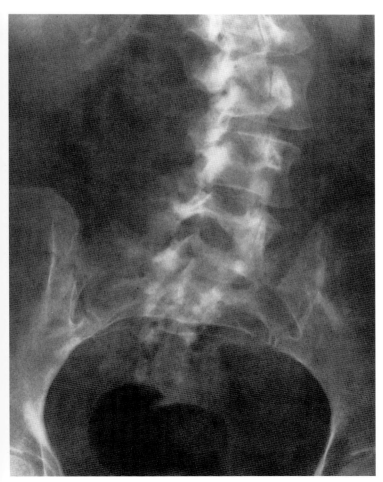

Fig. 12.**75** **Fluorosis.** Dense, uniform sclerosis of the lumbar spine.

Table 12.8 (Cont.) Differential Diagnosis of Disease with Generalized Involvement of Both Spine and Pelvis

Disease	Radiographic Findings	Comments
Hyperparathyroidism (primary or secondary) (Fig. 12.76)	Initially there is loss of bone density, subperiosteal and endosteal resorption of bone. Resorption is particularly prominent in symphysis pubis, ischia, and sacroiliac joints. Expanding focal bone lesions occur in pelvis. They are brown tumors or true cysts. Fractures and deformities of the pelvis follow. Generalized sclerosis of vertebral bodies or sclerotic bands adjacent to the endplates ("rugger jersey" spine) may be present.	"Rugger jersey" spine is more common in secondary hyperparathyroidism (renal osteodystrophy) than in primary hyperparathyroidism. A cyst will not heal after parathyroidectomy, but a brown tumor accumulates dense bone and may persist as a dense focus for years.

(continues on page 305)

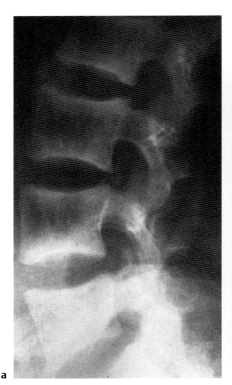

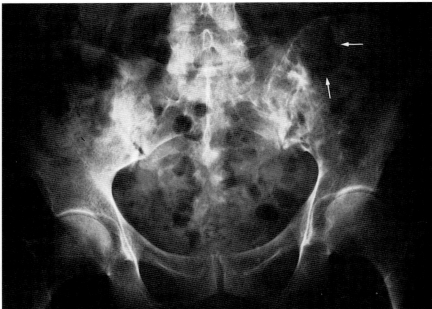

a

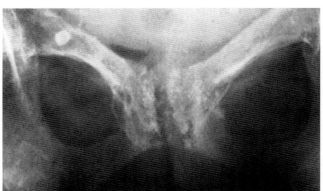

c

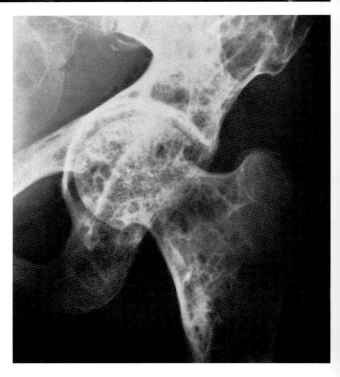

Fig. 12.**76 a–d Hyperparathyroidism a** Sclerotic bands adjacent to the vertebral endplates in renal osteodystrophy. **b** Large loculated cystic lesion in the left iliac bone (arrows) in primary hyperparathyroidism. **c** Erosion and sclerosis of the pubic symphysis (primary hyperparathyroidism). **d** Protrusio acetabuli and widespread cystic lesions in the pelvis and femur. Primary hyperparathyroidism.

Table 12.8   (Cont.)   Differential Diagnosis of Disease with Generalized Involvement of Both Spine and Pelvis

Disease	Radiographic Findings	Comments
Arthritides and arthritis like conditions involving spine and pelvis (Figs. 12.77–80)	For general radiographic findings and differential diagnostic aspects see Table 6.**2**.	

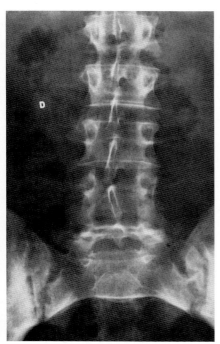

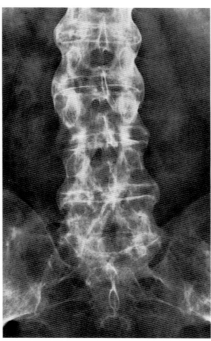

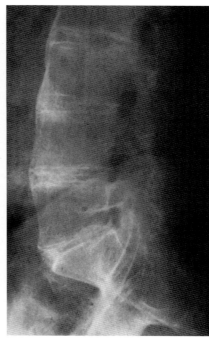

Fig. 12.**77   Ankylosing spondylitis.** Erosion and sclerosis of both sacroiliac joints. Narrowing and erosion of the apophyseal joints, no recognizable syndesmophytes.

a

b

Fig. 12.**78 a, b   Advanced ankylosing spondylitis.** Bamboo spine with syndesmophytes, squaring of vertebral bodies, fusion of sacroiliac and apophyseal joints, and narrow calcified disk spaces.

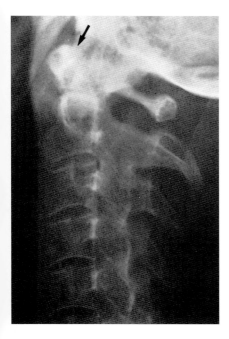

Fig. 12.**79   Ankylosing spondylitis.** Fusion of the apophyseal joints, squaring of vertebral bodies, and subluxation of the atlantoaxial joint (arrow).

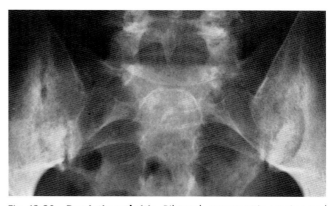

Fig. 12.**80   Psoriatic arthritis.** Bilateral, asymmetric erosion and sclerosis of the sacroiliac joints.

13 Clavicles, Ribs, and Sternum

Clavicles, ribs, and sternum are usually seen on the same plain films and will therefore be dealt with in the same chapter, although anatomically clavicles are part of the upper extremity. Many of the roentgenographic findings are incidental, seen in chest roentgenograms. In these high KV$_p$ exposures, bone details in the ribs and sternum are poorly visualized. Special views with lower KV$_p$ and better contrast are taken in the presence of local pain, a history of trauma, or a palpable lesion. The costal cartilage is not visualized unless calcification has taken place. Costal cartilage calcification is more common in females and tends to be central, whereas peripheral calcifications predominate in males.

Rib Anomalies

Rib deformities occur in 2.8% of the population. The so-called *cervical rib* may be a supernumerary rib *originating from the lowermost cervical segment.* An asymmetrically developed *hypoplastic first thoracic rib may mimic a cervical rib.* A true cervical rib is usually an asymptomatic incidental finding. It may occasionally compress the subclavian artery or brachial plexus. Congenitally *bifid, spurred, widened,* or *fused* ribs are relatively common variants (Fig. 13.1). It may be a manifestation of the rare *basal cell nevus syndrome (Gorlin's syndrome),* which consists of a combination of multiple basal cell epitheliomas, odontogenic cysts, brachydactyly, rib anomalies, scoliosis with vertebral anomalies, extensive calcification of the falx cerebri, and multiple calcified mesenteric cysts.

Thin or Small Ribs

Hypoplasia or *absence* of a rib is relatively common at Tl or T12. Eleven pairs of ribs are more common among females than males, and frequent among *Down's syndrome.*

A *regenerated rib* after resection (if periosteum is leaved intact) is usually thinner, shorter, and not as smoothly outlined as the original (Fig. 13.2). In *neurofibromatosis,* ribs may be thin due to hypoplasia. Intercostal neurofibromas cause superior and inferior erosions (ribbon rib; Fig. 13.3). Thinned or "ribbon" ribs may be a feature in *hyperparathyroidism,* due to sub-periosteal bone resorption, *osteogenesis imperfecta, severe osteoporosis,* long-standing *paraplegia* (poliomyelitis), *rheumatoid arthritis, scleroderma, trisomy 12–15* and *trisomy 17–18* syndromes, as well as in a number of rare *osteochondrodysplasias.*

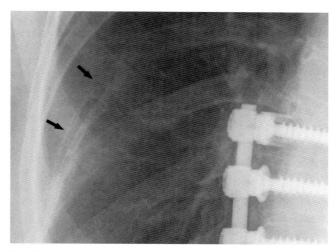

Fig. 13.**2** **Regenerated rib.** 7th rib on the right was removed because of skoliosis treatment. A regenerated rib is present two years after operation.

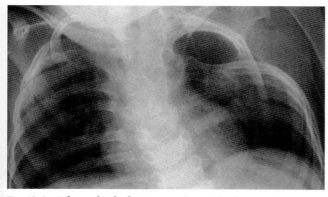

Fig. 13.**1** **Bilateral rib fusions** and vertebral anomalies cause severe deformity of the chest.

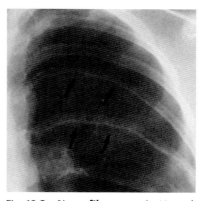

Fig. 13.**3** **Neurofibromatosis.** Hypoplastic ribs 5 and 6 on the left show inferior erosions (arrows). They are caused by intercostal neurinomas.

Wide Ribs

Several congenital conditions cause rib deformities as a reflection of generalized bone involvement.

In *achondroplasia* (Fig. 13.4), the ribs are *wide*, markedly *shortened*, and they do not extend normally around the chest. Among the *mucopolysaccharidoses*, rib widening is common (Fig. 13.5). In type IV (*Morquio's syndrome*), the ribs may have thinned posterior portions (Fig. 13.6). Rib changes similar to mucopolysaccharidoses are present also in various *mucolipidoses* (a congenital group of disorders in which excess material is stored in lysosomes and the clinical and radiologic findings resemble mucopolysaccharidoses). Patchy osteoporosis mimicking metastatic disease combined with rib widening may be present in *Gaucher's disease* and *Niemann–Pick disease*. Rib widening may be a feature in several other rare osteochondrodysplasias as well.

In *osteopetrosis* (Albers-Schonberg disease), the ribs and clavicles are uniformly dense. The sternal ends may be widened. Uniformly dense ribs are commonly caused by osteoblastic metastases, myelofibrosis, or Hodgkin lymphoma (see Chapter 2).

Anterior bulbous widenings and a coarse trabecular pattern are characteristic rib changes in *thalassemia*. Coarse trabeculation with cortical widening may also be seen in *sickle cell anemia* and *polycythemia*.

Cupping and widening of the sternal ends of ribs are characteristic of *rickets* (Fig. 13.7). Bulging, somewhat widened costochondral junctions are also seen in *scurvy*. In *Caffey's infantile cortical hyperostosis*, periosteal thickening and subperiosteal new bone formation are most frequently found in clavicles and ribs. The condition is accompanied by fever, soft-tissue swelling, and generalized symptoms of inflammation. Periosteal new bone formation in ribs also occurs in *leukemia*, especially in childhood.

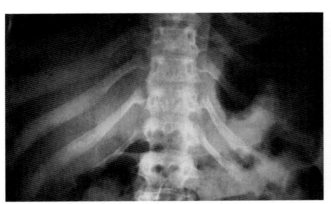

Fig. 13.4   **Achondroplasia.** The ribs are wide and short.

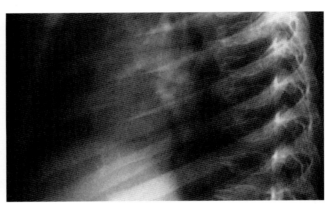

Fig. 13.6   **Morquio's syndrome.** Characteristic vertebral bodies and wide ribs laterally and anteriorly.

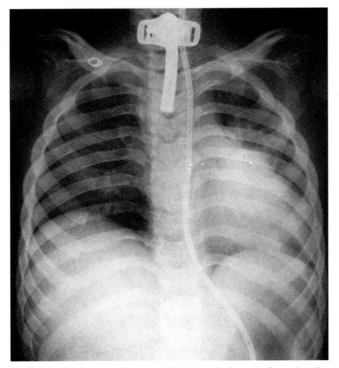

Fig. 13.5   **Hurler's syndrome.** The ribs are abnormally wide. The glenoid fossa and humeral epiphysis are also abnormal.

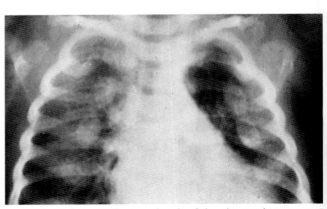

Fig. 13.7   **Rickets.** Wide sternal ends of the ribs, "rachitic rosary."

Localized Rib Lesions

Localized expansile lesions of the ribs occur most frequently due to *fibrocystic lesions*, e.g., *fibrous dysplasia* (Fig. 13.8), *bone cyst* (Fig. 13.9) or *nonossifying fibroma* (see Chapter 5). Expansion may also be due to *enchondroma* (Fig. 13.10), *osteochondroma* (exostosis) (Fig. 13.11), *expansile metastasis*, *myeloma* (Fig. 13.12), other neoplastic diseases, as well as a brown tumor of *hyperparathyroidism*, Langerhans cell histiocytosis (*eosinophilic granuloma*), *fracture* with extensive callus, and *osteomyelitis* (see Chapter 5). Cartilaginous expansion in *Tietze's syndrome* may occasionally cause expansion of the anterior end of the rib, but usually there is no associated bone abnormality. Long (>6 cm) solitary expansile lesions are encountered in sarcomatous tumors (*osteosarcoma, chondrosarcoma, Ewing's sarcoma*, Askin tumor is uncommon tumor of intercostals nerve.), *fibrous dysplasia*, *metastases*, and *plasmocytoma* or *myeloma*, but rarely in other bone tumors or in *Paget's disease*.

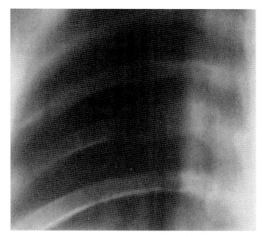

Fig. 13.**8** **Fibrous dysplasia** of a rib, seen as a local expansion in the posterior part of the rib.

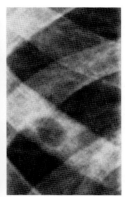

Fig. 13.**9** A small **unicameral bone cyst** of a rib. Eosinophilic granuloma or osteoid osteoma could have similar appearance.

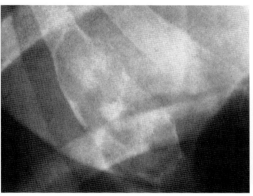

Fig. 13.**10** **Enchondroma.** An expansile lesion with ground glass appearance. Fibrous dysplasia could have similar appearance.

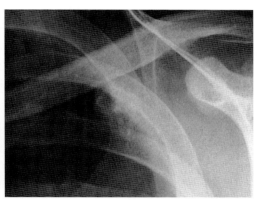

Fig. 13.**11** **Osteochondroma** of a rib.

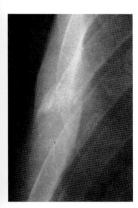

Fig. 13.**12** **Multiple myeloma** presenting as a lytic rib lesion.

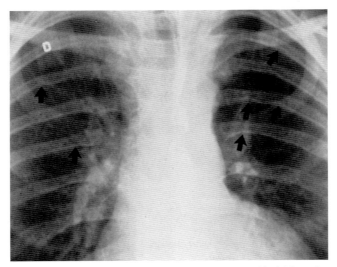

Fig. 13.**13** **Coarctation of the aorta** in a 6-year-old child. Multiple rib notches (arrows) and abnormal configuration of the left heart border.

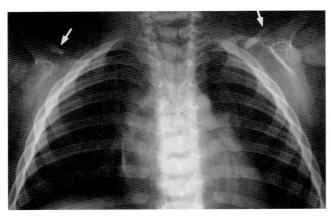

Fig. 13.**14** **Cleidocranial dysplasia.** Severe hypoplasia of clavicles (arrows), multiple spina bifidas, cone-shaped chest with relatively short ribs (long cartilaginous segments), relatively small scapulae.

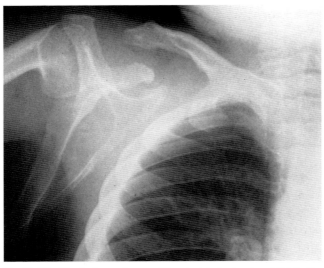

Fig. 13.**15** **Hurler's syndrome.** The clavicle is short and thick, the ribs are wide, and there is deformity of the scapula and humeral epiphysis.

Rib Notching

Rib notches (localized erosions of ribs) are considered characteristic of *coarctation of the aorta* (seen in 80% of cases). Rib notching due to coarctation occurs in ribs 3 to 9 (Fig. 13.**13**). The notches are usually located in the inferior margin of the ribs unless tortuous intercostal arteries are large enough to erode the superior surface of the adjacent rib. Rib erosions due to coarctation commonly appear after 6 to 12 years of age. Unilateral right-sided notching indicates coarctation proximal to the left subclavian artery and left-sided notching points to an anomalous origin of the right subclavian artery (take-off below coarctation). Several other conditions may cause rib notching, as follows:

- *obstruction of the abdominal aorta (thrombosis)*
- obstruction of the subclavian artery (*Blalock-Taussig procedure* for Fallot's tetralogy, *Takayasu's arteritis, arteriosclerosis obliterans*)
- pulmonary oligemia (*tetralogy of Fallot, absent pulmonary artery* or *pulmonary atresia* or *stenosis, pseudotruncus arteriosus, Ebstein's anomaly, pulmonary emphysema*)
- pulmonary or intercostal *arteriovenous malformation*
- *obstructions of the superior vena cava* or *subclavian vein*
- *neurofibromatosis* or intercostal neurinoma (Fig. 13.**3**)
- periosteal irregularities mimicking rib notches occur in *hyperparathyroidism, tuberous sclerosis, thalassemia, collagen diseases*, and sometimes without any known reason (idiopathic notching).

Notching of superior surface of ribs may occur in certain connective tissue diseases, such as rheumatoid arthritis, systemic lupus erythematosus, scleroderma and Sjögren's syndrome. Superior surface notching may occur in hyperparathyroidism, neurofibromatosis, restrictive lung disease, poliomyelitis, Marfan's syndrome, osteogenesis imperfecta and progeria.

Abnormal Clavicle

The clavicle is formed from three separate ossification centers. If one or more of them is absent, hypoplasia or absence of the clavicle occurs. This is a characteristic finding in *cleidocranial dysostosis* (hypoplasia or absence of clavicles, defective ossification of the calvarium, spina bifida, hypoplastic pelvic bones with separation of pubic symphysis). The chest may be cone-shaped and ribs may be short but otherwise normal in cleidocranial dysostosis (Fig. 13.**14**). Clavicular hypoplasia also occurs in *focal dermal hypoplasia* (*Goltz's syndrome*). In this condition, hypoplastic clavicles and ribs are associated with syndactyly, dental anomalies, and skin atrophy and pigmentations. *Holt-Oram syndrome* is characterized by finger-like or absent thumb and shoulder anomalies, including hypoplastic clavicles. Shortening and thickening of clavicles is a manifestation of *Hurler's syndrome* (Fig. 13.**15**), a more characteristic sign being hypoplasia of L2 and inferior beaking of the anterior margin of one or more vertebral bodies (see Chapter 12, Table 12.7). Thinning of clavicles and ribs occurs in *progeria*. In *trisomy 13/18*, tapering of the distal clavicle is one of the multiple anomalies. Unilaterally small clavicle and other shoulder bones may be caused by *brachial plexus damage at birth* (Fig. 13.**16**).

The most common *localized intraosseous lesions* of the clavicles are *osteomyelitis* (Fig. 13.**17**) and *trauma*. In patients

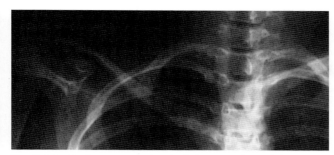

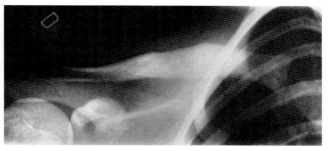

Fig. 13.**16**   **Birth trauma** to brachial plexus. Unilateral thinning of right clavicle and small shoulder bones, but the structure of bones is normal. There is also a healing fracture of the right first rib and upward dislocation of the sternal end of the left clavicle.

Fig. 13.**17**   **Chronic osteomyelitis** of the right clavicle. No destruction is seen, but there is slowly progressing sclerosis and thickening of bone.

with so called SAPHO (Fig. 13.**18**) (synovitis, acne, pustulosis, hyperostosis and osteomyelitis) syndrome there is hyperostosis in the medial end of the clavicle which mimics osteomyelitis. Other possibilities exist, and the differential diagnostic list of such a lesion is essentially the same as with a localized lesion in a rib.

Erosion and destruction of the outer end of the clavicle is most commonly caused by *rheumatoid arthritis* (see Chapter 6), *hyperparathyroidism* (Fig. 13.**19**) (see Chapter 1), *myeloma* (Fig. 13.**20**), and *rickets*. Other conditions to be considered as causes of bone erosion or defects in the lateral end of the clavicle include *scleroderma* and *gout* (intra-articular or periarticular calcium deposits occur in both), *lipoid dermatoarthritis* (reticulohistiocytoma), and a number of other conditions that rarely cause localized lesions in ribs and clavicles such as *posttraumatic osteolysis, metastasis, Ewing's sarcoma, amyloidosis, osteomalacia, progeria, pycnodysostosis, massive osteolysis* (Gorham-Stout), and *neurogenic osteolysis*.

Erosive changes in the medial end of the clavicle and the sternoclavicular joint are usually due to *rheumatoid* or, more rarely, *pyogenic arthritis*. A notch at the attachment of the costoclavicular ligament (inferior surface) or the sternocleidomastoid muscle (superior surface) should be distinguished from inflammatory erosion.

Widespread *sclerosis* of the clavicle may be due to *chronic osteomyelitis* (Fig. 13.**17**) or *Paget's disease*. Widespread sclerosis and even fusion of the clavicles with the sternum occurs in the rare, painful *sternocostoclavicular hyperostosis*, which may mimic sclerosing osteomyelitis Garre (see Table 5.4). Painful sclerosis of the clavicle may also be due to *osteoid osteoma*. Sclerosis of the sternal end of the clavicle, often associated with pain, can be due *to osteitis condensans claviculae*. Avascular necrosis (Friedrich's disease} involves only the caudal half of the sternal end of the clavicle. In small children, the middle portion of the clavicle may be seen "end-on" due to normal curvature and may mimic a sclerotic process or healed fracture.

Luxation or subluxation of the acromioclavicular joint (Fig. 13.**21**) usually produces downward and lateral displacement of the acromion in weight bearing. *Luxation of the sternoclavicular joint* (Fig. 13.**16**) is usually post-traumatic, but is also common after radical neck dissection.

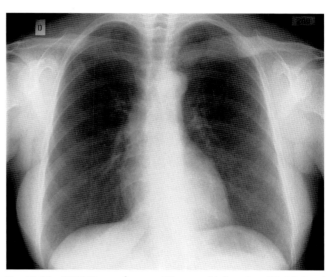

Fig. 13.**18**   **SAPHO syndrome.** 35-year-old female with bilateral thickening and sclerosis of medial halves of clavicles.

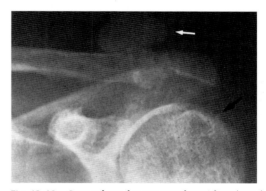

Fig. 13.**19**   **Secondary hyperparathyroidism**/renal osteodystrophy). There is erosion of the distal end of the clavicle and endosteal thinning of the cortex. Soft-tissue calcification (arrows) is also seen.

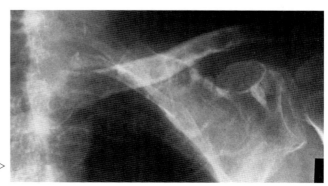

Fig. 13.**20**   **Multiple myeloma.** Multiple osteolytic lesions in the ▷ distal clavicle and in scapula, the head of the humerus, and ribs.

Abnormal Sternum

The sternum is visualized on lateral plain films, but is usually poorly shown in anteroposterior or oblique views. Fusion anomalies of the sternal segments (Fig. 13.**22**) are common and are sometimes seen in association with other anomalies, including congenital heart disease.

The most common anomaly is *fusion* of the *manubriosternal* synchondrosis, with or without a synchondrosis between the first and second segment of the body of the sternum. Fusion of the manubriosternal synchondrosis may also be the end result of *ankylosing spondylitis, rheumatoid arthritis, psoriatic arthritis, Reiter's syndrome, enteropathic arthritis,* healed *hyperparathyroidism, degenerative joint disease, trauma* or *surgery, pyogenic infection, fluorosis,* or, rarely, *relapsing polychondritis.* The same conditions may cause erosion and sclerosis of the sternal synchondrosis (Fig. 13.**23**). However, one should note that some irregularities of the joint surfaces are a normal finding.

A defect in the body of the sternum may represent a fusion anomaly if the hole has smooth cortical margins. Sclerosis and blurring of the margins of a sternal defect point to *osteomyelitis* (pyogenic or tuberculous) or to *metastatic* destruction. Infectious lesions tend to have sclerotic margins (Fig. 13.**24**), whereas the pattern of metastases (Fig. 13.**25**) and primary tumors (Figs. 13.**26** and 13.**27**) are similar to those in any other flat bone.

The xiphoid process is often radiolucent or contains only some calcified cartilage instead of bone. It is therefore usually poorly visualized.

Undue depression of the sternum, called *pectus excavatum*, is usually idiopathic without abnormalities other than an asthenic habitus. There are two major types of pectus excavatum: (1) a deep deformity in the central and distal parts of the sternum, while the manubrium is in a normal position and (2) a broad, flat deformity that also may involve the manubrium. The second type may interfere with cardiac function. Both types may show a shift or enlargement of the cardiac silhouette in the frontal view. Pectus excavatum can be associated with *congenital heart disease, homocystinuria, Marfan's syndrome* (Fig. 13.**28**), the *systolic click-late systolic murmur syndrome, congenital bowing of tibia, idiopathic mitral valve prolapse, Ehlers–Danlos syndrome* and *osteogenesis imperfecta.* Coexistent sternomanubrial protrusion may be present. Deformities may have a traumatic origin (Fig. 13.**29**).

Pectus carinatum, "pigeon breast," or undue prominence of the sternum is less common than pectus excavatum. This anomaly may be seen associated with *congenital heart disease, mucopolysaccharidosis IV (Morquio's syndrome), Noonan's syndrome* (Turner's phenotype with normal karyotype), and *spondyloepiphyseal dysplasia congenita.*

Cleft sternum is usually clinically obvious. The cleft may be located in the superior or inferior portion of the sternum or even be complete. Inferior and complete sternal clefts are often associated with other anomalies (defects in the ventral abdominal wall, diaphragm, pericardium, and heart).

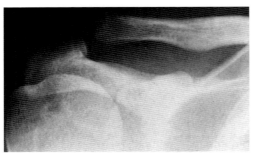

Fig. 13.**21** **Subluxation** of the acromioclavicular joint in weight bearing.

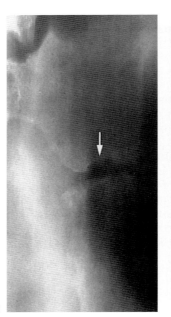

a

Fig. 13.**22** **Segmentation anomalies** of the sternum. There is a vertical cleft in the middle of the manubrium and a horizontal cleft between the first and second segments of the body (arrows).

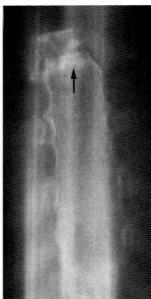

Fig. 13.**23 a, b** **Psoriatic arthritis** with, predominantly, a erosive and b sclerotic changes in the manubriosternal synchondrosis (arrows). Identical changes occur in ankylosing spondylitis, and rarely in rheumatoid arthritis.

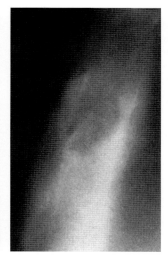

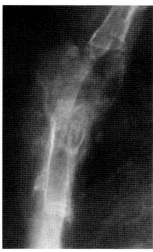

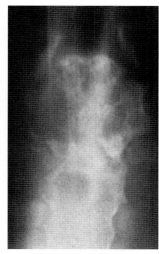

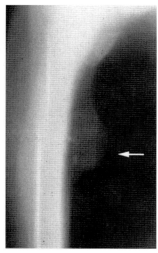

Fig. 13.**24   Sternal tuberculosis** (healed). A slightly expansile osteolytic lesion surrounded by sclerosis.

Fig. 13.**25   Metastatic adenocarcinoma** of the kidney. An expansile osteolytic lesion in the upper body of the sternum.

Fig. 13.**26   Non-Hodgkin's lymphoma.** Predominantly osteolytic, poorly marginated destruction of the manubrium with involvement of manubriosternal synchondrosis.

Fig. 13.**27   Benign osteochondroma** of sternum. A soft tissue mass projecting toward the mediastinum (arrow). The finding is radiographically nonspecific.

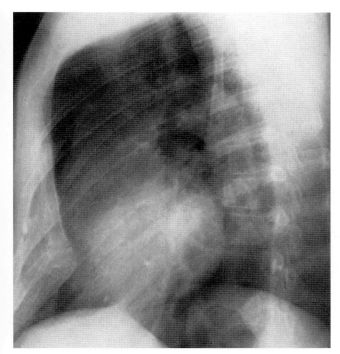

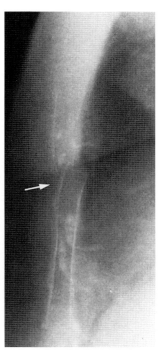

Fig. 13.**28   Pectus excavatum** associated with Marfan's syndrome. The patient also has an aneurysm of the ascending aorta.

Fig. 13.**29   Fracture of the body** of the sternum (arrow).

14 Extremities

Deformities of the long bones are either developmental, that is, caused by abnormal or asymmetric growth, or they may be the sequelae of fractures or associated with a disease that causes bone softening. In the latter case, the weight-bearing lower extremities are usually more affected than the upper extremities. The differential diagnosis of long bone deformities is discussed in Table 14.1.

Normally, the ends of long bones are wider than their diaphyses, and there is a progressive concentric decrease in the caliber of the shaft as one passes from the end toward the middle of a long bone. Abnormal modeling of the long bones can result from a variety of diseases affecting the growing bone and the end result is usually still evident in the adult. Less commonly, abnormal modeling of the long bones may only develop in adulthood. Such conditions are either associated with new periosteal bone formation (e.g. *Paget's disease* or healing *fractures* and *infections*) or caused by expansile nondestructive mass lesions within the bone. A widening of the bone shaft is termed *underconstriction* or *undertubulation*. Widening or splaying of the metaphyses may be associated with underconstriction of the shaft or may present as an isolated finding. A splayed distal femur metaphysis often assumes the shape of an Erlenmeyer flask and is accordingly termed *"Erlenmeyer flask" deformity* (Fig. 14.1). Conditions characterized by "Erlenmeyer flask" deformity include Gaucher's disease, Niemann-Pick disease, thalassemia, craniometaphyseal dysplasia, Pyle's disease, enchrondromatosis, hereditary multiple exstoses, osteogenesis imperfecta, osteopetrosis and lead poisoning. These disorders, as well as all other diseases with a more generalized, widened diametaphysis, are discussed in Table 14.2.

Overconstriction (or *overtubulation*) is the reverse of underconstriction. As one passes from the end of a long bone toward the middle, there is excessive concentric narrowing of the shaft. Overconstriction is usually the cause of a chronic disease affecting the growing bone. It is only rarely acquired in adulthood by marked periosteal resorption of the cortex, since abnormal cortical resorption in the adult occurs predominantly on the endosteal margins, this does not lead to overconstriction. Table 14.3 deals with the differential diagnosis of overconstricted long bones.

Transverse radiolucent and *sclerotic bands* or *lines* in the metaphyses are commonly found in the growing bones and do not necessarily indicate a pathologic process. They may persist into adult life. The differential diagnosis of radiolucent and sclerotic transverse bands is summarized in Tables 14.4 and 14.5, respectively.

Long tubular bones continue to increase in length until fusion of the epiphyseal plates. *Generalized elongation* or *overgrowth* of long bones is uncommon. The usual cause of overgrowth in association with normal length-width relationships is *gigantism*, either of hypothalamic or pituitary origin. Elongation of bones with narrow diametaphysis (overconstriction, overtubulation) is seen in *Marfan's syndrome* and *homocystinuria*. There are many individual variations in the width of bones, and it may be difficult to assess whether otherwise normal-looking bones are thin due to constitu-

tional reasons or to a specific pathologic entity. If deformation of bone is an associated finding, as in *neurofibromatosis*, other clinical or radiographic signs are usually present to suggest a specific diagnosis. *Generalized* or *localized shortening* of a tubular bone is more likely to occur, since a number of congenital or acquired diseases or their treatment will interfere with the growth of bone.

In Table 14.6, some conditions associated with generalized or localized shortening, hypoplasia, or deformity of the long bones of the extremities are presented. The majority of congenital bone dysplasias will not be mentioned here, since their differential diagnosis is more likely to be successful when based on the appearance of the hands and feet and the spine.

The metaphyses of the long bones, especially the knee, hip, and shoulder regions, are favored sites of several malignant bone tumors. Also, benign bone tumors and tumor-like processes are common in the extremities. The general description of these diseases in Chapter 5 is based on their appearance in typical locations and will not be repeated here. Similarly, inflammatory lesions of bone such as bone infection, arthritis, and associated calcifications have been presented in a systematic fashion above. The femoral head is the most important site of fragmentation or deformation for traumatic, inflammatory, vascular, metabolic, or unknown reasons. Therefore, the causes of an abnormal proximal femur are presented in Tables 14.10–14.12, although some overlapping with other chapters unavoidably occurs. Many

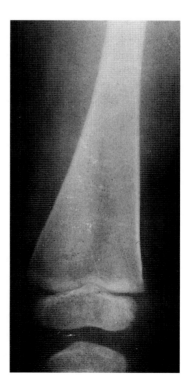

Fig. 14.**1** **"Erlenmeyer flask" deformity.** The splayed distal tibia metaphysis assumes the shape of an Erlenmeyer flask (Pyle's disease).

of the changes and diseases presented as typical of the femoral head also occur in other joints, especially in the shoulder.

Alignment of Joints of Extremities

Abnormalities of the alignment of the joints of the extremities may be the only sign of trauma, e.g., a dislocation without fracture. Malalignment may also be the result of a localized disease process characteristically seen in the knee joints. Since the alignment of the joint can be measured, it may be an objective starting point for a differential diagnostic approach, although it often represents a secondary phenomenon. Certain important facts concerning the alignment of the joints, and some terminological definitions, must be known in order to evaluate radiographs of the extremities appropriately and use Tables 14.7–14.13 properly. These will be presented here briefly.

It is difficult to judge abnormalities of alignment in the *shoulder* (Table 14.7) because of its very wide range of normal motion. Shoulder dislocations are best detected from the axillary view (see Fig. 4.33). In *anterior dislocation*, the humeral head is displaced medially and inferiorly (superimposed over scapula, Fig. 14.2). A defect called *Hill-Sachs deformity* (Fig. 14.3), a compression fracture of the humeral head, is best seen when the arm is abducted and internally rotated 60 degrees. Fracture of the anterior inferior rim of the glenoid, known as the *Bankart lesion*, is less commonly seen. Bankart lesion may affect cartilaginous labrum only. Then the diagnosis can be made by MRI or by CT arthrography. *Posterior dislocation* of the humeral head is less common than anterior dislocation. It is difficult to recognize on a routine view. An abnormal appearance of the humeral head because of rotation may be the only sign of abnormality. In the axillary view the humeral head is superimposed on the acromion and does not articulate with the glenoid fossa. A

compression fracture of the humeral head may be present. A *fracture of the lesser tuberosity* is so commonly associated with a posterior dislocation that its discovery on a routine view of the shoulder necessitates an axillary projection to determine its actual alignment. If the patient is capable of eversion of the humerus, the posterior dislocation is excluded. *Dislocation inferiorly,* towards the axilla, is rare and may be associated with a fracture of the greater tuberosity.

Normally, the *forearm* makes an angle of approximately 170 degrees with the humerus, deviating laterally. Medial deviation (*cubitus varus*) and lateral deviation (*cubitus valgus*) of the forearm may result from *trauma, connective tissue diseases, infections, neurotrophic diseases,* and *Turner's syndrome.*

The most common malalignment in the hip (Table 14.12) is an abnormal angle between the shaft of the femur and its neck. Normally this angle is between 120 and 130 degrees in an adult. In children before puberty, values between 130 and 140 degrees are encountered. An increase in an adult above 130 degrees is called *valgus deformity (coxa valga)*; a decrease below 120 degrees is a *varus deformity (coxa vara).* Valgus deformities are often related to congenital defects, while varus deformities may result from bone softening, such as osteomalacia or Paget's disease. A simple method of determining if varus or valgus deformity is present is shown in Fig. 14.4. Normally there is anterior angulation (anteversion) of the femoral neck between 10 and 15 degrees in the adult, as compared with the line tangential to the distal femoral condyles. This angle is as high as 35 degrees in an infant and decreases towards adulthood. Without inversion of the inferior extremities (approximately 20 degrees), the angle of the femoral neck may not be correctly measurable in anteroposterior films of the hip. Various lines used for the determination of the congenital dislocation of the hip in a neonate are presented in Figure 14.5.

When the tibia is angled laterally, too close approximation of the distal thighs results in *knock knees (genu valgum).* The

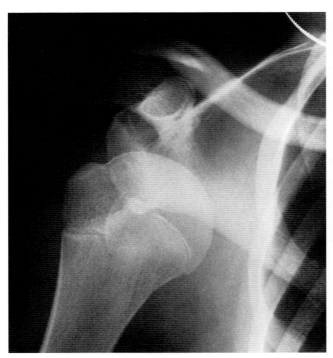

Fig. 14.**2**   **Anterior dislocation of the humeral head** with characteristic medial and inferior displacement.

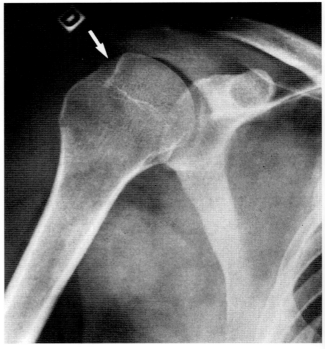

Fig. 14.**3**   **Compression fracture of the humeral head** after dislocation (Hill-Sachs defect, arrow).

opposite condition, separation of the distal thighs, is called *bowlegs (genu varum)*. These deviations cause excessive stress on the knee and lead to degenerative changes. Medial displacement of the distal femur is called *genu laxum*. One measurement used to determine the position of the patella in a lateral view at flexion between 20 to 70 degrees is presented in Fig. 14.6. The ratio of maximal length of the patella to the distance from the distal tip of the patella to the tuberosity of the tibia is normally between 0.8 and 1.2. *Patella alta* (high patella) may be associated with *recurrent subluxation, chondromalacia of the patella, rupture of the patellar ligament, osteomyelitis* of the femur, *poliomyelitis, avascular necrosis of the tibial tuberosity (Osgood–Schlatter disease)*, or the inferior ossification center of the patella (*Sinding–Larsen–Johansson disease*), and *cerebral palsy*. *Patella profunda* or *baja* (low patella) may occur as an inborn condition, as in *achondroplasia*, secondary to *rupture of the quadriceps muscle tendon*, or surgical *transposition of the tibial tuberosity*. It may also be secondary to *juvenile rheumatoid arthritis* or to paresis of the quadriceps muscle in *poliomyelitis*. *Incongruity of patellar motion*, e. g. lateral dislocation and tilting are more common and important abnormalities. Their demonstration is best done with cross sectional images using CT or MRI at flexion less than 30 degrees, since plain films are insensitive.

The patella may be absent or hypoplastic. This is usually due to *hereditary onycho-osteodysplasia* or *nail patella syndrome* (Fig. 14.7), which is characterized by iliac horns and several other abnormalities. Hypoplasia of the patella is occasionally reported in association with acrocephalosyndactyly, and aplasia of the patella in association with *birdheaded dwarfism, neurofibromatosis* and *popliteal pterygium syndrome*.

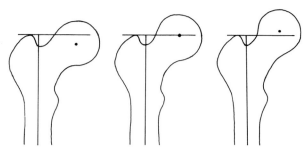

Fig. 14.**4 a–c** **Evaluation of the angle of the femoral neck,** **a** Coxa vara, **b** normal, and **c** coxa valga.

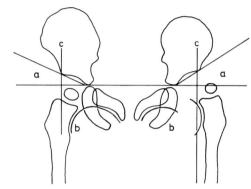

Fig. 14.**5** **Determination of congenital dislocation of the hip in a neonate.** The left side of the diagram represents normal relationships and the right side congenital dislocation, **a** Acetabular angle, **b** Shenton's line, and **c** Ombredanne line.

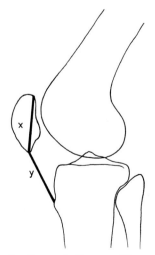

Fig. 14.**6** **Determination of the position of patella.** The measurements should be done at flexion between 20 to 70 degrees, y/x is normally between 0.8 and 1.2. Patella alta = y/x > 1.2, patella profunda = y/x < 0.8.

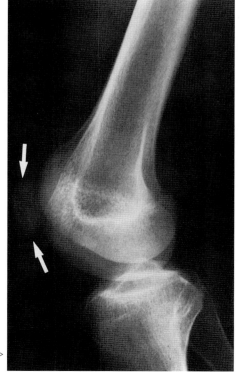

Fig. 14.**7** **Hereditary onycho-osteodysplasia.** Hypoplastic patella ▷ (arrows).

Table 14.1   Bowed or Deformed Long Bones

Disease	Radiographic Findings	Comments
Congenital bowing	Bowlegs: Lateral and usually some anterior bowing of the proximal two-thirds of the tibias and/or the distal segments of the femora. Spurring of the medial aspect of the proximal tibia shaft or the posterior aspect of the distal femur shaft may also be present.	Idiopathic bowlegs of infancy disappear spontaneously after 2 to 3 years. Bowed limbs at birth may also be found in different forms of dwarfisms (e.g., *achondroplasia* and *camptomelic* and *thanatophoric* dwarfism).
Osteodysplasty (Melnick-Needles syndrome)	Lateral bowing of the tibia characteristic. Sclerosis of the base of the skull and mastoids, tall vertebrae, ribbon-like appearance of the ribs, and metaphyseal flaring of short and long bones may also be evident.	Found only in females with small face, large ears, protruding eyes, micrognathia, malaligned teeth and short upper arms.
Infantile cortical hyperostosis (Caffey's disease)	Occasional sequelae of the disease in adulthood include bowing of the limbs, mandibular asymmetry and osseous bridging between adjacent bones.	The disease becomes evident in infants of less than 5 months of age. Usually the clinical and radiographic features subside slowly within a few months to a few years.
Osteogenesis imperfecta (Fig. 14.8)	Bowing deformities in slender overconstricted and osteoporotic long bones with tendency to fracture characteristic.	Inherited connective tissue disorder.
Hypophosphatasia	Bowing deformities and increased bone fragility are characteristically present both in the most severe form (seen in infants) and in the mildest form (seen in adults). In infancy, the disease resembles rickets (cupping and fraying of metaphyses), whereas in the adult the long bones are shortened and often demonstrate cortical thickening and pseudofractures.	Hypophosphatasia is a genetically determined metaphyseal dysplasia with failure to form primary spongiosa. Low serum alkaline phosphatase levels are characteristic.
Vitamin D resistent rickets (x-linked hypophosphatemia) (Fig. 14.9 a)	Bowing deformities occur in the long bones of the lower extremities. Pseudofractures (Looser's zones) may be associated and progress to complete fractures.	Extensive enteropathy and a general increase in bone density (especially in the axial skeleton) are characteristic features in adulthood. In the spine the disease may simulate ankylosing spondylitis without sacro-iliac joint involvement or DISH.
Madelung's deformity (dyschondrosteosis)	Radius is bowed and short and its distal articular surface demonstrates ulnar and volar angulation. The distal ulna is deformed and subluxed dorsally. The carpal bones are wedged between the deformed radius and ulna and assume a triangular configuration with the lunate at the apex. May be associated with short and bowed tibia, short fibula, and valgus deformity of the knee.	Rare hereditary mesomelic bone dysplasia with female preponderance. Process usually begins in adolescence with premature fusion of the medial aspect of the distal radial epiphysis resulting in asymmetrical growth. In the majority of cases, the patients are of short stature and the deformities are bilateral.
Blount's disease (tibia vara)	Medial tibia condyle is enlarged and deformed with an irregular, beak-like extension originating from the medial metaphysis and projecting medially and posteriorly. Medial aspect of proximal tibia epiphysis may also be deformed.	Osteochondrosis of the medial tibia metaphysis resulting in bowlegs. An infantile type (usually bilateral) is differentiated from an adolescent type (usually unilateral).
Weismann-Netter syndrome (Fig. 14.9 b)	Bilateral and symmetrical anterior and medial bowing of the tibia and fibula, producing a "sabre-shin" deformity. The fibula shaft is typically thickened ("tibialization" of the fibula).	Congenital nonprogressive condition that has also been reported in the elderly.
Enchondromatosis (Ollier's disease)	Deformity and shortening of tubular bones containing round, often expansile lesions or alternating columnar radiolucent and radiodense streaks. Enchondromas may contain punctate or stippled calcifications. Disease may be relatively localized, unilateral, or generalized.	Disease is usually diagnosed in the first decade of life. May be associated with multiple hemangiomas containing phleboliths (*Maffucci's syndrome*). In *hereditary multiple exostoses* bowing deformities typically are found in the radius and ulna.

(continues on page 320)

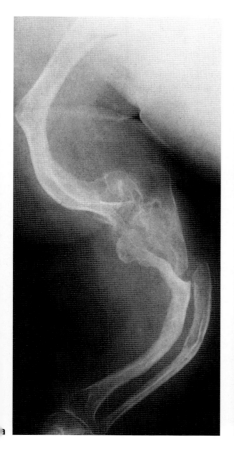 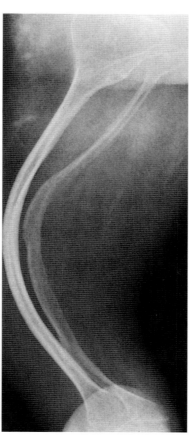

Fig. 14.**8 a, b** **Osteogenesis imperfecta.**
a Upper extremity; **b** lower extremity. Bowing deformities in slender over-constricted and osteoporotic long bones are associated with fractures, pseudarthrosis (proximal ulna) and splayed metaphyses.

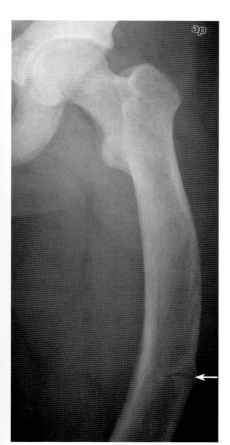

Fig. 14.**9 a** **Vitamin D resistent rickets (x-linked hypophosphatemia).** Increased bone density is seen in this adult with lateral bowing of the femur and a pseudofracture (arrow) in the lateral cortex.

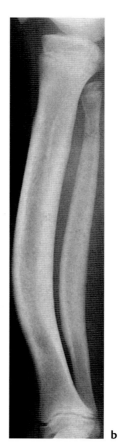

Fig. 14.**9 b** **Weismann–Netter syndrome.** Anterior bowing of the tibia and fibula producing a "sabre-shin" deformity is seen. Note also the characteristic underconstriction of the fibula ("tibialization" of the fibula).

Table 14.1   (Cont.) Bowed or Deformed Long Bones

Disease	Radiographic Findings	Comments
Osteomyelitis (Fig. 14.10)	Severe osteomyelitis may result in a deformed or bowed sclerotic tubular bone, particularly in the leg. Anterior bowing and cortical thickening of the tibia produces a "sabre-shin" appearance, characteristically found as late sequelae of both congenital and acquired *syphilis* and *yaws*. Bowing deformities confined to the distal half of the tibia associated with localized cortical thickening and solid periosteal reaction can be found in *tropical ulcer*.	*Echinococcus* rarely involves bones. Besides the spine, pelvis, and sacrum, the long bones may be affected with multiloculated cystic lesions, resulting occasionally in bone deformities.
Bowing fracture	Anteroposterior or lateral bending of radius, ulna or fibula. A fracture in the neighboring bone (e.g. radius or tibia) might be associated.	Usually in young children.
Fracture (healed)	Common cause of bone deformity usually associated with locally increased sclerosis.	All ages may be affected. Bowlegs in infancy are occasionally secondary to trauma.
Paralysis during growth	Bowed long tubular bones with narrowed, overconstricted shaft diameter due to decreased medullary cavity while the width of the cortex is relatively little affected.	In longstanding paralytic and pseudoparalytic conditions such as *old poliomyelitis*, *muscular dystrophy*, and *juvenile rheumatoid arthritis*.
Osteomalacia (Fig. 14.11)	Bowing deformities occur, besides in the pelvis, spine, and thorax, particularly in the lower extremities. The cortex is thinned as in osteoporosis, but bone deformities, pseudofractures and poor definition of the inner cortical margin and trabeculae help to differentiate osteomalacia from osteoporosis.	Bowing deformities are also a common feature in *rickets* of any etiology.
Hyperparathyroidism	Bone deformities similar to osteomalacia occur in an advanced stage.	In *renal osteodystrophy* (secondary hyperparathyroidism) bone deformities may be secondary to both osteomalacia and hyperparathyroidism.
Paget's disease (Fig. 14.12)	Bone deformities are common in the lower extremities involved by combined (sclerotic and lytic) phase of the disease. This results characteristically in coxa vara ("shepherd's crook" deformity of the upper femur) and anterior bowing of the tibia. In this stage, the involved long bones are widened, and both cortex and disorganized-looking trabeculae are thickened.	Common cause of bone deformities in the elderly patient. *Hereditary hyperphosphatasia* ("juvenile Paget's disease"), which occurs in children, presents characteristically with bowing and thickening of all long bones in the upper and lower extremities.
Fibrous dysplasia (Fig. 14.13)	Marked deformities of the long bones occur, particularly in the polyostotic form, where the bone involvement is generally more extensive. "Shepherd's crook" deformity (upper femur), cortical thickening, widening of the bone, and accentuated or abnormal trabeculation may be present, similar to Paget's disease. The presence of radiolucent or cyst-like lesions or "ground-glass" appearance of the involved bone are useful in differentiating fibrous dysplasia from Paget's disease.	In contrast to Paget's disease, fibrous dysplasia is usually diagnosed in children and young adults. Skin pigmentations ("café-au-lait" spots with irregular outline) and sexual prematurity in females may be present in the polyostotic form (*Albright's syndrome*).
Neurofibromatosis (Fig. 14.14)	Overgrowth of the long bones may result in bowed appearance. The fibula frequently is slender (overconstricted). Pseudarthrosis (especially of the tibia) is common with this presentation. Bowed long bones may occasionally also demonstrate cortical thickening and increased sclerosis.	Hereditary disease often associated with skin neurofibromas and smoothly marginated "café-au-lait" spots. *Congenital pseudarthrosis* of the radius and ulna may also be associated with bowing, but this condition is not related to neurofibromatosis.

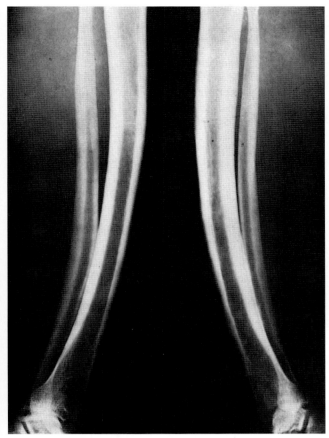

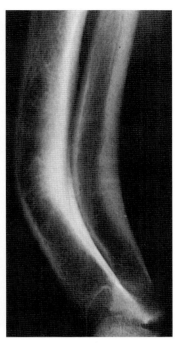

Fig. 14.**11   Healed rickets.** Late sequelae of severe rickets are seen in this adult with symmetrical bowing deformities of both legs including anterior and lateral bowing of the tibia and fibula and lateral bowing of the femur. Only lateral view of the right lower leg is shown.

Fig. 14.**10   Osteomyelitis (yaws).** Cortical thickening and symmetrical anterior bowing of both legs produces "sabre-shin" appearance of both tibias as sequelae of the disease.

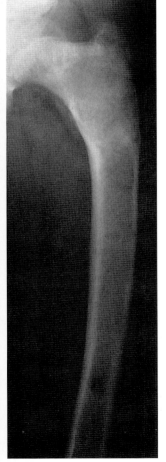

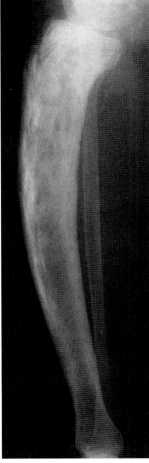

Fig. 14.**12   Paget's disease.** Anterior bowing of tibia that is markedly widened, sclerotic, and irregularly trabeculated in its proximal two-thirds is seen.

Fig. 14.**13   Fibrous dysplasia.** "Shepherd's crook" deformity of the femur that is widened in its proximal half. Characteristic "ground-glass" appearance is also evident beside sclerotic changes and ovoid radiolucencies.

Fig. 14.**14   Neurofibromatosis.** Long slender (overconstricted) tibia and fibula with thickened cortex and slight medial bowing are present.

14.12   **14.13**   **14.14**

Table 14.2 Wide Diametaphyses (Underconstriction or Undertubulation)

Disease	Radiographic Findings	Comments
Biliary atresia	Undertubulation and "Erlenmeyer flask" deformities combined with signs of osteoporosis and rickets are seen.	Congenital malformation resulting in progressive obstructive jaundice. Usually fatal within 2 years unless corrected surgically.
Rubella embryopathy	Undertubulation of the long bones with alternating radiolucent and sclerotic longitudinal streaks ("celery-stick pattern") and irregular metaphyses with radiolucent bands.	Osseous changes regress in those infants who grow normally, but may persist in those who fail to thrive.
Infantile cortical hyperostosis (Caffey's disease) (Fig. 14.15)	Periosteal new bone formation, cortical thickening and widening, primarily of the mandible, scapulae, clavicles, ribs and ulnae, are characteristic.	Disease develops in the first 5 months of life. Fever of abrupt onset, hyperirritability, and tender soft-tissue swelling over the affected bones are characteristic. The radiographic changes tend to regress spontaneously within one year.
Progressive diaphyseal dysplasia (Engelmann-Camurati disease) (Fig. 14.16)	Symmetrical involvement of the long bones with undertubulation and cortical thickening of the midshaft resulting in a spindle-shaped appearing bone.	Rare hereditary disease associated with progressive midshaft cortical thickening and neuromuscular dystrophy. Usually diagnosed between 4 and 12 years, causing a wide-based, waddling gate.
Mucopolysaccharidosis (Fig. 14.17)	Thickened undertubulated shafts, often with irregular wavy contours, are common findings. Metaphyseal flaring can be seen with Morquio's disease, whereas tapering of the small tubular bones suggests Hurler's disease.	Clinical and radiographic findings of different mucopolysaccharidoses and *mucolipidoses* are similar. A large dolichocephalic skull with J-shaped sella turcica, oval or hook-shaped vertebral bodies with gibbus formation in the thoracolumbar region, underdevelopment of the supra-acetabular region resulting in a widened acetabular roof, and coxa valga deformities with widened femoral necks, are characteristic.
Metatropic dwarfism	Long tubular bones are shortened and have "dumbbell" appearance that is caused by the markedly enlarged metaphyses at both ends.	Short-limb dwarfism, which is normal at birth with progressive kyphoscoliosis, finally resembling Morquio's disease. Flaring of the metaphyses with very short limbs are also seen in *thanatophoric dwarfism*, but this condition results in stillbirth or death in the neonatal period.
Pseudoachondroplasia (Fig. 14.18)	Initially the epiphyses are small and flattened and the metaphyses wide with dense, mushroom-shaped provisional zones of calcifications. In the adults the tubular bones are short and expanded at their end.	*Spondyloepimetaphyseal dysplasias* and *epimetaphyseal dysplasias* consist of a heterogeneous group of conditions that have metaphyseal flaring in common.
Osteogenesis imperfecta (Fig. 14.19)	Metaphyses of the long bones are often markedly widened and may contain irregular calcifications while the shaft is overconstricted and may show severe bending deformities and multiple fractures of different ages. Osteopenia is usually a dominant feature.	Radiographic findings are more severe in the congenital than tarda form of osteogenesis imperfecta.
Homocystinuria	Widened metaphyses and epiphyses with usually severe osteopenia and prominent growth lines are seen. In addition, Marfan-like changes (e.g., arachnodactyly) may be present.	Inborn error of the methionine metabolism.
Pyle's disease (familial metaphyseal dysplasia) (Fig, 14.20)	"Erlenmeyer flask" deformity or paddle-shaped enlargement of the metaphyses and, to a lesser degree, undertubulation of the long bones associated with cortical thinning and osteoporosis are characteristic. Thickened ribs and symmetrically enlarged proximal portions of the clavicles may be associated.	Rare hereditary disorder that can be differentiated from craniometaphyseal dysplasia by the lack of skull changes.
Craniometaphyseal dysplasia (Fig. 14.21)	Undertubulation and "Erlenmeyer flask" deformities characteristic and usually most pronounced in the distal femur, radius, and ulna. Osteoporosis may be associated. Skull may show sclerosis of the base and calvarium, lack of aeration of paranasal sinuses and mastoids, and thickening and sclerosis of the mandible.	Rare congenital and familial bone dysplasia. Clinical features include hypertelorism, a broad flat nose, and defective dentition.

(continues on page 324)

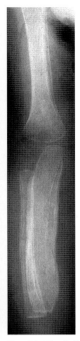

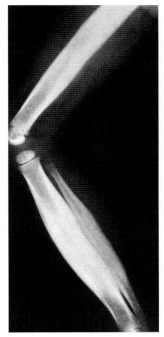

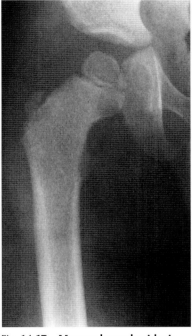

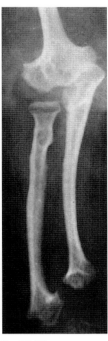

Fig. 14.**15 Infantile cortical hyperostosis** (Caffey's disease). Periosteal reactions progressing to cortical thickening are evident in the diaphyses of the long bones of the upper extremity, resulting in considerable widening especially of the ulna.

Fig. 14.**16 Progressive diaphyseal dysplasia** (Engelmann-Camurati disease). Spindle-shaped widening and sclerosis of the diaphyses of the long bones are characteristic.

Fig. 14.**17 Mucopolysaccharidosis (Morquio).** Widened femoral neck and mild coxa valga deformity associated with a widened acetabular roof, are characteristic.

Fig. 14.**18 Pseudoachondroplasia.** Metaphyseal flaring and irregular epiphyses are seen.

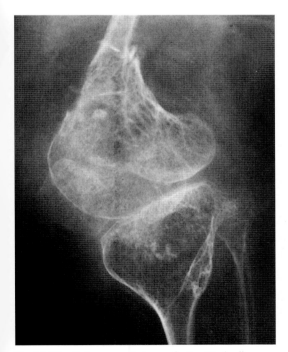

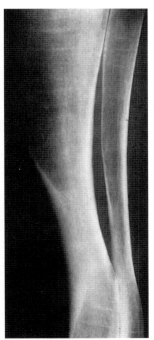

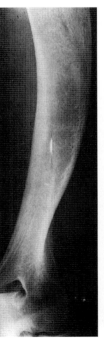

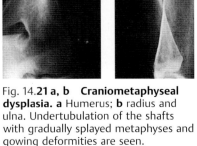

Fig. 14.**19 Osteogenesis imperfecta.** Markedly widened metaphyses containing small ("popcorn") calcifications are connected to overconstricted shafts. Severe osteopenia and a fracture in the distal femur are also present.

Fig. 14.**20 Pyle's disease.** Considerable widening of both proximal and distal ends of the tibia, and to a lesser degree of the fibula, is associated with a slight bowing deformity of the midshafts.

Fig. 14.**21 a, b Craniometaphyseal dysplasia. a** Humerus; **b** radius and ulna. Undertubulation of the shafts with gradually splayed metaphyses and gowing deformities are seen.

Table 14.2   (Cont.) Wide Diametaphyses (Underconstriction or Undertubulation)

Disease	Radiographic Findings	Comments
Hereditary multiple exostosis (diaphyseal aclasis) (Fig. 14.22)	Undertubulation and often bowing of the long bones of both upper and lower extremities with multiple osteochrondromas in the metaphyseal regions, but usually sparing the elbow, are characteristic. Shortening of ulna and fibula is often present, Shortening of the ulna may result in congenital dislocation of the radial head, false articulation between the distal ulna and radius, and ulnar deviation of the carpus.	The inherited disease is usually diagnosed in the first decade of life. Transformation to chondrosarcoma occurs in approximately 5% of cases, although higher malignant transformation rates have been described.
Enchondromatosis (Ollier's disease) (Fig. 14.23)	Undertubulation, deformity, and shortening of the involved bones are common. Longitudinal radiolucent streaks interspersed with normal to sclerotic-appearing streaks may extend from the metaphysis into the shaft, or expansile radiolucent lesions with or without stippled calcifications may be seen. The metaphyses are usually most severely involved and often show "Erlenmeyer flask" deformities.	The generalized form of the disease is usually discovered in the first decade of life. The disease may also be unilateral or present only with a few enchondromas, characteristically located near a joint. Malignant degeneration in this nonhereditary disease is reported in 5–25% of cases.
Bone cysts and benign tumors	Localized widening usually near the end of long bones is caused by a variety of benign expansile mass lesions.	For further differentiation, see Chapter 5.
Chronic osteomyelitis (Fig. 14.24 a)	Marked thickening of the involved area with scattered radiolucent, destructive lesions, solid periosteal new bone formation and sclerosis is characteristic.	In chronic *sclerosing osteomyelitis (Garré)*, diffuse uniform sclerosis of the involved bone may be seen (Fig. 14.**24 b**).
Healed fracture	Localized to generalized widening of the shaft often associated with a bone deformity. Elevated solid periosteal reaction may initially simulate a double cortex or even "bone-within-bone" appearance during the healing phase, particularly in infants and children, but will disappear with further bone remodeling. Cortex may be thickened by periosteal bone formation, but may become normal or even thinned at a later stage. A metaphyseal injury may result in an "Erlenmeyer flask" deformity.	Common cause of localized undertubulation and deformity of a long bone.
Thalassemia	Thinned cortices and a uniform reticular to cystic trabecular pattern in the widened diametaphyses with "Erlenmeyer flask" deformities characteristic, especially in the young patient.	A group of different hereditary hypochromic microcytic anemias, caused by the synthesis of abnormal hemoglobin polypeptide chains. Usually found in "Mediterranean" people and their descendants. Bone changes are caused by erythroid hyperplasia and are most pronounced in thalassemia major. Initially, all bones may be involved. With the conversion of red to yellow marrow in the tubular bones later in life the lesions may regress at these locations.
Sickle-cell anemia	Cortical thinning and coarsening of the trabecular pattern due to bone marrow hyperplasia occur, but are less pronounced than in thalassemia. Changes in the long bones are caused by osteomyelitis and/or infarction and include destructive changes and new bone formation that may result in irregular diametaphyseal widening. Cortical infarcts may result in cortical thickening or "splitting of the cortex." Layering of new bone along the inner cortex may produce a "bone-within-bone" appearance.	Sickle-cell anemia is a hereditary disorder limited almost exclusively to blacks, and caused by an abnormal hemoglobin HbS, where in position 6 of the β-globin chain, valine is substituted for glutamic acid.

(continues on page 326)

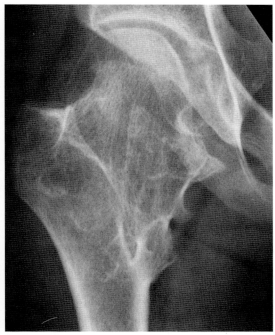

Fig. 14.**22   Hereditary multiple exostoses.** Deformed proximal femur with widened femoral neck containing several osteochondromas is characteristic.

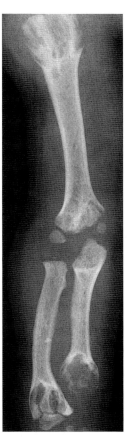

Fig. 14.**23   Enchondromatosis.** Undertubulation of the shortened and slightly bent long bones, and widened metaphyses containing longitudinal streaks of calcifications, are characteristic.

Fig. 14.**24 b   Sclerosing osteomyelitis Garre.** Circumferential localized cortical thickening and widening of the proximal tibia shaft is seen.

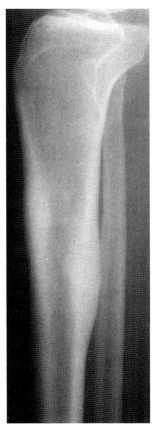

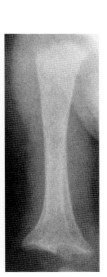

Fig. 14.**24 a   Congenital syphilis.** Widening of the humeral shaft and flaring of the metaphyses are caused by periosteal new bone formation. A destructive lesion is also present in the distal metaphysis.

Table 14.2 (Cont.) Wide Diametaphyses (Underconstriction or Undertubulation)

Disease	Radiographic Findings	Comments
Gaucher's disease (Fig. 14.25)	Lower extremities are involved more often. Characteristic is the combination of avascular necrosis of the femoral head and an "Erlenmeyer flask" deformity at the distal femur. The shaft of the long bones may be locally expanded. Bone resorption and reparation may result in generalized osteopenia, lytic lesions of varying sizes simulating metastases, and patchy areas of sclerosis. Similarly, the cortex may be thinned, with a scalloped inner margin, or thickened and "split." An inner layer of new bone formation may produce "bone-within-bone" appearance. Solid or lace-like periosteal reaction can occur, probably secondary to infarction.	Hereditary metabolic disease characterized by the accumulation of cerebrosides in the reticuloendothelial cells, resulting in hepatosplenomegaly. There is no sex predilection. The most common "adult" type occurs in Ashkenazic Jews, with the earliest manifestations appearing in childhood and progressing in the second and third decade of life. The acute type of Gaucher's disease is a rare, fatal neurodegenerative disorder with no ethnic predilection, that usually becomes manifest shortly after birth and has an average survival time of one year.
Niemann–Pick disease (Fig. 14.26)	Widening of the diametaphyses (undertubulation) and osteopenia with thinned cortices and coarsening of the trabecular pattern characteristic. Coxa valga occurs commonly. An "Erlenmeyer flask" deformity in the distal femur may simulate Gaucher's disease.	Hereditary metabolic disorder characterized by the accumulation of phospholipids (sphingomyelins) in the reticuloendothelial cells. Niemann–Pick disease can be differentiated radiographically from Gaucher's disease by the usual absence of avascular epiphyseal necroses, bone infarcts, and well-circumscribed radiolucent lesions.
Langerhans cell histiocytosis (histiocytosis X)	Expansile lytic lesion and periosteal new bone formation may produce irregular localized widening of the long bones.	The bone manifestations may be monostotic or disseminated.
Fibrous dysplasia (Fig. 14.27)	Localized widening by expansile lesion, usually at the metaphysis, or expansion of the entire shaft may occur. Lesions may be radiolucent, trabeculated, or have a "ground-glass" appearance and occasionally contain dense linear or irregular calcifications. The cortex is intact and can be thickened, but usually does not show periosteal new bone formation unless a fracture or pseudofracture has occurred. Marked deformities and pseudoarthrosis may be associated.	Fibrous dysplasia may be monostotic, monomelic or polyostotic. In the latter case, it is often unilateral and associated with irregular ("coast of Maine") "cafe-au-lait" spots in approximately one-third of the cases. Endocrine anomalies such as sexual precocity (almost exclusively in females), hyperthyroidism, acromegaly, Cushing's syndrome, gynecomastia, and parathyroid enlargement may be associated.
Paget's disease	Considerable widening of the involved bone with thickened cortex and coarse disorganized-appearing trabeculation. Bowing deformities, pathologic fractures, or pseudofractures may be associated.	The long bones are most commonly involved in the combined (sclerotic and lytic) phase. Localized expansion may occasionally also be seen in the much less common lytic phase.
Osteopetrosis (Fig. 14.28)	Besides a marked, uniform, and symmetrical increase in bone density "Erlenmeyer flask" deformities and widened proximal and distal diaphyses are commonly present. Occasionally, alternating transverse dense bands and lucent lines are found in widened diametaphyses.	*Pycnodysostosis*, a rare hereditary disorder, is also characterized by generalized osteosclerosis, but can be differentiated from osteopetrosis by the absence of "Erlenmeyer flask" deformities, no "bone-within-bone" appearance, and hypoplasia of the mandible.
Hypophosphatasia	"Erlenmeyer flask" deformity and cortical thickening of the long bones often with multiple fractures or pseudofractures and bowing deformities (especially femora) are characteristic for hypophosphatasia in adults.	Bony changes of hypophosphatasia in infants and childhood are more severe and similar to rickets.
Rickets (Fig. 14.29)	Irregular "frayed" metaphyses, which become widened and cupped with progression of the disease, are characteristic for the florid stage of the disease. "Erlenmeyer flask" deformities and undertubulation may be seen with healing.	Findings are similar in *vitamin D resistent rickets*.

(continues on page 328)

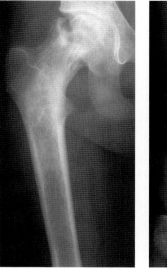
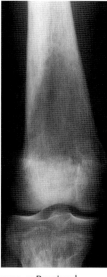
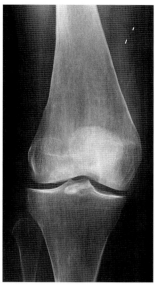

b

Fig. 14.**25 a, b**   **Gaucher's disease. a** Proximal femur: Avascular necrosis of the femoral head and increased patchy sclerotic areas in the proximal femur are seen. **b** Distal femur: "Erlenmeyer flask" deformity of the distal femur and osteolytic lesions in the distal femur and proximal tibia are seen. Irregular sclerosis in the proximal tibia metaphysis is caused by old bone infarcts.

Fig. 14.**26**   **Niemann-Pick disease.** Generalized osteopenia and flaring of the distal femur resulting in "Erlenmeyer flask" deformity are evident.

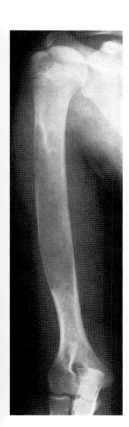
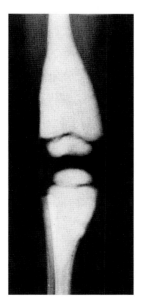
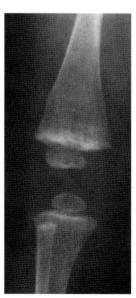

Fig. 14.**27**   **Fibrous dysplasia.** Widening (undertubulation) of the humerus shaft with thinned cortices and "ground-glass" appearancec is seen.

Fig. 14.**28**   **Osteopetrosis.** Splayed metaphyses are associated with a uniform dense osteosclerosis.

Fig. 14.**29**   **Healing rickets.** Splayed metaphyses with irregular sclerotic ends best seen in the distal femur are found in the healing stage of the disease.

Table 14.2   (Cont.) Wide Diametaphyses (Underconstriction or Undertubulation)

Disease	Radiographic Findings	Comments
Scurvy (healing)	Wide diametaphyses with cortical thickening that may persist for many years result from healing subperiosteal hemorrhages, which calcify and subsequently ossify.	
Lead poisoning (Fig. 14.30)	Besides the dense metaphyseal bands, "Erlenmeyer flask" deformities and, at a more advanced stage, undertubulation of the shaft may occur.	Mortality rate of chronic lead poisoning in children under 2 years of age may be as high as 25%.
Idiopathic hypercalcemia of infancy (Williams syndrome)	Osteosclerosis (particularly in the metaphyses) and "Erlenmeyer flask" deformities occur in the distal femora. Dense metaphyseal bands and cortical thickening are frequently associated. Soft tissue calcifications may also be present.	Clinical manifestations include an elfin face, mental and physical retardation and neonatal hypercalcemia. Supravalvular aortic stenosis and hypoplasia of major vessels are frequently associated. *Hypervitaminosis D* may produce a similar radiographic and clinical picture.

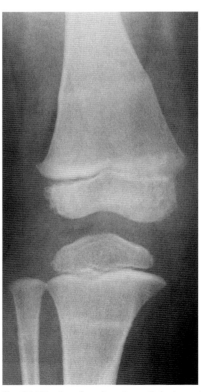

Fig. 14.**30**   **Lead poisoning.** Splaying of the metaphyses is associated with dense transverse metaphyseal bands.

Table 14.3   Narrow Diametaphyses (Overconstriction or Overtubulation)

Disease	Radiographic Findings	Comments
Hypopituitarism	Proportional dwarfism often with overconstricted tubular bones and delayed epiphyseal closure.	Hypogonadism and other endocrinological disturbances may concur.
Tubular stenosis (Kenny-Caffey disease)	Overconstricted tubular bones show symmetrical endosteal thickening and narrowed medulla. Sclerosis of the calvarium and coxa valga may be associated.	Proportional dwarfism. Tetany in early infancy from hypocalcemia.
Progeria	Excessive constriction of the long bones and generalized osteoporosis are common. Associated features include thin calvarium with wormian bone formation, small facial bones and small mandible, progressive resorption of tufts, clavicles and, occasionally, ribs, coxa valga, prominent knees and enlargement of the head of the radius and capitulum.	Progeria is characterized by dwarfism, cardiomegaly secondary to hypertension, coronary artery disease, and premature aging, with death occurring usually in the second or third decade. Onset of disease occurs at the end of first year of life.
Osteogenesis imperfecta (Fig. 14.31)	Long bones are slender and overconstricted. Bowing and fracture deformities are common. Osteoporosis with thinning of the cortex is characteristically present.	The hallmark of the disease is a marked susceptibility to fracture from minimal trauma. Blue sclera and a white ring surrounding the cornea ("Saturn's ring") are often present.
Marfan's syndrome	Elongation and thinning of all tubular bones, but most pronounced in the hands and feet (arachnodactyly). Bone mineralization is normal. Scoliosis and pectus deformity are common. Lumbar vertebra may be abnormally tall and demonstrate posterior scalloping.	Autosomal dominant growth disturbance caused by failure to produce normal collagen. Patients are tall, measuring usually over 6 feet in height. Laxity of ligaments leads to hyperextensible joints with recurrent dislocations. Bilateral subluxed lenses occur in over 50 % of cases. Aortic aneurysm or dissection is the most serious complication.
Homocystinuria	Marfan-like features including slender shafts of the tubular bones. In contrast to Marfan's syndrome, the long tubular bones have widened metaphyses and epiphyses and osteopenia is commonly present, resulting in biconcavity or compression fractures of the vertebral bodies.	Inborn error of metabolism resulting in high homocystine serum levels and homocystinuria.

(continues on page 330)

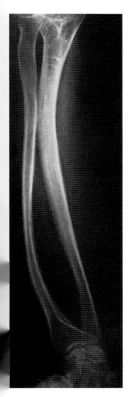

Fig. 14.**31   Osteogenesis imperfecta.** Markedly narrowed (overconstricted) and bowed shaft of the radius and to a lesser degree of the ulna, with only moderate osteoporosis is evident.

Table 14.3 (Cont.) Narrow Diametaphyses (Overconstriction or Overtubulation)

Disease	Radiographic Findings	Comments
Neurofibromatosis (Fig. 14.32)	Overtubulation may result in an extremely slender shaft (especially fibula) and is often associated with bowing deformities. Localized bony overgrowth and pseudarthroses are other characteristic features of neurofibromatosis, whereas shortening of the long bones is rare. Subperiosteal hematomas, cortical thickening, and intraosseous neurofibromas presenting as expansile cyst-like lesions are occasionally seen.	Approximately 50% of patients have bone involvement ranging from minimal to extensive and generalized.
Epidermolysis bullosa	Overconstriction of the shaft of the long bones occasionally associated with flexion contractures and subluxations. Resorption of terminal phalanges also occurs.	Rare hereditary disease characterized by skin blisters formation occurring either spontaneously or following minimal trauma. Flexion contractures and webbing between fingers may produce a claw-like hand. Healing of esophageal mucosal lesions may progress to stenotic webs.
Disuse atrophy	Osteoporosis with thin cortices and a decrease in size and number of trabeculae in the spongiosa are the hallmark of disuse atrophy. Concentric constriction of the shaft is commonly associated in children, but rarely seen in adults.	Found after disuse of the involved part of the skeleton for a long time. May be localized or generalized.
Juvenile rheumatoid arthritis	Overconstricted long tubular bones with narrow medullary cavity and osteopenia may be seen besides the more characteristic arthritic changes. Epiphyses, especially of large affected joints, are enlarged and appear ballooned.	See Chapter 6 for additional information.
Paralysis (infancy and childhood) (Fig. 14.33)	Paralysis in the growing bone results commonly in overconstriction of the shafts at the expense of the medullary cavity, whereas the cortex seems relatively little affected.	E.g., in *poliomyelitis, birth palsies, congenital malformations of the spinal cord* and *brain*.
Muscular dystrophy (Fig, 14.34)	Overconstriction of the diaphyses similar to paralysis (narrowed medullary cavity with relatively little affected cortices). Atrophic muscle bundles separated by increased fat layers and hypertrophy of the subcutaneous fat are often radiographically recognizable in these conditions.	E.g., *arthrogryposis multiplex congenita, amyotonia congenita (Oppenheim's disease), infantile muscular atrophy (Werdnig-Hoffmann disease)*, and others.

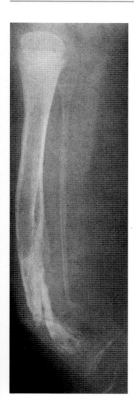

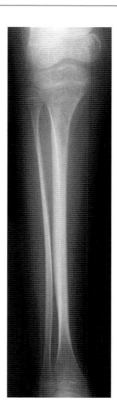

Fig. 14.**32 Neurofibromatosis.** A very slender fibula shaft is usually present in the disease. Osteopenia with chronic fractures in the distal tibia and fibula shafts resulting in bony deformities and pseudarthroses are also quite characteristic.

Fig. 14.**33 Poliomyelitis.** Markedly narrowed (overconstricted) shafts of both tibia and fibula at the expense of the medulla are seen, whereas the cortex is affected relatively little.

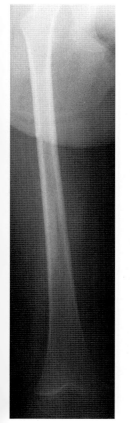

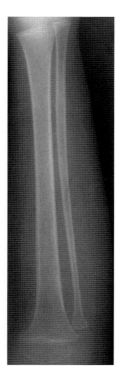

Fig. 14.**34 a, b Muscular dystrophy** (Werdnig-Hoffmann). **a** Femur; **b** tibia and fibula. Overconstriction of the shafts, coxa valga deformity, atrophic muscles separated by thick layers of adipose tissue, and hypertrophy of the subcutaneous fat are recognizable.

a

b

Table 14.4   Radiolucent Transverse Bands in the Metaphyses

Disease	Radiographic Findings	Comments
Normal variant in neonates	Striated appearance of metaphyses is not unusual.	Found in apparently healthy infants.
Osteogenesis imperfecta	Radiolucent metaphyses are part of the generalized osteopenia. Characteristic are slender long bones with thin cortices and bowing deformities.	Secondary shortening and thickening of the long bones may be secondary to "telescoping" fractures and subsequent excessive callus formation.
Leukemia (Fig. 14.35)	Transverse radiolucent bands are usually the earliest radiographic manifestation in childhood leukemia, whereas they are uncommon in adults. Scattered lytic and, rarely, sclerotic areas and periosteal reactions are found in more advanced cases.	Bony involvement in leukemia occurs in over 50% of cases in childhood and up to 10% in adults.
Metastases (especially from neuroblastoma)	Transverse radiolucent bands and other findings are indistinguishable from leukemia.	Approximately 80% of neuroblastomas are found in children under 2½ years of age. Presence of urinary vanillylmandelic acid and vanilphenylethylamine is diagnostic.
Juvenile rheumatoid arthritis	Osteopenia with transverse radiolucent bands. In contrast to adult rheumatoid arthritis, periostitis and joint fusions are common, and both joint space narrowing and erosions are late manifestations.	Occurs usually in children over 10 years of age with female predominance.
Prenatal infections (e.g., rubella, cytomegalic inclusion disease)	Transverse radiolucent metaphyseal bands may develop after neonatal period. Metaphyses are irregular but not cupped. Alternating longitudinal sclerotic and lucent streaks and coarse trabeculation are often seen in the diaphyses of the long bones.	Radiolucent metaphyseal bands can also be seen with other severe prenatal and postnatal infections and systemic diseases.
Osteoporosis in neonates and during childhood	Osteoporosis of any etiology developing in utero, infancy and early childhood is most pronounced in the metaphyses and may assume a striped appearance.	E.g. in neuromuscular disorders and paralysis, juvenile rheumatoid arthritis and malnutrition.
Scurvy	A radiolucent band (Trümmerfeld zone) is characteristically seen beneath the widened and sclerotic-appearing zone of provisional calcification in the metaphyses.	Radiographic signs of scurvy are summarized in Chapter 1.
Cushing's syndrome	Rare cause of band-like metaphyseal radiolucencies as part of generalized osteoporosis in the growing bone.	Caused by abnormally high (exogenous or endogenous) steroid blood levels. Endogenous overproduction of steroids in children is caused in over half of the cases by *adrenal carcinoma*.

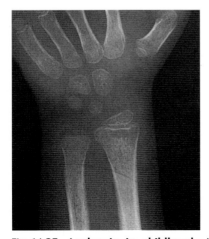

Fig. 14.**35** **Leukemia in childhood.** A transverse radiolucent band in the metaphyses of both the radius and ulna is seen.

Table 14.5   Sclerotic Transverse Bands or Lines in the Metaphyses

Disease	Radiographic Findings	Comments
Normal variant in young children	Relatively dense metaphyseal ends of long tubular bones, equal to the cortical density of the same bone, are commonly present.	In active children of less than 4 years of age.
Growth arrest lines (Fig. 14.36)	Single or multiple, sharply defined, fine sclerotic lines running across the metaphyses. Occur in infants and children, but may persist and remain recognizable in adults.	Normal finding, but may be related to malnutrition or severe disease during growth. Appear particularly prominent when associated with osteopenia. DD: *Reinforcement lines (bone bars)* developing in chronic osteopenia of adults as response to chronically weakened bone.
Osteopetrosis (Fig. 14.37)	Multiple transverse or longitudinal metaphyseal striations occur. At a more advanced stage, "bone-within-bone" appearance may result. "Erlenmeyer flask" deformity is commonly associated.	Hereditary disorder characterized by symmetrical generalized increase in bone density and failure of tubulation.
Cretinism (hypothyroidism)	Dense, transverse metaphyseal bands associated with shortened slender shafts, endosteal thickening, and irregular, fragmented epiphyses are characteristic.	Delayed appearance and fusion of all epiphyses (delayed bone age) is a hallmark of the disease.
Hypoparathyroidism and pseudohypoparathyroidism	Transverse sclerotic bands are found in the metaphyses of long bones. A slight generalized increase in bone density, ossification of tendinous and ligamentous insertions mimicking exostoses, and subcutaneous calcifications, are often also present.	Other associated findings may include marginal sclerosis of the iliac crests and vertebral bodies. In the skull, calvarial thickening, basal ganglia calcifications, and defective dentition, are characteristic. In pseudohypoparathyroidism, short metacarpals and metatarsals are also present.
Metaphyseal chondrodysplasia (Fig. 14.38)	Cupping and irregular mineralization of the metaphyses, which may demonstrate irregular sclerotic bands with radiolucent streaks. Diaphyses and epiphyses are normal, but the ossification of the latter may be delayed.	Several different and probably unrelated cartilage dysplasias with similar radiographic features are comprised in this rare entity (e.g. Schmid, Jansen, McKusick, and Schwachmann-Diamond types). Metaphyseal changes may resemble rickets but, in contrast to the latter, epiphyses are normal.

(continues on page 334)

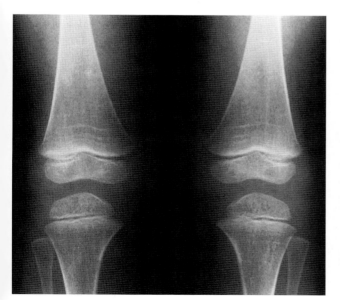

Fig. 14.**36   Growth lines.** Several fine and symmetric transverse lines in the distal femora are seen bilaterally. Osteopenia is also evident, caused by homocystinuria in this case.

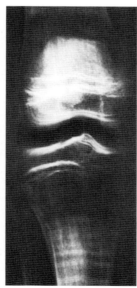

Fig. 14.**37   Osteopetrosis.** Multiple broad transverse striations are seen in the undertubulated distal femur and proximal tibia, both demonstrating "Erlenmeyer flask" deformities.

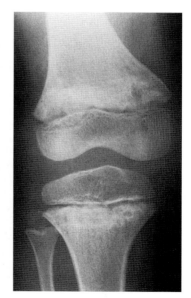

Fig. 14.**38   Metaphyseal chondrodysplasia** (McKusick). Irregular sclerotic and widened metaphyses are seen.

Table 14.5   (Cont.) Sclerotic Transverse Bands or Lines in the Metaphyses

Disease	Radiographic Findings	Comments
Idiopathic hypercalcemia of infancy (Williams syndrome) (Fig. 14.39)	Dense metaphyseal bands are characteristic of the severe, chronic form, often associated with cortical thickening and an overall increase in bone density. Sclerosis of the orbital rim and sphenoids may produce a striking "spectacle" appearance.	The severe chronic form of idiopathic hypercalcemia is associated with the triad of azotemia, mental and physical retardation, and osteosclerosis. Idiopathic hypercalcemia may result from hypersensitivity to vitamin D or an inborn error in the cholesterol metabolism. *Hypervitaminosis D* may produce identical findings.
Congenital syphilis (Fig. 14.40)	Transverse metaphyseal striping (sclerotic and lucent bands) may be the earliest finding. Destructive metaphyseal changes may be seen in more advanced cases, most characteristically located in the medial aspect of the proximal tibia metaphysis (Wimberger's sign).	Transverse striping of the metaphysis in infancy is not diagnostic for syphilis and can be seen with other severe diseases during the fetal period (e.g., *toxoplasmosis, rubella,* and *cytomegalic inclusion disease*), as well as with the administration of bismuth to the mother during pregnancy.
Erythroblastosis fetalis	Transverse metaphyseal bands and diffuse sclerosis of the diaphyses may be present.	Congenital hemolytic anemia resulting from Rhesus factor incompatibility.
Thalassemia Sickle-cell anemia	Transverse metaphyseal bands may occur.	More characteristic changes in thalassemia include splaying of the metaphysis ("Erlenmeyer flask" deformities), thinning of the cortices, and accentuated trabeculation. In sickle-cell anemia, bone changes are primarily caused by infarction and osteomyelitis and may result in "bone-within-bone" appearance, "cortical splitting," and new periosteal bone formation.
Radiation osteitis	A dense metaphyseal band can develop in the growing bone as a manifestation of repair.	Radiation-induced changes in the growing metaphyses include irregularities, fraying and sclerosis, and may superficially resemble rickets.
Healed radiolucent metaphyseal bands of different etiologies (e.g., treated rickets, renal osteodystrophy, scurvy, and leukemia) (Fig. 14.41)	Original disease characteristically produces radiolucent metaphyseal bands that may become dense under proper therapy.	Occasionally alternating radiolucent and sclerotic metaphyseal bands may already be seen in childhood leukemia before treatment.
Stress fractures (Fig. 14.42)	A band-like focal sclerosis is seen at the end of tubular bones (e.g. femoral neck and tibia plateau).	Present clinically with activity-related pain that is relieved by rest. *Fatigue fractures* resulting from abnormal stress in normal bone can be differentiated from *insufficiency fractures* resulting form normal stress in osteopenic bone.
Lead poisoning (Fig. 14.43 a)	Dense metaphyseal bands exceeding the cortical density of the same bone, found in the growing skeleton. Interference with normal modeling may result in splaying of the involved metaphysis ("Erlenmeyer flask" deformity). Separation of the cranial sutures and lead particles seen in the gastrointestinal tract support the diagnosis.	Bone changes become radiographically evident approximately 3 months after chronic lead poisoning. *Bismuth, phosphorus,* and *mercury poisoning* as well as *vitamin D intoxication* may also produce one or several dense bands in the metaphysis similar to lead poisoning. Occasionally, dense metaphyses are seen in an apparently healthy child under the age of 4.
Drug or hormone therapy (Fig. 14.43 b)	Rare cause of transverse sclerotic bands.	E.g., with high dosages of steroids, parathormone, methotrexate, and other drugs.

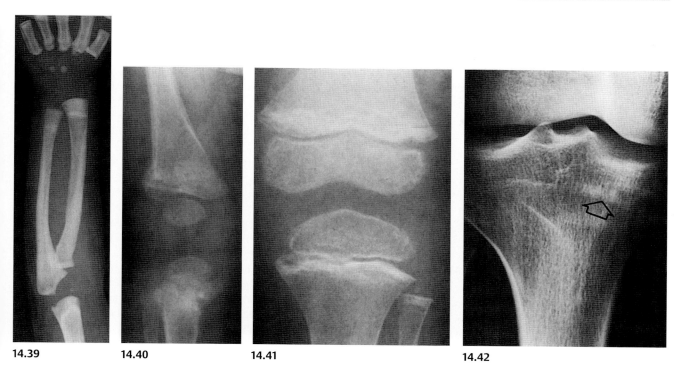

14.39   14.40   14.41   14.42

Fig. 14.**39** **Idiopathic hypercalcemia of infancy** (Williams syndrome). Transverse metaphyseal bands are seen in the distal radius and ulna. Cortical thickening and a marked generalized osteosclerosis is also present.

Fig. 14.**40** **Congenital syphilis.** Irregular transverse metaphyseal striping is associated with destructive metaphyseal lesions.

Fig. 14.**41** **Leukemia.** Sclerotic metaphyseal bands are seen in this child already prior to the initiation of proper treatment.

Fig. 14.**42** **Stress fracture.** A band-like focal sclerosis (arrow) is seen in the proximal tibia.

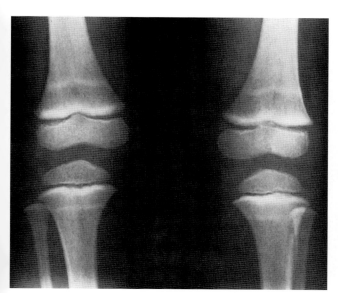

Fig. 14.**43 a** **Lead poisoning.** Dense and symmetrical metaphyseal bands in the metaphyses of both the distal femora and the proximal tibias are seen.

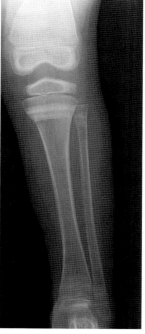

Fig. 14.**43 b** **Methotrexate therapy in acute lymphoblastic leukemia.** Dense metaphyseal bands only developped after initiation of therapy. Note also the sclerotic outline of the epiphyses and the "Erlenmeyer flask" deformity of the distal femur.

Table 14.6   Short Bone in Extremities

Abnormality	Usual Causes	Comments
Symmetrically short limbs	*Achondroplasia* (most common) (Fig. 14.**44**) Other *short limb dwarfism syndromes*. Syndromes with *growth disturbance of bone*.	For differential diagnosis, analyze various portions of bone and eventual associated findings.
Localized shortening of bone (resulting from an insult to a growing bone)	*Osteomyelitis*	Epiphyseal damage causes shortening and may produce a "ball-and-socket" metaphyseal deformity.
	Trauma	Shortening is due to impacted fracture or epiphyseal damage in a growing bone.
	Scurvy	In severe scurvy, a fracture through a radiolucent Trummerfeld zone may cause premature fusion.
	Hypervitaminosis A	May rarely cause asymmetric shortenings due to premature fusion of the ossification centers. Splayed metaphyses.
	Rickets (all etiologies)	Infantile or juvenile rickets may leave shortening and deformation of long bones after healing.
	Enchondromatosis (Ollier's disease)	Rounded expansile radiolucencies in the metaphyses may be associated with deformities and shortening of bone.
	Radiation therapy	Sufficient dosages cause an arrest of bone growth in infants and children. More important sequelae tend to occur in spine and pelvis, mimicking achondroplasia or osteochondrodystrophy.
	Bone infarcts (e.g., sickle-cell anemia)	The majority of infarcts occur in HbSS genotype, and are located between the shaft and metaphysis of femur, proximal tibia, and distal humerus. The radiographic pattern is indistinguishable from osteomyelitis, which may be superimposed.
	Neoplasm	Bone tumor like *Ewing's sarcoma* may invade the growth plate.
	Hereditary multiple exostoses (Fig. 14.**55**)	

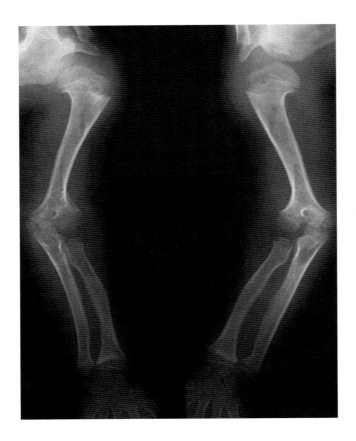

Fig. 14.**44**   **Achondroplasia.** Bilaterally short, deformed upper extremities.

Table 14.7   Abnormal Scapula

Abnormality	Usual Causes	Comments
Hypoplasia	*Achondroplasia*	Hypoplastic scapula may be a feature in several bone dysplasias but other radiographic characteristics are more diagnostic.
	Nail-patella syndrome	Hypoplastic scapula and thickening of the glenoid rim may be associated with this condition.
Malposition	*Sprengel's deformity* (Fig. 14.**45**)	Elevation of scapula. Scapula is connected to the cervical spine by an *omovertebral bone* in one third of cases. In the absence of an omovartebral bone, a fibrous fascial shealt extends from the superior angle of the scapula to the spinous process, the lamina or the transverse process of 1 or more lower cervical vertebrae. The scapula may be hypoplastic.
	Brachial plexus damage (Fig. 14.**46**)	Winging of scapula, downward subluxation of the humerus, and various secondary deformities may occur. The radiographic pattern depends on the site and number of nerve roots involved.

(continues on page 338)

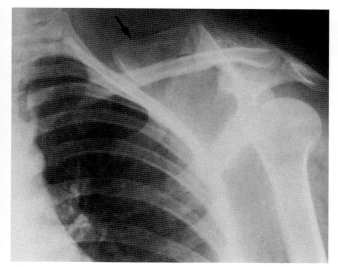

Fig. 14.45   Sprengel's deformity. An anomalous omovertebral bone on the left (arrow) is connected to the scapula. The scapula is elevated and hypoplastic.

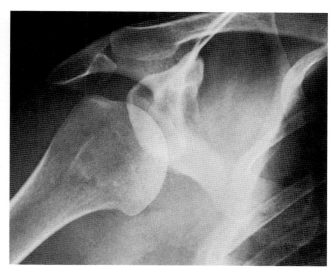

Fig. 14.46   Brachial plexus (C5 root) damage. Winging of the scapula and depression of the shoulder joint secondary to posttraumatic paralysis of the rhomboideus muscle.

Table 14.7   (Cont.) Abnormal Scapula

Abnormality	Usual Causes	Comments
Deformation	*Glenohumeral dysplasia* (Fig. 14.**48**)	Deformation or absence of the rim of the glenoid fossa Flattening of the humeral head. Deformation of the humeral head is more obvious than deformity of the scapula. Hurler's syndrome: See Fig. 13.**15**.
	Arthritis *Syringomyelia*	Severe deformation of these structures may be seen in several *arthritides* and in *syringomyelia* (neurotrophic joint), but changes in the humeral head are more characteristic (see Table 14.**8**).
	Benign bone tumors (Fig. 14.**47**)	*Osteochondroma* or *enchondroma* may cause deformation. (Destructive lesion of scapula is likely due to *eosinophilic granuloma, metastasis, Ewing's sarcoma*, or *osteomyelitis*, but they are rare) .
	Fracture	

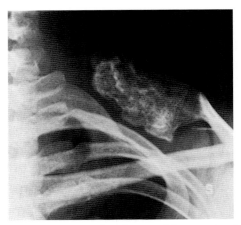

Fig. 14.**47   Osteochondroma** of the scapula which has an appearance somewhat similar to Sprengel's deformity (Fig. 14.**45**).

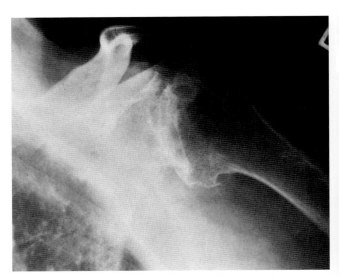

Fig. 14.**48   Glenohumeral dysplasia** with absence of the glenoid rim and flattening of the humeral head. Secondary osteoarthritis is also present.

Table 14.8   Humeral Head Deformity

Etiology	Abnormality	Comments
Congenital	Glenohumeral dysplasia (Fig. 14.**48**)	Usually bilateral and asymptomatic.
Traumatic	Fracture of greater tuberosity	A displaced fracture of the greater tuberosity is an obvious cause of a grooved defect. *Fracture of the lesser tuberosity* is usually associated with a posterior dislocation of the head of the humerus.
	Hill-Sachs deformity (repeated dislocation) (see Fig. 14.**3**)	An irregularity and/or area of condensed bone on the *posterior superior* border of the articular surface, best seen in an abducted and internally rotated humerus. It is a compression fracture caused by (repeated) anterior dislocations.
Arthritis	Rotator cuff tear (Fig. 14.**49**)	Upward subluxation of the humeral head indicates rotator cuff (supraspinatus tendon) tear. Longstanding elevation may erode the inferior surface of the acromion.
	Periarthrosis humeroscapularis (periarthritis humeroscapularis, bursitis calcarea)	Deposition of calcium in the wall of the subdeltoid bursa.
	Rheumatoid arthritis Ankylosing spondylitis	Erosions and grooves appear first *near the attachment of the joint capsule.* Often associated with erosion of the distal clavicle and inferior acromion, upward subluxation of the humerus, subchrondral cysts, and distention of the subdeltoid bursa.
	Gout	Grooved defects have sclerotic margins. Otherwise similar to rheumatoid arthritis, unless gout tophi are calcified.
	Multicentric reticulohistiocytosis	Rheumatoid arthritis-like erosions associated with cutaneous xanthomas.
	Infectious arthritis	May mimic rheumatoid arthritis, but changes occur much more rapidly.
Tumor	Pigmented villonodular synovitis	Erosions are near the capsular attachment, as in rheumatoid arthritis, but no osteoporosis or narrowing of the joint space is present. May contain hemosiderin and therefore appears calcified.
	Other tumors, see Chapter 5.	

(continues on page 340)

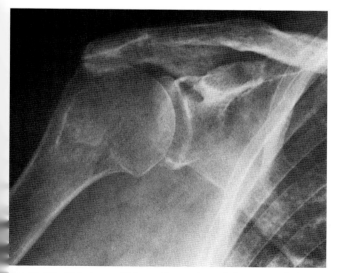

Fig. 14.49   Rotator cuff tear. Narrowing of the space between the humeral head and the acromion with erosion on adjacent bone surfaces. Osteoarthritic spurs and a cyst (geode) in the glenoid fossa are present as additional findings.

Table 14.8   (Cont.) Humeral Head Deformity

Etiology	Abnormality	Comments
Vascular	*Aseptic necrosis* (Fig. 14.**50**) (most common causes: sickle cell disease, steroid therapy) (see also hip, Fig. 14.**63**)	Beginning in the center of the articular surface, cortical breaks, rarefaction, and sclerosis continue until the humeral head is flattened and deformed. The glenoid fossa is intact, which indicates a primary epiphyseal disturbance.
	Hemophilia	Mimics Hill-Sachs deformity, but radiolucent defects also occur in the glenoid fossa.
Neurotrophic	*Syringomyelia* (Figs. 14.**51–52**)	Fragmentation of articular surface without reactive changes and intra-articular scattered bone fragments are a typical finding in Charcot joint. Bone fragments may migrate to midhumerus along dissection of chronically distended joint capsule.

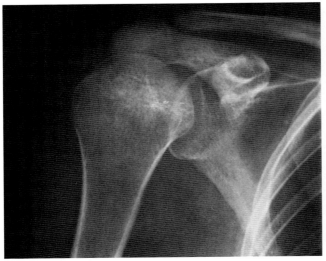

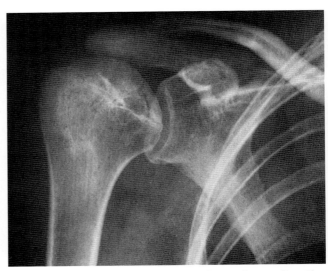

Fig. 14.**50 a, b   The course of avascular necrosis** of the humeral head due to steroid therapy, **a** Subchondral resorption of bone and small depressed fractures of the articular surface (arrows),

b Sclerosis of the humeral head with an obvious fracture line. Flattening of the articular surface.

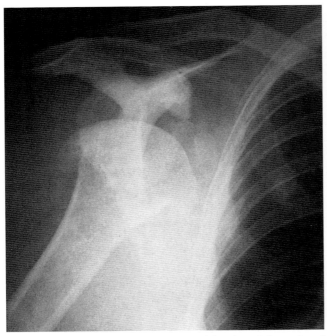

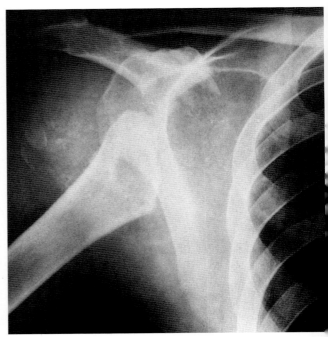

Fig. 14.**51   Syringomyelia.** The humeral head is deformed and subluxed downwards. No obvious bone fragmentation is seen in this case.

Fig. 14.**52   Syringomyelia.** The whole humeral head is destroyed. Bone fragments are present in the joint capsule.

Table 14.9   Forearm Deformity

Deformity	Usual Causes	Comments
Proximal radioulnar dislocation	Traumatic *Chassaignac subluxation* ("nursemaid's elbow", occurs in children under 6 years of age). *Traumatic dislocation of radial head* without fracture (occurs in children over 6).	The head of the radius should be in direct relation to the capitellum no matter what position the elbow is in, A "nursemaid's elbow" is usually a result of jerking upward on a child's arm. Dislocation may be partial and not detectable radiologically.
	Fracture of the ulna with dislocation of the head of the radius usually in anterolateral direction (*Monteggia fracture*) (Fig. 14.**53**).	A fracture through ulna with significant foreshortening of the forearm is always accompanied by either a fracture or dislocation of the radius.
Deformity or hypoplasia of radius or ulna	Syndromes with hypoplastic radius (see Table 14.**1**) or aplasia of radius (Fig. 14.**54**).	Hypoplasia of the radial head predisposes to dislocation.
	Enchondromatosis (Ollier's disease)	Shortening of ulna secondary to enchondromas.

(continues on page 342)

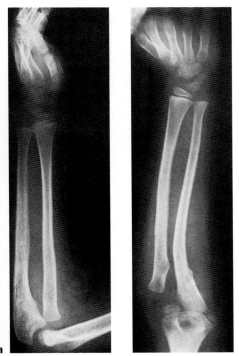

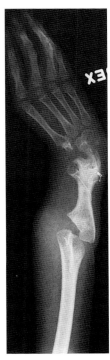

Fig. 14.**53 a, b   Monteggia fracture.** Fracture of the ulna with anterolateral dislocation of the radius.

Fig. 14.**54   Fanconi's anemia.** Absence of radius, short and deformed ulna, carpal bone fusion, and the absence of the first metacarpal and the thumb.

Table 14.9   (Cont.) Forearm Deformity

Deformity	Usual Causes	Comments
	Hereditary multiple exostoses (diaphyseal aclasis) (Fig. 14.**55**)	There is a characteristic *shortening of the ulna* and fibula. Ulnar shortening causes curvature of the radius and often dislocation of the radial head, see Table 14.**6**.
	Osteogenesis imperfecta	Secondary to bowing of bones.
	Madelung's deformity (Fig. 14.**56**)	Premature fusion of the ulnar part of the epiphysis of radius, manifest at adolescence as a characteristic deformity: 1 ulnar and volar angulation of the distal radial articular surface; 2 decreased carpal angle; and 3 dorsal subluxation of the distal ulna. May occur as an isolated unilateral or bilateral anomaly. When associated with other anomalies such as a short, curved tibia, short fibula, and valgus deformity of the knee, the condition is called *dyschondrosteosis*. Juvenile trauma may produce a similar deformity in the wrist called *pseudo-Madelung*. A somewhat similar deformity may be present in *mucopolysaccharidosis I (Hurler's syndrome)*.
	Congenital radioulnar fusion (Fig. 14.**57**)	A rare anomaly which results in relative hypoplasia of the involved bones secondary to a lack of muscular stress.
	Isolated anomaly	Hypoplasia or aplasia of the radius may be also associated with other anomalies, including *nail–patella syndrome*.
	Generalized growth disturbance of bones (Fig. 14.**58**)	

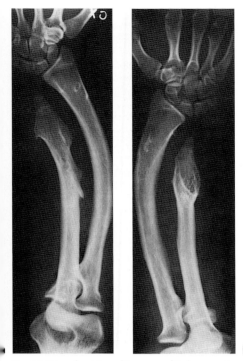
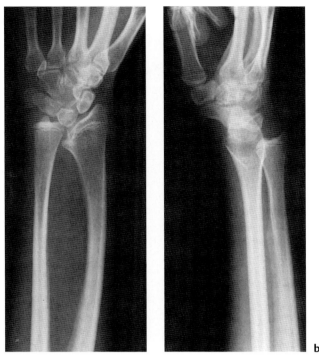

Fig. 14.**55 a, b   Hereditary multiple exostoses.** Shortening of the ulna with exostoses. Bowing of the radius but no dislocation of the radial head.

Fig. 14.**56 a, b   Madelung's deformity.** Ulnar and volar angulation of the distal radial articular surface, decreased (v-shaped) carpal angle, and dorsal subluxation of the distal ulna.

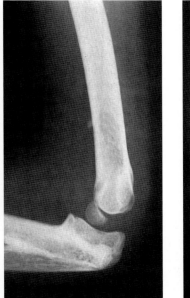
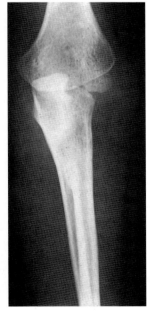
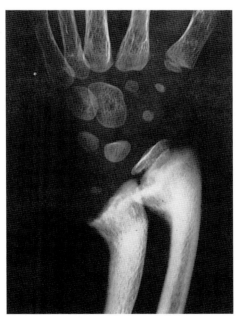

Fig. 14.**57 a, b   Proximal radioulnar fusion** in a 4-year-old girl. The radial head has grown together with the olecranon. Both radial and ulnar shafts are thin.

Fig. 14.**58   Severe deformity, sclerosis,** and ulnar deviation of distal radius and ulna in a child with renal osteodystrophy (renal rickets).

Table 14.10   Abnormal Femoral Epiphysis in a Child or Adolescent

Disease	Radiographic Findings	Comments
Legg–Perthes disease (osteochondrosis of the femoral epiphysis, avascular necrosis of the femoral head) (Fig. 14.59)	Changes in order of appearance: 1. slight widening of the joint space and lateral displacement of the femur, epiphyseal ossification center may be smaller than that of the other side; 2. subchrondral fracture, subcortical radiolucent crescent; 3. flattening of the femoral head; 4. sclerosis of the epiphysis; 5. radiolucent metaphyseal defects; and 6. reossification and remodeling resulting in either a spherical or deformed shape.	Peak age of 4 to 8 years, male:female ratio is 4:1 Bilateral in 10% to 15% of cases. MRI allows earlier detection than plain films of the presence and extent of the process of avascular necrosis.
Congenital dislocation of hip ("Perthes' luxation")	Untreated dislocation results in a deformed, dislocated femoral head and coxa valga.	Avascular necrosis of the femoral head is unusually frequent in children with congenital dislocation of the hip, either secondary to treatment or on a constitutional basis.
Hemophilia	Epiphyseal changes are similar to Perthe's disease, but no metaphyseal changes occur.	Probably due to increased pressure from intra-articular hemorrhages.
Infection Arthritis	See Chapter 6	Increased intra-articular pressure may cause avascular necrosis of the femoral head.
Slipped capital femoral epiphysis (epiphysiolysis capitis femoris) (Fig. 14.60)	Salter-Harris type 1 fracture through the proximal epiphyseal cartilage plate. The direction of slipping depends on the angulation between the shaft of the femur and its neck. The most common combination is an angulation of 140 degrees (coxa valga) and slipping toward the posteroinferior direction. Avascular necrosis of the epiphysis may complicate slipping (with or without operative treatment).	Usually occurs between ages 9 and 17, bilateral in 20% to 30%. Is either *idiopathic* or *secondary* to *trauma, renal osteodystrophy,* or *rickets.* Rare causes: *scurvy, lues, metaphyseal dysostosis, hyperparathyroidism, congenital coxa vara, pseudohypoparathyroidism, hemophilia* and *Gaucher's disease.*
Osteochondritis dissecans (osteochondrosis dissecans, segmental avascular necrosis)	A small, dense segment of bone with its articular cartilage lies in depression in the joint surface, demarcated by a crescenting radiolucent zone. It usually occurs in the uppermost (weight-bearing) region of the femoral head. Secondary osteoarthrosis may occur in older age.	MRI is helpful in defining the lesion and the viability of the fragment.
Chondrodysplasia punctata (chondrodystrophia calcificans congenita, Conradi's syndrome)	Multiple discrete punctate areas of calcification in the epiphyses of hips, knees, shoulders, and wrists, which may disappear at the age of three years.	For other anomalies in this rare entity see Table 15.1.
Multiple epiphyseal dysplasia (Fairbank's disease)	The epiphyseal ossification centers of hips, knees, and ankles are mottled and irregular.	May be a tarda form of chondrodysplasia punctata, which manifests usually between 5 and 14 years of age. A number of other anomalies occur (see Table 15.1). Rare.
Mucopolysaccharidosis (especially Morquio's syndrome) (Fig. 14.61)	Defective, irregular ossification of the femoral capital epiphyses. Femoral neck is short and thick.	Spinal changes are more characteristic (Table 12.7).
Diastrophic dysplasia (dwarfism)	Bone ends are enlarged. The femoral heads may be larger than acetabula.	
Cretinism (congenital hypothyroidism) (Fig. 14.62)	Delayed and spotty ossification of epiphyses, which may be nonhomogeneous, stippled, or fragmented. The femoral neck is shortened and there is coxa vara.	
Rickets (all etiologies)	Irregularity of the provisional zone of calcification and widening of the epiphyseal plate.	Residual deformity of the femoral head and other epiphyses may persist after treatment.

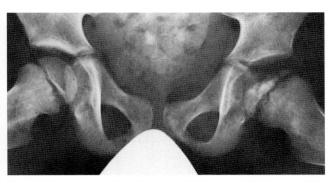

Fig. 14.**59** **Legg-Perthes disease,** left hip, age 8. Widening of the joint space; smaller femoral epiphysis with flattening, fragmentation, and sclerosis.

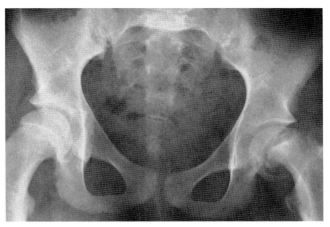

Fig. 14.**60** **Slipped capital femoral epiphysis** on the left with posteroinferior slipping. There is also coxa valga of the right side.

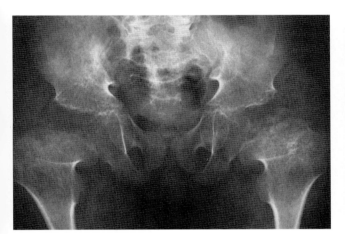

Fig. 14.**61** **Morquio's syndrome,** age 7. Fragmented, irregular femoral capital epiphyses with short and thick femoral necks. Deformed acetabula.

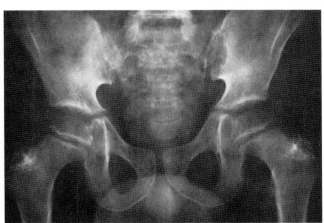

Fig. 14.**62** **Cretinism,** age 20. Unfused, slightly deformed femoral epiphyses and generalized delay of ossification. The femoral neck angles are within normal limits in this case.

Table 14.11   Abnormal Femoral Head in Adult

Disease	Radiographic Findings	Comments
Trauma	Fragmented or irregular femoral head after intracapsular femoral neck fracture, traumatic dislocation of the femoral head, or surgical correction of slipped femoral epiphysis	Avascular necrosis follows if the blood supply from the femoral neck or the ligamentum teres is inadequate.
Sickle-cell disease	Radiographic evidence of avascular necrosis (AVN) of the femoral head in up to 60 % of patients.	Sludging of sickled erythrocytes results in functional vascular occlusion.
Necrosis of femoral head, vide variety of causes such as: **Femoral neck fracture** **Steroid therapy** **Cushing's disease** **HIV infection** **Thromboembolic disease** **Pancreatitis** **Fat embolism (alcoholism)** **Connective tissue disease** **Dysbaric AVN (Caisson disease)** **Gaucher's disease** **Gout** **Radiation therapy** (Fig. 14.63 a)	Radiographic changes of avascular necrosis of the femoral head include cortical breaks and rarefaction of bone followed by sclerosis, flattening and deformation. No late remodeling occurs in adult avascular necrosis (cf. Legg-Perthes). MRI allows early detection of avascular necrosis of bone .	Underlying mechanism is unclear, and may be similar in most conditions. May be due to microscopic emboli in end-arteries, steroid-induced osteoporosis, with microfractures or compression of the vascular bed by an increase in the marrow fat cell mass. Avascular necrosis of the femoral head has also been reported in association *adult myxedema, sarcoidosis, amyloidosis, histiocytosis* and *polyvinylpyrrolidone therapy*, as well as during *pregnancy*. HIV-patients on protease inhibitors have an even greater risk of developing AVN.
Femoroacetabular impingement (FAI) (Fig. 14.63 b)	Articular cartilage and/or labrum damage resulting from repetitive forceful hip flexion is caused by either an abnormal femoral head and neck relationship (Cam type), or an overextended acetabular coverage of the femoral head (Pincer type) or both.	Usually diagnosed in athletes or highly active individuals. Significant athletic activity before skeletal maturity increases the risk of FAI.
Osteoarthritis, primary or secondary	(See Ch. 6)	The most common cause of hip joint abnormality in the elderly.
Neurotrophic joint	(See Ch. 6)	

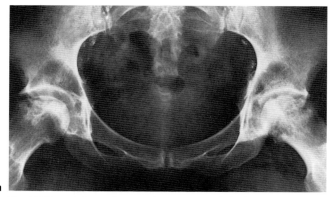

a

Fig. 14.**63 a**   **Bilateral avascular necrosis** of the femoral head following therapy of Hodgkin's disease. There is subchondral demineralization of the joint surface, flattening, fragmentation, and sclerosis of the femoral head.

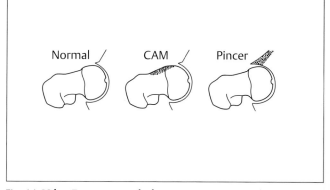

Fig. 14.**63 b**   **Femoroacetabular impingement (FAI). CAM:** Femoral waist deficiency is evident by bone apposition at the anterosuperior junction of the femoral head and neck resulting in the loss of the spherical contour of the head. **PINCER:** Overcoverage of the femoral head anterosuperiorly is caused by either acetabular retroversion and/or acetabular protrusion.

Table 14.12   Abnormal Angle of the Femoral Neck

Disease	Radiographic Findings	Comments
Primary congenital coxa vara	1 decreased angle of the femoral neck; 2 epiphyseal plate almost vertical, with inferior metaphyseal fragmentation; 3 short and thick neck of femur; and 4 delayed ossification, dysplastic acetabulum and other deformities may occur.	A deformity that is sometimes associated with aplasia of fibula.
Secondary congenital coxa vara (Figs. 14.64–14.65)	As above.	Associated with various *osteochondrodysplasias*.
Osteogenesis imperfecta	Coxa vara with bowing, overconstricted long bones, and fractures.	
Osteopetrosis	Coxa vara with marble bones. Fractures are common.	
Cretinism (Fig. 14.66)	Coxa vara with short femoral neck.	
Rickets, renal osteodystrophy	Coxa vara with other signs characteristic of hyperparathyroidism.	Softening of bone and metaphyseal disturbance cause deformity.
Old Legg–Perthes, old slipped capital femoral epiphysis (Fig. 14.67)	Unilateral coxa vara associated with deformity of the femoral head	
Fibrous dysplasia	Upper femur is commonly involved. Expanding, trabeculated, lucent or ground-glass lesion. The "shepherd's crook" deformity of the proximal femur occurs in polyostotic fibrous dysplasia. Pathologic fractures may be present.	

(continues on page 348)

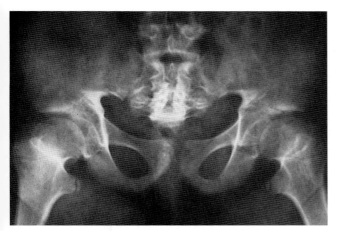

Fig. 14.**64   Achondroplasia with bilateral coxa vara,** short and thick neck of femur and small sacrum.

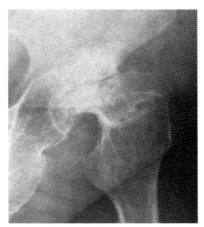

Fig. 14.**65   Achondroplasia.** Coxa vara with almost complete destruction of the femoral head and hypoplastic acetabulum. Severe secondary osteoarthritic changes. Age 38.

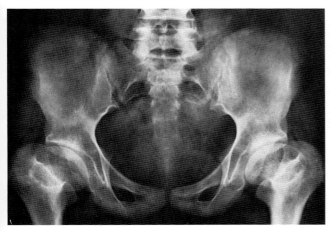

Fig. 14.**66   Cretinism with bilateral coxa vara.** Iliac apophyses are still unfused. Age 31.

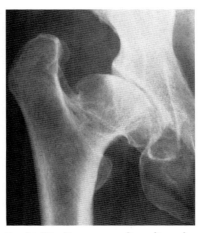

Fig. 14.**67   Coxa vara after slipped capital femoral epiphysis.** Growth disturbance has resulted in a short femoral neck. Secondary osteoarthritis. Age 51.

Table 14.12   (Cont.) Abnormal Angle of the Femoral Neck

Disease	Radiographic Findings	Comments
Malunited fracture **Osteomyelitis of the femoral neck** **Paget's disease**	May cause "shepherd's crook" deformity of the upper femur.	
Rheumatoid arthritis	Usually unilateral coxa valga. Severe erosion of the superior aspect of the femoral head may give a coxa vara appearance. Protrusio acetabuli may be present.	
Juvenile rheumatoid arthritis (Fig. 14.68)	Bilateral coxa valga, with or without deformity of the femoral head. Protrusio acetabuli may be present.	
Bilateral paralytic disorders (meningomyelocele, muscular dystrophy, poliomyelitis) (Fig. 14.69)	Bilateral coxa valga, often associated with obvious mineral loss from bones or hypoplastic bones.	Lack of muscular force. In unilateral paralytic disorders, coxa valga may be unilateral.
Rare congenital syndromes or idiopathic (Fig. 14.70)	Bilateral coxa valga and often other more diagnostic radiographic findings.	Bilateral coxa valga is a constant finding in *progeria*.
Congenital dislocation of hip	Untreated dislocated hip will assume a coax valga configuration.	

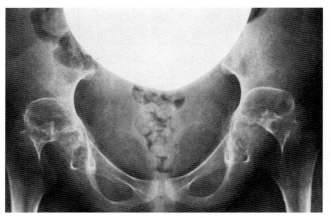

Fig. 14.**68**   **Juvenile rheumatoid arthritis,** age 12. Bilateral destruction of the femoral head and acetabulum, coxa valga and protrusio acetabuli.

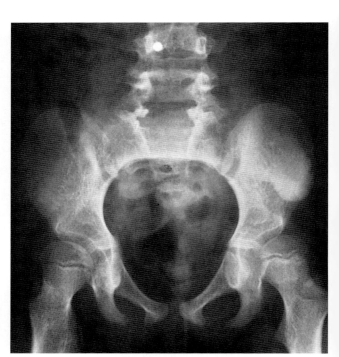

Fig. 14.**69**   **Bilateral coxa valga** in a patient with meningomyelocele.

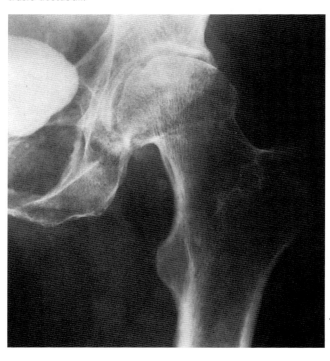

◁ Fig. 14.**70**   **Coxa valga** (bilateral) in a patient with acromegaly, an incidental finding. There are also osteoarthritic changes in the hip joint.

Table 14.13   Abnormal Angulation of the Knee

Abnormality	Usual Causes	Comments
Genu varum (bow legs) bilateral	Idiopathic or physiologic *prenatal bowing* (Fig. 14.**71**)	No obvious pathology. May straighten without treatment.
	Tibia vara *(Blount's disease)* (Fig. 14.**72**)	Aseptic necrosis of the medial tibial metaphysis. The infantile type is usually bilateral. It may also occur at adolescence and be unilateral. The medial metaphysis is irregular. A beak-like projection from the metaphyseal plate pointing medially and distally is characteristic.

(continues on page 350)

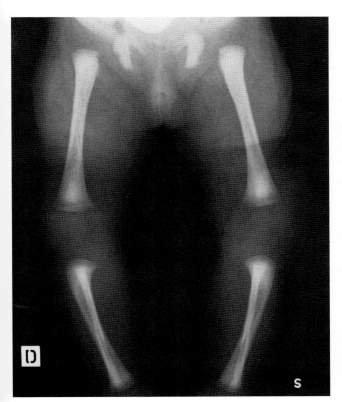

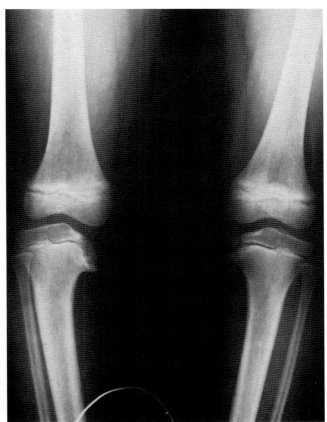

Fig. 14.**71**   **Prenatal bowing of knees** (physiologic) in a patient with congenital hypothyroidism. Delayed ossification of femoral epiphyses.

Fig. 14.**72**   **Bilateral Blount's disease** (tibia vara), age 6. The medial tibial metaphysis of both knees is irregular and shows a characteristic beak.

Table 14.13   (Cont.) Abnormal Angulation of the Knee

Abnormality	Usual Causes	Comments
bilateral	*Rickets* (all causes) (Fig. 14.**73**)	Bowing of legs with typical changes of rickets. Deformity may remain after treatment of the disease.
	Turner's syndrome (Fig. 14.**74**)	Depression of the medial tibial plateau is the most common skeletal sign in this disorder. Medial tibial exostoses or overgrowth of medial tibial condyles may be present.
	(*Campomelic dysplasia* [dwarfism], *metaphyseal dysplasia, dyschondrosteosis,* and *spondyloepiphyseal dysplasia* are rare causes of bilateral genu varum.)	

(continues on page 351)

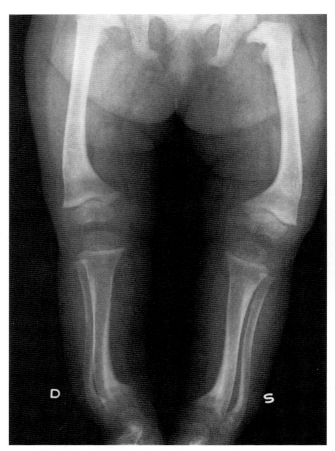

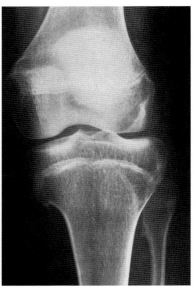

Fig. 14.**74** **Turner's syndrome,** age 20, Depression of the medial tibial plateau and medial tibial (and fibular) exostoses are characteristic.

Fig. 14.**73** **Rickets,** age 2. A mixed pattern of genu valgum and genu varum is produced by severe bowing of distal femora. Bowing and characteristic metaphyseal changes are also seen at ankles. There is bilateral coxa vara.

Table 14.13   (Cont.) Abnormal Angulation of the Knee

Abnormality	Usual Causes	Comments
Genu varum, genu laxum unilateral	*Trauma* *Osteoarthritis*, primary or secondary *Neurotrophic knee* (Fig. 14.**75**, 14.**77**) *Achondroplasia* (Fig. 14.**76**) *Dysplasia epiphysealis hemimelica (Trevor's disease)*	Fracture of the medial condyle of femur or tibia. Osteoarthritis of the knee predominantly affects the medial compartment and the patellofemoral joint and results in a genu varum deformity, often associated with medial displacement of the femur (genu laxum). A rare, unilateral overgrowth of the epiphysis, usually in the knee or ankle. A single osteochondroma may rarely have a similar effect. If the overgrowth appears on the lateral side, the end result is genu varum; if it appears on the medial aspect, genu valgum results.

(continues on page 352)

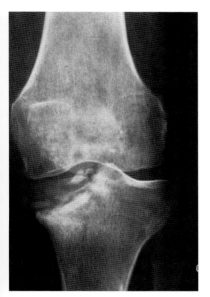

Fig. 14.**75**
Neurotrophic knee, diabetes. Depression of the medial tibial plateau due to bone destruction. A mild genu varum deformity.

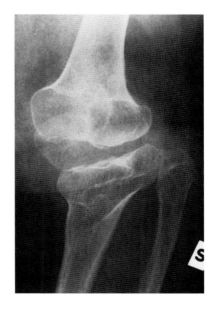

Fig. 14.**76**
Achondroplasia, age 38. Severe depression of the medial tibial plateau and medial displacement of the femur (genu laxum).

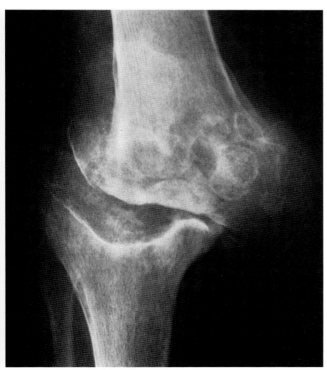

Fig. 14.**77   Genu laxum in a severely deformed neurotrophic knee.** Medial displacement of the deformed distal femur and destruction of the proximal tibia and loose bodies.

Table 14.13   (Cont.) Abnormal Angulation of the Knee

Abnormality	Usual Causes	Comments
Genu valgum (knock knee)	*Physiologic* or due to regional muscular weakness or bowing bones (Fig. 14.**78**)	Due to the wide pelvis, a certain degree of genu valgum is physiologic in women.
	Flatfeet	Malalignment of the tarsus may produce genu valgum as a secondary, compensatory phenomenon.
	Rickets	Instead of bow knees, a knock-knee deformity may arise secondary to rickets.
	Hereditary osteo-onychodysplasia (nail-patella syndrome)	The lateral femoral condyle is small and results in genu valgum and lateral subluxation of the hypoplastic patella.
	Dysplasia epiphysealis hemimelica (Trevor's disease)	
	Juvenile rheumatoid arthritis (Fig. 14.**79**)	Asymmetric growth of the epiphyses may result in knock knees.
	Secondary osteoarthritis confined to the lateral compartment of the knee joint (Fig. 14.**80**)	Common causes include *rupture of the lateral meniscus* and *rheumatoid arthritis*.

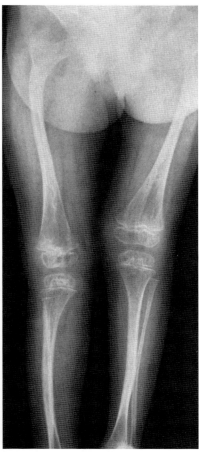

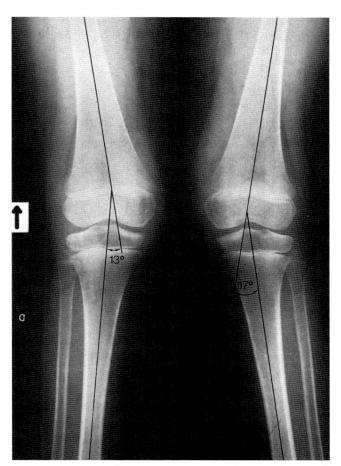

Fig. 14.**78** **Osteogenesis imperfecta.** There is bilateral coxa vara and left-sided genu valgum. The bones are slender and bowed and the metaphyses widened ("Erlenmeyer flask" deformity).

Fig. 14.**79** **Juvenile rheumatoid arthritis** with bilateral genu valgum deformity.

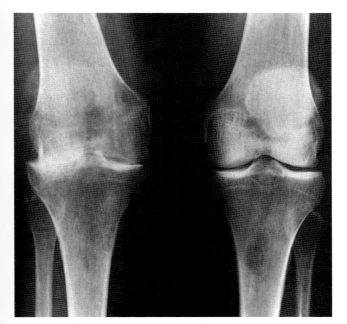

Fig. 14.**80** **Rheumatoid arthritis** with secondary osteoarthritis of the right knee. The lateral compartment is more affected and results in genu valgum deformity on the right side.

15 Hands and Feet

There are 106 bones in the hands and feet, which is more than 50% of the total number of bones (206) in the entire skeleton. These bones, therefore, reflect fairly accurately both normal skeletal development and congenital or acquired disorders of the peripheral skeleton. Minor changes are better visualized in the hands and feet than in the more central skeleton. These provide early diagnostic sign in generalized arthritic and metabolic diseases.

Several measurements are useful in the examination of the radiograph of the hand and wrist: (1) *Metacarpal sign:* A line tangential to the heads of the fourth and fifth metacarpals normally extends distal to the head of the third metacarpal. A positive metacarpal sign is present when the line passes through the head of the third metacarpal (Fig. 15.1). Positive metacarpal sign occurs in such disorders as *pseudo- and pseudopseudohypoparathyroidism* (Figs. 15.2), gonadal dysgenesis *(Turner's syndrome), basal cell nevus syndrome, multiple epiphyseal dysplasia, Beckwith–Wiedemann syndrome, juvenile rheumatoid arthritis, sickle-cell anemia with infarction, trauma, and neonatal hyperthyroidism.*

(2) *Metacarpal index:* The ratio of the length to width at mid-shaft of metacarpals two to five varies from 5.4 to 7.9. In *arachnodactyly (Marfan's syndrome),* it is more than eight (Fig. 15.3). (3) *Carpal angle:* The angle between two lines: the first tangent to the proximal surfaces of the scaphoid and lunate, the second tangent to the proximal margins of the triquetrum and lunate (Fig. 15.4) in a normal white population, it ranges from 120 to 150 degrees. It is decreased in *Madelung's deformity, Turner's, Morquio's* and *Hurler's syndromes* and increased in *arthrogryposis, epiphyseal* and *spondyloepiphyseal dysplasias,* and *trisomy 21.*

Congenital Anomalies

Many anomalies of the hands and feet are isolated without any association with a syndrome, but when detected, a possible constitutional condition should be sought. A detailed discussion of various bone dysplasias of infancy is beyond the scope of this text. Radiographs of the hand have

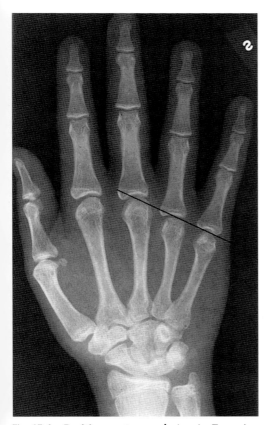

Fig. 15.**1 Positive metacarpal** sign in Turner's syndrome. The terminal tufts have a drumstick appearance.

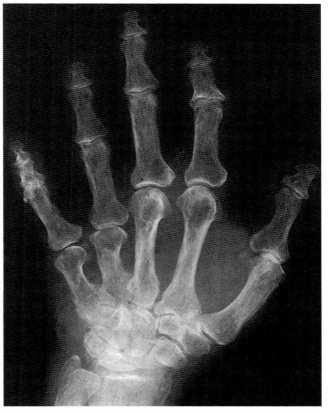

Fig. 15.**2 Pseudopseudohypoparathyroidism.** Short metacarpals and phalanges, with strongly positive metacarpal sign due to very short metacarpals 4 and 5.

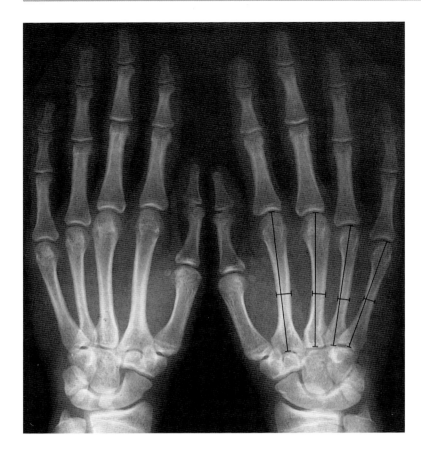

Fig. 15.**3**   **Metacarpal index** over eight in arachnodactyly.

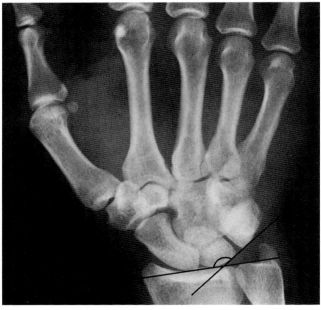

Fig. 15.**4**   **Normal carpal angle.**

such an important role in the differential diagnosis of many constitutional conditions that it was felt imperative to include a short summary of hand, wrist and foot anomalies and associated conditions (Tables 15.**1** and 15.**2**). For the proper understanding of these tables, less common terms used are explained here*:

Brachydactyly	=	shortening of phalanx or phalanges (Figs. 15.**5** and 15.**6**)
Brachymetacarpaly	=	shortening of metacarpal(s) (Figs. 15.**7** and 15.**8**)
Camptodactyly	=	permanent flexion of finger(s) (Figs. 15.**13** and 15.**14**)
Clinodactyly	=	curvature of (usually fifth) finger in a mediolateral plane (Figs. 15.**9** and 15.**10**)
Diastrophic	=	twisted
Dysplasia	=	intrinsic growth disturbance
Polydactyly	=	supernumerary digits (Fig. 15.**11**)
Symphalangism	=	end-to-end fusion of contiguous phalanges (absent joint)
Syndactyly	=	soft-tissue or bony union between adjacent digits (Fig. 15.**9**)

The foot, as much as the hand, may yield useful information in the study of generalized congenital disorders. In certain conditions, the radiographic finding may be most characteristic in the foot. Many congenital syndromes involve some foot abnormality, but Table 15.**2** is limited to those disorders in which the foot findings are an important part of the syndrome or are unique or unusual.

---

*   Some other features mentioned in Tables 15.**1** and 15.**2** are further illustrated in Figs. 15.**12**–15.**15**.

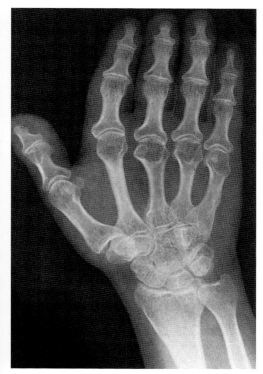

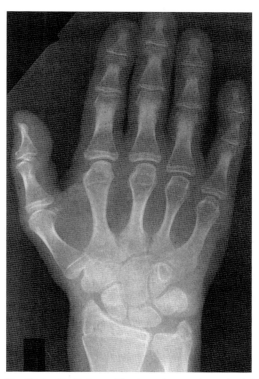

Fig. 15.**5** **Achondroplasia.** Short metacarpals and phalanges with wide epiphyses.

Fig. 15.**6** **Cretinism.** Short metacarpals and slightly shortened phalanges. Fusion of epiphyseal plates at the age of 26.

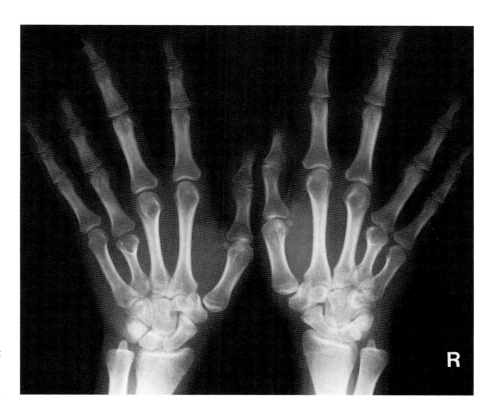

Fig. 15.**7** **Brachymetacarpaly.** Short metacarpals IV and V on the right and IV on the left. Incidental finding without constitutional abnormalities.

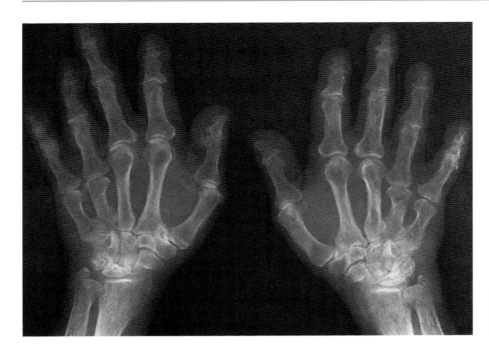

Fig. 15.**8** **Pseudohypoparathyroidism.** Short metacarpals 4 and 5, as well as short distal phalanges and abnormally shaped carpal bones.

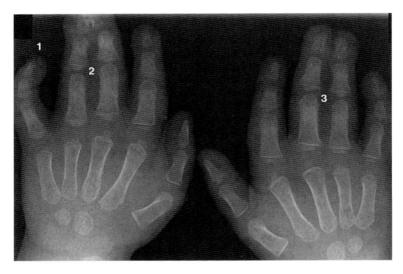

Fig. 15.**9** **Multiple anomalies in the hands** of a 2-year-old child: 1 clinodactyly, 2 syndactyly with bony fusion of distal phalanges of fingers 3 and 4, 3 syndactyly with only soft-tissue fusion of fingers 3 and 4.

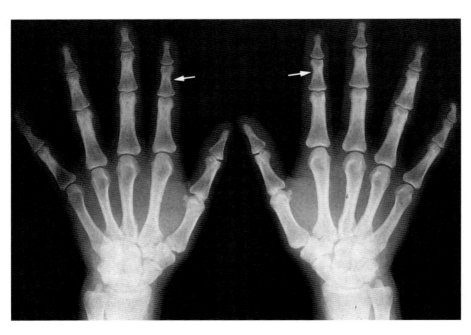

Fig. 15.**10** **Kirner's deformity** in the distal phalanges of both fifth fingers evident as incurving (curvature with dorsal apex). Incidentally the patient also has hyperparathyroidism with subperiosteal tunneling and frank erosion of the radial side of the second phalanx of the index fingers (arrows).

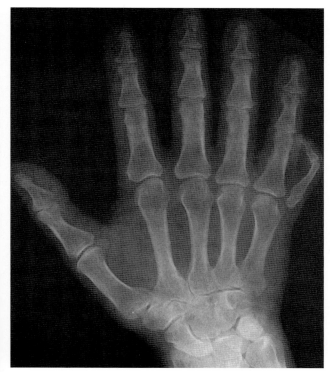

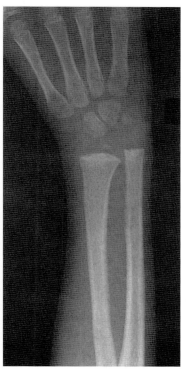

Fig. 15.**11**   **Polydactyly.** A supernumerary, rudimentary 6th finger.

Fig. 15.**12**   **Aplasia** of 1st metacarpal and thumb. A case of **Fanconi's anemia.**

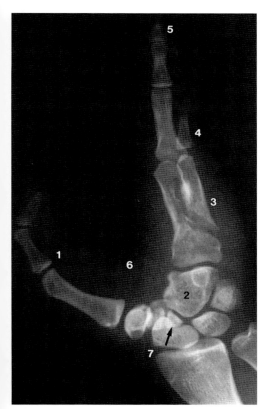

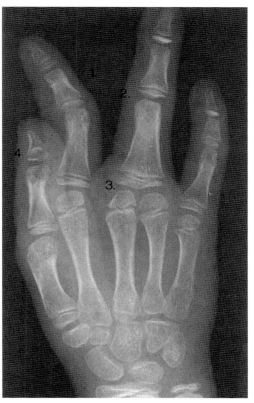

Fig. 15.**13**   **Severe anomalies in a cleft hand:** 1 Camptodactyly of the thumb. 2 abnormal shape of capitate with fusion of capitate and hamate, 3 partial fusion of two metacarpals with fracture of the union, 4 uniphalangeal hypoplastic finger, 5 short distsal phalanx, 6 aplasia of two metacarpals and fingers, and 7 os centrale (arrow)

Fig. 15.**14**   **Anomalies in the hand bones.** 1 Camptodactyly of the index finger, 2 hypertrophic finger with wide proximal phalanx articulating with two adjacent metacarpals, one of which has an abnormal, cone-shaped epiphysis (3), and 4 short distal phalanx of the thumb with a cone-shaped epiphysis.

Table 15.1 Hand and Wrist Anomalies and Associated Dysplasias

Legend: + = Frequent occurrence；○ = Occasional occurrence

Column groups: Columns 1–27 = **Syndromes usually evident at birth**; Columns 28–45 = **May manifest later**.

Row groups (left margin, under "Anomalies"): **Hand and Fingers** (Arachnodactyly → Ulnar deviation of fingers); **Thumb** (Duplication → Triphalangeal thumb); **Wrist** (Os centrale → Hypoplasia of radius).

Anomaly	Achondroplasia	Acrocephalosyndactyly (Apert's syndrome)	Acrocephalopolysyndactyly (Carpenter's syndrome)	Arthrogryposis multiplex congenita	Asphyxiating thoracic dysplasia	Cleidocranial dysplasia	Chondrodysplasia punctata	Chondroectodermal dysplasia (Ellis–van Creveld syndrome)	Cornelia de Lange syndrome	Diastrophic dysplasia (dwarf)	Down's syndrome (trisomy 21)	Fanconi's anemia	Focal dermal hypoplasia syndrome (Goltz's syndrome)	Hand–foot–uterus syndrome	Holt–Oram syndrome	Laurence–Moon–Biedl syndrome	Oculodento-osseous syndrome	Orodigitofacial syndrome	Otopalatodigital syndrome	Poland's syndrome	Prader–Willi syndrome	Rubinstein–Taybi syndrome	Russell–Silver syndrome	Thanatophoric dysplasia (dwarf)	Trisomy 13–15	Trisomy 18	Symphalangism–surdity syndrome	Acrodysostosis	Basal cell nevus syndrome	Dyschondrosteosis	Hereditary multiple exostoses	Homocystinuria	Hurler's syndrome (mucopolysaccharidosis I)	Klinefelter's syndrome	Marfan's syndrome	Morquio's syndrome (mucopolysaccharidosis IV)	Multiple epiphyseal dysplasia (Fairbank's disease)	Myositis ossificans progressiva	Onycho-osteodysplasia	Progeria	Pseudohypoparathyroidism	Pseudopseudohypoparathyroidism	Rothmund's syndrome	Turner's syndrome	Werner's syndrome
Hand and Fingers																																													
Arachnodactyly																												○				○			+										
Brachydactyly	+	+	+		+	+	○		+	+	+	+	+	+	+		+	+	+	+		+	+	+				+			+		+				+			+	+	+	+		
Camptodactyly										○			+		+	+			○								+					○					○								
Clinodactyly			+	+				+		○	+		+	+		○	+	+	+	○	○	○	+		○	○						○	+	○	○		○	○						○	
Cone-shaped epiphyses	○	○		○	○		+						+						+									+		○	○									○					
Hemihypertrophy (hand)																					+																								
Hypoplasia metacarpal (III, IV, and/or V)			○	○		○																		○				+	○	○			○				○			○	+	+		+	
Hypoplasia metacarpals (all)	+			+	+			+			+												+					+					+			+									
Kirner's deformity									○													○																					○		
Polydactyly		+		○	+			+					+			+		○		+		○			+	○																			
Small hands	+	+	+		+				+	+	+		○								+		+																					○	+
Symphalangism																											+																		
Syndactyly		+	+		○		○						○	+			+	+		+			○		○	○																			
Tapering (proximal) metacarpals																																	+			+									
Ulnar deviation of fingers (III, IV, V)																											+																		
Thumb																																													
Duplication	○	○											○																																
Aplasia									+				+														○																	○	
Short metacarpal									+	+			+		+	+											○		+											+		○	○	○	
Long metacarpal													+																																
Wide metacarpal									+	+			+																											+					
Short proximal phalanx		+																				+						+												+					
Triangular proximal phalanx		+																				+																							
Short distal phalanx		+					○		+				+						+			+														+									
Broad distal phalanx		+	+																			+		○																					
Clasped thumb			+																																										
"Hitchhiker thumb"		○								+												+																							
Triphalangeal thumb															+												○																		
Wrist																																													
Os centrale (Fig. 15.13, p. 359)													+	+					○																										
Irregular carpal margins										+																															+	+			
Extra distal carpals										+									○																										
Abnormally shaped navicular			○							○			+	+	+				○																								○		
Navicular fused to other carpals			○							○				+	+				○																			○							
Absent or hypoplastic navicular										+									○																										
Abnormally shaped capitate			○							○			○		○				+														+		+		+								
Absent or hypoplastic capitate																																					+								
Some carpal fusion			+					+		○				+	+				○								+		○																○
Decreased carpal angle	○																													+		+												+	
Increased carpal angle			+							○																											+								
Small carpus			+							+									○																			+							
Hypoplasia of radius									+			○			○										○	○						+												○	

Modified from ME Kricun, J Edeiken, *The hand and wrist in systemic disease*, Baltimore: Williams and Wilkins, 1973

Table 15.**2**   Foot Anomalies in Some Congenital Bone Dysplasias

+ = Frequent occurrence
○ = Occasional occurrence

Group	Feature	Acrocephalosyndactyly (Apert's syndrome)	Acrocephalopolysyndactyly (Carpenter's syndrome)	Arthrogryposis multiplex congenita	Chondrodysplasia punctata	Chondroectodermal dysplasia (Ellis–van Creveld syndrome)	Cornelia de Lange syndrome	Diastrophic dysplasia (dwarf)	Down's syndrome (Trisomy 21)	Fanconi's anemia	Focal dermal hypoplasia (Goltz's syndrome)	Hand–foot–uterus syndrome	Laurence–Moon–Biedl syndrome	Oculodento-osseous syndrome	Otopalatodigital syndrome	Prader–Willi syndrome	Rubinstein–Taybi syndrome	Russell–Silver syndrome	Trisomy 13–15	Trisomy 18	Symphalangism–surdity syndrome	Dyschondrosteosis	Myositis ossificans progressiva	Pseudohypoparathyreoidism	Pseudopseudohypoparathyreoidism	Turner's syndrome
		Syndromes usually manifest at birth																			*May manifest later*					
Metatarsal and toes	Cone-shaped epiphyses											○			○							○				
	Hemihypertrophy																	+								
	Hypoplasia metatarsal (III, IV, and/or II)																				○			+	+	○
	Polydactyly		+			○	+				○		+				+	+								
	Symphalangism											+		+							+					
	Syndactyly	+	+			○	○		○	○	○	○		○	○	○	○									
Great toe	Short metatarsal	+	+									+			+					+		+				
	Short proximal phalanx						+								+							+				
	Short distal phalanx						+					+			+			+								
	Broad distal phalanx																+									
	Uniphalangeal great toe	+																				+				
Tarsus	Short calcaneus											+														
	Tarsal fusion (including cuneiform)	+	+	+	○							+			+						+					+
	Clubfoot		+		○		○	+											○	+						
	Small feet											+														

Compiled from AK Poznanski, Foot manifestations of the congenital malformation syndromes. Semin Roentgenol 1970;5:354–66.

Terminal Phalanx Pattern

The distal ends of the toes are usually poorly delineated in ordinary radiographs, but the distal phalanges of fingers are well visualized. A variety of acquired and congenital diseases, as well as localized lesions, cause changes in the radiographic appearance of the terminal phalanges. The radiographic changes around the distal interphalangeal joints are similar to elsewhere in the skeleton and joints, but the pattern may be different in the terminal tufts. A list of various patterns of distal phalangeal abnormalities with their common or typical causes is presented in Table 15.**3**.

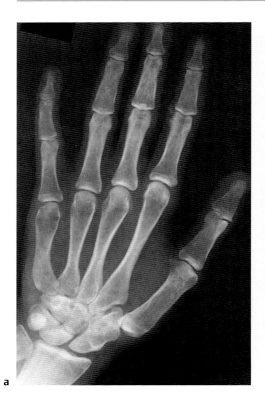

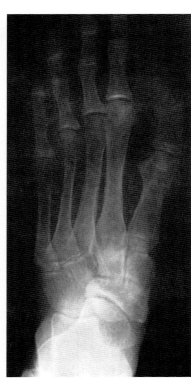

Fig. 15.**15 a, b   Otopalatodigital syndrome. a** The distal row of carpal bones and the scaphoid are fused. Metacarpal bones 2–4 have narrow diaphyses, while the fifth has an abnormally wide diaphysis but normal length. Finger bones show no gross abnormality. **b** The foot shows fusion of the navicular with the first cuneiform and of the cuboid with the third cuneiform. The first metatarsal is short relative to the others. The great toe has an abnormal shape (clinodactyly).

Table 15.3   Differential Diagnosis of Abnormal Terminal Phalanx

Type of Change	Common or Typical Causes
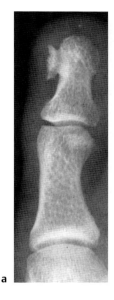 **Atrophic** **Exaggerated**	a) Normal variants b) Subungual exostosis (Fig. 15.**16a**) Causes of clubbing of the fingers (bronchogenic carcinoma, cirrhosis of liver, congenital heart disease, pulmonary hypertrophic osteoarthropathy, pachydermoperiostosis, pulmonary interstitial fibrosis) Acromegaly (Fig. 15.**16b**) Basal cell nevus syndrome

(continues on page 364)

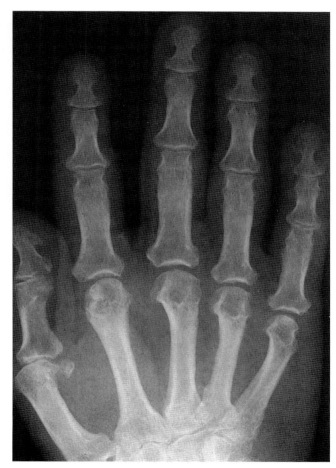

Fig. 15.**16a**   **Subungual** exostosis projects characteristically from the distal and dorsomedial aspects of the terminal phalanx of the great toe.

Fig. 15.**16b**   **Acromegaly** with exaggerated terminal phalangeal tufts, wide metacarpophalangeal joint spaces, increased soft tissue, and premature osteoarthritis.

Table 15.3   (Cont.) Differential Diagnosis of Abnormal Terminal Phalanx

Type of Change	Common or Typical Causes
Acro-osteosclerosis	Idiopathic Rheumatoid arthritis (and other connective tissue disorders) (Fig. 15.**17**) Chronic active hepatitis Sarcoidosis (Osteopetrosis, melorheostosis, osteopoikilosis, Figs. 15.**18** and 15.**19**)
Smoothly delineated lytic lesion	Epidermoid inclusion cyst Enchondroma Glomus tumor Sarcoidosis Bone cyst Arthritis Cystic osteomyelitis Tuberous sclerosis Osteoid osteoma
Poorly defined lytic lesion at phalangeal tuft	Osteomyelitis (panaritium ossale) (Fig. 15.**20**) Leprotic osteomyelitis (rare) Aneurysmal bone cyst (rare)
Poorly defined lytic lesion, including the base	Metastasis (especially bronchogenic carcinoma, Fig. 15.**21**) Carcinoma of nail bed Subungual sarcoma Psoriatic arthropathy Giant cell tumor (rare) Myeloma (rare) Sarcoidosis (rare) Fibrous dysplasia

(continues on page 366)

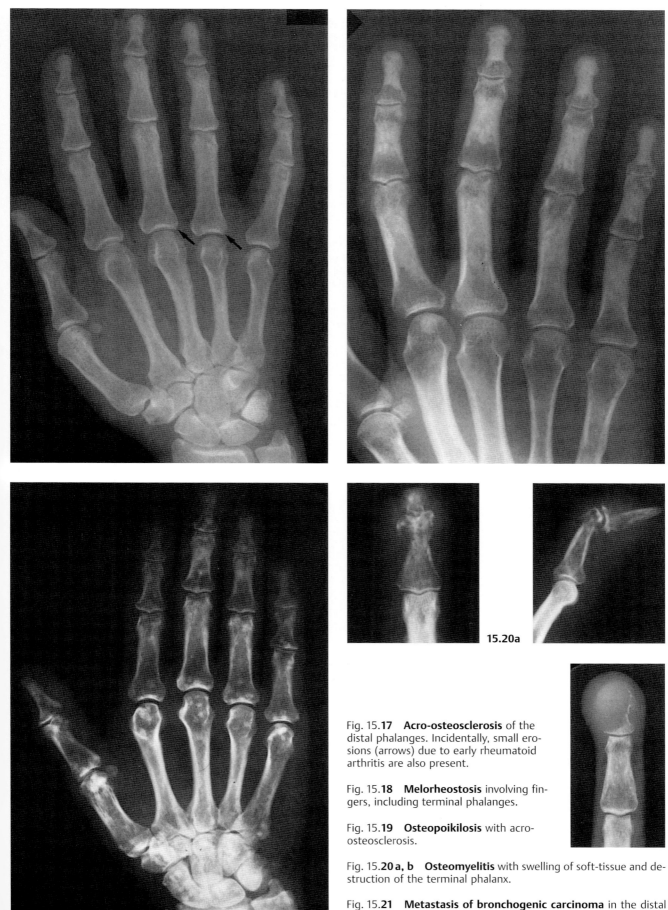

15.18

15.20a

15.20b

15.21

Fig. 15.**17** **Acro-osteosclerosis** of the distal phalanges. Incidentally, small erosions (arrows) due to early rheumatoid arthritis are also present.

Fig. 15.**18** **Melorheostosis** involving fingers, including terminal phalanges.

Fig. 15.**19** **Osteopoikilosis** with acro-osteosclerosis.

Fig. 15.**20 a, b** **Osteomyelitis** with swelling of soft-tissue and destruction of the terminal phalanx.

Fig. 15.**21** **Metastasis of bronchogenic carcinoma** in the distal phalanx. A relatively well-demarcated osteolytic lesion and soft-tissue swelling is seen.

Table 15.3   (Cont.) Differential Diagnosis of Abnormal Terminal Phalanx

Type of Change	Common or Typical Causes
"Morning star"	Psoriatic arthritis (Fig. 15.**23**) Hyperparathyroidism (Fig. 15.**24**) Sjogren's syndrome
Acro-osteolysis (*with possible soft-tissue calcification)	Collagen vascular disease* (especially scleroderma and dermatomyositis) (Fig. 15.**25**) Sjogren's syndrome Hyperparathyroidism* (Fig. 15.**22**) Arteriosclerosis obliterans Diabetic gangrene Buerger's disease Burn, frostbite, radiation* (Fig. 15.**26**) Pachydermoperiostosis Neurotrophic disease (syringomyelia, leprosy) (Fig. 15.**27**) Epidermolysis bullosa* Psoriatic arthritis Pycnodysostosis Familial acro-osteolysis Progeria Pseudoxanthoma elasticum Congenital indifference to pain* Porphyria Vinylchloride exposure Lesch–Nyhan syndrome Multicentric reticulohistiocytosis Rothmund's syndrome*

(continues on page 368)

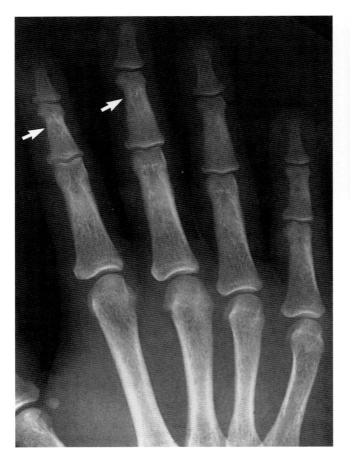

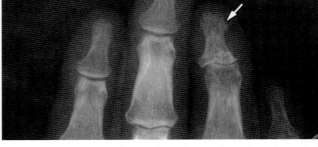

Fig. 15.**23   Psoriatic arthritis.** "Morning star" erosion of terminal phalangeal tuft of the fourth finger (arrow).

Fig. 15.**22   Secondary hyperparathyroidism** (renal osteodystrophy). Rarefaction of terminal tufts and subperiosteal erosion in phalanges (arrows).

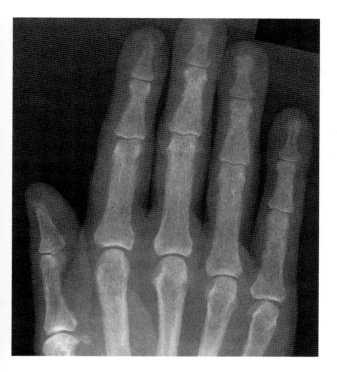

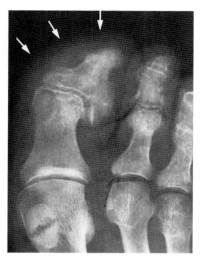

15.26

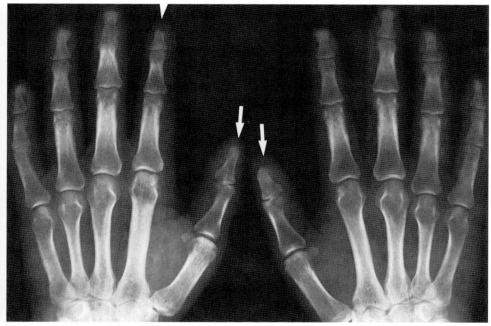

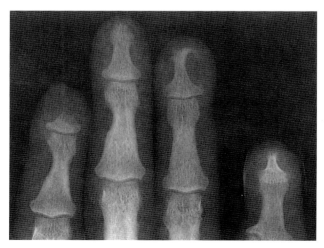

Fig. 15.**24** **Hyperparathyroidism.** Erosion in the index finger has a "morning star" pattern, but unlike psoriatic arthritis, there is widespread demineralization and subperiosteal erosion elsewhere in the fingers. The other tufts only show rarefaction.

Fig. 15.**25** **Scleroderma.** Acro-osteolysis and soft-tissue atrophy in some fingers (arrows), but no other obvious bone changes.

Fig. 15.**26** **Frostbite.** Localized acro-osteolysis in the great toe with a large soft-tissue ulcer (arrows).

Fig. 15.**27** **Leprosy.** Acro-osteolysis in distal phalanges of the second, fourth and fifth fingers.

15.27

Table 15.3   (Cont.) Differential Diagnosis of Abnormal Terminal Phalanx

Type of Change	Common or Typical Causes
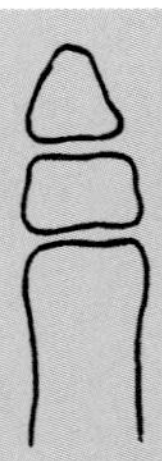 **Short distal phalanges (absent tufts) Brachy-telephalangy**	Several congenital syndromes with short phalanges (see Table 15.1) Associated with hypoplastic nails Maternal use of anticonvulsants (phenytoin) Frostbite Trauma
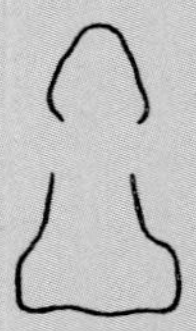 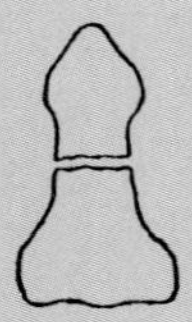 **Midtuft erosion** **Pseudoepiphysis in small distal phalanges**	Chemical acro-osteolysis (vinyl chloride exposure) Hyperparathyroidism (primary or secondary) (Fig. 15.28) Hajdu–Cheney syndrome (congenital acro-osteolysis) Juvenile rheumatoid arthritis (Fig. 15.29) Cleidocranial dysostosis
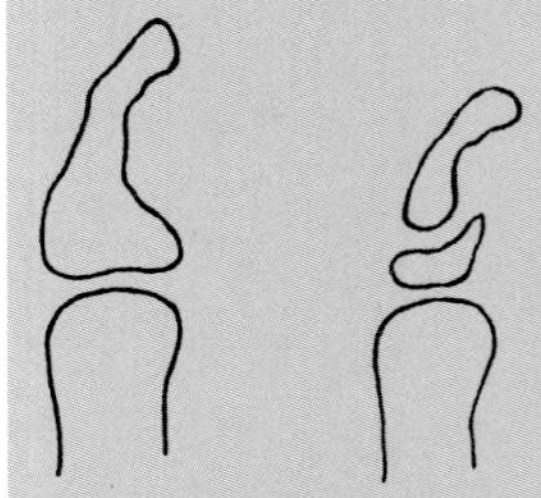 **adult juvenile** **Kirner's deformity**	Curvature with apex dorsal of the distal phalanx of the 5th finger ("incurving") Isolated anomaly (see Fig. 15.10) or in congenital syndromes (Russell–Silver syndrome, Cornelia de Lange syndrome)
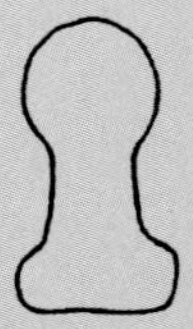 **Drumstick (rounded, broad tuft)**	Turner's syndrome (Fig. 15.30)

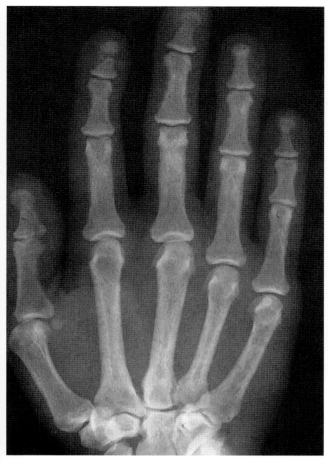

Fig. 15.**28**   **Renal osteodystrophy** with midtuft erosions and sub-periosteal erosions in the phalanges.

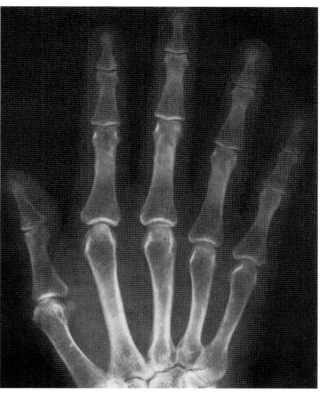

Fig. 15.**30**   **Tuner's syndrome.** Drumstick tufts and positive metacarpal sign.

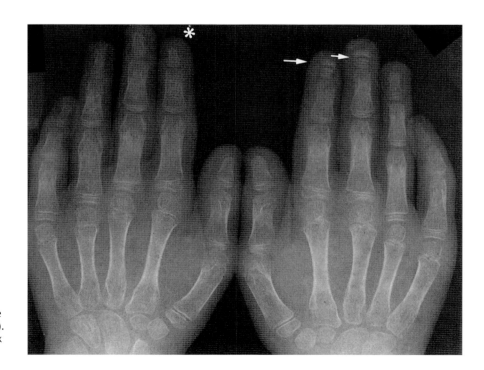

Fig. 15.**29**   **Juvenile rheumatoid arthritis.** Midtuft erosions are seen in the 2nd and 3rd fingers on the right (arrows). There is acro-osteolysis in the left index finger (asterisk).

Orthopedic Foot Problems

The feet are subject to a number of deformations or painful conditions, not necessarily as a result of the congenital syndromes listed in Tables 15.1 and 15.2.

In the analysis of a deformed foot, one should be aware of a number of important lines and angles of the foot. Some useful lines and angles that should be evaluated from the weight-supporting dorsoplantar and lateral views are presented here (Fig. 15.31).

The *midtarsal joint line* (A-A) is a continuous line along the anterior margin of the talus and calcaneus on the lateral view and talus and cuboid on the anteroposterior view. A lack of continuity indicates a mobile talus, altered position of the talus and calcaneus relative to the navicular and cuboid at the midtarsal joint, e.g., a *midtarsal fault*.

The *calcaneal pitch* (B) is an index of the height of the foot framework; low: 10 to 20 degrees; medium: 20 to 30 degrees; and high, over 30 degrees. Low pitch is indicative of a change in the position of the calcaneus and talus at the ankle joint, e.g., a *hindfoot fault* as seen in flatfoot.

Böhler's angle of the calcaneus (C, normal: 20 to 40 degrees) indicates the integrity of the plantar arch of the calcaneus. It is decreased by a *calcaneal fracture*.

The diagonal axis of the talus (D-D) is a fair indicator of the proper relation of the talus to the calcaneus, normally nearly horizontal. It is not horizontal in most foot deformities.

The *talocalcaneal angle* in the dorsoplantar view (E) ranges from 20 degrees to 50 degrees in infants and young children and from 15 degrees to 30 degrees from age five on. A line through the axis of the talus points to the head of the first metatarsal bone. The axial line of the calcaneus points to the fourth metatarsal bone. The talocalcaneal angle is increased in *flatfoot* and is reduced or reversed in *clubfoot*.

The *midtalar* and *midcalcaneal* lines from the lateral view meet near the anterior margin of the cuboid, forming an angle of 25 to 50 degrees (F). The *midtalar/ midcalcaneal angle* is reduced in *clubfoot* or *rockerbottom deformity* and in-creased in *flatfoot* and *pes cavus*. The angle formed by lines along the inferior margin of the calcaneus and the fifth metatarsal bone (G) ranges from 150 degrees to 175 degrees and is unaffected by age. The apex of this angle faces downward in *flatfoot* and *rockerbottom deformity*.

In order to give a meaningful roentgenographic report on a deformed foot, the radiologist must also know the orthopedic terminology:

1. Valgus (eversion, pronation) = bent outward from the midline of the body, distal to the point or joint of reference
2. Varus (inversion, supination) = bent inward toward midline of the body, distal to the point or joint of the reference
3. Adduction = displacement on a transverse plane toward the axis of the body
4. Abduction = displacement on a transverse plane away from the axis of the body
5. Heel valgus (Fig. 15.32b) = the outward slant of the heel, as seen from the rear, is increased above 10 degrees (associated with an increased talocalcaneal angle from the dorsoplantar view)
6. Heel varus (Fig. 15.32c) = the normal valgus angle (5 to 10 degrees) is decreased or the heel slants inward (associated with a decreased talocalcaneal angle in the dorsoplantar view)
7. Equinus = fixed plantar flexion of the hindfoot (anterior end of calcaneus down). From the lateral view, the calcaneus makes an angle of more than 90 degrees anteriorly with the tibia

Heel valgus or varus cannot be determined directly from the routine AP and lateral radiographs, but can be inferred from the talocalcaneal angle on the AP view. Table 15.4 lists the more common foot deformities, with their diagnostic and differential diagnostic criteria. The overall appearances of various congenital foot deformities are presented diagrammatically in Fig. 15.33a–g.

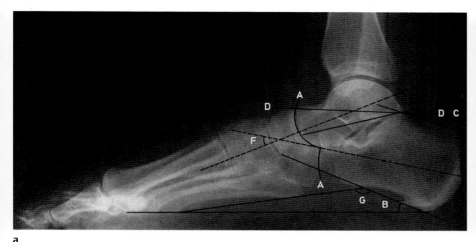

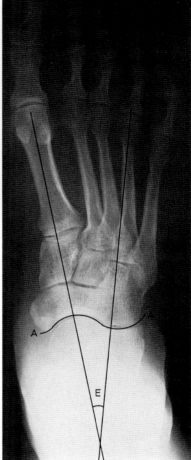

Fig. 15.**31 a, b   Some useful lines and angles in the evaluation of an orthopedic foot problem.** A–A = midtarsal joint line, B = calcaneal pitch, C = Böhler's angle of the calcaneus. D = diagonal axis of the talus, E = talocalcaneal angle, F = midtalar-midcalcaneal angle, and G = inferior cortex of calcaneus-fifth metatarsal angle.

b

Fig. 15.**32 a–c   a** Normal heel position (as seen from the rear); **b** Heel valgus, seen in metatarsus varus (adductus). **c** Heel varus, seen in clubfoot.

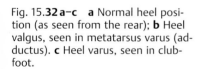

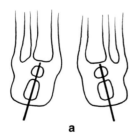

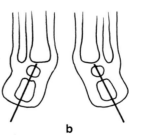

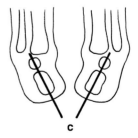

a   **b**   **c**

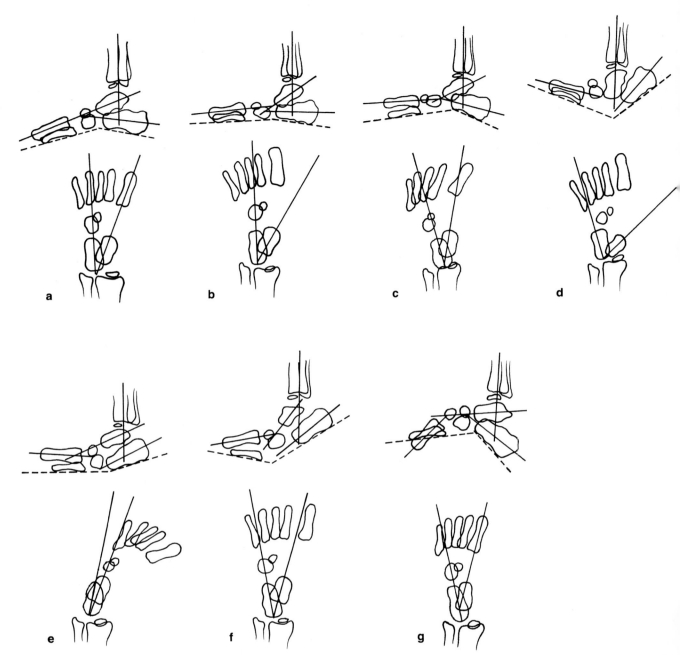

Fig. 15.**33 a–g The appearance of various congenital foot deformities** with special reference to the midtalar-midcalcaneal angle (AP, normally 15°–30°, infants 30°–50° and lateral 25°–50°), the inferior cortex of calcaneus-fifth metatarsal angle (lateral, normally 150°–175°) and the orientation of the metatarsals. **a** Normal foot, **b** flatfoot, **c** metatarsus varus (adductus), **d** congenital vertical talus (rockerbottom deformity), **e** clubfoot, **f** overcorrected clubfoot, and **g** pes cavus

Table 15.4   Differential Diagnosis of a Deformed Foot

Deformity	Radiographic Characteristics	Comments
Hallux valgus (hallux abductus valgus) (Figs. 15.34, 15.35)	1 Abduction of the hallux (angle between the first metatarsal and great toe 10 degrees to 20 degrees = mild; 20 degrees to 30 degrees = moderate; 30 degrees to 45 degrees = severe) with valgus rotation of the hallux. 2 Deviation or subluxation of the metatarsophalangeal joint. 3 Medial prominence and cratering of the medial epicondyle of the first metatarsal head. 4 Adduction of the first metatarsal, intermetatarsal angle (between metatarsal I and II) over 10 degrees. 5 Relative lateral displacement of sesamoid bones. Adduction of the first metatarsal bone may be structural (abnormal metatarsal base called *congenital metatarsus primus adductus*: abnormal, elongated anterodistal margin of the cuneiform) or positional (hypermobile gap of the first metatarsal segment of the adducted forefoot).	The most common foot deformity: Diversion of the big toe into abduction followed by inflammatory reaction over the medial epicondyle of the metatarsal head. Associated with shoe incompatibility and/or predisposing foot anatomy. The valgus (eversion) component of the deformity occurs due to the rotating effect of imbalanced muscle action on the proximal phalanx. Progressive deformity is more likely to occur in positional abnormalities. Hallux valgus may be a feature of *rheumatoid arthritis* and of *Ehlers-Danlos syndrome* (joint laxity, subcutaneous calcifications). In the absence of soft-tissue calcification (in gout), the erosions and degenerative changes of the first metatarsal head due to hallux valgus alone and in connection with gout may be similar.
Morton's metatarsus atavicus (Morton's syndrome)	The first metatarsal is short and the second is broad.	Also called Dudley Joy Morton. Causes pain while walking usually bilateral.
Morton's neuroma	Plain film findings are usually normal.	A neuralgia most often in the region of either the head of the fourth metatarsal, since the third and fourth or the fourth and fifth metatarsal bones are too close together and compress the plantar nerve. MRI or ultrasound are suggested for diagnosis.

(continues on page 374)

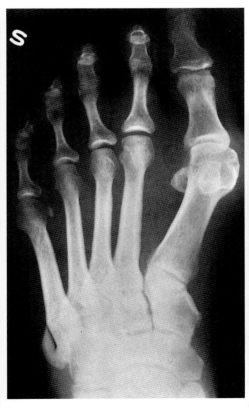 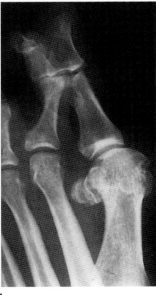 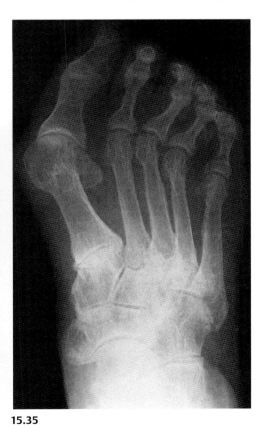

a   b   15.35

Fig. 15.**34 a, b** **Mild hallux valgus** with lateral displacement of sesamoid bones, medial prominence, and cratering of the medial epicondyle of the first metatarsal head, best seen in the oblique projection, and structural adduction of the first metatarsal.

Fig. 15.**35** **Severe hallux valgus.** Incidentally, renal osteodystrophy is also present.

Table 15.4   (Cont.) Differential Diagnosis of a Deformed Foot

Deformity	Radiographic Characteristics	Comments
Flatfoot (Pes planus) (Figs. 15.37, 15.38)	Dorsoplantar view: 1 talocalcaneal angle is increased; 2 forefoot is abducted; 3 the heel is valgus: the long axis of the talus runs medial to the first metatarsal while the long axis of the calcaneus remains near the fourth metatarsal base. Lateral view: 1 the foot dorsiflexes to normal angle (or even more); 2 the talocalcaneal angle is increased due to plantar flexion of the talus; 3 the long axes of the talus and the fifth metatarsal angulate toward the plantar.	*Acquired flatfoot* can be differentiated from *congenital flatfoot* through a careful study of the position and shape of the calcaneus and an evaluation of the midtarsal joint: 1 In acquired foot collapse the calcaneal pitch is 10 degrees or more, in congenital it is less. 2 In acquired flatfoot the calcaneus has a downwards concave form, in congenital it is downward convex or flat. 3 In acquired flatfoot the midtarsal joint line is altered (talus juts forward), in congenital pes planus the joint line is pseudonormal, although the talus is displaced medially. In *rigid flatfoot*, pronation and supination are limited and the condition is painful, unlike flexible flatfoot.

(continues on page 376)

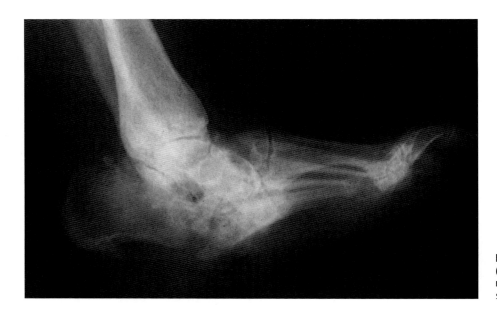

Fig. 15.**36   Diabetic arthropathy** (neurotrophic foot) with an acquired rockerbottom deformity due to destruction and malposition of bones.

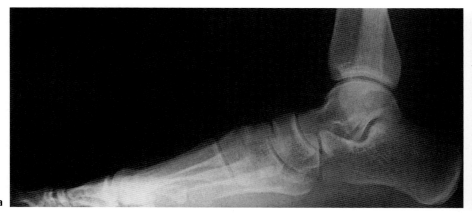

a

Fig. 15.**37 a, b   Acquired flatfoot. a** The calcaneal pitch is low and the midtarsal joint line is slightly discontinuous. **b** Flattening of the transverse arch is seen as an increased distance between metatarsal heads in dorsoplantar projection.

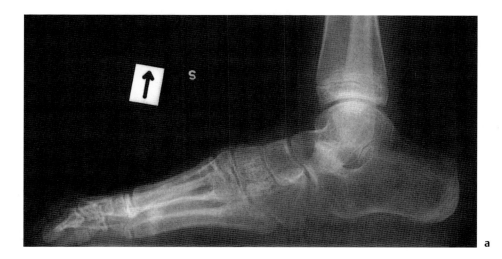

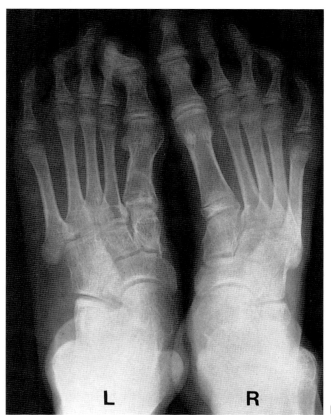

Fig. 15.**38 a, b Congenital left flatfoot** in a 13-year-old with scleroderma and bone deformities in the left foot. The calcaneal pitch is less than 10 degrees, calcaneus is convex downwards, and the midtarsal joint line appears normal in the lateral view, although the talus is displaced medially in the dorsoplantar view.

Table 15.4   (Cont.) Differential Diagnosis of a Deformed Foot

Deformity	Radiographic Characteristics	Comments
Metatarsus varus (adductus) (Fig. 15.39)	Dorsoplantar view: 1 the heel is in normal position or in valgus (long axis of talus either near the base of the first metatarsal or medial to it) ; 2 forefoot is adducted and in varus (overlapping metatarsals). Lateral view; 1 normal or greater than normal dorsiflexion of the foot; 2 the talocalcaneal angle is normal or slightly increased; 3 the first metatarsal is higher than the fifth.	A congenital foot type in which the forefoot is adducted. Often overlooked in infancy.
Congenital vertical talus (Fig. 15.40)	Dorsoplantar view: Severe heel valgus (increased talocalcaneal angle, the talar axis falls far medial to the first metatarsal). Lateral view: 1 the heel is in the equinus position (plantar flexed, calcaneus tilted front end down); 2 talus is in extreme plantar flexion the talocalcaneal angle is increased; 3 the forefoot dorsiflexes at midtarsal level, producing a convex plantar surface (rockerbottom deformity); 4 dorsal dislocation of the navicular (becomes visible after its ossification center has appeared).	*Severe flatfoot* also has vertical talus but no heel equinus. *Treated clubfoot* has persistent heel equinus but not a plantar flexed talus. In *triple arthrodesis* reduction of plantar flexion is often attemted by placing the anterior talus into the inferior aspect of the navicular, thus the navicular projects dorsal to the talus. A *neurotrophic foot* in an adult may show a rockerbottom deformity due to bone destruction and malposition (Fig. 15.36).
Clubfoot (Talipes equinovarus) (Fig. 15.41)	Dorsoplantar view: 1 the talocalcaneal angle is markedly reduced, the talus and calcaneus may be parallel; 2 the forefoot is in varus and adducted. The bases of metatarsals may be overlapping or appear in lateral profile if varus is severe. Lateral view: 1 the heel is in the equinus position; 2 the forefoot is plantar flexed (cavus), more than hindfoot, even in forced dorsiflexion; 3 long axes of the talus and calcaneus are parallel.	*Flat-top talus* is a late complication of clubfoot, causing incongruity of the ankle joint.

(continues on page 378)

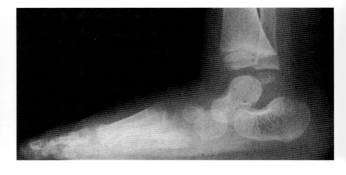

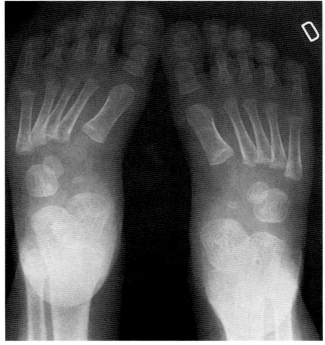

Fig. 15.**39 a, b   Metatarsus varus** in a 2-year-old, left more than right. a The long axis of the talus is medial to the first metatarsal (heel valgus) and the metatarsals are overlapping in the dorsoplantar view. b Lateral view shows a slightly increased talocalcaneal angle. The first metatarsal is much higher than the fifth.

a

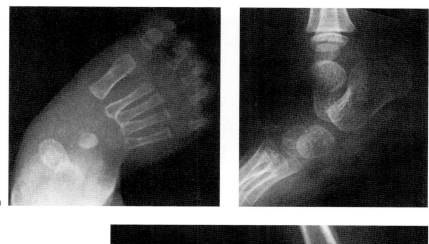

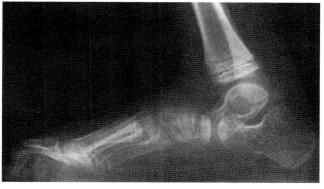

Fig. 15.**40 a–c   Congenital vertical talus. a** Dorsoplantar view at the age of 4 months. The talus is adducted and the talocalcaneal angle is very wide. **b** Lateral view at the age of 6 years. The talus is tilted front end down and the talocalcaneal angle is increased. Calcaneus is in relatively normal position due to treatment and consequently there is no more rockerbottom deformity left. **c** An untreated case with rockerbottom deformity.

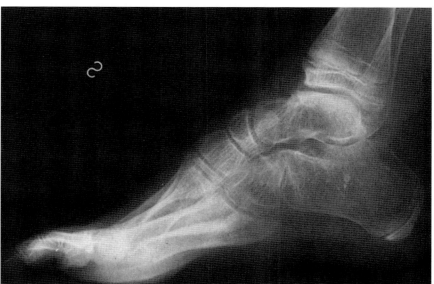

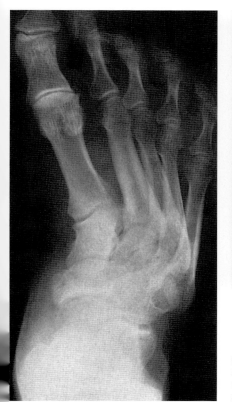

Fig. 15.**41 a, b   Clubfoot,** age 27. **a** Dorsoplantar view: markedly reduced talocalcaneal angle and overlapping metatarsals. **b** Lateral view: plantar flexion of the forefoot, and the long axes of the talus and calcaneus are parallel. The top of the talus is flat, a late complication.

Table 15.4   (Cont.) Differential Diagnosis of a Deformed Foot

Deformity	Radiographic Characteristics	Comments
Pes cavus (cavus deformity) (Fig. 15.42)	Dorsoplantar view: normal findings unless associated with other abnormalities. Lateral view: 1 increased talocalcaneal angle; 2 midtalar -first metatarsal lines form an angle, apex upward; 3 heel varus, heel valgus, equinus or calcaneus deformity may be present.	Abnormally high longitudinal arch of the foot, often associated with neuromuscular disease.
Tarsal coalition (Figs. 15.43–46)	*Calcaneonavicular coalition* may not become visible until ossified, then seen as fusion or abnormal articulation between the anterior process of the calcaneus and the navicular, best seen in a 45 degree medial oblique view of the foot. *Talocalcaneal coalition* usually takes place at the sustentaculum tali joint or near the os trigonum posteriorly. Sustentacular talar coalition is best seen from the tangential view of the heel (Harris view) with varying angles of the central beam parallel to the articular surfaces of the sustentaculum tali joint. A common secondary sign of talocalcaneal coalition is an osseous excrescence at the dorsal aspect of the talus, called talar beak.	Bony, cartilaginous or fibrous bridging of either the calcaneus and navicular or the calcaneus and talus, are common causes of *peroneal spastic flatfoot*. Tarsal coalition may not be seen before age 10 because tarsal ossification centers are small and coalition is still cartilaginous. Tarsal coalition in many multiple malformation syndromes involves the cuneiforms. Fusion of tarsal (and carpal) bones may be secondary to *rheumatoid arthritis* or an *inflammatory lesion*. Talar beak may be also secondary to degenerative changes in the talonavicular joint, or a plain anatomical variant once considered to be secondary to wearing high heeled shoes (Fig. 15.**46**).

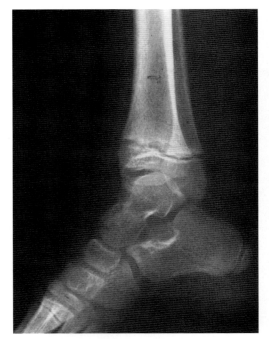

Fig. 15.**42   Pes cavus type deformity** in an 8-year-old with meningomyelocele.

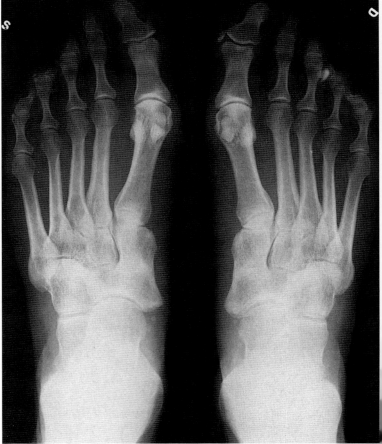

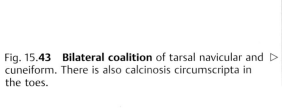

Fig. 15.**43   Bilateral coalition** of tarsal navicular and ▷ cuneiform. There is also calcinosis circumscripta in the toes.

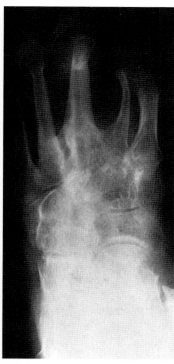

15.44a

15.44b

15.45a

15.45b

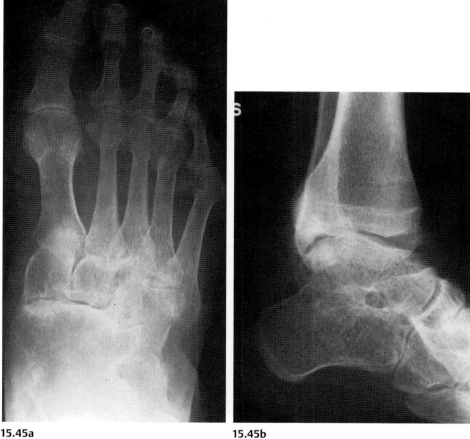

Fig. 15.**44 a, b   Tarsal coalition** in a foot with multiple malformations. The coalition involves calcaneus, cuboideum, cuneiforms and several metatarsals.

Fig. 15.**45 a   Midtarsal fusion** and **b talocalcaneal fusion** secondary to rheumatoid arthritis.

Fig. 15.**46   "Talar beak"** without associated abnormality.

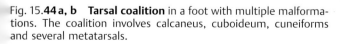

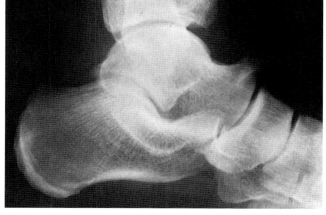

15.46

Tumors and Infections

Tumors involving hands and feet have radiographic characteristics not dissimilar to the general descriptions given in Chapter 5 and will not be discussed in detail here. The most common *benign bone tumor* of the small tubular bones of the hand is an *enchondroma*. It is also frequent in the foot. Whereas solitary enchondromas are usually seen between the ages of 10 and 50, *enchondromatosis* (Fig. 15.**47**) is already present in the very young. An epidermoid inclusion cyst may mimic an enchondroma (Fig. 15.**9**). The most common tumor in the foot is an *osteochondroma*. A *subungual exostosis* arises from the distal phalanx beneath the nail bed, usually on the medial aspect of the big toe. *Solitary bone cysts* appear frequently in the lateral aspect of the anteroinferior portion of the calcaneus (Fig. 15.**48 a**). A pseudocystic radiolucency in this location may mimic a true cyst (Fig. 15.**48 b**).

A calcified fleck in the cystic cavity is considered to be characteristic of *lipoma of the calcaneus* (Fig. 15.**48 c**). Malignant primary or metastatic bone tumors are rare in hands and feet. Also, soft-tissue tumors are rare. A *hemangioma* may be identified due to associated phleboliths and it may cause gigantism of the involved area. *Neurofibromatosis* may cause elephantoid-like soft-tissue changes and bone deformation. *Villonodular synovitis* may present as bone erosion and soft-tissue tumor.

Arthritides and inflammatory lesions of the bones are discussed in Chapter 6. Many of the characteristic features are seen in hands and feet, and are not repeated here.

Local trauma is the most common cause of *osteomyelitis* of the hands and feet, more common than hematogeneous (Fig. 15.**49**). In children, the calcaneus is an important site of primary hematogeneous osteomyelitis. It is relatively common (8.8 % of all hematogeneous infections), but may run an indolent course. *Osteomyelitis* in a diabetic (Fig. 15.**50**) and *neurotrophic (diabetic)* arthropathy with extensive demineralization may have identical patterns in the foot. *Tuberculosis* of the small tubular bones also causes pronounced demineralization, followed by bone destruction, minimal sclerosis, but no sequestra (Fig. 15.**51**). It is more common in fingers *(spina ventosa)* than in toes. Disseminated *fungal infections* may involve hands and feet. Their radiographic features are nonspecific and may mimic tuberculosis, pyogenic osteomyelitis, or a malignant neoplasm. Localized cyst-like rarefactions and sclerosis may also be present in noninflammatory conditions such as *tuberous sclerosis*, which especially affects the distal phalanges. The rare *granulomatous disease of childhood* occurs predominantly in hands and feet. It lacks local inflammatory signs, causing bone destruction without either sclerosis, abscess, or sequestra. *Sarcoidosis* can cause a variable spectrum of bone changes in hands and feet including cyst-like defects, acroosteolysis or acroosteosclerosis, periosteal reaction, and abnormal trabecular pattern of the small tubular bones.

Several infectious diseases that are rare in temperate regions are endemic and common in tropical areas. Many of them cause destructive changes in the underlying bone, although they primarily affect the skin and soft tissues. Often they are inoculated through the hands or feet. Since tropical diseases are rarely considered as a major differential diagnostic possibility in temperate or cold climates. They often involve the hands and feet and are summarized in Table 15.**5**.

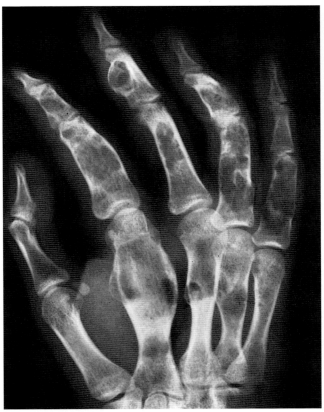

Fig. 15.**47** **Enchondromatosis of the hand.** Multiple, expansile radiolucent lesions cause marked deformity of the bones. Faint calcifications are seen within the tumors.

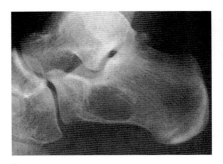
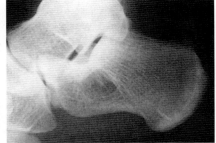
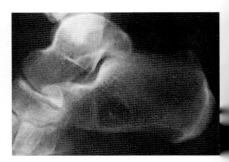

a   b   c

Fig. 15.**48 a–c** **a** Calcaneal cyst. **b** A **pseudocystic** lucency mimicking calcaneal cyst. **c Lipoma** of the calcaneus.

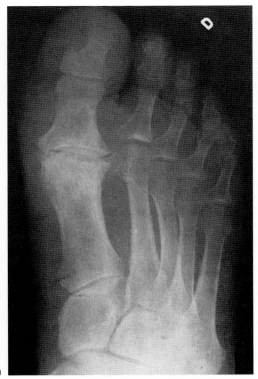

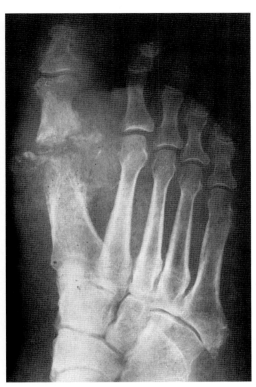

b

Fig. 15.**49 a, b   Pyogenic osteomyelitis** complicating an osteoarthritic first metatarsophalangeal joint. **a** Periarticular soft-tissue swelling and early destructive changes are seen in the sclerotic head of the first metatarsal, three weeks after penetrating trauma.

b Extensive destruction of the joint and adjacent bone eight months later.

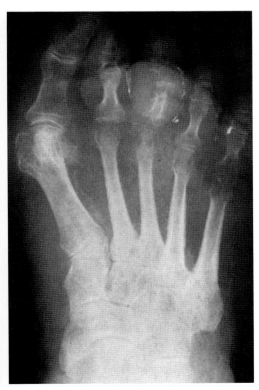

Fig. 15.**50   Diabetic foot.** Extensive bone destruction in the third toe and metatarsophalangeal joint due to **osteomyelitis**.

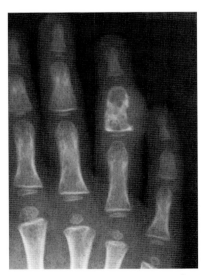

Fig. 15.**51   Tuberculous osteomyelitis** of the middle phalanx of the fourth finger. Radiolucent bone destruction and some sclerosis, but no sequestra.

Table 15.5   Tropical Diseases Involving Hands and Feet

Disease	Radiographic Findings	Comments
Yaws (Figs. 15.52, 15.53)	*Primary yaws:* skin eruption , no bone lesions. *Secondary yaws:* a sequence of osteoporosis, small, coalescent foci of bone rarefaction and florid periosteal reaction. *Tertiary yaws:* like secondary yaws but larger foci of destruction, some sclerosis and more ragged periostitis. Growth disturbances occur in children.	A nonvenereal infection caused by *Treponema pertenue.* Enters through skin abrasion, usually in childhood, and causes osteoperiostitis of feet, hands, legs, and forearms. Bone changes are seen in about one-sixth of the cases.
Leprosy (Fig. 15.54)	Three types of bone changes: 1 *Osteitis leprosum,* a localized cortical or subperiosteal bone destruction within the phalanges, especially the fingers. 2 *Nonspecific osteitis* modified by neurotrophic and vascular factors in patients with sensory loss: erosion of subungual tufts due to infection or acute osteitis. The phalanges in fingers and distal metatarsal bones may be eroded, fragmented or completely dissolved. 3 *Disuse osteoporosis.*	A *Mycobacterium leprae* infection. Disability is due primarily to involvement of peripheral nerves, which is minimal in the *tuberculoid* type, but extensive in the more virulent *lepromatous* type. About 15% of cases have bone changes. *Mimics diabetic neuropathy, congenital indifference to pain, syringomyelia, scleroderma, psoriasis, Raynaud's disease and frostbite.* May affect tarsal bones and result in Charcot-type joint.
Tropical ulcer	About 20% develop a nonspecific periosteal reaction of the underlying anterior tibia. A malignant change may occur in chronic cases.	A chronic ulcer, caused by the *fusiform bacilli* and *Vincent's spirochetes,* usually in mid-or lower leg.
Smallpox (variola) osteomyelitis	Within 10 days tubular bones show a transverse band of metaphyseal destruction with possible sequestration of the epiphysis. Periosteal new bone appears along the shaft. Original shaft may appear sequestered after 2 to 3 weeks, but becomes incorporated in the slowly remodeling involucrum. Growth disturbances, ankyloses, and secondary osteoarthritis are common,	Occurs in about 5% of young children with smallpox, 1–6 weeks after the onset of the disease. Metaphysitis of elbows, hands, wrists, ankles, and feet causes tenderness and swelling.
Mycetoma (Madura foot)	*Superficial:* Soft-tissue swelling in the confines of the plantar aponeurosis. *Deep:* Bone changes develop after several months: 1 endosteal cavitation, no sequestration; 2 parosteal erosion; 3 periosteal new bone; 4 amorphous expansion of bone. Usually affects tarsal and metatarsal bones, which appear moth-eaten,	Direct inoculation of fungus (actinomyces or maduromyces) via a thorn prick into the bare foot, causing either a superficial or deep plantar mycetoma. Sinus tracts discharge grains. Endemic in thorny, semidesert areas.
Filariasis	Enormous soft-tissue swelling. No underlying bone involvement; calcified coils of worms are rarely seen in soft tissues of extremities.	Infection of lymphatics by *Wuchereria bancrofti* worms. Lymphangitis and granulomatous or allergic reaction results in subcutaneous edema followed by lymphedema.

(continues on page 384)

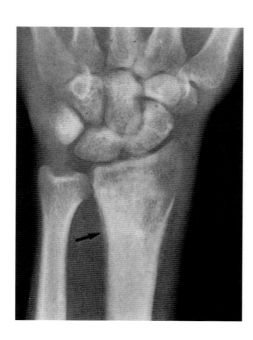

Fig. 15.**52   Secondary yaws** in distal radius seen as a bone rarefaction and periosteal reaction (arrow).

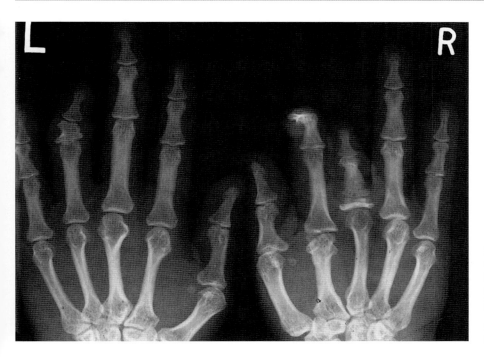

Fig. 15.**53** **Tertiary yaws.** Growth disturbances have resulted in short middle phalanx of the left fourth finger and rudimentary proximal phalanx of the right middle finger. There is flexion contracture of the distal interphalangeal joint in the right index finger.

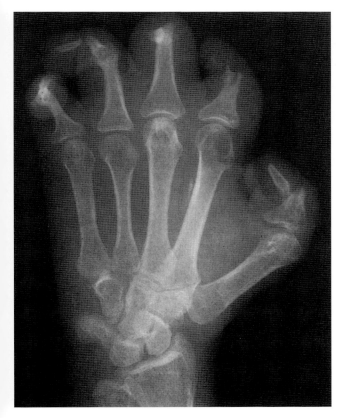

Fig. 15.**54** **Leprosy.** Bone destruction in fingers (non-specific osteitis).

Table 15.5 (Cont.) Tropical Diseases Involving Hands and Feet

Disease	Radiographic Findings	Comments
Guinea worm (dracunuliasis)	Serpiginous, coiled calcifications in subcutaneous tissues of the feet and ankles, also elsewhere.	The worm, *Dracunculus medinensis*, may cause an inflammatory reaction. Dead worms may calcify.
Loiasis	Fine, coiled, lacelike or filamentous calcifications between metacarpal and metatarsal bones.	Loa-loa infection is characterized by hot erythematous swellings, especially in upper limbs.
Kaposi's sarcoma	Soft-tissue nodules, osteoporosis of underlying bones, cortical erosions and small bone cysts. No new bone production or periosteal reaction.	A low-grade chronic malignancy, primarily affecting the skin as bluish-red, rubbery, highly vascular nodules. Feet, legs, hands, and arms usually affected. Common in equatorial regions and South Africa. High incidence in AIDS *(acquired immune deficiency syndrome).*
Ainhum (Fig. 15.55)	Constriction of soft tissue between proximal and middle phalanx of the fifth toe. Pressure may cause erosion, fracture, or dissolution of the underlying bone.	A nonspecific concentric inflammation of the deep fascial layers of the fifth toe. Affects African blacks and their descendants, mainly elderly men.
Sickle cell dactylitis (hand-foot syndrome) Fig. 15.56)	Bone destruction followed by periosteal new bone formation (bone within bone) secondary to bone infarction of the metacarpal, metatarsals, and/or phalanges.	Affects infants and young children with sickle-cell anemia. Hands and feet are tender and swollen. May be complicated by (salmonella) osteomyelitis. Osteomyelitis by itself may produce an identical picture.

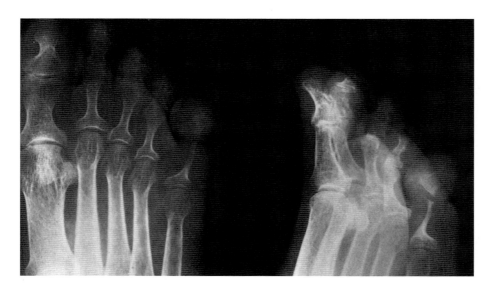

Fig. 15.**55** **Ainhum.** Dissolution of bone due to soft-tissue constriction of the middle phalanx of the fifth toe.

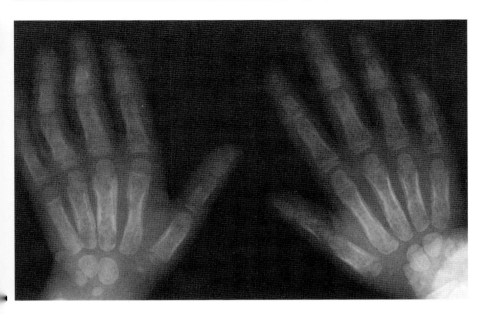

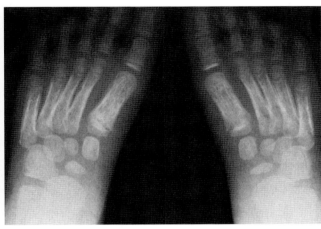

Fig. 15.**56 a, b**   **Sickle-cell dactylitis.** Bone destruction and periosteal reaction in both hands and feet. Radiographic changes are similar to osteomyelitis but occur symmetrically in multiple bones.

Traumatic Lesions

Fractures and other traumatic lesions of the hands and feet are an everyday problem. The most common location in the upper extremity is the wrist, and in the lower extremity, the ankle. The multiplicity of bones in hands and feet creates a wide variety of different lesions.

The alignment abnormalities of a lunate or perilunate dislocation should not remain unrecognized, since severe osteoarthrosis and permanent limitation of motion will ensue in untreated cases.

In a *perilunate dislocation*, the lunate maintains a normal relationship with the distal radius, and the surrounding carpal bones dislocate dorsally (Fig. 15.**57**). It is often associated with fractures of the ulnar styloid, the scaphoid bone, and the triquetrum. The lateral view shows dislocation that might be overlooked on an anteroposterior projection.

Lunate dislocation involves volar displacement of the lunate. The distal carpal row moves toward the radius to fill the space left by the lunate. This type of dislocation is clearly identified on the lateral projection (Fig. 15.**58**). *Scaphoid subluxation* may be a residual deformity from an incomplete reduction of a carpal dislocation, or it may result from a localized rupture of the lunate-scaphoid ligament. On an anteroposterior view, the scaphoid appears shortened, and there is a gap of more than 2 mm between lunate and scaphoid.

The epiphyses in the hands and feet may be duplicated, stippled, fragmented, or remain divided without fracture. In juvenile patients it is advisable to make a comparison with the opposite extremity in case of uncertainty. Among accessory ossicles of the wrists the os centrale (Fig. 15.**13**) and os triangulare (accessory ossicle between ulna and carpal bones) are of interest, since they are common in certain congenital malformation syndromes. Ossicles should not be confused with fractures. Fusion of the carpal bones can be a congenital anomaly. The most common is fusion of the lunate and the triquetrum (Figs. 15.**59**, 15.**63 b**). In the foot, major fractures and dislocations are usually not a problem to detect if one pays attention to the normal lines of alignment and the structural integrity of the bones. *Avulsion* fractures are generally thin and easily overlooked. They are usually seen only in tangential projection. Chip fractures of the foot should be sought at the site of clinical symptoms. Small avulsion fractures between the major bones are common. Sesamoids and accessory ossicles may have similar locations, but they are smooth in outline and frequently symmetrical (Fig. 15.**60**).

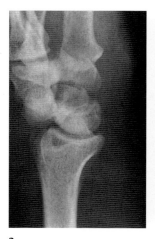
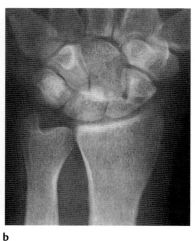

a   b

Fig. 15.**57 a, b**   **Perilunate dislocation** of the wrist with the lunate in normal relationship with the distal radius. Navicular fracture is associated (perilunate transschaphoid dislocation).

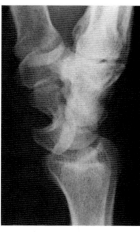
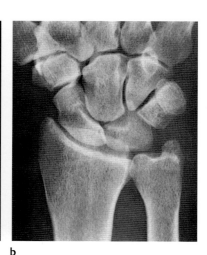

a   b

Fig. 15.**58 a, b**   **Lunate dislocation** with volar displacement of the lunate. **a** The shape of the lunate is abnormal in the AP projection, whereas the lateral view **b** shows abnormal location and alignment of the lunate.

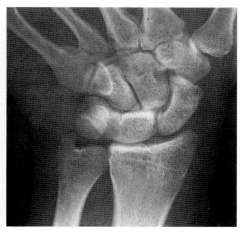

Fig. 15.**59**   **Fusion anomaly** of the lunate and triquetrum.

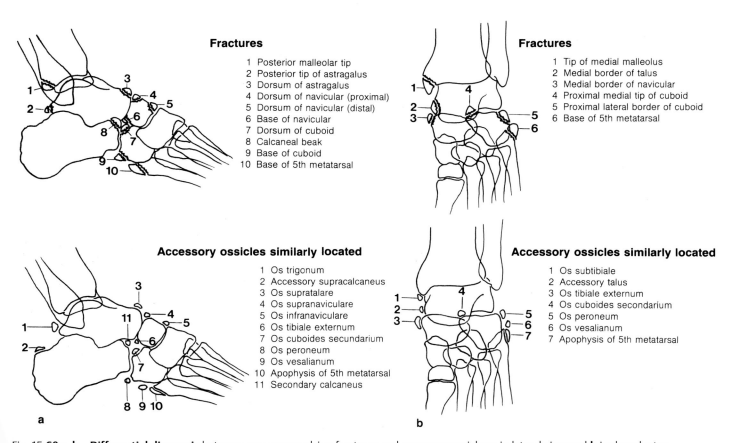

Fractures

1 Posterior malleolar tip
2 Posterior tip of astragalus
3 Dorsum of astragalus
4 Dorsum of navicular (proximal)
5 Dorsum of navicular (distal)
6 Base of navicular
7 Dorsum of cuboid
8 Calcaneal beak
9 Base of cuboid
10 Base of 5th metatarsal

Fractures

1 Tip of medial malleolus
2 Medial border of talus
3 Medial border of navicular
4 Proximal medial tip of cuboid
5 Proximal lateral border of cuboid
6 Base of 5th metatarsal

Accessory ossicles similarly located

1 Os trigonum
2 Accessory supracalcaneus
3 Os supratalare
4 Os supranaviculare
5 Os infranaviculare
6 Os tibiale externum
7 Os cuboides secundarium
8 Os peroneum
9 Os vesalianum
10 Apophysis of 5th metatarsal
11 Secondary calcaneus

Accessory ossicles similarly located

1 Os subtibiale
2 Accessory talus
3 Os tibiale externum
4 Os cuboides secundarium
5 Os peroneum
6 Os vesalianum
7 Apophysis of 5th metatarsal

a   b

Fig. 15.**60 a, b**   **Differential diagnosis** between common avulsion fractures and accessory ossicles **a** in lateral view and **b** in dorsplantar view.

Secondary Osteoarthritis

When *osteoarthritis* involves a nontypical joint of the hand or foot, one should look for an underlying factor. Any condition that limits normal motion results in exaggerated stress and predisposes to secondary osteoarthritis. In the wrist it is often an *old fracture*, especially of the scaphoid. In the foot, primary osteoarthritis usually involves only the first metatarsophalangeal, the first tarsometatarsal and the talonavicular joints. *Osteoarthrosis of one of the metatarsophalangeal joints* other than the first is likely to be secondary to trauma or avascular necrosis (*Freiberg's disease,*

Fig. 15.61). Avascular necroses occur relatively frequently in the lunate (*Kienböck*, Fig. 15.62), scaphoid (*Preiser*, Fig. 15.63), and the tarsal navicular (*Köhler*, Fig. 15.64). If all metatarsophalangeal joints are involved, *epiphyseal dysplasia* may be the underlying cause. Extensive osteoarthritis of the talonavicular joint points to abnormal subtalar motion (due to *tarsal coalition* or *subtalar arthritis*). Dramatic progression of denegerative changes with destruction in the ankle, tarsal joints, or, occasionally, in metatarsophalangeal joints is suggestive of a *neurotrophic process* (Charcot joint, Fig. 15.36). Neurotrophic changes in the hands are most commonly due to *syringomyelia*.

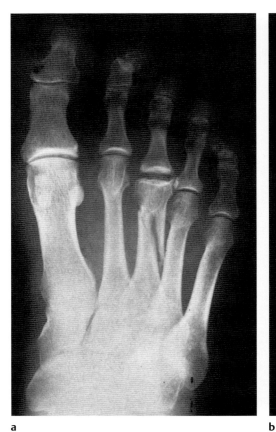

a

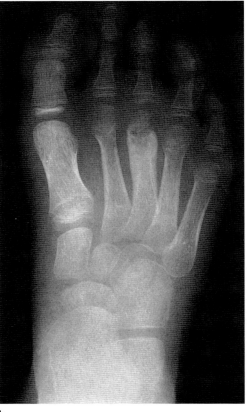

b

Fig. 15.**61 a**   **Avascular necrosis** of the third metatarsal head, incidentally associated with a fracture of the diaphysis of the third metatarsal. **b** Early avascular necrosis of the third metatarsal in a 7-year-old associated with epiphyseal destruction and periosteal reaction. Later a typical appearance of Freiberg's disease developed.

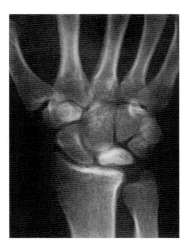

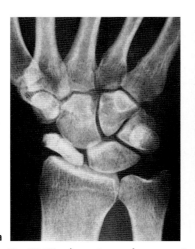

a

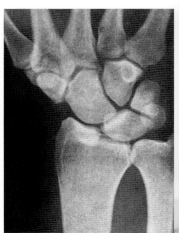

Fig. 15.**62**   **Avascular necrosis** of the lunate, evident as dense sclerosis of this bone.

Fig. 15.**63 a, b**   **a Avascular necrosis** of the scaphoid. **b fusion of the scaphoid into the radius** with abnormal alignment of the carpus. An unusual anomaly, somewhat mimicking avascular necrosis.

Soft-Tissue Changes

In a small percentage of films the definitive clue to diagnosis lies in the soft tissues. Often, careful analysis of the soft-tissue densities of the radiographs gives important supplementary information and helps in the differential diagnosis. Ultrasound examination using a high-frequency transducer is often helpful. At certain sites the information may be important enough to warrant a special soft-tissue exposure. The various causes of soft-tissue calcification have been presented in Chapter 7.

Apart from edema due to systemic diseases such as cardiac, renal, or hepatic failure, myxedema and malignancy, a *generalized increase of soft tissue in hands and feet* may represent overgrowth due to *acromegaly* (Fig. 15.65) or infiltration of the skin by edema and fibrous tissue in *idiopathic osteoarthropathy (pachydermoperiostosis)*.

In the absence of edema, myxedema, local infection, and the rare condition of pachydermoperiostosis, any increase in the heel pad thickness is a reliable indicator of acromegaly. Heel pad thickness of less than 21 mm in men and 18 mm in women in non-weight bearing practically excludes acromegaly. On the other hand, heel pad thickness of over 25 mm with a body weight of 60 kg and 30 mm with a body weight of 120 kg almost certainly indicates acromegaly.

A diffuse increase in soft tissue, usually due to edema, of the whole hand or foot may be due to *venous or lymphatic obstruction, Sudeck's atrophy, shoulder-hand syndrome, neurotrophic disorder* (in the hand, most likely syringomyelia, in the foot, diabetic neuropathy), or *myxedema* (Fig. 15.66). Transient edema may follow a *cerebrovascular accident*.

A *generalized decrease* of soft-tissue thickness in hands and feet is most commonly due to *collagen vascular diseases* (Fig. 15.67), *epidermolysis bullosa*, disuse from *muscle or neurologic abnormalities*, and, rarely, *lipodystrophy*.

Clubbing of Fingers

Bulbous configurations of the ends of fingers, called finger clubbing, is most commonly due to *bronchogenic carcinoma, cirrhosis of the liver, congenital heart disease, pulmonary hypertrophic osteoarthropathy, or pulmonary interstitial fibrosis* with or without *pneumoconiosis*. Several uncommon causes of finger clubbing include *pachydermoperiostosis, polycythemia*, and some *chronic infections*. It may rarely be idiopathic.

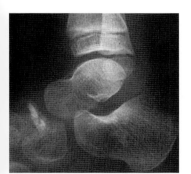

Fig. 15.**64**   **Avascular necrosis** of the navicular, which is shrunken and sclerotic.

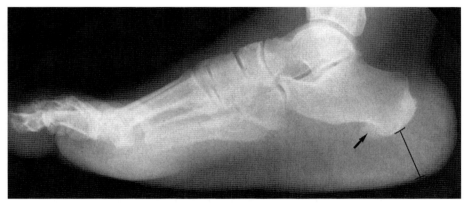

Fig. 15.**65**   **Acromegaly.** Generalized incearse of soft tissues of the foot, best seen as increased thickness of the heel pad. Calcaneal "spur" is also demonstrated (arrow).

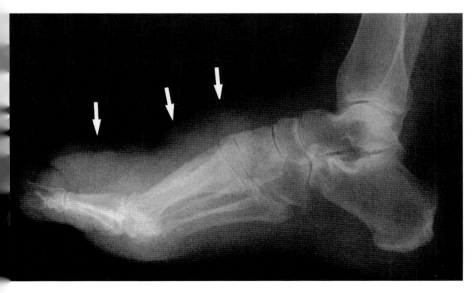

Fig. 15.**66**   **Localized myxedema** of the dorsum of the foot seen as increased soft-tissue thickness without bone lesions (arrows).

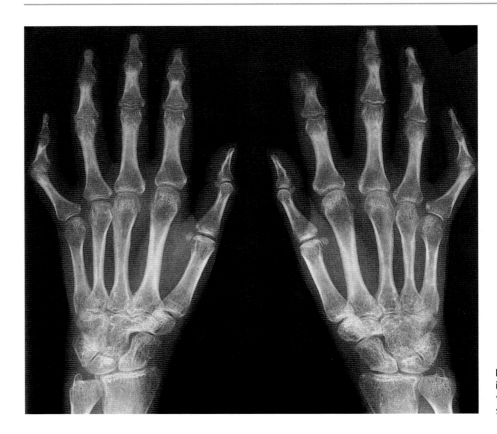

Fig. 15.**67** **Scleroderma.** Generalized soft-tissue atrophy associated with both acro-osteolysis and acrosclerosis.

Soft-Tissue Masses

An isolated soft-tissue mass in the hand or foot may represent a benign or malignant *soft-tissue tumor* or an underlying arthritis. Subcutaneous nodules in *rheumatoid arthritis* are more common in the extensor surface of the forearms, but may occur in hands. *Tuberculosis* (cold abscess) may rarely cause a localized mass in a digit, whereas other granulomatous diseases (e.g., sarcoidosis and leprosy) tend to cause more generalized swelling of a digit. Metabolic arthritides *gout* (see Figs. 6.**63**–6.**69**) *amyloidosis, lipoid dermatoarthritis*, and *hyperlipidemia* may produce discrete soft-tissue masses. These should be distinguished from soft-tissue masses and mucoid cysts adjacent to the joint margins in *osteoarthrosis*, commonly seen in the distal interphalangeal joints of fingers. Localized swelling of soft tissue may also be due to inflammation of the subcutaneous tissues, called *cellulitis*. Radiolucent areas in a localized subcutaneous swelling indicate either gas-forming organisms such as *Clostridia (gas gangrene)* or access of air into tissues through an open wound (subcutaneous emphysema).

Articular effusions cause expansion and/or increased density of the soft tissues of the joint involved. *Rheumatoid arthritis, viral infections* (particularly viral hepatitis), *sarcoidosis*, and several *gastrointestinal disorders* (Whipple's disease, ulcerative colitis, Crohn's disease, Henoch–Schönlein purpura, and small-bowel bypass surgery) may develop monoarticular or polyarticular effusions without bone lesions. Other causes of monoarticular effusions are gout, fungal infections, tuberculosis, hemophilia, and villonodular synovitis. Secondary erosion of underlying bone often follows. Unlike rheumatoid arthritis, *psoriatic arthritis* and *Reiter's syndrome* affect joints in a random fashion, involving tendons as well as joint capsules. The entire finger may become swollen (sausage finger). Overgrowth or other causes of enlargement of digits involving both soft tissues and possibly also osseous structures is called localized gigantism. Causes of localized gigantism are presented in Table 15.**6**.

Table 15.6   Localized Gigantism in Hands or Feet

Disease	Radiographic Findings	Comments
Macrodystrophia lipomatosa (Fig. 15.68)	Overgrowth of both soft tissues and osseous structures; second and third digits of either hand or foot are most frequently involved. Soft-tissue overgrowth is most marked along the volar aspect. The phalanges are long, broad and often splayed. Changes are most severe at the distal ends of the digits.	A rare form of congenital localized gigantism. The condition may be static or progressive, but growth ceases with puberty. Polydactyly or syndactyly is often associated, clinodactyly is almost invariable.
Maffucci's syndrome	Multiple enchondromas in the bones of hands and feet, with the addition of hemangiomas seen as phleboliths, and soft-tissue masses.	Radiographic features are similar to those of Ollier's disease (multiple enchondromas), with the addition of soft-tissue masses.
Klippel–Trenaunay–Weber syndrome	Localized gigantism with both soft-tissue and osseous overgrowth. May affect an entire extremity or only the distal digits. Other osseous anomalies are common.	A triad of cutaneous capillary hemangiomas, varicose veins and localized gigantism. Arteriovenous malformations are common.
Neurofibromatosis	Enlarged digits may be bilateral, not necessarily involving contiguous digits. Distal phalanges are not most severely affected. Premature fusion of the growth plates may occur.	Macrodactyly resulting from plexiform neurofibromas combined with mesodermal dysplasia.
Hemangioma Lymphangioma	Soft-tissue enlargement in the involved region.	Phleboliths may be present in a hemangioma.
Ollier's disease	Multiple enchondromas	Large enchondromas may cause an appearance of localized gigantism even in the absence of soft-tissue tumor.
Dactylitis (Fig. 15.69)	Soft-tissue mass in a digit secondary to infection, infarction gout, sarcoidosis, or Still's disease.	See Chapter 6.

(continues on page 392)

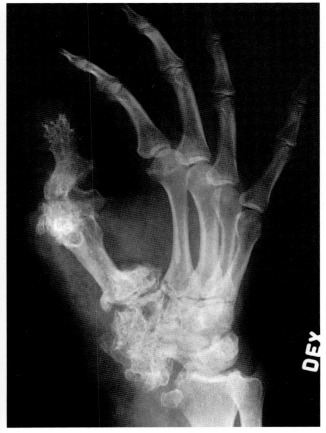

Fig. 15.**68** **Macrodystraphia lipomatosa** involving the soft tissues and bones of the thumb, first metacarpal and trapezium.

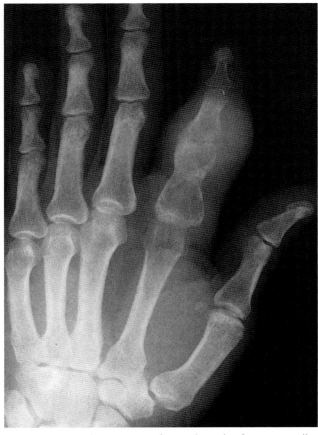

Fig. 15.**69** **Dactylitis in sarcoidosis.** The index finger is swollen, and the proximal phalanx contains coarse, expansile bone lesions.

Table 15.6 Localized Gigantism in Hands or Feet

Disease	Radiographic Findings	Comments
Osteoid osteoma	Bone changes in metatarsals, metacarpals or phalanges are variable, depending on the location of the tumor. Soft-tissue swelling may be prominent.	See Chapter 5.
Melorrheostosis (Fig. 15.70)	Characteristic osseous excrescences along the length of the involved bone simulate candle wax flowing down the side of a lit candle.	Growth disturbance may cause increased circumference and inequality of limb length. Soft-tissue changes include tense, erythematous skin and subcutaneous edema.
Localized myxedema (Fig. 15.66)	Soft-tissue swelling without bone involvement.	A rare cause of localized enlargement of a limb.

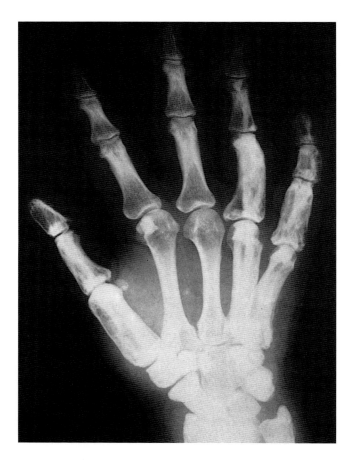

Fig. 15.**70** **Melorrheostosis.** The first, fourth, and fifth metacarpals and finger bones are thickened. The sclerotic changes follow the length of the bones. There is also soft-tissue swelling.

Tendons, Capsules, and Bursae

A properly exposed radiograph is able to delineate some tendon sheaths and joint capsules. Inflammation in these locations manifests itself as either an increased density or an increased width. Ultrasound examination is more sensitive and will show decreased echogenicity and/or expansion due to edema, effusion and inflammation.

Tenosynovitis of the *extensor pollicis brevis* and the *abductor pollicis longus* can cause obliteration of tissue planes in the radial aspect of the wrist.

In rheumatoid arthritis the *extensor carpi ulnaris* tendon is frequently involved and recognized by swelling of the ulnar side of the wrist in anteroposterior projection. Distension of the capsules of interphalangeal and metacarphophalangeal joints may further document synovitis.

The anatomy of the Achilles tendon is sharply defined on a lateral projection of the ankle due to a triangular fat pad anterior to it (Kager's triangle). The normal diameter of the Achilles tendon is 9 mm or less. Any cause of *tendinitis, edema,* or *hemorrhage* results in an increased diameter of the Achilles tendon, with or without loss of sharpness of the posterior margin of Kager's triangle. Causes of an increased diameter of the Achilles tendon include hemorrhage due to *rupture, stress tendinitis,* edema due to *venous stasis, infection* of adjacent tissues, or *inflammation* (rheumatoid arthritis, ankylosing spondylitis, Reiter's syndrome, and gout). Inflammation of the retrocalcaneal bursa between the bone and the Achilles tendon may cause an erosion of the posterior calcaneus. This is characteristic for an inflammatory arthritis. Any of the *metabolic arthritides* (gout, amyloidosis, lipoid dermatoarthritis and hyperlipidemia) may increase the diameter of the Achilles tendon or produce localized swelling. In asymptomatic hypercholesterolemic patients, increased thickness (over 9 mm) of the Achilles tendon is virtually diagnostic of familial hypercholesterolemia (Fig. 15.71), since nonfamilial hypercholesterolemia does not produce xanthomatous thickening of the Achilles tendon.

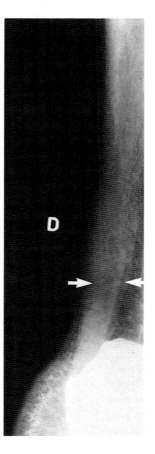

Fig. 15.**71   Thickening of the Achilles tendon** measuring 13 mm in diameter in familial type IIA hypercholesterolemia.

The extent of tendon involvement is dependent on the patient's age and serum cholesterol concentration. Ultrasound examination is more sensitive than radiography in detecting subtle xanthomas in the Achilles tendon of a patient with familial hypercholesterolemia.

Chest

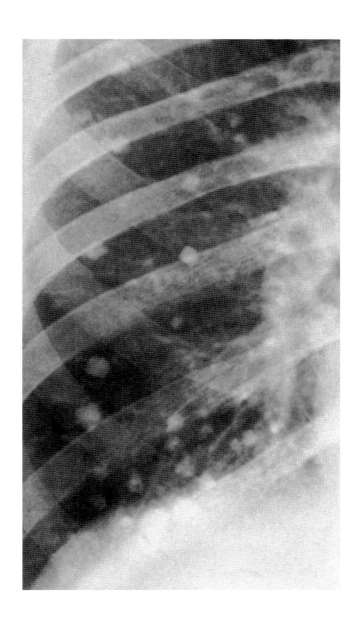

16 Cardiac Enlargement

Most of the diseases involving the heart will cause either generalized or localized enlargement of the heart or great vessels. A small heart is usually constitutional (asthenia, senility, wasting) and only rarely reflects a disease (Fig. 16.**1**). Exceptions to this are *adrenal insufficiency, constrictive pericarditis, dehydration,* or an *asthmatic paroxysm* with emphysema, where a relatively small heart may be considered to reflect the effects of the disease process itself.

The size of the heart can be estimated in several ways. A simple approach is the *cardiothoracic index:* the ratio between the total transverse diameter of the cardiac shadow and the internal diameter of the chest (Fig. 16.**1a**). After the age of 5 years, this ratio normally varies, between 0.4 and 0.5. In smaller children and neonates, the ratio may be as high as 0.6, and during the second month after birth even 0.65.

The cardiac volume can be estimated with a fair degree of accuracy by measuring the *relative volume* of the heart according to the following equation:

$$\text{Relative cardiac volume} = \frac{L \times B \times S \times 0.44}{\text{body surface area (m}^2)}$$

where L = longest diameter of the heart in posteroanterior view; B = broad diameter of the heart (perpendicular to L); and S = longest sagittal diameter of the heart in lateral view (Fig. 16.**1b, c**). Factor 0.44 applies to the film-focus distance of 2 m. If this distance is 1.5 m, a factor of 0.42 should be used instead. The surface area of the body is available from charts if the height and weight of the body are known (Fig. 16.**2**). The relative volume of the heart shows great interindividual variation. Values between 350 cc/m² and 500 cc/m² are considered normal for men. In women they tend to be slightly smaller. A single measurement of the relative volume has therefore little diagnostic value, but it may be useful in the follow-up of an individual patient, since many interindividual variables are then excluded. Interindividual variation of interthoracic pressure and other factors still have a great effect (Fig. 16.**3**). Enlargement of in-

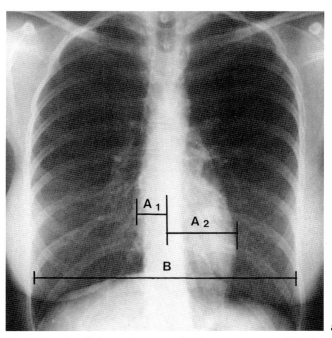

Fig. 16.**1a   Small heart in an asthenic woman,** age 20. The method of measuring the cardiothoracic index is shown.

$$\text{Cardiothoracic index} = \frac{(A_1 + A_2)}{B}$$

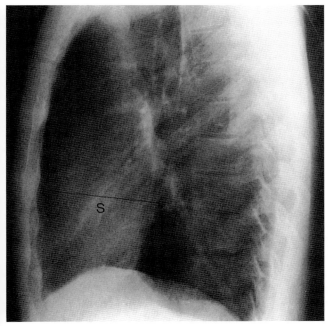

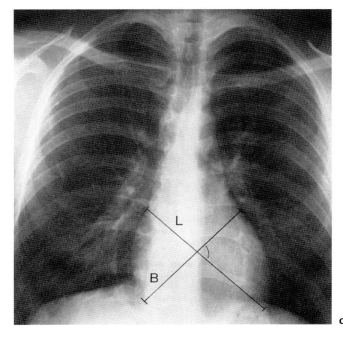

Fig. 16.**1b, c**

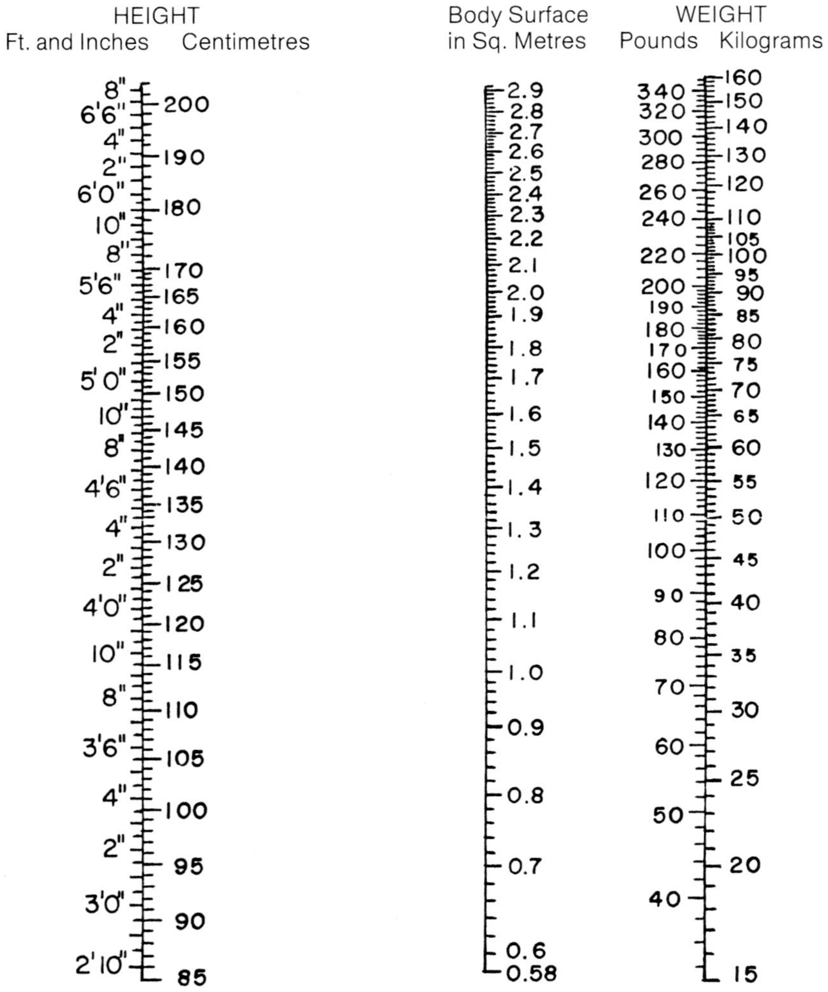

HEIGHT
Ft. and Inches Centimetres

Body Surface
in Sq. Metres

WEIGHT
Pounds Kilograms

Fig. 16.2 Nomogram for the determination of body surface area of adults (adapted from Documenta Geigy, Scientific Tables, Basel). Join patients weight and weight with a line. In the mid column you find the body surface.

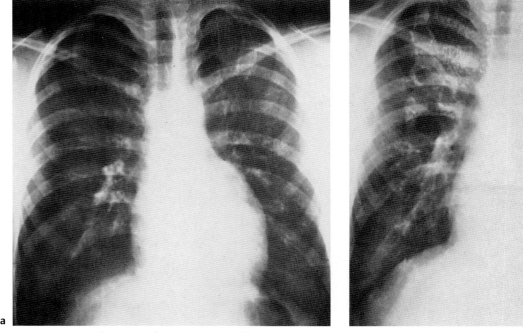

a

Fig. 16.3 **Great change in the appearance of heart size is produced by the Valsalva effect.** The two exposures were taken a few minutes apart.

dividual chambers of the heart may cause typical configurations, as seen in Fig. 16.4. When there is enlargement of several chambers, the pattern is more complicated and its interpretation may be difficult. In addition to evaluating the configuration of the margins of the heart itself, one has to observe carefully the location and relative size of the pulmonary trunk and aorta as well as of the pulmonary vasculature. The effect of abnormalities of the thoracic cage has to be taken into account as well. The heart may appear enlarged in the frontal projection if the sagittal diameter of the thoracic cage is decreased. This is the case in the *straight back syndrome* and in *pectus excavatum*.

Left ventricle:
- cardiac apex bulges down and left
- positive Hoffman–Rigler sign on lateral view: the posterior border of the left ventricle extends 1.8 cm or more posteriorly to the posterior border of the inferior vena cava at a level 2 cm cephalad to their crossing.

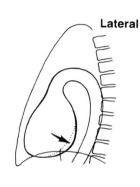
Lateral
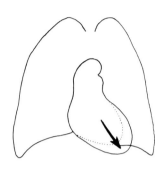

Left atrium:
- esophagus displaced posteriorly
- prominent left auricle
- dense left atrial shadow, double contour on the right
- elevated left main bronchus
- left lower lobe collapse in an extreme case, due to obstructed left lower lobe bronchus

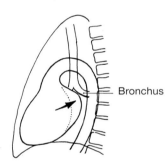
Bronchus
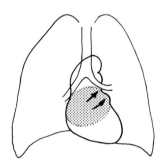

Right ventricle:
- cardiac enlargement toward left with elevated apex
- filling of retrosternal space
- may displace right atrium toward right
- may displace left ventricle backwards
- often poorly seen except for pulmonary stenosis, tetralogy of Fallot, etc.

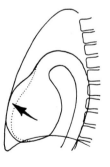
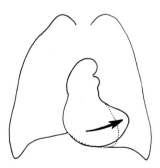

Right atrium:
- right heart border beyond ¹/₃ of the right hemithorax
- may fill the retrosternal space
- rare as a solitary finding

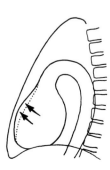
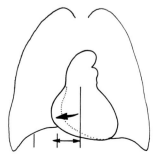

Fig. 16.4 Typical manifestations of the enlargement of individual cardiac chambers

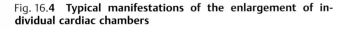

Evaluation of a suspected congenital heart disease is a difficult task and often it is impossible to name a specific diagnosis without ultrasound examination, catheterization or angiography. A dynamic MRI examination is also diagnostic. When analyzing plain films, the following morphological features should be evaluated in each case:

1 Cardiac enlargement – which chambers are enlarged?
2 The size of the aorta- small, wide, narrow, dilated?
3 The vascular pedicle – narrow or wide?
4 Right-sided aortic arch?
5 A notch in the aortic arch, resulting in a number 3 appearance?
6 Pulmonary vascularity: are the main trunks of the pulmonary artery wide or unusually narrow; is there pulmonary oligemia or hyperemia?
7 The pulmonary artery segment in the left cardiac shadow: large and convex or small and concave.
8 Rib notching (see Fig. 16.**40**).

The following clinical information is important in evaluating suspected congenital heart disease:

1 Is the patient cyanotic or not?
2 Is there right- or left-sided dominance in electrocardiography?
3 Are there typical murmurs?

By using the radiographic and clinical information, it is possible to classify congenital heart diseases of childhood into various groups as presented in Table 16.**1** or often to predict the correct diagnosis, unless multiple defects exist.

In a neonate, only two congenital heart diseases can be diagnosed with great certainty because of their characteristic appearance in chest roentgenogram, namely, *total anomalous pulmonary venous return* (snowman heart) (see Fig. 16.**48**) and *pulmonary stenosis with atrial septal defect* (prominent main pulmonary trunk with oligemic lungs). In other cases further clinical information is very helpful in narrowing down the differential diagnostic possibilities. Nowadays ultrasound and Doppler ultrasound examinations have largely replaced plain radiographic analysis of the heart.

Based on the time of appearance of cardiac failure and cyanosis, the patients can be divided into the following groups:

1 Cardiac failure manifests early (at birth or during the first week) but there is no cyanosis: *hypoplasia of the left heart; atresia of the aortic* (and *possibly mitral) valve; coarctation of aorta.*
2 Cardiac failure develops later: *ventricular septal defect; patent ductus arteriosus; truncus arteriosus; total anomalous pulmonary venous return (TAPVR).*
3 Cyanosis develops at birth or within a week: *transposition of great vessels; hypoplastic right heart; Ebstein's anomaly; tricuspid atresia; obstructive type of TAPVR.*
4 Cyanosis develops later during childhood: *tetralogy of Fallot; pulmonary stenosis with atrial septal defect.*

Table 16.**3** gives the approximate relative frequency of the congenital heart diseases. In Table 16.**5**, the diseases are grouped according to their dominant, most common or earliest findings. The differential diagnostic groupings in Table 16.**2** may be helpful in narrowing the differential diagnosis in congenital heart diseases in children.

In the adult patient with suspected congenital heart disease, the following features are of particular importance: the position of the diaphragm (high or low); degree of inspiration; calcifications; Kerley B-lines; the appearance of the branches of the pulmonary artery; possible arteriovenous malformations in the lung parenchym anomalous veins across the lung field.

Evaluation of Blood Flow and Blood Pressure in Lungs

When blood circulation through the lungs is increased, both arteries and veins are full of blood. This occurs in left-to-right shunting (Table 16.**1**) and to a milder degree in hyperkinetic conditions (*hypervolemia, anemia, polycytemia, pregnancy, hyperthyroidism*). A clear oligemia may be a result of a right-to-left shunt or narrow or obliterated pulmonary arterial channels (*narrow pulmonary artery, thromboembolic disease* or*emphysema*). Pulmonary blood flow can increase two to three times before the arterial pressure increases. When the precapillary pressure increases, the peripheral branches of the pulmonary arteries appear narrow, but the central trunks are wide.

An increase in the pulmonary venous pressure causes characteristic changes in the distribution of blood in the lungs. On upright films of an adult untreated patient, such changes relatively accurately reflect the pulmonary venous and left atrial pressure as diagrammatically presented in Fig. 16.**5**. These changes, together with the less sensitive changes in the size and configuration of the heart, are the cornerstone of the radiographic diagnosis of congestive heart failure. The findings in the most common conditions involving left ventricular strain are presented in Table 16.**4**. Although the radiologic evaluation of the pulmonary venous pressure is relatively accurate, the evaluation of venous pressure of the right side is difficult on roentgenograms and is better assessed from the filling of the veins of the patient's neck. Occasionally a prominent azygos vein may be seen (see Fig. 16.**6a**). In conditions such as acute myocardial infarction, even the central venous pressure readings do not reliably reflect the patient's hemodynamic condition.

Pericardial effusion mimics generalized cardiomegaly. Although it sometimes may cause a characteristic (bottle-like) configuration of the heart shadow, most of the cases are difficult to diagnose on plain films, and as much as 200 ml of pericardial fluid usually goes undetected in the primary reading. Ultrasound examination CT or MRI are far more sensitive than plain films in detecting pericardial effusion.

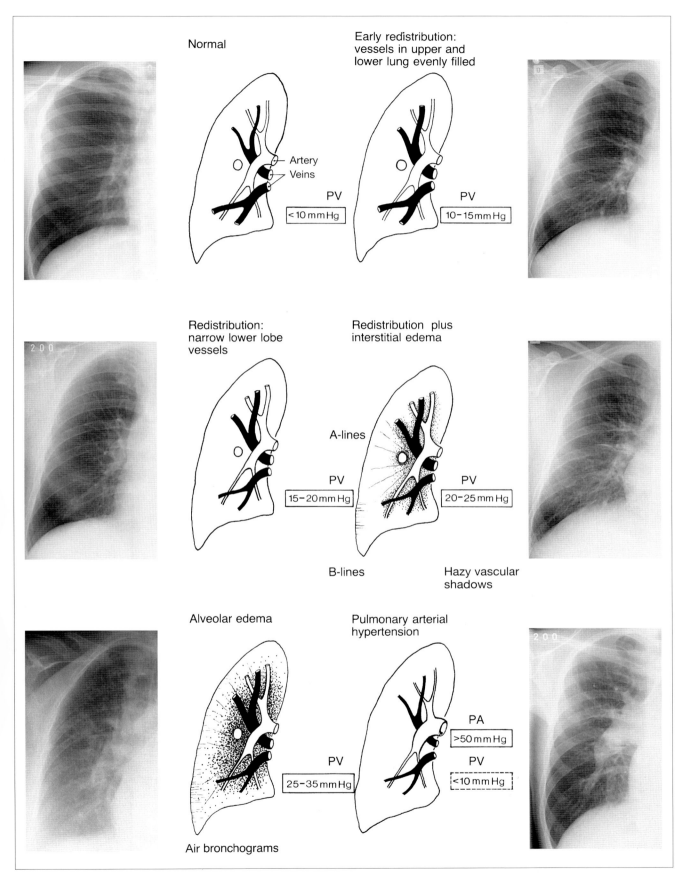

Normal

Early redistribution: vessels in upper and lower lung evenly filled

Artery
Veins

PV
<10 mm Hg

PV
10–15 mm Hg

Redistribution: narrow lower lobe vessels

Redistribution plus interstitial edema

A-lines

PV
15–20 mm Hg

PV
20–25 mm Hg

B-lines

Hazy vascular shadows

Alveolar edema

Pulmonary arterial hypertension

PA
>50 mm Hg

PV
25–35 mm Hg

PV
<10 mm Hg

Air bronchograms

Fig. 16.**5** **Manifestations of increased pulmonary venous (PV) and arterial (PA) pressure.**

Table 16.1 Pulmonary Vasculature in Congenital Heart Disease

Pulmonary vasculature	Cyanosis	Diseases
Increased	Cyanotic	Mixed lesions with major malformations: 　　Complete transposition 　　Truncus arteriosus (Type I) 　　Single ventricle 　　Common atrioventricular canal 　　Total anomalous pulmonary venous return
	Acyanotic	Left to right shunts: 　　Atrial septal defect 　　Ventricular septal defect 　　Patent ductus arteriosus 　　Aorticopulmonary defect 　　Partial anomalous pulmonary venous return
Normal	Acyanotic	Coarctation of aorta Aortic stenosis Subaortic stenosis Pulmonary arterial stenosis Congenital mitral stenosis Endocardial fibroelastosis
Decreased	Cyanotic	Tetralogy of Fallot Trilogy of Fallot Truncus (pseudotruncus) arteriosus Tricuspid atresia Ebstein's anomaly Pulmonary stenosis with ASD or transposition

Table 16.2 Some General Differential Diagnostic Features of Congenital Heart Disease

Unusually small ascending aorta and aortic arch	Atrial septal defect Ventricular septal defect Uncorrected transposition of great vessels
Enlarged ascending aorta and aortic arch	Patent ductus arteriosus Valvular congenital aortic stenosis Coarctation of aorta Truncus arteriosus
Concave pulmonary artery segmented in posteroanterior view	Tetralogy of Fallot Tricuspid atresia Ebstein's anomaly Pseudotruncus arteriosus Uncorrected transposition of great vessels
Prominent pulmonary artery segment (a moderate prominence is normal under age 20 or in pregnancy)	Patent ductus arteriosus Atrial septal defect Ventricular septal defect Eisenmenger's complex Valvular pulmonary stenosis (poststenotic dilatation) Cor pulmonale
Enlarged left atrium in a child	Patent ductus arteriosus Ventricular septal defect Congenital mitral stenosis

Table 16.3 Relative Frequency of Various Entities Among Congenital Heart Diseases
(Significant congenital heart diseases occur in approximately 1% of babies)

Common	
Ventricular septal defect	20–25%
Patent ductus arteriosus	12–15%
Tetralogy of Fallot	11–15%
Pulmonary stenosis without ventricular septal defect	10–15%
Atrial septal defect	7–14%
Transposition of great vessels	5–9%
Coarctation of aorta	5–9%
Congenital aortic stenosis	3–6%
Rare	
Tricuspid atresia	1.2–3%
Truncus arteriosus	1–3%
Single ventricle	2–3%
Corrected transposition	1.2–3%
Common atrioventricular canal	2%
Total anomalous venous return	2%
Aortic atresia	2%
Pulmonary atresia	1–1.7%
Endocardial fibroelastosis	1%
Ebstein's anomaly	1%

The rest are very rare (less than 1%).

Table 16.4 Radiologic Findings in Common Conditions which Cause Left Ventricular Strain

Pulmonary Veins	Size of the Left Ventricle	
	Normal	**Enlarged**
Normal	No heart disease Aortic valve stenosis Arterial hypertension	Athlete's heart Aortic regurgitation Myocardial damage
Venous congestion	Acute myocardial infarction Mitral stenosis Hypervolemia Constrictive pericarditis	Congestive heart failure Mitral regurgitation
Both arteries and veins distended	Atrial septal defect Patent ductus arteriosus Ventricular septal defect Arteriovenous malformation	Possible enlargement of the left ventricle depends on the magnitude of shunting.

Table 16.5 Predominantly Left Ventricular or Generalized Cardiac Enlargement

Disease	Radiographic Findings	Comments
Athlete's heart (no disease)	Generalized cardiomegaly with left ventricular prominence, no pulmonary vascular changes.	Associated with bradycardia (large stroke volume); secondary to excessive training.
Arteriosclerotic heart disease (myocardial ischemia)	Chest roentgenogram is usually unrevealing. Variable degrees of generalized or left ventricular enlargement may occur.	Calcification of the coronary arteries indicates coronary atherosclerosis.
Acute myocardial infarction (Figs. 16.6–16.8)	Chest roentgenogram is often unrevealing. Some cardiac dilatation, with variable degrees of pulmonary venous congestion, occurs frequently. Acute pulmonary edema may ensue.	Myocardial aneurysm may develop early in the infarcted muscle or later in the scar. It is seen as a bulge or an unusual prominence in the left ventricular border, which occasionally calcifies.
Postmyocardial infarction syndrome (Dressler's syndrome)	Rapid increase in the heart size due to pericardial effusion, always accompanied by either pleural effusion and/or pulmonary infiltrates in the left base or bilaterally.	Can occur a few days or up to two months following an acute infarction. Left-sided or bilateral pleural effusion is the most common finding (80 %) and may occur alone. Pericardial effusion is present in 70 % and pulmonary infiltrates in 60 % of cases. Response to steroid therapy is striking.

(continues on page 406)

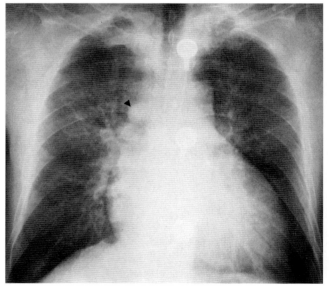 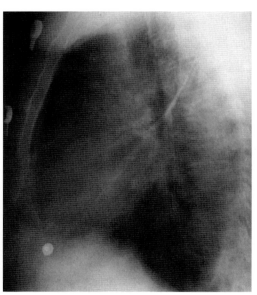

Fig. 16.**6 a, b Acute myocardial infarction. a** dilatation of the heart, pulmonary edema, and congestion of the azygos veins (arrowhead). **b** Lateral view reveals pleural effusion in the pleural fissures.

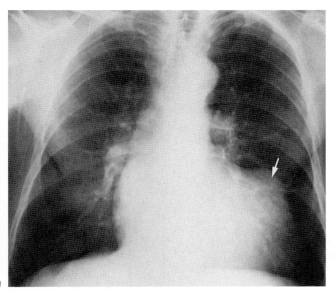
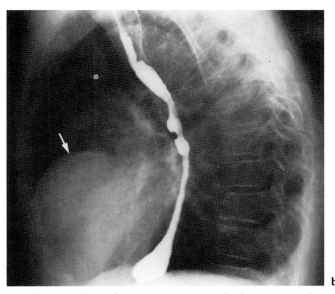

b

Fig. 16.**7 a, b** **Left ventricular aneurysm after myocardial infarction.** A bulge in the cardiac contour is seen in both projections (arrows). Pulmonary vasculature indicates mild venous congestion.

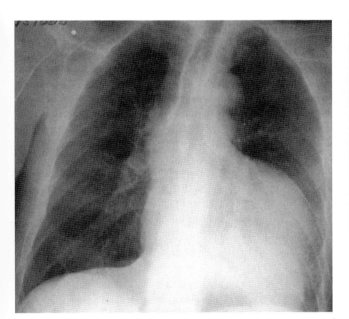
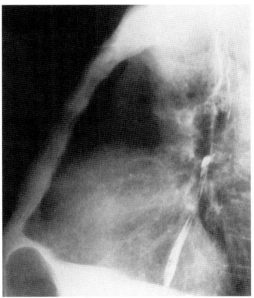

b

Fig. 16.**8 a, b** A large **left ventricular aneurysm** bulges posteriorly, a complication of myocardial infarction. A double density is seen in the AP projection.

Table 16.5 (Cont.) Predominantly Left Ventricular or Generalized Cardiac Enlargement

Disease	Radiographic Findings	Comments
Congestive myocardial failure		
Left-sided failure (Fig. 16.9)	Cardiac enlargement, related to the severity of failure and the precongestive heart size. The increase of pulmonary venous pressure can be evaluated as presented in Fig. 16.5). Pleural effusions (bilateral or right-sided).	Pulmonary signs of congestive failure without significant cardiac enlargement. Pericardial calcification is seen in 50%. Often the cardiac configuration resembles that of mitral stenosis. Unilateral left-sided effusion is likely due to causes other than congestive failure.
Right-sided failure (Fig. 16.10)	Dilatation of the right ventricle and atrium. Widening of the superior vena cava and azygos vein. Liver enlargement.	If right heart failure develops following left heart failure, pulmonary venous congestion from left-sided failure diminishes.
Chronic arterial hypertension (hypertensive heart)	Left ventricular hypertrophy may produce no radiographic changes or some rounding of the left margin. Left ventricular dilatation causes typical signs of left ventricular enlargement. The aortic knob enlarges concomitantly. Congestive failure may supervene.	Hypertension is most often essential but may be associated *with renal* or *renovascular disease, coarctation of the aorta, adrenal diseases with adrenal hyperfunction, collagen diseases (lupus erythematosus, polyarteritis nodosa),* or *hyperthyroidism.*
Aortic valve insufficiency (Aortic regurgitation) (Fig. 16.11)	Dilated left ventricle, concave left cardiac border, some dilatation of the ascending aorta and sometimes calcification of the aortic annulus or even the valves. Congestive failure may supervene in advanced cases. Radiographic findings may be subtle although findings in ultrasonography may be obvious.	Insufficiency of the aortic valve can be secondary to: 1 Primary damage of the valve (e.g., *rheumatoid endocarditis, bacterial endocarditis, congenital valvular deformity, lues, ankylosing spondylitis and Reiter's disease, mucopolysaccharidosis, spontaneous or traumatic rupture of the valve,* or *degenerative phenomena*); 2 Diseases of the aortic wall or annulus fibrosus (e.g., *cystic medial necrosis, Marfan's syndrome, dissecting aneurysm, lues, arterial hypertension*); or 3 Congenital malformation of the aortic root (e.g., *aneurysm of the sinus of Valsalva, congenital coronary fistula,* or *high ventricular septal defect with prolapse of the noncoronary cusp*). Congenital aortic insufficiency is usually due to a bicuspid valve. *Acute* aortic insufficiency occurs in *bacterial endocarditis, rupture of the valve* or *dissecting aneurysm.*

(continues on page 408)

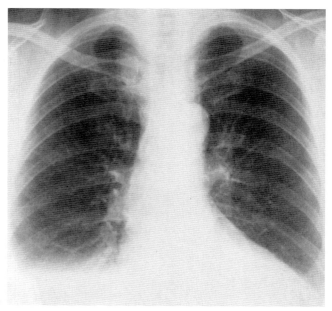
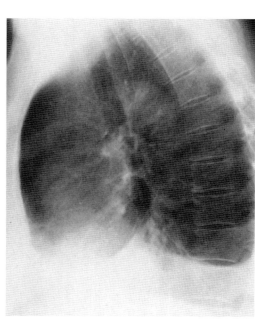

a
b

Fig. 16.**9 a, b** **Chronic left heart failure.** There is left ventricular enlargement, pulmonary venous congestion and bilateral pleural effusion, more on the right side.

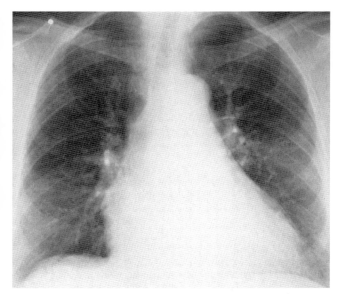

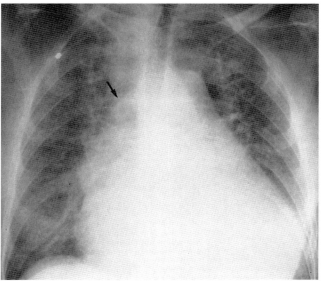

b

Fig. 16.**10 a, b Congestive left heart failure developing into both left- and right-sided failure. a** Left ventricular enlargement and pulmonary venous congestion. **b** Enlargement of the heart, in-cluding the right side, widening of the mediastinum (superior vena cava, and severe pulmonary venous congestion). The azygos vein is also congested (arrow).

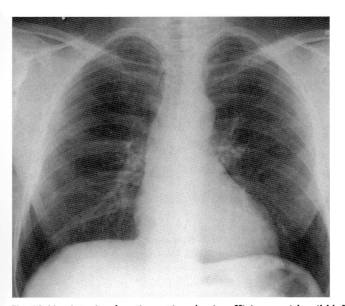

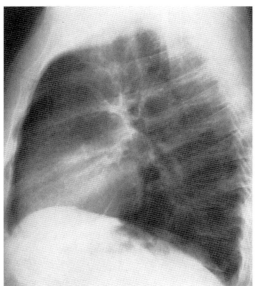

b

Fig. 16.**11 Arteriosclerotic aortic valve insufficiency with mild left ventricular enlargement**, no congestive heart failure, and a nor-mal-looking aorta.

Table 16.5   (Cont.) Predominantly Left Ventricular or Generalized Cardiac Enlargement

Disease	Radiographic Findings	Comments
Combined aortic valve insufficiency and stenosis (Fig. 16.12)	Dilatation of the left ventricle and ascending aorta is more prominent and left atrium may enlarge. May mimic pure aortic stenosis.	Rheumatoid heart disease usually causes a combination of aortic valve stenosis and insufficiency.
Subvalvular aortic stenosis (idiopathic hypertrophic subaortic stenosis)	Enlarged left ventricle, often enlarged left atrium. Poststenotic aortic dilatation is absent.	Narrowing of the left ventricular outflow tract by muscular hypertrophy. Essentially ultrasonographic diagnosis.
Supravalvular aortic stenosis	The heart may be enlarged or normal, the aorta is normal or small.	Congenital fibrous ring or thickening above the sinuses of Valsalva. Frequently associated with idiopathic hypercalcemia of infancy.
Aortic stenosis		See Table 16.**9**
High-output heart	Cardiac enlargement, dilatation of the main pulmonary artery, prominent pulmonary vasculature (both arteries and veins).	*Associated conditions:* Pregnancy or athletic (physiological). Severe anemia including sickle-cell anemia, leukemia, or primary polycythemia. Beriberi (vitamin B deficiency). Hypervolemia (fluid overload). Extrapulmonary arteriovenous fistula. Mild forms occur in extreme obesity, thyrotoxicosis, and pyrexia. Advanced Paget's disease is a rare cause of high-output heart.
Myocardiopathy (Figs. 16.13 and 16.14)	Diffuse enlargement of the heart, predominantly of the left ventricle. The aorta appears small as compared with the size of the heart. Pulmonary venous congestion may develop. Moderate left atrial enlargement and fullness of the main pulmonary artery occurs. Superimposed pericardial effusion may further enlarge the cardiac shadow.	The many causes of myocardiopathy may be classified into five groups: 1 Idiopathic, unassociated with extracardiac disease: *non-specific myocardosis; endocardial fibroelastosis (neonate or child); postpartum cardiopathy.* 2 Infectious: *Coxsackie B and other viral infections; Chagas' disease (South American trypanosomiasis) ; rheumatic, septic, diphtheric, toxoplasmic.* 3 Infiltrative: *amyloidosis (especially primary), generalized glycogen storage disease (Pompe's disease, infant); leukemia.* 4 Endocrine: *hypothyroidism; acromegaly; Cushing's disease; thyrotoxicosis.* 5 Miscellaneous causes: *ischemic; uremia; collagen diseases; nutritional deficiency (beriberi, alcoholism, potassium or magnesium depletion); toxicity (drugs, chemicals, cobalt); sarcoidosis; neuromuscular dystrophy.* A combination of cardiac enlargement and normal pulmonary vasculature is usually due to one of the following four entities: 1 Myocardiopathy; 2 Aortic stenosis; 3 Aortic coarctation, or 4 Athlete's heart.

(continues on page 410)

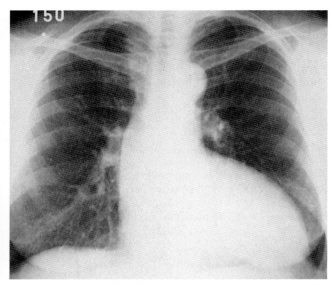

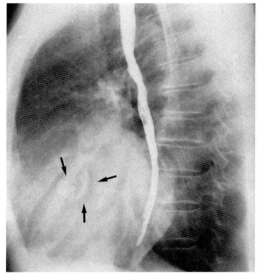

Fig. 16.**12 a, b Combined aortic valve stenosis and insufficiency of rheumatic origin.** Extensive enlargement of the left ventricle and dilated ascending aorta. Aortic valve calcification is
demonstrated (arrows)

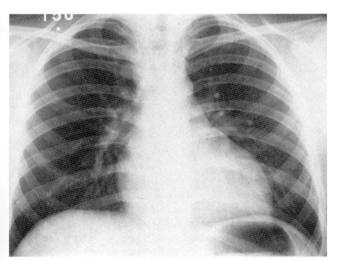

Fig. 16.**13 Uremic myocardiopathy.** Left ventricular enlargement without congestive failure. The aorta is relatively small.

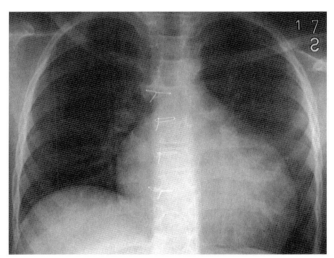

Fig. 16.**14 Diabetic cardiomyopathy** in a child aged 10. The
heart is large, and left ventricles is very prominent. Pulmonary
vasculature is normal.

Table 16.5 (Cont.) Predominantly Left Ventricular or Generalized Cardiac Enlargement

Disease	Radiographic Findings	Comments
Mitral insufficiency **Coarctation of aorta** **Patent ductus arteriosus** **Ventricular septal defect**	Left ventricular enlargement is a feature in these conditions as well as in a number of rare congenital heart diseases.	Since other characteristics are more useful for differential diagnosis they will be discussed elsewhere.
Pericardial defect **(Fig. 16.15)**	1 Displacement of the heart to the left without displacement of trachea. 2 Unusual configuration of the left heart border (bulging aortic, pulmonary arterial and left ventricular segments). 3 Bulging through a partial defect may mimic left ventricular aneurysm, but shows no paradoxal pulsations.	Either total (in 3/4) or partial absence of pericardium, usually on the left side, which usually is symptomless and discovered incidentally. Displacement of the heart may simulate left ventricular enlargement. A deep notch between the aorta and pulmonary artery is characteristic.
Acute glomerulonephritis in children	Generalized cardiomegaly Pleural effusions Pulmonary interstitial or alveolar edema	Cardiac dilatation occurs in over 50% of acute cases in children. The mechanism is unknown. The radiographic changes subside together with healing of the underlying disease.
Pericardial effusion **(Figs. 16.16–16.17)**	Enlarged cardiac shadow mimics generalized cardiomegaly. Large effusions tend to obliterate normal cardiac markings. There is less posterior displacement of the barium-filled esophagus in the lateral view than could be expected from the apparent heart size. Rapid changes occur in the cardiac silhouette in consecutive films, in the absence of pulmonary vascular enlargement. Postural alterations change cardiac contours. The pulmonary vasculature is decreased and the superior vena cava may be prominent if tamponade of the right atrial inflow occurs.	Common causes of pericardial effusion are: *Pericarditis* (especially Coxsackie virus, but also in other infections) *Congestive heart failure* *Collagen diseases (LED)* *Cardiac surgery or trauma* *Renal failure* *Postmyocardial infarction syndrome* *Tumor invasion* (from lung or mediastinal lymphoma) or metastases (from lung, breast, or melanoma) *Radiation therapy* *Still's disease*
Transposition of great vessels **(Fig. 16.18)**	"Egg-on-side" cardiomegaly that appears during the first week after birth together with congestive heart failure. Concave pulmonary artery segment, although vascularity in the lungs is increased unless transposition is associated with pulmonary stenosis, the latter occurs in 15%. Narrow vascular pedicle in frontal projection (aorta and pulmonary artery are superimposed), seen in 50%.	A rare anomaly, but the most frequent form of congenital heart disease associated with cyanosis present since birth. Due to lack of spiralization of the spiral septum, the aorta remains anterior and originates from the right ventricle. The pulmonary artery is behind the aorta and originates from the left ventricle. Pulmonary and systemic circulation are connected through a defect in the atrial and/or ventricular septum or through a patent ductus arteriosus.
Tricuspid atresia		See Table 16.7
Anomalous left coronary artery	Radiographic changes are identical to other myocardiopathies such as endocardial fibroelastosis (see under myocardiopathy in this Table, above).	Left coronary artery originating from the pulmonary artery is the most common significant anomaly of the coronary circulation.

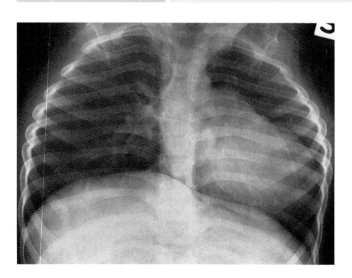

Fig. 16.**15 Pericardial defect**, age 5. The heart (not mediastinum) is displaced to the left. The aortic, pulmonary, and left ventricular segments are sharply bulging, a characteristic pattern.

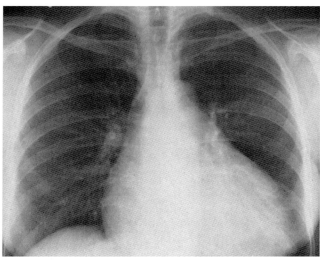 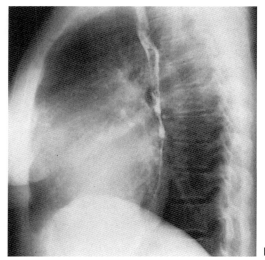

Fig. 16.**16 a, b**   **Pericardial effusion.** The cardiac shadow is large, but the esophagus in the lateral view is not proportionally displaced posteriorly.

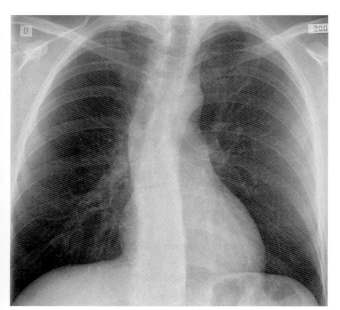 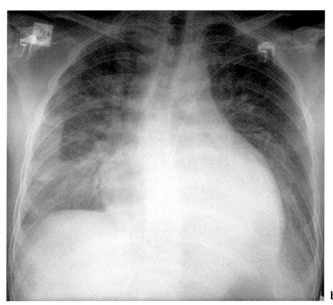

Fig. 16.**17 a, b**   **Still's disease.** Fig. 16.**17 a** was taken one month before Fig. 16.**17 b**. Massive increase in heart size is due to pericardiac effusion which also caused emerging heart tamponade and pulmonary constriction.

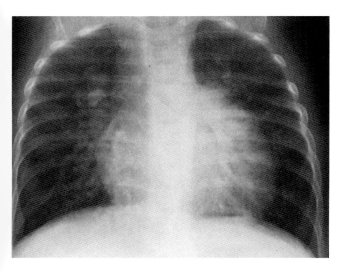

Fig. 16.**18**   **Transposition of great vessels.** "Egg-on-side" cardiomegaly and a concave pulmonary segment associated with increased vascularity of lungs. Narrow vascular pedicle.

Table 16.6 Predominantly Left Atrial Enlargement

Disease	Radiographic Findings	Comments
Mitral stenosis (acquired or congenital) (Figs. 16.19 and 16.20)	1. Left atrial enlargement 2. Possible calcification of the mitral valve, not to be confused with the heavy calcification of the mitral anulus 3. Pulmonary venous congestion 4. Prominent main pulmonary artery segment, enlarged hilar vessels 5. A small aortic knob 6. Right ventricular enlargement, normal-sized left ventricle 7. Dilatation of the central pulmonary arteries and narrowing of peripheral arteries (pulmonary arterial hypertension) 8. Pulmonary parenchymal changes due to hemosiderosis (granular opacities) (see Fig. 21.**17**), multiple up to 8 mm ossifications, or pulmonary fibrosis (pulmonary infarctions)	Obstruction of flow from the left atrium into the left ventricle during diastole, resulting in increased pressure and enlargement of the left atrium. The increased pressure is transmitted to the pulmonary veins and eventually to the pulmonary arteries and the right heart. The usual cause is a *rheumatic* valvular lesion. *Congenital mitral stenosis* can be identical to the rheumatic one (short chordae tendineae, fibrotic valves and fused commissures). A rare congenital form of mitral stenosis is the *parachute deformity* (all chordae tendineae originate from a single papillary muscle). The latter is associated with other anomalies. In the early phase, congenital mitral stenosis and a left-to-right shunt may appear similar but in mitral stenosis the vascular shadows are hazier due to venous and lymphatic congestion. Enlarged confluence of right pulmonary veins may mimic left atrial enlargement or tumor.

(continues on page 414)

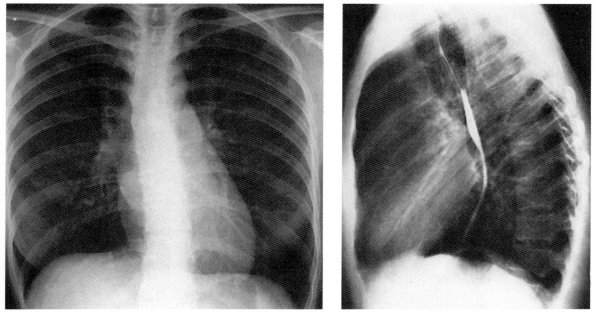

b

Fig. 16.**19 a, b** **Mitral stenosis, early.** The left atrium is enlarged and seen as a double density in the PA projection. It displaces the esophagus posteriorly. Pulmonary vasculature is unremarkable.

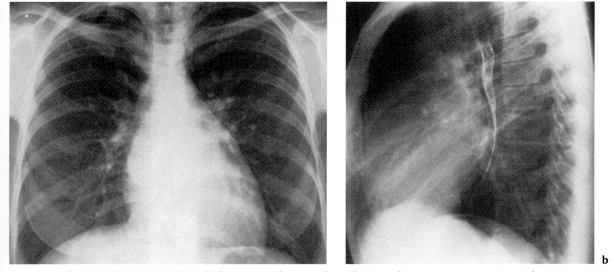

b

Fig. 16.**20 a, b** **Mitral stenosis.** Enlarged left atrium, right ventricle, and main pulmonary artery segment, pulmonary venous congestion and a small aortic knob.

Table 16.6 (Cont.) Predominantly Left Atrial Enlargement

Disease	Radiographic Findings	Comments
Mitral insufficiency (mitral regurgitation) (Figs. 16.21–16.24)	1 Enlarged, sometimes enormous left atrium 2 Enlarged left ventricle 3 Small or normal aortic knob 4 Normal pulmonary vasculature, sometimes venous congestion and prominent pulmonary artery are present.	Most commonly caused by *rheumatic valvulitis*, but may also be caused by functional dilatation of the mitral ring secondary to other cardiac diseases (*congestive heart failure, acute rheumatic fever, aortic valve disease, coarctation of aorta*), or from *papillary muscle dysfunction*. Regurgitation of blood during ventricular systole leads to overfilling and dilatation of the left atrium and dilatation of the left ventricle. In most cases both valvular conditions (stenosis and insufficiency) coexist, giving a mixed pattern, Mitral disease is often associated with aortic disease or tricuspid disease or both, which results in a complicated radiographic pattern.
Myxoma of the left atrium	The heart may have a configuration of mitral stenosis. Calcification of the tumor is rare, but helpful in differential diagnosis if present.	Myxoma is the most common tumor of the heart, which usually occurs in the left atrium.
Patent ductus arteriosus **Ventricular septal defect** **Myocardiopathy** **Congenital coronary fistula** **Trilogy of Fallot** **Tricuspid atresia**	Left atrial enlargement may be a significant feature in these conditions.	Other radiographic changes are more diagnostic and these entities are presented elsewhere in this Chapter.

(continues on page 416)

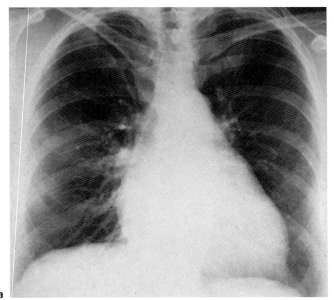 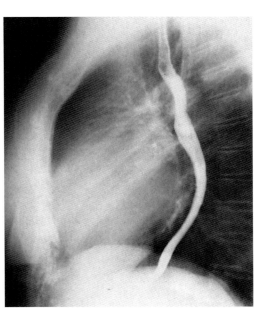

a   b

Fig. 16.**21 a, b** **Mitral insufficiency.** Enlarged left atrium and left ventricle, small aortic knob. Normal pulmonary vasculature.

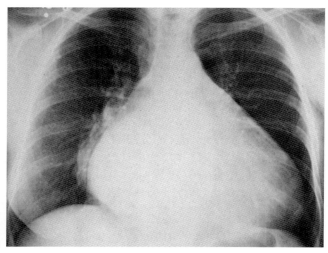
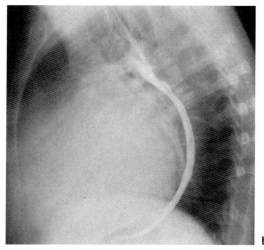

Fig. 16.**22 a, b**   **Mitral insufficiency.** Enormous left atrium, dilatation of the left ventricle and generalized cardiomegaly with small aortic knob.

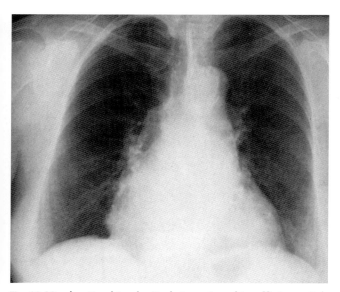
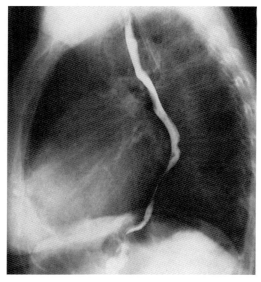

Fig. 16.**23 a, b**   **Combined mitral stenosis and insufficiency.** Enlargement of left atrium and both ventricles. Pulmonary venous congestion.

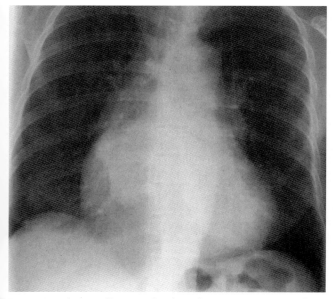
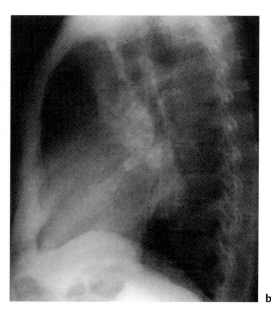

Fig. 16.**24 a, b**   **Confluence of right pulmonary veins mimicking enlarged left atrium.** The patient has aortic and mitral insufficiency and pulmonary venous congestion. The bulge caused by an enlarged right pulmonary venous confluence is more localized than an enlargement of the left atrium and may mimic a tumor, **a** Oblique and **b** lateral views.

Table 16.6 (Cont.) Predominantly Left Atrial Enlargement

Disease	Radiographic Findings	Comments
Constrictive pericarditis (Fig. 16.25)	Pulmonary venous congestion without cardiac enlargement. Left atrium is usually prominent. Calcification of the pericardium may be seen. The pattern mimics mitral stenosis.	Lack of calcification does not exclude constrictive pericarditis. Conversely, calcified pericardium is associated with constrictive pericarditis only in about 50 % of cases.
Single ventricle (cor triloculare biatriatum) (Fig. 16.26)	Plain film findings are not diagnostic. Left atrium is often enlarged and pulmonary vasculature increased, sometimes suggestive of ventricular septal defect.	A single functional ventricle usually associated with other anomalies, most often pulmonary artery stenosis.

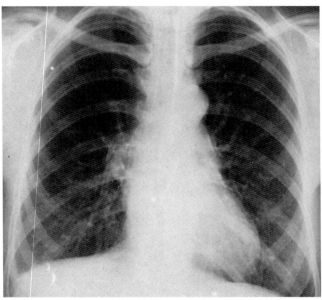
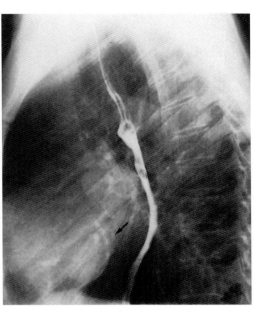

Fig. 16.**25 a, b Constrictive pericarditis.** Enlarged left atrium displaces barium-filled esophagus in the lateral view. Pulmonary venous congestion in the absence of generalized cardiomegaly mimics mitral stenosis. Pericardial calcification (arrow).

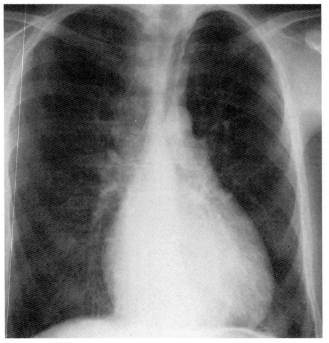
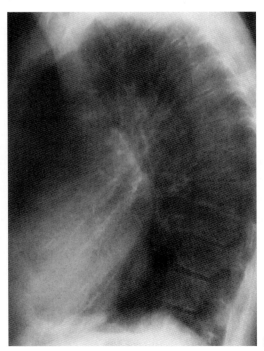

Fig. 16.**26 a, b Single ventricle.** Mild cardiomegaly, prominent left atrium, small aorta, and increased pulmonary vascularity.

Table 16.7   Predominantly Right Ventricular Enlargement

Disease	Radiographic Findings	Comments
Tetralogy of Fallot (Figs. 16.27 and 16.28)	Changes depend on the degree of pulmonary stenosis and the size of the septal defect. 1 Right ventricular enlargement causes elevation of the cardiac apex but heart is not particularly big. 2 Pulmonary blood vessels are either oligemic or normal-looking. 3 The main pulmonary artery segment is concave or small. 4 The size of the aorta is normal or enlarged. Right-sided aortic arch is present in 25%. 5 Short straight lines in lungs represent enlarged bronchial arteries.	The most common cyanotic congenital heart disease. Primary changes are infundibular pulmonary stenosis and a high ventricular septal defect. Overriding of the aorta and right ventricular hypertrophy are secondary structural defects. Mixing of venous blood with arterial blood leads to cyanosis after closure of ductus arteriosus. The smaller the pulmonary artery, the bigger the aorta. A typical radiographic appearance is present only in one-third of cases. If pulmonary stenosis is minimal, the clinical picture is as in ventricular septal defect. If foramen ovale persists, the condition is called *pentalogy of Fallot*.

(continues on page 418)

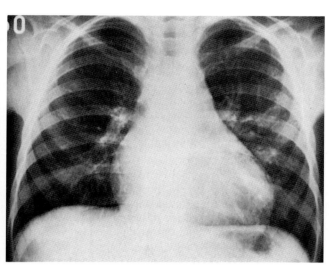
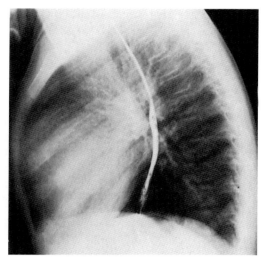

Fig. 16.**27 a, b   Tetralogy of Fallot** in a child. The right ventricle is enlarged but the main pulmonary segment is concave, and the pulmonary blood vessels normal-looking or slightly oligemic.

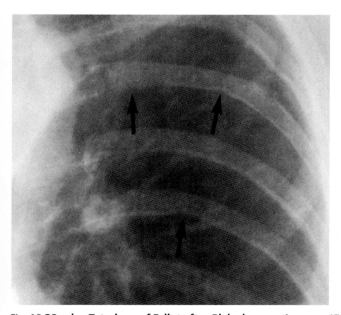
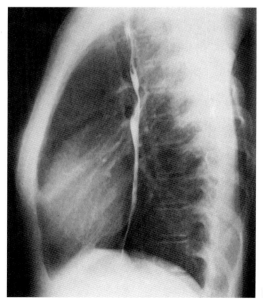

Fig. 16.**28 a, b   Tetralogy of Fallot after Blalock operation,** age 17, Relatively small heart but apex still elevated and pulmonary artery segment very small. Rib notching post-Blalock operation (arrows).

Table 16.7 (Cont.) Predominantly Right Ventricular Enlargement

Disease	Radiographic Findings	Comments
Tricuspid atresia (mimics right ventricular enlargement) (Fig. 16.29)	"Pure" tricuspidal atresia 1 Normal or slightly enlarged heart size. 2 The left heart border is rounded and elevated, simulating right ventricular enlargement. 3 Concave main pulmonary artery segment. 4 Pulmonary oligemia with eventual reticular densities representing bronchial arteries. 5 Right-sided aortic arch (in 20%). 6 Left atrial enlargement (in 50%).	Congenital obliteration of the tricuspid valve that results in early cyanosis. Blood that should flow into the right ventricle is deviated through an atrial septal defect or foramen ovale into the left atrium and into the enlarged left ventricle. The roentgenographic appearance may mimic tetralogy of Fallot but electrocardiography shows left axis deviation (right axis deviation in Fallot's tetralogy). Usually associated with pulmonary artery obstruction (infundibular stenosis or pulmonary valvular atresia).
	If associated with transposition of great vessels (in more than 25% of cases) the appearance is different: 1 The aorta is small. 2 Pulmonary vasculature is increased. 3 The abnormally located right auricular appendage bulges in the left upper cardiac border.	Tricuspid atresia with transposition of great vessels may be present with or without pulmonary arterial obstruction.
Truncus arteriosus (common aorticopulmonary trunk) (Fig. 16.30)	1 Right ventricular enlargement in a slightly enlarged heart 2 Absence of the usual main pulmonary artery (concave pulmonary artery segment) 3 Hypervascular lungs (types I–III). If pulmonary arteries are hypoplastic, lungs are hypovascular (type IV). 4 Right-sided aortic arch in one-fourth of cases	A usually fatal failure of the development of the spiral septum. Several forms of the takeoff of pulmonary arteries from the common trunk, including absence of pulmonary arteries (type IV), which results in a radiographic picture similar to the tetralogy of Fallot.
Pseudotruncus arteriosus	1 Large right ventricle 2 Concave main pulmonary artery segment 3 Pulmonary oligemia (bronchial arteries may be seen) 4 Right-sided aortic arch The plain film appearance of pseudotruncus is identical to tetralogy of Fallot.	The term pseudotruncus arteriosus is used to designate atresia of the pulmonary valve or the main pulmonary trunk, associated with a ventricular septal defect. There is an intracardiac right-to-left shunt (VSD) and a left-to-right shunt at patent ductus arteriosus.
Chronic left heart failure (myocardiopathy, mitral insufficiency) **Mitral stenosis**	Right ventricular enlargement occurs often in these conditions secondary to pulmonary arterial hypertension.	See Tables 16.5 and 16.6
Cor pulmonale **Left-to-right shunt** **Pulmonary stenosis**	Increased flow or pressure causes enlargement of the right ventricle in these conditions.	Enlargement of the main pulmonary artery segment is a more sensitive sign and easier to appreciate. Hence, these conditions are discussed under the enlargement of pulmonary artery segment (Table 16.10).

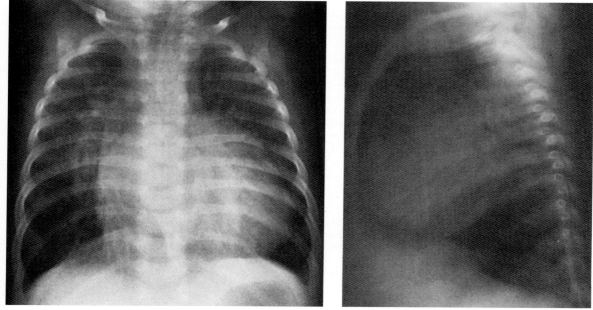

Fig. 16.**29 a, b   Tricuspid atresia,** age 2 months. The heart is enlarged and rounded. The pulmonary artery segment is concave, and the left atrium is enlarged. The reticular vascular pattern represents enlarged bronchial arteries.

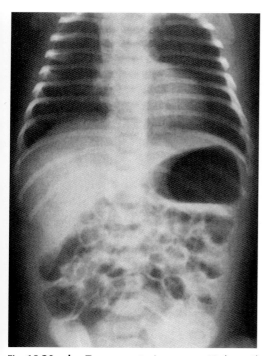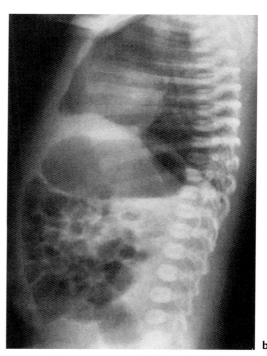

Fig. 16.**30 a, b   Truncus arteriosus,** age 10 days, Absence of pulmonary artery (concave segment), elevated cardiac apex, hypovascular lungs, and right-sided aortic arch.

Table 16.8 Right Atrial Enlargement or Prominent Right Heart Border

Disease	Radiographic Findings	Comments
Pericardial cyst or lipoma (Figs. 16.31 and 16.32)	A localized bulge usually at the cardiophrenic angle; no cardiovascular abnormality.	Fat or fluid content can be demonstrated with CT
Hypoplasia of the lung and/or pulmonary artery (Fig. 16.33)	Displacement of the normal-sized heart shadow towards right. Vessels of the lung may be abnormally small (arterial hypo-plasia). The diaphragm may be elevated, the hemithorax smaller, and an abnormal vein (scimitar syndrome) may be seen across the tower lung field (pulmonary hypo-plasia).	
Tricuspid stenosis and insufficiency	1 Rounding of the right cardiac border 2 Prominent superior vena cava 3 Elevated right hemidiaphragm due to enlarged liver.	Usually a rheumatic lesion of the tricuspid valve. Tricuspid stenosis and insufficiency produce identical roentgenographic findings. The condition is almost always associated with mitral and/or aortic valvular diseases that are responsible for overall cardiac enlargement. The rare solitary tricuspid stenosis may occur in *carcinoid syndrome, lupus erythematosus,* or *endomyocardial fibrosis.*

(continues on page 422)

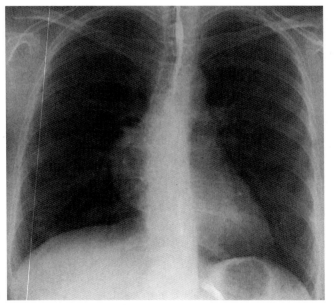 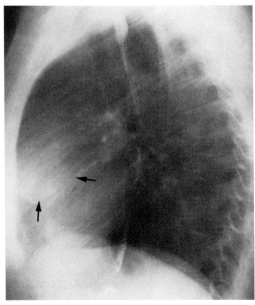

a   b

Fig. 16.**31 a, b**   **Pericardial cyst.** A soft-tissue mass in the right heart border mimics right atrial enlargement, but in the lateral view **b** it is seen to be more anterior than the right atrium (arrows).

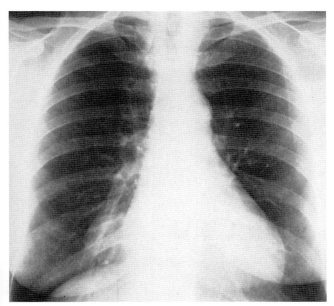
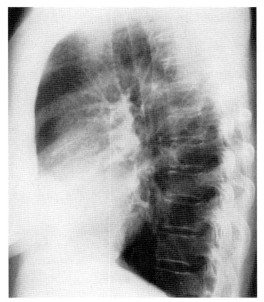

Fig. 16.**32 a, b   Pericardial lipoma.** A low-density mass in the right anterior cardiophrenic angle.

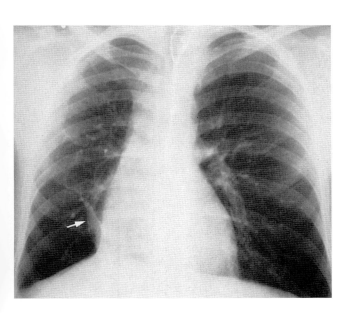

Fig. 16.**33 Hypoplasia of the right lung with partial anomalous venous return.** The mediastinum and right heart border are displaced to the right. The heart size is normal. Anomalous vein drawing into the inferior vena cava (scimitar sign) is seen in the right lower lung field (arrow).

Table 16.8 (Cont.) Right Atrial Enlargement or Prominent Right Heart Border

Disease	Radiographic Findings	Comments
Ebstein's anomaly (Figs. 16.34 and 16.35)	1 Large globular or box-like heart 2 Great enlargement of the right atrium 3 Concave pulmonary artery segment, small pulmonary arterial branches 4 A bulge below the left hilum simulates left atrial enlargement, but is caused by a dilated and left-displaced right ventricular outflow segment. 5 Narrow vascular pedicle	Downward displacement of the basket-like, incompetent, and stenotic tricuspid valve. As a result, a large portion of the right ventricle belongs to right atrium. There is always a right-to-left shunt through an atrial septal defect, which helps in the impaired emptying of the right atrium.
Left-to-right shunt into the right atrium (most commonly ASD)		See Table 16.10
Pulmonary stenosis or atresia, right heart failure of any cause, tetralogy of Fallot, and other causes of right ventricular enlargement	Whereas conditions that cause primary enlargement of the right atrium are rare, extensive enlargement of the right ventricle may cause secondary enlargement of the right atrium.	These diseases are presented under right ventricular enlargement, generalized cardiomegaly, and enlargement of the pulmonary artery segment (Tables 16.5, 16.7, 16.10).

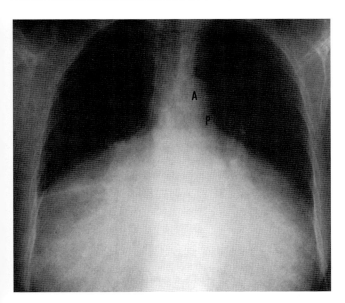

Fig. 16.**34** **Ebstein's anomaly.** Massive enlargement of the right atrium and large globular heart. The pulmonary artery (P) is disproportionally small compared with the aorta (A), and the vascular pedicle is narrow.

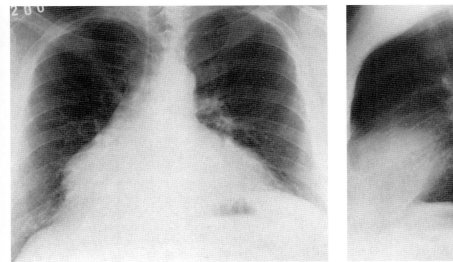

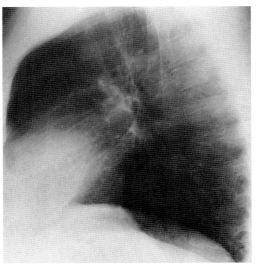

b

Fig. 16.**35 a, b** **Ebstein's anomaly.** The right heart border is dilated due to an enlarged right atrium, which is seen in the lateral view as a high-density area.

Table 16.9 Prominent or Malpositioned Ascending Aorta and/or Aortic Arch

Disease	Radiographic Findings	Comments
Atherosclerosis Hypertensive heart disease	1 Moderate dilatation of aorta with eventual intimal calcification 2 Moderate prominence of the ascending orta, seen as a bulge above the right heart border	Some degree of unfolding and sclerosis of aorta is considered physiologic in old age. In the region of the ligamentum arteriosum, kinking of an elongated aorta can produce a configuration similar to that of *congenital pseudocoarctation*, or simulate aortic aneurysm.
Aneurysm of the aorta (Fig. 16.36) Aneurysm of sinus of Valsalva (Fig. 16.37)	Aneurysm of the aorta: 1 A sharply marginated saccular or fusiform mass of homogenous density 2 Curvilinear calcification of the outer wall of the aneurysm 3 Dilatation of aorta	Conditions associated with aneurysm of the ascending aorta or aortic arch include: *atherosclerosis; cystic medial necrosis; lues; trauma; mycotic infection*. In luetic aortic insufficiency, the ascending aorta is usually dilated and calcified, whereas *rheumatoid aortic insufficiency* causes no calcification of the aortic wall and less dilatation. Dilatation of the ascending aorta and occlusive disease of several major aortic branches in younger women suggests Takayasu's arteritis. *Traumatic aneurysms* (even weeks or years after a closed trauma) usually occur just distal to the origin of the left subclavian artery.
	Aneurysm of the sinus of Valsalva: 1 Small aneurysms are intracardiac and cannot be detected on plain films. 2 Large aneurysms produce a smooth bulge of the right cardiac border, rarely of the left supracardiac area. 3 Curvilinear calcification is common in acquired aneurysm, 4 Acute signs of left-to-right shunt may indicate rupture.	*Congenital* aneurysms are usually small and asymptomatic. Large symmetric aneurysms occur in *cystic medial necrosis* with or without Marfan's disease. Acquired aneurysms are usually asymmetric and calcify. They are secondary to *lues, atherosclerosis* or (rarely) *non-syphilitic infection*. Aortic insufficiency is a common complication.
Dissecting aneurysm of the ascending aorta (Fig. 16.38)	1 Progressive widening of the aortic shadow. 2 Increased (over 4 mm) distance between the outer aortic wall and pre-existing intimal calcifications, which separate the original vascular lumen from the dissection.	Contrast enhanced CT arteriography confirms the presence of dissecting aneurysm. Predisposing factors of dissecting aneurysm include: *atherosclerosis; hypertension; cystic medial necrosis (including Marfan's disease); aortic stenosis, coarctation, or trauma; Ehler–Danlos syndrome (cutis laxa)*.

(continues on page 426)

Fig. 16.**38 a, b** Dissecting aortic aneurysm involving the aortic arch, There is progressive widening of the aortic shadow from film **a** to film **b**, taken two weeks apart. No intimal calcification is present (age 39).

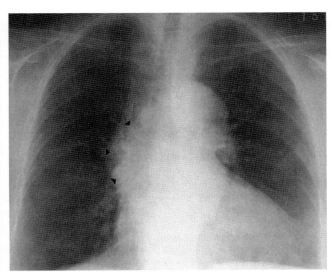
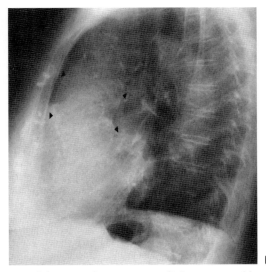

Fig. 16.**36 a, b   Luetic aneurysm of the ascending aorta.** The diameter of the ascending aorta is well demonstrated by calcifications (arrowheads). A prominent bulge is seen above the right heart border. There is also left ventricular enlargement.

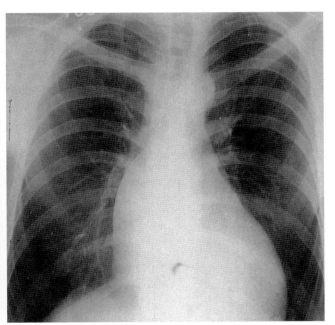
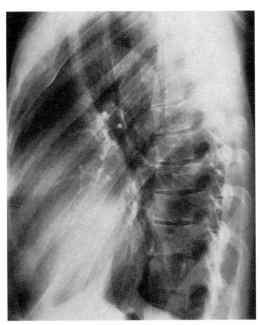

Fig. 16.**37 a, b   Sinus of Valsalva aneurysm and aortic Insufficiency in Marfan's syndrome. a** A large smooth bulge is seen over the right heart border and **b** behind the sternum. There is also left ventricular enlargement

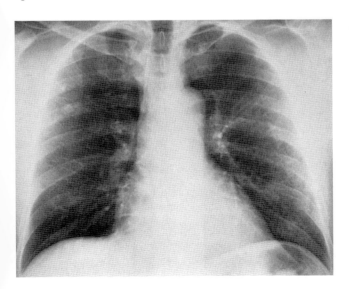
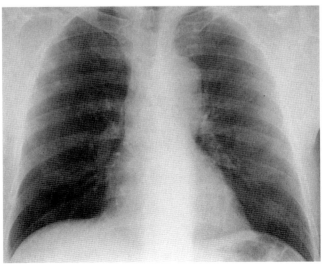

Table 16.9   (Cont.) Prominent or Malpositioned Ascending Aorta and/or Aortic Arch

Disease	Radiographic Findings	Comments
Aortic valvular stenosis (congenital or acquired) (Fig. 16.39)	1 There is little or no enlargement of the heart but the left lower border may present convex bulging. 2 Poststenotic dilatation of the ascending aorta while the aortic knob is normal or small. 3 Calcifications of the diseased aortic valve increase with age, but may be undetected on high kVp films. 4 Dilatation of the left ventricle is a late finding and often followed by congestive failure.	Congenital valvular stenosis is usually associated with bicuspic valves. Radiographic changes are similar to acquired stenosis. Acquired aortic stenosis usually develops on a rheumatic basis and it is often associated with other valvular, especially mitral, involvement. Aortic stenosis may also develop on atherosclerotic basis, but it is usually a combination of stenosis and insufficiency (see Table 16.5).
Aortic insufficiency	See Table 16.5	
Coarctation of the aorta (Figs. 16.40–16.42)	1 Dilated or prominent ascending aorta. 2 The narrowed segment appears as a notch in the contour of the descending aorta just below the knob. 3 Dilated left subclavian artery often produces a bulge above the aortic knob. 4 Poststenotic dilatation immediately below the narrowed segment may produce a figure "3" appearance of the descending aorta. 5 Dilatation of the internal mammary arteries may be visualized on the lateral film as a soft-tissue density. 6 Cardiac enlargement is rarely marked; it usually involves the left ventricle.	Notching of the inferior margins of the ribs (3 to 9) is the most common diagnostic finding in patients over 6 years.
Congenital pseudo-coarctation of the aorta	Two bulges in the region of the aortic knob, mimicking coarctation, in the absence of other findings typical of coarctation.	Buckling or kinking of the aortic arch in the region of ligamentum arteriosum without obstruction or other hemodynamic abnormality. Asymptomatic if no other abnormalities exist.

(continues on page 428)

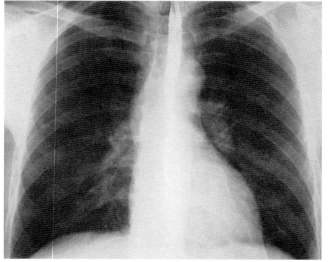
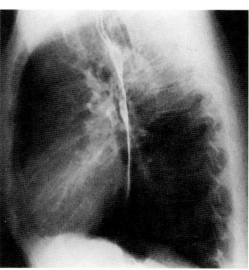

a   b

Fig. 16.**39 a, b   Aortic valvular stenosis of rheumatic origin**, age 32. The heart size is normal but the ascending aorta is too wide in the PA projection, considering the patient's age,

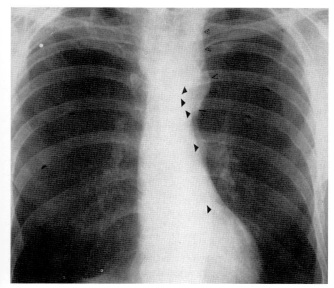

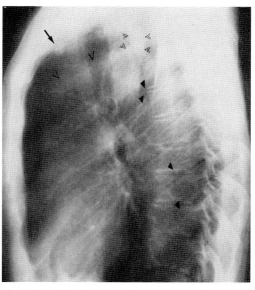

b

Fig. 16.**40 a, b   Coarctation of the aorta,** age 59. The aortic knob (∧∧) is prominent. The narrowing of proximal descending aorta is demonstrated on plain films (▲▲). Dilated left subclavian artery (⩕⩕) and rib notching (–) are characteristic. There is no continuity of aortic outline between the precoarctation and postcoarctation segments in the posteroanterior view. Dilated internal mammary artery (arrow) is seen behind the manubrium on the lateral film.

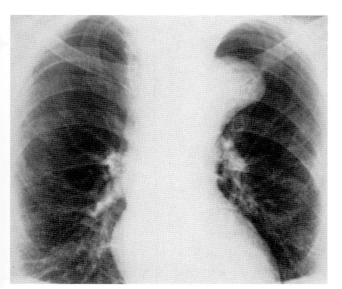

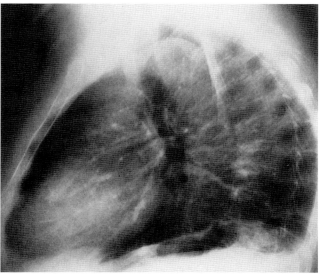

b

Fig. 16.**41 a, b   Poststenotic dilatation of the aorta in a patient with coarctation of aorta and Turner's syndrome** (age 43). Fusion of the manubriosternal joint and pectus carinatum are also seen.

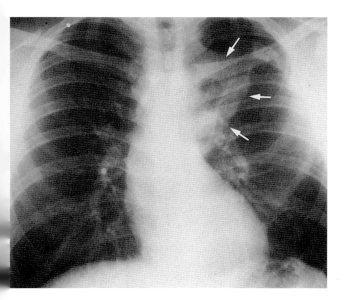

Fig. 16.**42   Coarctation of aorta, postsurgical.** The prosthetic segment is seen as a wide loop, which, however, has a normal diameter (arrows).

Table 16.9 (Cont.) Prominent or Malpositioned Ascending Aorta and/or Aortic Arch

Disease	Radiographic Findings	Comments
Tricuspid atresia without transposition of great vessels and Truncus arteriosus	Aortic enlargement is a feature of these rare congenital disorders.	See Table 16.7
Aortic arch malformations (Fig. 16.43)	Several types occur: 1 Right-sided aortic arch with mirror branching of the major arteries. 2 Right-sided aortic arch with an aberrant left subclavian artery and persistent left ligamentum arteriosum. 3 Anomalous right subclavian artery. 4 Double aortic arch (left, right, and posterior indentation of the esophagus)	Anomalous right subclavian artery is the most frequent anomaly. *Indentation of the posterior esophagus* occurs in all but the right-sided arch with mirror branches. In the latter anomaly the aorta is *anterior to esophagus* and trachea. It is almost always associated with cyanotic congenital heart disease (tetralogy of Fallot, truncus arteriosus, transposition of great vessels).
Corrected transposition of great vessels	Reversed positions of the great vessels and reversed functions of the ventricles. A smooth bulge of the upper left cardiac border is caused by the left-sided ascending aorta.	Uncomplicated corrected transposition is very rare. Associated defects include ventricular septal defect, a single ventricle or pulmonary stenosis. They modify the radiographic appearance.

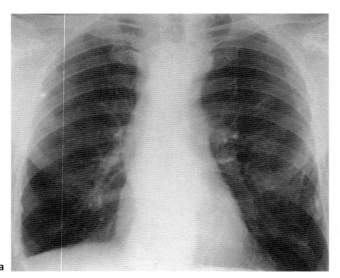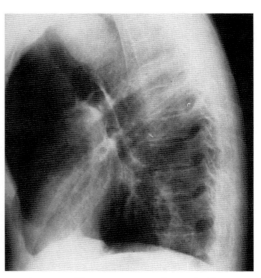

a   b

Fig. 16.**43 a, b Right-sided aortic arch.** The aorta passes behind the esophagus and is seen as a round mass in the upper mediastinum. Hence, there is no associated congenital heart anomaly. Extensive pleural calcifications (asbestosis), an incidental finding.

Table 16.10   Dilatation of the Main Pulmonary Artery Segment

Disease	Radiographic Findings	Comments
"Idiopathic" (No disease)	Convexity or moderate prominence of the pulmonary artery segment without abnormality.	Physiologic feature in young persons that may persist. Cardiac rotation in pectus excavatum causes a relative prominence of the pulmonary artery segment. In lordotic view and oblique projections the pulmonary artery segment appears prominent.
Pregnancy High output heart Congestive heart failure	Moderately enlarged pulmonary artery segment due to increased flow or increased blood volume in pulmonary circulation.	See Table 16.5
Cor pulmonale and Pulmonary arterial hypertension (Fig. 16.44)	1 Fullness and increased convexity of the main pulmonary artery segment. 2 Prominence of the main branches of the pulmonary artery. 3 Abrupt decrease of the caliber of the peripheral pulmonary arterial branches may be present, indicating pulmonary hypertension. 4 Normal heart size, later right ventricular enlargement. 5 If right heart failure supervenes, further cardiac dilatation and distention of the superior vena cava appears, together with eventual pleural fluid.	Cor pulmonale may develop secondary to a variety of conditions, easily overlooked in chest X-rays 1 Diffuse lung disease: *chronic obstructive emphysema*; *interstitial fibrosis* of various causes. 2 Diffuse pulmonary arterial diseases: *pulmonary thromboembolism*; (e.g., recurrent emboli, sickle cell anemia); *arteritis* (e.g., polyarteritis nodosa, Wegener's granulomatosis, schistosomiasis); *primary pulmonary hypertension*. 3 Chronic heart disease: *left ventricular failure; mitral valve disease; left-to-right shunt*. 4 Extrapulmonary causes of hypoventilation (*kyphoscoliosis, obesity, neuromuscular disorders, ankylosing spondylitis*).
Pulmonary embolism or thrombosis	Fullness of the main pulmonary artery segment with or without dilatation of the right ventricle is occasionally present in pulmonary embolism or infarction. In most cases the heart appears normal.	In serial films, changes in the main pulmonary artery segment are more frequently observable.

(continues on page 430)

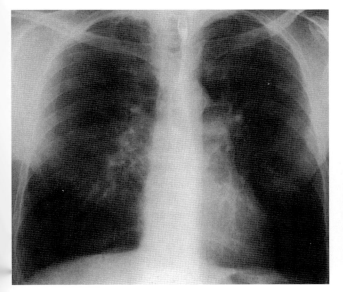
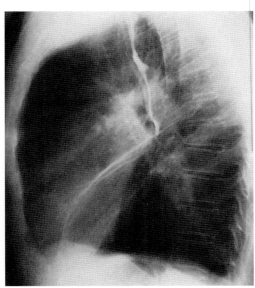

b

Fig. 16.**44 a, b   Cor pulmonale.** Wide pulmonary artery segment and main branches. Narrow peripheral pulmonary arteries. Severe chronic obstructive emphysema. The heartsize is otherwise normal but the right ventricle is prominent. Left lower lobe atelectasis is also seen.

Table 16.10 (Cont.) Dilatation of the Main Pulmonary Artery Segment

Disease	Radiographic Findings	Comments
Atrial septal defect (Fig. 16.45)	The size of the defect will determine the amount of blood shunted into the pulmonary circulation. 1 Enlargement of the main pulmonary artery segment and pulmonary arterial branches. 2 Dilatation of the right ventricle and the right atrium. 3 The aortic knob is relatively small. 4 The left atrium and left ventricle are normal.	The most common defect type is the so called ostium secundum near the foramen ovale. The less common ostium primum defect is just above the mitral valve and may be associated with abnormal mitral and tricuspid valves and a ventricular septal defect (*atrioventricularis communis, endocardial cushion defect*). This defect is most frequently found in association with *Down's syndrome* (mongolism). A defect above the foramen ovale is rare, but often associated with right-sided *anomalous-pulmonary venous return*. Abrupt narrowing of the peripheral arteries and wide central arteries including almost aneurysmatic dilatation of the main pulmonary artery is characteristic of *pulmonary hypertension (Eisenmenger's physiology)*, that may even reverse the shunt.
Ventricular septal defect (Fig. 16.46)	1 Prominent main pulmonary artery segment. 2 Increased pulmonary vascularity. 3 Enlarged left atrium and left ventricle. 4 Small aortic knob. 5 The right ventricle may be enlarged. The larger the shunt, the larger the left atrium and left ventricle and the smaller the aortic knob.	The most common congenital heart disease. The size and location of the defect determine its hemodynamic effect. A low muscular defect is usually small and rarely has clinical significance. A high ventricular septal defect near the aortic valve results both anatomically and functionally in an overriding aorta. Increased flow into the right ventricle in such a situation causes right ventricular enlargement and enlargement of the pulmonary artery. If pulmonary hypertension develops, right ventricular enlargement increases but the left ventricle may appear smaller. A defect high in the ventricular septum can cause prolapse of the non-coronary cusp with resultant aortic insufficiency and dilatation of the ascending aorta.

(continues on page 432)

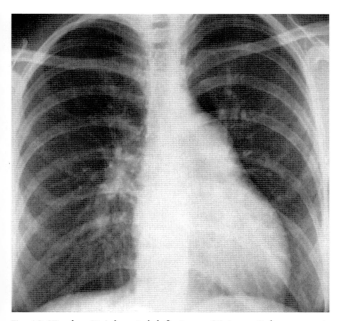
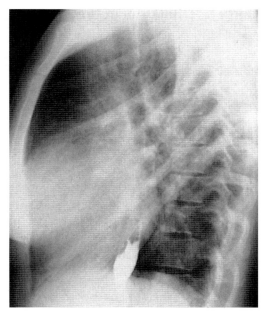

b

Fig. 16.**45 a, b   Atrial septal defect,** age 24. Large Pulmonary artery segment and pulmonary arterial branches. Dilated right Ventricle is seen as prominence of the anterior border of the heart.

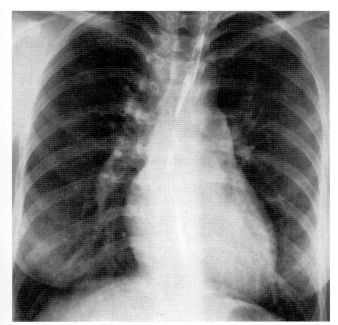
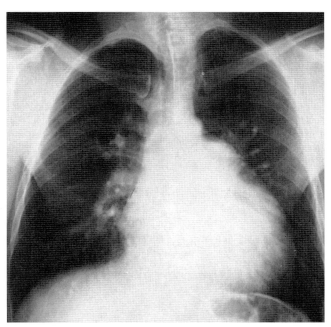

b

Fig. 16.**46 a, b   Ventricular septal defect. a** Prominent pulmonary artery segment, increased pulmonary vasculature, small aorta, and minimal left ventricular enlargement. Age 20.

b Another patient, grossly dilated pulmonary artery segment, large left ventricle, pulmonary arterial hypertension (wide but rapidly tapering pulmonary arteries).

Table 16.10 (Cont.) Dilatation of the Main Pulmonary Artery Segment

Disease	Radiographic Findings	Comments
Patent ductus arteriosus (Fig. 16.47)	Radiographic changes depend on the age and volume of shunted blood: 1 The main pulmonary artery segment and the central pulmonary arteries are enlarged. Often the right hilar shadow is larger than the left. 2 The pulmonary vascularity is increased. 3 The left atrium and left ventricle are enlarged and produce moderate cardiomegaly. 4 Aorta proximal to the shunt may enlarge. A convex bulge below the aortic knob represents the origin of the ductus. This "infundibulum sign" is present in one-third of patients.	If the ductus arteriosus remains open for over 3 months after birth, it is called patent ductus arteriosus. It is the most common extracardiac left-to-right shunt. A young patient with increased pulmonary vascularity and a large aortic knob is a typical radiographic presentation of patent ductus arteriosus. The ductus may calcify. In the rare *aorticopulmonary window*, the shunt is in the ascending aorta and the knob does not enlarge. Pulmonary hypertension is a frequent late complication of an untreated patent ductus arteriosus.
Total anomalous pulmonary venous return (TAPVR) (Fig. 16.48)	Nonobstructive TAPVR 1 If pulmonary veins drain directly into the right atrium the plain film appearance may be identical to the atrial septal defect. 2 If there is persistent left vena cava or vena verticalis, the heart and mediastinum have a number 8 or snowman appearance. 3 The hypoplastic aorta and enlarged pulmonary artery form a shelf-like density superimposed on the left abnormal veins. 4 The right atrium and right ventricle are dilated. The left heart is hypoplastic.	All venous blood returns to the right atrium, either directly or through a systemic vein (superior or inferior vena cava, portal vein). Atrial septal defect is a life-saving anomaly in this condition. Thus there is a combined left-to-right and right-to-left shunt. Obstruction of the pulmonary vein (e.g., drainage into the portal vein) is associated with pulmonary venous congestion and normal heart size.
Partial anomalous venous return (PAVR) (see Fig. 16.33)	There may be no abnormality in the chest roentgenogram. Hypervascularity, right heart enlargement, and an anomalous vessel crossing downward on the right side of the heart may be present.	PAVR is more common than TAPVR and usually asymptomatic.

(continues on page 434)

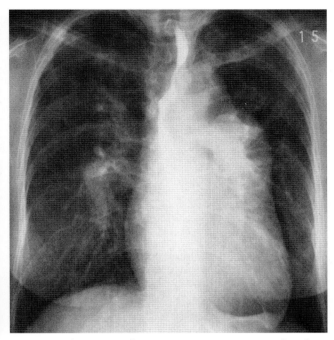

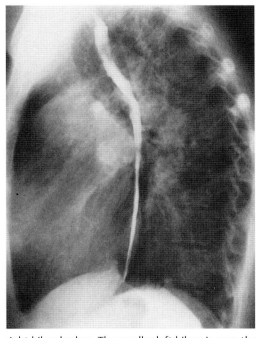

b

Fig. 16.**47 a, b** **Patent ductus arteriosus,** age 40, with pulmonary arterial hypertension. Very large main pulmonary artery and

right hilar shadow. The smaller left hilum is seen through the wide pulmonary artery segment. Left heart is only slightly enlarged.

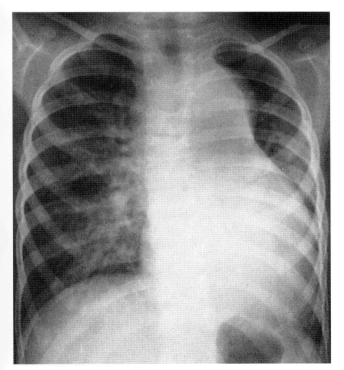

Fig. 16.**48** **Total anomalous pulmonary venous return with persistent left vena cava,** which produces a snowman appearance. Increased pulmonary vasculature.

Table 16.10 (Cont.) Dilatation of the Main Pulmonary Artery Segment

Disease	Radiographic Findings	Comments
Isolated pulmonary stenosis (see also coarctation of the pulmonary arteries) (Fig. 16.49)	In the majority of cases the chest findings are entirely normal except for the prominence of the main pulmonary artery. The left pulmonary artery is often more enlarged than the right.	Pulmonary stenosis may occur in *rubeola syndrome* (transplacental infection), *carcinoid syndrome*, or *rheumatic heart disease*. Congenital pulmonary valvular stenosis is a relatively common anomaly. Poststenotic dilatation of the pulmonary arterial segment is absent in the less common *infundibular* pulmonary stenosis (5% of pulmonary stenoses).
Pulmonary stenosis with atrial septal defect (Fallot's trilogy)	A prominent main pulmonary segment associated with pulmonary oligemia. This is an important sign to differentiate Fallot's trilogy from tetralogy of Fallot, pseudotruncus arteriosus, and tricuspid atresia. Secondary tricuspid insufficiency following right ventricular enlargement may enlarge the right atrium. The pulmonary valve calcification is rarely seen.	In most cases of pulmonary stenosis there is an open foramen ovale, less frequently a true atrial septal defect. Pulmonary stenosis associated with a ventricular septal defect is usually called tetralogy of Fallot even if the aorta may not be overriding.
Mitral valve disease Tricuspid atresia Truncus arteriosus (type I, common origin of aorta and pulmonary artery)	Enlargement of the main pulmonary artery segment occurs in these conditions.	These entities are discussed in Tables 16.**6** and 16.**7**.
Congenital coronary fistula	Plain films reveal a nonspecific left-to-right shunt with prominent pulmonary artery segment, dilated pulmonary vessels and a dilated left atrium. The aortic knob is normal.	A communication between a coronary vessel and a cardiac chamber or a pulmonary artery. The right coronary artery is more commonly involved and usually terminates in the right heart or pulmonary trunk.
Cor triatriatum sinistrum	Plain roentgenographic findings are not characteristic, but include: Prominent main pulmonary artery segment Prominent hilar vessels Enlargement of the right ventricle Occasionally there is pulmonary venous congestion and rarely left atrial enlargement	A transverse incomplete fibromuscular membrane divides the left atrium into two chambers with a hemodynamic effect similar to that of mitral stenosis. Patent foramen ovale and atrial septal defect are commonly associated.
Common atrioventricular canal (endocardial cushion defect)	Cardiomegaly with findings indicative of a nonspecific left-to-right shunt. Pulmonary hypertension often develops in adults.	Different combinations of ostium primum atrial septal defect, cleft mitral and/or tricuspidal valves and ventricular septal defect occur. Pulmonary stenosis is a common associated anomaly.
Coarctation of pulmonary arteries	An unusual combination of small hilar arteries and large posthilar central branches is suggestive of this diagnosis. An associated pulmonary valvular stenosis is present in over half of the cases.	A rare anomaly in which single or multiple constrictions occur in the branches of the pulmonary artery. The vessels immediately distal to the narrowing are prominent because of poststenotic dilatation.

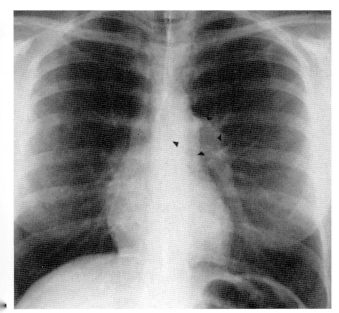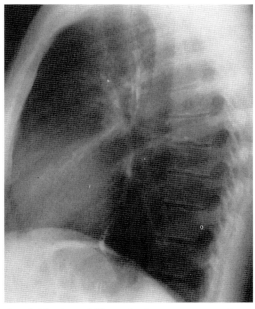

Fig. 16.**49 a, b   Isolated pulmonary valvular stenosis. a** Heart size and pulmonary vascularity are normal, but the main pulmonary artery and its left main branch are enlarged in the PA projection, **b** The lateral film only shows some prominence of the anterior heart border (right ventricular hypertrophy).

17 Mediastinal or Hilar Enlargement

The mediastinum is defined as the extrapleural space within the thorax lying between the lungs. The soft-tissue structures that compose the margins of the mediastinum and abut against the lungs usually cast discernible shadows on roentgenograms. These lung-mediastinal interfaces are keys to the radiologic analysis of the mediastinum. Well-penetrated high kVp films are essential to visualize the interfaces lying behind the lateral margins of the mediastinum and heart. Opacification of the esophagus may further help in delineating the suspected lesion.

Although careful analysis of the mediastinum on plain films is not a replacement for computed tomography of known or suspected mass lesions, it is important in detecting early or unsuspected lesions from routine chest roentgenograms. Differentiation of mediastinal disease from cardiac, pericardial, pleural, and pulmonary lesions is better done with CT.

Useful lines and signs in anteroposterior projection; Fig. 17.**1**: The *paraspinal line* may be displaced by pleural fluid, a paravertebral abscess, hemorrhage from a dorsal spine fracture, or extravertebral extension of a neoplasm. The more prominent the aorta, the wider the space between the left paraspinal line and the spine. Visualization of *normal paraesophageal* and *posterior junction* lines are due to the lack of interposed soft-tissue or esophageal distention.

The *paratracheal* and *parabronchial lines* become wider (over 2 to 3 mm) with pleural thickening or fluid, mediastin-

itis, and hemorrhages. An uneven outline is likely due to paratracheal lymphadenopathy or tumor. The normal azygos vein is seen as a spindle shaped dense widening of the right paratracheobronchial line at the level of the tracheal bifurcation, and its transverse diameter may vary with posture and Valsalva maneuver, which can be used to differentiate the azygos vein from an enlarged lymph node. In upright position it is normally less than one centimeter wide. Increased systemic venous pressure (congestive heart failure, acute pulmonary hypertension due to embolism, constrictive pericarditis), portal thrombosis, ascending thrombosis of the vena cava, or absence of the subhepatic portion of the vena cava, may cause dilatation of the azygos vein.

The anterior borders of the upper lobes join immediately behind the manubrium to form the *anterior junction line* slightly to the left of midline. It is not seen in infants and young children because of the presence of the thymus. Enlargement of the aorta, hemorrhage, adenopathy, or tumor may interpose between the lungs at this point.

On the left side the paraesophageal line is not consistently visualized, but the *para-aortic* line is continuous with the profile of the aortic arch. This line is often curved due to elongation of the aorta. A discontinuity may represent coarctation of the aorta (see Fig. 16.**40**). Coarctation may also cause convexity of the profile of the left subclavian artery above the aortic knob. The angles between the aorta and the subclavian artery as well as the indentation be-

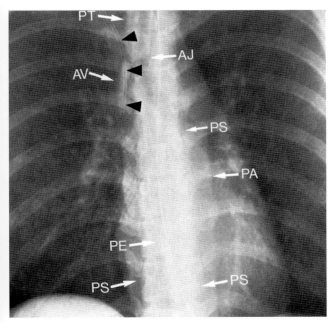

Fig. 17.**1 a** **Mediastinal lines** as seen in anteroposterior projection. The location of superior vena cava, trachea, and esophagus are demonstrated by a CVP line and tracheal and esophageal tubes. PT = paratracheal line, AV azygos vein, AJ anterior junction line, PS = paraspinal line, PA para-aortic line, PE paraesophageal line. Central venous catheter (arrowheads).

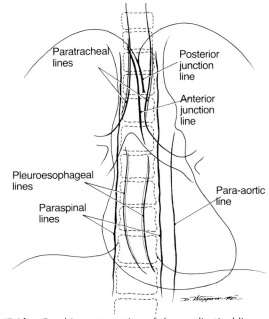

Fig. 17.**1 b**   Graphic presentation of the mediastinal lines.

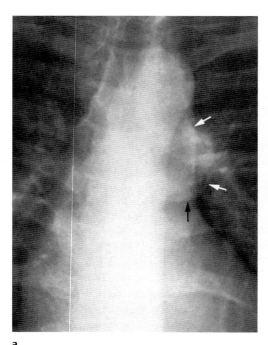

a

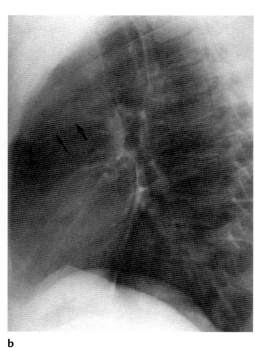

b

Fig. 17.**2 a, b   Hilum overlay sign, a** A double profile of the main pulmonary artery segment, which appears enlarged (arrows), **b** Lateral film shows that there is a mass (lymphoma) in the anterior mediastinum (arrow), which projects over the left hilum in posteroanterior projection.

tween the aorta and the superior surface of the pulmonary artery may be obliterated by lymphadenopathy or tumor. A double profile of the main pulmonary artery segment, if not explained by the left main artery, is likely due to a neoplasm, usually anterior to the pulmonary artery (*hilum overlay sign*, Fig. 17.**2**).

Widening of the whole mediastinum in anteroposterior projection and disappearance of the normal mediastinopulmonary interfaces occurs especially in hemorrhage and in *postoperative bleeding*, but it may occur with extensive infiltrating *neoplasm*, mediastinal *amyloidosis*, mediastinal *fibrosis*, and *inflammation*. Since the cephalic border of the anterior portion of the mediastinum ends at the level of the clavicles while that of the posterior portion extends much higher, a lesion clearly visible above the clavicles on the frontal view must lie entirely within the thorax. The more cephalad an upper mediastinal mass extends while still remaining visible, the more posteriorly it lies. A thoracic lesion in anatomic contact with the neck or extending into it will be obliterated along its upper lateral borders by the cervical soft tissues (*cervicothoracic sign*, Fig. 17.**3**). Thoracoabdominal mass lesions may be visible through the diaphragm, since they are in contact with the posterior lower lobes. Lack of downward convergence of the lower border of such a lesion (*iceberg sign*, Fig. 17.**4**) indicates that a considerable portion of the mass is in the abdomen. An iceberg sign is common in thoracoabdominal *aneurysms, esophagogastric lesions*, and *azygos continuations of the inferior vena cava*. Also, a *retroperitoneal tumor* may extend into the thorax and widen the inferior paravertebral shadow.

In about 9% of infants and young children the normal thymus may produce a *sail shadow* projecting from the upper mediastinum on the frontal film (Fig. 17.**5**). The sail shadow is differentiated from right upper lobe consolidation by its well defined vertical lateral border, and from encapsulated pleural effusion by its sharp inferior angle. The lateral borders of the normal thymus may be indented by adjacent ribs, causing a subtle wavy margin on the frontal projection that is not seen in thymic tumors or in other anterior mediastinal masses. In an infant, *pneumomediastinum* may dis-

sect the thymus from the rest of the mediastinum and elevate it like a 'spinnaker sail.'

If a thymus in the neonate less than 4 days of age is not visible in anteroposterior or lateral radiographs of the chest (the retrosternal area is lucent, the anterior borders of the heart and great vessels are clearly defined, and in the frontal projection the mediastinum is narrow), thymic aplasia should be suspected. Absence of the thymus and parathyroids (immunologic deficiency and tetany) is called *DiGeorge syndrome* (Fig. 17.**6**). Hypoplastic mandible, deformities of the ear and anomalies of the aortic arch may be associated. Thymic aplasia or hypoplasia may be seen also in severe, *combined immunodeficiency syndromes*.

In lateral view, the mediastinum also has significant profiles (Fig. 17.**7**). Effacement of the aortic arch and tracheal wall profiles indicates interposed soft tissue. The *posterior tracheal band* is a 3-mm-wide band extending from the upper mediastinum to the lower lobe bronchi. It is well visualized in patients who have a sizable azygoesophageal recess filled by the right lung. *Carcinoma of the esophagus*, other *mediastinal neoplasms, bleeding*, or *infection* may obliterate a previously well-visualized posterior tracheal band or cause its general or localized widening (Fig. 17.**8**). The posterior margin of the inferior vena cava is always seen in good-quality lateral films. Its absence is rare (Fig. 17.**9**).

Differentiation of enlarged hilar blood vessels from hilar lymphadenopathy may be easier if one remembers that blood vessels tend to be parallel with bronchi, whereas lymph nodes actually surround them and may produce accentuated cross-sectional shadows of main bronchi in the lateral view. Mediastinal contrast enhanced CT greatly helps differentiation of blood vessels from other structures.

The lines and signs presented above are helpful in localizing a lesion. Division of the mediastinum into anterior, middle, and posterior mediastina is more useful than strictly anatomical subdivision. This artificial division of the mediastinum into anterior, middle, and posterior portions varies among different authors. The division used in this presentation is shown in Fig. 17.**10**. The shape, size, and radiographic structure of mediastinal mass lesions in conventional films

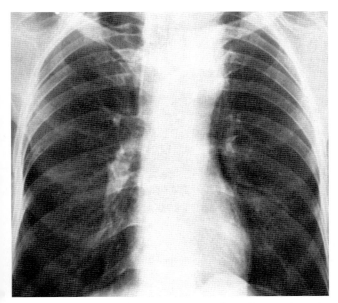

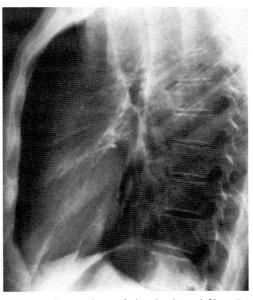

Fig. 17.**3 a, b Cervicothoracic sign, a** In frontal projection, the upper mediastinal mass extends over the clavicles and joins into the soft tissues of the neck, indicating posterior position of the mass, as shown also in **b** by the lateral film. Carcinoma of the esophagus.

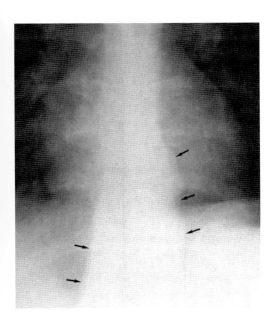

Fig. 17.**4 Iceberg sign.** Nodular widening of the paravertebral soft tissues (arrows), more so on the left. Para-aortic metastases of a testicular carcinoma extending beyond the diaphragm.

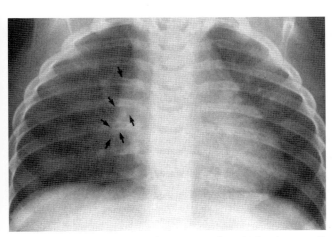

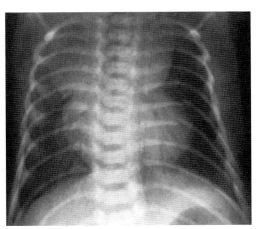

Fig. 17.**5 a, b** Thymic sail shadow, **a** A small "sail" that has a well-defined border and sharp inferior angle (arrows), **b** Thymus presenting as an upper mediastinal mass with a sharp inferior angle on the right side.

often provide insufficient information for definitive diagnosis and computed tomography is required for better anatomical definition. Different types of lesions tend to occur at different anteroposterior subdivisions of the mediastinum. Associated pulmonary or pleural changes provide further information for differential diagnosis.

The most common lesions which cause mediastinal widening are summarized in Table 17.1 according to their usual location. Enlarged lymph nodes in this context refer to masses which are recognizable on plain radiographs, on which normal-sized lymph nodes are not seen unless they are calcified. The question of how to define the boundary between normal and enlarged individual lymph nodes, commonly encountered in CT or more resently in PET-CT, will therefore not be discussed. In Table 17.2, diseases which cause hilar and/or mediastinal lymph node enlargement are discussed, while diseases causing diffuse mediastinal widening are presented in Table 17.3.

Table 17.1   The Most Common Lesions in the Anterior, Middle and Posterior Mediastinum

Anterior Mediastinum	Middle Mediastinum	Posterior Mediastinum
Aneurysm of ascending aorta	Aneurysm of aortic arch	*Aneurysm or tortuosity of descending aorta*
Lymphoma (most common)	Azygos vein enlargement	*(most common)*
Pericardial cyst	Bronchogenic cyst	Lymph node enlargement
Retrosternal thyroid	Esophageal lesions	Neurogenic tumor
Teratoid lesion	Hiatal hernia	Paraspinal manifestations of spinal lesions
Thymic lesion	*Lymph node enlargement* (most common)	
	Thyroid tumor	
	(Hilar vascular dilatation)	

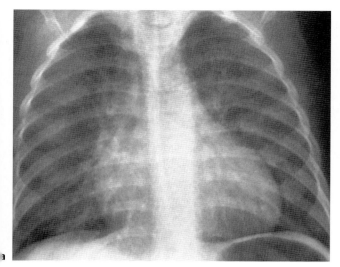

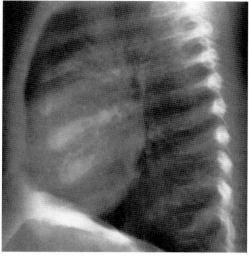

Fig. 17.**6 a, b   DiGeorge syndrome.** Absence of thymus is suggested **a** by the narrow upper mediastinum, presence of the ante-rior junction line in a small child, and **b** radiolucency of the retro-sternal space in the lateral view.

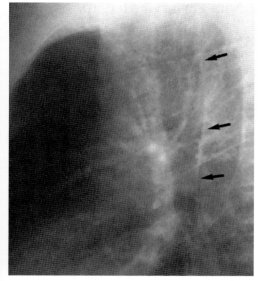

Fig. 17.**7   Normal posterior tracheal band** (arrows)

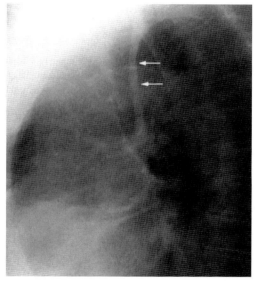

Fig. 17.**8   Thickening of the posterior tracheal band** (arrows).

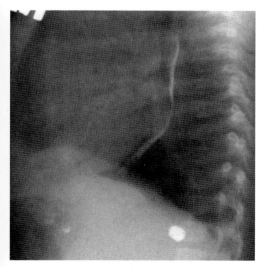

Fig. 17.**9   Congenital absence of the proximal IVC.** The silhouette of the inferior vena cava, normally present in the lateral film, is lacking. Blood is conducted via the azygos vein.

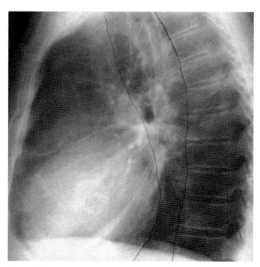

Fig. 17.**10   Division of the mediastinum** into three (artificial) compartments. "Anterior mediastinum" refers to front of the trachea or of the posterior cardiac silhouette. "Posterior mediastinum" refers to area posterior to the anterior paraspinal line. "Middle mediastinum" refers to the compartment between these two artificial lines.

Table 17.2 Hilar and/or Mediastinal Lymph Node Enlargement

Disease	Radiographic Findings	Comments
Neoplastic diseases (malignant or benign)		
Bronchogenic carcinoma (Fig. 17.11)	Unilateral hilar node enlargement involving bronchopulmonary and tracheobronchial nodes, in some cases paratracheal and posterior mediastinal nodes.	Influence of cell type: 1 A hilar mass as the sole roentgenographic abnormality is characteristic of an undifferentiated small-cell carcinoma; 2 Generalized mediastinal widening almost certainly indicates spread from an undifferentiated carcinoma; 3 Hilar or mediastinal lymph node enlargement is rare in *alveolar cell* (bronchiolar) *carcinoma*.
Hodgkin's disease (Fig. 17.12)	Bilateral but asymmetric enlargement, especially of paratracheal and tracheobronchial nodes, frequently also anterior mediastinal and retrosternal nodes. Bronchopulmonary nodes are less frequently enlarged than the more central ones. Unilateral involvement is very rare.	Mediastinal lymph node enlargement is seen on the initial chest roentgenogram in approximately 50% of patients. May be associated with pulmonary involvement or pleural effusion in advanced cases.
Non-Hodgkin's lymphoma	Bilateral, asymmetric node enlargement similar to Hodgkin's disease.	May occasionally present as parenchymal consolidation without associated lymph node enlargement.
Leukemia	Usually symmetric enlargement of mediastinal and bronchopulmonary nodes.	Occurs in 25% of patients, more commonly in lymphocytic than in myelocytic leukemia. Pleural effusion and parenchymal involvement may be associated.

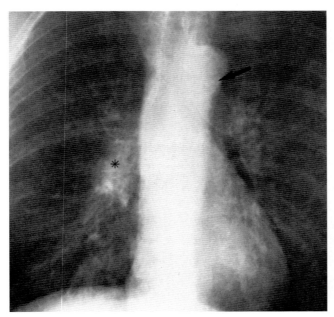

Fig. 17.**11** **Small cell carcinoma** with mediastinal lymph node metastases and lymphangitis carcinomatosa. Enlarged right tracheobronchial lymph nodes (asterisk) and subtle obliteration of the notch between aorta and main pulmonary artery by metastatic lymph nodes (arrow).

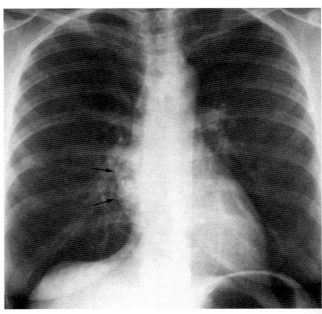

Fig. 17.**12** **Hodgkin's disease.** Enlarged anterior mediastinal and hilar lymph nodes. Intrapulmonary mass lesion in the left lung.

Fig. 17.**13 a–d** **Bronchopulmonary amyloidosis. a, b** Hilar and azygos nodes are enlarged, with a pattern similar to sarcoidosis. Even small pulmonary densities occur. **c, d** The same patient, 6 years later. Unlike sarcoidosis, the hilar and mediastinal lymph nodes continually grow. Miliary parenchymal changes have also increased.

Table 17.2 (Cont.) Hilar and/or Mediastinal Lymph Node Enlargement

Disease	Radiographic Findings	Comments
Immunoblastic lymph-adenopathy (a hyperimmune disorder of B lympho-cytes)	Bilateral, asymmetric node enlargement similar to Hodgkin's disease.	Lungs are occasionally affected in a pattern similar to Hodgkin's disease.
Heavy-chain disease (a plasma cell dyscrasia)	Symmetric enlargement of mediastinal lymph nodes.	Hepatosplenomegaly is common, lung involvement rare.
Bronchopulmonary amyloidosis (a plasma cell dyscrasia) (Fig. 17.13)	Symmetric hilar and mediastinal lymph node enlargement. Enlarged nodes may be densely calcified.	Sometimes associated with diffuse pulmonary involvement.

(continues on page 444)

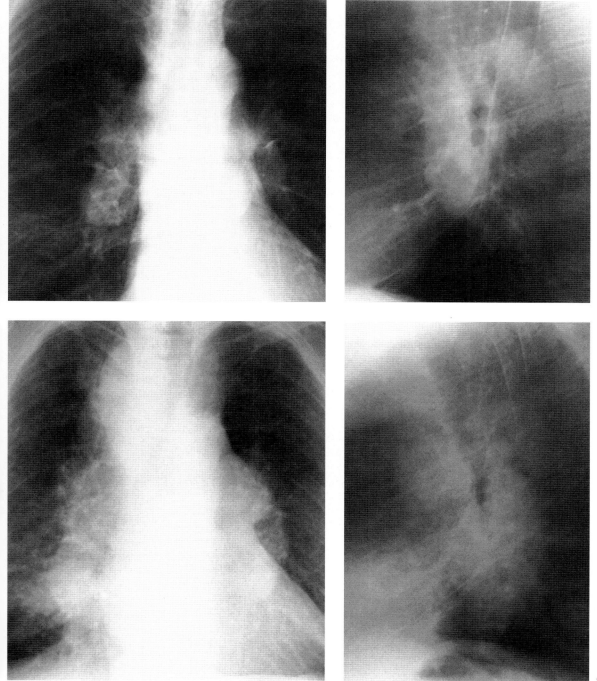

b

d

Table 17.2 (Cont.) Hilar and/or Mediastinal Lymph Node Enlargement

Disease	Radiographic Findings	Comments
Lymph node metastases (Fig. 17.14)	Unilateral or bilateral enlargement of either hilar or mediastinal nodes or both.	May be associated with lymphangitic changes in the lungs (see Table 17.3).
Post-transplantation lymphoproliferative disorder (PTLD)	Hilar and mediastinal lymph node enlargement often associated with pulmonary nodules measuring up to 5 cm in diameter. Rarely pleural and/or pericardial effusion/thickening is also evident.	Lymphocyte proliferation developing 1 month to 1 year after transplant. Histologic range from benign hyperplastic proliferation to malignant lymphoma. Related to Epstein-Barr virus-infected B-cells.
Castleman's disease (giant lymph node hyperplasia)	Hilar or mediastinal nodes or both. Large circumscribed mediastinal mass is the most common presentation.	This rare benign condition may be associated with fever, anemia and gammaglobulinemia. Two types can be differentiated. Type 1: the hyaline vascular type (90%), almost always local, with no systemic symptoms; Type 2 the plasma-cell type, which may be multicentric and associated with systemic symptoms.
Bacterial and mycoplasma infections		
Primary tuberculosis (Fig. 17.15)	Mostly unilateral hilar (60%) or hilar and paratracheal (40%) lymph node enlargement. Bilateral node enlargement is a rare presentation.	Hilar node enlargement differentiates primary from secondary (reunification) tuberculosis. In the latter, there is no observable lymphadenopathy.
Tularemia (*Francisella tularensis*)	Unilateral hilar node enlargement with characteristically oval pneumonic consolidations and pleural effusion.	Ipsilateral hilar node enlargement occurs in 25–50% of tularemic pneumonias. Is a potential bioterrorism agent.
Pertussis (whooping cough)	Unilateral hilar node enlargement.	Often associated with ipsilateral segmental pneumonia and atelectasis.
Anthrax (*Bacillus anthracis*)	Symmetric enlargement of all lymph nodes or generalized mediastinal widening.	Often associated with pleural effusion, rarely with pulmonary hemorrhages. Has been used as a bioterrorism weapon
Plague pneumonia (caused by *Yersinia pestis*)	Symmetric hilar and paratracheal node enlargement.	Nonsegmental homogeneous consolidations may occur in lungs mimicking alveolar edema. May be used as a bioterrorism weapon.
Mycoplasma pneumoniae	Unilateral or bilateral hilar lymph node enlargement associated with segmental pneumonia, predominantly in lower lobes.	Most common in children. Together with parenchymal disease.
Viral, rickettsial infections	Unilateral or bilateral hilar node enlargement.	
Rubeola	Bilateral hilar node enlargement may be associated with diffuse interstitial pneumonia.	If pneumonia in rubeola is segmental, it is due to secondary bacterial infection.
Echovirus pneumonia	Bilateral hilar node enlargement and associated increase of bronchovascular markings.	Respiratory infections occur predominantly in infants.
Varicella pneumonia	Bilateral hilar node enlargement associated with patchy, diffuse air-space consolidation.	Pulmonary consolidation may mask hilar node reaction. Mainly occurs in adults with varicella.
Psittacosis (ornithosis)	Unilateral or bilateral hilar node enlargement associated with variable radiographic presentations of pneumonia.	Roentgenographic resolution of pneumonia is slow.
Epstein-Barr (infectious mononucleosis) (Fig. 17.16)	Bilateral, symmetric, predominantly hilar lymph node enlargement.	Splenomegaly. Roentgenographic changes in the lungs are rare.
AIDS (acquired immunodeficiency syndrome) (Figs. 17.15 and 17.17)	Bilateral lymph node enlargement.	Lymphadenopathy is common in AIDS patients (up to 80%); most often related to chest infections, less commonly caused by AIDS-associated lymphoma.

(continues on page 446)

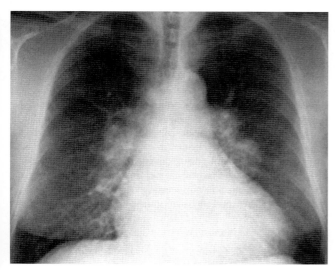

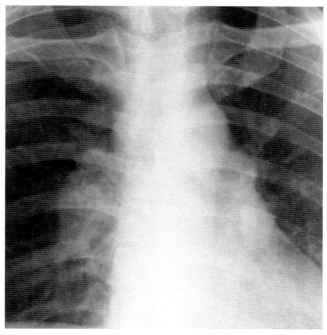

Fig. 17.**14** **Metastatic melanoma** with lymphangitis carcinomatosa and bilateral hilar lymph node enlargement.

Fig. 17.**15** **Primary tuberculosis** in a patient with AIDS. Right hilar lymph node enlargement.

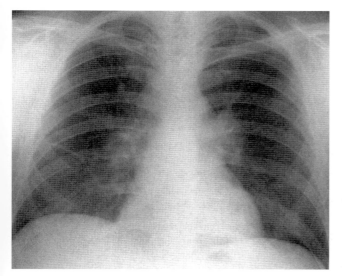

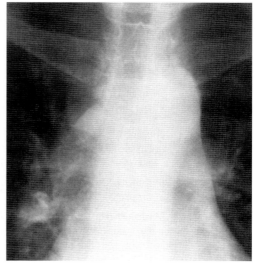

Fig. 17.**16** **Infectious mononucleosis.** Enlargement of bronchopulmonary nodes and the azygos node—a pattern characteristic of sarcoidosis.

Fig. 17.**17** Benign mediastinal lymphadenopathy in **AIDS.** Lymph nodes on the right side are predominantly enlarged, both in the hilar and the upper mediastinal regions.

Table 17.2 (Cont.) Hilar and/or Mediastinal Lymph Node Enlargement

Disease	Radiographic Findings	Comments
Fungal infections		
Histoplasmosis (Fig. 17.18)	Unilateral or bilateral, hilar, mediastinal, and occasionally intrapulmonary lymph node enlargement, with or sometimes without associated pneumonia. Hilar node enlargement is a common feature in all other fungal infections, too.	*Several forms of presentation:* 1 Benign type: one or more ill-defined nonsegmental opacities in lungs, 2 Pneumonic type: simulates an acute nonsegmental air-space pneumonia of bacterial origin, 3 Histoplasmoma: one or few "coin" lesions, which may calcify ("target" lesion). Hilar lymph node calcification is common, although nodes may not be enlarged, 4 Lymph node enlargement without associated pulmonary changes, particulary common in children, 5 Acute diffuse nodular histoplasmosis with or without pulmonary manifestations (pneumonia or miliary nodules).
Coccidioidomycosis	Unilateral or bilateral enlargement of hilar and/or paratracheal nodes, with or without associated pulmonary parenchymal disease.	Enlargement of paratracheal lymph nodes may indicate an imminent dissemination.
Sporotrichosis	Unilateral hilar node enlargement.	The associated parenchymal changes are variable.
Parasitic diseases		
Tropical eosinophilia (caused by filariasis)	Occasionally bilateral hilar lymph node enlargement.	Micronodular densities and increased linear markings in the lungs.
Pneumoconiosis		
Silicosis (Fig. 17.19)	Symmetric, predominantly bronchopulmonary lymph node enlargement, usually associated with diffuse nodular disease of the parenchyma. Eggshell calcification of lymph nodes occurs in 5% of silicosis patients.	When present, eggshell calcification of lymph nodes is almost pathognomonic of silicosis. Occasionally it is seen in sarcoidosis and irradiated Hodgkin's disease. Lymph node enlargement is present in some cases of *coal miner's lung*.
Chronic berylliosis	Symmetric bronchopulmonary lymph node enlargement occurs in a minority of cases,	The roentgenographic pattern in chest varies and is neither specific nor diagnostic.
Other diseases		
Sarcoidosis (Fig. 17.20) (The most common cause of bilateral hilar node enlargement)	Symmetric enlargement of bronchopulmonary, tracheobronchial and paratracheal lymph nodes is characteristically seen in 75% to 90% of patients. The outer borders of the enlarged hila are usually lobulated and there is often a lucent zone between the heart and enlarged tracheobronchial nodes. Enlargement of the azygos node is also typical.	Typical patterns are: 1 Lymph node enlargement without pulmonary abnormality 2 Combined diffuse pulmonary disease and lymph node enlargement (in up to 20%) 3 Homogeneous alveolar-looking densities (rare) 4 Uneven pulmonary fibrosis. With the onset of diffuse lung disease, the lymph node size diminishes, which aids in differentiating sarcoidosis from lymphoma and tuberculosis.
Extrinsic allergic alveolitis (occupational exposure to organic dust <5 μm in size)	Rarely a combination of symmetric enlargement of bronchopulmonary nodes associated with diffuse interstitial pattern.	May mimic sarcoidosis, but hilar node enlargement in extrinsic allergic alveolitis is rare except for mushroom-worker's lung, where it is fairly common.

(continues on page 448)

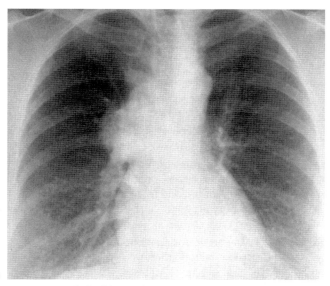

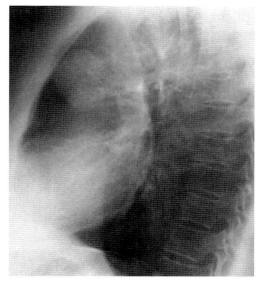

b

Fig. 17.**18** **Calcified histoplasmoma** of the right anterior mediastinum. Hilar nodes are not enlarged.

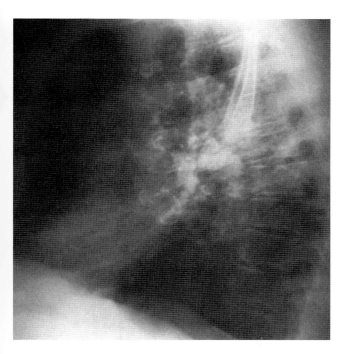

Fig. 17.**19** **Sillcosis.** Enlarged hilar and mediastinal lymph nodes with eggshell calcification.

Fig. 17.**20 a, b** **Sarcoidosis.** Characteristic distribution of lymph node enlargement: bronchopulmonary and tracheobronchial nodes (including the azygos node) leaving a lucent zone between the nodes and the heart.
▽

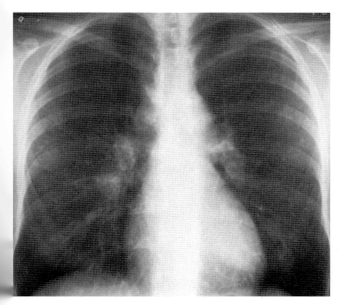

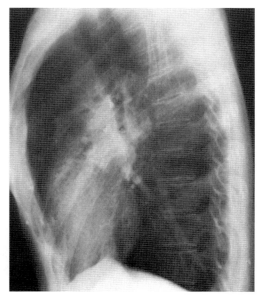

b

Table 17.2 (Cont.) Hilar and/or Mediastinal Lymph Node Enlargement

Disease	Radiographic Findings	Comments
Langerhans' cell histiocytosis (Histiocytosis X)	Symmetric hilar and mediastinal lymph node enlargement is a rare manifestation of Langerhans'-cell histiocytosis.	Lymph node enlargement in the presence of diffuse interstitial pulmonary disease favors sarcoidosis.
Goodpasture syndrome	Symmetric hilar node enlargement occurs predominantly in the acute stage.	The degree of diffuse alveolar and interstitial disease is dependent on the number of hemorrhagic episodes.
Cystic fibrosis (Fig. 17.21)	Unilateral or bilateral hilar node enlargement occurs in about half of chest X-rays of adult patients with cystic fibrosis. Can resemble sarcoidosis or lymphoma.	Areas of atelectasis and bronchiectasis with diffuse increase of pulmonary markings, hyperinflation, and pulmonary arterial hypertension predominate.
Drug induced	Bilateral hilar or mediastinal lymph node enlargement.	May occur during diphenylhydantoin or trimethadione therapy.
Pseudoenlargement	Enlargement of hilar vascular shadows may mimic hilar adenopathy. Blood vessels tend to parallel the bronchi, lymph nodes surround them.	Seen often in cardiovascular diseases (e.g., shunts, cardiac failure, valvular pulmonic stenosis, cor pulmonale, pulmonary embolism).

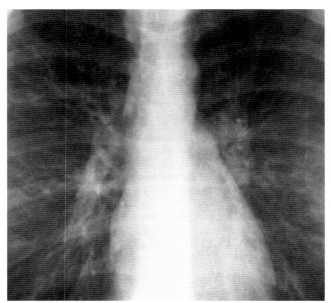 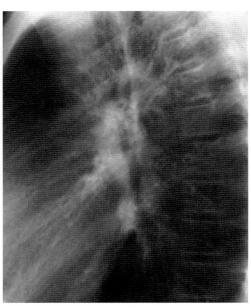

a   b

Fig. 17.**21 a, b Cystic fibrosis,** age 14. Hilar lymph nodes appear enlarged, but most of the increased density may be vascular, as shown by the lateral view. Pulmonary parenchymal changes are evident.

Table 17.3   Mediastinal Widening

Disease	Radiographic Findings	Comments
Mediastinal pseudo-widening	Expiratory film. Scoliosis.	Apparent mediastinal widening in expiratory films occurs especially in infants and children.
Normal thymus (see Fig. 17.5)	Anterior mediastinal mass in a neonate.	For differential diagnostic characteristics, see the introductory text of this chapter.
Foregut cysts (bronchogenic, neurenteric, etc.) (Fig. 17.22)	Round or oval, usually single well-defined density but can be multilocular. *Bronchogenic* cysts are usually found in contact with the trachea or central bronchi. Rarely they contain air. *Neurenteric* cysts are located in the posterior mediastinum.	Bronchogenic cyst may slowly grow and compress tracheobronchial tree or esophagus. Cysts in the hilar area are usually asymptomatic. Neurenteric cysts are frequently associated with spinal anomalies. The cystic structure of the mass is demonstrated with contrast enhanced CT.
Mesothelial cyst (pericardial or pleuropericardial cysts and diverticula) (see Fig. 16.31)	Smoothly marginated, round or oval density in the anterior or middle mediastinum, most commonly in the right pericardiophrenic angle.	Lateral bulge and smooth, sharp contour differentiate a cyst from right middle lobe lesion or fat in the cardiophrenic angle. Better definition is achieved with CT.

(continues on page 450)

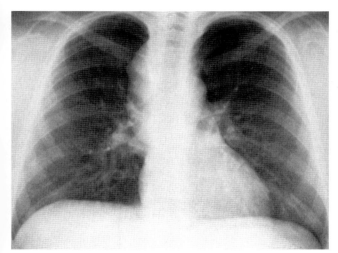 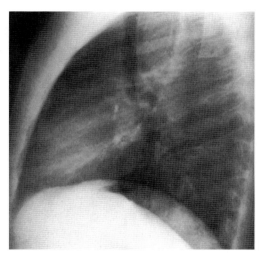

b

Fig. 17.**22 a, b   Bronchogenic cyst.** An oval well-delineated mass in the right middle mediastinum with anterior tracheal displacement.

Table 17.3 (Cont.) Mediastinal Widening

Disease	Radiographic Findings	Comments
Diverticula of the pharynx or esophagus (Fig. 17.23)	A cyst-like structure near pharynx or esophagus. Communication with esophagus is demonstrated by barium swallow.	Small diverticula are not visible without barium. Larger cysts may displace contiguous esophagus. Aspiration pneumonia may be a complication of a pharyngeal diverticulum (Zenker's diverticulum).
Meningocele	A sharply circumscribed, solitary or multiple density in the posterior mediastinum.	Spine or rib deformities are frequent.
Thyroid masses and tumors (Figs. 17.24 and 17.25)	A smooth or lobulated mass usually in the superior, anterior mediastinum, but may protrude behind the trachea and esophagus. Sometimes calcified.	Calcifications occur both in benign and malignant thyroid masses. Respiratory symptoms and dysphagia may occur.
Thymoma (Figs. 17.26 and 17.27)	Smooth or lobulated anterior mediastinal lesion, rarely calcifies.	Myasthenia gravis is frequently associated. Thyroid and thymic tumors are often roentgenographically indistinguishable. The site of origin is better predicted using CT.

(continues on page 452)

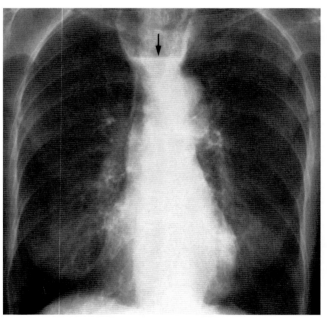

Fig. 17.**23** **A large Zenker's diverticulum** presenting as a cystic expansion of the upper mediastinum with an air-fluid level (arrow).

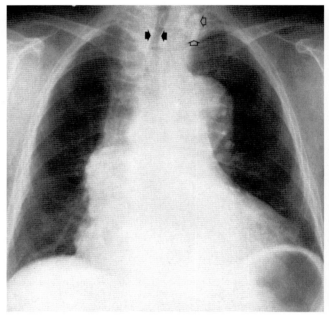

Fig. 17.**24** **Enlarged thyroid.** Upper mediastinal mass with narrowed trachea (closed arrowheads) and calcification (open arrowheads). The ascending aorta is seen as a hump overlying the right hilus.

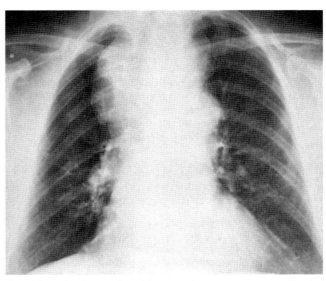
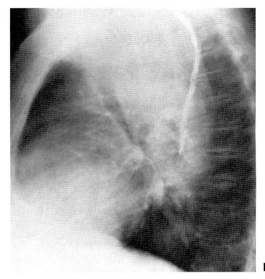

Fig. 17.**25 a, b** **Large thyroid** presenting as an upper mediastinal mass, which in the lateral view extends down into the middle mediastinum between the trachea and esophagus.

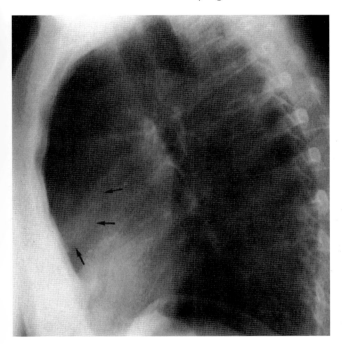

Fig. 17.**26** **Thymoma.** A smooth anterior mediastinal mass that was visible only in the lateral view (arrows).

Fig. 17.**27 a, b** **a A large thymoma** mimics an enlarged main pulmonary segment in posteroanterior projection, but the lesion is behind the sternum in the lateral view (**b**).
▽

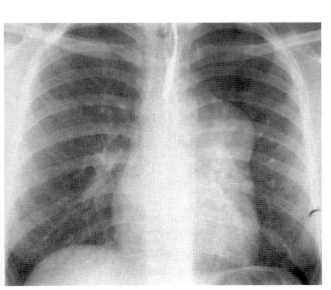
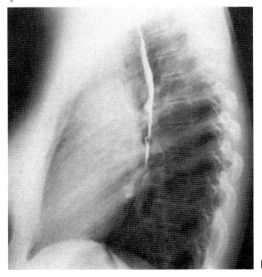

Table 17.3   (Cont.) Mediastinal Widening

Disease	Radiographic Findings	Comments
Teratoma Germinal cell neoplasms (dermoid cyst, seminoma, choriocarcinoma, endodermal sinus tumor) (Figs. 17.28 and 17.29)	Smoothly delineated mass, almost invariably in the anterior mediastinum. Calcification, bone, teeth or fat may be identified in teratomas and dermatoid cysts.	Usually manifest in adolescence or early adulthood. Teratomas are most common, they tend to be symptomatic in children. Cystic tumors are usually benign and solid ones malignant. Fat, soft-tissue and bone components are often demonstrated by CT.
Parathyroid tumors	Most tumors are too small to be seen on plain films, but may be detectable with ultrasound examination. Large ones occur in the anterior, upper mediastinum and may displace the esophagus.	Roentgenographic and laboratory evidence of hyperparathyroidism may be present independent of the size of the tumors.
Lipoma Liposarcoma mediastinal lipomatosis (see 16.32)	A smooth bulge to either side of the mediastinum, usually anterior. Fat density may be distinguishable even on plain films. CT scans show uniform fat density.	Lipomas are usually asymptomatic. Symmetric widening of the upper mediastinum and large epicardial fat pads (lipomatosis) occurs in long term corticosteroid therapy.
Fibroma Fibrosarcoma Hemangioma hemangiosarcoma hemangioendothelioma, lymphangioma (Fig. 17.30) hygroma leiomyoma (Fig. 17.31)	Most occur in the anterior mediastinum as well circumscribed densities with no distinctive features. Fibrosarcomas occur more commonly in the posterior mediastinum.	Demonstration of phleboliths is diagnostic of a hemangioma type tumor. Hygroma occurs in infants as a cervicomediastinal mass.

(continues on page 454)

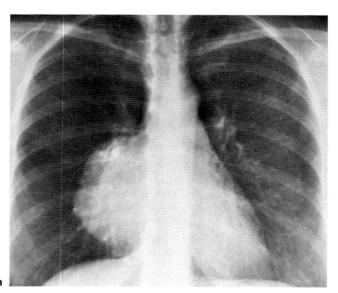
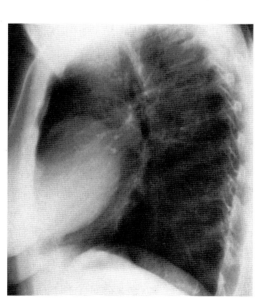

a   b

Fig. 17.**28**   **A large mediastinal teratoma,** radiographically similar to pericardial cyst.

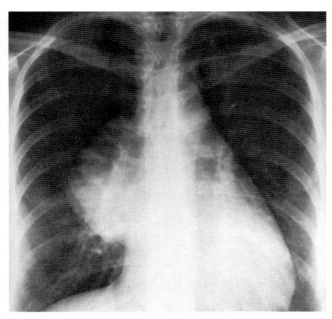
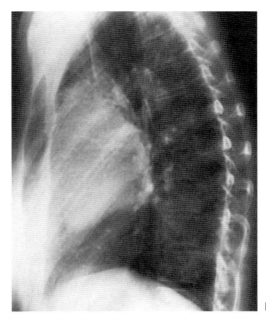

Fig. 17.**29**   **Malignant epidermoid tumor** at the right heart border. The tumor is slightly lobulated but otherwise indistinguishable from the teratoma in Fig. 17.**28**.

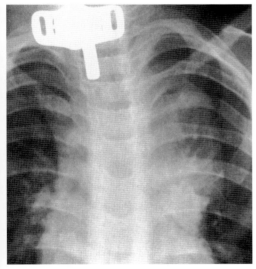

Fig. 17.**30**   **Cavernous lymphangioma** (cystic hygroma), in a 4-year-old child, appears as a smooth left-sided upper mediastinal mass.

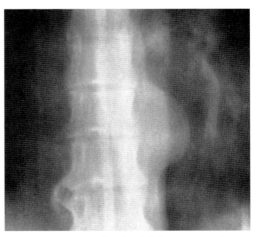

Fig. 17.**31**   **Paramediastinal leiomyoma.** A smooth bulge attached to the paraspinal ligament without bone erosion.

Table 17.3 (Cont.) Mediastinal Widening

Disease	Radiographic Findings	Comments
Lymphoma (Hodgkin's or non-Hodgkin's) Leukemia (Figs. 17.32 and 17.33)	Middle or anterior mediastinal mass. Solitary, tabulated, or symmetrical widening of the mediastinum. Leukemic masses tend to be smaller than those due to lymphoma.	The most common mediastinal mass lesion (25%). Constitutional and local symptoms are frequent, the latter especially in lymphoma.
Metastatic lymph node enlargement (Fig. 17.34)	Usually in the middle mediastinum, commonly unilateral, involving paratracheal and bronchopulmonary nodes.	The common primary cause is bronchogenic carcinoma. May originate from GI/GU tract (prostate, kidney, etc.).
Esophageal neoplasms (see Fig. 17.3)	Widening of the posterior tracheal band or obliteration of the retrotracheal lucency. Benign tumors are rare (e.g. leiomyoma) and may present as a rounded mass along the course of the esophagus.	Malignant esophageal neoplasms rarely become large enough to be seen as mass lesions, but if the upper two-thirds of the esophagus are involved, abnormality of the posterior tracheal band is a fairly sensitive indicator.

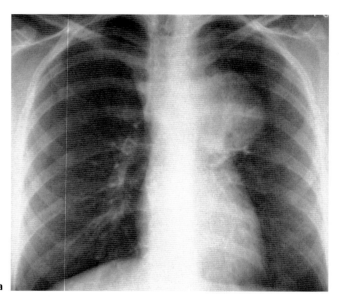
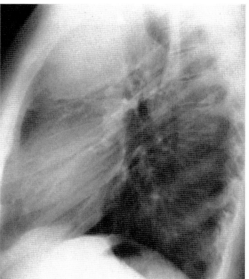

a
b

Fig. 17.**32 a, b** **Hodgkin's lymphoma.** A solitary anterior mediastinal mass is seen.

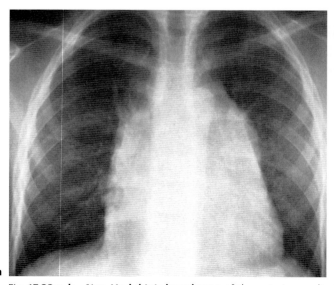
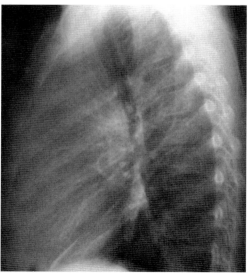

a
b

Fig. 17.**33 a, b** **Non-Hodgkin's lymphoma** of the anterior mediastinum causing bilateral anterior mediastinal widening.

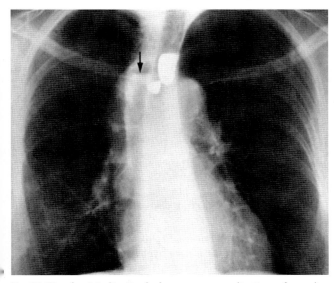

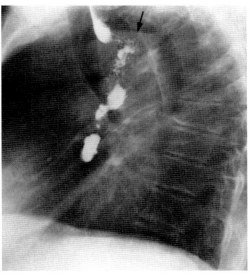

Fig. 17.**42 a, b** **Mediastinal abscess,** a complication of esophageal carcinoma. **a** Widening of mediastinum toward the right. An airfluid level superimposed on the right clavicle (arrow), **b** Extra-esophageal location of the air-fluid level shown with barium in the esophagus.

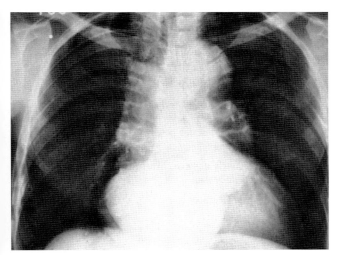

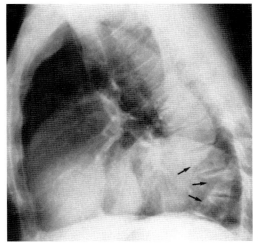

Fig. 17.**43 a, b** **Aneurysm of the thoracic descending aorta** simulating a mediastinal tumor. The aneurysm has eroded three thoracic vertebral bodies anteriorly (T9 to T11, arrows).

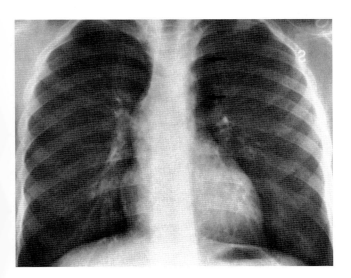

Fig. 17.**44** **Persistent left superior vena cava** without other vascular anomalies. An accessory silhouette, continuous with the left heart border and lateral to the aortic shadow (arrows).

Table 17.3 (Cont.) Mediastinal Widening

Disease	Radiographic Findings	Comments
Dilatation of the superior vena cava (Fig. 17.45)	Smooth widening of the right middle paramediastinal area extending from hilum upwards.	Secondary to elevated central venous pressure (heart failure), or compression/obstruction due to a mediastinal mass.
Dilatation of the azygos vein	A smooth mass at the right tracheobronchial angle. Its diameter changes with change in body position or intrathoracic pressure.	Associated with heart failure, vena cava obstruction, or azygos continuation of the inferior vena cava.
Pneumomediastinum (Fig. 17.46)	Smooth, usually minor widening of mediastinum associated with air in the mediastinum. Air tends to migrate upward in to the neck.	Commonly spontaneous. May be associated with pneumothorax and subcutaneous or interstitial emphysema. If there is air only in the pericardium, it does not rise above the pulmonary artery:
Mediastinal hemorrhage or hematoma (Fig. 17.47)	Focal or more commonly diffuse mediastinal widening.	Trauma or mediastinal surgery (most commonly coronary bypass) are the most frequent causes. Rupture of an aortic aneurysm is likely if there is no history of trauma. Hemorrage may be due fracture of thoracic vertebra.
Hernia through foramen of Morgagni	A round "bump" at the right anterior cardiophrenic angle; can be bilateral. May contain intestine (colon) or liver.	In liver herniation, the abdominal portion of the liver appears small. Congenital cardiac malformation may be associated.
Esophageal hiatus hernia (Fig. 17.48)	A retrocardiac mass of variable size, usually containing an air–fluid level.	Readily identified by giving a barium swallow. More common in elderly patients.
Herniation through foramen of Bochdalek	Round or oval retrocardiac density, usually unilateral. 80–90% occur on the left side. If large it may contain bowel loops, which displace ipsilateral lung.	The most common congenital defect of the diaphragm. A large Bochdalek hernia is a rare cause of acute respiratory distress in a neonate.
Diaphragmatic eventration	A broad-based mass, more laterally on PA chest X-ray than mediastinal lesions.	Usually easy to differentiate from a mediastinal lesion.
Diaphragmatic rupture.	Usually on the left side after trauma	

(continues on page 462)

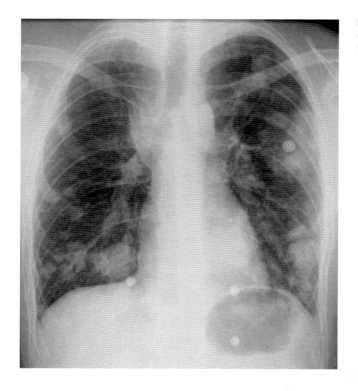

Fig. 17.**45 Dilatation of superior vena cava** by metastasis of synovial sarcoma of right glenohumeral joint (partially visible) in 28-years-old male.

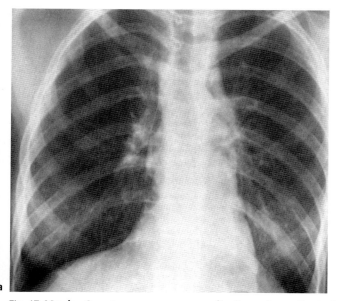 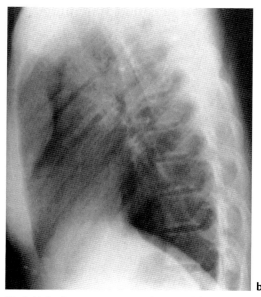

Fig. 17.**46 a, b** **Spontaneous pneumomediastinum** in a patient with Hodgkin's disease. **a** Minor widening of the mediastinum in frontal projection, **b** Air outlines the retrosternal mass.

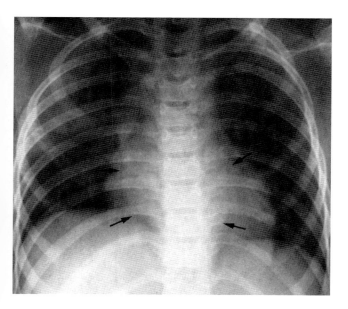

Fig. 17.**47** **Traumatic mediastinal hematoma.** Bilateral increase of softtissue density is seen behind the heart (arrows). It does not extend into the posterior costophrenic sinuses, thus suggesting middle mediastinal location.

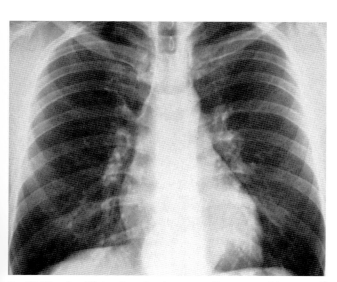 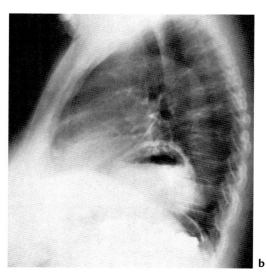

Fig. 17.**48 a, b** **Hiatus hernia.** A retrocardiac mass with an air–fluid level.

Table 17.3 (Cont.) Mediastinal Widening

Disease	Radiographic Findings	Comments
Megaesophagus (Fig. 17.49)	A broad vertical opacity at the right side of the mediastinum, turning toward the left side just above diaphragm. Air in the lumen and air–fluid level are common.	Achalasia is the most common cause. Chaga's disease can be radiographically indistinguishable. A stricture in the gastroesophageal junction with prestenotic dilatation (e.g. in scleroderma) may produce a similar radiographic appearance. Esophageal carcinoma does not usually cause extensive widening and/or muscular thickening of the esophagus.
Post surgery (Figs. 17.50 and 17.51)	Bizarre patterns may be produced, especially by colonic or stomach interposition for the treatment of esophageal carcinoma.	Refer to patient history for surgery information.

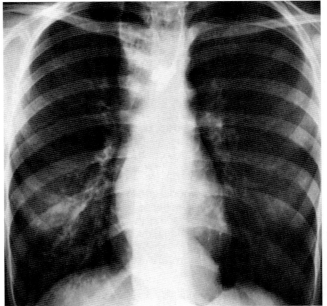
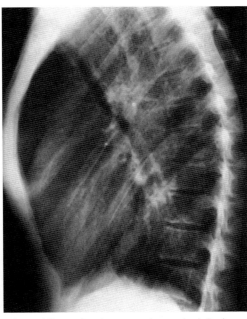

a   b

Fig. 17.**49 a, b**   **Achalasia** (megaesophagus). A vertical opacity in the right middle mediastinum curving to the left above the diaphragm.

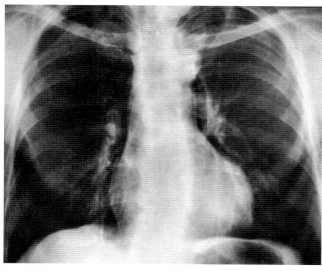
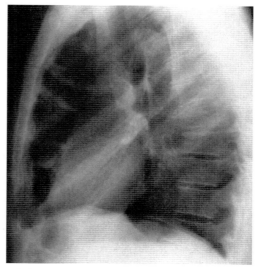

a   b

Fig. 17.**50 a, b**   **a Colonic interposition** for the treatment of esophageal obstruction mimicking pneumomediastinum. **b** Typical colonic haustra are seen in the anterior mediastinum.

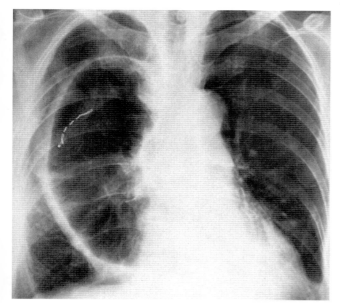
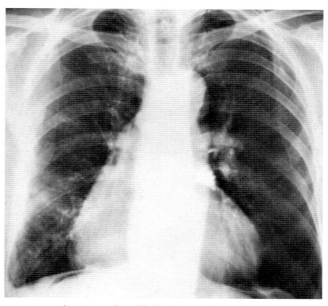

b

Fig. 17.**51**   **Stomach surgically interposed** in the mediastinum for the treatment of distal esophageal carcinoma may **a** mimic pneumomediastinum if gasfilled or **b** a mediastinal mass, if not distended with gas.

18 Pleura and Diaphragm

Up to 15 ml of pleural fluid is present in normal healthy humans. This amount is not visualized in normal chest roentgenograms, but it can be demonstrated using a horizontal roentgen beam and lateral decubitus projection, which is the most sensitive plain film technique for such a purpose. As much as 250–600 ml of pleural fluid is required for roentgenographic demonstration in the erect subject.

Lowering or flattening of diaphragm may be caused by increased air pressure, emphysema of any origin and air trapping for any reason. Elevation is caused by a number of conditions which are discussed on Table 18.2. Diaphragm may show one or several humps. They may be congenital or caused by disease which usually is extrapulmonary.

Roentgenologic Signs of Pleural Effusion

Gravity and elastic recoil of lung tissue cause collection of fluid between the inferior surface of the lung and the hemidiaphragm, particularly in the deepest posterior sinus. The layer of fluid that spreads upward in a mantle-like fashion around the lung becomes thinner until the parietal and visceral layers of the pleura meet again. This is influenced by capillary attraction. Since there is less elastic recoil in the mediastinal surface of the lung, less fluid accumulates along this surface than around the convexity. Thus in posteroanterior projection, the density of the fluid will be high laterally and will curve gently downward and medially, with a smooth *meniscus-shaped* upper border (Fig. 18.1). The height of fluid accumulation is identical posteriorly, laterally, and anteriorly, but the thin layer of fluid viewed

en face will not cast a discernible shadow. Frequently, small amounts of fluid may accumulate between the inferior surface of the lower lobe and the diaphragm without "spilling over" into the costophrenic sinuses. Such infrapulmonary fluid collections may be confirmed by using the lateral decubitus position with a horizontal beam. In this position, the fluid accumulates into the lowermost lateral pleural space. The typical radiographic findings caused by free pleural effusion are: (1) obliteration of the normally sharp costophrenic angles (first posterior, then lateral and finally anterior); (2) extension of the fluid up the chest wall resulting in a meniscus-shaped density. In the presence of pneumothorax, the fluid layer laterally is strictly horizontal in the absence of capillary attraction (Fig. 18.2); (3) thickening of the interlobar pleural septa (wet pleura), commonly present in congestive heart failure. (4) Replacement atelectasis of the ipsilateral lung, enlargement of the ipsilateral hemithorax, displacement of the mediastinum to the contralateral side, and concave depression of the ipsilateral hemidiaphragm are changes typical of massive pleural fluid accumulation. If one hemithorax is totally opacified, but the mediastinum shows no shifting and the hemidiaphragm is not markedly depressed, the findings are not caused primarily by a space-occupying process of pleural effusion but are due to primary reduction of the volume of the ipsilateral lung, e.g., pulmonary disease. The most likely cause of such a finding is an endobronchial obstruction, such as bronchogenic carcinoma. Films taken in the supine position are insensitive in detecting pleural effusion, which layers behind the lung. Increased density of the hemithorax and a

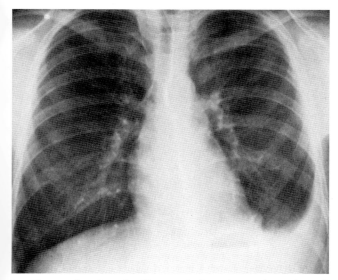

Fig. 18.**1 Left pleural effusion** (tuberculous pleuritis) with characteristic meniscus shape. No other abnormality.

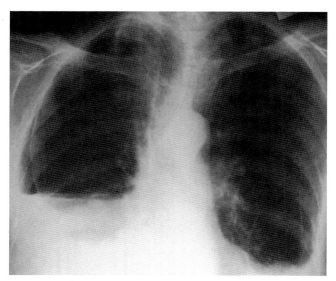

Fig. 18.**2 Bilateral, freely mobile pleural effusions** with and without pneumothorax. On the left side, the pleural fluid has a meniscus shape, while on the right side it is strictly horizontal due to pneumothorax.

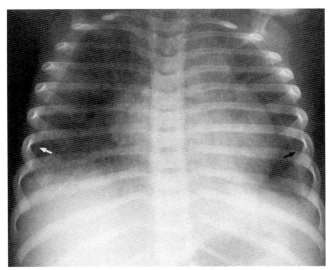

Fig. 18.**3 Bilateral pleural effusion** in a newborn (due to heart failure) as seen in supine position. There is a slight increase in the density of the right hemithorax, where the amount of fluid is greater and there is more replacement collapse of the lung, The layer of fluid in the pleural space is widest near the pulmonary apices. Major fissures are demonstrated because fluid enters into the lateral aspect of the fissures (arrows).

layer of fluid in the surrounding pleural space may be seen (Fig. 18.**3**).

Atypical distribution of pleural fluid may indicate localized parenchymal disease as well as pleural disease. In the region of parenchymal disease, the elastic recoil is decreased and fluid is attracted to those areas of the thorax where retraction force is greatest, e.g., where lung tissue is normal. Pleural fluid may simulate atelectasis or consolidation (Figs. 18.**4** and 18.**5**). Lateral decubitus view may help in visualizing the underlying parenchymal changes by re-

distributing the fluid. Infrapulmonary (subpulmonary) pleural effusion (Fig. 18.**6**) without blunted costophrenic angles may represent a phenomenon of altered pulmonary recoil, but it is also seen with apparently normal lung. Although the lateral decubitus view is the best way of demonstrating an infrapulmonary fluid collection, it is important to know the following signs commonly present in erect films to raise suspicion of infrapulmonary effusion:

1. Infrapulmonary fluid is more common on the right; it can be bilateral.
2. In posteroanterior projection, the peak of the pseudodiaphragmatic configuration is lateral to that of the normal hemidiaphragm.
3. On the left side, there is an increased distance between the lung base and the gastric air bubble (this also occurs with gastric tumors and interposition of the liver or spleen) (Fig. 18.**6**). An indentation on the gastric air bubble represents the depressed diaphragm.
4. The posterior costophrenic gutter is usually blunted, although other signs of fluid in costophrenic angles are lacking.
5. In the lateral projection, the contour of the fluid is usually flattened anterior to the major fissure. This segment descends abruptly to the anterior costophrenic angle.
6. There may be a triangular mediastinal collection of fluid seen in the anteroposterior view.

Loculated or encysted pleural fluid may occur anywhere in the pleural space secondary to pleural adhesions. Samples of loculated pleural fluid are presented in Figures 18.**7** and 18.**8**. Encapsulated fluid in the lower half of the major fissure may mimic atelectasis and consolidation of the right middle lobe. However, encapsulated fluid does not obscure the minor fissure or right heart border as do atelectasis or consolidation of the middle lobe. Furthermore, encapsulated fluid has a spindle-shaped form, whereas the shadow of the diseased middle lobe has straight or slightly concave borders. Encapsulated fluid does not move in response to postural changes. Thus, encapsulated fluid and pleural thickening may have identical appearance.

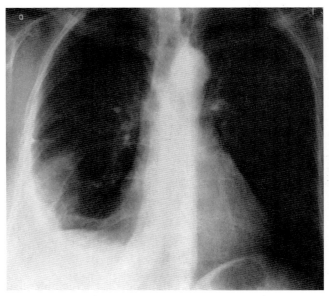

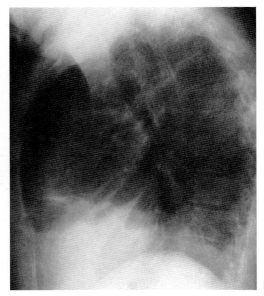

a

Fig. 18.**4 a, b Right pleural effusion** (metastatic breast carcinoma, post left mastectomy) may mimic consolidation or atelecta-

b

sis in anteroposterior projection. The densities are created by fluid in the fissures surrounding the middle lobe.

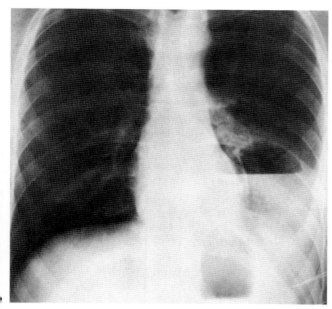

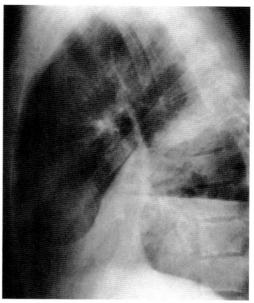

b

Fig. 18.**5 a, b** **Atypical accumulation of pleural effusion** around a left lower lobe abscess containing an air–fluid level.

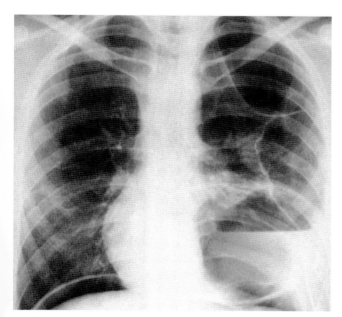

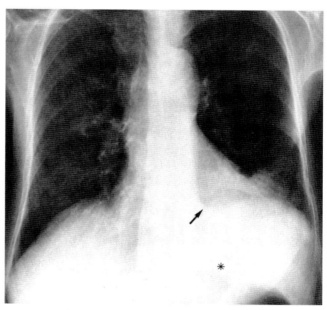

Fig. 18.**5 c** **Post thoracentesis.** There is inadvertent pneumothorax and pneumoperitoneum. The fluid within the abscess remains, while the pleural collection has disappeared.

Fig. 18.**6** **Infrapulmonary pleural effusion** on the left (chronic leukemia). The peak of the pseudodiaphragmatic configuration is more lateral than normal and there is increased distance between the lung base and the gastric air bubble (asterisk). A triangular rnediastinal collection of fluid is seen (arrow).

Pleural fluid tends to have an identical roentgenographic appearance independent of its nature (transudate, exudate, pus, blood). Transudate contains protein more than 30 g/l and exudate less than 30 g/l. Transudate is often present with heart or liver failure, nephrotic syndrome or Meigs syndrome. Infections, malignancies, collagen vascular diseases, etc often causes presence of exudate. Differential diagnosis of pleural fluid (effusion) therefore often has to be based on other radiographic manifestations of disease in the chest, patient history, and pleural tap.

Positive diagnosis is often, but not always, obtained from laboratory studies of the pleural fluid. In Table 18.1, emphasis has been put on associated radiologic findings as criteria for differential diagnosis.

Pleural effusion unassociated with other roentgenographic evidence of disease in the thorax is a nonspecific finding and the differential diagnosis depends on additional clinical information or roentgenographic findings elsewhere in the body.

Common causes of pleural fluid with the otherwise normal-looking chest are:

1 infection of the pleura (*tuberculosis, viral diseases*) or of the abdomen (*pancreatitis, subphrenic abscess*);
2 extrathoracic carcinoma, either metastatic to the pleura or mediastinal nodes (most commonly due to *breast carcinoma*) or via diaphragmatic lymphatics (*carcinoma of the pancreas* or *retroperitoneal lymphoma*);
3 collagen diseases (*rheumatoid arthritis, systemic lupus erythematosus*);
4 *cirrhosis* with *ascites*;
5 closed *chest trauma* or *abdominal surgery*.

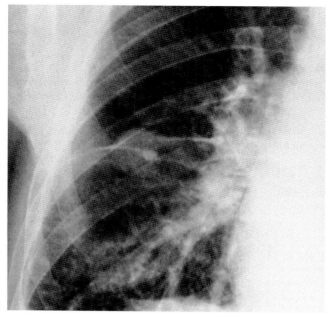

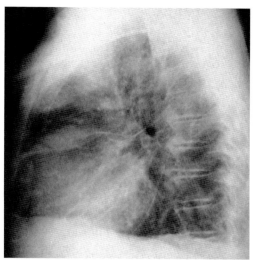

b

Fig. 18.**7 a, b   Encapsulated fluid in the minor fissure;** a pseudotumor, The lobulated effusion has a typical spindle-shaped form. Severe heart failure with interstitial pulmonary edema.

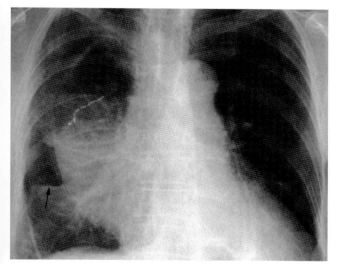

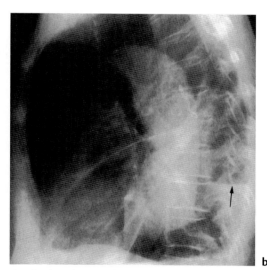

b

Fig. 18.**8 a, b   Loculated right posterior hydropneumothorax** post surgery for esophageal carcinoma. An air–fluid level is seen around the right lower lobe (arrows), secondary to the rupture of the displaced stomach which is seen as a density over the right heart border.

Table 18.1 Differential Diagnosis of Pleural Effusion

Disease	Radiographic Findings	Comments
Neoplasms		
Bronchogenic carcinoma	A common radiological manifestation of bronchial carcinoma at presentation is a pleural effusion. Obstructive pneumonitis associated with ipsilateral pleural effusion and eventual hilar or mediastinal lymphadenopathy.	The volume of effusion is usually large. Following aspiration it rapidly accumulates. It is commonly blood stained and contains malignant cells.
Lymphoma (Fig. 18.9)	Pleural effusion is associated with single or multiple areas of consolidation and hilar or mediastinal lymph node enlargement. Approximately one-third of patients have pleural fluid.	Includes leukemia, Hodgkin's disease, and non-Hodgkin's lymphoma. Pleural effusion alone may occur especially in retroperitoneal lymphoma.
Metastatic neoplasm (see Fig. 18.4)	Diffuse pulmonary densities and pleural effusion together with normal heart size.	Hematogeneous spread results generally in nodular densities. Lymphangitic spread results in linear densities (A and B lines) with eventual lymph node enlargement. Pleural effusion may be the only presenting finding. Breast cancer is the most common origin. Other primaries include pancreas, stomach, ovary and kidney.
Mesothelioma (Fig. 18.10)	Massive pleural effusion associated with nodular diffuse pleural thickening. Volume of ipsilateral hemithorax may be reduced despite massive opacification,	In the diffuse variety of mesothelioma, pleural effusion is a characteristic finding. History of asbestosis is common. The local variety of mesothelioma presents as a peripheral mass and pleural effusion is rare.
Ovarian neoplasms (Meigs' syndrome)	Pleural fluid and/or ascites associated with benign ovarian tumour.	Pleural fluid and/or ascites secondary to ovarian neoplasms other than benign primary ovarian tumors or GI malignancies is called pseudo-Meigs' syndrome.
Carcinoma of pancreas	Effusion may occur by transport of fluid into thorax through diaphragmatic lymphatics, in such case pleural fluid is the only presenting sign in the chest roentgenogram.	Pleural fluid is negative for malignant cells unless metastatic deposits occur in pleura.
Multiple myeloma	Expanding soft-tissue lesion(s) arising from the chest wall is sometimes associated with pleural fluid.	Pleural effusion as a first sign of multiple myeloma is rare.
Primary neoplasms of the chest wall	May present an identical pattern compared to multiple myeloma.	Rare condition. Most are sarcomas.
Infections		
Bacterial pneumonia	Variable findings including pleural effusions may be seen. Some more specific presentations are described below.	The pattern of pulmonary parenchymal disease is more diagnostic in pneumonia but not a specific finding.
Tularemia (*Francisella tularensis*)	Spherical or oval pulmonary densities. Enlarged lymph nodes and pleural effusion occurs in one third of patients.	Pleural effusions are more common in the typhoidal form (50–77%) than in the non-typhoidal form (8–26%). History of animal exposure is suggestive. Is a potential bioterrorism agent.
Q fever (*Coxiella burnetii*)	Q fever pneumonia has a nonspecific appearance on chest radiographs. A small pleural effusion may occur.	Zoonosis with a world wide distribution. Has caused epidemics in Eastern Europe. Is a potential bioterrorism agent.
Staphylococcus aureus	Pneumonia followed by empyema in infants and children is typical. Abscesses or pneumatoceles are common.	A confluent, destructive segmental pneumonia followed by empyema. Empyema occurs in 90% of cases in children and in 50% of adults.
Tuberculosis (see Fig. 18.1)	Pleural effusion is often the only manifestation, associated parenchymal disease is rare.	A manifestation of primary tuberculosis more common in adults than in children.
Clostridium perfringens	A combination of pleural effusion, gas in soft tissues, and eventual segmental broncho-pneumonia.	Gas in soft tissues occurs more commonly in postoperative conditions or is associated with trauma.
Invasive fungal infections	A combination of cavitary pneumonia, pleural effusion (empyema), and chest wall involvement is highly suggestive of actinomycosis or nocardiosis.	Pleural effusion in other fungal infections of the chest is rare. Occasionally, (in 2%) histoplasmosis may present with pleural effusion indistinguishable from tuberculous pleuritis. Aspergillus may invade empyema cavity but is a rare cause of pleural effusion.

(continues on page 472)

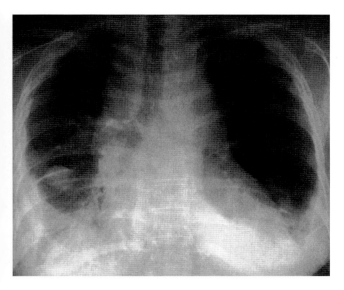

Fig. 18.**9** **Bilateral pleural effusion** in non-Hodgkin's lymphoma involving the mediastinum. Loculated fluid is seen in the minor fissure.

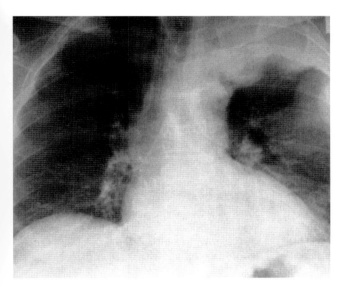

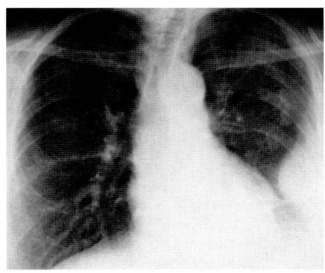

b

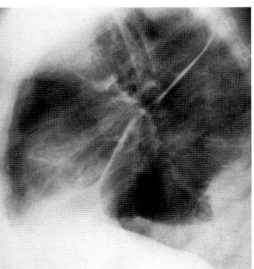

Fig. 18.**10 a–c** **Mesothelioma** (two cases). **a** A characteristic pattern of diffuse mesothelioma. Nodular thickening of pleura and pleural fluid are seen. **b, c** The tumor is seen as a local, slightly irregular, bulge in both AP and lateral projections, i.e., the tumor is more extensive than can be expected from a single view. Moderate amount of pleural fluid.

Table 18.1   (Cont.) Differential Diagnosis of Pleural Effusion

Disease	Radiographic Findings	Comments
Viral infections and *Mycoplasma pneumoniae*	A combined interstitial and air-space pneumonia is a common presentation. Pleural effusion only is uncommon.	Occasionally, pleural effusion may be the only presenting sign.
Amebiasis *(Entamoeba histolytica)*	A rare combination of lower lobe consolidation, pleural effusion, and enlarged liver in a patient with diarrhea.	The organism may infiltrate from the liver abscess through diaphragm into pleura, lung and pericardium and cause this rare combination.
Echinococcus (Hydatid disease)	Hydropneumothorax occurs when an echinococcal cyst ruptures into the pleural space.	
Abdominal inflammation	Ipsilateral pleural effusion associated with evidence of abdominal disease.	Pleural effusion occurs commonly in pancreatitis (characteristically left-sided) and in subphrenic abscesses.
Miscellaneous		
Systemic lupus Erythematosus	Bilateral pleural effusion, nonspecific cardiac enlargement, and basal atelectasis or pneumonia are suggestive.	Pulmonary changes are nonspecific. Cardiac enlargement is usually due to pericardial effusion.
Rheumatoid arthritis	A long-standing pleural effusion with or without pulmonary interstitial disease.	Pleural effusion may be the only presenting sign. The glucose content of the effusion is typically low.
Wegener's granulomatosis	A combination of pleural effusion and single or multiple pulmonary nodules, which may cavitate, associated with renal disease.	Effusion may be present in about half of the cases.
Waldenstrom's macroglobulinemia	Pleural effusion associated with diffuse reticulonodular pattern in the lungs.	Anemia, monoclonal IgM gammopathy, and lymphocytic or plasma cell infiltration of the bone marrow. Pleural effusion is present in roughly 50% of cases.
Pulmonary embolism and infarction (Fig. 18.11)	Variable patterns may include line shadows, segmental consolidation, elevation of the hemidiaphragm, small pleural effusions, and increased or decreased peripheral pulmonary vasculature.	Pleural effusion may occasionally be the only presenting sign. Pulmonary CT angiography is nowadays a common practice. Positive ventilation-perfusion scan is highly suggestive.

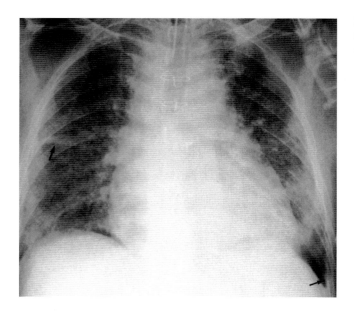

Fig. 18.**11** **Pulmonary embolism.** Bilateral small pleural effusions (arrows), pulmonary edema pattern, and an enlarged heart are seen.

Table 18.1   (Cont.) Differential Diagnosis of Pleural Effusion

Disease	Radiographic Findings	Comments
Congestive heart failure (see Fig. 16.9)	Cardiac enlargement associated with pleural effusion and clinical signs of cardiac decompensation, see Chapter 16.	Pleural effusion is right-sided or bilateral.
Postmyocardial infarction syndrome	See Chapter 16. Left-sided or bilateral pleural effusion is common (80%), often accompanied by pericardial effusion and/or pulmonary infiltrates.	Can occur a few days, or up to two months, after acute myocardial infarction.
Constrictive pericarditis	Signs of systemic venous hypertension associated with pericardial calcification (in about 50%) and pleural effusion (in about 50%).	
Obstruction of superior vena cava or azygos vein	Clinical signs of the superior vena cava syndrome, associated with mediastinal widening and pleural effusion.	May be caused by a tumor or, rarely, a benign process such as sclerosing mediastinitis.
Asbestosis	Three types of pleural changes occur alone or in combination with others: 1 Pleural plaques which calcify in about one third of cases; 2 pleural thickening and 3 pleural effusions. Associated pulmonary manifestations may produce a "shaggy heart" sign.	High incidence of associated bronchogenic carcinoma and mesolhelioma.
Open or closed chest trauma (including surgery) (Fig. 18.12)	A wide variety of changes: fractured ribs, pulmonary hemorrhage or hematoma, mediastinal hematoma, aortic aneurysm, pneumothorax, pneumomediastinum.	The history or associated findings usually allow a precise diagnosis. After abdominal surgery and closed chest trauma, pleural effusion may be the only presenting finding.

(continues on page 474)

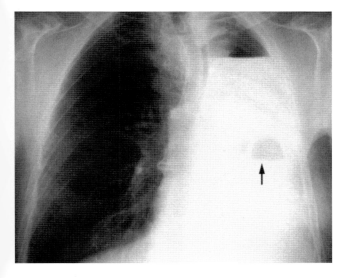

Fig. 18.**12   Surgical removal of the left lung.** There is gradual filling of the empty hemithorax with fluid. Displacement of the mediastinum to the left and of the gastric air bubble upward (arrow) indicate passive accumulation of fluid into the left hemithorax. Active accumulation of fluid (such as metastatic) would displace neighbouring organs away from the fluid-filled hemithorax.

Table 18.1 (Cont.) Differential Diagnosis of Pleural Effusion

Disease	Radiographic Findings	Comments
Chylothorax (Fig. 18.13)	After thoracic surgery and inadvertent injury to the thoracic duct, chylothorax (chylous effusion) may develop, often after a delay of a few days.	Chylous effusion may also be secondary to malignancy, parasites (filariasis) and lymphangiomyomatosis.
Sarcoidosis	Pleural effusion is rare (incidence 0.7 to 4%) in sarcoidosis and should be diagnosed only after exclusion of other more common causes of pleural effusion.	Miliary pulmonary shadows associated with pleural effusion is more likely due to disseminated metastases or tuberculosis.
Nephrotic syndrome Diminished plasma osmotic pressure	Commonly infrapulmonary effusion.	Biochemical assay of serum and urine shows proteinuria, hypoproteinemia and generalised edema.
Hydronephrosis	Pleural effusion without chest disease is a rare manifestation of hydronephrosis.	May be related to transport of fluid via diaphragmatic lymphatics.
Uremia, dialysis (Fig. 18.14)	Pleural effusion associated with pericardial effusion and/or pulmonary manifestations of uremia.	May mimic congestive heart failure.
Myxedema	Pleural effusion without distinctive features.	Pericardial effusion is more common.
Cirrhosis of the liver with ascites	Presents as pleural effusion without chest disease.	Ascites and other signs of cirrhosis are usually present.
Lymphedema	Pleural effusion associated with clinical findings of lymphedema.	Hypoplasia of the lymphatic system.
Familial Mediterranean fever (familial recurrent polyserositis)	Pleural effusion associated with osteoporosis, arthritis, and often pericarditis.	Hereditary, limited to Armenians, Arabs, and Sephardic (non-Ashkenazi) Jews. Typical manifestations include episodes of fever, with abdominal, thoracic or joint pain due to inflammation of the peritoneum, pleura, and synovial membrane. Amyloidosis may complicate the condition.
Drug-induced pleural effusion	Pleural effusion associated with interstitial lung disease or a lupus-like pattern.	Drugs: nitrofurantoin, hydralazine, procainamide.

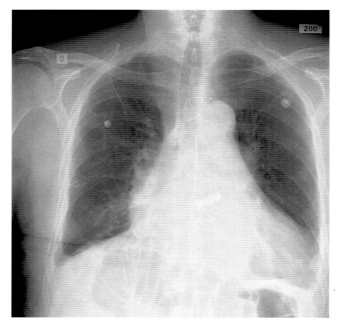

Fig. 18.**13** **Chylothorax** due to lacerated ductus thoracicus after thoracic aorta surgery in 70-years-old male.

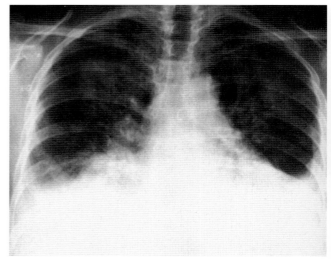

Fig. 18.**14** **Uremia.** Bilateral massive pleural effusions and patchy alveolar infiltrates (pulmonary edema).

Table 18.2 Differential Diagnosis of Diaphragmatic Elevation

Disease	Radiographic Findings	Comments
Normal variation	Usually right hemidiaphragm is 1–2.5 cm higher than left. Poor inspiration and obesity may cause apparent elevation.	In 10% of population diaphragms are at the same level or left hemidiaphragm is higher than right.
Eventration	Abnormal elevation of all or a portion of an attenuated but otherwise intact diaphragmatic leaf.	More common on right side. Diaphragm muscle is permanently elevated, but retains its continuity.
Phrenic nerve palsy (Fig. 18.15)	The affected side does not move correctly. In inspirium affected side tends to rise instead of lowering.	May be due bronchogenic carcinoma, mediastinal metastasis, neurologic disease, injury to the phrenic nerve at any location.
Pulmonary infarction secondary to pulmonary embolism. (Fig. 18.16)	Chest X-ray signs are nonspecific. They may include subpleural consolidation, segmental collapse or plate atelectasis, pleural reaction with small effusion, elevation of hemidiaphragm of the affected side. Rarely cavitation of the infarct.	Patients with pulmonary embolic disease leads to infarction in about one third of cases. Pulmonary CT angiography is diagnostic.

(continues on page 476)

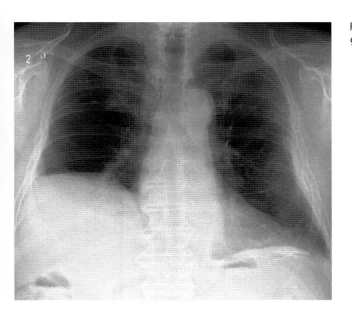

Fig. 18.**15 Phrenic nerve palsy.** The right hemidiaphragm is grossly elevated.

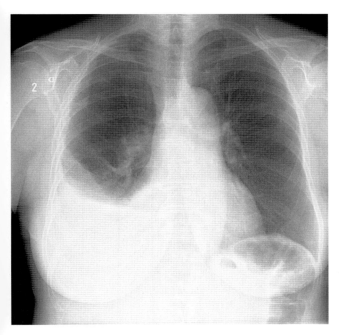

Fig. 18.**16 Pulmonary infarction.** Slightly elevated right hemidiaphragm, distorted branches of right lower lobe arteries and dilated main trunk of right pulmonary artery.

Table 18.2 (Cont.) Differential Diagnosis of Diaphragmatic Elevation

Disease	Radiographic Findings	Comments
Pulmonary collapse because of bronchial obstruction (Fig. 18.17)	Elevated hemidiaphragm. The cause of obstruction may not be seen.	Occlusion of a bronchus for any reason.
Subphrenic inflammatory disease	Elevated hemidiaphragm and restricted motion	Common causes: *pancreatitis* *subpherenic abscess* *hepatic abscess* *splenic abscess* *cholecystitis* *perforated ulcer*
Increased abdominal volume (Fig. 18.18)	Usually bilaterally elevated diaphragm	Common causes: *ascites* *pregnancy* *hepatomegaly (splenomegaly)* *large tumour* *obesity*
Old haemothorax Old empyema Post thoracotomy	Decreased lung volume associated with pleural thickening	
Post surgery	Combination of pneumothorax and air–fluid level. The volume of pneumothorax tends to decrease and eventually disappears	After pulmectomy or lobectomy the space fills with pleural fluid and hemidiaphragm raises.
Diaphragmatic hernias	May mimic unilateral diaphragmatic elevation	On lateral view Morgagni hernia is situated on the anterior portion and Bochdalek hernia on posterior location.
Diaphragmatic trauma Diaphragmatic splinting	More commonly on the left side.	May mimic elevated diaphragm as soft tissues herniate into the hemithorax. Stomach and/or bowel herniates on the left and liver on the right side.
Subpulmonic effusion (see Fig. 18.6)	This is not true elevation of diaphragm but pleural fluid collection between lung base and diaphragm. The distance between diaphragm and stomach air bubble is increased	Radiographic with horizontal X-rays on suspected side reveals fluid.
Rib fracture	Pain induced limited mobility of the diaphragm.	May be associated with hemo- or pneumothorax

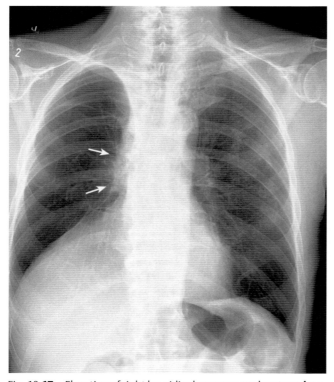

Fig. 18.**17** Elevation of right hemidiaphragm secondary to **pulmonary collapse** (epidermoid carcinoma).

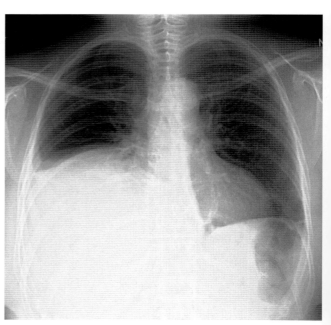

Fig. 18.**18** Elevated right hemidiaphragm due to **breast carcinoma metastases to the liver**.

19 Intrathoracic Calcifications

Calcifications in chest roentgenograms appear commonly. They are most frequently found in asymptomatic individuals as signs of "burned-out" disease or as the result of physiological calcification, such as calcification of the cartilagenous portions of the ribs or calcifications of the tracheobronchial tree. The causes of calcification of the soft tissues surrounding the thoracic cage are the same as those causing generalized calcification of periarticular soft tissues, and the reader should consult Chapter 7, Table 7.3.

Calcification of the aorta and other arteries is a common feature of old age in western countries and may have little diagnostic significance unless associated with other changes such as aneurysmatic dilatation of the artery. Atherosclerotic calcifications also commonly occur in the mitral and aortic annuli of the heart. Arteriosclerotic calcification of the coronary arteries is likewise common, but due to its high kVp, the routine chest radiograph rarely reveals such small calcifications in the heart or elsewhere. Multidetector CT is used for better visualization of cardiac calcifications. The lung is the most frequent visceral site of *metastatic calcifications*, which are most commonly associated with renal failure. Metastatic calcifications of the lungs are, however, rarely demonstrated radiographically. *Granulomatous calcifications* (Fig. 19.1) of the pulmonary parenchyma are common and diagnostically important, since demonstration of a calcified central nidus or laminated calcification in a pulmonary nodule is the most reliable sign of benignancy.

Diffuse or *miliary calcification* of the pulmonary parenchyma may be caused by several conditions but is less common than nodular calcification. Miliary calcifications of healed disseminated infections, mitral stenosis, or alveolar microlithiasis usually have distinctive features. *Calcification of pulmonary metastases* is uncommon. The most common primary neoplasm with calcified pulmonary metastases is osteosarcoma, but calcification may rarely occur in metastases of any mucinous adenocarcinoma. An eccentric calcification in a pulmonary mass can occasionally be found in a bronchogenic carcinoma engulfing a pre-existing granulomatous calcification.

Calcifications occur frequently in the thyroid, and may present as an upper mediastinal mass. Unfortunately, calcification of the thyroid mass is not a reliable sign of benignancy of the lesion. Other mediastinal tumors often have distinctive calcifications, e.g., demonstration of a bone or a tooth within a mass lesion is diagnostic for a *dermoid cyst*.

Calcification of the pleura may have the form of *continuous sheets* or *multiple calcified plaques*. The former type is usually unilateral and secondary to an old *pleural infection* (especially empyema or tuberculosis), or *hemothorax*. In such a case, calcium is usually deposited on the thickened visceral pleura and there is a thick layer of soft-tissue density between the calcification and the thoracic wall. Calcified or noncalcified plaques of the parietal pleura are typical of *asbestosis*, and the changes are usually bilateral. Associated pulmonary fibrosis is often lacking. If distinct calcification of apparently thickened pleura is lacking, nonpleural masses abutting the pleura should be considered. Such a finding may also be caused by intercostal fat or unusually prominent chest musculature. The latter is most common in the region from the 5th to 9th ribs in adults with inwardly concave lateral chest walls.

Hilar calcifications most commonly represent healed granulomatous infection of lymph nodes. They are usually stippled or amorphous and are irregularly distributed throughout the node. Ring calcification of the periphery of the lymph nodes (*"eggshell" calcification*) is unusual and characteristic of silicosis, but may very rarely also be found in sarcoidosis and in *irradiated Hodgkin's lymphoma*.

  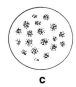 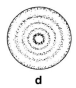 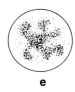

a   b   c   d   e

Fig. 19.**1** **Diagram of benign calcifications occurring in peripheral pul monary nodules: a** central nidus, **b** target lesion, **c** multiple punctate foci, **d** laminated, **e** conglomerate or "popcorn." Types **a** and **c** occur in granulomas or hamartomas. Type **b** is characteristic of histoplasmosis. Type **d** occurs only in granulomas and type **e** is characteristic of hamartomas.

Table 19.1 Differential Diagnosis of Cardiovascular Calcifications

Location of the calcification	Causes or associated condition	Comments
Aortic wall (Figs. 19.2 and 19.3)	Atherosclerosis Aneurysm Aortitis	Increased diameter of the aorta indicates an aneurysm. Increased distance between intimal calcification and the outer wall of the aorta suggests dissecting aneurysm. Heavy calcification of the dilated ascending aorta is characteristic of syphilitic aortitis.
Sinus of Valsalva (usually best seen in the lateral view) (Fig. 19.2)	Aneurysm of the sinus of Valsalva or, rarely, arteriosclerosis	Calcification may occur in the wall of the sinus and in the adjacent aorta. Heavy in syphilitic aneurysms. A thrombus in the aneurysm may calcify.
Coronary arteries (Fig. 19.4)	Arteriosclerosis of the coronary arteries (common) Coronary artery aneurysm (very rare)	The most common site of visible calcification is the proximal left circumflex artery. Easier to recognize in the lateral view as parallel linear or tubular calcifications.
Aortic annulus or aortic valves (Fig. 19.5)	Calcified annulus only: arteriosclerosis Valves with or without calcified annulus: Rheumatic aortic valve disease Arteriosclerosis Endocarditis Congenital defect of valve Hypercalcemia	Calcification of the annulus is usually heavy and distinct, whereas valvular calcifications are stippled and often superimposed by annulus, and not seen on plain films. If aortic valve disease appears before the age of 50 it is likely to be of rheumatic origin.

(continues on page 480)

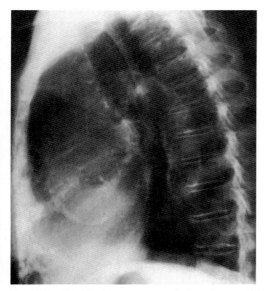

Fig. 19.**2** **Calcified aneurysm** of the sinus of Valsalva. Widespread atherosclerotic calcification of the thoracic aorta, multiple calcified paratracheal lymph nodes and heavily calcified rib cartilages are present.

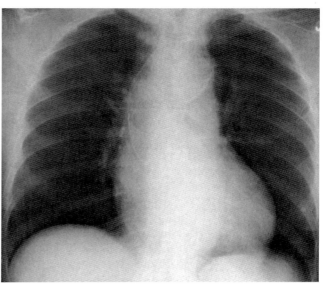

Fig. 19.**3** **Syphilitic aortitis** with aneurysmal dilatation and heavy calcification of the ascending aorta.

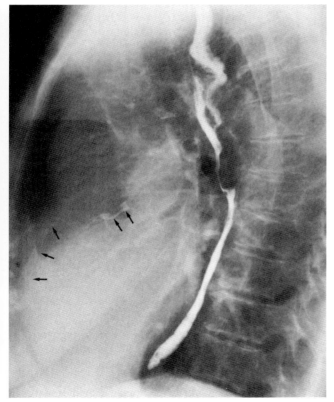

Fig. 19.**4** **Coronary artery calcifications** (arrows).

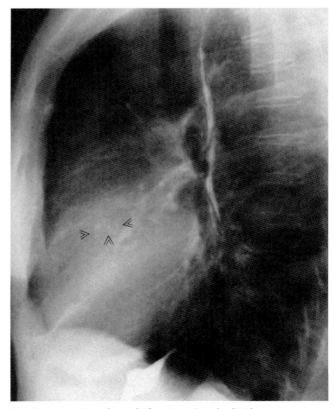

Fig. 19.**5** **Aortic valve calcifications** (marked). Rheumatic stenosis and insufficiency of the aortic valve.

Table 19.1 (Cont.) Differential Diagnosis of Cardiovascular Calcifications

Location of the calcification	Causes or associated condition	Comments
Mitral annulus (Fig. 19.6)	Arteriosclerosis	A dense curved or annular calcified band around the mitral valve. Usually insignificant, but rigid annulus may cause functional insufficiency of the mitral valve.
Mitral valve	Rheumatic mitral valve disease	Calcification may be indistinct and easily missed. The amount of calcification does not reflect the degree of functional disturbance.
Myocardium (Fig. 19.7)	Myocardial infarct Myocardial aneurysms due to infarct or rarely other causes such as syphilis Myocardial damage such as trauma, myocarditis, rheumatic fever (rare) Congenital (rare) Hyperparathyroidism (rare) Vitamin D overdosage (rare)	Calcification is usually smaller than the infarct. Most common at the apex with or without aneurysm.
Left atrium (rare) (wall or intra-atrial)	Rheumatoid mitral valve disease. Left atrial myxoma or thrombus	Calcification of the wall of the left atrium is seen as a thin, ring-like density in the frontal view. If the left atrial appendage is calcified, it is always due to a calcified thrombus. A calcified wall and a calcified thrombus may be difficult to differentiate from each other on the lateral view.
Ductus arteriosus (rare)	Patent ductus arteriosus	Difficult to differentiate from aortic calcification. May also occur with a closed ductus.
Pericardium (Fig. 19.8)	Pericarditis caused by: Tuberculosis Rheumatoid fever Bacterial pneumonia Myocardial infarction Viral infection Syphilis Histoplasmosis Asbestosis Trauma	The most common site of calcification is at the atrioventricular groove. Gross calcification of pericardium is associated with constrictive pericarditis in 50% of cases. The so-called annular constrictive pericarditis (rigid atrioventricular groove) may mimic mitral valve disease. Extensive calcification of the circumflex coronary may mimic atrioventricular groove calcification. It may be difficult to differentiate between myocardial and pericardial calcifications.

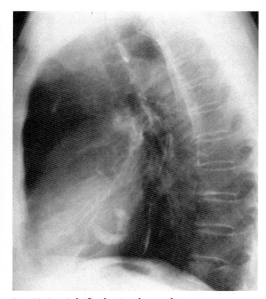

Fig. 19.**6   Calcified mitral annulus.**

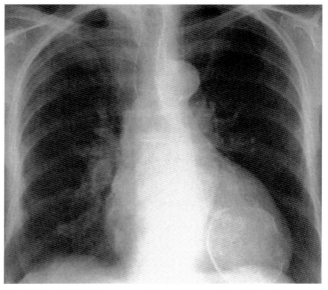

Fig. 19.**7   Calcified myocardial aneurysm** after infarction.

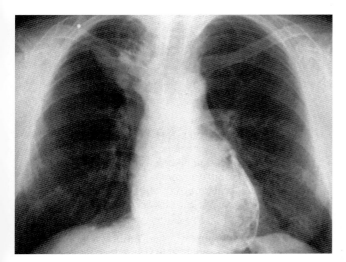

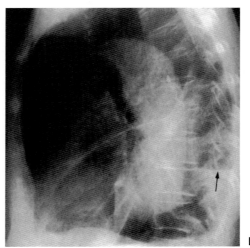

b

Fig. 19.**8 a, b   Calcified pericardium** (tuberculous pericarditis). Tuberculous granulomas and scarring in the right apex and an elevated right hilum are also evident.

Table 19.2 Differential Diagnosis of Pulmonary Calcifications Solitary calcified pulmonary nodule of any size (single or occasionally multiple)

Causes or associated condition	Comments
Bronchogenic cyst (rare)	Two-thirds occur medially in the lungs, one-third in the mediastinum. Usually several centimeters wide, smooth, and well-defined. Rarely the thin cyst wall may calcify. Once infected, cyst may contain air.
Pulmonary arteriovenous fistula (rare)	Up to 6 cm slightly lobulated well-defined, multiple in one-third of cases. Contains occasionally calcified phleboliths. Feeding artery and vein often identifiable.
Tuberculoma (common) (Figs. 19.9 and 19.10) Histoplasmoma (common in endemic areas) (Fig. 19.11) Coccidioidomycosis (rare)	A 0.5–5 cm round or oval lesion, with central calcification (calcific nidus, lamellated calcification or multiple punctate calcifications). A sizable target calcification is characteristic of histoplasmoma. A small lesion may be entirely calcified. Often associated with calcified regional lymph nodes and "satellite" lesions. May be multiple. If the calcification is eccentric, bronchogenic carcinoma growing around a granuloma is a possibility.
Bronchial adenoma (rare)	Approximately 20–25% of bronchial adenomas present as sharply circumscribed pulmonary nodules having a diameter of a few centimeters. Their calcification is rare.
Hamartoma (Fig. 19.12) Chondroma (rare)	These constitute about 5% of solitary peripheral nodules. Usually less than 4 cm in diameter and sharply marginated. "Popcorn" calcification of the cartilaginous portion is virtually diagnostic but calcification occurs in a minority of cases. May be multiple or grow slowly.
Hematogenous metastases (Fig. 19.13)	Calcification is rare; the most common primary tumor is an osteosarcoma. Rarely, a calcification is seen in pulmonary metastases of chondrosarcoma, synovial cell sarcoma, giant cell tumor of bone and mucinous carcinoma of colon, ovary, breast, thyroid, and (treated) choriocarcinoma.
Bronchopulmonary amyloidosis	A rare cause of usually multiple pulmonary nodules of variable size, which may show peripheral calcification or ossification.
Thrombus of pulmonary artery	Thrombi in the pulmonary arteries following embolism may rarely calcify. It is not associated with a mass lesion.

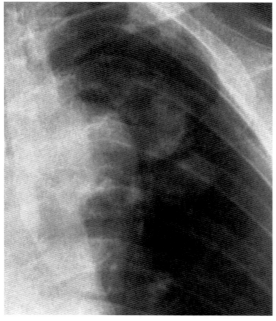

Fig. 19.**9 Multiple tuberculomas** in the left upper lobe. Both central nidus and multiple punctate calcifications are seen.

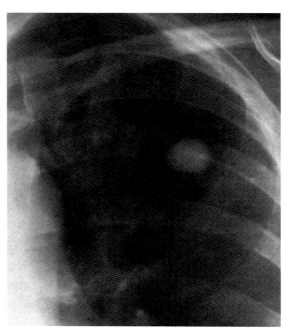

Fig. 19.**10 Adenocarcinoma** arising from a tuberculous scar. The calcified nidus is eccentric.

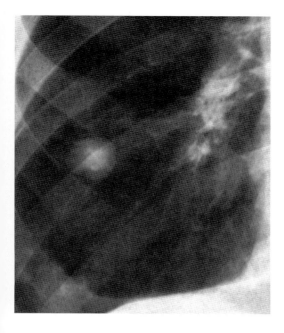

Fig. 19.**11** **Histoplasmoma** with central target calcification.

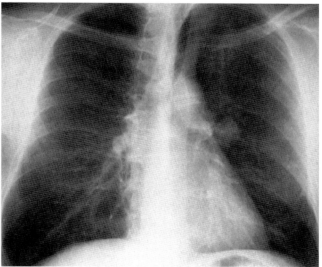

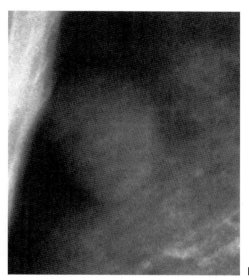

b

Fig. 19.**12 a, b** **Hamartoma.** A smooth 4-cm soft-tissue nodule with a faint conglomerate calcification in the center, better seen on the close-up lateral view (**b**).

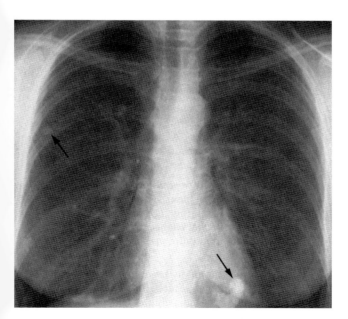

Fig. 19.**13** **Calcified metastatic osteosarcoma.** One calcified lesion is seen in each lung (arrows).

Table 19.3 Differential Diagnosis of Multiple Pulmonary Calcifications measuring less than 1 cm

Causes or associated condition	Comments
Histoplasmosis (healed) (Fig. 19.14)	Widespread densities of 3 to 4 mm in diameter throughout the lung fields containing punctate calcifications. Seen following disseminated histoplasmosis. Spleen may contain punctate calcifications, too.
Varicella (healed) (Fig. 19.15)	Miliary and larger densities with punctate calcifications a year or more after pulmonary chickenpox infection.
Mitral stenosis (Fig. 19.16)	Ossified and/or calcified nodules of up to 8 mm in diameter, predominantly in the right middle and lower lung fields. A rare but characteristic finding in mitral stenosis.
Pneumoconiosis due to inorganic dust, especially silicosis	Miliary and larger pulmonary densities, fairly sharply defined. May calcify. Hilar (eggshell) calcification may be present, too.
Alveolar microlithiasis (Fig. 19.17)	Extremely sharply defined, less than 1 mm, sandlike densities diffusely involving both lungs with an overall greater density in the lower than upper zones are diagnostic.
Metabolic (metastatic) calcification (primary or secondary hyperparathyroidism, hypervitaminosis D, milk alkali syndrome, intravenous calcium therapy)	A very rare cause of alveolar calcification that mimics alveolar disease. Calcium may precipitate, especially at sites of pneumonic exudation. May occur within 3 weeks of open-heart surgery in children, and slowly regress.

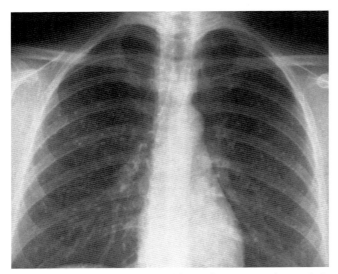

Fig. 19.**14** **Healed disseminated histoplasmosis.** Miliary calcifications.

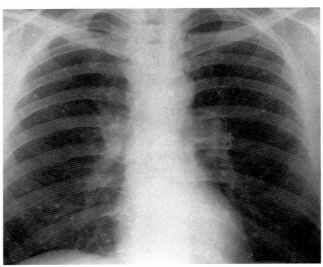

Fig. 19.**15** **Healed varicella pneumonia.** Miliary and larger densities with punctate calcifications.

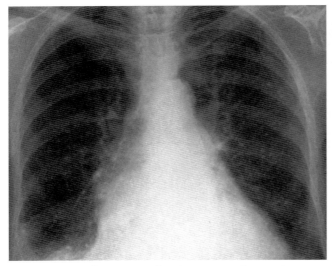

Fig. 19.**16** **Mitral stenosis** with pulmonary ossification, best seen in the right lower lung field.

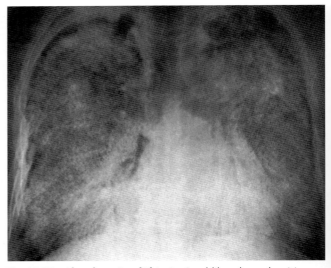

Fig. 19.**17** **Alveolar microlithiasis.** Sand-like, sharp densities are seen throughout the lungs, primarily in the lower lobes. Apices show pleural thickening, bullous cavities and scarring consistent with old tuberculosis.

Table 19.4 Differential Diagnosis of Pleural Calcifications

Causes or associated condition	Comments
Sequela of hemothorax pyothorax tuberculous pleuritis (Fig. 19.18)	Calcification and thickening of the visceral pleura or discrete plaques in the lower and middle fields. A thick layer of soft-tissue density is interposed between the calcific layer and the thoracic wall. Usually unilateral.
Asbestosis (Fig. 19.19) Talcosis	Pleural plaques and thickening originate from the parietal pleura. Usually bilateral and commonly diaphragmatic in position. Pulmonary parenchymal changes may be absent. Pleural calcifications are present in less than 50 % of cases.

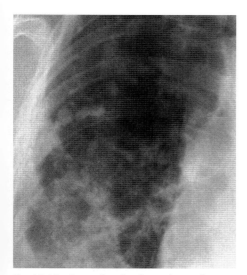

Fig. 19.**18 Sequela of tuberculous pleuritis.** Vertical sheet-like calcifications and discrete plaques are seen on the right side. A layer of soft tissue between the calcification and thoracic wall is seen laterally.

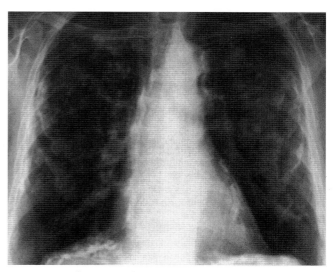

Fig. 19.**19 Asbestosis.** Bilateral pleural plaques and calcifications are seen along the chest wall, diaphragm and mediastinum. Calcifications tend to follow the course of the ribs. Parenchymal changes are not prominent.

Table 19.5 Differential Diagnosis of Hilar or Mediastinal Calcifications

Causes or associated condition	Comments
Thyroid mass	Most commonly seen in the upper anterior mediastinum or less frequently in the upper posterior mediastinum. Calcification within the mass is frequent. Calcification occurs in both benign and malignant masses.
Dermoid tumors **Teratoma (Fig. 19.20)** **Thymoma** **Neurogenic tumors (neurilemoma, neurofibroma, ganglioneuroma, neuroblastoma, paraganglioma)**	Calcification may be present around the lesion, particularly of dermoid cysts, but it has little differential diagnostic value. If bone is demonstrated within the lesion, the diagnosis of dermoid cyst is made with certainty. Neurogenic tumors may contain speckled calcification and are usually seen in the posterior mediastinum. If rib destruction is associated in a child, neuroblastoma is likely.
Radiation therapy (Figs. 19.21 and 19.22)	Lymph node calcification in the mediastinum occurs after radiation therapy of mediastinal lymphoma or metastases, and rarely after chemotherapy.
Tuberculosis **Histoplasmosis (Fig. 19.23)**	Amorphous or irregular calcification of involved nodes. Often associated with the Ghon lesion (parenchymal scar with calcification).
Granulomatous mediastinitis **Sclerosing mediastinitis** **(Idiopathic mediastinal fibrosis)**	Associated with tuberculosis or histoplasmosis, rarely silicosis or nocardiosis (granulomatous) or idiopathic. Mediastinal widening appears dense due to fine diffuse calcification that may be present even in absence of calcifications in plain films.
Silicosis (Fig. 19.24) **sarcoidosis (rarely) (Fig. 19.25)** **coccidioidomycosis (very rarely)**	Ring calcification of the periphery of lymph nodes, usually affecting bronchopulmonary lymph nodes.
Calcified tracheal cartilage (Fig. 19.26)	A common finding in elderly patients; no diagnostic significance.

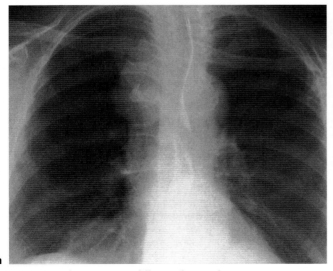
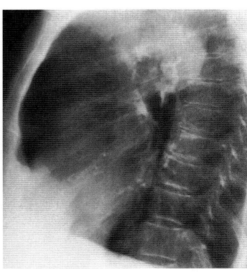

a   b

Fig. 19.**20 a, b Upper middle mediastinal teratoma** containing characteristic calcified structures. The patient also has an anterior diaphragmatic hernia on the right side and a posterior diaphragmatic hernia on the left side.

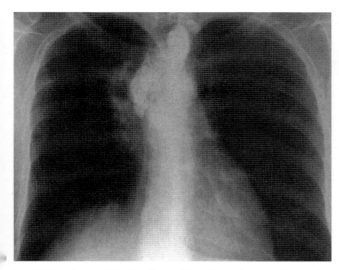

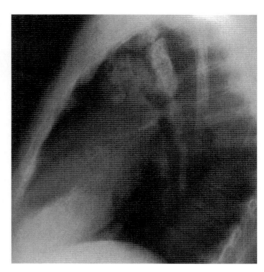

b

Fig. 19.**21 a, b   Calcified enlarged lymph nodes** after irradiation of Hodgkin's disease.

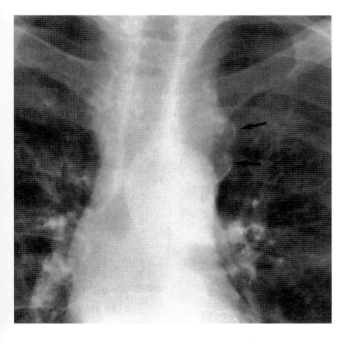

Fig. 19.**22   Eggshell calcifications** after irradiation of mediastinal metastases of seminoma are seen on the left, above the aortic knob.

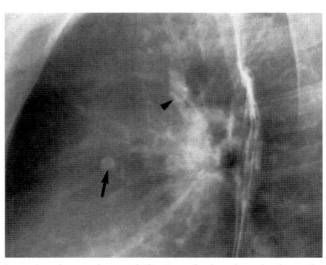

b

Fig. 19.**23 a, b   Calcified Ghon complex.** Laminated calcification of a granuloma in the anterior segment of the right upper lobe

(arrow) and amorphous calcification of a lymph node above the right hilum (arrowhead).

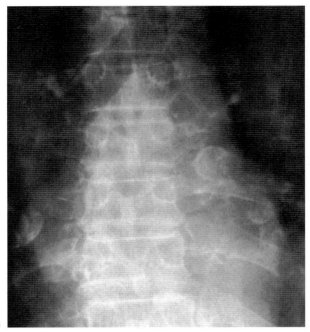
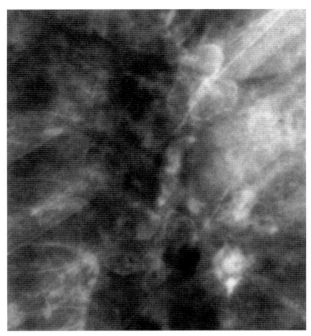

a

b

Fig. 19.**24 a, b**   **Silicosis.** Hilar lymph nodes contain characteristic "egg-shell" calcifications.

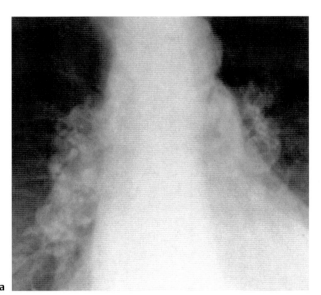
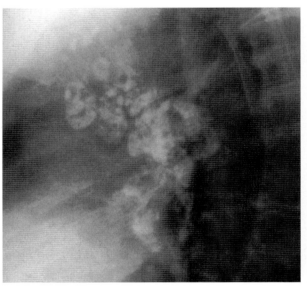

a

b

Fig. 19.**25 a, b**   **Sarcoidosis.** Enlarged hilar and mediastinal lymph nodes are extensively calcified, some of them showing the egg-shell pattern. A rare finding in sarcoidosis.

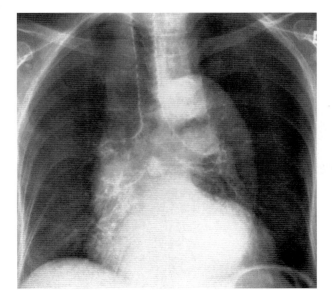

Fig. 19.**26**   **Extensive calcification of cartilaginous rings of the trachea and bronchi.** Granulomatous calcification of a subcarinal lymph node is also seen. Age 81.

20 Alveolar Infiltrates and Atelectasis

An increase in the radiologic density of the lung may be caused by a pulmonary or an extrapulmonary process. Differentiation between these two entities should be attempted first whenever an increased density is observed in the lung (Figs. 20.1–20.3).

Normal and *pathologic structures of the chest wall* can cause an opacification in a lung field and simulate at times pulmonary disease. In women, the density of the lower lung fields is altered on the frontal examination by the presence and size of the breasts. Similarly, the pectoralis muscle, particularly when strongly developed, or an overlying scapula may produce a localized increase in lung density. Whereas the recognition of normal soft tissue and bony structures does not usually cause any difficulty because of their constant anatomic location, a pathologic condition such as a tumor or a hematoma of the chest wall is more likely to be confused with a pulmonary process. Radiographic evaluation in two projections and/or clinical examination of the patient should, however, allow easy differentiation between a chest wall and a pulmonary lesion.

A unilateral increase in lung density is found when the frontal chest radiograph is taken in a slightly *rotated position*.

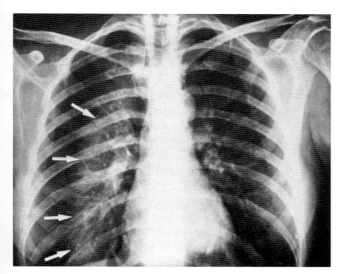

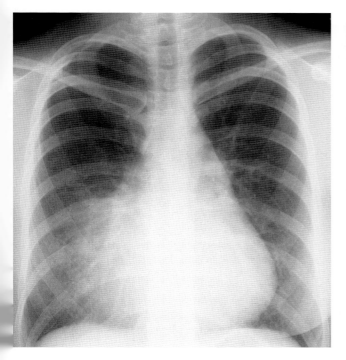

Fig. 20.**1**   Artifact caused by long hair combed in a ponytail simulating an infiltrate in right lung (arrows).

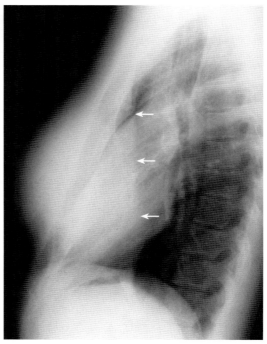

Fig. 20.**2 a, b   Pectus excavatum deformity.** A large opacity is evident in the lower portion of the right hemithorax contiguous with the thoracic spine mimicking a right middle lobe infiltrate (**a**). This is however a normal finding in patients with severe pectus deformity (**b**) caused by the posteriorly displaced sternum (arrows) resulting in compression of the adjacent right lung parenchyma and displacement of the heart toward the left.
▽

b

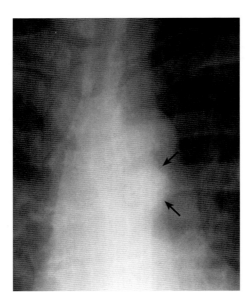

Fig. 20.**3**   **Osteophytosis in a costovertebral joint.** A round opacity (arrows) is overlying the left seventh rib posteriorly in the area of the costovertebral joint caused by advanced degenerative changes including marked hyperostosis in this articulation that could be mistaken for either a pulmonary or calcified mediastinal lesion.

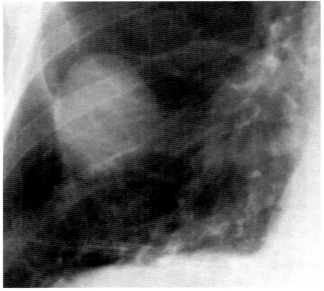

a

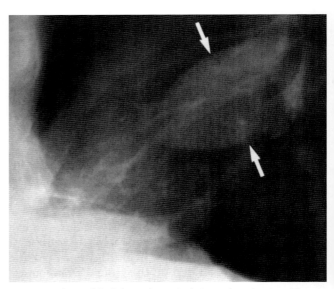

Fig. 20.**4**   **Loculated pleural effusion in major fissure** (lower half). **a** Anteroposterior projection: A homogeneous and well defined density projects into the right lower lung field. Smaller (thinner) fluid accumulations in that location are usually poorly defined and may mimic a right middle lobe atelectasis. **b** Lateral projection: The encapsulated fluid accumulation is spindle-shaped, with characteristically convex borders (arrows). Its long axis parallels the major fissure, which can often be seen exiting the density at one or both poles.

The lung, on which the spine is superimposed because of the rotation, usually demonstrates an increase in density. This is produced by the musculature around the spine that absorbs a significant portion of the roentgen beam passing through. A similar effect may also be found by incorrect centering of the roentgen beam or in patients with scoliosis. It is easy to recognize when the chest radiograph is centered off midline, as there is a variable distance between the lateral chest walls and the film margins: the side more distant from the midline is less exposed and appears lighter. On a supine chest film a pleural effusion layering out posteriorly may also mimic a unilateral underexposed (light) film.

Common causes for a bilateral and symmetrical increase in lung density of a healthy person are poor inspiration and underexposure of the film.

Pleural abnormalities may occasionally be difficult to differentiate from pulmonary lesions. A loculated effusion in the minor fissure could be mistaken for a neoplasm, although its location and radiographic appearance (a sharply demarcated and spindle-shaped lesion in both frontal and lateral projection) are quite characteristic. Furthermore the extremities of the loculated interlobar effusion blend imperceptibly with the interlobar fissure when viewed tangentially. Loculated fluid accumulation in the lower half of the major fissure is occasionally difficult to differentiate from a *right middle lobe atelectasis*. The encapsulated fluid has convex borders in the lateral projection and does not obscure the right heart border in the anteroposterior projection (Fig. 20.4). Furthermore, the minor fissure may be visible as a separate entity in one or both projections.

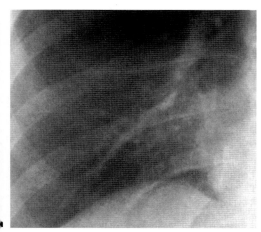

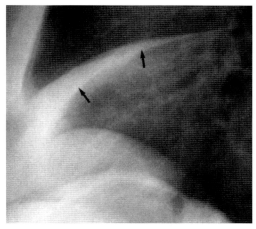

Fig. 20.**5** **Right middle lobe atelectasis. a** Anteroposterior projection: A poorly defined pulmonary density obliterates the adjacent right heart border (positive "silhouette sign"; see Fig. 20.**8**, for negative "silhouette sign" with right lower lobe atelectasis). **b** Lateral projection: A well defined triangular density with characteristic concave inferior border (arrows) is evident. Furthermore, the minor fissure cannot be seen in either projection as a separate shadow, since this fissure constitutes the superior border of the triangular density.

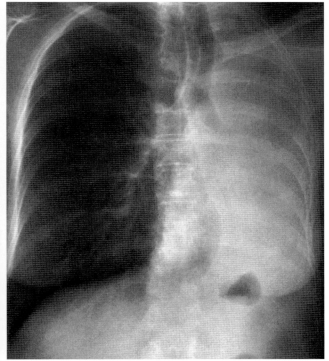

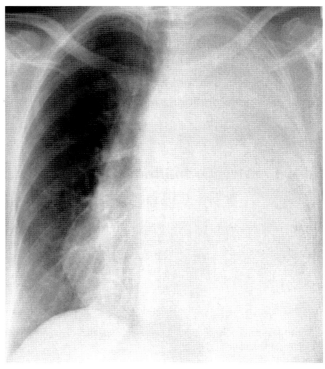

Fig. 20.**6** **Complete opacification of one hemithorax (atelectasis versus pleural effusion). a** Total atelectasis of the left lung caused by bronchogenic carcinoma. Opacification of the left hemithorax is associated with signs of loss of volume: shifting heart and mediastinum toward the atelectasis, approximation of ribs, and elevation of ipsilateral diaphragm. **b** Large left pleural effusion caused by ovarian carcinoma. Opacification of the left hemithorax is associated with signs of mass effect: shifting of heart and mediastinum away from the pleural effusion and depresston of the ipsilateral diaphragm.

An atelectasis involving the entire right middle lobe has straight or concave margins in the lateral projection, and tends to obliterate the adjacent right heart border (positive "silhouette sign") in the anteroposterior projection (Fig. 20.5). The minor fissure is never seen as a separate linear density.In the upper half of the major fissure, an encapsulated fluid accumulation may, particularly on the frontal view, be confused with a pulmonary mass. On the lateral view, however, the encapsulated fluid has a characteristic elliptical shape with the long axis of the density paralleling the course of the major fissure. The encapsulated fluid blends at both ends with the fissure, provided the latter is visible. An infrapulmonary effusion may atypically extend into the posteromedial gutter, simulating a *lower lobe atelectasis.*

Opacification of a hemithorax by either massive atelectasis or effusion should not be difficult to differentiate, since the former is associated with radiographic signs of loss of volume (e.g., shifting of the heart and mediastinum toward the atelectasis, approximation of ribs, and elevation of the ipsilateral hemidiaphragm), where as the latter is an expanding process displacing the adjacent organs away from the effusion (Fig. 20.6). Complete Opacification of a hemi-

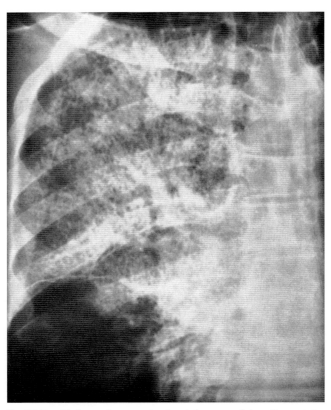

Fig. 20.7 Air bronchogram in the right upper lobe. Air containing bronchi are visible, since they are surrounded by an alveolar infiltrate caused by pneumococcal pneumonia.

thorax with signs of volume loss similar to an atelectasis is also found after *pneumonectomy.*

In *alveolar lung disease* as defined in this chapter, the air in the alveolar and peripheral airways is replaced by fluid or tissue, resulting radiographically in opacities ranging in size from a few millimeters to several centimeters. Alveolar infiltrates may involve a segment or even a whole lobe, in which case boundaries of the resulting parenchymal consolidation are sharply demarcated. On the other hand, a large number of superimposed and partly confluent alveolar infiltrates may produce nonhomogeneous and rather poorly defined lung densities.

Air bronchograms are commonly found in alveolar lung disease, where the air-containing bronchi become clearly visible because of the surrounding infiltrates (Fig. 20.7). However, an air bronchogram is not diagnostic of alveolar disease, since an increase in the density of the peribronchial tissue is occasionally caused by interstitial or atelectatic lung disease. Whereas the absence of an air bronchogram in a lung density does not rule out alveolar disease, its presence is diagnostic for lung parenchyma involvement as opposed to pleural or extrapleural disease. The radiographic demonstration of an air bronchogram leads strongly away from a diagnosis of a malignant pulmonary neoplasm, with the exceptions of alveolar cell carcinoma and lymphoma. Air in the lung can be replaced by either fluid, cells, or solid substances under the following conditions: 1 the osmotic pressure of the blood is too low (e.g., hypoproteinemia); 2 the blood pressure in the capillaries is too high (e.g., heart failure); 3 the capillary permeability is increased (e.g., inhalation of noxious gases); 4 the barrier between blood and air space is defective (e.g., bleeding); 5 liquid or solid materials are aspirated; 6 abnormal material is secreted (e.g., cystic fibrosis) or deposited (e.g., alveolar proteinosis); and 7 cells are growing (e.g., neoplasm) or invading (e.g., infection and inflammation) the air space. In an atelectasis the resorbed air is not replaced by any material. All the aforementioned conditions may radiographically produce opacities within the lung parenchyma and their differentiation depends on size, location, and distribution, the association of other radiographic findings, and knowledge of the patient's clinical history and physical examination. The differential diagnosis of alveolar infiltrates and atelectasis is discussed in Table 20.1.

Table 20.1 Alveolar Infiltrates and Atelectasis

Disease	Radiographic Appearance	Comments
Bronchial adenoma (Fig. 20.8)	Centrally located tumors arising from major bronchi (80%) often present as recurrent segmental and lobar atelectasis and/or obstructive pneumonia. Pulmonary, hilar and bony metastases (lytic and blastic) occur occasionally with carcinoids.	90% in patients between 30 and 50 years old. Slightly more common in females. Histologically 3 types: 1 carcinoid adenomas (90%) including oncocytoid type; 2 cylindromas (7%) and 3 mucoepidermoid tumors (3%).
Papillomas and other benign endobronchial tumors	Atelectasis and obstructive pneumonia	Rare. Papillomas may originate in larynx or trachea. They may be multiple and commonly occur in children.
Bronchogenic carcinoma (Fig. 20.9)	Persistent atelectasis and obstructive pneumonia (usually segmental, but may also be lobar or, less commonly, involve a whole lung) is most common radiologic presentation. Ipsilateral hilar enlargment and when further advanced, mediastinal widening is often associated with the parenchymal disease. Pleural effusions are simultaneously present in approximately 10% of all cases. *Pancoast* or *superior pulmonary sulcus tumors* present as unilateral apical mass, often with destruction of the adjacent rib.	Approximately 75% occur in males in their 5th and 6th decades. Inhalation of carcinogens (cigarette smoke, asbestos, etc.) are predisposing factors. Incidence in cigarette smokers ten times higher than in non-smokers. Carcinomas also originate in tuberculous scars with higher than purely coincidental incidence. Histologically adenocarcinomas (50%), squamous cell carcinomas (30%), small cell carcinomas (15%) and large cell carcinomas (5%) are distinguished. Pancoast tumors often present clinically with Horner's syndrome.

(continues on page 494)

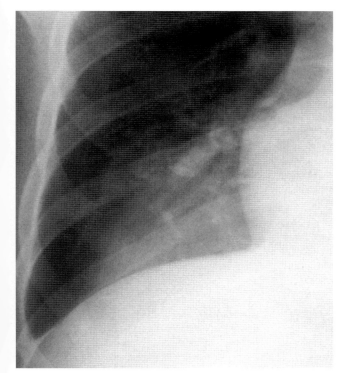

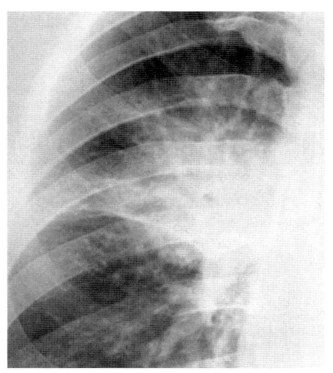

Fig. 20.**8 Bronchial adenoma** (carcinoid type) causing right lower lobe atelectasis. Note that the right cardiac border is not obliterated by the atelectatic right lower lobe, since these anatomical structures are not contiguous (negative "silhouette sign").

Fig. 20.**9 Bronchogenic carcinoma** in the right upper lobe causing obstructive pneumonitis.

Table 20.1   (Cont.) Alveolar Infiltrates and Atelectasis

Disease	Radiographic Appearance	Comments
Bronchioloalveolar carcinoma (alveolar cell carcinoma) (Fig. 20.10)	Peripheral homogeneous consolidation ranging in size from 1 cm in diameter to the involvement of an entire lobe. Air bronchograms are often present. Diffuse bilateral involvement with fluffy confluent infiltrates occurs in a more advanced stage. Hilar enlargement and pleural effusions are occasionally associated with the pulmonary involvement.	Most commonly found in middle-aged patients, without sex predilection.
Lymphoma (Fig. 20.11)	Perihilar infiltrate is the most common parenchymal manifestation. Peripheral consolidations and atelectasis secondary to endobronchial lymphoma are less common. Air bronchograms are often encountered. Hilar and/or mediastinal involvement is usually present with lung parenchyma involvement.	Primary pulmonary lymphoma is rare and radiographically indistinguishable from *pseudolymphoma*, a rare benign condition not associated with hilar or mediastinal adenopathy. Any alveolar lung infiltrate in a patient with known lymphoma is more likely to represent an infectious than a lymphomatous process.
Kaposi's sarcoma (Fig. 20.12)	Bilateral, symmetric, poorly defined nodular opacities are characteristic. Nodules measure up to 3 cm and tend to coalesce. Pleural effusions (50%) and hilar or mediastinal adenopathy (10%) may be associated.	Occurs almost exclusively in HIV-infected male homosexuals and rarely in other HIV-infected patients.
Amyloidosis (tracheobronchial form)	Endobronchial amyloid deposition may cause atelectasis and obstructive pneumonia involving a segment to an entire lung.	Pulmonary manifestations occur in primary amyloidosis or in conjunction with multiple myeloma.
Arteriovenous malformation	Homogeneous, sharply defined and often somewhat lobulated density with lower lobe predilection. Identification of feeding and draining vessel not always possible. Multiple lesions in approximately one-third of patients.	Approximately half of the patients have arteriovenous fistulas elsewhere (*hereditary hemorrhagic telangiectasia* or *Rendu–Osler–Weber's disease*).
Pneumonia, bacterial		
Staphylococcus aureus (Fig. 20.13)	Patchy consolidations without air bronchograms characteristic. Bilateral in over 60%. Both pneumatocele and abscess formations occur frequently and may contain air-fluid levels. Pneumatoceles have characteristically thin walls that differentiate them from abscesses. Pleural effusion (or empyema) is found in 50% of adults and is even more common in children.	Common in hospital patients and compromised hosts. Pneumatoceles are cyst-like lesions resulting from a check-valve-obstructed communication with a bronchus. They are particularly common in children.
Streptococcus pyogenes	Similar to staphylococcal pneumonia: patchy or homogeneous consolidations without air bronchograms and a high incidence of accompanying pleural effusion. Differentiating features are a lower tendency to form abscesses and pneumatoceles.	Streptococcal pneumonias are often found in mixed or secondary infections.

(continues on page 496)

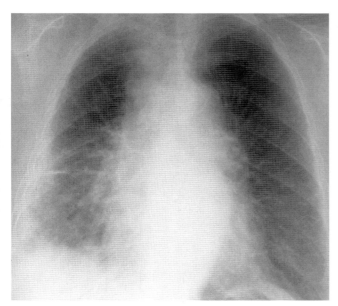

Fig. 20.**10 Bronchioloalveolar carcinoma.** Poorly defined, confluent nodular opacities are seen in the right lower lobe. A small right pleural effusion is also present. Furthermore smaller, poorly defined nodules are scattered throughout the remaining right lung and left lower lung zone.

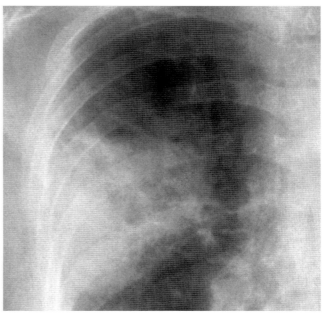

Fig. 20.**11 Non-Hodgkin lymphoma.** A large consolidation is seen in the right upper lobe.

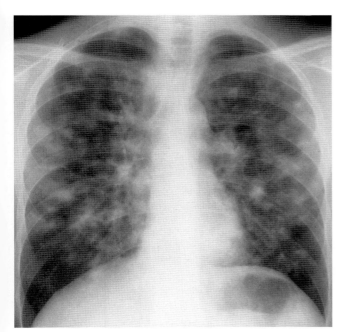

Fig. 20.**12 Kaposi's sarcoma.** Bilateral, symmetric, poorly defined, partly coalescent nodules are seen.

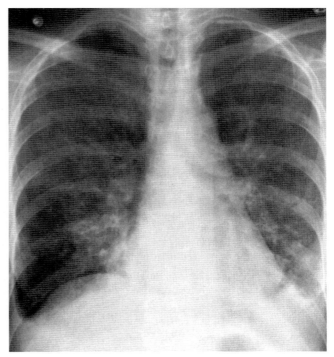

Fig. 20.**13 Staphylococcal pneumonia** presenting as bilateral patchy infiltrates in the lower lobes with small pleural effusions.

Table 20.1   (Cont.) Alveolar Infiltrates and Atelectasis

Disease	Radiographic Appearance	Comments
Pneumonia, bacterial (cont.)		
Pneumococcus (Streptococcus pneumoniae) (Fig. 20.14)	Homogeneous consolidation with air bronchograms characteristic. Usually confined to one lobe. Another presentation observed with apparently increasing frequency consists of patchy bronchopneumonia-like infiltrates that may be bilateral. Small pleural reactions occur in 20% of cases. Cavitation is rare.	Common in alcoholics and compromised hosts, but also occurs in otherwise healthy people. In children, the disease may present as a spherical, well-circumscribed pulmonary density.
Klebsiella (Fig. 20.15)	Large well-defined homogeneous consolidation with air bronchograms similar to pneumococcal pneumonia. Differentiating features from the latter are: 1 upper lobe predilection, 2 tendency to expand involved lobe, 3 abscess formation and pleural effusion common.	Common in alcoholics and in elderly patients with chronic pulmonary disease.
Legionella (Fig. 20.16)	Poorly defined round or diffuse infiltrates central or peripheral in location, usually beginning in one lobe and spreading in two-thirds of cases to the other lung. Pleural effusion may be present. Cavitation and hilar adenopathy does not occur.	Legionnaires' disease is an acute Gram-negative bacterial pneumonia found in local outbreaks or as sporadic cases. Clearing of pneumonic infiltrates within one month.
Pseudomonas (Fig. 20.17)	Bilateral patchy infiltrates with predilection for the lower lobes, progressing rapidly to extensive homogeneous consolidations with air bronchograms, are characteristic. Abscess formation is common. Small but radiographically not very conspicuous effusions are usually present.	Almost invariably in compromised hosts who acquire the disease in the hospital. Organism resistant to almost all antibiotics.
Haemophilus influenzae (Fig. 20.18)	Patchy, poorly defined infiltrates, predominantly in the lower lobes, unilateral or bilateral. Pleural effusions occur frequently and may be the dominant feature, especially in children.	Most common organism cultured from purulent expectorations of patients with chronic pulmonary disease, although its pathogenicity is still in doubt, since it is also commonly found in the flora of healthy people.

(continues on page 498)

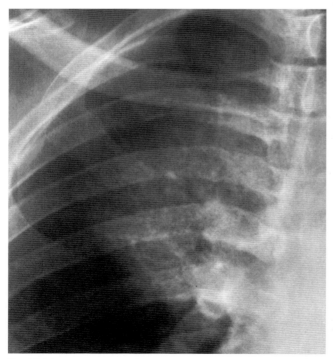

Fig. 20.**14 Pneumococcal pneumonia** presenting as consolidation with air bronchogram in the anterior segment of the right upper lobe. The pneumonic process obliterates the lateral border of the adjacent ascending aorta (positive "silhouette sign"). See also Fig. 20.**5**.

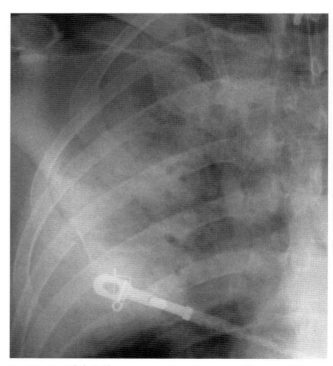

Fig. 20.**15 Klebsiella pneumonia.** An expansile consolidation with air bronchograms is involving the entire right upper lobe.

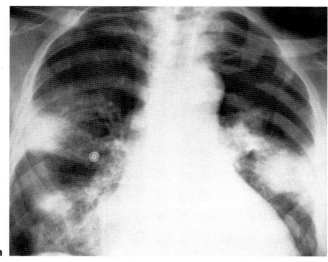

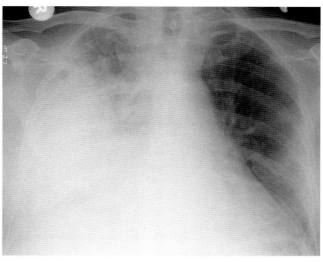

Fig. 20.**16 a, b** **Legionella pneumonia (Legionnaires' disease)** (two cases). **a** Bilateral poorly defined, peripheral infiltrates are seen. **b** Besides bilateral small patchy infiltrates a large consolidation is seen in the right lung.

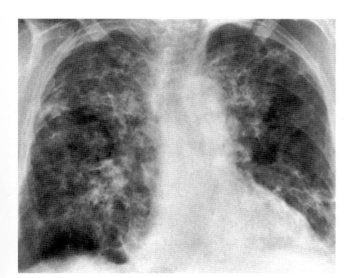

Fig. 20.**17** **Pseudomonas pneumonia.** Extensive bilateral patchy infiltrates with small effusions are seen.

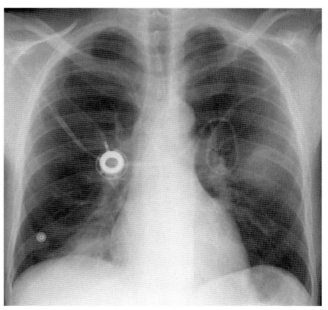

Fig. 20.**18** **Haemophilus influenza pneumonia.** Poorly defined infiltrates are seen in both lower lobes (right posterior basal segment and left superior segment).

Table 20.1 (Cont.) Alveolar Infiltrates and Atelectasis

Disease	Radiographic Appearance	Comments
Pneumonia, bacterial (cont.)		
Bordetella pertussis	Infiltrates conglomerate, often contiguous to the cardiac silhouette, producing a "shaggy heart sign." Mild hilar lymph node enlargement is occasionally associated.	Most common in nonimmunized children, but can occur in immunized adults.
Francisella (Pasteurella) tularensis	Unilateral or bilateral patchy to homogeneous consolidations, sometimes oval in shape. Ipsilateral hilar enlargement and pleural effusion are commonly associated.	Organism usually found in rodents and other small mammals. Tularemia often caused by occupational exposure (hunter, laboratory worker, butcher).
Yersinia (Pasteurella) pestis	Unilateral or bilateral homogeneous consolidations with air bronchograms. Hilar and paratracheal lymph node enlargement may be the dominant radiographic feature. Pleural effusions occur.	Organism still widespread among wild rodents. *Bacillus anthracis* (cattle, sheep and goats) may cause similar radiographic chest findings. Both anthrax and plague pneumonia are nowadays extremely rare diseases.
Other Gram-negative aerobic bacteria (Fig. 20.19)	Noncharacteristic, often nonhomogeneous infiltrate(s) in lower lobes. Cavitation occurs with varying frequency with most organisms. Pleural effusion may be present.	Organisms: *Bacillus proteus, Escherichia coli, Salmonella, Brucella, Enterobacter, Serratia,* and others.
Bacteroides and other anaerobic bacteria	Homogeneous infiltrate(s) preferentially in posterior segments with abscess formation early in the course characteristic. Pleural effusion (empyema) is very common.	Anaerobes are common organisms of normal flora of mouth and respiratory tract. Often found in "aspiration pneumonias" in alcoholics and people with poor oral hygiene. Course protracted over weeks to months.
Tuberculosis (Mycobacterium tuberculosis) (Figs. 20.20 and 20.21)	*Primary:* Consolidation with only slight predilection for upper lobes. Hilar and/or paratracheal lymph node enlargement is usually present. Pleural effusion is common in adults.	Primary tuberculosis is often found in children.
	Postprimary: Patchy, inhomogeneous infiltrate in apical or posterior segments of upper lobes or superior segment of lower lobes is characteristic. Bilateral involvement is common, but often asymmetric. Pleural effusion and lymph node enlargement are rare. Cavitation occurs and may result in bronchogenic spread characterized by multiple patchy infiltrates.	In adults. Reactivation of an old focus, after BCG vaccination, or exogenous reinfection (rare), or as direct continuation of the original (primary) infection.

(continues on page 500)

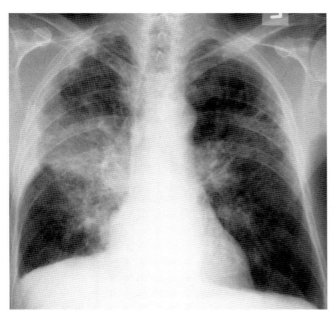

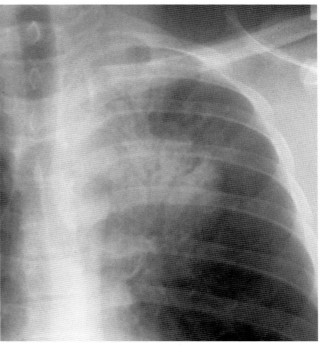

Fig. 20.**19** **Serratia marcescens pneumonia.** Bilateral infiltrates with numerous small cavities and a larger consolidation in the right mid lung are seen. Small bilateral effusions, partially loculated along the right lateral chest wall, are also present.

Fig. 20.**20** **Primary tuberculosis in AIDS.** A left upper lobe consolidation with air bronchogram and left hilar adenopathy is seen.

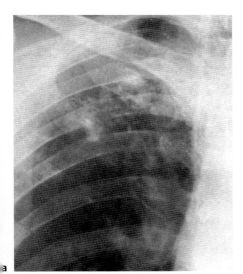

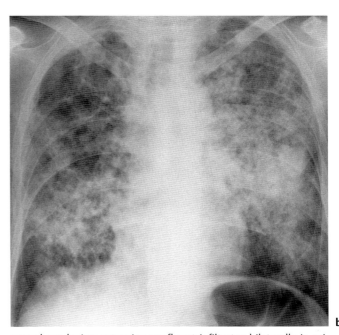

a

b

Fig. 20.**21 a, b** **Postprimary tuberculosis** (two cases). **a** A non-homogeneous infiltrate is seen in the apical and posterior segment of the right upper lobe. **b** Cavitary tuberculosis with bronchogenic spread producing extensive confluent infiltrates bilaterally is evident.

Table 20.1 (Cont.) Alveolar Infiltrates and Atelectasis

Disease	Radiographic Appearance	Comments
Pneumonia, bacterial (cont.)		
Atypical mycobacteria (mycobacterium avium intracellulare or kansasii) (Figs. 20.22 and 20.23)	Similar to tuberculosis, but greater tendency for cavitation, while pleural effusions and hilar adenopathy are less common. Strong association with preexisting pulmonary disease (e.g., emphysema, chronic bronchitis) and relatively common in AIDS.	Atypical mycobacteria can be isolated from the sputum of healthy people. Tuberculin test is negative and there is no response to antituberculous therapy.
Actinomycosis Nocardiosis (Figs. 20.24 and 20.25)	Homogeneous consolidation with lower lobe predilection. Cavitation and pleural effusion (empyema) are common. Extension through pleura into chest wall is frequent and often associated with rib destruction.	Whereas actinomycosis affects otherwise healthy people, nocardiosis is virtually limited to compromised hosts (e.g., diseases of reticuloendothelial system, immunosuppressive therapy, and alveolar proteinosis).
Pneumonia, fungal **Histoplasmosis**	*Primary:* Nonhomogeneous consolidations, most often in a lower lobe with hilar lymph enlargement are characteristic. A pleural effusion is rarely associated. *Postprimary:* Consolidations that clear in one area and appear in another are characteristic. Preferentially located in the upper lobes. Cavitation may occur. Lymph node enlargement is uncommon.	Clinical and radiographic features often resemble tuberculosis.
Coccidioidomycosis	Patchy homogeneous consolidations preferentially in lower lobes and often associated with hilar and/or mediastinal lymph node enlargement and less commonly with a pleural effusion. Cavitation (usually thin-walled) occurs predominantly in the upper lobes, and unlike tuberculosis, involves also the anterior segments.	The disease is asymptomatic in the majority of infected patients or causes mild influenza-like symptoms. Endemic in southwest desert of USA, northern Mexico and in parts of Central and South America.
Blastomycosis	Nonspecific homogeneous or patchy consolidation, rarely associated with lymph node enlargement, pleural effusion and cavitation.	Caused by *Blastomyces dermatitidis* and found in North, Central, and South America and Africa. Also referred to as North American blastomycosis.
Cryptococcosis (Fig. 20.26)	Well-defined segmental or lobar consolidation preferentially in lower lobes. Cavitation and lymph node enlargement are rare.	Peripheral mass lesion is a more common radiographic presentation of this disease. Also referred to as torulosis or European blastomycosis.
Mucormycosis (phycomycosis)	Homogeneous consolidation, frequently with cavitation.	In patients with diabetes, lymphoma, or leukemia.
Geotrichosis	Consolidation in upper lobes, frequently associated with thin-walled cavities.	
Sporotrichosis	Segmental consolidations, commonly associated with hilar lymph node enlargement. Thin-walled cavities are not unusual. Spreading of the disease through pleura into the chest wall may occur.	The disease may also present radiographically as single large mass or as numerous small nodules.
Aspergillosis (Fig. 20.27)	Single or multiple consolidations. Abscess formation can occur.	Exceedingly rare in healthy patients (primary aspergillosis) but not unusual in compromised hosts ("aspergillosis with chronic debilitating disease"). Other manifestations of the disease include aspergillomas within pulmonary cavities and hypersensitivity aspergillosis (mucoid impaction especially in asthmatics, often simulating bronchogenic carcinoma radiographically).
Candidiasis (moniliasis)	Patchy infiltrates. Cavitation may occur.	Candida is a common saprophyte of upper respiratory tract. Common in elderly or persons with chronic debilitating disease.

(continues on page 502)

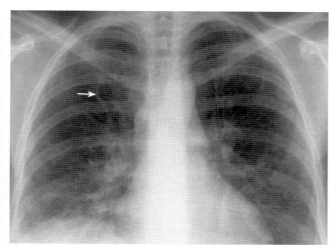

Fig. 20.**22** **Atypical mycobacterial pneumonia.** Bilateral poorly defined nodular opacities predominantly involving the mid and lower lung zones are seen. A pneumatocele (arrow) is also evident in the right upper lobe.

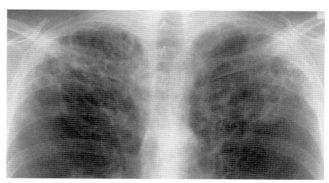

Fig. 20.**23** **Atypical mycobacterial pneumonia.** Bilateral upper lobe infiltrates with numerous small thin-walled cavities are evident.

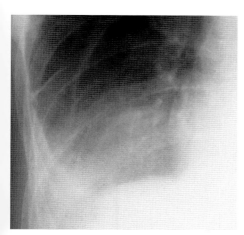

Fig. 20.**24** **Pulmonary actinomycosis.** A right lower lobe consolidation with pleural reaction and extension into the adjacent ribs is seen.

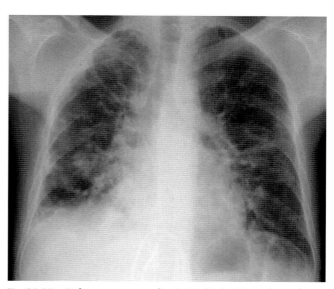

Fig. 20.**25** **Pulmonary nocardiosis.** Multiple bilateral poorly defined nodular opacities often with cavitation are seen. A partially loculated right pleural effusion is also present.

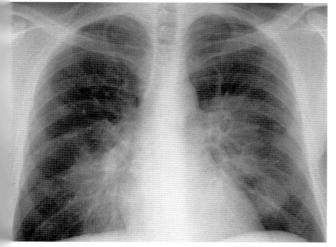

Fig. 20.**26** **Cryptococcal pneumonia.** Bilateral, well defined homogeneous consolidations are seen in the lower lobes.

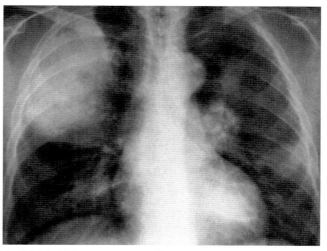

Fig. 20.**27** **Pulmonary aspergillosis** in a patient with dermatomyositis treated with steroids, presenting with bilateral, rapidly increasing consolidations.

Table 20.1   (Cont.) Alveolar Infiltrates and Atelectasis

Disease	Radiographic Appearance	Comments
Pneumonia, myco-plasma and viral Mycoplasma Influenza Parainflueuza Coxsackie Adenovirus Psittacosis (Figs. 20.28, 20.29 and 20.30)	Patchy infiltrates, often preceded by fine reticular pattern and commonly located in one or both lower lobes, are characteristic. Small pleural effusions may be present. Cavitation does not occur and hilar lymph node enlargement is extremely rare in adults.	Common in children and young adults. *Rubeola (measles)* and *echovirus pneumonias*, almost exclusively found in infants and young children, are commonly associated with hilar lymph node enlargement. *Respiratory syncytial* virus infections are particularly common in infants and small children presenting with severe respiratory symptoms and only minimal radiographic findings (e.g., overinflation).
Mononucleosis (Epstein–Barr virus)	Similar to mycoplasma and aforementioned viral pneumonias, but hilar lymph node enlargement occurs.	Common disease in the 15–25-year age group, but pulmonary manifestations are rare. Usually associated with generalized lymphadenopathy and splenomegaly, the latter being often the most conspicuous radiographic feature.
Varicella (zoster) (Fig. 20.31)	Bilateral fluffy nodular infiltrates that may coalesce near the hilum when extensive and produce a "pulmonary edema"-type infiltrate. Lymph node enlargement and pleural effusions are rarely present.	Clinical symptoms and radiographic findings of chickenpox pneumonia occur 2–3 days after skin manifestation.
Cytomegalic inclusion disease (cytomegalovirus) (Fig. 20.32)	Patchy, often bilateral interstitial and alveolar infiltrates in advanced stage. Pleural effusion and cavitation do not occur.	In compromised hosts. Cytomegalovirus often coexistent with Pneumocystis carinii pneumonia.
SARS (Severe Acute Respiratory Distress Syndrome) (Fig. 20.33)	Unilateral or, slightly less common, bilateral, often multifocal airspace disease with lower lobe predilection. Pleural effusions are uncommon at initial presentation.	Highly contagious viral pneumonia with 10% mortality rate.
Pneumonia, rickettsial Q-fever (Coxiella burnetii)	Homogeneous consolidation involving an entire segment (usually in a lower lobe) is characteristic. Pleural reaction may be present.	Disease clinically simulates influenza. Chest radiographs abnormal in less than 50% of patients.

(continues on page 504)

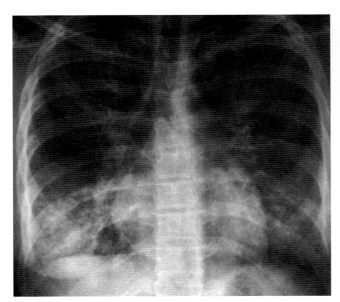

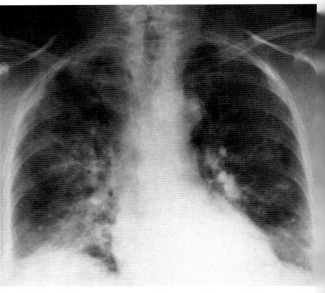

Fig. 20.**28**   **Mycoplasma pneumonia** presenting as mixed interstitial and alveolar infiltrates in the right middle lobe and both lower lobes.

Fig. 20.**29**   **Influenza pneumonia** presenting as bilateral patchy infiltrates.

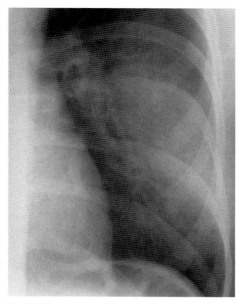

Fig. 20.**30** **Psittacosis pneumonia.** A homogeneous "ground-glass" opacity in the left lower lobe is associated with mild left hilar adenopathy. This is a relatively unique presentation of the disease that often presents in a less characteristic, viral pneumonia pattern.

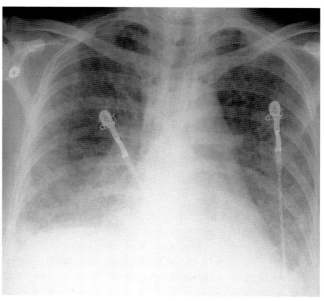

Fig. 20.**31** **Varicella pneumonia.** Bilateral fluffy nodular infiltrates are seen that coalesce in the lower lobes.

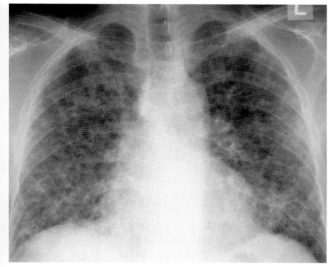

Fig. 20.**32** **Cytomegalic inclusion disease.** Bilateral reticulonodular and early alveolar infiltrates are seen, mainly involving the mid and lower lung zones.

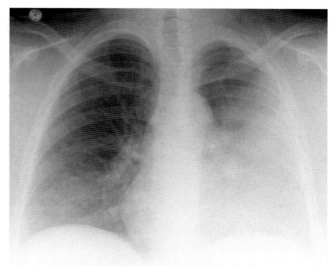

Fig. 20.**33** **SARS.** A poorly defined consolidation involving the lingula and left lower lobe is seen.

Table 20.1 (Cont.) Alveolar Infiltrates and Atelectasis

Disease	Radiographic Appearance	Comments
Pneumonia, parasitic **Pneumocystis carinii (Fig. 20.34)**	Begins as interstitial perihilar infiltrates that are commonly bilateral, and progresses to patchy areas of airspace consolidation with air bronchograms. At an advanced stage, the disease mimics pulmonary edema. Pleural effusion is uncommon.	Common in immunosuppressed patients. Most frequent pneumonia, with very poor prognosis in the acquired immune deficiency syndrome (AIDS) found in homosexual males, intravenous drug abusers, and after receiving contaminated blood transfusions (e.g., in hemophiliacs).
Toxoplasmosis (Toxoplasma gondii)	Combined interstitial and alveolar disease. Hilar lymph node enlargement is common.	Clinically, toxoplasmosis often resembles infectious mononucleosis in the adult.
Amebiasis (Entamoeba histolytica)	Homogeneous consolidation in right lower lobe with pleural effusion. Cavitation is rare.	Organism invades the lung via diaphragm from a liver abscess. Hematogenous origin is very rare.
Roundworm **Ascariasis**	Patchy consolidations, often bilaterally.	Pulmonary disease represents allergic response caused by larvae passing through lungs. Eosinophilia is invariably present.
Strongyloidiasis	Patchy consolidations similar to ascariasis. Small pleural effusions might be present.	Pulmonary changes caused by migration of larvae from the capillaries into the alveoli causing alveolar hemorrhage, edema, inflammation and infarction. Pulmonary manifestations often associated with hemorrhagic gastroenterocolitis.
Ancylostomiasis (Hookworm disease)	Pulmonary manifestations similar to strongyloidiasis but less common.	Anemia is often the predominant clinical feature. Eosinophilia is also present.
Flatworm **Paragonimiasis (Paragonimus westermanii)**	Patchy consolidations often containing small cystic lesions with relatively thick walls simulating infected cystic bronchiectasis. These ring shadows contain characteristically a localized crescent shaped opacity in one location along their inner borders. Pleural effusions and pneumothorax can occur.	Hemoptysis is usually the dominant clinical feature. Organisms enter lungs through diaphragm and pleura and spread via bronchial tree. Acquired by eating raw crabs or crayfish.
Chronic granulomatous disease of childhood (Fig. 20.35)	Bilateral patchy infiltrates and granulomas often associated with hilar and mediastinal adenopathy are the most common presentation.	A heterogeneous group of inherited diseases with enzyme deficiencies in white blood cells presenting with chronic and recurrent infections in the lungs, abdomen and skeleton.
Sarcoidosis (Fig. 20.36)	Consolidations with air bronchograms can be produced by the confluence of numerous, indistinctly defined, small nodular lesions.	This rare manifestation of sarcoidosis is usually associated with more characteristic changes such as a diffuse reticulonodular pattern and hilar and mediastinal lymph node enlargement.
Silicosis and coal miner's disease (both in advanced stage) (Fig. 20.37)	Homogeneous, usually bilateral consolidations, preferentially in the upper lobes *(progressive massive fibrosis)*. Cavitation secondary to central ischemic necrosis or superimposed tuberculous caseation can occur. Emphysema and hilar lymph node enlargement are usually present. "Eggshell" calcifications are characteristic but only rarely seen.	Progressive massive fibrosis is caused by the confluence of numerous individual nodules. Its lateral border is characteristically better defined than its medial border. It commonly develops in the midzone or periphery of the lung and migrates later toward the hilum.

(continues on page 506)

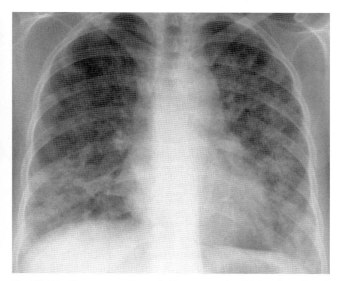

Fig. 20.**34** **Pneumocystis carinii pneumonia.** Bilateral confluent patchy infiltrates are seen sparing only the lung apices.

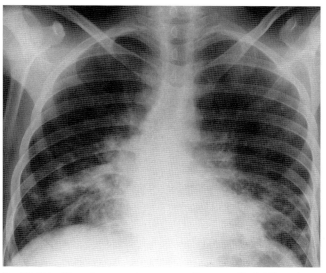

Fig. 20.**35** **Chronic granulomatous disease of childhood.** Bilateral poorly defined nodular opacities are seen in the perihilar areas and lower lung fields. Mild hilar adenopathy is also present.

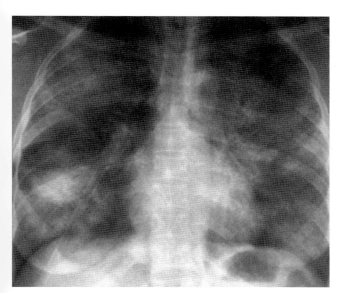

Fig. 20.**36** **Sarcoidosis.** Bilateral consolidations with air bronchograms are mimicked by the confluence of numerous, indistinctly defined, small nodular lesions.

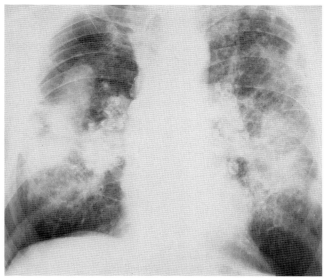

Fig. 20.**37** **Coal miner's disease.** Bilateral large oblong opacities (progressive massive fibrosis [PMF]) in the mid lung are associated with dense pulmonary nodules, fibrosis (honeycombing), compensatory emphysema and enlarged hili with "eggshell" calcifications.

Table 20.1   (Cont.) Alveolar Infiltrates and Atelectasis

Disease	Radiographic Appearance	Comments
Asbestosis (Fig. 20.38)	Combination of parenchymal and pleural changes in mid and lower-lung fields results in partial obliteration of the heart border ("shaggy heart" sign) and diaphragm. Parietal pleural plaques, which may be calcified, may be present and are characteristic.	High incidence of associated malignancies such as mesothelioma, bronchogenic and alveolar cell carcinomas.
Talcosis	Pulmonary (reticulonodular pattern with homogeneous, poorly defined infiltrates) and pleural changes (plaques) similar to asbestosis.	
Aspiration of solid foreign body	Localized , gravity-dependent consolidation and atelectasis, most often in lower lobes. Abscess formation is common.	If the foreign body produces a check-valve mechanism, hyperinflation and air trapping can be seen distally to it. The foreign body occasionally can be identified when radiopaque or outlined by air.
Aspiration, acute	Confluent patchy infiltrates to homogeneous consolidations, often bilateral.	Aspiration of gastric contents *(Mendelson's syndrome)* usually results in bilateral infiltrates that clear in 7 to 10 days.
Aspiration, chronic	One or more segmental consolidation (s) slowly clearing in one area and appearing in consolidation(s) another.	Encountered with Zenker's diverticulum, esophageal stenosis, tracheoesophageal fistula and neuromuscular disorders. Acute and chronic aspiration pneumonias are also found in alcoholics.
Lipoid pneumonia (exogenous)	Relatively homogeneous consolidations in one or more segments preferentially in lower lobes. Interstitial thickening, evident as linear densities in the periphery of the lesion, may be found.	Aspiration of oil (e.g., oily nose drops). *Endogenous lipoid pneumonias* (e.g., cholesterol pneumonia, and primary or secondary inflammatory pseudotumors, the latter in association with pre-existing lung disease) must be differentiated.
Lymphocytic interstitial pneumonia (Fig. 20.39)	Bilateral reticulonodular or, less commonly, ground glass opacities and consolidations with preferential involvement of the lower lung zones. Hilar and mediastinal lymphadenopathy may be associated in patients with AIDS.	Patients usually have underlying diseases such as rheumatoid arthritis, Sjögren's syndrome or AIDS, in which children typically are affected.
Mucoid impaction (hypersensitivity aspergillosis) (Fig. 20.40)	Mucous plugs often recognizable as "broad band"-like, V- or Y-shaped densities preferentially in upper lobes. Atelectasis or obstructive pneumonitis often present distally to the plug, simulating a neoplasm. May clear in one area and reappear in another.	Usually associated with asthma and/or chronic bronchial disease (e.g., bronchiectasis, cystic fibrosis). Peripheral eosinophilia commonly found in mucoid impaction caused by hypersensitivity (allergic) aspergillosis. *Bronchocentric granulomatosis (Liebow)* presents clinically and radiographically similar to mucoid impaction and may be considered a variant of that entity.

(continues on page 508)

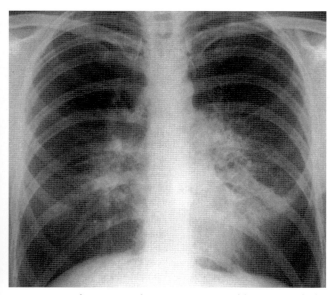

Fig. 20.**38** **Pulmonary asbestosis** causing obliteration of the heart border ("shaggy heart" sign).

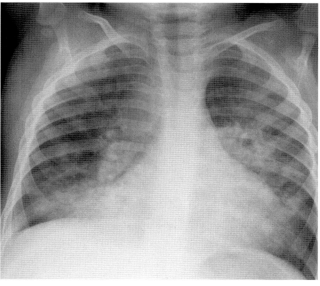

Fig. 20.**39** **Lymphocytic interstitial pneumonia in transplacental AIDS.** Bilateral consolidations in the mid and lower lung zones are associated with hilar and right mediastinal adenopathy.

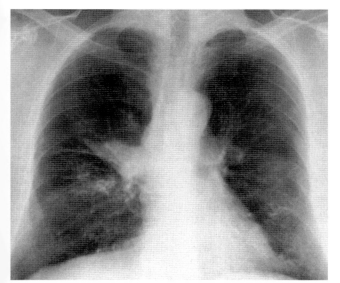

Fig. 20.**40 a, b** **Mucoid impaction (hypersensitivity aspergillosis)** in a patient with chronic lung disease. **a** Atelectasis and obstructive pneumonitis in the right middle lobe caused by a mucous

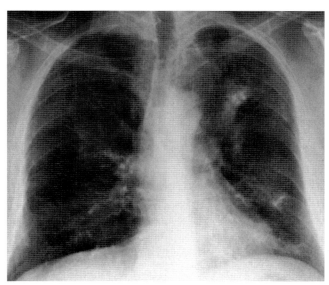

b

plug are followed several months later by obstructive pneumonitis secondary to a plug in the left upper lobe seen in **b**.

Table 20.1 (Cont.) Alveolar Infiltrates and Atelectasis

Disease	Radiographic Appearance	Comments
Loeffler's syndrome (Fig. 20.41 and 20.42)	One or several poorly defined transient consolidations in the lung periphery are characteristic ("reversed pulmonary edema pattern").	Blood eosinophilia is almost invariably present. May be idiopathic, drug-induced (e.g., penicillin, sulfonamides) or parasite-induced. A chronic form ("chronic eosinophilic pneumonia") that is radiographically indistinguishable but persists for weeks without steroid treatment, can be differentiated from (acute) Loeffler's syndrome.
Bronchiolitis obliterans organizing pneumonia (BOOP) Cryptogenic organizing pneumonia (COP) (Fig. 20.43)	Four distinctive patterns are discerned: 1. Multiple bilateral patchy consolidations. 2. Diffuse bilateral reticulonodular infiltrates. 3. Focal consolidation. 4. Multiple large nodules.	May be idiopathic (cryptogenic) or associated with connective tissue disease, drugs, infection and aspiration. Present clinically as a subacute illness with cough (90%), dyspnea (80%), fever (60%), and weight loss (50%).
Connective tissue disease (Fig. 20.44)	Nonspecific patchy peripheral consolidations often associated with pleural effusions.	In systemic lupus erythematosus and polyarteritis nodosa, for example.
Wegener's granulomatosis (Fig. 20.45)	Patchy infiltrates or a relatively homogeneous consolidation involving part of a segment to an entire lobe are well-recognized but not very common manifestations of this disease. Pleural reactions can occasionally be associated.	Most commonly found in middle-aged men, slightly less common in women. Pulmonary nodules which may cavitate are the characteristic radiographic presentation of this disease.
Pulmonary infarct (Fig. 20.46)	Pleural based consolidation(s), preferentially in lower lobes, which is often associated with pleural effusion and the elevation of ipsilateral diaphragm. *Hampton's hump* is characteristic but not common: The infarct appears as a truncated cone with its base contiguous to the visceral pleura.	Time of resolution varies between a few days (when only edema and/or hemorrhage is present) to several weeks (when associated with necrosis). Characteristically, a resolving infarct gradually diminishes but maintains the original shape and homogeneity ("melting ice cube" sign).
Pulmonary edema (cardiogenic and non-cardiogenic)	Nonsymmetrical, atypical presentation as areas of localized consolidations occurs in patients with pre-existing lung disease.	For differential diagnosis see Chapter 22.

(continues on page 510)

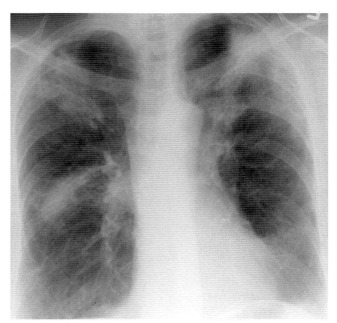

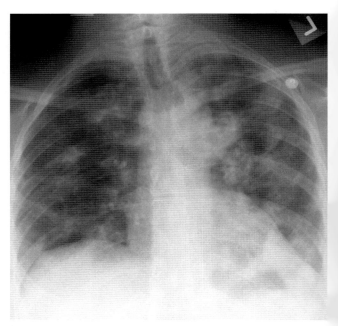

Fig. 20.**41** **Loeffler's syndrome.** Bilateral, poorly defined, patchy infiltrates are seen in the periphery of the mid and upper lung zones in this patient with chronic obstructive pulmonary disease (COPD).

Fig. 20.**42** **Chronic eosinophilic pneumonia.** Multiple, bilateral, poorly defined, patchy infiltrates are evident.

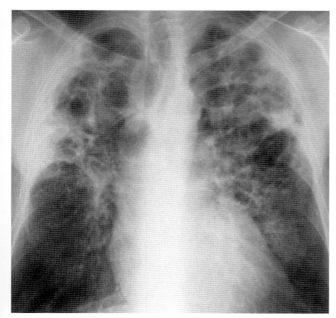

Fig. 20.**43 Bronchiolitis obliterans organizing pneumonia (cryptogenic organizing pneumonia).** Bilateral patchy infiltrates mainly involving the mid and upper lung zones are superimposed on chronic pulmonary changes including fibrosis ("honeycombing"), cystic bronchiectasis and bullous emphysema as well as chronic pleural disease.

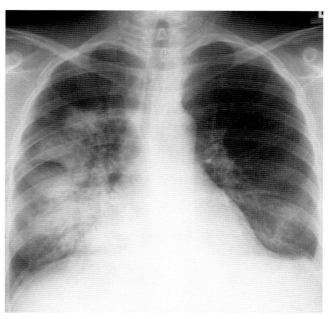

Fig. 20.**44 Lupus pneumonitis.** A large dense, poorly defined consolidation in the right perihilar and mid-lung zone is associated with an early left lower lower infiltrate and small left pleural reaction. Because of the patient's hemoptysis and absence of infection the underlying cause was considered to be extensive alveolar hemorrhage.

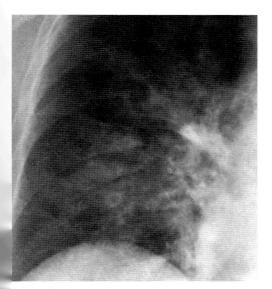

Fig. 20.**45 Wegener's granulomatosis.** An air-space consolidation involving mainly the right lower lobe is seen. Similar but less severe infiltrates were also present in the left lower lobe,

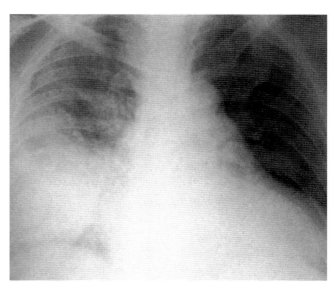

Fig. 20.**46 Pulmonary infarct** of the right middle and lower lobe in a patient with arteriosclerotic heart disease presenting as large consolidation.

Table 20.1 (Cont.) Alveolar Infiltrates and Atelectasis

Disease	Radiographic Appearance	Comments
Pulmonary hemorrhage (nontraumatic) (Fig. 20.47)	Usually bilateral alveolar densities clearing 2–3 days after single bleeding episode.	E.g. in *bleeding diathesis, idiopathic pulmonary hemosiderosis,* and *Goodpasture's syndrome.*
Pulmonary contusion	Patchy infiltrates to extensive homogeneous consolidations apparent within 6 hours after trauma. Resolution begins rapidly and is completed within 3–7 days.	Usually in lung adjacent to the traumatized area but occasionally in the opposite lung (contre coup effect).
Bronchial fracture (Fig. 20.48)	Opacification (atelectasis) of a lobe or even an entire lung. May not become evident until months after traumatic episode, when bronchial stenosis develops at fracture side. Besides a pneumothorax, a localized to extensive pneumomediastinum is a common initial finding. Fractures of the first three ribs are very often associated in the adult.	Pneumothorax is usually the most striking finding but not present in 30% of cases, when fracture is incomplete or affects a bronchus within the mediastinum.
Lung torsion	Exudation of blood causes opacification of the entire lung, that is rotated 180 degrees. Alteration in pulmonary vasculature characteristic.	Almost invariably in children.
Radiation pneumonitis (Fig. 20.49)	Consolidation often with air bronchograms developing 1 month to 1 year (most commonly 2–4 months) after cessation of radiation therapy. Localization corresponds to irradiated area. The fibrotic stage is usually present at 9–12 months and characterized by significant loss of volume, dense strands, and opacification of the involved area. Radiation-induced pleural effusions are unusual but pleural thickening is relatively common.	Radiation effect depends on total dose, number of fractions, and time elapsed between first and last treatment. A dose of at least 20 Gy is usually required, whereas doses of 60 Gy administered over 6 weeks almost always cause a severe radiation pneumonitis.

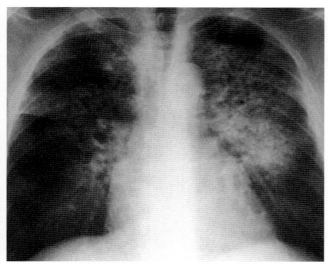

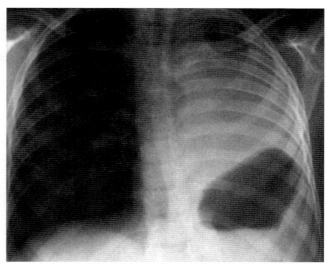

Fig. 20.**47** **Pulmonary hemorrhage in idiopathic pulmonary hemosiderosis.** Bilateral alveolar densities with predominantly perihilar distribution are seen.

Fig. 20.**48** **Bronchial fracture.** Atelectasis of the left lung is evident.

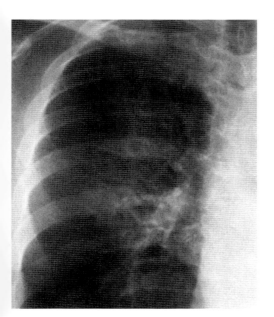

Fig. 20.**49** **Radiation pneumonitis.** An infiltrate in the anteromedial portions of the right upper and mid lung field is seen, corresponding to the radiation ports for breast carcinoma.

21 Interstitial Lung Disease

Interstitial lung disease is diagnosed radiographically when a *reticular*, *nodular*, or *honeycomb pattern* or any combination thereof is recognizable.

The *reticular pattern* consists of a network of linear densities (Fig. 21.1 a). Depending on the mesh size, one can distinguish between fine, medium, and coarse reticular patterns, although this distinction has no obvious differential diagnostic significance. Kerley lines refer to septal lines that are thickened either by fluid accumulation, cellular infiltration, or connective tissue proliferation within the interlobular septa. Acute or transient Kerley lines are usually found with hydrostatic pulmonary edema (elevated microvascular pressure caused by left ventricular failure, renal disease and fluid overload), and occasionally with pneumonia and pulmonary hemorrhage. Acute Kerley lines are frequently associated with prominent interlobar fissures caused by subpleural edema. Permanent Kerley lines are most often present in chronic and severe pulmonary venous hypertension (especially mitral stenosis) that eventually results in fibrosis and hemosiderin deposition within the interlobular septa. Lymphatic obstruction appears to be a major factor in the development of Kerley lines associated with malignancies (e.g., lymphangitic carcinomatosis, bronchogenic carcinoma, and lymphoma), since at least histologically, ipsilateral hilar involvement with tumor is almost invariably present under such conditions. Finally, fibrosis of the interlobular septa can be associated with any form of pulmonary fibrosis, but is most frequently observed with pneumoconiosis.

Different kinds of Kerley lines are distinguished: Kerley A lines are straight lines measuring 2–6 cm in length and approximately 1 mm in thickness. They are located in radiating fashion midway between the hilum and pleura and appear to cross over bronchoarterial bundles showing no anatomic relationship with the latter. Kerley A lines are usually best seen in the mid and lower lung fields. Kerley B lines are thinner and shorter than Kerley A lines (up to 2 cm) and lie in the lung periphery perpendicular to the lateral pleural surface (Fig. 21.1 b). They are most numerous at the base of the lungs. *Plate-like (discoid) atelectases and localized fibrotic strands* can be differentiated from Kerley lines by their lack of a characteristic anatomic location and by the great variation in length and width of these densities.

A nodular pattern (Fig. 21.1 c) consists of numerous punctate densities essentially ranging in diameter from 1 mm (barely visible as an individual lesion) to 5 mm, although a few slightly larger nodular lesions can be interspersed. A purely nodular pattern is found with the hematogenous spread of certain infections and tumors, but can also be encountered with other diseases (Table 21.1). More often, however, nodular and reticular patterns are combined in the same patient, resulting in a *reticulonodular appearance* of the interstitial disease.

A *ground-glass appearance* (Fig. 21.1 d) is caused by a hazy increase in lung density that is not associated with obscuration of underlying vascular markings. It is found, besides in interstitial diseases, also with air-space disease (e.g. pneumocystis carinii pneumonia) and increased capillary blood volume (e.g. congestive heart failure). In interstitial disease it is produced when the fine reticulogranular pattern has progressed to such an extent that the overall density of the involved lung is increased, but the individual interstitial lesion is no longer recognizable.

A *honeycomb pattern* is characterized by round or oval cystic lesions with a diameter up to 1 cm (Fig. 21.1e). In a given patient, they are relatively uniform in size and usually bunched together in grape-like clusters. Honeycombing is the only dependable radiographic sign of *interstitial fibrosis*. It may present radiographically in a reticulonodular pattern, too, but this presentation is also found with many other disorders, including various acute abnormalities that can resolve completely with time. *Cystic bronchiectases* may produce a radiographic picture similar to honeycombing. However, they can usually be differentiated from honeycombing by their larger and less uniform size and by the presence of tiny meniscus-like fluid levels at the bottom of these cystic lesions. Diseases that cause a characteristic honeycomb pattern are summarized in Table 21.2.

The majority of interstitial lung diseases involve both lungs, or stated differently, the interstitial disease is usually diffuse, although some areas may be more affected and others more or less spared. Truly *localized interstitial lung disease* is relatively rare and most often of an infectious etiology. *Mycoplasma* and *viral pneumonias* can present in their early stages as localized interstitial diseases of fine reticular appearance before the extension of the inflammation into the air spaces causes a consolidation. Localized fibrotic changes are often found in the chronic stage of a disease (e. g., *tuberculosis* and *radiation pneumonitis*). Finally, fibrotic scars may be the sequelae of virtually any disease capable of damaging the lung parenchyma severely enough.

Both congenital and acquired *bronchiectases* can be mistaken radiographically for localized interstitial lung disease (Fig. 21.1f). In approximately 50% of cases, they are limited to one lung. Cylindrical bronchiectases present as tubular opacities with parallel walls of 1 mm or slightly larger thickness. When these bronchiectatic segments become filled with retained secretion, they appear as homogeneous band-like densities ("gloved-finger" shadows). Varicose and cystic (saccular) bronchiectases are often evident on plain radiography as cystic lesions up to 2 cm in diameter and often containing a small air-fluid level at the bottom. This appearance is virtually diagnostic, although under very rare circumstances both pulmonary papillomatosis and paragonimiasis may mimic cystic bronchiectases. Bronchiectases are often associated with loss of volume and crowding of the lung markings in the affected area together with compensatory overinflation of the spared lung (Fig. 21.2).

Table 21.3 summarizes all disorders that demonstrate radiographically a diffuse reticular or reticulonodular pattern characteristic of interstitial lung disease.

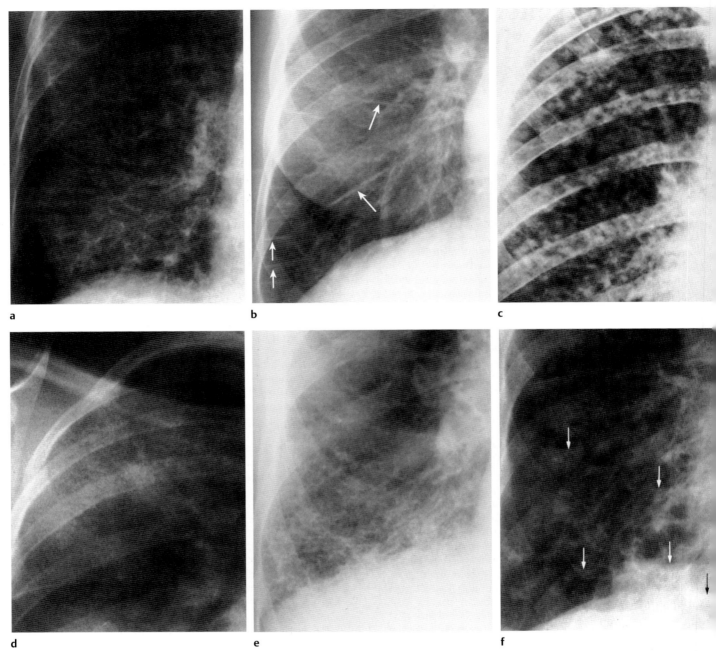

a   b   c

d   e   f

Fig. 21.**1 a–f   Patterns of interstitial lung disease. a** Reticular pattern (Pneumocystis carinii pneumonia). **b** Kerley A lines (long arrows, touched up) and Kerley B lines (short arrows) (mitral stenosis). **c** Nodular pattern (silicosis). **d** Ground-glass appearance produced by the summation of innumerable tiny reticulogranular densities (sarcoidosis). **e** Honeycomb pattern (idiopathic interstitial fibrosis). **f** Bronchiectases evident as cystic lesions varying considerably in size and characteristically containing small air–fluid levels (arrows).

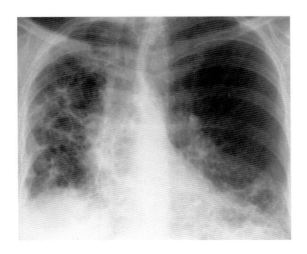

Fig. 21.**2   Bronchiectases.** Extensive, predominantly cystic bronchiectases in the right lung and left lower lobe are associated with loss of volume in the affected lung and compensatory overinflation of the nonaffected left upper lobe.

Table 21.1   Disseminated Pulmonary Nodules Measuring Less than 1 cm in Diameter ("Miliary" is defined as 1–3 mm in diameter)

Disease	Characteristics of Nodules
Bronchioloalveolar carcinoma (alveolar cell carcinoma) (Fig 21.3)	Often poorly defined, confluent nodules of varying size. Roentgenographic pattern of disseminated alveolar cell carcinoma may be fairly uniform throughout both lungs or vary regionally.
Metastases (e.g., carcinomas from thyroid, lung, breast, or gastrointestinal tract; or melanomas, sarcomas and lymphomas) (Fig. 21.4)	Usually well defined and of varying size.
Pneumonias	
Staphylococcus aureus	Miliary and larger, often poorly defined; can form microabscesses.
Salmonella	Miliary.
Pseodomonas pseudomallei	4 to 10 mm, poorly defined (early acute stage of disease).
Listeriosis (newborn)	Intrauterine infection with high mortality rate.

(continues on page 516)

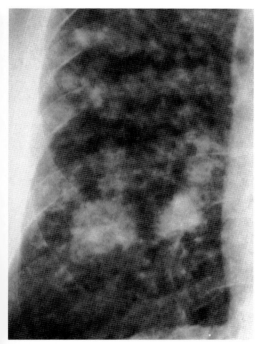

Fig. 21.**3 Bronchioloalveolar carcinoma.** Poorly defined, confluent nodules are seen bilaterally, but only shown for the right side.

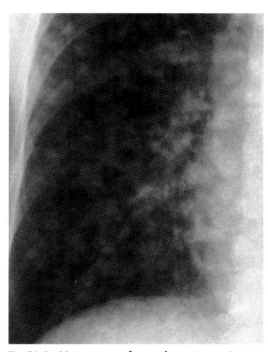

Fig. 21.**4 Metastases from breast carcinoma.** Numerous nodules measuring only a few millimeters in diameter are present bilaterally, but are only shown for the right lower lung field.

Table 21.1 (Cont.) Disseminated Pulmonary Nodules Measuring Less than 1 cm in Diameter ("Miliary" is defined as 1–3 mm in diameter)

Disease	Characteristics of Nodules
Tuberculosis (Fig. 21.5)	Miliary, discrete (DD: tuberculomas that are larger than 5 mm and can calcify).
Histoplasmosis (Fig 21.6)	2 to 4 mm, discrete. Can result in nodular calcifications 1 to several years later.
Coccidioidomycosis, blastomycosis, and Cryptococcosis (Fig. 21.7)	Miliary and larger (up to 3 cm). Calcification extremely rare.
Candidiasis	Miliary (rare manifestation)
Varicella (chickenpox) pneumonia (Fig. 21.8)	Miliary and larger, poorly defined. Healing may result in punctate calcifications years later,
Schistosomiasis	Miliary
Filariasis	Miliary and slightly larger (up to 5 mm). Predominantly in the mid- and lower-lung fields.

(continues on page 518)

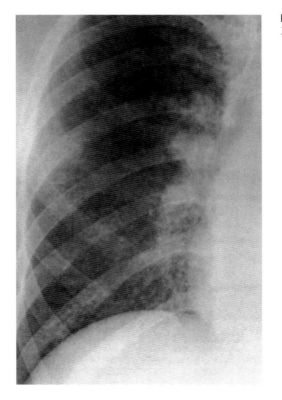

Fig. 21.**5 Miliary tuberculosis.** Numerous discrete nodules measuring 1 to 3 mm in diameter are seen bilaterally, but are only shown for the right side.

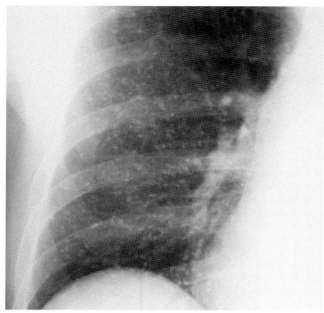

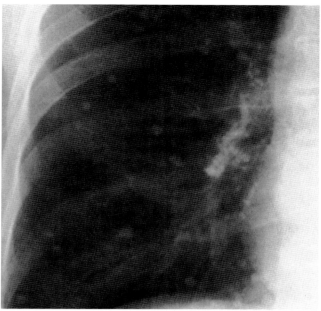

b

Fig. 21.**6**   **Histoplasmosis (two cases).** Bilateral miliary (**a**) and larger (**b**) scattered calcified nodules are present, but only shown for the right side.

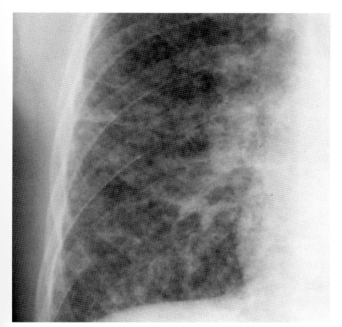

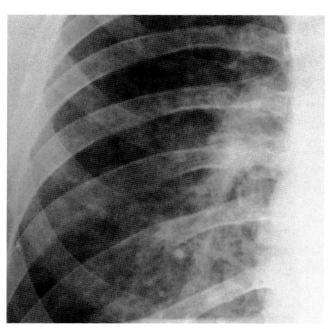

Fig. 21.**7**   **Aspergillosis.** Diffuse bilateral poorly defined small nodular densities are present, but only shown for the right lower lung field.

Fig. 21.**8**   **Varicella (chickenpox) pneumonia.** Poorly defined nodular densities are seen bilaterally, but are only shown for the right lower lung field.

Table 21.1 (Cont.) Disseminated Pulmonary Nodules Measuring Less than 1 cm in Diameter ("Miliary" is defined as 1–3 mm in diameter)

Disease	Characteristics of Nodules
Sarcoidosis (Fig. 21.9)	Miliary and larger, often indistinctly defined.
Pneumoconiosis (inorganic dust) (e.g., silicosis, coal miner's lung, berylliosis) (Figs. 21.10 and 21.11)	Miliary and larger. Fairly well defined in silicosis and poorly in berylliosis. Calcification occurs.
Pneumoconiosis caused by radiopaque dusts (iron, tin, barium, antimony and rare-earth compounds) (Figs. 21.12 and 21.13)	Finely granular stippling uniformly distributed over both lung fields. Density of the tiny nodules depends on the atomic number of the inhaled element.
Silo filler's disease (NO_2 inhalation)	Miliary nodulation only manifest 2–5 weeks after initial exposure (third phase of disease).
Extrinsic allergic alveolitis (e.g., farmer's lung, bird-fancier's lung, mushroom-worker's lung, bagassosis, and others) (Figs. 21.14 and 21.15)	Miliary and larger, usually poorly defined (acute stage). Often less evident in apices and bases.
Rheumatoid lung	Miliary and larger (in early stage).
Wegener's granulomatosis	Multiple nodules ranging from a few millimeters up to 10 cm.

(continues on page 520)

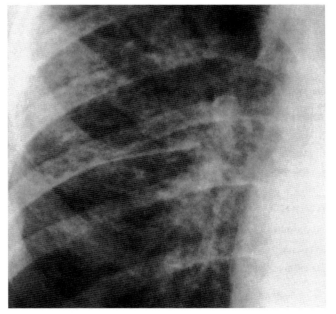

Fig. 21.9 Sarcoidosis. Multiple small nodules of variable sizes are seen bilaterally, but are only shown for the right mid lung field.

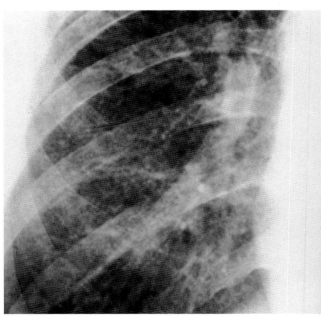

Fig. 21.10 Silicosis. Numerous fairly well defined miliary nodules are seen bilaterally besides diffuse reticular changes and early honeycombing, but are only shown for the right side.

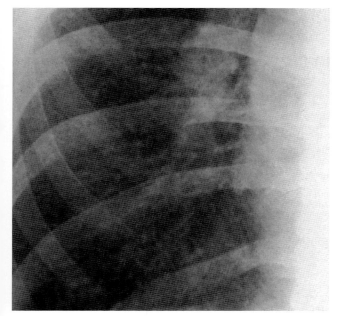

Fig. 21.**11** **Berylliosis.** Numerous relatively poorly defined miliary nodules and bilateral hilar enlargement are present, but are only shown for the right side. Findings simulate sarcoidosis radiographically.

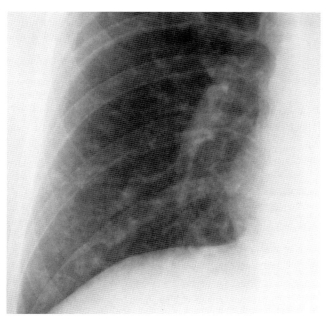

Fig. 21.**12** **Siderosis.** Bilateral small nodules with preferential involvement of the mid and lower lung zones are seen in this arc welder that are not associated with hilar adenopathy or fibrosis and resolved after exposure was discontinued. Only the right lower lung field is shown.

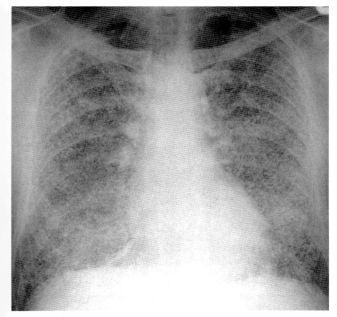

Fig. 21.**13** **Stannosis** (inhalation of tin oxide). Multiple tiny nodules of high density are distributed evenly throughout both lungs, sparing only the apices.

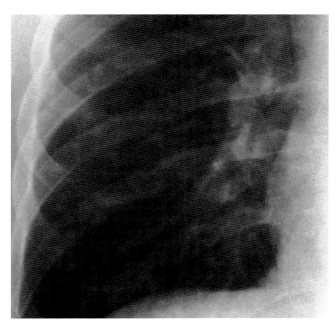

Fig. 21.**14** **Farmer's lung.** Bilateral poorly defined nodules are present.

Table 21.1   (Cont.) Disseminated Pulmonary Nodules Measuring Less than 1 cm in Diameter ("Miliary" is defined as 1–3 mm in diameter)

Disease	Characteristics of Nodules
Langerhans cell histiocytosis (eosinophilic granuloma) (Fig. 21.16)	Miliary and larger with mid and upper lung fields predominance. This presentation is seen in the active stage, which may completely resolve or progress to the chronic fibrotic stage.
Gaucher's disease	Miliary and larger.
Niemann–Pick syndrome	Miliary and larger.
Interstitial edema (cardiogenic)	Symmetrical, miliary nodulation, preferentially located in the lower-lung fields. May occasionally be the dominant feature.
Hemosiderosis and pulmonary ossification secondary to mitral stenosis (Fig. 21.17)	Punctate densities (hemosiderosis) and densely calcified 2 to 8 mm nodules (pulmonary ossification), predominantly in the mid and lower lung fields, usually more numerous on the right side. Hemosiderosis-like pulmonary calcifications are occasionally seen in chronic renal failure (see Fig. 22.**29**).
Bronchiolitis acute or obliterans	Miliary and larger
Amyloidosis (diffuse alveolar septal form)	Miliary and larger
Talc granulomatosis secondary to intravenous drug abuse	Discrete, 1 mm and smaller, may slowly increase in size and number over months and years.
Alveolar microlithiasis (Fig. 21.18)	Discrete and extremely sharply defined, less than 1 mm in diameter.
Oily contrast material embolism (e.g., secondary to lymphography) (Fig. 21.19)	Finely granular and relatively dense stippling preferentially located in the posterior (dependent) parts of the lungs and most obvious a few hours after lymphography.

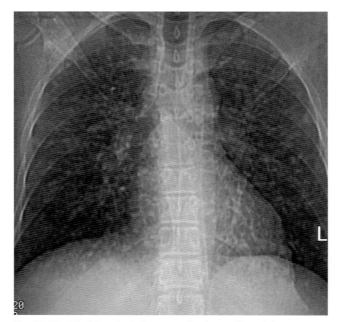

Fig. 21.**15   Bird-fancier's lung.** Multiple small nodules are scattered throughout both lung fields.

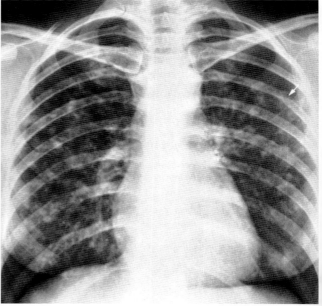

Fig. 21.**16 Langerhans cell histiocytosis (eosinophilic granuloma).** Multiple poorly defined nodules are seen bilaterally. Note also the lytic involvement of the left fifth rib with pathologic fracture (arrow).

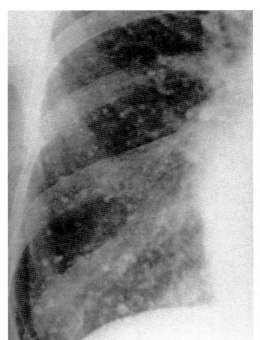

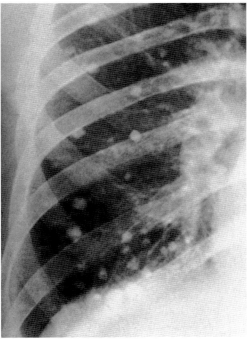

Fig. 21.**17** **Mitral stenosis** (two cases). **a** Punctate densities (hemosiderosis), and **b** larger calcified nodules (pulmonary ossification) are seen bilaterally, but only shown for the right side.

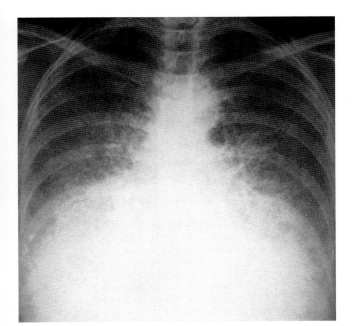

Fig. 21.**18** **Alveolar microlithiasis.** Innumerable, extremely sharply defined, tiny densities measuring less than 1 mm in diameter are seen bilaterally.

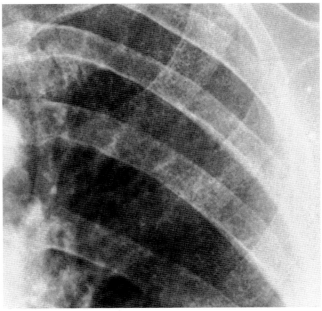

Fig. 21.**19** **Oily contrast material embolism after lymphography.** Finely granular and relatively dense stippling is seen throughout both lungs, but only shown for the left upper lung field.

Table 21.2 Honeycombing

Disease	Comments
Pneumoconiosis (silicosis, coal miner's lung, asbestosis, beryllio-sis, and others.) (Fig. 21.20)	Usually associated with other manifestations (nodules; conglomerate masses, hilar enlargement, etc). Lung volume normal or increased (emphysema).
Sarcoidosis (Fig. 21.21)	Persisting hilar and mediastinal lymphadenopathy often present. Lung volume normal or increased (emphysema).
Tuberculosis (Fig. 21.22)	A localized honeycombing pattern in the upper lobes can be simulated by tuberculous bronchiectasis and fibrosis.
Langerhans cell histiocytosis (eosinophilic granuloma) (Fig. 21.23)	Honeycombing characteristically more prominent in upper and mid lung fields and sparing the lung bases. Lung volume normal. Spontaneous pneumothorax occurs relatively frequently.

(continues on page 523)

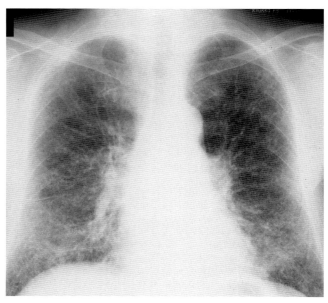

Fig. 21.**20** **Silicosis.** Diffuse bilateral interstitial lung disease with extensive fibrosis (honeycombing) is present.

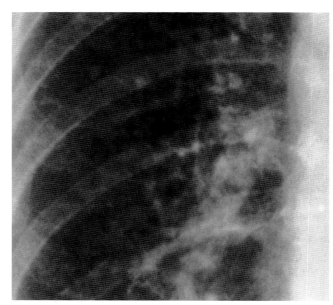

Fig. 21.**21** **Sarcoidosis.** Reticulonodular disease with early honey-combing is seen bilaterally, but only shown for the right mid lung field.

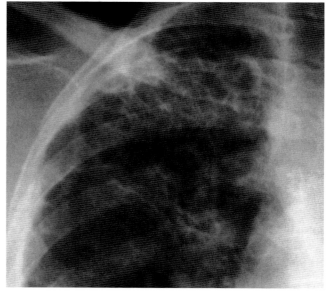

Fig. 21.**22** **Tuberculous bronchiectasis.** A honeycomb pattern is simulated by the bronchiectatic changes in both upper lobes, but more pronounced on the right side shown here.

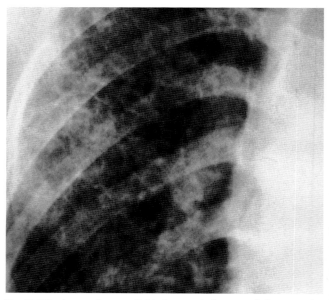

Fig. 21.**23** **Langerhans cell histiocytosis (eosinophilic granulo-ma).** Pulmonary fibrosis evident as honeycombing is predomi-nantly involving the mid and upper lung fields.

Table 21.2   (Cont.) Honeycombing

Disease	Comments
Connective tissue disease (especially scleroderma and rheumatoid lung) (Figs. 21.24 and 21.25)	Honeycombing usually most prominent at the bases. Progressive loss of lung volume is characteristically associated, particularly in scleroderma.
Idiopathic pulmonary fibrosis ("usual" interstitial pneumonia [UIP], Hamman–Rich syndrome) (Fig. 21.26)	Honeycombing usually most prominent at the bases. Progressive loss of lung volume characteristic. (Radiographically indistinguishable from scleroderma).
	Diffuse interstitial fibrosis, similar to the idiopathic form, may represent the end stage of a variety of pulmonary conditions (e.g., *drug induced*, especially by busulfan, bleomycin, methotrexate), *inhalation of noxious gases* and *organic dusts* (e.g., farmer's lung), *chronic or recurrent pulmonary edema,*especially in mitral valve disease, and others. Radiographically, however, an unequivocal honeycombing pattern is rarely found in these conditions.

(continues on page 524)

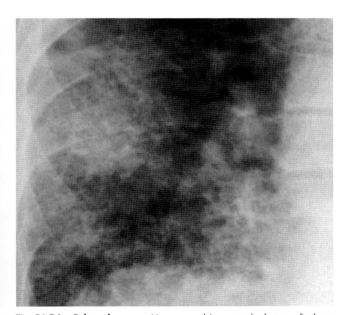

Fig. 21.**24 Scleroderma.** Honeycombing and loss of lung volume, evident by the high diaphragms bilaterally, are present, but only shown for the right lower lung field.

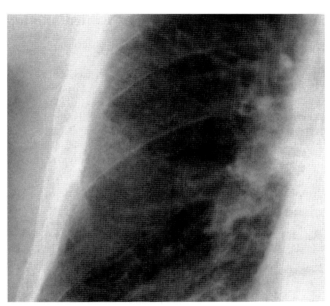

Fig. 21.**25 Rheumatoid lung disease.** Reticulonodular disease with honeycombing is present, but only shown for the right lower lung field.

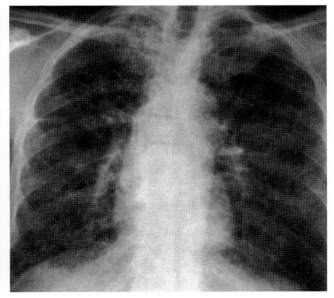

Fig. 21.**26 Idiopathic pulmonary fibrosis.** Extensive bilateral fibrosis with honeycombing and loss of lung volume is seen.

Table 21.2 (Cont.) Honeycombing

Disease	Comments
Desquamative interstitial pneumonitis (DIP) (Fig. 21.27)	Honeycombing indistinguishable from idiopathic pulmonary fibrosis (base predominance and loss of volume) is found in end-stage DIP. Ground-glass opacification and loss of definitions of basal vascular markings are often associated and quite characteristic.
Lipoid pneumonia (exogenous)	Rare. Localized honeycombing usually located in a lower lobe.
Amyloidosis	Rare. Honeycombing preferentially in lower lobes. Hilar and mediastinal adenopathy may be associated.
Ankylosing spondylitis with upper lobe pulmonary fibrosis	Rare. Exclusively located in upper lobes. Resembles upper lobe fibrosis and bronchiectasis secondary to tuberculosis.
Tuberous sclerosis	Rare. Predominantly lower lobe involvement. Diffuse honeycombing represents the end stage of pulmonary manifestations. Lung volume is normal or increased (associated emphysema). Chylous pleural effusions are often associated. Sclerotic bone lesions may be evident.
Lymphangiomyomatosis (lymphangioleiomyomatosis) (Fig. 21.28)	Rare, nonfamilial disease exclusively found in females of childbearing age, with pulmonary and pleural manifestations indistinguishable from tuberous sclerosis.
Neurofibromatosis	Rare. Pulmonary fibrosis and bullae are often combined. Skin nodules, scoliosis, rib notching and mediastinal masses may also be evident.
Gaucher's disease	Rare. Splenomegaly and bony changes (e.g. osteopenia, compression fractures in the thoracic spine and osteonecrosis in long bones) may be associated.
Niemann–Pick disease	Rare. Splenomegaly and bony changes in the thoracic spine similar to Gaucher's disease.

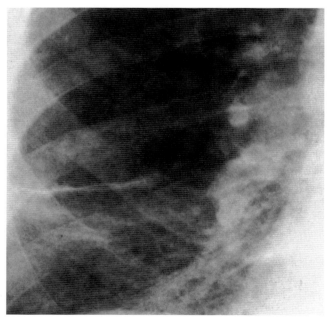

Fig. 21.27 Desquamative interstitial pneumonitis. Interstitial disease producing ground-glass appearance and honeycombing is particularly pronounced in the lower lung fields, but only shown for the right side. A loss of definition of the basal vascular markings is also evident.

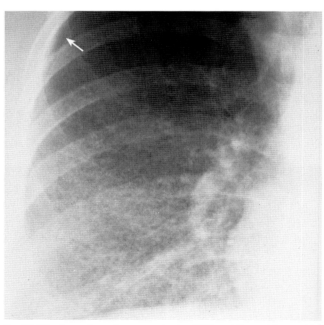

Fig. 21.28 Lymphangiomyomatosis. Diffuse bilateral interstitial disease with a fine honeycomb pattern is evident in the mid and lower lung zones, but only shown for the right side. A small pneumothorax (arrow) is also associated.

Table 21.3   Diffuse Reticular or Reticulonodular Disease

Disease	Radiographic Findings	Comments
Lymphangitic carcinomatosis (e.g., from breast, lung, pancreas, stomach, thyroid, cervix and prostatic carcinoma) (Fig. 21.29)	Usually uniform linear or reticular pattern with or without nodular component throughout both lungs but often more obvious in the lower-lung fields. Simulates interstitial pulmonary edema. Both hilar lymph node enlargement and pleural effusions are relatively common. Rapidly progressive loss of lung volume characteristic.	Caused by invasion of lymphatics from hematogenous metastases or, much less common, retrograde invasion into lungs from bronchopulmonary lymph nodes. Severe dyspnea is characteristic, which may even precede the radiographic manifestations.
Lymphoma (Hodgkin's and non-Hodgkin's lymphoma) (Fig. 21.30)	Interstitial infiltrate often most conspicuous in the perihilar area and usually associated with hilar and mediastinal lymphadenopathy, Pleural effusion may be present.	This pulmonary manifestation occurs probably by direct extension from hilar and mediastinal adenopathy. *Leukemia* and *macroglobutinemia Waldenström* can produce similar radiographic changes, but these are rare presentations in both disorders.

(continues on page 526)

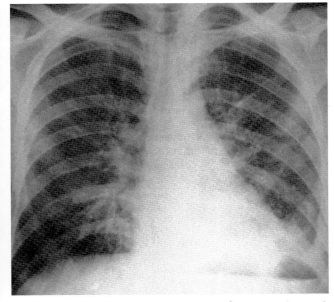

Fig. 21.**29 Lymphangitic carcinomatosis from gastric carcinoma.** Bilateral perihilar reticulonodular densities that are most prominent in the lower-lung fields are seen. Note also the left pleural effusion, whereas hilar lymph node enlargement cannot be appreciated in this case.

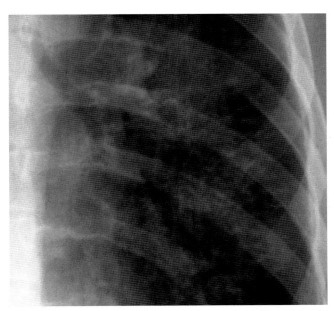

Fig. 21.**30 Non-Hodgkin's lymphoma.** Besides hilar and mediastinal lymph node enlargement, a reticular infiltrate in the left perihilar area is seen.

Table 21.3 (Cont.) Diffuse Reticular or Reticulonodular Disease

Disease	Radiographic Findings	Comments
Pneumonias *Mycoplasma* **(Fig. 21.31)**	Diffuse bilateral reticulonodular pattern, usually most conspicuous in lower lobes.	This presentation is less common than the localized form beginning with a fine reticular infiltrate that progresses rapidly to a consolidation.
Influenza **Respiratory syncytial virus (especially in infants and young children)** **Rubeola (measles)** **Varicella (Fig. 21.32)**	Mild increase in interstitial markings, particularly perihilar and at the bases to extensive reticulonodular involvement. Hilar lymph node enlargement occurs only in children.	Pulmonary findings in these viral infections similar to mycoplasma pneumonias. Localized or diffuse manifestations may progress to patchy consolidations.
Cytomegalovirus (Fig. 21.33)	Reticulonodular pattern with nodules measuring up to 2 mm preferentially in periphery of middle and lower lobes.	This early-stage manifestation is followed by patchy consolidations.
Pneumocystis carinii (Fig. 21.34)	Fine reticulonodular pattern particularly in perihilar areas.	This early-stage manifestation is followed by patchy consolidation simulating pulmonary edema.
Atypical mycobacteria (Fig. 21.35)	Multiple thin-walled cavities, preferentially located in the upper lobes, may produce a reticular pattern. Small nodules measuring lass than 1 cm may also be associated.	Radiographic presentation similiar to tuberculosis, but with a much greater tendency for cavitation. Usually found in patients with pre-existing pulmonary disease (e.g., emphysema and pneumoconiosis) or AIDS.
Toxoplasmosis	Reticular pattern that may be focal and indistinguishable from mycoplasma and viral pneumonia. Hilar lymph node enlargement is common.	Represents the early pulmonary manifestation of a generalized disease,
Coccidioidomycosis **Blastomycosis** **Cryptococcosis**	Disseminated, predominantly nodular disease that may progress to a reticulonodular pattern.	Rare presentation of these fungal diseases.
Schistosomiasis	Reticulonodular pattern, which can be associated with signs of pulmonary arterial hypertension (dilatation of pulmonary artery and its branches with rapid tapering toward periphery).	Interstitial changes produced by migration of ova through vessel wall with subsequent granuloma formation. Embolized ova can cause obliterative arteriolitis resulting in pulmonary hypertension.
Filariasis (Fig. 21.36)	Fine reticular to reticulonodular pattern, often with nodules up to 5 mm, predominantly in mid and lower lung fields. Hilar lymph node enlargement can occur.	Disease confined to tropics *(tropical pulmonary eosinophilia)*. Patients with pulmonary disease do not usually have characteristic cutaneous and lymphatic changes such as elephantiasis.

(continues on page 528)

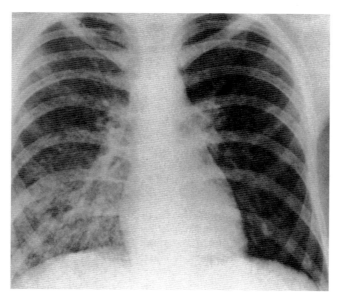

Fig. 21.**31** **Mycoplasma pneumonia.** Diffuse bilateral reticulonodular infiltrates are seen. The findings are most pronounced in the right lower lobe, where an early alveolar component is also present.

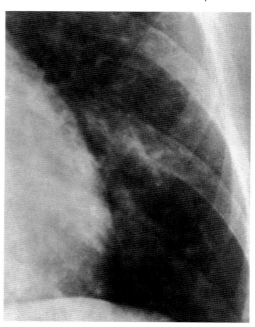

Fig. 21.**32** **Varicella pneumonia.** A bilateral reticulonodular infiltrate with numerous poorly defined nodules is predominantly involving the lower lobes, but only shown for the left side.

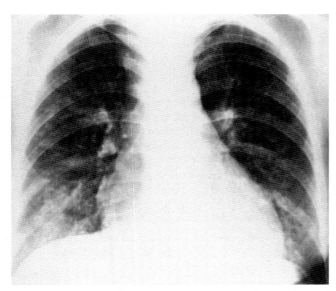

Fig. 21.**33** **Cytomegalovirus pneumonia** in patient with renal transplant. Reticulonodular and alveolar infiltrates are seen in both lower-lung fields.

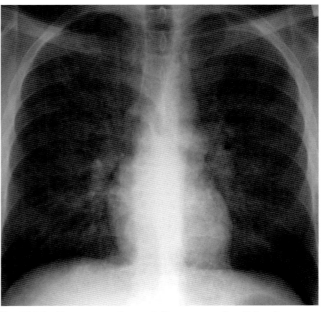

Fig. 21.**34** **Pneumocystis carinii pneumonia.** Extensive symmetrical reticulonodular infiltrates involving predominantly the perihilar areas are seen in this patient with AIDS.

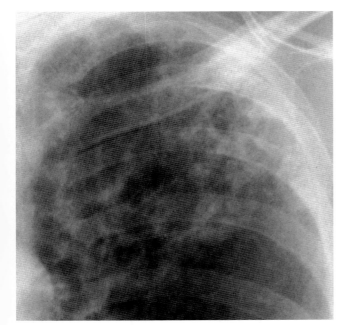

Fig. 21.**35** **Atypical mycobacterial infection.** Bilateral symmetrical reticulonodular to cystic infiltrates in the upper lobes are present in this patient with AIDS, but only shown for the left side.

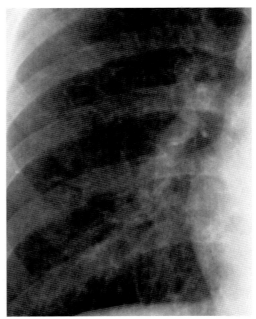

Fig. 21.**36** **Filariasis.** A fine reticuionodular pattern is seen in both lung fields, but only shown for the right side.

Table 21.3   (Cont.) Diffuse Reticular or Reticulonodular Disease

Disease	Radiographic Findings	Comments
Oily contrast material embolism (e.g., after lymphography)	Finely reticulogranular pattern caused by the oily contrast lodged in the terminal arterial branches. Rarely progresses to pulmonary edema.	Fat embolism after trauma, on the other hand, can only be diagnosed radiographically when the condition progresses to bilateral alveolar infiltrates with preferential involvement of the lung bases.
Interstitial edema (cardiogenic)	Increased interstitial markings, especially in the mid and lower lung fields, thickening of interlobular septa (Kerley A and B lines), loss of sharp definition of vascular structures, and perihilar haze, are characteristic.	Cardiomegaly (especially left atrial enlargement) and pulmonary venous hypertension (recognizable as redistribution of blood flow from the lower to the upper lobes) are usually present.
Fibrosis secondary to chronic left heart failure (Fig. 21.37)	Coarse, often poorly defined reticulation predominantly in mid and lower lung fields.	Results from recurrent episodes of interstitial and alveolar edema and hemorrhage. Differentiation between cardiogenic interstitial edema and fibrosis is often impossible on a single examination.
Acute bronchiolitis	Overinflation of the lungs is most characeristic. Often associated with reticulonodular densities with "miliary" appearance.	Viral (occasionally mycoplasma or bacterial) infection most commonly affecting children under 3 years of age and adults with pre-existing chronic respiratory disease.
Chronic bronchitis/bronchiolitis (Fig. 21.38)	Coarse increase in interstitial markings often associated with some emphysema.	May also be referred to as "dirty chest." Bronchiectases may also be associated.
Bronchiolitis obliterans	Hyperinflation, often associated with reticulonodular pattern, especially in the lower lobes.	End stage of lower respiratory tract damage of a variety of diseases.
Bronchiolitis obliterans organizing pneumonia (BOOP) Cryptogenic organizing pneumonia (COP) (Fig. 21.39)	Interstitial disease associated with patchy areas of consolidations that are commonly found bilaterally in the periphery of the mid and lower lung fields.	Clinically similar to idiopathic pulmonary fibrosis, but more responsive to steroid therapy and with better prognosis.
Cystic fibrosis (Fig. 21.40)	Coarse reticular pattern with cyst-like lesions often containing small air–fluid levels (bronchiectases). Overinflation is characteristically associated. Pulmonary fibrosis along the cardiac border may produce a "shaggy heart" sign. Recurrent pneumonias or atelectases are common. Signs of pulmonary arterial hypertension in the advanced stage.	Autosomal recessive transmission. Lack of pancreatic enzymes results in poor fat digestion and frequent small bowel obstructions (meconium ileus of the neonate).
Familial dysautonomia (Riley–Day syndrome)	Pulmonary findings indistinguishable from cystic fibrosis.	Autosomal recessive transmitted and almost exclusively found in Jews. Presents clinically with widespread neurologic disturbances.
Oxygen toxicity	"Spongy" lung caused by fibrosis, atelectasis and focal areas of emphysema.	Usually developing in premature infants receiving a high (up to 100 %) percentage oxygen therapy for *respiratory distress syndrome* (hyaline membrane disease) or *Wilson–Mikity syndrome* (pulmonary dysmaturity). In the latter condition, similar radiographic findings are occasionally found before oxygen is given. Oxygen therapy in the adult may produce similar findings.

(continues on page 530)

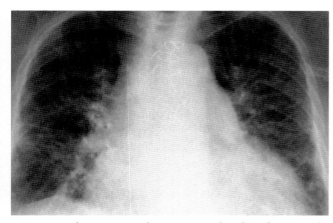

Fig. 21.**37 Fibrosis secondary to mitral valve disease.** The coarse and relatively poorly defined reticular pattern involving mainly the mid and lower lung fields persisted unchanged over a period of several years after mitral valve replacement.

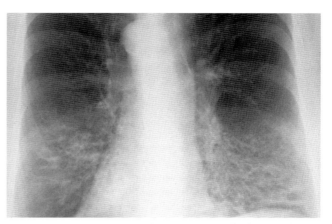

Fig. 21.**38 Kartagener syndrome (immotile/dysmotile cilia syndrome).** Situs inversus is associated with interstitial disease including bronchiectases mainly involving the lower lobes. Underdeveloped paranasal sinuses and sinusitis were also associated.

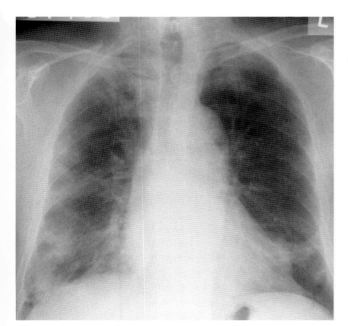

Fig. 21.**39 Bronchiolitis obliterans organizing pneumonia (Cryptogenic organizing pneumonia).** Bilateral small nodular densities and patchy peripheral infiltrates are seen.

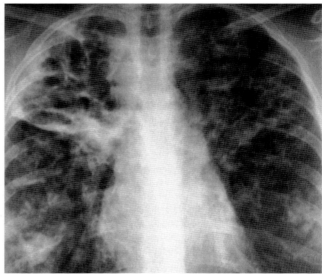

Fig. 21.**40 Cystic fibrosis.** A coarse reticulonodular pattern with cystic bronchiectases and fibroses is seen, involving predominantly the upper lobes. Note also the overinflated middle and lower lobes and the hilar prominence secondary to pulmonary arterial hypertension.

Table 21.3 (Cont.) Diffuse Reticular or Reticulonodular Disease

Disease	Radiographic Findings	Comments
Pneumoconiosis **Silicosis** **(Fig. 21.41)**	Well-circumscribed nodular lesions ranging from 1 to 10 mm are usually the dominant radiographic feature, but are commonly associated with a reticular pattern that may even precede the nodules. Hilar lymph node enlargement is frequent, but the characteristic eggshell calcification occurs only in 5%. Progressive massive fibrosis (PMF) may develop in the upper lobes and present as bilateral homogenous opacifications that occasionally cavitate due to central ischemic necrosis or superimposed tuberculous caseation.	Exposure to highly concentrated silicon dioxide dust usually over 10 to 20 years before first radiographic manifestations. *Caplan's syndrome:* association of necrobiotic (rheumatoid) nodules, ranging from 0.5 to 5 cm in diameter, rheumatoid arthritis, and silicosis.
Coal miner's lung	Radiographic findings similar to silicosis, although nodules are somewhat less well defined and hilar lymph node enlargement is less conspicuous.	Exposure to coal dust, which always contains small amounts of free silica but massive deposition of carbon, is assumed to be mainly responsible for the disease. *Progressive massive fibrosis (PMF)* and *Caplan's syndrome* (association with necrobiotic lung nodules and rheumatoid arthritis) occur with even higher frequency than in silicosis.
Asbestosis **(Fig. 21.42)**	Reticulonodular changes initially predominantly in lower lobes, later generalized. Pleural plaques with or without calcifications involving the parietal and diaphragmatic pleura are usually the dominant radiographic feature. Early interstitial changes combined with pleural thickening can produce "ground-glass" appearance. Conglomerate masses are occasionally found in an advanced stage and tend to show a lower zonal predominance. A combination of parenchymal and pleural changes may partially obscure the heart border ("shaggy heart" sign). Hilar lymph node enlargement does not occur.	Manifestations occur usually only 20 years after onset of exposure. Mesotheliomas and bronchogenic carcinomas are associated with a high incidence.
Talcosis	Pulmonary and pleural manifestations similar to asbestosis, but large opacities (conglomerate lesions) are more common.	Incidence of pleural and bronchogenic neoplasms also increased.
Berylliosis	Reticular to reticulonodular pattern with relatively poorly defined nodules that may calcify. Hilar lymph node enlargement occurs. Radiographic differentiation from sarcoidosis is usually not possible, unless the pulmonary nodules are calcified. Emphysematous changes, particularly in the upper lobe, result in a pneumothorax in 10%.	Berylliosis is not only found in workers exposed to beryllium (e.g., phosphorescent industry), but can also be attracted at home from contaminated work clothes or atmospheric pollution from a nearby plant.
Aluminum (bauxite) pneumoconiosis	Reticular or reticulonodular pattern often associated with loss of lung volume and pleural thickening. Emphysematous bullae are common, resulting in a spontaneous pneumothorax.	Occurs a few months to several years of exposure in workers processing bauxite or inhaling fine aluminum powder.
Pneumoconiosis caused by radiopaque dusts (iron [siderosis], tin [stannosis], barium [baritosis], antimony, and rareearth compounds)	Density of fine reticulonodular changes reflects atomic number and particle size of inhaled element.	Since these substances are not fibrogenic, no significant clinical symptoms are found in these pneumoconioses.
Silo filler's disease (NO₂ inhalation) (Fig. 21.43)	Bilateral reticulonodular infiltrates preferentially in the mid and lower lung fields that may progress rapidly to patchy alveolar densities and even massive pulmonary edema.	Pulmonary manifications resolve completely within a few days if not fatal. After an asymptomatic period of 2–5 weeks (second phase), the third phase of the disease becomes radiographically manifest as "miliary nodulation," representing bronchiolitis obliterans fibrosa.

(continues on page 532)

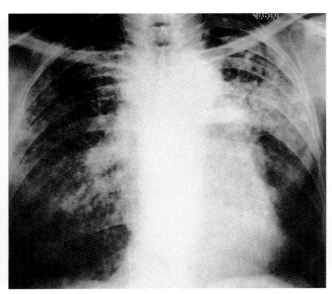

Fig. 21.**41** **Silicosis.** Fibrosis causing a reticulonodular pattern and honeycombing in the mid and upper lung fields and emphysematous changes at the bases are seen.

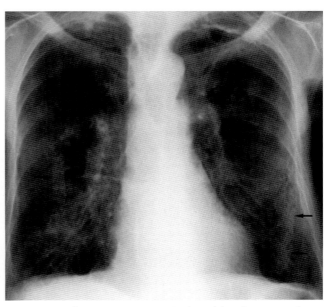

Fig. 21.**42** **Asbestosis.** Coarse reticulonodular changes and emphysema combined with pleural plaques and calcifications (arrows) are characteristic.

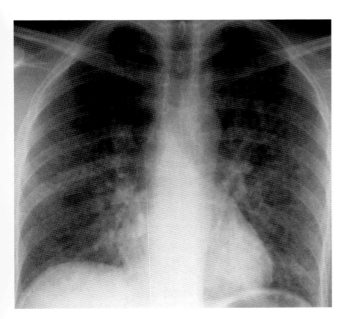

Fig. 21.**43** **Silo filler's disease.** Bilateral reticuionodular infiltrates with preferential involvement of the mid and lower lung fields are seen.

Table 21.3 (Cont.) Diffuse Reticular or Reticulonodular Disease

Disease	Radiographic Findings	Comments
Extrinsic allergic alveolitis due to organic dust (e.g., farmer's lung, bird-fancier's lung, mushroom-worker's lung, bagassosis [sugar cane], and others) (Fig. 21.44)	Radiographic presentation ranges from diffuse poorly defined nodules, one to several millimeters in diameter and often associated with patchy infiltrates (acute stage) to coarse reticulation (chronic stage), Hilar lymph node enlargement is rare and never a dominant feature.	Clinical symptoms (dyspnea, often associated with dry cough and malaise) occur a few hours after exposure to relevant antigen.
Drug-induced pulmonary disease (amiodarone, nitrofurantoin, busulphan, bleomycin, methotrexate, ganglionic blockers, and many others) (Figs. 21.45 and 21.46)	Diffuse reticular to reticulonodular pattern, that might progress to patchy infiltrates and even pulmonary edema.	May be an allergic reaction to the drug, in which case it is associated with eosinophilia (e.g., nitrofurantoin), or a toxic effect causing interstitial infiltrates that may progress to fibrosis (e.g., chemotherapeutics). A variety of other drugs (e.g., penicillin, sulfonamides) cause a Loeffler's syndrome-like pattern.
Connective tissue diseases (rheumatoid lung, scleroderma, systemic lupus erythematosus, dermatomyositis) (Fig. 21.47)	Generalized reticular to reticulonodular disease, usually more prominent at the bases. Co-existing pleural effusion not common, except in lupus.	Pulmonary connective tissue manifestations of *polyarteritis nodosa* (another connective tissue disease) are highly variable and include increased interstitial markings, poorly defined nodules of varying size, and patchy consolidations.

(continues on page 534)

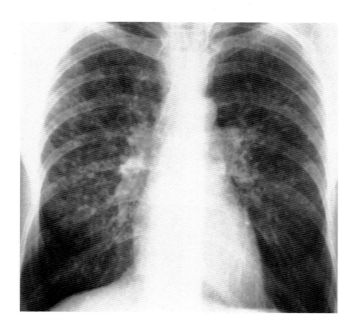

Fig. 21.44 Farmer's lung. A reticulonodular pattern is seen in both lungs with sparing of the bases and apices. The poorly defined nodules are indicative of the acute stage of the disease.

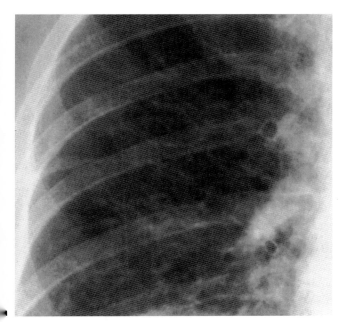

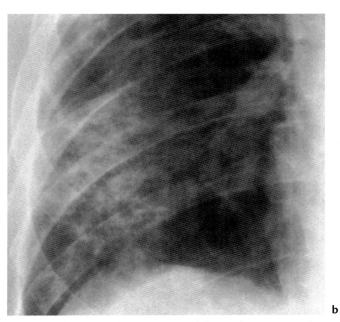

b

Fig. 21.**45 Bleomycin-induced pulmonary disease** (two cases). **a** Early stage: Bilateral interstitial infiltrates of predominantly reticular nature are present, but only shown for the right mid and lower lung fields. **b** Advanced stage: Intestitial disease has progressed to patchy infiltrates.

Fig. 21.**46 Amiodarone-induced pulmonary disease.** Bilateral interstitial and early alveolar infiltrates are present in the lower lung zones, but only shown for the right side.

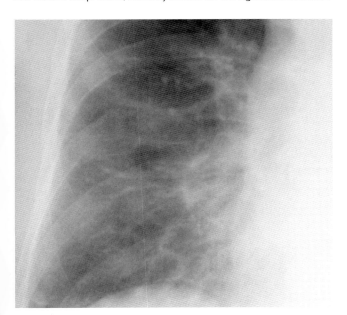

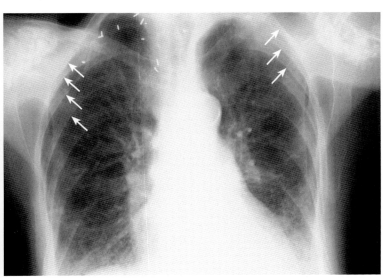

Fig. 21.**47 Scleroderma.** Interstitial lung disease with honeycombing at the lung bases is associated with extensive soft tissue calcifications in both shoulder regions and thinning of several ribs (arrows) in the upper chest bilaterally.

Table 21.3 (Cont.) Diffuse Reticular or Reticulonodular Disease

Disease	Radiographic Findings	Comments
Sjögren's syndrome (Fig. 21.48)	Reticulonodular, similar to connective tissue disease.	Syndrome consists of keratoconjunctivitis sicca, xerostomia and recurrent parotid gland swelling. 90% of the cases occur in women.
Idiopathic pulmonary hemosiderosis and Goodpasture's syndrome (Fig. 21.49)	Fine reticular pattern predominantly in mid- and lower-lung fields, found a few days after acute bleeding episode, evident as patchy consolidations. Persistence of a reticular to reticulonodular pattern after numerous bleeding episodes indicates irreversible interstitial changes resulting eventually in pulmonary fibrosis. Hilar enlargement and pleural effusions occur occasionally.	Clinical manifestations are repeated episodes of pulmonary hemorrhage resulting in anemia and pulmonary insufficiency. Goodpasture's syndrome additionally includes renal disease. Male predominance.
Langerhans cell histiocytosis (eosinophilic granuloma) (Fig. 21.50)	Poorly defined nodules up to 10 mm in diameter and fine reticular changes predominantly in the mid and upper lung fields. Disease may progress to honeycombing pattern. Hilar enlargement and pleural effusions are very rare and never a dominant feature.	Approximately one-third of patients are asymptomatic when initially diagnosed on a screening chest radiograph. Diagnosed most frequently in the 3rd and 4th decade with caucasian female predominance and often history of heavy cigarette smoking.
Sarcoidosis (Fig. 21.51)	Pulmonary manifestations vary from purely nodular to purely reticular, but a reticulonodular pattern is the most common presentation. Majority of cases is associated with significant hilar and mediastinal lymph node enlargement, which commonly precedes the lung involvement and may regress spontaneously in the presence of the latter.	Approximately half of patients are asymptomatic when first diagnosed on a screening chest radiograph. High incidence in black women living in the USA, usually diagnosed between 20 and 40 years of age.
Desquamative interstitial pneumonitis (DIP) (see Fig. 21.27)	Increased interstitial markings and reticulonodular densities, sometimes having a confluent or groundglass appearance are characteristic. Manifestations bilaterally symmetrical, and usually predominant in the lower lung fields, where they may cause a loss of definition of the vascular markings.	Etiology of DIP is unknown. May progress to pulmonary fibrosis (honeycombing) or regress spontaneously. *Lymphoid (LIP)* (Fig. 21.**52**) and *giant cell interstitial pneumonias (GIP)* are rare related conditions with similar radiographic features.
Idiopathic pulmonary fibrosis ("usual interstitial pneumonia" [UIP], Hamman–Rich syndrome) (Fig. 21.53)	Generalized coarse reticular or reticulonodular pattern. Honeycombing especially at the bases and loss of lung volume on serial films are often found.	Middle-aged and elderly men are most commonly affected. *Bronchiolitis obliterans with diffuse interstitial pneumonia (BIP)* represents a similar condition, but is associated with obliterating bronchiolitis.
Interstitial fibrosis secondary to pulmonary disease (Fig. 21.54)	Localized or generalized interstitial thickening. May be associated with fibrotic strands or scars.	Common cause of interstitial lung disease, though the offending agent is not always recognized. May be the sequela of recurrent infections, chronic aspiration, lung trauma, radiation, or thromboembolic disease (e.g., in sickle-cell anemia, where the lower lung fields are preferentially involved).
Familial and developmental disorders (tuberous sclerosis, lymphangiomyomatosis, neurofibromatosis, Gaucher's disease, Niemann–Pick disease, lipoid proteinosis) (Fig. 21.55)	Diffuse interstitial changes of a reticulonodular nature, with lower-lobe predilection. May progress to honeycombing and emphysema.	Associated findings on chest radiograph: Tuberous sclerosis: chylous effusions, osteoblastic lesions. Lymphangiomyomatosis: chylous effusions. Neurofibromatosis: skin nodules, scoliosis, rib notching, mediastinal masses. Gaucher's and Niemann–Pick disease: splenomegaly, osteopenia with compression fractures in vertebral bodies. Lipoid proteinosis: thickened vocal cords.

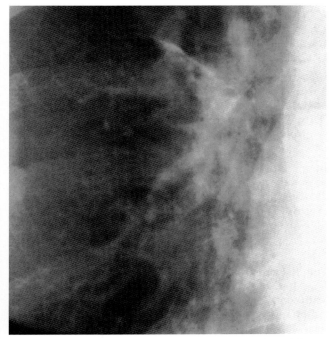

Fig. 21.**48** **Sjögren's syndrome.** Symmetrical reticulonodular infiltrates, predominantly involving the perihilar areas, but only shown for the right side.

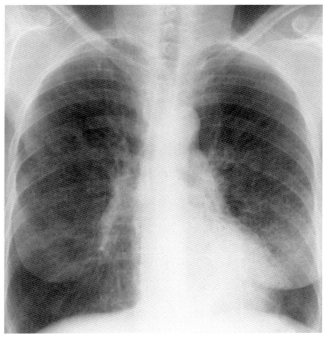

Fig. 21.**49** **Goodpasture's syndrome.** Bilateral interstitial disease of reticulonodular nature is seen mainly involving the mid and lower lung zones.

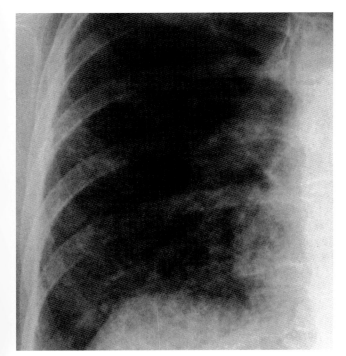

Fig. 21.**50** **Langerhans cell histiocytosis (eosinophilic granuloma).** Diffuse fine reticulonodular infiltrates with early honeycombing, involving both lungs symmetrically, but only shown for the right side.

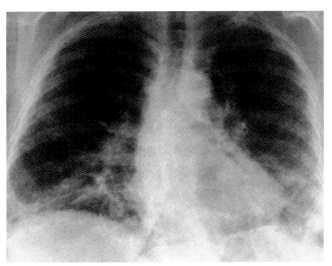

Fig. 21.**51** **Sarcoidosis.** Extensive bilateral reticulonodular disease with a few larger and poorly defined opacities at the bases is evident.

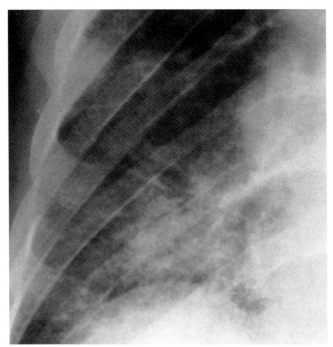

Fig. 21.**52 Lymphoid interstitial pneumonia (LIP).** Bilateral interstitial infiltrates in the mid and lower lung fields, with progression to consolidation in the central areas, are present, but only shown for the right lower lung field.

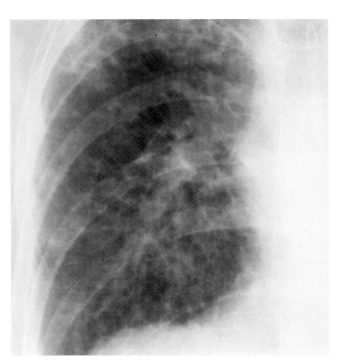

Fig. 21.**53 Idiopathic pulmonary fibrosis.** Bilateral reticulonodular disease with honeycombing is present, but only shown for the right side.

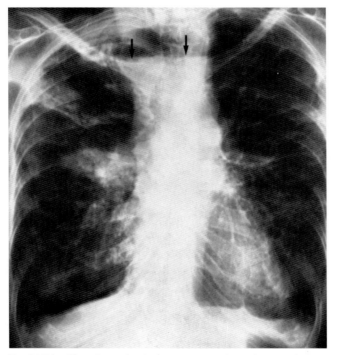

Fig. 21.**54 Chronic aspiration pneumonia in patient with Zenker diverticulum.** Diffuse coarse interstitial thickening is noted throughout both lung fields besides several areas of opacification resulting from more recent episodes of aspiration. Note also the large air–fluid level (arrows) in the Zenker diverticulum projecting just above the medial ends of both clavicles.

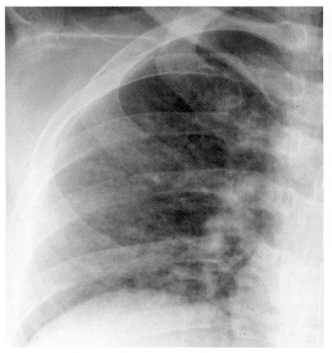

Fig. 21.**55 Tuberous sclerosis.** Bilateral interstitial lung disease of fine reticulonodular nature with beginning honeycombing at the bases is present, but only shown for the right side.

22 Pulmonary Edema and Symmetrical Bilateral Infiltrates

Pulmonary edema is caused by the accumulation of excessive fluid in both the interstitial and alveolar spaces. The two main factors responsible for the leak of fluid from the capillary space into the interstitial and subsequently the alveolar compartments are an *elevated capillary blood pressure* and *increased capillary permeability*. A decrease in either serum osmotic pressure or interstitial fluid pressure can contribute to the development of pulmonary edema, although these abnormalities are unlikely to cause edema by themselves. Other factors contributing to the development of pulmonary edema include a decrease in alveolar pressure and surface tension as well as obstruction of the lymphatics draining the lung interstitium, but their significance in this pathophysiologic mechanism is not clearly determined yet.

The most common cause of pulmonary edema resulting from an increased capillary pressure (*hydrostatic pulmonary edema*) is left ventricular failure (cardiogenic edema). Pulmonary veno-occlusive disease (e.g. idiopathic, congenital pulmonary vein anomalies, invasion or compression of pulmonary veins) may also induce hydrostatic pulmonary edema. An elevated pulmonary capillary pressure associated with a decreased serum osmotic pressure is responsible for pulmonary edema associated with renal failure and fluid overload. Neurogenic pulmonary edema results from a combination of both elevated capillary blood pressure and increased capillary permeability.

Pulmonary edema caused by increased capillary permeability is frequently referred to as *adult respiratory distress syndrome (ARDS)*. It is associated with sepsis, overwhelming pneumonia, aspiration, inhalation of noxious gases, pulmonary contusion, fractures (e.g. long bones and pelvis), near-drowning, burns, blood transfusions, major surgery (e.g. coronary bypass), prolonged hypotension, disseminated intravascular coagulation, and drug overdose.

Pulmonary edema is radiographically characterized by a bilateral, diffuse increase in interstitial markings with a loss of definition and by fluffy confluent opacities representing the alveolar process. This radiographic pattern is found most commonly in cardiogenic pulmonary edema, where the increased capillary blood pressure causes an abnormal plasma leak into the interstitial and alveolar spaces (Fig. 22.1). The edema accumulates predominantly in the most dependent portions of the lungs. In the upright position, this is in the mid- and, particularly, lower lung fields, whereas in the bedridden patient with the radiograph taken in the supine position, the edema appears more evenly distributed throughout both lungs. An unusual distribution pattern of the pulmonary edema might, however, be found with a pre-existing chronic lung disease (e.g. emphysema), where the edema spares the most severely damaged parts of the lungs (Fig. 22.2). Bronchogenic spread of various exogenous and endogenous materials and organisms may also cause diffuse alveolar infiltrates that may or may not be associated with interstitial disease. Finally, the infiltration of the alveolar and interstitial space with inflammatory or neoplastic cells can produce a radiographic appearance that also simulates pulmonary edema.

An unusual presentation of pulmonary edema takes the form of the *"bat's wing"* or *"butterfly pattern,"* in which the hilar and perihilar areas of the lungs are fairly dense and uniformly consolidated and the peripheral 2–3 cm of the lung parenchyma are relatively uninvolved (Fig. 22.3). This pat-

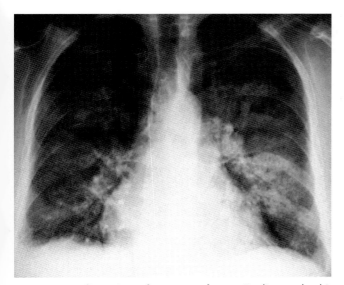

Fig. 22.**1 Cardiogenic pulmonary edema.** Cardiomegaly, bilateral interstitial and alveolar infiltrates involving predominantly the mid- and lower lung fields, and small pleural effusions are seen. This acute edema was caused by a left atrial myxoma that has suddenly enlarged secondary to intratumoral bleeding.

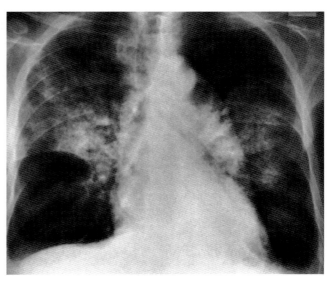

Fig. 22.**2 Cardiogenic pulmonary edema** in chronic obstructive pulmonary disease. Asymmetric distribution of the pulmonary edema that spares the parts of the lungs with the most severe emphysematous changes is seen.

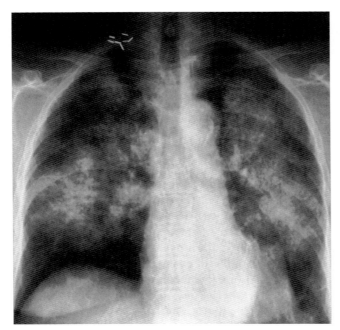

Fig. 22.**3 Pneumocystis carinii pneumonia** in compromised host. The pulmonary infiltrates, consisting of an interstitial (reticulonodular) and alveolar component, assume a *"bat's wing"* or *"butterfly pattern,"* sparing the peripheral 2–3 cm of the lung parenchyma.

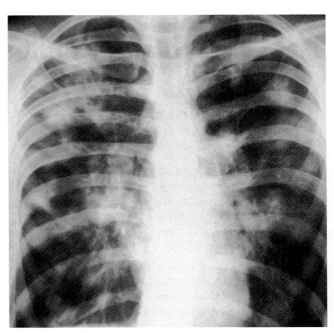

Fig. 22.**4 Loeffler's syndrome** (acute eosinophilic pneumonia). Bilateral patchy consolidations in the lung periphery parallel to the lateral chest wall are characteristic (*"reversed pulmonary edema pattern"*). The more central appearing infiltrates are anatomically located in the anterior or posterior lung periphery.

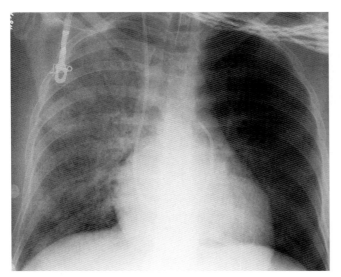

Fig. 22.**5 Aspiration.** A *unilateral pulmonary edema pattern* with air bronchograms is seen in the right lung. The aspiration occurred with the patient lying on his right side.

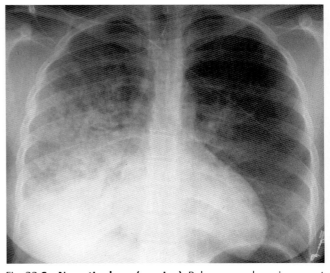

Fig. 22.**6 Narcotic abuse (cocaine).** Pulmonary edema is present bilaterally, but much more severe on the right side.

tern is relatively frequently seen with uremia, alveolar proteinosis, and pneumocystis carinii pneumonia, and with conditions causing pulmonary hemorrhage, such as idiopathic pulmonary hemosiderosis and polyarteritis nodosa. However, it is not at all pathognomonic of these conditions and can be found with virtually every disease known to produce a pulmonary edema pattern.

The *"reversed pulmonary edema pattern"* represents virtually a photographic negative of the "bat's wing" or "butterfly" pattern and is characterized by homogeneous consolidations in the lung periphery running more or less parallel to the lateral chest wall. This pattern is commonly found in acute (Loeffler's syndrome) and chronic eosinophilic pneumonia (Fig. 22.4).

An edema pattern caused by *pulmonary hemorrhage* frequently appears somewhat more dense than usual, although this finding largely depends on the employed radiographic technique. It may be observed with lung contusion, bleeding or clotting disorders, idiopathic pulmonary hemosiderosis, Goodpasture syndrome, systemic lupus erythematosus and chronic renal failure.

Unilateral pulmonary edema (Fig. 22.5 and 22.6) can be divided into ipsilateral and contralateral types. The former refers to conditions in which the pathogenetic mechanism

Table 22.1   Pulmonary Edema and Symmetrical Bilateral Alveolar Infiltrates

Disease	Radiographic Findings	Comments
Bronchioloalveolar carcinoma (alveolar cell carcinoma) (Fig. 22.7)	Alveolar infiltrates combined with reticulonodular and linear densities.	Pleural effusions in approximately 10%. Hilar and mediastinal lymph node enlargement uncommon.
Lymphangitic carcinomatosis (Fig. 22.8)	Interstitial and alveolar infiltrates similar to cardiogenic pulmonary edema, but with severe loss of lung volume and without cardiomegaly. Pleural effusions are commonly associated.	This represents an advanced stage of the disease that is virtually always associated with severe dyspnea.

(continues on page 540)

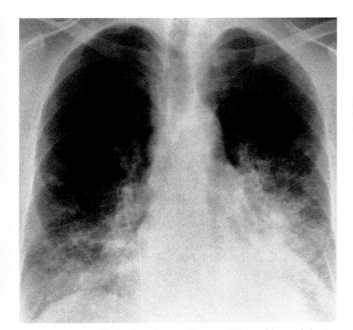

Fig. 22.**7   Bronchioloalveolar carcinoma.** Bilateral lower lobe infiltrates combined with poorly defined nodular densities are seen.

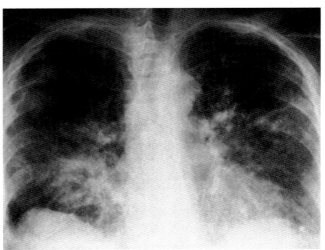

Fig. 22.**8   Lymphangitic carcinomatosis** from breast carcinoma (advanced stage). Mixed interstitial and alveolar pulmonary infiltrates with small pleural effusions are seen appearing similar to cardiogenic pulmonary edema. However, there is no cardiomegaly. Note also the marked loss of lung volume characteristically associated with advanced carcinomatosis.

leading to the asymmetry is on the side of the edema and include prolonged lateral decubitus position in cardiac decompensation, unilateral aspiration, pulmonary contusion, rapid thoracentesis, and unilateral bronchial or pulmonary venous obstruction. Contralateral pulmonary edema refers to accumulation of excess water in the normal lung opposite the diseased lung. The most common cause is chronic obstructive pulmonary disease (COPD), but it is also associated with acute pulmonary thromboembolism, Swyer–James syndrome, and unilateral lung destruction, fibrosis and pleural disease.

The differential diagnosis of pulmonary edema and of symmetrical bilateral alveolar infiltrates is discussed in Table 22.1. Occasionally an extensive diffuse interstitial disease simulates a pulmonary edema pattern when individual lesions, such as nodules, are so numerous that they become confluent and/or superimpose on each other while located in different planes. Therefore, the reader should also refer to Tables 21.1 and 21.2 of the preceding Chapter 21 for a complete differential diagnosis of a pulmonary edema pattern.

Table 22.1   (Cont.) Pulmonary Edema and Symmetrical Bilateral Alveolar Infiltrates

Disease	Radiographic Findings	Comments
Lymphoma and leukemia (Fig. 22.9)	Bilateral interstitial and alveolar infiltrates involving preferentially the perihilar areas and lower-lung fields. Appearance of symmetrical lung involvement may vary from predominantly interstitial edema to homogeneous consolidations.	In a lymphoma or leukemia patient these findings are, however, more often caused by intervening pneumonias, drug reaction, or hemorrhages, rather than by the underlying malignancy itself.
Kaposi's sarcoma (Fig. 22.10)	Numerous poorly defined metastases may mimic extensive bilateral infiltrates (opportunistic infections).	Common in male homosexual AIDS patients.
Pneumonia, bacterial (e.g., staphylococcus, Gram-negative bacteria, anaerobics, and tuberculosis) (Fig. 22.11)	Patchy confluent infiltrates often associated with areas of homogeneous consolidations. Cavitary lesions are relatively common and their demonstration is useful for the differentiation from other conditions presenting with a pulmonary edema pattern.	Bronchogenic spread by inhalation (e.g., staphylococcus), aspiration (e.g., anaerobic bacteria) or communication between abscess or cavity and bronchial system (e.g., tuberculosis).
Pneunomia, fungal (e.g., histoplasmosis, coccidioidomycosis, blastomycosis, aspergillosis, candidiasis)	Bilateral confluent infiltrates similar to aforementioned bacterial pneumonias, but cavitation less common. Hilar lymph node enlargement occurs only rarely, but when present, might be useful for differential diagnosis from nonfungal pneumonias.	This form is virtually limited to compromised hosts. An overwhelming exposure to the fungus rarely may produce this radiographic appearance in histoplasmosis.
Pneumonia, mycoplasma and viral (influenza, parainfluenza, coxsackie, adenovirus, psittacosis, varicella, SARS) (Fig. 22.12)	Diffuse reticular pattern with superimposed patchy alveolar infiltrates. Cavitation does not occur and hilar lymph node enlargement is extremely rare in the adult.	SARS (*severe acute respiratory distress syndrome*) presenting with a pulmonary edema pattern (15%) is associated with the highest mortality rate. *Rickettsial infections* (e.g. Q-fever and Rocky Mountain spotted fever) may occasionally mimic viral pneumonias.
Cytomegalovirus (cytomegalic inclusion disease, CID) (Fig. 22.13)	Diffuse reticulonodular and alveolar infiltrates, preferentially involving the periphery of the middle and lower lobes.	In compromised hosts (e.g., renal transplants).
Pneumocystis carinii (Fig. 22.14)	Diffuse reticulonodular and alveolar infiltrates. Characteristically, the infiltrates are most pronounced in the perihilar areas, sparing the lung periphery.	Common presentation in compromised hosts and in the *acquired immune deficiency syndrome* (AIDS), where it is by far the most frequent complication. Despite certain differences in their characteristic locations, pneumocystis carinii and cytomegalovirus pneumonias can usually not be differentiated radiographically and, furthermore, often occur in the same patient.

(continues on page 542)

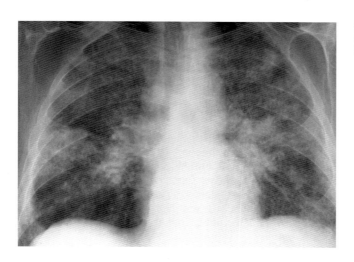

Fig. 22.**9   Non-Hodgkin's lymphoma** (histiocytic). Bilateral interstitial and alveolar infiltrates are seen besides hilar and mediastinal lymph node enlargement.

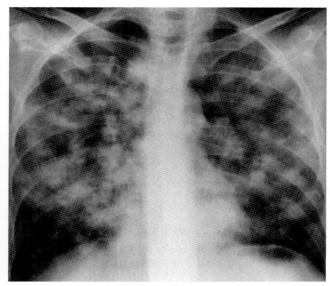

Fig. 22.**10   Kaposi's sarcoma.** Bilateral, poorly defined, confluent nodular densities are seen in this AIDS patient. Open lung biopsy revealed no evidence of an opportunistic infection.

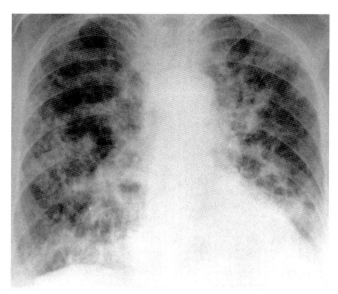

Fig. 22.**11   Pseudomonas pneumonia.** Extensive bilateral patchy infiltrates are seen.

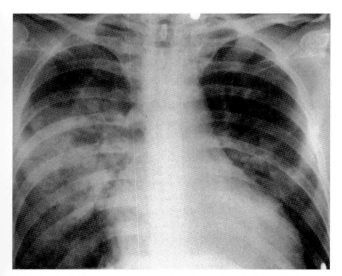

Fig. 22.**12   Influenza pneumonia.** Bilateral well defined airspace consolidations are seen, with considerably more extensive involvement of the right lung.

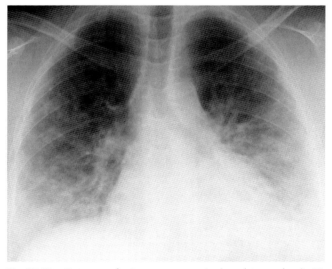

Fig. 22.**13   Cytomegalovirus pneumonia** (renal transplant). Bilateral reticulonodular and alveolar infiltrates, predominantly involving the mid and lower lung fields are evident.

Fig. 22.**14   Pneumocystis carinii pneumonia** (AIDS). Extensive bilateral reticulonodular interstitial disease is associated with early alveolar infiltrates with preferential perihilar and lower lung zone involvement.

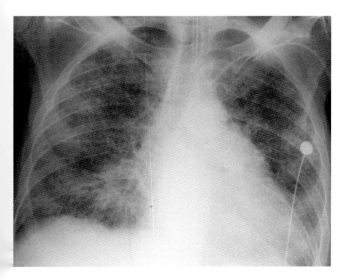

Table 22.1 (Cont.) Pulmonary Edema and Symmetrical Bilateral Alveolar Infiltrates

Disease	Radiographic Findings	Comments
Malaria	Bilateral alveolar infiltrates.	Rare complication with Plasmodium falciparum in high blood concentrations.
Worm infestations (ascaris, strongyloidiasis, filariasis, paragonimiasis)	Bilateral confluent patchy infiltrates often with fine reticulonodular component.	Eosinophilia in peripheral blood invariably present in these conditions.
Oxygen therapy	Prolonged oxygen therapy in high concentration results in bilateral alveolar infiltrates (intra-alveolar hemorrhages) followed by hyaline membrane formation, and alveolar and interstitial fibroblastic proliferation. At this stage the bilateral infiltrates appear nonhomogeneous with "bubbly" appearance.	Similar process occurs in *premature infants* receiving oxygen therapy. A resembling radiographic appearance (diffuse bilateral infiltrates with "bubbly" appearance) may however, also be found in the *Wilson–Mikity syndrome* (pulmonary dysmaturity) of premature infants before oxygen therapy. *Transient tachypnea* of the newborn is caused by retained fetal lung fluid that clears rapidly in 1–4 days.
Noxious gas inhalation (e.g., silo filler's disease [nitrogen dioxide], or inhalation of carbon monoxide, smoke, and organophosphates [insecticides]) (Figs. 22.15 and 22.16)	Bilateral patchy parenchymal densities (transient pulmonary edema) developing within hours after exposure and clearing within a few days if not fatal.	This is the acute phase after exposure. Depending on the inhaled gas, other pulmonary complications such as atelectasis and pneumonic infiltrates can develop within days (e.g., in smoke inhalation) or weeks (e.g., in silofiller's disease, where a "miliary nodulation" pattern can be found).
Extrinsic allergic alveolitis (e.g., farmer's lung)	Bilateral reticulonodular pattern with poorly defined nodules and superimposed patchy, confluent infiltrates.	Develops within a few hours after exposure.
Berylliosis, acute	Diffuse confluent alveolar infiltrates. May be rapidly fatal.	Following overwhelming exposure to beryllium dust.
Aspiration of gastric content (Mendelson's syndrome) (Fig. 22.17)	Bilateral patchy infiltrates to homogeneous consolidations. Pulmonary distribution often asymmetric (depending on position of patient at time of aspiration). Resolves in 7–10 days with proper treatment (steroids and antibiotics).	Found with vomiting related to anesthesia, seizure, coma, alcohol and barbiturate poisoning. *Aspiration of hypertonic contrast agents* may cause pulmonary edema due to influx of fluid into the alveolar space.
Near-drowning (Fig. 22.18)	Symmetrical pulmonary edema that may occasionally be delayed for up to 2 days. Resolution occurs usually in 3–5 days, but may only be complete in 10 days.	There is radiographically no difference between fresh and saltwater aspiration.
Fluid overload/ overtransfusion (hypervolemia, hypoproteinemia)	Bilateral patchy infiltrates. Rapidly clearing with appropriate treatment.	Pulmonary edema also may be the result of an *incompatible blood transfusion*.

(continues on page 544)

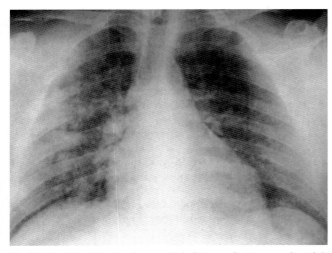

Fig. 22.**15 Silo filler's disease** (inhalation of nitrogen dioxide). Bilateral patchy infiltrates are seen throughout both lungs.

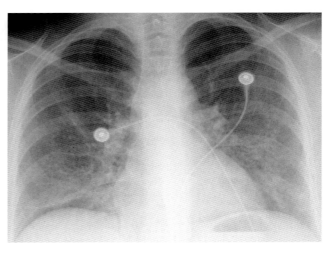

Fig. 22.**16 Smoke inhalation.** Early interstitial and alveolar edema is seen bilaterally in the mid and lower lung zones.

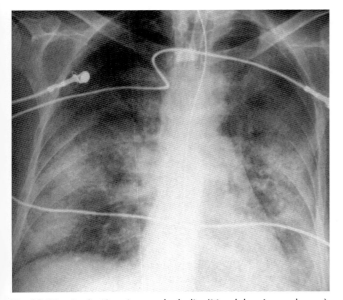

Fig. 22.**17 Aspiration** in an alcoholic (Mendelson's syndrome). Extensive bilateral alveolar infiltrates producing homogeneous consolidations with air bronchograms are seen.

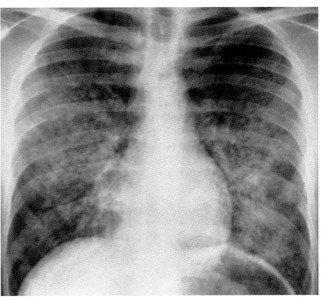

Fig. 22.**18 Near-drowning** in fresh water. Pulmonary edema developed 12 hours after admission. The initial radiograph performed at the time of admission was essentially negative.

Table 22.1 (Cont.) Pulmonary Edema and Symmetrical Bilateral Alveolar Infiltrates

Disease	Radiographic Findings	Comments
Narcotic abuse (Fig. 22.19)	Bilateral patchy densities to massive confluent consolidations. May be delayed up to 10 hours after admission and resolves rapidly within 1 to 2 days.	Most often a complication of heroin or methadone overdose. If the edema pattern persists after 2 days, aspiration or superimposed bacterial pneumonia should be suspected.
Drug-induced pulmonary disease (Fig. 22.20)	Pulmonary manifestations vary from minimal interstitial disease to patchy consolidations and massive pulmonary edema. The time required for both the development and resolution of the pulmonary disease depends on the mechanism involved and is extremely variable, ranging from a few minutes to several months. Resolution may not always be complete.	Pulmonary disease is caused by either drug hypersensitivity or drug toxicity. The following manifestations can be found: spasmodic asthma, noncardiogenic edema, hypersensitivity pneumonitis with or without peripheral eosinophilia, interstitial and alveolar pneumonitis, systemic lupus erythematosus, and pulmonary vasculitis.
Adult respiratory distress syndrome (ARDS) (Fig. 22.21)	Bilateral alveolar pulmonary infiltrates characteristically delayed up to 12 hours after clinical onset of respiratory failure. May progress to extensive bilateral consolidations within 48 hours. Absence of pleural effusions is characteristic. Interstitial emphysema, pneumomediastinum, and pneumothorax can result from positive pressure ventilation. Slow resolution begins after one week, when the infiltrates become inhomogeneous and demonstrate a reticular and cystic component (DD: superimposed pneumonia with microabscesses).	Mechanisms of lung capillary leak resulting in ARDS are not clear. Hypovolemic shock plays an important role, but other factors (e.g., endotoxins, vasoactive agents) must be involved also. ARDS has been associated with sepsis, disseminated intravascular coagulation (DIC), vasoactive substance released from traumatized tissue or blood constituents, prolonged respirator care and cardiopulmonary bypass. *Respiratory distress syndrome (hyaline membrane disease)* in infants is characterized by overinflated lungs with granular appearance, air bronchograms, interstitial pulmonary emphysema, and atelectatic areas.
Disseminated intravascular coagulation (DIC) (Fig. 22.22)	Minimal scattered parenchymal densities to massive pulmonary edema. In the latter case, both pulmonary manifestations and the course of the disease are indistinguishable from the adult respiratory distress syndrome.	Refers to uncontrolled clotting within blood vessels resulting in coagulation failure due to fibrinogen deficiency, thrombocytopenia and excessive fibrinolysis ("consumption coagulopathy"). Always secondary to another disorder such as shock, sepsis, cancer, obstetric complications, burns, and liver disease.

(continues on page 546)

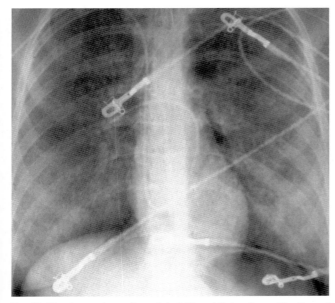

Fig. 22.**19** **Drug abuse (heroin).** Diffuse bilateral opacification of the lungs with confluent alveolar infiltrates is seen.

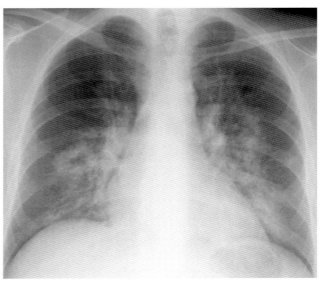

Fig. 22.**20** **Drug-induced pulmonary disease** (methotrexate). Bilateral patchy perihilar infiltrates are seen.

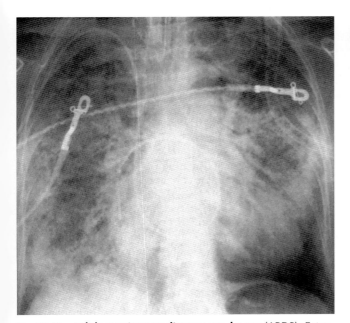

Fig. 22.**21** **Adult respiratory distress syndrome** (ARDS). Extensive bilateral consolidations with air bronchograms and scattered cystic radiolucencies are seen in this patient one week after episode of severe hemorrhagic shock.

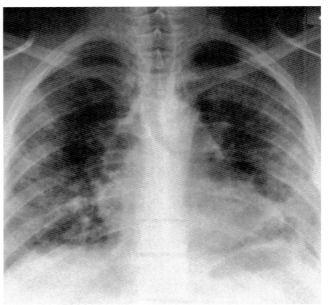

Fig. 22.**22** **Disseminated intravascular coagulation** (DIC). Symmetric bilateral patchy densities are seen in this patient with septic abortion.

Table 22.1   (Cont.) Pulmonary Edema and Symmetrical Bilateral Alveolar Infiltrates

Disease	Radiographic Findings	Comments
Pulmonary contusion (Fig. 22.23)	Parenchymal densities caused by hemorrhages are seldom symmetrical (involvement is greater on the side of maximum impact, that may be evident by rib fractures). In contrast to fat embolism, hemorrhages are invariably apparent within the first 6 hours and resolve rapidly within one week.	Most common complication of blunt chest trauma.
Pulmonary hemorrhage, nontraumatic (e.g., bleeding-diathesis, idiopathic pulmonary hemosiderosis, Goodpasture's syndrome, polyarteritis nodosa, Wegener's granulomatosis) (Fig. 22.24)	Bilateral alveolar infiltrates clearing within 2 to 3 days after single bleeding episode. Reticular changes may, however, persist for several more days in these areas, especially in idiopathic pulmonary hemosiderosis and Goodpasture's syndrome.	Pulmonary hemorrhage in idiopathic pulmonary hemosiderosis, Goodpasture's syndrome, polyarteritis nodosa, and Wegener's granulomatosis is caused by severe damage to the alveolar-capillary membranes secondary to an alteration in the immune system. Hemorrhagic pulmonary edema based on a similar mechanism also can be found in *acute glomerulonephritis*.
Thromboembolic disease (Fig. 22.25)	Bilateral consolidations preferentially in lower lobes. Associated findings include enlarged hilar arteries with abrupt peripheral tapering, pulmonary oligemia (Westermark sign), loss of lung volume (elevated diaphragms), small pleural effusions, and prominent azygos vein.	This is a rare pulmonary manifestation of extensive thromboembolism with infarction. The radiographic findings usually are rather minimal considering the severity of clinical symptoms.
Fat embolism (Fig. 22.26)	Bilateral peripheral alveolar infiltrates that predominantly involve the lower lung fields. Usually only apparent 1–2 days after trauma. Resolution requires 1 week or longer. Absence of cardiomegaly, pulmonary venous hypertension, and interstitial edema differentiates this condition from cardiogenic edema.	Fat embolism after trauma goes unrecognized in the majority of cases because of mild clinical symptoms and minimal radiographic changes. However, the presence of petechial skin rash and cerebral pathology together with the described radiographic lung manifestations is virtually diagnostic. *Oily contrast material embolism* (e.g. after lymphography) progresses only exceptionally to this stage.
Amniotic fluid embolism	Widespread pulmonary consolidations, often rapidly fatal	Predisposing factors include tumultuous labor, intrauterine fetal death, old age of mother, and multiparity. Pathogenesis derives from 3 factors associated with the entrance of amniotic fluid into the maternal circulation: 1 embolic obstruction of pulmonary vasculature by particulate matter in the amniotic fluid, 2 anaphylactoid reaction to particulate matter in the amniotic fluid, and 3 coagulation failure secondary to disseminated intravascular coagulation (DIC).

(continues on page 548)

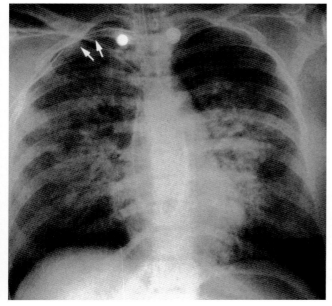

Fig. 22.**23** **Pulmonary contusion.** Bilateral, patchy infiltrates are present. A small right apical pneumothorax is also present (arrows).

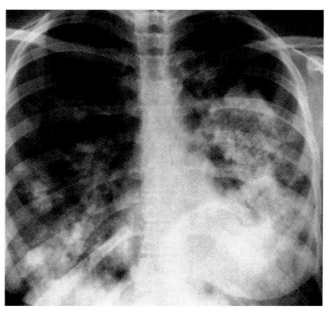

Fig. 22.**24** **Goodpasture's syndrome.** Bilateral, patchy and largely confluent infiltrates are seen in the mid and lower lung fields.

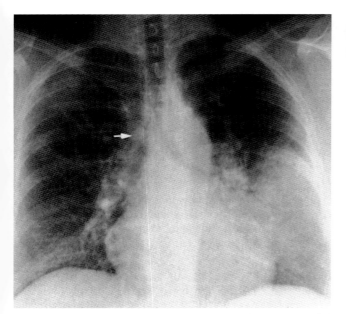

Fig. 22.**25** **Thromboembolic disease.** Bilateral, prominent hili (pulmonary arteries) and perihilar densities are seen. The area of consolidation along the left chest wall proved to be a large infarct. Note also the distended azygos vein (arrow).

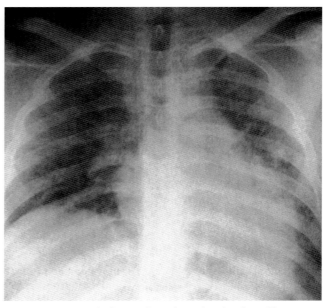

Fig. 22.**26** **Fat embolism.** Bilateral patchy alveolar infiltrates are seen that are confluent in many areas.

Table 22.1   (Cont.) Pulmonary Edema and Symmetrical Bilateral Alveolar Infiltrates

Disease	Radiographic Findings	Comments
Neurogenic disorders (e.g., head trauma, seizures, increased intracranial pressure) (Fig. 22.27)	Edema is frequently asymmetric. Resolution occurs within several days following surgical relief of increased intracranial pressure.	Related to increased intracranial pressure, but mechanism is not clear. May be caused by the combination of increased capillary pressure and abnormal capillary permeability in both lungs.
Cardiovascular disease causing pulmonary venous hypertension (see Figs. 22.1 and 22.2)	Bilateral, symmetrical, interstitial and alveolar densities are the usual presentation. May be preceded by a predominantly interstitial phase with Kerley A and B lines. Pulmonary venous hypertension, evident by redistribution of blood flow from the lower to upper lung fields almost invariably present. Cardiomegaly is usually present if the edema is caused by left heart failure. An asymmetric edema pattern can be found in emphysema, where the edema spares the most severely damaged parts of the lung. A more unilateral distribution is observed in patients lying preferentially on one side.	Most common cause of the pulmonary edema pattern. Cardiogenic causes include left ventricular failure, mitral valve disease, left atrial myxoma, cor triatriatum and hypoplastic left heart syndromes. Noncardiogenic causes include partial occlusion of the pulmonary veins by thrombosis, fibrosis or tumor, and an anomalous pulmonary venous return. Impairment of the lymphatic drainage of the lung interstitium may also contribute to the development of pulmonary edema.
Renal failure/uremia (Fig. 22.28)	Bilateral symmetrical infiltrates similar to cardiogenic pulmonary edema, but may show "butterfly pattern" and can appear quite dense.	The occasionally observed greater radiographic density of the pulmonary edema in renal failure can be explained by the fibrogeneous nature of the edema with hemorrhage, cellular infiltration, and organization ("uremic pneumonia"). Calcification of the underlying lung parenchyma can also contribute to the overall increased density of the edema in chronic renal failure (Fig. 22.29).
Radiation pneumonitis	Infiltrates confined to areas of irradiation.	Lung manifestations usually begin to appear 1–6 months after cessation of treatment.
High altitude	Patchy, irregular pulmonary edema. Rapid clearing after oxygen administration or return to lower altitude.	Symptoms develop between 12 hours to 3 days after arrival at high altitude (3500 m above sea level and higher).
Rapid lung re-expansion	Unilateral, unless both lungs are re-expanded.	Following thoracentesis of a large (50% and more) pneumothorax or hydrothorax that has been present for several days.
Alveolar proteinosis (Fig. 22.30)	Bilateral confluent alveolar infiltrates, often with "butterfly distribution." Very slow and often asymmetric progression or resolution of infiltrates is characteristic. Fatal in approximately one-third of cases.	Predominantly in men between 20 and 50 years of age. Patients susceptible to opportunistic fungal infections, especially nocardiosis.
Alveolar microlithiasis (see Fig. 21.18)	Superimposition and summation of discrete and extremely sharply defined microliths measuring less than 1 mm diameter produce symmetrical bilateral opacification that is usually most pronounced in the lower lung fields.	Rare disorder of obscure etiology with familial occurrence in over 50%. Usually found in patients under the age of 50, but may already be observed in infants.
Sarcoidosis	A predominantly alveolar pattern is extremely rare, more often it is mixed with a reticulonodular component.	Hilar and mediastinal lymph node enlargement is often present.

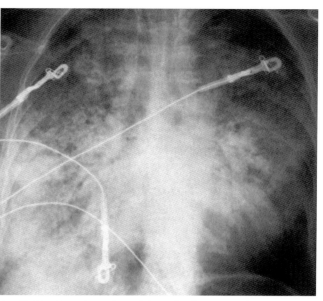

Fig. 22.**27** **Neurogenic pulmonary edema.** Extensive bilateral opacification of both lungs, that is denser on the left than right side, is caused by alveolar pulmonary edema. Note also that the tip of the endotracheal tube has been placed erroneously in the left main bronchus.

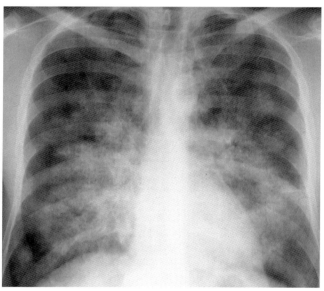

Fig. 22.**28** **Uremia.** A dense bilateral pulmonary edema pattern is seen.

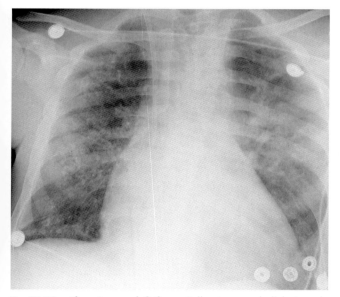

Fig. 22.**29** **Chronic renal failure.** Following renal dialysis only mild pulmonary edema in the left perihilar area is present. The sharply demarcated punctate and reticular opacities in the right lung sparing its periphery are caused by extensive parenchymal calcifications.

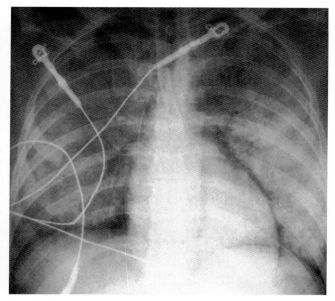

Fig. 22.**30** **Alveolar proteinosis.** Bilateral patchy and confluent alveolar infiltrates sparing the lung periphery ("butterfly pattern") are seen. Characteristic is a slow progression and resolution of the infiltrates over months.

23 Pulmonary Nodules and Mass Lesions

A variety of lesions located outside the lung parenchyma can simulate pulmonary nodules and mass lesions. Extrapulmonary lesions projecting into the lung fields and simulating intrapulmonary conditions are either surrounded by air (e.g., skin lesions) or have a density that is significantly greater than that of the surrounding soft tissue. The latter is the case, for example, in calcified and ossified lesions.

Nipple shadows frequently simulate pulmonary coin lesions on the frontal chest radiograph but can be differentiated from them easily by repeating the chest radiograph with arms elevated over the head. With the latter technique, it is possible to separate a nipple shadow that by chance was superimposed on a true intrapulmonary nodule. Similarly, skin tumors (e.g., *neurofibromas*) must be differentiated from intrapulmonary mass lesions (Fig. 23.1 and 23.2). When skin tumors are multiple, some of them are likely to project outside the lung fields, thus facilitating the correct diagnosis. Focal rib lesions can be diagnosed by confirming with oblique views that the lesion cannot be seen separately from the bone in different projections. Cloth and film artifacts must also be excluded.

Pleural and extrapleural mass lesions protruding into the lung can be difficult to differentiate from a pulmonary lesion abutting the visceral pleura. When the lesions are seen tangentially, both pleural and extrapleural lesions are said to form an obtuse angle with the chest wall.

However, pulmonary mass lesions abutting the pleural surface (e.g., "Hampton's hump" in pulmonary infarction)

may also form an obtuse angle. Furthermore, larger pleural and extrapleural lesions often resemble the shape of a female breast when viewed in profile. In these cases an obtuse angle with the chest wall is found only on the upper margin of the lesion, whereas it becomes acute on its lower end. Pleural and extrapleural lesions, therefore, can be more reliably differentiated from pulmonary lesions by demonstrating a triangular soft-tissue density at the side where the lesion blends into the chest wall (Fig. 23.3). This triangular soft-tissue density is caused by gradual separation of the pleura from the chest wall by the mass lesion. Demonstration of this sign requires viewing the lesion in profile. It cannot be seen when a tumor originates from the visceral pleura and grows exclusively into the lung parenchyma. It might be hidden at the inferior margin of the breast-shaped pleural or extrapleural lesion.

Pleural and extrapleural lesions usually have a well-demarcated surface when projected in profile, since they are covered with pleura, whereas pulmonary lesions may have smooth or shaggy margins. Since pleural and extrapleural lesions often have a long, flat appearance, they may only produce a vague and indistinct increase in the lung density when seen en face. Pleural lesions are often lobulated or multiple, whereas extrapleural lesions are often associated with a rib fracture or rib destruction.

Mass lesions and loculated pleural effusions within the interlobar fissures must also be differentiated from parenchymal lung lesions. This is usually possible because of the

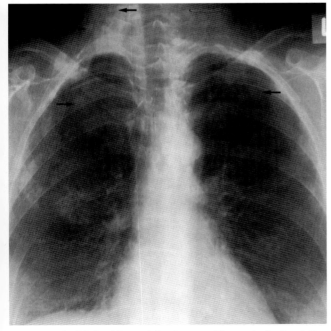

Fig. 23.**1** **Multiple skin nodules** in neurofibromatosis simulating intrapulmonary nodules. Multiple nodular lesions (arrows) are seen. Some of them are projecting into the lung fields, while others are clearly outside the lungs.

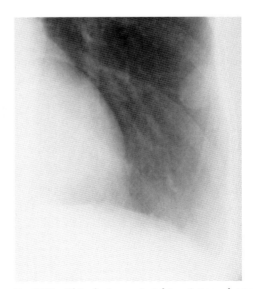

Fig. 23.**2** **Skin lesion mimicking intrapulmonary nodule.** An ovoid density projects into the left lower lung field.

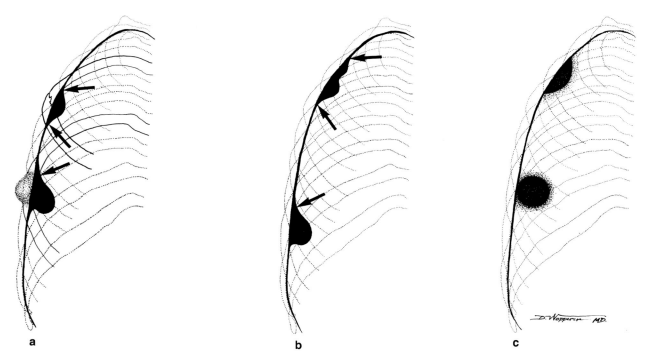

a   b   c

Fig. 23.3 Differential diagnosis of extrapleural, pleural, and pulmonary lesions, when seen in profile. **a** Extrapleural lesions are often associated with rib lesions (fracture or destruction) and lift up the parietal and visceral pleurae from the chest wall, which is evident as a triangular density at the upper and lower margin of the lesion (arrows). **b** Pleural lesions are often lobulated and also demonstrate the "pleural lift-up sign" at their margins (arrows), unless they originate from the visceral pleura and grow primarily into the lung parenchyma, **c** Pulmonary lesions abutting the pleural surface do not separate the pleura from the chest wall and may be well or poorly demarcated. An acute angle between a lesion and the chest wall at both its superior and inferior margins is also characteristic of a pulmonary mass. See text for more detailed discussion.

characteristic anatomic location, oblong shape, and well-defined margins of such pleural lesions. When viewed tangentially their ends blend imperceptibly with the corresponding interlobar fissure.

The *margins of true pulmonary nodules* may be smooth, lobulated or spiculated. In general, smooth margins suggest benignity and spiculation malignancy, whereas lobulation is found with approximately equal frequency in benign and malignant lesions. *Satellite lesions* are defined as small nodu-

lar opacities in close proximity to a larger, usually solitary lesion. They usually indicate an infectious etiology such as a tuberculoma.

The differential diagnosis of solitary or multiple pulmonary nodules and masses is summarized in Table 23.1, while the differential diagnosis of disseminated pulmonary nodules measuring less than 1 cm in diameter has already been summarized in Table 21.1 of Chapter 21.

Table 23.1   Pulmonary Nodules and Mass Lesions

Disease	Radiographic Findings	Comments
Bronchogenic cyst (Fig. 23.4)	Solitary, sharply circumscribed, round mass measuring up to several centimeters in diameter, most commonly in the medial third of the lungs with predilection for lower lobes. Cavitation occurs with infection, resulting in communication with the bronchial system. Calcification of cyst wall and cyst content is very rare.	Approximately two-thirds of bronchogenic cysts are pulmonary and the rest mediastinal in origin. Congenital and acquired (e.g., following lung abscess or trauma) cysts are radiographically indistinguishable from each other. Acquired cysts have no site predilection.
Intralobar bronchopulmonary sequestration (Fig. 23.5)	Well-defined, homogeneous mass usually contiguous with the diaphragm and characteristically located in the posterobasal segment of a lower lobe (left to right ratio, 3 : 1), whereas the upper lobes are rarely affected. Air–fluid levels are seen within the lesion when communication with the bronchial system occurs, usually because of infection. Angiographically, large feeding arteries from the thoracic and/or abdominal aorta are characteristic. Drains to pulmonary veins.	Asymptomatic until sequestered tissue becomes infected. This often occurs only in adulthood, when the anomaly is usually first recognized. *Congenital cystic adenomatoid malformation* (type III) may also present as large bulky mass (see Fig. 24.**7**).

(continues on page 554)

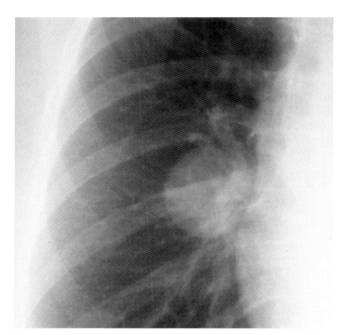

Fig. 23.**4 Bronchogenic cyst.** A solitary, sharply circumscribed round lesion projects into the right hilum.

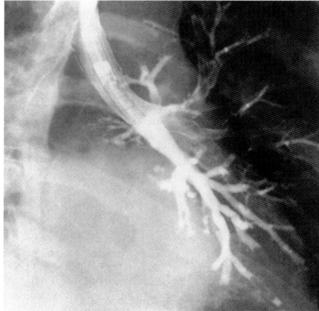

Fig. 23.**5 Intralobar bronchopulmonary sequestration.** A homogeneous mass contiguous to the diaphragm is seen in the left lower lobe displacing the opacified bronchi laterally (bronchography).

Table 23.1   (Cont.) Pulmonary Nodules and Mass Lesions

Disease	Radiographic Findings	Comments
Extralobar bronchopulmonary sequestration (Fig. 23.6)	Well-defined homogeneous mass that is related to the left diaphragm (above or below) in 90 % of patients, and in the remaining cases related to the right diaphragm or the mediastinum. Cavitation is rare, since the lesion is enclosed by its own visceral pleura. Blood supply derives from a systemic artery (usually from the abdominal aorta or one of its branches) and drainage occurs via the inferior vena cava, the azygos or hemiazygos system, or the portal vein.	Frequently associated with other more severe congenital anomalies (e.g. diaphragmatic hernias, eventrations and foregut communications), which may result in death during infancy.
Arteriovenous fistulas (Fig. 23.7)	Solitary or less common, multiple, well-defined round or slightly lobulated lesion(s) measuring up to several centimeters. Change in size and shape with Vasalva and Mueller maneuvers. Predilection for medial third of lungs and lower lobes. Feeding artery and/or draining vein can often be identified as band-like density extending from hilum to lesion. Calcifications (phleboliths) are rarely seen.	Approximately half of the cases are associated with *hereditary hemorrhagic telangiectasia (Rendu-Osler-Weber disease)* with arteriovenous fistulas in the skin, mucous membranes, and other organs. A *pulmonary artery branch aneurysm* (Fig. 23.**8**) can also present as a central pulmonary nodular lesion.
Pulmonary vein varicosity	One to several round, well-defined densities measuring up to a few centimeters in diameter. Characteristic central location, best seen on lateral radiograph projecting posterior and inferior to the hilar structures. Change shape and size with Valsalva and Mueller maneuvers (similar to arteriovenous fistulas).	Congenital or acquired tortuosity and dilatation of a pulmonary vein just before its entrance into the left atrium.
Bronchial adenoma (Fig. 23.9 and 23.10)	Twenty percent present as solitary, well-circumscribed and often slightly lobulated peripheral lung lesions measuring usually 1 to 3 cm (occasionally up to 10 cm) in diameter. Calcifications/ossifications are rarely visible on chest radiographs, but may be identified on CT in about 30 % of cases. Eighty percent are centrally located in the bronchial lumen presenting with segmental or lobar atelectasis and obstructive pneumonia. Cavitation is extremely rare. Hilar, mediastinal and bony metastases (lytic and/or blastic) are occasionally associated.	Locally invasive, low-grade malignant tumors with tendency for recurrence and occasional metastases to extrathoracic sites. Four types: carcinoid (90 %), cylindroma (6 %), mucoepidermoid carcinoma (3 %) and pleomorphic adenoma (1 %). Age ranges from 12 to 60 years (mean age 35 to 45 years) without sex predilection, but very rare in blacks. Clinical manifestations include hemoptysis (50 %), atypical asthma, persistent cough and recurrent obstructive pneumonia.

(continues on page 556)

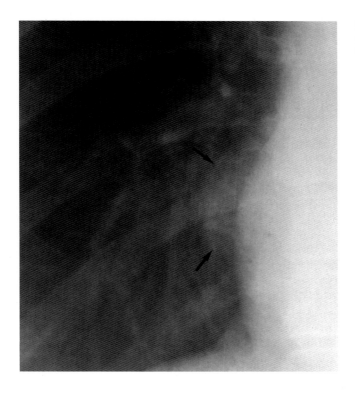

Fig. 23.6   Extralobar bronchopulmonary sequestration. A well-defined mass (arrows) is seen abutting the right border of the mediastinum posterior to the heart.

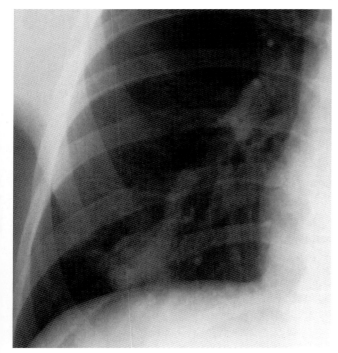

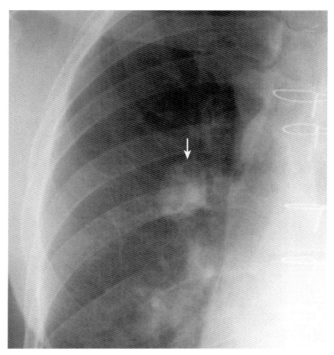

Fig. 23.7 Arteriovenous fistula. A slightly lobulated mass that is connected with the hilum by a bandlike density (feeding artery) is seen in the right lower lobe.

Fig. 23.8 Aneurysm of the right upper lobe artery in Behçet's syndrome. A nodular lesion (arrow) projects above the right hilum.

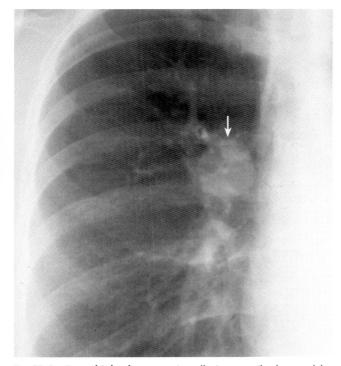

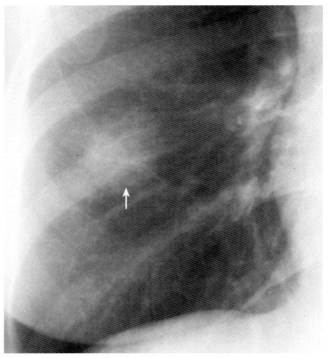

Fig. 23.9 Bronchial adenoma. A well circumscribed, round lesion (arrow) projects into the upper pole of the right hilum.

Fig. 23.10 Bronchial adenoma. A solitary, slightly lobulated lesion (arrow) is seen in the right middle lobe.

Table 23.1 (Cont.) Pulmonary Nodules and Mass Lesions

Disease	Radiographic Findings	Comments
Hamartoma (Fig. 23.11 and 23.12)	Solitary, well-circumscribed, and often lobulated lesion in the lung periphery measuring up to 4 cm in diameter. Calcifications occur in less than 10% of cases and are virtually diagnostic when they resemble popcorn (multiple punctate calcifications throughout the lesion). Rarely, radiolucent areas (fat) can be seen within the lesion.	Peak incidence in the sixth decade (similar to bronchogenic carcinoma) with only 6% occurring in patients under 30. *"Multiple pulmonary fibroleiomyomatous hamartomas"* can be considered a related condition that is extremely rare.
Papilloma	Solitary, or more commonly multiple, well-defined nodules that frequently cavitate. When they are centrally located in the bronchial lumen, they may present as segmental atelectatis and obstructive pneumonitis.	Most common laryngeal tumor in children, but rare in adults. Bronchopulmonary papillomas develop only rarely in the absence of laryngeal or tracheal lesions.
Mesenchymal tumors (e.g., leiomyoma, lipoma, hemangioma, teratoma, chemodectoma, and neurogenic tumors)	Rare, usually solitary, well-defined lesions.	Except for hemoptysis in hemangiomas, these lesions are in the majority of cases asymptomatic. Malignant counterparts of these mesenchymal tumors may very rarely also originate in the lung, but represent usually hematogenous metastases from a sarcoma located in another organ.
Bronchioloalveolar carcinoma (alveolar cell carcinoma) (Fig. 23.13)	Local form (75%). Well-circumscribed focal mass in peripheral/subpleural location, often associated with linear strands ("rabbit ears" or "tail sign") extending from the lesion to the pleura (desmoplastic reaction). Larger lesions (> 4 cm) may become ill-defined with spiculated margins ("sunburst" appearance). Tumor may surround aerated bronchus ("open bronchus sign"). The earliest stage may present with ground-glass haziness and bubble-like hyperlucencies (pseudocavitation) caused by dilatation of intact airspace from desmoplastic reaction. Diffuse form (25%) presents as airspace consolidation with air bronchograms and poorly marginated borders or multiple bilateral poorly or well-defined nodules. Pleural effusions are associated in 10% of cases.	Considered to be a variant of bronchogenic adenocarcinoma with mucinous (80%) and nonmucinous (20%) subtypes. Occurs in patients between 40 and 70 years of age without sex predilection. May be asymptomatic or presenting with cough (50%), shortness of breath (15%), weight loss (12%), hemoptysis (10%) and/or fever (8%). Risk factors include smoking, pulmonary fibrosis (e.g. scleroderma) and localized scarring (e.g. secondary to tuberculosis or infarction). Localized form tends to be slowly progressive with 70% surgical cure rate of tumors < 3 cm. Tumor spread occurs most frequently by tracheobronchial dissemination of detached cells to the ipsilateral or contralateral lung.

(continues on page 558)

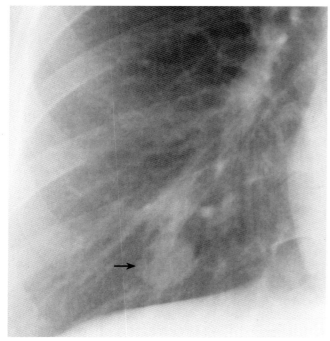

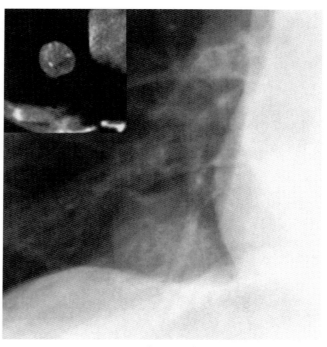

Fig. 23.**11** **Hamartoma.** A round lesion (arrow) containing several small radiolucent foci (fat) is seen in the right lower lobe.

Fig. 23.**12** **Hamartoma.** A solitary nodule in the right lower lobe projects into the right cardiophrenic angle. Insert: popcorn calcifications are seen within the lesion with computed tomography.

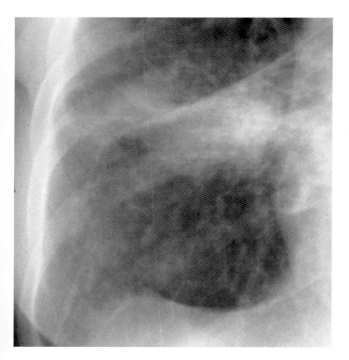

Fig. 23.**13** **Bronchioloalveolar carcinoma.** A poorly-defined mass with a few linear strands extending from the lesion toward the pleura is seen in the right middle lobe. Reticulonodular densities in the lower-lung field suggest spreading of the disease beyond the primary lesion.

Table 23.1   (Cont.) Pulmonary Nodules and Mass Lesions

Disease	Radiographic Findings	Comments
Bronchogenic carcinoma (Figs. 23.14, 23.15, and 23.16)	Relatively poorly-defined nodule or mass with slight upper lobe predilection is a common presentation. Adenocarcinomas and large cell carcinomas tend to be located in the lung periphery, whereas squamous cell carcinomas and small cell carcinomas are typically located centrally. Central lesions commonly present with segmental or lobar atelectasis and obstructive pneumonitis. The "Golden S sign" is found when a central convex tumor bulge on the interlobar fissure is associated with atelectasis producing a concave deformity of the distal interlobar fissure. Cavitation occurs in 20% of squamous cell carcinomas and 6% of large cell carcinomas. The presence of one or a few eccentric tumor calcifications is rare and may be caused by either a tumor engulfing a calcified granuloma, dystrophic calcifications in tumor necrosis, or calcified mucus in adenocarcinomas. The demonstration of diffuse, laminated, or central calcifications virtually rules out a bronchogenic carcinoma. Air bronchograms are typically also absent except in bronchioloalveolar carcinomas that are dealt with separately in this table. Ipsilateral hilar and mediastinal tumor involvement is common and may even be the only initial presentation of small cell carcinomas. Pleural effusions (15%) and chest wall involvement (10%) including erosions in the adjacent ribs and spine may also be evident. Distant bony metastases tend to be predominantly osteolytic, but occasionally are osteoblastic in adenocarcinomas and small cell carcinomas.	Most common cause of cancer-related death in men and women. Histologically 4 types are differentiated: 1. Adenocarcinomas (50%); 2. Squamous cell carcinomas (30%); 3. Undifferentiated small cell carcinomas (15%); 4. Undifferentiated large cell carcinomas (5%). Clinically son-small cell carcinomas are frequently differentiated from small cell carcinomas. Presents in patients ranging in age from 40 to 80 years (mean 55 to 60 years) with a male/female ratio of 1.5:1. May be asymptomatic (especially with peripheral tumors) or present with cough (75%), hemoptysis (50%), pneumonitis (40%) and/or pleurisy (10%). Initial symptoms may also be related to distant metastases (e.g. CNS, bone, liver, or adrenals) or paraneoplastic syndromes. Approximately 85% of all tumors are attributable to cigarette smoking. Other risk factors include exposure to second hand smoke, radon gas, asbestos, and arsenic, previous radiotherapy, pulmonary fibrosis and scars related to infarcts and tuberculosis. *Pancoast (superior sulcus) tumors (5%)* arise in the apex of the lung, present as unilateral apical mass or pleural cap that is commonly associated with soft tissue invasion and bone destruction. Symptoms include pain and weakness of the ipsilateral shoulder and arm, swelling of the arm and Horner syndrome (exopthalmos, ptosis, myosis, and anhidrosis).
Metastases (Fig. 23.17)	Solitary or multiple, usually well-circumscribed lesions ranging from a few millimeters to several centimeters in diameter with some lower lobe predilection. Cavitation occurs in 4%, whereas calcification is virtually limited to metastases from osteosarcomas, other bone-forming sarcomas, and mucinous adenocarcinomas.	Hematogenous metastases are multiple in 75%. Contrary to the lymphatic tumor spread in the lung, hematogeneous metastases seldom cause clinical symptoms. Metastases with an unknown primary tumor commonly originate from breast, kidney, or thyroid carcinomas. Nodules from *Kaposi's sarcoma* in AIDS patients are usually poorly defined (Fig. 23.**18**).

(continues on page 560)

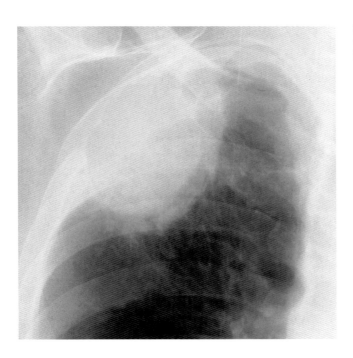

Fig. 23.**14** **Bronchogenic carcinoma.** A large peripheral mass with invasion of the adjacent chest wall and partial destruction of the right third and fourth rib is seen.

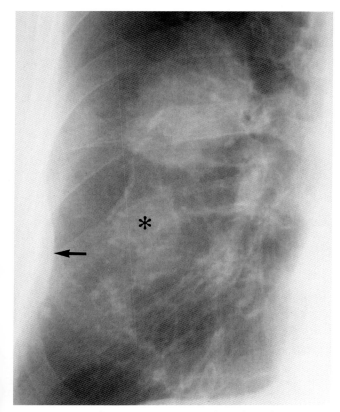

Fig. 23.**15** **Bronchogenic carcinoma.** A large bronchogenic carcinoma has developed adjacent to the right hilum in this patient with asbestosis evident from interstitial thickening in the paracardiac area, emphysematous changes, pleural plaques (arrow) and posterior pleural calcifications seen face on (asterisk).

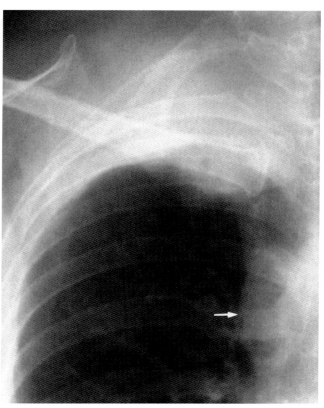

Fig. 23.**16** **Bronchogenic carcinoma** (Pancoast tumor). A right apical mass with destruction of the right second rib posteriorly and right paratracheal lymph node metastases (arrow) is seen.

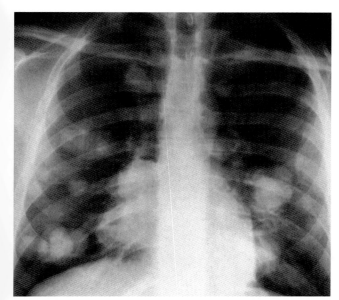

Fig. 23.**17** **Hematogenous metastases** from renal cell carcinoma. Multiple, well-circumscribed nodules of different sizes with slight lower lobe predilection are seen bilaterally.

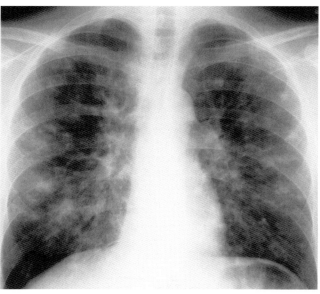

Fig. 23.**18** **Kaposi's sarcoma.** Multiple poorly defined nodular opacities are scattered throughout both lungs of this male homosexual with AIDS.

Table 23.1   (Cont.) Pulmonary Nodules and Mass Lesions

Disease	Radiographic Findings	Comments
Lymphoma (Fig. 23.19)	Single or, more commonly, multiple nodular lesions with well-circumscribed or shaggy borders. Air bronchograms can often be found, since bronchial obstruction is very rare. In the majority of cases hilar and/or mediastinal lymphoma manifestations are associated. Cavitation is rare.	A manifestation of primary and secondary non-Hodgkin's lymphoma. Secondary Hodgkin's disease presents more commonly as a large mass than as multiple pulmonary nodules.
Multiple myeloma (plasmacytoma)	Solitary or multiple pulmonary masses of varying sizes.	An extrapleural mass originating from a destructive rib lesion and protruding into the lung parenchyma is a more common manifestation.
Post-transplantation lymphoproliferative disorder (PTLD)	Solitary, or more commonly, multiple, well circumscribed nodules measuring up to 5 cm in diameter and randomly distributed throughout the lungs. Patchy, predominantly peribronchial air space disease is occasionally associated. Mediastinal and hilar lymph node is present in over 50% of cases.	Lymphocyte proliferation developing 1 month to 1 year after bone marrow or solid-organ transplant. Ranges histologically from benign hyperplastic proliferation to frank malignant lymphoma. Related to Epstein–Barr virus-infected B-cells.
Amyloidosis (nodular form)	Single or, more often, multiple nodules up to several centimeters in diameter. Cavitation and calcification occur.	Nodular, parenchymal form seldom causing clinical symptoms Prognosis is better than both the tracheobronchial (obstructive) and diffuse interstitial forms.
Abscess and septic emboli (Figs. 23.20 and 23.21)	Solitary or multiple round lesions ranging from 1 cm to several cm in diameter. Predilection for lower lobes and posterior segments of upper lobes. Cavitation is very common. An airborne abscess often presents originally as a poorly-defined lesion that becomes progressively better demarcated with time, whereas septic emboli present initially as well-circumscribed lesions that become more fuzzy with healing.	Staphylococcus is the most common organism. A single abscess is usually present with inhalation or aspiration of the organism, whereas multiple abscesses suggest pyemia with septic emboli. Common sources for the latter are endocarditis and septic thrombophlebitis (e.g., in drug abusers, patients with indwelling catheters or arteriovenous shunts for hemodialysis, and with pharyngeal or pelvic infections).
Tuberculoma	Usually solitary and well-circumscribed lesion ranging usually from 0.5 to 4 cm in diameter. Calcifications and "satellite" lesions (small densities in immediate vicinity) are found frequently. Cavitation is extremely uncommon. Hilar lymph node calcification and scarring are often present.	Tuberculomas are late manifestations of either primary or postprimary tuberculosis. Predilection for upper lobes and posterior segments. In *atypical mycobacterial infection* multiple bilateral small nodules measuring under 1 cm are common, but occasionally larger nodules are seen (Fig. 23.**22**).
Histoplasmoma (Fig. 23.23)	One or several well-circumscribed, round lesion(s) up to 3 cm in diameter. Predilection for lower lobes, calcification common and often in the center ("target" appearance). "Satellite" lesions may be present. Cavitation is rare.	Hilar lymph node calcifications are commonly associated.

(continues on page 562)

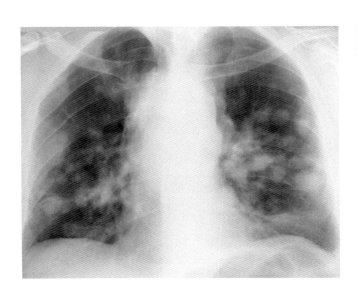

Fig. 23.**19 Non-Hodgkin's lymphoma.** Multiple, relatively poorly-defined nodules are seen bilaterally. Note also the hilar and, particularly, mediastinal lymphadenopathy.

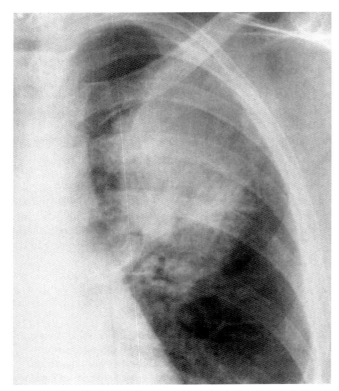

Fig. 23.**20 Pulmonary abscess.** A poorly-defined mass lesion is seen in the left upper lobe.

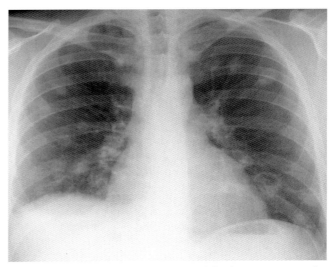

Fig. 23.**21 Septic emboll.** Multiple nodular lesions are seen bilaterally, some of which have cavitated and contain air–fluid levels.

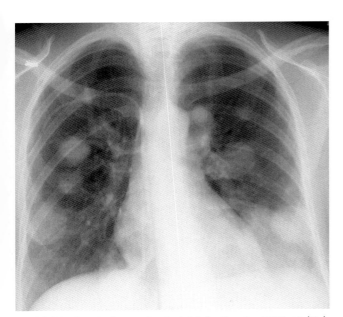

Fig. 23.**22 Atypical mycobacterial infection in AIDS.** Multiple, bilateral, well circumscribed, large nodules of varying sizes are seen. This is an unusual presentation of the disease.

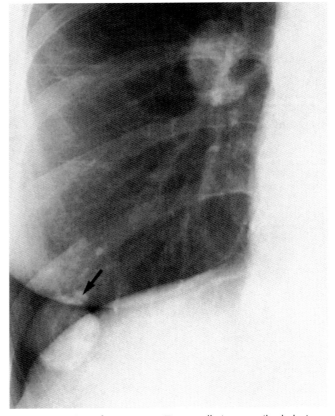

Fig. 23.**23 Histoplasmomas.** Two well-circumscribed lesions, one projecting into the right hilum and the other into the right costophrenic angle, are seen. Note also the small satellite lesion (arrow) at the periphery of the right lower lobe lesion.

Table 23.1   (Cont.) Pulmonary Nodules and Mass Lesions

Disease	Radiographic Findings	Comments
Coccidioidomycosis **(Fig. 23.24)**	Solitary or multiple, well-circumscribed nodules up to 3 cm in diameter. Upper lobe predilection. Cavitation is relatively common, calcifications rather rare.	Even patients with cavitary disease are often asymptomatic.
Actinomycosis **Nocardiosis** **Blastomycosis** **Cryptococcosis** **(Figs. 23.25 and 23.26)**	Usually single, large mass lesion measuring up to 10 cm in diameter. Except for blastomycosis, cavitation is relatively common and the lower lobes are preferentially involved. Disease may extend through the pleura into the chest wall and involve the ribs.	In cryptococcosis, the lesion is characteristically pleural-based, but an effusion is uncommon. Empyema is a common complication of actinomycosis and nocardiosis only.
Echinococcal disease **(Fig. 23.27)**	Usually solitary, sharply circumscribed, spherical or oval mass preferentially in a lower lobe (slightly more common on the right), and ranging up to 10 cm in diameter. Large lesions may have bizarre, polycystic, lobulated outlines. Calcification virtually never occurs in lung lesions.	Cyst wall is composed of 3 layers: pericystic (fibrous reaction formed by host), exocystic (chitinous outer cyst membrane), and endocystic (thin inner lining of syncytial cells). Air entering between the pericystic and exocystic layers produces a crescent-shaped, peripheral radiolucency: the "double arch" sign, found in 5%. After rupturing into a bronchus, an air–fluid level is found with the endocyst floating on the surface, producing the "water lily" sign or "camelot sign."
Hypersensitivity aspergillosis with mucoid impaction **(Fig. 23.28)**	Solitary or, less common, multiple, round, oval or elliptical opacities caused by plugs in dilated, usually second-order bronchi. Upper lobes are preferentially involved. Opacifications may also have a "Y" or "V" configuration when a bronchial bifurcation is plugged.	Hypersensitivity aspergillosis is usually associated with asthma or pre-existing chronic bronchial disease. Other forms of secondary aspergillosis include aspergillomas in cavitary lesions and single or multiple, occasionally cavitary consolidations in patients with chronic debilitating diseases. Primary aspergillosis is exceedingly rare and presents as homogeneous consolidation that may progress to abscess formation. *Bronchocentric granulomatosis (Liebow)* may be considered a variant of hypersensitivity aspergillosis and appears both clinically and radiographically in a similar fashion (Fig. 23.**29**).

(continues on page 564)

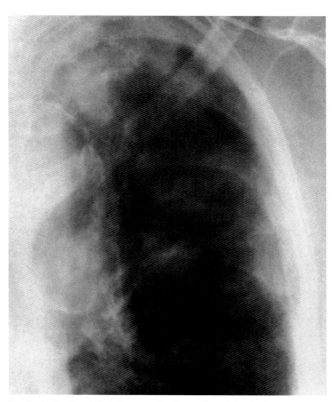

Fig. 23.**24   Coccidioidomycosis.** Several nodular lesions are seen in the left upper lobe in this patient with preexisting, unrelated chronic pulmonary and pleural changes.

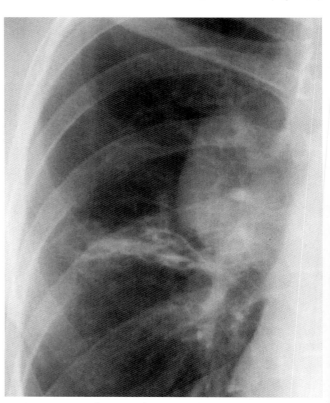

Fig. 23.**25   Nocardiosis.** A large ovoid mass projects into the upper pole of the right hilum in this patient with AIDS. Interstitial infiltrates caused by atypical mycobacterial infection are also evident.

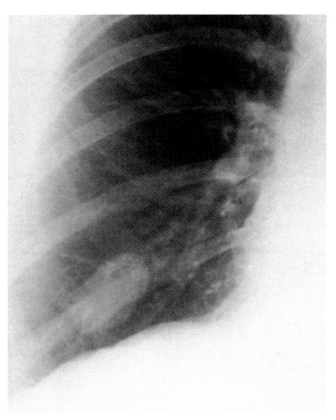

Fig. 23.**26** **Cryptococcosis.** A large, well-defined mass is seen in the left lower lobe in this patient with AIDS. There is also mild left hilar adenopathy, which is unusual for this disease.

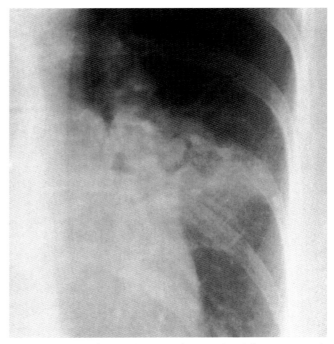

Fig. 23.**27** **Echinococcus.** A solitary, oval-shaped and slightly lobulated lesion is seen in the right lower lobe.

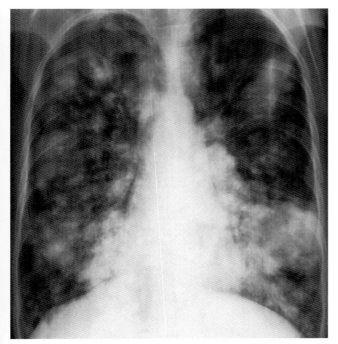

Fig. 23.**28** **Hypersensitivity aspergillosis** complicating cystic fibrosis. Multiple round opacities and areas of consolidations are seen throughout both lungs. This is an unusually extensive involvement by hypersensitivity aspergillosis. More often the disease presents as solitary lesion.

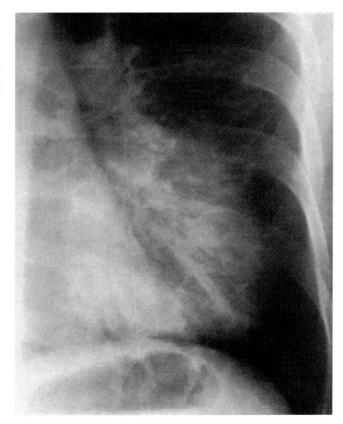

Fig. 23.**29** **Bronchocentric granulomatosis Liebow.** A poorly defined mass lesion silhouetting the left cardiac border is seen in the lingula.

Table 23.1 (Cont.) Pulmonary Nodules and Mass Lesions

Disease	Radiographic Findings	Comments
Congenital bronchial atresia	Well-circumscribed, somewhat elliptical mass, caused by mucus accumulated in a bronchus peripheral to the point of stenosis or atresia. Usually located in an upper lobe, most commonly in the apicoposterior segment of the left side.	This anomaly rarely causes symptoms and usually is discovered in a screening chest radiograph in children or young adults.
Inflammatory pseudo-tumor (Fig. 23.30)	Solitary nodule or homogeneous area of consolidation, ranging up to 7 cm in diameter and often mimicking a primary carcinoma.	May represent the sequela of an unresolved pneumonia, although a history of acute respiratory illness is not always available. An inflammatory pseudotumor should not be confused with a so-called "pseudotumor" of a pleural fissure resulting from loculated fluid accumulation.
Pseudolymphoma	Nodular lesions less common than parenchymal consolidations that characteristically contain air bronchograms. In contrast to pulmonary lymphoma, hilar and mediastinal lymph nodes are never involved.	May represent a modified form of an inflammatory pseudotumor.
Lipoid pneumonia (Fig. 23.31)	Peripheral, usually well-defined mass measuring up to several centimeters in diameter and preferentially being located in the posterior segments. Occasionally, a shaggy outline is found caused by linear shadows (thickened interlobular septa) radiating from the periphery of the lesion.	Caused by chronic aspiration of vegetable, animal, or mineral oils. May mimic peripheral bronchogenic carcinoma.
Pulmonary infarct (Fig. 23.32)	Solitary or multiple homogeneous consolidations abutting the pleural surface. Nodular densities are less common. A "Hampton's hump" (pleural-based semicircular consolidation) is characteristic but rare. Resolution occurs through a gradual decrease in size ("melting ice cube sign").	Other signs of pulmonary thromboembolism are often associated, and include: 1 loss of lung volume with elevation of the ipsilateral diaphragm, 2 oligemia resulting in increasing radiolucency of affected lung areas (Westermark sign), 3 pleural effusions, 4 enlargement of the hilar pulmonary artery and azygos vein and 5 acute cardiac enlargement (cor pulmonale).
Pulmonary hematoma (Fig. 23.33)	Single or multiple, well-circumscribed, round or oval lesions, usually measuring between 2 and 6 cm. Peripheral subpleural location immediately underlying the point of maximum impact is characteristic. Air-fluid level may be present. Lesion may initially be masked by surrounding lung contusion.	Results from bleeding into a parenchymal laceration or a traumatic cyst. Gradual decrease in size over several weeks or months.

(continues on page 566)

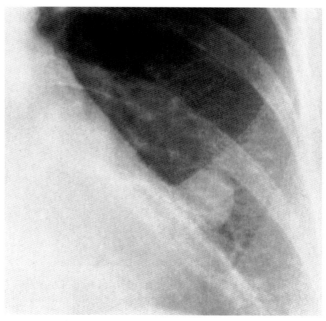

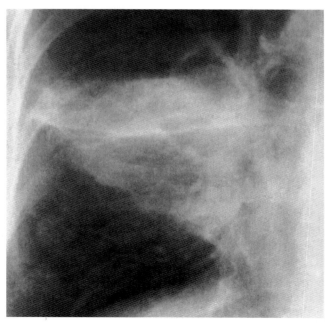

a

Fig. 23.**30 a, b   Inflammatory pseudotumors** (two cases). A solitary nodule in the left lower lobe is seen in **a** and a larger mass lesion involving the right middle lobe is present in **b**. Both cases underwent surgery, since a bronchogenic carcinoma was suspected.

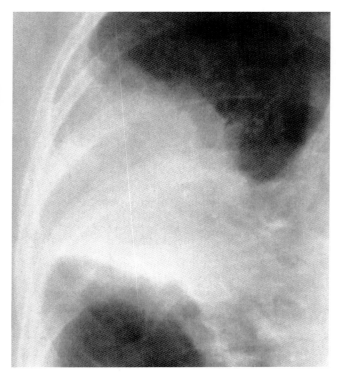

Fig. 23.31 Lipoid pneumonia. A peripheral mass with somewhat shaggy outline is seen.

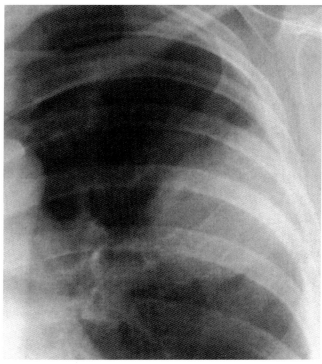

Fig. 23.32 Pulmonary infarct. A solitary, well-defined mass ("Hampton's hump") abutting the diaphragmatic pleura is seen.

Fig. 23.33 Pulmonary hematoma. A mass lesion in the right upper lobe is seen in this patient after he was shot.

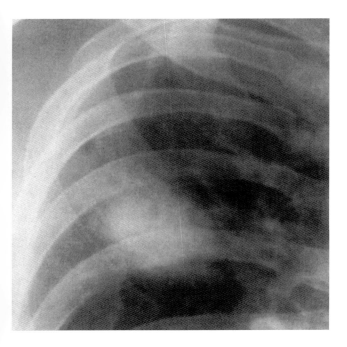

Table 23.1   (Cont.) Pulmonary Nodules and Mass Lesions

Disease	Radiographic Findings	Comments
Progressive massive fibrosis (PMF) (Fig. 23.34)	Large, often bilateral, but usually asymmetric, spindle-shaped, mass lesions in the upper half of the lungs. The lateral border paralleling the rib cage is usually better defined than the medial border. May contain calcifications and cavitate (due to either ischemic necrosis or superimposed tuberculosis). Tend to migrate toward the hila over the years.	PMF is associated with *pneumoconiosis* (especially coal miner's lung and silicosis) although radiographic evidence of the underlying pneumoconiosis may occasionally not be obvious. Similar conglomerate masses of fibrosis may occasionally be found with sarcoidosis where they may contain air bronchograms.
Sarcoidosis (Fig. 23.35)	Multiple, well-circumscribed nodules measuring up to 2 cm and conglomerate masses of fibrosis. Commonly associated with reticulonodular interstitial disease or fibrosis (honeycombing). Hilar and mediastinal lymphadenopathy may also be present.	This is a relatively rare manifestation of sarcoidosis.
Wegener's granulomatosis (Fig. 23.36)	Solitary or, more often, multiple, fairly well-circumscribed nodules ranging from less than 1 cm to 10 cm in diameter. Cavitation is common. Alveolar infiltrates may be associated. Pleural effusion is not unusual. Hilar lymph node enlargement is very rare.	Multiple nodules simulating metastases are the most common pulmonary presentation of Wegener's granulomatosis. In the limited form, lungs are the only affected organ, whereas in the full-blown form of Wegener's granulomatosis, kidneys, nose, and paranasal sinuses are involved also. The radiologic manifestations of the *lymphomatoid variant of Wegener's granulomatosis* in the lung are virtually identical to those of Wegener's granulomatosis, but the paranasal sinuses are characteristically not involved with the former.
Polyarteritis nodosa (Fig. 23.37)	Poorly-defined nodules with patchy consolidations. The fleeting nature of pulmonary manifestations is characteristic.	Renal and gastrointestinal symptoms usually predominant. Poor prognosis. Some cases have histories of drug reactions: *"hypersensitivity angiitis."* *Churg–Strauss syndrome* is a variant of polyarteritis nodosa presenting with allergic asthma, eosinophilia and systemic small vessel vasculitis with granulomatous inflammation.
Rheumatoid necrobiotic nodules (Fig. 23.38)	Solitary or, more commonly, multiple, well-circumscribed peripheral nodules measuring a few millimeters to several centimeters. Lower lobe predilection. Cavitation common.	Necrobiotic nodules are a rare manifestation of rheumatoid lung disease. Nodules may wax and wane in concert with subcutaneous nodules. *Caplan's syndrome:* necrobiotic nodules and rheumatoid arthritis in pneumoconicosis. Calcifications can occur in these nodules.

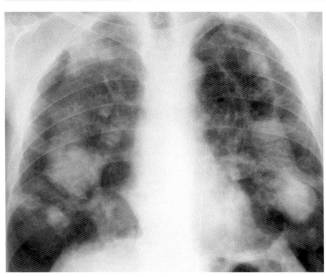

Fig. 23.**34 Progressive massive fibrosis** (PMF) in coal miner's lung. Besides smaller areas of fibrosis, one larger, spindle-shaped opacity is seen in each lung, extending from the mid-lung fields into the upper lobes. The lateral borders of these opacities characteristically are better defined than are the medial borders, Note also that cavitation in the upper half of the left mass has occurred, probably due to ischemic necrosis, but superimposed tuberculosis cannot be ruled out radiographically.

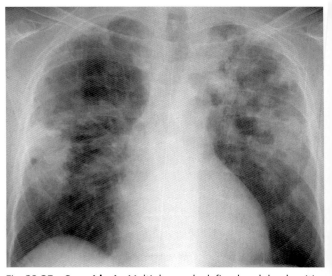

Fig. 23.**35 Sarcoidosis.** Multiple poorly defined nodular densities are seen bilaterally in the mid and upper lung zones associated with interstitial lung disease including honeycombing and mild hilar lymphadenopathy. Beginning formation of conglomerate fibrotic masses in the lung periphery is caused by the coalescence of the nodular lesions.

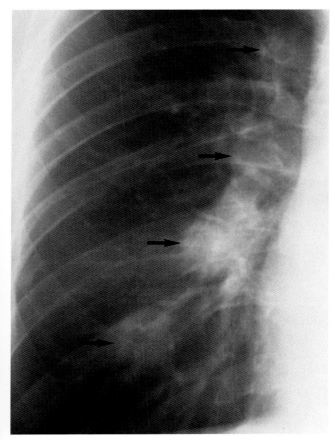

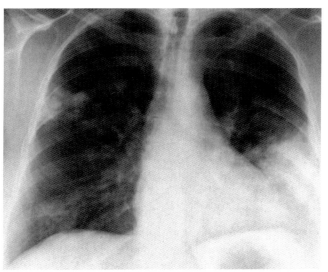

Fig. 23.**36** **Wegener's granulomatosis.** Four fairly well-circumscribed nodules (arrows) are seen in the right lung. Incipient central cavitation is recognizable in the lowest nodule.

Fig. 23.**37** **Polyarteritis nodosa.** Poorly defined nodules with patchy consolidations are seen involving both lungs.

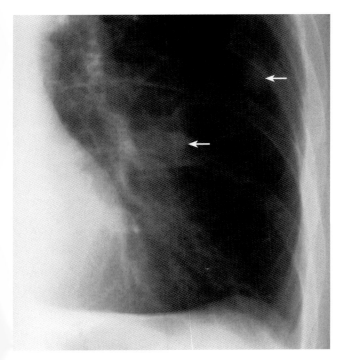

Fig. 23.**38** **Rheumatoid necrobiotic nodules.** Two nodules (arrows) are associated with slightly increased interstitial markings.

24 Pulmonary Cavitary and Cystic Lesions

Pulmonary cavitary and cystic lesions are characterized by their central air content. Cavities usually result from central necrosis within a lesion and the subsequent expulsion of the necrotic material into the bronchial system. Rupture of a fluid-filled cyst or infection of a bulla may produce a similar radiographic appearance. Cavities often contain fluid that appears as an air–fluid level on radiographs performed with horizontal beam. Air–fluid levels occur when a lesion with a liquid content ruptures into the tracheobronchial system and part of its content is expelled, or when both gas and pus are produced by bacteria. A cavitary lesion with an air–fluid level is, however, not pathognomonic of a pulmonary lesion (e.g., a lung abscess), but also can be encountered in the event of a *loculated hydropneumothorax* (e.g., loculated empyema secondary to the bronchopleural fistula). Radiologic differentiation of these two entities is, however, made possible by the fact that a pulmonary cavity tends to be spherical and, consequently, the length of the air–fluid level is very similar on frontal, lateral, and decubitus films. A loculated hydropneumothorax, however, is virtually never spherical, since it must conform in shape to the adjacent chest wall and, consequently, the length of the air–fluid level varies widely between different projections (Fig. 24.1).

Cystic lesions can be mimicked by plastic (radiolucent) spheres inserted in the past into the extrapleural space to collapse the adjacent lung for the treatment of tuberculosis. Since these spheres were often not water-tight, small amounts of fluid could collect in them, mimicking small air-fluid levels on upright films. Nowadays, cystic lesions with or without air–fluid levels can be simulated by both *hiatal* and *diaphragmatic hernias* (congenital or posttraumatic), when they contain the stomach or loops of bowel. Characteristic of these hernias is, however, a considerable change in the size and shape of the lesions between subsequent radiographs.

Cavitary lesions can be differentiated from each other by their size, location, wall thickness, number and by the nature of both their inner lining (smooth or irregular) and content (fluid versus mass).

The cavity wall thickness can be described as hairline (1 mm or less), thin (2 to 4 mm) and thick (5 mm and more) (Fig. 24.2). Hairline cavities are invariably associated with benign conditions such as bullae, blebs and pneumatoceles. The vast majority of thin-walled cavities are also found with a variety of benign lesions including chronic infections such as coccidiodomycosis, whereas thick-walled cavities are equally divided between benign and malignant conditions such as lung abscess, primary and metastatic carcinoma, and Wegener's granulomatosis. However an extremely thick cavity wall exceeding 15 mm is highly suspicious of a malignant neoplasm.

A solitary cavitary lung lesion is frequently found in a pulmonary abscess, a malignant neoplasm or a lung cyst (congenital or posttraumatic). Multiple cavitary lung lesions suggest Wegener's granulomatosis and septic emboli or metastatic disease. The inner lining of a cavity is usually nodular in a bronchogenic carcinoma, shaggy in an acute lung abscess and smooth in most other lesions.

Fluid in the presence of gas can be diagnosed in a cavitary lesion by the demonstration of an air–fluid level on radiographs taken with horizontal beam. The intracavitary fluid

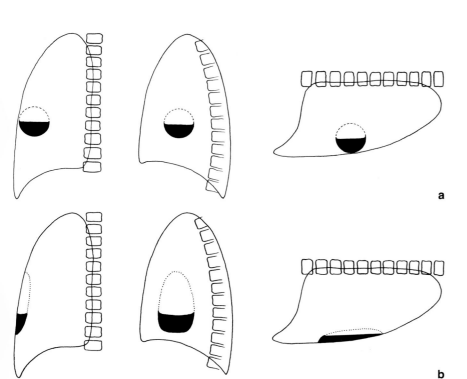

Fig. 24.**1 a, b   Differentiation between air–fluid levels, a** in a peripheral pulmonary cavity and **b** in a loculated hydropneumothorax. **a** A pulmonary cavity tends to be spherical and therefore an air–fluid level in such a lesion has the same length in anteroposterior, lateral, and decubitus films. **b** A loculated hydropneumothorax must conform to the chest wall and is therefore never spherical. The length of the air–fluid level varies considerably between different projections as shown here in the anteroposterior, lateral, and decubitus films.

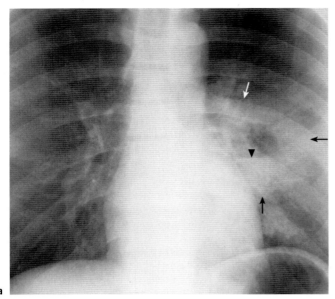

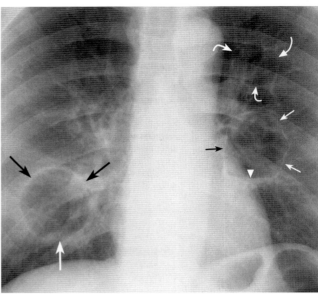

a

Fig. 24.2 Cavitary lesions with variable wall thickness. a A lung abscess (arrows) presenting as poorly defined thick-walled cavitary lesion with air–fluid (pus) level (arrowhead) is seen in the left lower lobe. **b** Four years later a pneumatocele with hairline wall (small ar- rows) and tiny fluid level (arrowhead) has replaced the abscess. A second pneumatocele (curved arrows) is seen more cephalad. A thin-walled cyst (large arrows) representing another healing ab- scess is now seen in the right lower lobe.

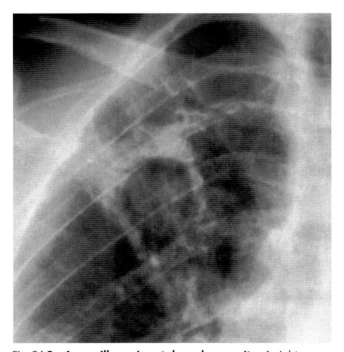

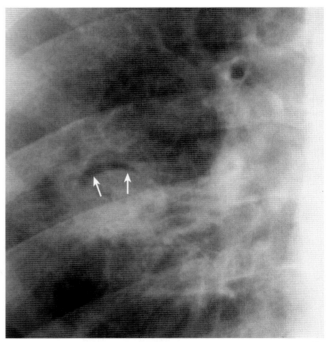

Fig. 24.3 Aspergilloma in a tuberculous cavity. A right upper lobe cavity is seen containing a mass lesion. Note also the pericavi- tary infiltrates indicating still-active tuberculosis.

Fig. 24.4 Aspergilloma in old abscess cavity. The aspergilloma is separated from the wall of the cavity by a crescent-shaped air space (arrows).

may be serous or sanguinous or represent pus or liquefied necrotic tissue. Besides fluid, a mass can also be found within a cavitary lesion. With regard to the size of the cavity, the mass can be quite small or occupy most of the cavitary space. In the latter case, the mass is only separated from the wall of the cav- ity by a crescent-shaped air space. Most commonly, intracavi- tary mass lesions represent *mycetomas*, especially *aspergil- lomas* (Figs. 24.3 and 24.4). They can be found in infectious (particularly tuberculous), tumoral, bronchiectatic, and cys-

tic cavities that do not contain any fluid. Similar intracavitary masses can be produced by necrotic tumor fragments in carci- nomas, sequestered necrotic lung tissue in klebsiella or, rarely, in pneumococcal pneumonias, a blood clot, or by the collapsed membrane of a ruptured echinococcal cyst floating on top of the fluid ("water-lily" or "camelot" sign).

The differential diagnosis of various cavitary and cystic le- sions measuring 1 cm or more in diameter is given in Table 24.1.

Table 24.1   Solitary or Multiple Cavitary and Cystic Pulmonary Lesions

Disease	Radiographic Findings	Comments
Bronchogenic cyst (congenital or traumatic)	Solitary thin-walled lesion with or without air–fluid level.	Congenital cysts are characteristically located in medial third of the lungs with lower lobe predilection.
Intralobar bronchopulmonary sequestration (Fig. 24.5)	Solitary, unilocular, or multilocular cystic mass that may or may not contain air–fluid levels. Cyst walls are thick or thin.	Lesion is usually contiguous with the diaphragm and characteristically located in a posterobasal segment of a lower lobe (left to right ratio 3 : 1). Masking of lesion by surrounding pneumonia is possible.
Congenital cystic adenomatoid malformation (Fig. 24.6 and 24.7)	Multilocular cystic mass with or without air–fluid levels, similar to bronchopulmonary sequestration, but involves at least an entire lobe without predilection. The volume of the affected lung is usually increased or, less commonly, decreased. Three types are differentiated. Type I: Single or multiple large cysts exceeding 20 mm in diameter. DD: *Congenital lobar emphysema* involving LUL (40%), RML (35%), RUL (20%), or two lobes (5%). Type II: Multiple cysts measuring 5 to 12 mm in diameter. Type III: Solitary large bulky mass with 3 to 5 mm small microcysts.	Involves characteristically one lobe, but occasionally two lobes or both lungs are affected. Usually diagnosed in infancy, but may occasionally be diagnosed first in older children or adolescents. May be part of a wider spectrum that includes also bronchogenic cysts and sequestrations. DD: *Diaphragmetic hernia* containing bowel loops (Fig. 24.8) and extensive cystic bronchiectases (Fig. 24.9).

(continues on page 572)

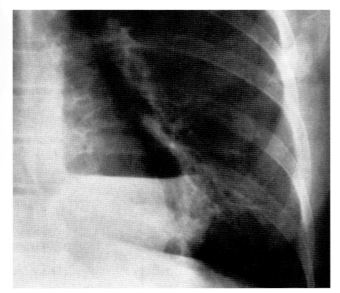

Fig. 24.**5** **Intralobar sequestration.** A cystic mass with a large air–fluid level is seen in the posterobasal segment of the left lower lobe.

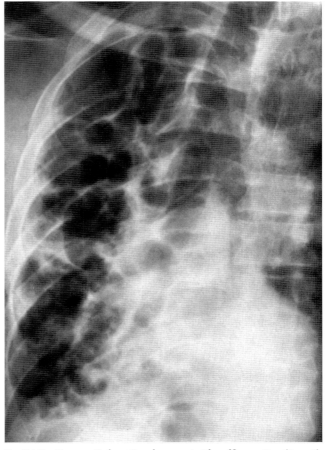

Fig. 24.**6** **Congenital cystic adenomatoid malformation (type I).** A multilocular cystic mass has replaced the right lung. Note also the significant loss of volume that helps to differentiate this condition from a large diaphragmatic hernia containing bowel loops.

Table 24.1 (Cont.) Solitary or Multiple Cavitary and Cystic Pulmonary Lesions

Disease	Radiographic Findings	Comments
Pulmonary papillomatosis	Multiple, well-defined nodules that frequently cavitate and then resemble cystic bronchiectases.	Most common laryngeal tumor in children, but rare in adults. Pulmonary papillomas seldom develop in the absence of laryngeal or tracheal lesions.
Bronchogenic carcinoma (Fig. 24.10)	Solitary, usually thick-walled cavity with irregular inner lining. A smooth, thin-walled cavity is a rare presentation. Necrotic tumor tissue may simulate mycetoma. Air–fluid levels are uncommon.	Cavitation occurs in up to 10% of cases of bronchogenic carcinoma, most commonly in squamous cell carcinomas, especially in the upper lobes, and undifferentiated large cell carcinomas, rarely in adenocarcinomas, and never in small cell carcinomas
Metastases, hematogenous (Fig. 24.11)	Multiple nodules of different sizes with thin or thick-walled cavities developing in a varying percentages of lesions (few to almost all).	Cavitation less common than in bronchogenic carcinoma. Metastases frequently originate from squamous cell carcinoma of the head and neck (thin-walled cavities), or gynecologic tumors and sarcomas (thick-walled cavities).
Lymphoma (Fig. 24.12)	One or more consolidations with usually thick-walled cavities that have an irregular inner lining and may contain an air–fluid level.	A manifestation of primary and secondary non-Hodgkin's lymphoma and secondary Hodgkin's disease. In secondary pulmonary involvement the disease is associated with simultaneous or past presentations in other organs (e.g., peripheral and mediastinal lymph nodes).

(continues on page 574)

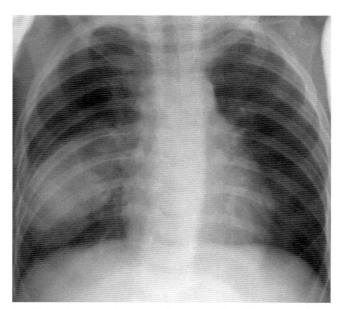

Fig. 24.**7 Congenital cystic adenomatoid malformation (type III).** A large bulky mass occupies the right middle lobe. The microcysts within the lesion cannot be appreciated.

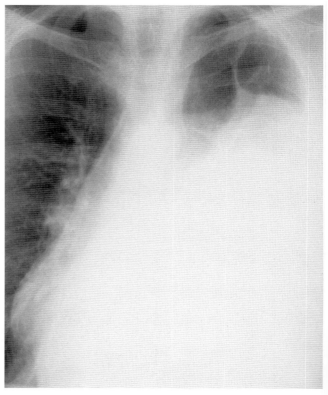

Fig. 24.**8 Diaphragmatic hernia.** The hernia occupies most of the left hemithorax with air filled bowel loops seen in its apex. Note also the shift of the heart toward the contralateral side caused by the mass effect of the hernia.

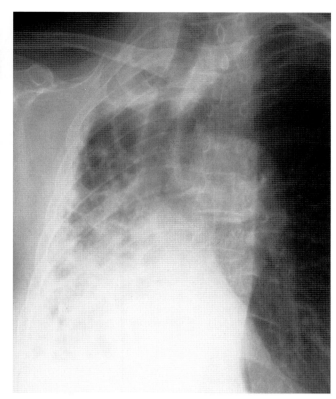

Fig. 24.**9** **Cystic bronchiectasis in chronic tuberculosis.** Multiple cystic lesions with marked loss of volume are seen in the shrunken fibrotic right lung resulting in shift of heart and mediastinum towards the ipsilateral side.

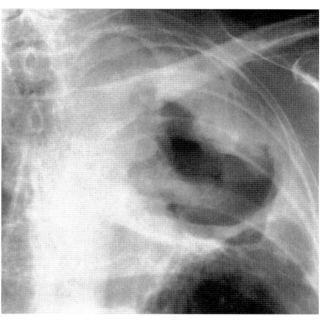

Fig. 24.**10** **Bronchogenic carcinoma** (squamous cell type). A left upper lobe mass containing a large cavity with irregular nodular inner lining is seen.

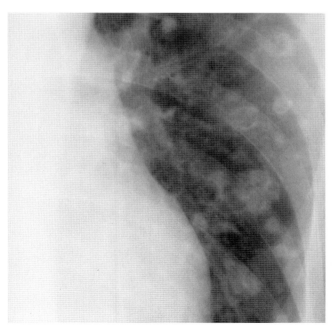

Fig. 24.**11** **Hematogenous metastases from carcinoma of the hypopharynx.** Multiple, different-sized nodules are present bilaterally with a large number demonstrating central cavitation. The finding is best appreciated in the left mid and lower lung field shown here.

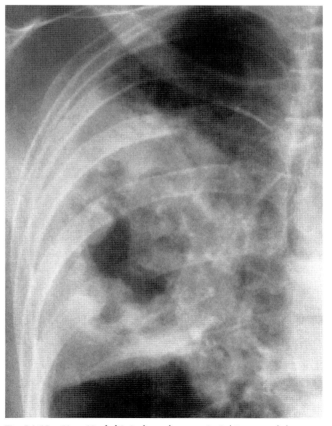

Fig. 24.**12** **Non-Hodgkin's lymphoma.** A right upper lobe consolidation with irregular central cavitation is seen.

Table 24.1   (Cont.) Solitary or Multiple Cavitary and Cystic Pulmonary Lesions

Disease	Radiographic Findings	Comments
Abscess, bacterial		
Staphylococcus (Fig. 24.13 and 24.14)	Single or multiple thick-walled cavities with often shaggy inner linings and air–fluid levels occur in approximately half of the patients with staphylococcus pneumonia. Pleural effusion (empyema) with or without bronchopleural fistula (pyopneumothorax) and pneumatoceles are common, particularly in children.	*Pneumatoceles* are thin-walled cystic spaces that may contain air–fluid levels, commonly found in children. Probably caused by check-valve obstruction of a communication between a peribronchial microabscess and the lumen of a bronchus.
Klebsiella (Fig. 24.15)	Single thick-walled cavity with shaggy inner border in upper lobe is characteristic. Besides an air–fluid level, one or several pieces of necrotic lung parenchyma floating like icebergs in the cavity fluid is occasionally seen indicating pulmonary gangrene.	A radiographically similar upper lobe abscess is a common finding in *Proteus pneumonias* and a rare manifestation in *pneumococcal pneumonias*.
Pseudomonas Anaerobic bacteria	Bilateral consolidations with multiple cavities predominantly in lower lobes and posterior segments characteristic. Diameter of cavities ranges from less than 1 cm to several centimeters, but majority measures less than 3 cm. Air–fluid levels are not a dominant feature and are often only conspicuous in large cavities exceeding 3 cm in diameter. Pleural effusions (empyema) are commonly associated.	Usually in patients with debilitating diseases. A Pseudomonas pneumonia is commonly acquired in the hospital. Mode of infection by inhalation (Pseudomonas) or aspiration (anaerobics) and via bloodstream. Similar radiographic findings are found in *Escherichia coli* and *Salmonella pneumonias*.
Tuberculosis (Figs. 24.16 and 24.17)	One or more thin- or thick-walled cavities with a generally smooth inner lining. High predilection for apical and posterior segment of upper lobes and superior segment of lower lobes. Air–fluid levels are rarely present.	Persistent thin-walled cavitation after chemotherapy does not necessarily indicate active disease. With *atypical mycobacterial infections* cavities (usually multiple) are even more common (Fig. 24.**18**).

(continues on page 576)

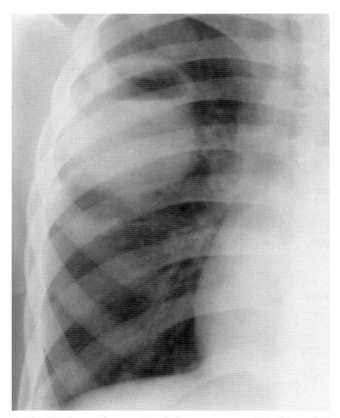

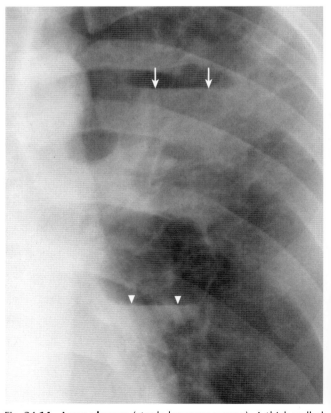

Fig. 24.**13** **Lung abscess** (staphylococcus aureus). A thin-walled cavity with relatively smooth inner lining and air–fluid (pus) level is seen in the right upper lobe.

Fig. 24.**14** **Lung abscess** (staphylococcus aureus). A thick-walled cavity with shaggy inner lining, air–fluid level (arrows) and surrounding infiltrate is seen in the left upper lobe. A pneumatocele with small air–fluid level (arrowheads) in the left lower lobe is the sequela of an old abscess shown in Fig. 24.**2a** 2.5 years earlier.

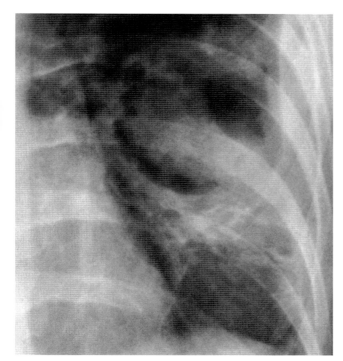

Fig. 24.**15 Klebsiella pneumonia.** A thick-walled cavity with shaggy inner border containing a large mass of necrotic lung is evident.

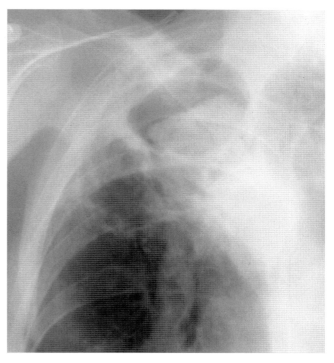

Fig. 24.**16 Tuberculous cavity with aspergilloma.** Chronic tuberculosis with a large cavity containing an aspergilloma is seen in the shrunken fibrotic and infiltrated right upper lobe surrounded by extensive apical pleural thickening.

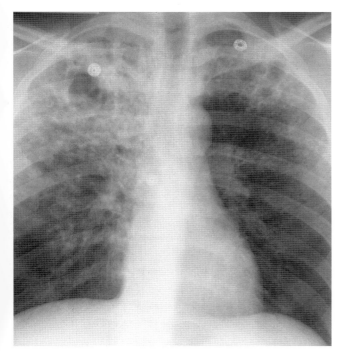

Fig. 24.**17 Cavitary tuberculosis.** Bilateral interstitial and alveolar infiltrates with several thin-walled cavities are seen in both upper lobes and the superior segments of the lower lobes.

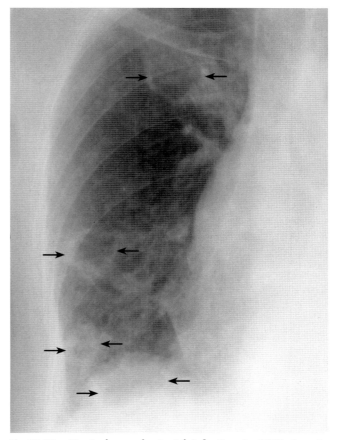

Fig. 24.**18 Atypical mycobacterial infection in AIDS.** Four irregular thin-walled cavities (arrows) are associated with reticulonodular disease.

Table 24.1   (Cont.) Solitary or Multiple Cavitary and Cystic Pulmonary Lesions

Disease	Radiographic Findings	Comments
Actinomycosis Nocardiosis (Fig. 24.19)	Solitary, large, thick-walled cavitary lesion with lower lobe predilection. Extension through pleura into chest wall with rib involvement occurs.	Empyema is commonly associated with actinomycosis and nocardiosis
Fungal diseases		
Histoplasmosis	One or more cavities usually located in upper lobes and indistinguishable from tuberculosis.	Tuberculosis and histoplasmosis may even coexist in the same patient.
Coccidioidomycosis (Fig. 24.20)	Solitary or multiple, thin- or thick-walled, cavitary lesions. Air–fluid levels may be present. Cavitation occurs predominantly in upper lobe nodules, but, unlike tuberculosis, they are characteristically located in the anterior segments.	Very thin-walled cystic lesions, predominantly in the upper lobes, may be the sequelae of an asymptomatic or flu-like coccidioidomycosis infection.
Mucormycosis (Fig. 24.21)	Homogeneous consolidation with frequent cavitation.	Almost invariably in patient with underlying disease (e.g., diabetes, lymphoma, and leukemia).
Blastomycosis Cryptococcosis (Fig. 24.22)	Solitary mass lesion or, less commonly, multiple nodules, often with air bronchograms (> 50%), and occasionally with cavitation (15%) and hilar/ mediastinal lymphadenopathy (20%).	Opportunistic invaders in immunocompromised patients and diabetics.
Aspergillosis Candidiasis (moniliasis)	Cavitation occurs in patchy infiltrates.	Virtually limited to debilitated patients. Both organisms can also be found as fungus balls in cavitary lesions of various origins.
Parasitic diseases		
Amebiasis	Solitary, thick-walled, right lower lobe cavity with as irregular inner surface characteristic. Right pleural effusion almost invariably present.	Pulmonary manifestation is a direct extension from a liver abscess through the diaphragm. Besides the right lower lobe, other lobes contiguous to the diaphragm and covering the liver surface can be involved occasionally.
Echinococcus (Fig. 24.23)	Solitary or less common, multiple cystic lesions with lower lobe predilection. Cystic membrane may float on top of air–fluid level ("water-lily" sign) or lie at the bottom of a dry cyst.	After rupturing into bronchus, part or, less commonly, all of the liquid content is expelled into the bronchial system.
Paragonimiasis	Usually multiple, relatively thin-walled cysts ranging from less than one to several centimeters in diameter. Local elevation or hump on inner lining characteristic.	This presentation of paragonimiasis has been limited to an endemic area in Thailand.

(continues on page 578)

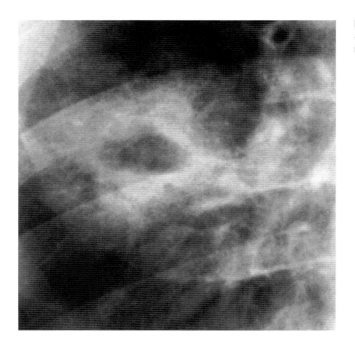

Fig. 24.19 Actinomycosis. A poorly-defined consolidation with central cavitation containing an air–fluid level is seen in the superior segment of the right lower lobe.

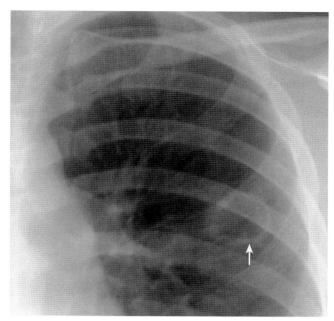

Fig. 24.**20** **Coccidioidomycosis.** A solitary thin-walled cavity (arrow) is seen in the anterior segment of the left upper lobe.

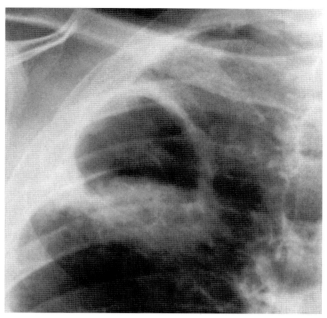

Fig. 24.**21** **Mucormycosis** in patient with diabetes. A relatively thin-walled cavity containing a mass with slightly convex upper border (mycetoma) at its base is seen in the right upper lobe.

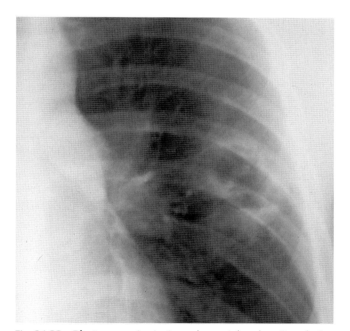

Fig. 24.**22** **Blastomycosis.** An irregular peripheral cavitary lesion is associated with left hilar and mediastinal lymphadenopathy.

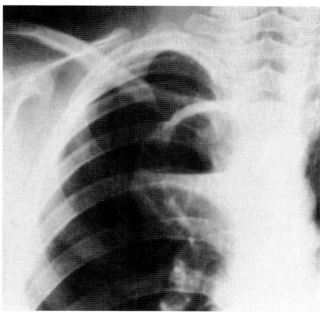

Fig. 24.**23** **Echinococcus.** A solitary cystic lesion with an air–fluid level is seen in the right upper lobe adjacent to the mediastinum.

Table 24.1   (Cont.) Solitary or Multiple Cavitary and Cystic Pulmonary Lesions

Disease	Radiographic Findings	Comments
Progressive massive fibrosis (PMF) in pneumoconiosis (Fig. 24.24)	Usually thick-walled cavity with irregular inner surface in a mid and upper lung zone mass in silicosis or coal miner's lung.	Cavitation in PMF is caused more often by superimposed tuberculosis than by ischemic necrosis.
Rheumatoid necrobiotic nodules	Usually multiple, thick- or thin-walled cavitary lesions measuring a few millimeters to several centimeters with smooth inner surface and lower lobe predilection.	Both cavitary and noncavitary lesions decrease during remission and increase with exacerbation of the rheumatoid arthritis. Cavitary lesion may fill in and become homogeneous again.
Wegener's granulomatosis (Fig, 24.25)	Multiple, bilateral, thick-walled cavitary nodules with irregular inner surface characteristic. Solitary or thin-walled cystic lesions are occasionally seen. Air–fluid levels rarely occur.	Cavitation occurs in almost half of all patients. When multiple nodules are present, rarely all cavitate.
Pulmonary hematoma and traumatic cyst (pneumatocele) (Fig. 24.26)	Presents initially either as homogeneous well-circumscribed mass (hematoma) that eventually may partially evacuate into the bronchial system producing a cavitary lesion or as thin-walled cyst with or without air–fluid (blood) level measuring up to 10 cm and more in diameter.	Lesions may be seen radiographically immediately after a blunt chest trauma, but more often they are only evident hours or days later. Complete evacuation of a hematoma into the bronchial system can also produce a traumatic cyst or pneumatocele, respectively.
Septic emboli (Fig. 24.27)	Multiple, thin- or, less commonly, thick-walled, peripheral, round or wedge-shaped cavitary lesions, sometimes with air–fluid levels.	Often in patients under 40 years of age with endocarditis, septic thrombophlebitis (e.g. in intravenous drug abusers and patients with indwelling catheters or arteriovenous shunts for hemodialysis), pharyngeal and pelvic infections (e. g., septic abortion) and osteomyelitis. Cavitation in *nonseptic emboli* and *infarcts* is very rare.
Bronchiectasis, cystic (Fig. 24.28)	Multiple, relatively thin-walled cystic lesions measuring up to 3 cm in diameter, often with a tiny air–fluid level at the bottom of the ring shadow. Lower lobe predilection.	Change in size of the small air–fluid levels, evident as menisci at the bottom of the cystic lesions, between examinations is virtually diagnostic.

(continues on page 580)

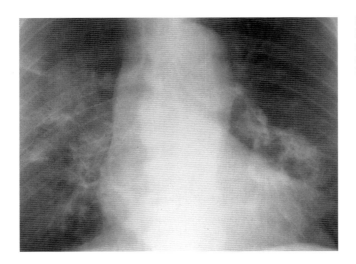

Fig. 24.**24** **Progressive massive fibrosis (PMF)** in coal miner's lung. Besides bilateral perihilar interstitial lung disease and several smaller nodular densities, a larger opacity consistent with PMF is seen in each lung adjacent to a slightly enlarged hilum. The opacity in the left lung depicts massive cavitation due to ischemic necrosis.

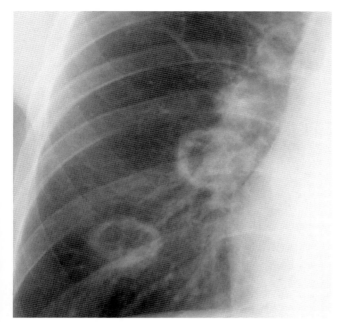

Fig. 24.**25** **Wegener's granulomatosis.** Four cavitating nodules are seen in the right lung.

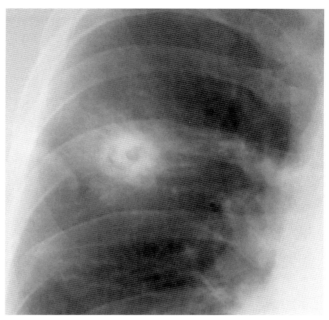

Fig. 24.**26** **Pulmonary hematoma.** A dense nodular lesion is seen in the right mid-lung field containing two irregular radiolucent foci caused by partial evacuation of the hematoma into the bronchial system.

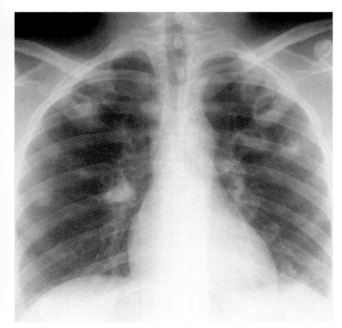

Fig. 24.**27** **Septic emboli.** Several round and sharply outlined nodules are seen bilaterally. Most of the nodules have cavitated and some contain air–fluid levels.

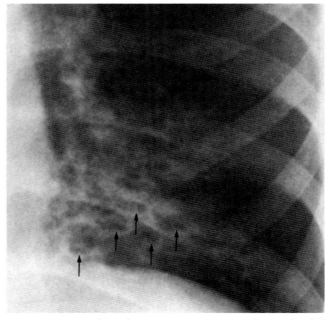

Fig. 24.**28** **Cystic bronchiectasis** in Kartagener's (immotile cilia) syndrome (situs inversus with dextrocardia, sinusitis, often with polyposis, and bronchiectasis). Cystic bronchiectasis, some of the lesions with tiny meniscus-like fluid levels at the bottom (arrows), are seen in the left lower lobe.

Table 24.1   (Cont.) Solitary or Multiple Cavitary and Cystic Pulmonary Lesions

Disease	Radiographic Findings	Comments
Blebs and bullae (Fig. 24.29)	Cystic spaces greater than 1 cm and confined by thin or even hairline wall that may be incompletely visible. The adjacent lung can be compressed, faking locally a thicker wall. Usually multiple lesions with upper lobe predilection. Pneumothorax is a common complication.	Radiographic evidence of diffuse emphysema may be present. Air–fluid levels develop with infection or, less commonly with hemorrhage. A *solitary bulla* may develop as a sequela of a lung abscess or tuberculosis. It may also represent a bronchogenic cyst whose fluid content has been expelled or is posttraumatic in origin.
Pneumatoceles (Fig. 24.30)	Solitary or multiple thin-walled cystic lesions commonly associated with staphylococcal pneumonia.	Found in 50 % of children with staphylococcal pneumonias. Less common in other pneumonias (e.g., *streptococcal* and *Pneumocystis carinii* in AIDS patients). Results from check-valve obstruction of a communication between a peribronchial micro-abscess and the lumen of a bronchus.
Cystic fibrosis (Fig. 24.31)	Thin-walled cystic lesions with or without air–fluid levels associated with diffuse, coarse, reticular changes, hyperinflation, and pulmonary arterial hypertension.	Ring shadows are caused by a combination of cystic bronchiectasis, bullae, microabscesses, and honeycombing.
Sarcoidosis (Fig. 24.32)	Cystic lesions and cavitary nodules are rarely found superimposed on more characteristic diffuse, reticulonodular lung changes.	Mycetomas may occur in these cavitary lesions. (Fig. 24.**33**)

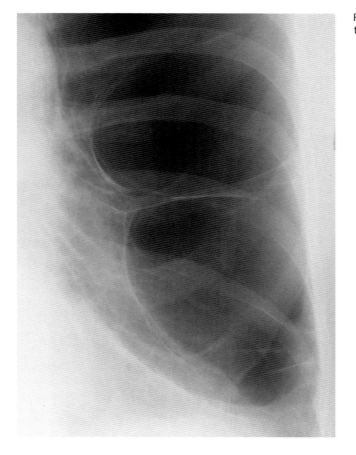

Fig. 24.**29** **Bullae.** Two large bullae with hairline wall are seen in the left lower lobe compressing the adjacent lung.

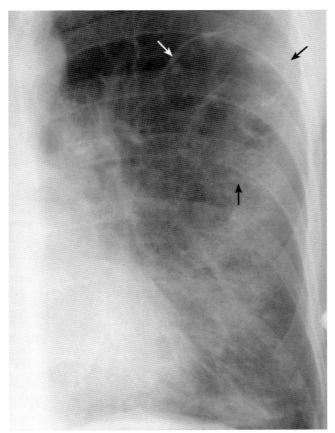

Fig. 24.**30 Pneumatocele in pneumocystis carinii pneumonia (PCP).** An irregular cystic lesion with hairline wall (arrows) has developed in this AIDS patient with advanced PCP.

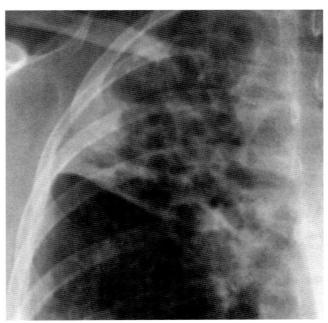

Fig. 24.**31 Cystic fibrosis.** Multiple cystic lesions associated with coarse reticular and patchy densities are seen in the right upper lobe. Similar changes were also present in the left upper lobe.

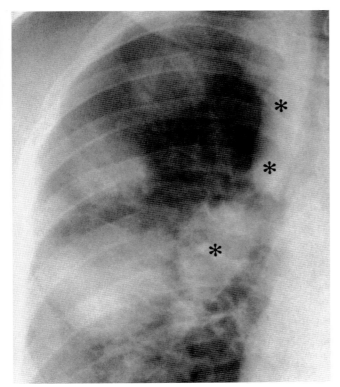

Fig. 24.**32 Sarcoidosis.** Relatively poorly defined nodular densities are seen in the right lung. The nodule projecting just beneath the right clavicle has cavitated. Hilar and paratracheal lymphadenopathy (asterisks) is also evident. Similar changes were also present in the left hemithorax.

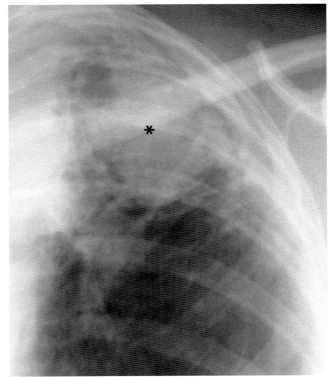

Fig. 24.**33 Sarcoidosis.** A cavitary lesion in the left apex containing a large aspergilloma (asterik) is associated with interstitial lung disease including fibrosis (honeycombing) and significant pleural thickening.

25 Hyperlucent Lung

The roentgenographic density of the lungs is determined by the absorption of roentgen rays by gas, blood, and tissue. The major blood vessels have a density of 1.0 g/ml, whereas the density of lung parenchyma at total capacity is only 0.08 g/ml. This allows visualization of blood vessels in the lungs without using contrast medium. The density of lung parenchyma increases with the increasing amount of capillary blood and interstitial tissue or fluid. The increase in the amount of contained gas decreases the lung density. A decrease of lung density manifests as increased darkening on the chest radiograph.

The sensitivity of the assessment of bilateral changes in lung density with roentgenograms is limited due to technical variables, variations in the amount of extrathoracic soft tissue, and observer error. CT is able to detect bilateral pulmonary hyperlucency earlier, when plain films are still apparently normal. An apparent *bilateral decrease of pulmonary density* may be caused by three factors or combinations thereof: (1) reduction of the caliber of peripheral pulmonary vessels; (2) reduction of the size of pulmonary hila; and (3) generalized pulmonary overinflation. Four combinations of these changes are possible:

1. *Small peripheral vessels, no overinflation; small hila.*
This combination is indicative of a reduction in pulmonary blood flow and is pathognomonic of usually cyanotic congenital cardiac anomalies with a right to left shunt (tetralogy of Fallot with pulmonary atresia, persistent truncus arteriosus Type IV, Ebstein's anomaly) or of isolated pulmonic stenosis without poststenotic dilatation.

2. *Small peripheral vessels; no overinflation; enlarged hilar pulmonary arteries.*
This combination results from various causes of pulmonary artery hypertension (pulmonary artery stenosis, widespread embolic disease to small arteries, pulmonary arteritis, primary pulmonary hypertension, etc.).

3. *General pulmonary overinflation; small peripheral vessels; normal or enlarged hilar pulmonary arteries.*
This combination is pathognomonic of bilateral pulmonary hyperinflation due to an airway disease such as emphysema.

4. *Generalized overinflation of lungs; vascular markings throughout the lungs of normal caliber; normal hilar shadows.*
This combination is pathognomonic of bilateral acute airway disease such as an asthmatic attack or bronchiolitis. The diseases that manifest as combinations 1 and 2 are presented in Chapter 1 and only airway diseases appearing as diffuse, bilaterally hyperlucent lungs, e.g., a general excess of air in the lungs, are included in Table 25.1.

Unilateral hyperlucency of a lung is easier to perceive than a bilaterally increased radiolucency. However, asymmetry of the roentgenographic density of the two lungs may be due to factors unrelated to lung disease. If the patient is rotated, the density of the lung on which the spine is superimposed will be uniformly greater than the density of the other lung. A similar effect may be produced by scoliosis or by incorrect centering of the roentgen beam. Other nonpulmonary causes of asymmetry of the roentgenographic density are the asymmetry of soft tissues surrounding the chest (e.g., caused by a mastectomy, unilateral hypoplasia, or as absence of thoracic musculature) or a grossly asymmetric thoracic cage. It may also occasionally be difficult to decide whether the side of lower or higher density is abnormal in the case of asymmetric density. Diffuse unilateral alveolar consolidation (e.g., pneumonia), unilateral pulmonary edema, or the effect of pleural effusion on supine film should be easy to exclude as causes of asymmetric density by using the general diagnostic signs of parenchymal disease (see Chapter 20) or pleural disease (Chapter 18).

Localized pulmonary hyperlucency may involve the whole lung, a lobe, or a segment. A pulmonary air cyst (bulla or bleb) must be one to a few centimeters in diameter in order to be visible, since the change in density and vasculature can only be compared with the remainder of the lung at that size.

The diagnostic evaluation of localized pulmonary hyperlucency is based on the same variables as is generalized hyperlucency: (1) the amount of air in the involved area, (2) the presence and caliber of blood vessels in the hyperlucent area, and (3) possible changes in the central pulmonary arteries or hilar nodes. The localized decrease of blood flow in the hyperlucent area may cause a compensatory increase of flow in the remaining or contralateral lung. Hilar changes in localized pulmonary hyperlucency may be insignificant or absent in the case of small hyperlucent lesions. When the whole lung is involved (unilateral hyperlucent lung) or when there is compensatory ipsilateral hyperinflation due to lobar atelectasis, the altered caliber or course of the major pulmonary arterial branches or possible hilar adenopathy may provide important diagnostic information.

A fourth important diagnostic variable in localized hyperlucency, the presence or absence of air trapping, is obtained by comparing inspiratory and expiratory films. Lobar air trapping is virtually diagnostic of obstructive emphysema (e.g., foreign body or tumor). Diseases characterized by a unilateral hyperlucent lung or by localized pulmonary hyperlucency and their differential diagnostic features are presented in Table 25.2.

Table 25.1   Bilateral Diffuse Pulmonary Hyperlucency (Overinflation)

Disease	Radiographic Findings	Comments
Chronic obstructive emphysema (Figs. 25.1 and 25.2)	1 *General signs of overinflation*: hyperlucent lungs; low, flat, or concave diaphragm; increased posteroanterior chest diameter; increased retrosternal space. 2 Limitation of diaphragmatic excursions to less than 2 cm, and air trapping evident by comparing inspiratory and expiratory films. 3 Rapid peripheral tapering of pulmonary vessels and their unequal distribution, often with the presence of bullae. Small heart. (*Emphysema with decreased pulmonary markings*.) 4 Prominent pulmonary vessels of an irregular and indistinct contour and often with cor pulmonale. Bullae uncommon. (*Emphysema with increased pulmonary markings*).	Pattern 3 is common in panlobular emphysema ("pink puffer") and pattern 4 in centrilobular emphysema ("blue bloater"). The "increased markings" emphysema (pattern 4) is often overlooked and regarded merely as chronic bronchitis or recurrent bronchopneumonitis, since signs of overinflation are less prominent. Signs of overinflation may be superimposed and partially obscured by left-sided heart failure. Usually associated with *chronic bronchitis*. In the absence of chronic bronchitis, emphysema may be associated with rare heritable connective tissue diseases (*Marfan's syndrome, osteogenesis imperfecta, cutis laxa*) or with α₁-*antitrypsin deficiency* and predominantly lower lobe emphysema.
Primary bullous disease of the lung (vanishing lung) (Fig. 25.3)	Bullae (air-filled, thin-walled, sharply demarcated avascular spaces within the lung) more commonly occur in the upper lobes and may grow. There is hyperinflation (as in chronic obstructive emphysema), but no diffuse oligemia of the remaining pulmonary parenchyma.	Primary bullous disease of the lung involves males and is asymptomatic unless the remaining healthy lung parenchyma is severely compressed. Spontaneous pneumothorax from ruptured bullae is common. Bullae are a common feature of chronic obstructive emphysema, with which bullous disease can be fortuitously associated.
Asthma (status asthmaticus, prolonged asthmatic attack) (Fig. 25.4)	Severe overinflation of lungs with air trapping. Lowered diaphragm, but it is still convex. The vascular markings throughout the lungs are of normal caliber. Tubular shadows or "tram lines" may represent edema or thickening of bronchial walls.	Between the episodes, the chest roentgenogram is often normal. Severe status asthmaticus and diffuse emphysema can be differentiated by the lack of pulmonary oligemia and the concave configuration of the upper surface of the diaphragm in the former.

(continues on page 586)

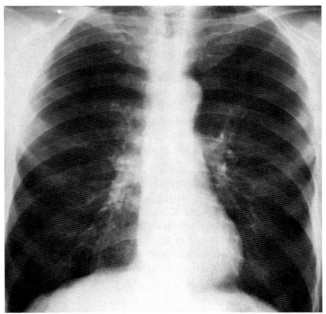
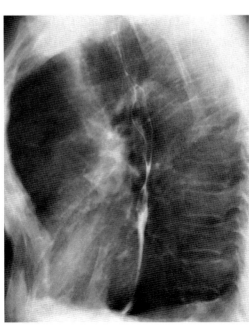

a   b

Fig. 25.**1 a, b   Emphysema with decreased pulmonary markings.** Hyperlucent lungs, flat diaphragm, increased retrosternal space. Rapid peripheral tapering of pulmonary vessels.

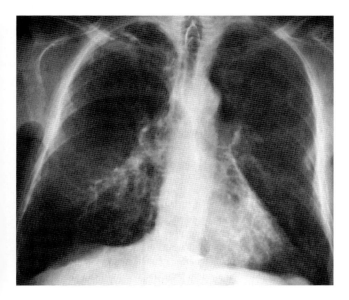

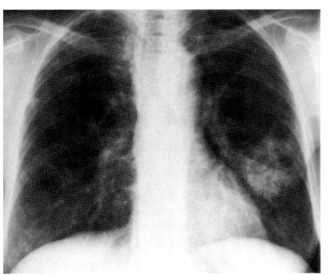

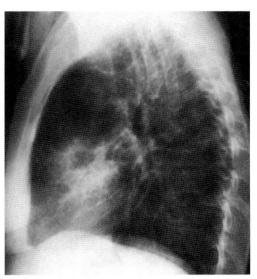

Fig. 25.2 Emphysema with left-sided heart failure. General signs of overinflation, prominent pulmonary vessels with indistinct, irregular contours. Small bullae are seen behind the heart. Left ventricular enlargement.

b

Fig. 25.**3 a, b Primary bullous disease of the lung.** Thin-walled bullae are seen in the mid- and upper-lung fields. The diaphragm is not flattened. Vascular markings in the remaining lung are normal.

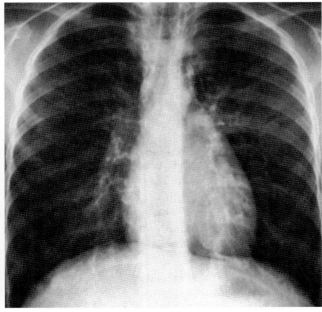

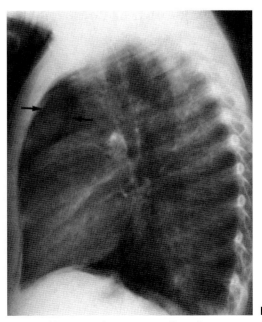

b

Fig. 25.**4 a, b Asthma complicated by mediastinal emphysema** (arrows). The lungs are overinflated but the diaphragm is concave.

Increased linear markings, especially in the upper- and middle-lung fields, are considered to represent thickened bronchial walls.

Table 25.1   (Cont.) Bilateral Diffuse Pulmonary Hyperlucency (Overinflation)

Disease	Radiographic Findings	Comments
Acute bronchiolitis (Fig. 25.5)	Severe overinflation of the lungs may be the only finding. Often accentuated lung markings and small miliary nodules (reticulonodular pattern), particularly in lower zones. Local areas of atelectasis occur in 15 %.	Usually a viral infection of small airways. Affects children below the age of three years and adults with a pre-existing chronic respiratory disease. Childhood bronchiolitis may cause unilateral or lobar emphysema (*MacLeod's syndrome*) in later life through *bronchiolitis obliterans*, overdistention and emphysematous destruction.
Diffuse infantile bronchopneumonia	Diffuse or patchy overinflation. Enlargement of peribronchial lymph nodes. Consolidation usually follows, eventually associated with patchy atelectasis.	This type of bilateral pneumonia is a common complication of *whooping cough, measles,* and *influenza,* but is rarely seen in *bacterial pneumonia.* The pattern of roentgen findings may change suddenly.
Cystic fibrosis (Fig. 25.6)	Overinflation of lungs. Accentuation of linear markings (bronchial walls). Atelectasis. Recurrent local pneumonias.	Tenacious mucus obstructs air passages. Parenchymal overinflation is largely compensatory, but true emphysema may occur in adults. Excessive concentration sodium chloride concentration in the sweat is diagnostic.
Tracheal or laryngeal obstruction or compression: foreign body vascular ring tumor scabbard trachea tracheobronchomegaly relapsing polychondritis	All these rare conditions may be visible as overinflation of lungs with associated findings in the trachea (e.g., compression of the trachea and of the esophagus by the vascular ring, collapse of the flaccid trachea during expiration in tracheobronchomegaly) or in lungs (recurrent pneumonias, parenchymal scarring).	*Vascular ring:* The most common tracheal tumors are: *squamous cell carcinoma, adenoid cystic-carcinoma, osteochondroma,* and *papilloma* (especially in children). *Tracheobronchomegaly (Mounier–Kuhn syndrome):* Dilatation of deficient cartilage rings and bulging of intercartilaginous portions. Tracheal diameter is over 3 cm. Affects primarily middle-aged men. *Scabbard trachea:* Flattening of trachea from side to side so that the coronal diameter is equal to or less than two-thirds of the sagittal diameter when measured 1 cm above the aortic arch. Almost exclusively affects men. Emphysema is common. *Localized tracheomalacia* (or stenosis) may be a late complication of endotracheal intubation or tracheostomy. *Relapsing polychondritis* involves cartilage in the ear, nose, tracheobronchial tree and joints

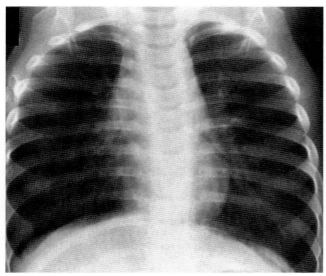

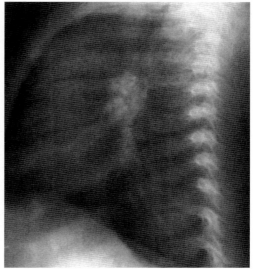

b

Fig. 25.**5 a, b**   **Acute bronchiolitis**, age 1. Severe overinflation of both lungs with flat diaphragm and bulging of lung toward intercostal spaces.

Fig. 25.**6**   **Cystic fibrosis.** Overinflated lungs contain accentuated linear markings and small patchy infiltrates.

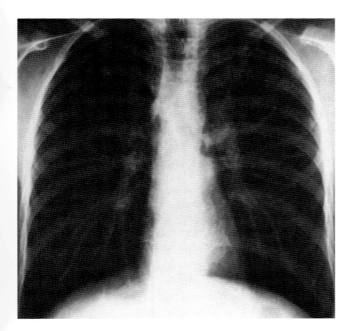

Table 25.2 Unilateral, Lobar, or Localized Hyperlucency of the Lung

Disease	Radiographic Findings	Comments
Hypogenetic lung syndrome	Small and, therefore, often hyperlucent right lung, small or absent pulmonary artery, small right hilus. May be associated with scimitar sign (abnormal, curved, broad vein descending toward the diaphragm).	A rare anomaly, often associated with dextrocardia and a mirror-image bronchial tree. The right lung is supplied by systemic arteries (in part or wholly).
Absence (proximal interruption) of pulmonary artery	Reduced volume, hypoplasia and increased radiolucency of one lung, usually the right. Small ipsilateral hilar shadow. Absence of air trapping in combined inspiratory and expiratory films.	The anomaly is usually on the side opposite the aortic arch. When on the left, there is a high incidence of associated cardiovascular anomalies.
Anomalous origin of left pulmonary artery from the right pulmonary artery	Various degrees of obstructive overinflation and/or atelectasis of the right lung. Posterior displacement of barium-filled esophagus due to interposition of the anomalous artery between lower trachea or the right main bronchus and the esophagus.	Manifests shortly after birth with symptoms of airway obstruction.
Congenital bronchial atresia	Overinflation of the apicoposterior segment of the left upper lobe. A smooth lobulated soft-tissue mass (mucus) distal to the point of atresia. Diminution of vascular markings of the affected segment.	A usually asymptomatic, rare anomaly with a characteristic radiographic pattern. May rarely affect other segmental bronchi. Collateral air drift from the anterior segment is responsible for overinflation.
Congenital (neonatal) lobar emphysema (Fig. 25.7)	Severe overinflation of a pulmonary lobe, most commonly the left upper, right middle, or right upper lobe. Contralateral displacement of the mediastinum and ipsilateral depression of the diaphragm. Congenital cardiac anomaly in 50 %.	A life-threatening condition that manifests at birth or within a few weeks. Bronchial obstruction is either due to vascular compression or a bronchial cartilage defect, or is unexplained. Since operation is often obligatory, differentiation from other causes of lobar overinflation (foreign body, tumorous bronchial obstruction, congenital, avascular lung cyst, hypoplasia of the contralateral lung, or pneumothorax) should be made.
Bronchial adenoma (and other benign pulmonary neoplasms)	Air trapping in *expiration* and possibly oligemia, whereas the volume of the affected parenchyma is usually smaller than normal at full inspiration. Obstructive pneumonitis and atelectasis may follow and are the most common finding. A soft-tissue mass may be visualized.	In most cases, benign bronchial obstruction is complete and results in atelectasis, but occasionally a check-valve effect causes peripheral air trapping.
Bronchogenic carcinoma (Fig. 25.8)	A hilar mass with atelectasis is the common manifestation. Air trapping may be present in an expiratory film, but overinflation is rare.	The affected area may be slightly hyperlucent due to diminished blood flow. Overinflation is also a rare finding in *endobronchial lymphomas* and in *tracheobronchial amyloidosis*.
Primary tuberculosis	Overinflation of the anterior segment of the upper lobe or the medial segment of the middle lobe. Ipsilateral hilar node enlargement.	Partial bronchial obstruction is caused by lymph node compression or by a granulomatous scar. Atelectasis may follow hyperlucency.
Staphylococcal pneumonia	Acute, usually bilateral, pneumonia in a child followed by pneumatoceles, pneumothorax, or pleural effusion.	Common in infants and children. In adults, Staphylococcal pneumonia more likely produces lung abscesses with pleural effusion or empyema. Similar changes may develop secondary to *streptococcal pneumonia*.

(continues on page 590)

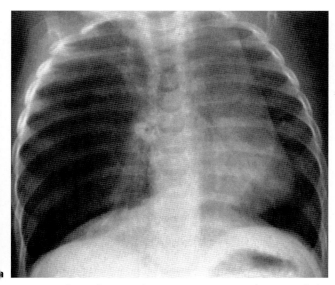

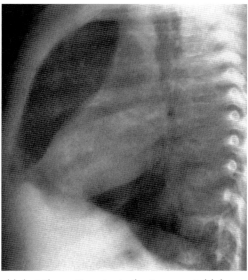

Fig. 25.**7 a, b** **Lobar emphysema.** Massive emphysema of the right middle lobe, collapse of the rest of the right lung and displacement of the mediastinum. This patient was already 8 months old, but the pattern is similar to neonatal lobar emphysema. No underlying cause was found at operation.

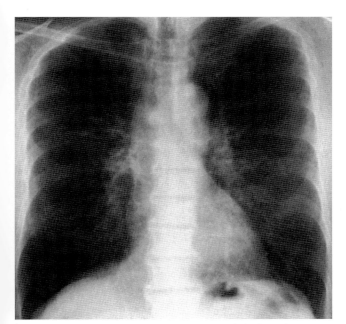

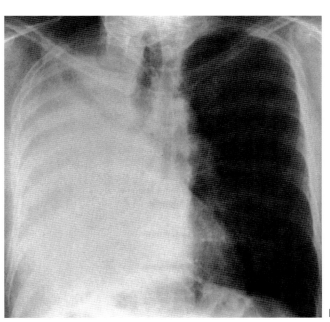

Fig. 25.**8 a, b** **Bronchogenic carcinoma, a** Slight hyperlucency in the right lung. A subtle density is present in the right hilum. **b** Three weeks later, there is total atelectasis of the right lung, shifting of the mediastinum to the right, and hyperlucency of the left lung.

Table 25.2   (Cont.) Unilateral, Lobar, or Localized Hyperlucency of the Lung

Disease	Radiographic Findings	Comments
Pulmonary thromboembolism (Fig. 25.9)	Widening and abrupt obstruction of a major pulmonary artery. Local oligemia (Westermark's sign). Moderate loss of volume of the involved segment, but may still be hyperlucent due to oligemia.	Pulmonary embolism can cause a variety of radiographic findings, and often no definite diagnostic sign is present. Westermark's sign is useful if films prior to emboli are available.
Foreign body aspiration (Figs. 25.10 and 25.11)	Air trapping in the expiratory film. Local oligemia may be present. Lower lobe predominance, most commonly on the right side.	Foreign body may be identifiable if radiopaque.
Local obstructive emphysema	Changes similar to chronic diffuse obstructive emphysema (Table 25.1) but localized as assessed roentgenologically.	Function tests indicate generalized disease. Radiographically, lower lobes are more commonly involved.
Unilateral hyperlucent lung (MacLeod's syndrome or Swyer–James syndrome) (Fig. 25.12)	Unilateral hyperlucent lung (rarely, the lobe) with normal or reduced volume. Oligemia of the affected lung, small hilus. Air trapping on expiration (diagnostic).	A complication of pulmonary infection in childhood (bronchiolitis obliterans), morphologically similar to emphysema. *Congenital aplasia of the pulmonary artery* is the major differential diagnostic entity. It is not associated with air trapping.

(continues on page 592)

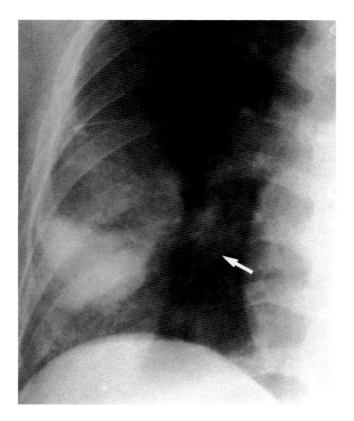

Fig. 25.**9**   **Pulmonary thromboembolism.** Abrupt obstruction of the right lower lobe artery (arrow), under which there is a hyperlucent, oligemic area. The density lateral to it is a pulmonary infarct.

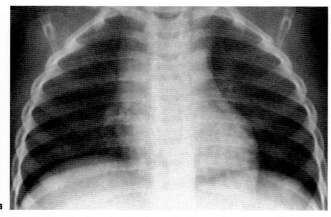

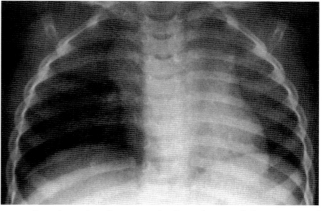

Fig. 25.**10 a, b   Foreign body aspiration. a** Inspiratory film is normal, but **b** expiratory film shows obstructive emphysema of the right middle and lower lobes, indicating obstruction of the right intermediate bronchus between the branchings of the upper and medial lobes. Note the widening of the mediastinum in expiration, a normal finding in small children.

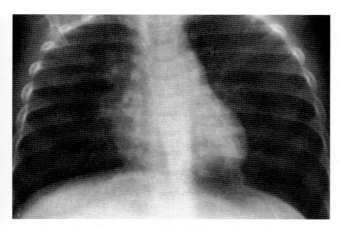

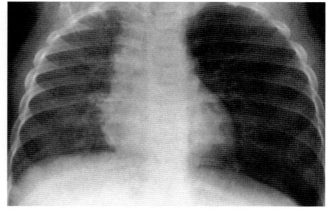

Fig. 25.**11 a, b   Obstruction of the left main bronchus** (a piece of carrot). **a** Inspiratory film shows minor hyperlucency that is accentuated on the expiratory film (**b**).

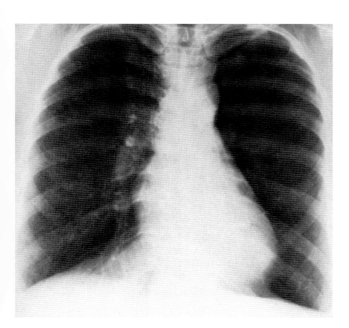

Fig. 25.**12   Swyer–James or MacLeod's syndrome.** Slight hyperlucency of the left lung is caused by oligemia of the left lung and by air trapping (note flat diaphragm).

Table 25.2   (Cont.) Unilateral, Lobar, or Localized Hyperlucency of the Lung

Disease	Radiographic Findings	Comments
Bulla, pneumatocele, bleb (Figs. 25.13 and 25.14)	Sharply defined, air-containing spaces with hairline walls, can range from 1 cm to the volume of a hemithorax. Vascular markings are absent. Adjacent lung may be compressed. Overinflation and air trapping are usual.	Predominantly unilateral. Unlike in unilateral emphysema, vascular markings are absent. May be a complication of destructive (usually staphylococcal) pneumonia, but may arise de novo. The words bulla, cyst, and pneumatocele usually refer to an air-filled, thin-walled space within the lung. A bleb usually represents a collection of air within the layers of visceral pleura, often associated with the development of the pneumothorax.
Sarcoidosis (advanced pulmonary) (Fig. 25.15)	Compensatory emphysema typically is associated with advanced pulmonary fibrosis evident as honeycombing. Blebs, bullae and bronchiectases may also be evident. Reticulonodular infiltrates usually preceed pulmonary fibrosis.	Hyperlucent lung in early sarcoidosis is rare. Bronchial obstruction by enlarged nodes occasionally is observed. In advanced pulmonary fibrosis, cor pulmonale and pulmonary hypertension may also be evident.

(continues on page 594)

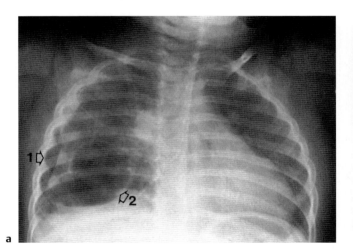

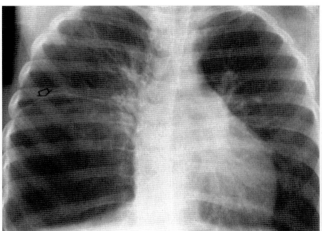

a

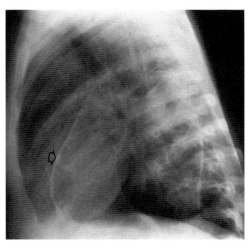

c

Fig. 25.13 a–c   Pneumatocele and pneumothorax, secondary to staphylococcal pneumonia, **a** A small right pneumothorax (1) and a pneumatocele in the right lower lobe (2) are seen, **b, c** Same patient, two years later. The right lower lobe pneumatocele has grown into a giant bulla involving one half of the right hemithorax.

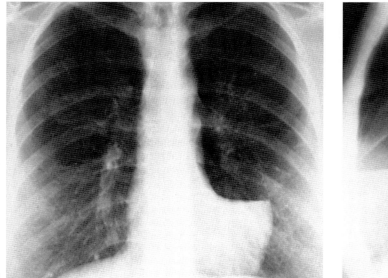

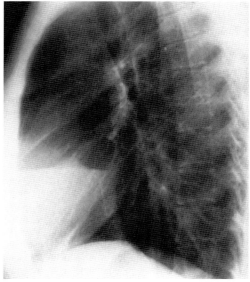

Fig. 25.**14 a, b**   **Intrapulmonary cyst.** The cyst compresses the left cardiac margin and in this case produced a peculiar cardiac silhouette, since it contains an air–fluid level.

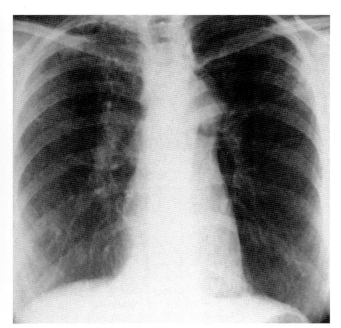

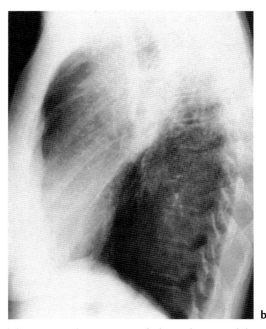

Fig. 25.**15 a, b**   **Advanced pulmonary fibrosis with compensatory emphysema in sarcoidosis.** There is shrinking of upper lobes, upward retraction of the pulmonary hili, and resulting emphysema of the lower lobes.

Table 25.2   (Cont.) Unilateral, Lobar, or Localized Hyperlucency of the Lung

Disease	Radiographic Findings	Comments
Postlobectomy (post-pneumonectomy)	Reorientation of vessels in the operated lung. Reduced volume of the hemithorax (elevated hemidiaphragm, shifted mediastinum). Distorted or small ipsilateral hilus. Blunted costophrenic angle due to adhesions (late).	Bronchopleural fistula and empyema are common complications, often associated with displacement of the heart and mediastinum to the contralateral side. Excessive fluid accumulation may be due to empyema or delayed bleeding. A decrease in the level of pleural fluid or persistent pneumothorax suggests a bronchopleural fistula. After a *pneumonectomy*, the empty hemithorax is slowly (within 3 weeks to 9 months) filled with fluid. *Herniation of the contralateral lung* is seen often after pneumonectomies.
Compensatory emphysema (without surgery) (Figs. 25.16–25.18)	Collapse of one lobe results in expansion of the neighboring lobe(s). May be produced by bronchial obstruction or any cause of lobar collapse.	Common causes are endobronchial tumors, post-inflammatory lobar collapse, or atelectasis secondary to anesthesia.
Pneumothorax (Figs. 25.19 and 25.20)	Absent lung markings. A sharp line of visceral pleura outlines the partially collapsed lung. If unclear, better demonstrated by an expiratory film. Often an air-fluid level (hydropneumothorax or hemopneumothorax) is present. Pleural scarring may produce a loculated pneumothorax. Enlargement of the ipsilateral hemithorax, displacement of the mediastinum toward the contralateral side, often with extensive collapse of the lung, are signs of *tension pneumothorax*.	Spontaneous pneumothorax is most commonly a result of rupture of a subpleural cyst, bleb, or bulla, and is most common in men in the third and fourth decades. It may be a complication of tuberculosis, asthma, eosinophilic granuloma, interstitial pulmonary fibrosis, staphylococcal pneumonia or penetrating trauma. Chronic pneumothorax indicates a bronchopleural fistula.
Asymmetric thoracic soft tissues: mastectomy hypoplasia or absence of thoracic musculature		

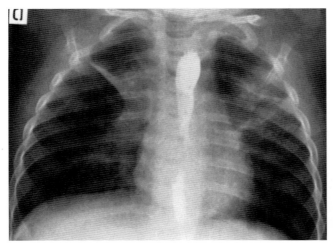

Fig. 25.**16 Congenital stricture of the right upper lobe bronchus** (age 10 months). There is partial collapse of the right upper lobe with expansion and hyperlucency of the right middle lobe. Pneumonia is present on the left side.

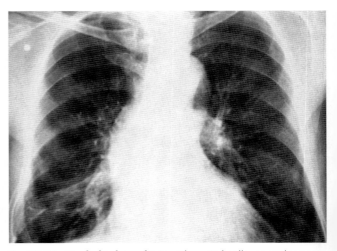

Fig. 25.**17 Healed tuberculosis** with partial collapse and scarring of the right middle lobe, and compensatory expansion and hyperlucency of the right upper lobe.

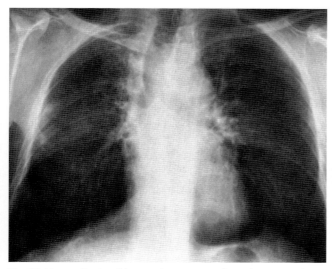

Fig. 25.**18**   **Radiation fibrosis** (carcinoma of esophagus) and partial collapse of both upper lobes with upward retraction of the hili, and compensatory emphysema of the lower lobes.

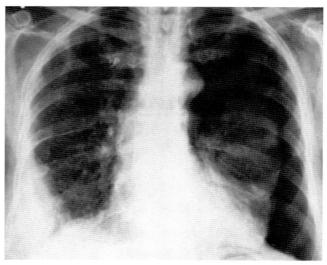

Fig. 25.**19**   **Posttraumatic left-sided pneumothorax** with right-sided pleural effusion and left subcutaneous emphysema. The collapsed lung has an increased density, whereas the rest of the left hemithorax is devoid of lung markings.

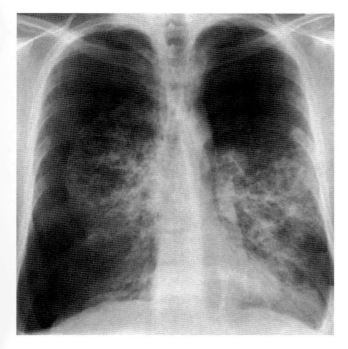

Fig. 25.**20**   Bilateral **pneumothorax** complicating a pneumonia (Pneumocystis carinii and atypical mycobacteria) in an AIDS patient. Hyperlucent pneumothorax surrounds the collapsed and consolidated pulmonary lobes.

Abdomen

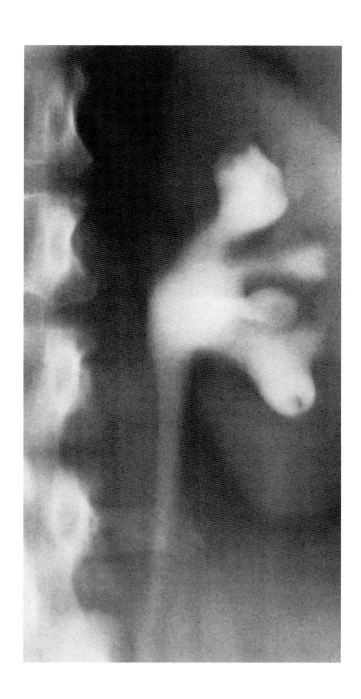

26 Abnormal Abdominal Gas Patterns and Dilatation and Motility Disorders in the Gastrointestinal Tract

The muscular activity of the alimentary canal is responsible for the transport of food and fluid through the gut to provide mixing with the digestive juices and absorption into the blood stream. The smooth muscle of the gut is arranged in three coats: an inner muscular mucosa, a circular muscle coat, and an outer longitudinal coat. The latter two layers affect the tone and cause the peristaltic contractions in the gut.

The alimentary tract is divided into functional units by a series of sphincters and valves: the pharyngoesophageal sphincter (cricopharyngeus), the lower esophageal sphincter, the pyloric sphincter, the ileocecal valve, and the internal and external anal sphincters. Normal motility in the gastrointestinal tract is characterized by coordinated contractions and relaxations of the different muscle layers in the bowel wall and various sphincters. This is regulated by a combination of *myogenic, neural,* and *hormonal factors.* Besides a disorder affecting one of these systems, irritation of the bowel by *inflammation* or *vascular insufficiency,* or *obstruction* of the bowel lumen can result in a variety of motility disturbances affecting the alimentary canal.

Depending on the mechanism involved, a motility disorder in the gastrointestinal tract may be localized or generalized, the lumen dilated or narrowed, and the peristaltic contractions increased or decreased, and physiologically coordinated or not.

Gas in the bowel, whether normal or abnormal, serves as a natural contrast agent and allows various segments of the bowel to be identified by their wall patterns (Fig. 26.1). Small bowel loops wider than 3 cm in diameter are considered distended. Differentiation between widely dilated ileum and colon may be difficult, but the fixed lateral position of the ascending and descending colon as well as stool in the colon are helpful. The watchspring appearance of the valvulae conniventes of the small bowel and the interrupted haustral pattern of the large bowel, which are characteristic in adults and older children, are not evident in the neonate. Under normal circumstances, a single large air–fluid level is found in the stomach when the radiograph is taken with a horizontal beam (e. g., on upright or decubitus films). Small fluid levels in the duodenum and small bowel are uncommon in the healthy subject and because of its solid contents absent in the colon.

For all practical purposes an obstructive pattern has to be distinguished from adynamic ileus. Radiographic findings of purely *mechanical obstruction* reflect the increased peristalsis throughout the entire gastrointestinal tract. Distended loops of bowel containing an increased amount of gas and fluid up to the point of obstruction are evident, with a horizontal beam, as numerous relatively small air–fluid levels at different heights (stepladder formation) that change in location upon subsequent radiographic examinations. Beyond the point of obstruction, it is characteristic that little or no gas, fluid, or fecal material are present (Fig. 26.2). On the other hand, *adynamic ileus* is characterized by distension of the entire gastrointestinal tract with increased gas, fluid, and

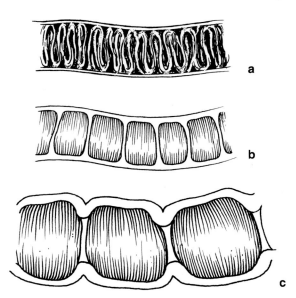

Fig. 26.**1 a–c Wall patterns** of **a** jejunum, **b** ileum, and **c** colon.

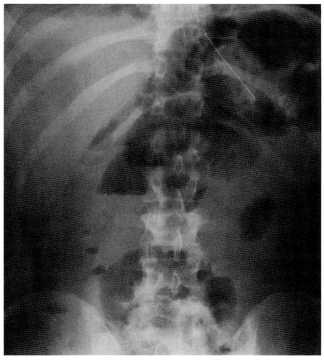

Fig. 26.**2 Mechanical small bowel obstruction** (upright film). Distended loops of small bowel with an inverted U-shape and multiple air–fluid levels at different levels (stepladder formation) are seen. Small gas collections retained between folds resemble a string of beads. Note also the absence of gas and fecal material in the colon.

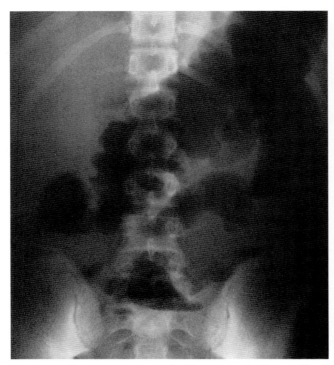

Fig. 26.3   Adynamic ileus (upright film). Distended loops of both small and large bowel with multiple, relatively long air–fluid levels located at similar heights in the mid-abdomen are seen.

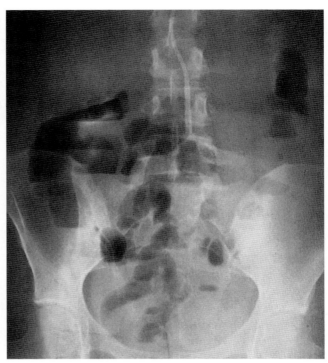

Fig. 26.4   Diarrhea (gastroenteritis) (upright film). Multiple small air–fluid levels at different heights are seen in nondistended small and large bowel loops. Note particularly the air–fluid levels in the descending colon.

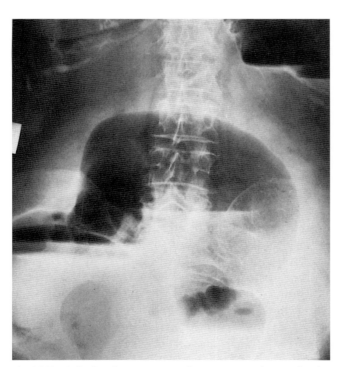

Fig. 26.5   Colonic obstruction with competent ileocecal valve (upright film). A markedly distended colon with multiple air–fluid levels is seen. Note the absence of gas or fluid in the small bowel. The colonic obstruction was caused by herniation of the sigmoid into a left femoral hernia.

solids dispersed throughout the entire bowel. Relatively long air–fluid levels at similar heights with little change between subsequent radiographic examinations are seen (Fig. 26.3). Besides air–fluid levels, air and fecal material are present in the colon and particularly the rectosigmoid area.

Unfortunately these classical patterns in their pure form are rarely encountered in clinical practice, since the mechanical obstruction may be early, incomplete, intermittent, or associated with adynamic ileus, thus obscuring the radiographic findings. Correlation with clinical findings therefore appears essential to arrive at a correct diagnosis. In cases in which the diagnosis remains indefinite, barium examinations or computed tomography are required either to rule out a mechanical obstruction or to identify the point of obstruction.

Acute gastroenteritis with *diarrhea* can produce a picture with multiple stepladder air–fluid levels, but they are characteristically not associated with bowel dilatation, and are located in both small and large bowel, the latter being useful to differentiate this condition from small bowel obstruction (Fig. 26.4).

Colonic air–fluid levels that may or may not be associated with small bowel air–fluid levels, depending on the competency of the ileocecal valve, are also found with colonic obstruction (Fig. 26.5). In this condition, the proximal colon is dilated to the point of obstruction, while the colon distal to it is collapsed. In adynamic ileus, the colon is dilated in its entire length. Long fluid levels may be found in the proximal colon, while they are rare in the distal colon. Furthermore, colonic air–fluid levels can also be the result of a cleansing enema that has immediately preceded the radiographic examination.

In the following section, functional disturbances are discussed separately for different segments of the alimentary canal.

Pharyngeal and Esophageal Dilatation and Motility Disorders

Pharyngeal dysfunction is manifested radiographically by the inability of the pharynx to clear the swallowed barium completely. The barium remains trapped in the valleculae and inferior recesses of the piriform sinus. This condition is often associated with aspiration and can be found with an obstructive lesion at the level of the cricopharyngeal muscle or the cervical esophagus and in a variety of neuromuscular diseases. Failure of the cricopharyngeus to relax properly during swallowing can produce a marked dysphagia that is termed *cricopharyngeal achalasia*. In this idiopathic disorder, the hypertrophic cricopharyngeal muscle is radiographically evident as a large hemispheric filling defect on the posterior aspect of the esophagus at the level of C5–6. A similar radiographic picture is sometimes found in patients after *laryngectomy* in whom the hypertrophy of the cricopharyngeus is induced by developing esophageal speech. Unilateral palsy results in asymmetric deformity of the pharynx that should not be confused with neoplastic involvement

Abnormal contractions are not uncommon in the esophagus. A contraction originating in the middle or lower third of the esophagus, spreading simultaneously upward and downward and producing radiographically an hourglass deformity has been termed *secondary contraction*. Such contractions are rare and usually found with esophagitis.

Tertiary contractions or segmental spasms are usually limited to the lower two-thirds of the esophagus. They are irregular contractions, radiographically producing a "corkscrew" appearance, or occurring as multiple areas of severe narrowing alternating with areas of saccular distension producing a "shish kebab" appearance (Fig. 26.6). They are often found in asymptomatic people without any organic lesions. They may be found in the elderly without esophageal symptoms, but are often associated with other radiographic abnormalities such as dilatation *(presbyesophagus)*. However, if the contractions are associated with intermittent dysphagia, chest pain, and thickening of the esophageal wall, then the syndrome is called *idiopathic diffuse esophageal spasm*. It is most commonly found in middle-aged patients, the sex ratio being equal. In *thyrotoxicosis*, diffuse esophageal spasms can occasionally be seen combined with abnormal relaxation of the upper esophageal sphincter.

"Felinization" of the esophagus caused by transient contractions of the longitudinally oriented muscularis mucosae produces characteristic transverse ridges (Fig. 26.7). This is a normal finding in the esophagus of cats. In humans a *feline esophagus* is most often associated with reflux esophagitis, but it is a rare finding in this condition. Occasionally a feline esophagus is also encountered in healthy subjects.

Dilatation of the esophagus is found in many diseases and may or may not be associated with a motility disorder. The lumen of the normal esophagus rarely exceeds 2 cm in diameter. The differential diagnosis of a dilated and dysfunctional esophagus is discussed in Table 26.1.

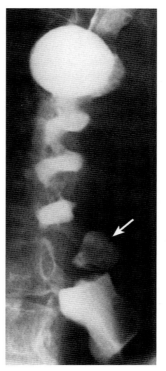

Fig. 26.**6** **Tertiary contractions.** A characteristic "corkscrew" appearance of the distal esophagus is seen. Note also the coincidental small pulsion diverticulum (arrow) and hiatal hernia.

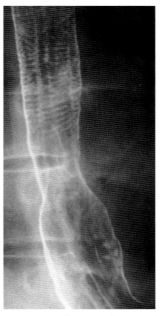

Fig. 26.**7** **Feline esophagus.** Thin transverse folds are seen in the esophagus of a patient suffering from gastroesophageal reflux.

Table 26.1   Dilatation and Motility Disorders of the Esophagus Including Hypopharynx

Disease	Radiographic Findings	Comments
Achalasia (Fig. 26.8)	Moderate to extensive dilatation of the whole thoracic esophagus tapering smoothly to a beak-like narrowing at the diaphragmatic hiatus. Peristalsis is replaced by intermittent, disorganized contractions. Small spurts of barium enter the stomach in the erect position.	Achalasia develops usually in the middle-aged, the sex ratio being equal. A positive *methylcholine test* is characteristic: 5–10 mg intramuscular or subcutaneous results in tetanic contraction of esophagus and retrosternal pain. Extensive dilatation often causes right paracardial and mediastinal mass on chest radiographs, often with air–fluid levels. The air bubble in the gastric fundus is usually small or absent.
Presbyesophagus	Mild to moderate dilatation, decreased peristaltic activity, and tertiary contractions are seen, especially in the lower esophagus. Failure of lower esophageal sphincter relaxation may be associated.	In elderly patients, usually without symptoms. Rarely dysphagia while eating solids.
Obstructive lesion, extrinsic or intrinsic (Fig. 26.9)	Mild to moderate prestenotic dilatation of esophagus, with normal peristaltic waves. Eventually the esophagus may become aperistaltic. Radiographic appearance at the site of lesion is greatly variable, depending on location and type of obstruction.	Obstruction with prestenotic dilatation may be caused by extrinsic or intrinsic mass, stricture, web, Schatzki's ring, or foreign body.
Esophagitis	Commonly involves lower esophagus, Its caliber is only rarely increased and much more often decreased. Abnormal contractions and segmental spasm are commonly associated, whereas peristalsis is often decreased or even absent, Functional changes may precede mucosal abnormalities.	Most often caused by reflux (peptic esophagitis, usually in association with hiatal hernia), but may also be of infectious (e.g., candidiasis), caustic, or radiogenic origin.
Chagas' disease (Trypanosoma cruzi) (Fig. 26.10)	Moderate to extensive dilatation of entire esophagus with intermittent uncoordinated contractions. Radiographically indistinguishable from achalasia.	Virtually limited to South America. Cardiomegaly secondary to myocarditis, megacolon and megaureter is often associated. Methacholine test often positive and therefore not useful for differential diagnosis from achalasia.

(continues on page 604)

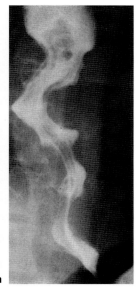

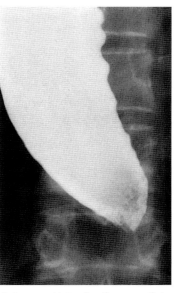

a

b

Fig. 26.**8 a, b**   **Achalasia** (two cases). Extensive dilatation of the esophagus, **a** with disorganized contractions and **b** with aperistal- sis is seen. Note also the smooth tapering of the distal esophagus to a beaklike narrowing at the diaphragmatic hiatus.

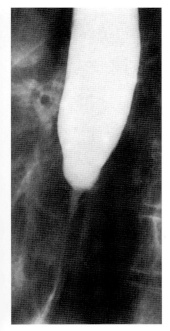

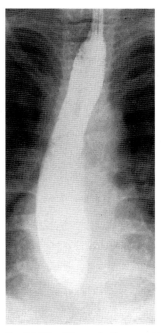

Fig. 26.**9**   **Peptic esophagitis.** A stricture of the distal esophagus with significant prestenotic dilatation is seen.

Fig. 26.**10**   **Chagas' disease.** Dilatation of the entire esophagus with smooth tapering at its distal end is seen.

Table 26.1 (Cont.) Dilatation and Motility Disorders of the Esophagus Including Hypopharynx

Disease	Radiographic Findings	Comments
Scleroderma (Fig. 26.11)	Mild to moderate dilatation of the lower esophagus (below aortic arch) that is hypotonic and hypokinetic, since only the smooth muscle portion is affected. Barium empties by gravity into the stomach in upright position through the patulous lower esophageal sphincter, but pools in the esophagus in supine position. High incidence of gastroesophageal reflux leading to peptic esophagitis and stricture formation.	Abnormal esophageal motility is rarely found with other connective tissue diseases such as *Raynaud's disease, systemic lupus erythematosus, rheumatoid arthritis,* and *dermatomyositis,* that may also be associated with pharyngeal dysfunction.
Amyloidosis	Mild to moderate dilatation of the esophagus with decreased peristalsis.	Esophageal involvement is usually associated with other gastrointestinal manifestations. May be found with primary or secondary amyloidosis.
Neuromuscular diseases (e.g., cerebral disease, Parkinson's disease, multiple sclerosis, amyotrophic lateral sclerosis, familial dysautonomia, muscular dystrophy, myasthenia gravis)	Mild to moderate dilatation with decreased or absent peristalsis, primarily involving the proximal esophagus that contains predominantly striated muscle. Pharyngeal dysfunction is usually much more conspicuous.	Aspiration and barium retention in hypopharynx is seen in neuromuscular disorders, but is also commonly found with a local mass lesion or a foreign body stuck in the hypopharynx. Delayed opening of the cricopharyngeal muscle is an additional feature of familial dysautonomia (Riley–Day syndrome).
Endocrine diseases (diabetes, myxedema)	Mild dilatation, decreased incidence and velocity of peristaltic waves, and nonperistaltic and nonpropulsive contractions are found.	Especially in patients with diabetic neuropathy. Clinical symptoms are, however, infrequent.
Drugs (IV anesthetics, atropine, anticholinergic drugs, curare)	Mild dilatation and depression of motor activity may involve the entire esophagus (anesthetics), the striated muscle of the proximal esophagus (curare), or the smooth muscle of the distal esophagus (atropine and anticholinergic drugs).	Changes in *chronic alcoholism* (particularly in association with peripheral neuropathy) are caused by vagal neuropathy and are similar to atropine medication. *Postvagotomy syndrome* (following vagal denervation of distal esophagus). Mild dilatation of esophagus and failure of lower esophageal sphincter to relax. Findings return spontaneously to normal within months.

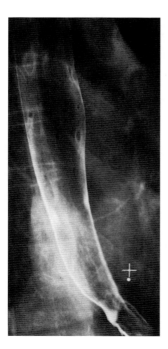

Fig. 26.**11** **Scleroderma.** Moderate dilatation of a hypotonic and hypokinetic esophagus with a wide open lower esophageal sphincter is seen. Barium empties characteristically into the stomach by gravity in the upright position but pools in the esophagus in the supine position.

Gastric Dilatation

Gastric dilatation is a relatively common condition caused by *mechanical obstruction* or *functional disturbance.* In *gastric outlet obstruction,* the dilated stomach may contain up to 5 liters of fluid and a varying amount of air, resulting in a large air–fluid level when the radiograph is taken with horizontal beam. Little or no gas is characteristically found in the bowel beyond the point of obstruction. Gastric dilatation is also found with a duodenal or high small bowel obstruction. In these cases, however, the duodenum and small bowel are also dilated up to the point of obstruction.

The leading cause of gastric outlet obstruction in adults is *peptic ulcer disease* (Fig. 26.12). The narrowing of the lumen in this condition can be caused by spasm, edema, inflammation and scarring. The obstructive lesion is usually in the duodenal bulb or pyloric channel and rarely in the distal antrum.

Gastric carcinoma is the second most common cause of gastric outlet obstruction. The annular constricting lesion is usually located in the antrum. In contrast to patients with peptic ulcer disease, who have characteristically a long history of ulcer pain, primary and secondary gastric malignancies causing outlet obstruction are either not associated with pain, or the pain is of less than one year's duration.

Prolapsing antral polyps and *bezoars* are rare causes of gastric outlet obstruction, usually intermittent.

In *Crohn's disease, sarcoidosis, tuberculosis, syphilis, corrosive gastritis, pancreatitis, cholecystitis,* and other inflammatory disorders, narrowing of the gastric lumen by spasm, inflammation or stricture formation is only rarely severe enough to cause gastric outlet obstruction. *Gastric volvulus* is a rare cause of mechanical obstruction that can result in dilatation of the stomach. The axis of rotation may be around a line extending from the cardia to the pylorus ("organoaxial" volvulus) or around an axis running transversely across the middle of the stomach from the lesser to the greater curvature ("mesenteroaxial" volvulus) (Figs. 26.13–26.15). The majority of cases are associated with diaphragmatic abnormalities such as eventrations or diaphragmatic hernias. Twisting beyond 180 degrees is usually required for complete obstruction.

Hypertrophic pyloric stenosis is not a rare cause of gastric dilatation in the adult (Fig. 26.16). Hypertrophy of the pyloric muscle may be idiopathic or result from previous gastritis or ulcer disease. On barium examination, elongation and concentric narrowing of the pyloric canal is found. In its midportion a triangular niche, the apex of which points inferiorly, is present in about 5% of cases and has to be differentiated from pyloric ulcer. On the other hand, a benign ulcer on the lesser curvature near the incisura, with concentric narrowing of the distal antrum, is found in over half of the patients with this condition.

Infantile hypertrophic pyloric stenosis is by far the most common gastric lesion during the first weeks of life. A palpable, olive-sized mass in the epigastrium combined with projectile vomiting is virtually diagnostic for this condition, which is strikingly more common among males. Radiographically, the elongated, narrowed, and downward-curved pyloric channel, with symmetric and concave indentation of the duodenal bulb by the hypertrophied muscle mass, is characteristic. Other congenital lesions that rarely result in gastric obstruction include an *antral web, gastric duplication,* and *annular pancreas.*

Dilatation of the stomach without mechanical obstruction is a common *postoperative complication,* but may also be

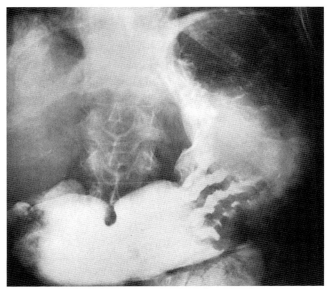

Fig. 26.**12 Gastric outlet obstruction** caused by scarring secondary to chronic ulcer disease. A markedly dilated stomach with a large quantity of retained fluid diluting the barium is seen.

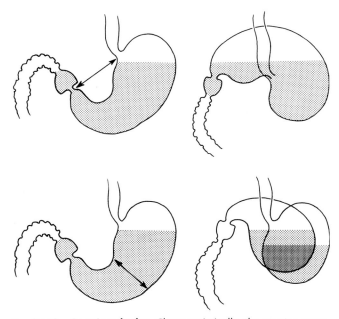

Fig. 26.**13 Gastric volvulus.** Characteristically, the greater curvature is above the lesser curvature, cardia and pylorus are at the same level, and the pylorus and bulbus duodeni point downwards. **a** *Organoaxial volvulus.* Axis of rotation occurs along a line extending from the cardia to the pylorus. **b** *Mesenteroaxial volvulus.* Axis of rotation occurs around a line running across the middle of the stomach from the lesser to the greater curvature.

found after severe *trauma,* in patients *immobilized by cast,* in *inflammatory disease* of the abdomen (e.g., acute pancreatitis, peritonitis, appendicitis, subphrenic abscess), in patients with *severe abdominal pain* (e.g., renal and biliary colics), and various *neurogenic disorders* including postvagotomy state (Fig. 26.17). In *scleroderma,* gastric dilatation, decreased motor activity, and delayed emptying are seen, but the stomach is less frequently involved than other parts

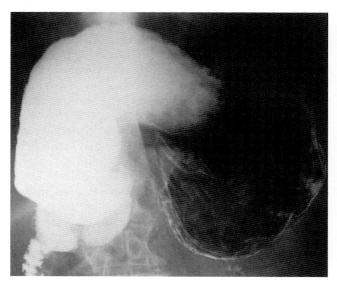

Fig. 26.**14** **Organoaxial volvulus.** A markedly distended upside-down stomach with gastric outlet obstruction is seen.

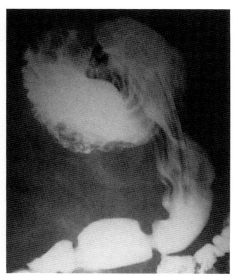

Fig. 26.**15** **Organoaxial volvulus with partial diaphragmatic hernia.** The twisted proximal portion of the stomach is located in a diaphragmatic hernia, whereas the antrum and duodenal bulb are directed downwards and backwards as seen in this lateral projection.

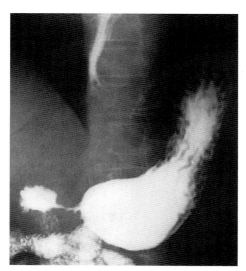

Fig. 26.**16** **Pyloric hypertrophy** in the adult. Elongation and concentric narrowing of the pyloric canal is seen causing mild dilatation of the stomach.

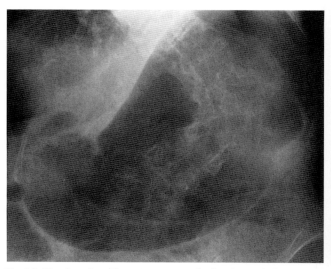

Fig. 26.**17** **Gastric dilatation.** A markedly distended stomach without mechanical obstruction is seen in this paralyzed scoliotic patient.

of the gastrointestinal tract. *Diabetes* and a variety of *drugs* (e.g., anticholinergic drugs and morphine derivatives) are common causes for gastric atony, whereas it is a relatively rare finding in *hypokalemia, uremia, porphyria,* and *lead poisoning.* Finally, a greatly distended stomach is also encountered with *aerophagia* (e.g., in psychopaths) or may be *idiopathic* in the absence of any other obvious cause. Table 26.**2** summarizes the various causes of gastric dilatation.

Dilatation of the Duodenum

Duodenal dilatation secondary to obstruction may be caused by *adhesions* or an *extrinsic mass* such as a neoplasm of the pancreas, aortic lymphadenopathy, and mesenteric metastases (e.g., in the ligament of Treitz) (Fig. 26.**18**). Obstruc-

tions caused by *intrinsic mass* lesions are rare in the adult, since primary duodenal tumors, either benign or malignant, occur infrequently. Duodenal obstruction may also be secondary to *post-bulbar ulcer* and *inflammatory disease* (e.g., Crohn's disease). *Congenital lesions* (e.g., annular pancreas, duodenal duplication, stenosis, and atresia) may cause obstruction in infancy but rarely in adulthood. The double-bubble sign in the newborn is virtually diagnostic of a high-grade duodenal obstruction. This appearance reflects large amounts of gas in both a markedly dilated stomach (left bubble) and in the duodenum proximal to the obstruction (right bubble).

In *midgut volvulus,* the third portion of the duodenum is obstructed, but spontaneous remissions occur. The condition is associated with malrotation and incomplete mesenteric

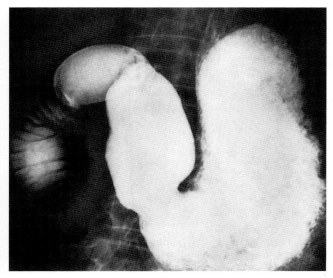

Fig. 26.18 Pancreatic carcinoma. Almost complete obstruction between the second and third portion of the duodenum is seen, with markedly prestenotic dilatation of the duodenum and stomach.

fixation of the gut, allowing the jejunum to twist around the mesenteric root at the site of the origin of the superior mesenteric artery. The duodenojejunal junction (ligament of Treitz) is located inferiorly and to the right of its expected position, and a malpositioned cecum (e.g., in the upper left quadrant) is often present also.

In *superior mesenteric artery syndrome,* the third portion is compressed by this artery or the mesenteric root, respectively. Both of these anatomical structures cross the duodenum anteriorly. It is characteristic for this syndrome that the duodenal dilatation diminishes considerably in prone position. This syndrome is most often found in thin patients. Duodenal compression by the superior mesenteric artery has also been observed in patients with severe burns or lying in a body cast.

Duodenal dilatation is, however, much more often the result of functional disturbances than mechanical obstruction. A localized duodenal ileus is often associated with *acute pancreatitis* or *cholecystitis. Scleroderma* can also present with localized duodenal dilatation and delayed emptying, but more often additional radiologic and clinical findings, quite characteristic of this disorder, are associated (Fig. 26.19). Similarly, a variety of *drugs* (atropine, spasmolytics, and opioids) may induce dilatation of the duodenum, but in this case it is rarely an isolated finding. An *idiopathic mega-duodenum* may result from an abnormality in the myenteric plexus (Fig. 26.20). Causes of duodenal dilatation are summarized in Table 26.3.

Small Bowel Dilatation

Normally only minimal amounts of gas are found in the small bowel of a healthy adult. Bedridden patients have in general an increased amount of gas in the small bowel, since the supine position facilitates the passage of gas from the stomach into the duodenum and subsequently into the small bowel.

An increase of both gas and fluid in the small bowel is found with mechanical obstruction, adynamic ileus, and

Table 26.2 Gastric Dilatation

Cause	Disorder
Gastric outlet obstruction	Peptic ulcer disease Gastric carcinoma and other primary and secondary malignancies Prolapsing antral polyps and benign tumors Bezoars Spasm and edema secondary to an acute inflammatory condition Stricture formation secondary to a chronic inflammatory condition Gastric volvulus Hypertrophic pyloric stenosis (infantile and adult types) Congenital lesions (antral web, gastric duplication, annular pancreas)
Functional disturbance without obstruction	Postoperative (especially following abdominal surgery) Posttraumatic (especially with involvement of back) Immobilization (cast syndrome) Inflammatory disease (e.g., pancreatitis, peritonitis, appendicitis, subphrenic abscess) Pain (e.g., renal and biliary colics) Neuromuscular disorders Scleroderma Diabetes (especially in diabetic ketoacidosis) Drugs (e.g., atropine and anticholinergic drugs) Postvagotomy Electrolyte imbalance (e.g., hypokalemia, hypercalcemia, hypocalcemia) Coma (uremic and hepatic) Porphyria Lead poisoning Aerophagia Idiopathic

Table 26.3 Duodenal Dilatation

Cause	Disorder
Mechanical obstruction (prestenotic duodenal dilatation) (Fig. 26.21)	Extrinsic mass (pancreatic carcinoma and pseudocyst, aortic or mesenteric lymphadenopathy and metastases, hematoma) Intrinsic mass (carcinoma, intramural hematoma, gallstone) Postbulbar ulcer Inflammatory disease (Crohn's disease, tuberculosis, strongyloidiasis, sprue) Radiation therapy Superior mesenteric artery syndrome Midgut volvulus (infants and older) Annular pancreas (infants) Duodenal atresia, stenosis, web and duplication (infants) Congenital peritoneal or duodenal (Ladd's) bands (infants)
Functional disturbance	Pancreatitis Cholecystitis Drugs Scleroderma Idiopathic

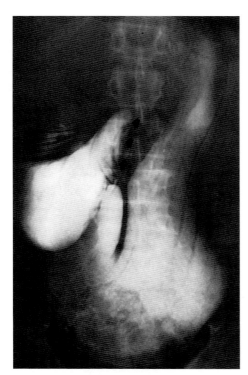

Fig. 26.**19 Scleroderma.** A markedly dilated and atonic stomach and duodenum are seen. Barium is held up where the superior mesenteric artery crosses the third portion of the duodenum (arrows).

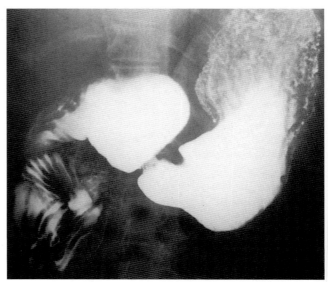

Fig. 26.**20 Idiopathic (congenital) megaduodenum.** A markedly dilated duodenal bulb and descending duodenum is complicated by intermittent retrograde small-bowel intussusceptions.

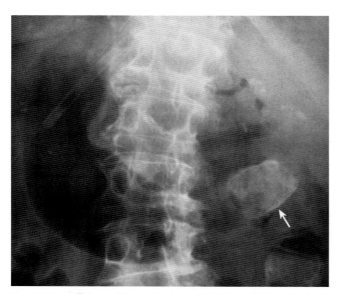

Fig. 26.**21 Gallstone ileus.** Marked dilatation of the duodenal sweep due to an obstructing gallstone (arrow) near the ligament of Treitz is seen.

gastroenteritis (diarrhea). The radiographic plain film findings of these three entities are different and produce characteristic patterns.

Small bowel obstruction is characterized by distended gas and fluid-filled loops of small bowel preferentially located in the mid-abdomen. Valvulae conniventes are often seen in the jejunum producing a characteristic spring-coil appearance. Small gas collections retained between folds may resemble a string of beads, whereas loops of small bowel containing only fluid have a sausage-like appearance. The small bowel gas pattern changes characteristically between sub-

sequent radiographic examinations. A minimal amount of gas and fecal material is present in the colon and if the colon is locally somewhat distended, haustral markings are recognizable. In the upright or decubitus films taken with a horizontal roentgen beam, the small bowel loops have an inverted U-shape with multiple small air–fluid levels at different heights producing a stepladder appearance (Fig. 26.**22**).

Mechanical *small-bowel obstruction* may be associated with a *compromised mesenteric blood supply* and in particular with compression of the venous drainage. In such cases, both the intestinal wall and mucosal folds of the involved bowel segment become rapidly edematous or hemorrhagic and appear radiographically thickened. General paresis of the gut occurs rather quickly under these circumstances, thus masking the radiographic signs of an underlying obstruction and mimicking adynamic ileus.

In *nonobstructive bowel distension* (paralytic ileus in the widest sense), the gas- and fluid-distended loops of jejunum and ileum tend to be large and contain characteristically long air–fluid levels at similar heights. The distended small bowel segments do not have a preferred location. Mucosal folds and markings are often effaced or when edematous, may appear thick. Subsequent abdominal surveys demonstrate little change in the gas pattern. The colon characteristically contains large amounts of gas and stool and may occasionally demonstrate long air–fluid levels. Gastric dilatation is often conspicuous and much more frequently seen than in mechanical obstruction (Fig. 26.**23**).

The diarrheal bowel pattern is found in acute gastroenteritis. Increased gas and fluid is found throughout the entire bowel. Besides numerous small air–fluid levels throughout the small bowel without a preferred location, small air–fluid levels in stepladder configuration are characteristically also found in the colon (see Fig. 26.**4**). Immedi-

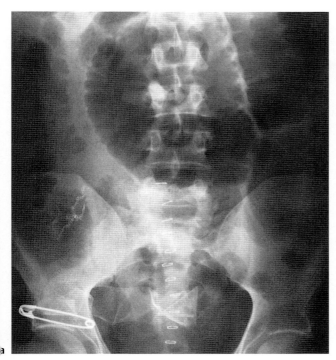
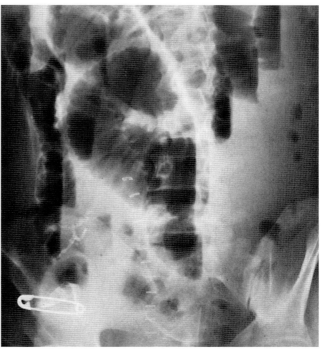

Fig. 26.22 Distal small bowel obstruction in Crohn's disease in **a** supine and **b** left lateral decubitus projections. Dilated loops of small bowel with multiple air–fluid levels at different heights and smaller air collections resembling a string of beads are seen. Note also the spring coil appearance of the valvulae conniventes in the jejunum. The colon is collapsed and contains only a minimal amount of gas.

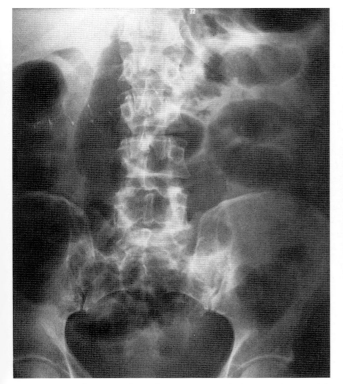
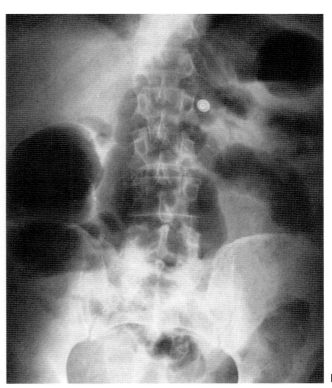

Fig. 26.23 Adynamic ileus (postoperative) in **a** supine and **b** upright projections. Dilatation of the entire gastrointestinal tract is caused predominantly by air with only a few fluid levels evident on the upright film. Mucosal and haustral markings are largely effaced.

ately after defecation, the colon may be completely empty and barely recognizable on the radiographs. A rapidly changing small and large bowel pattern is the hallmark of diarrhea.

The differential diagnosis of various diseases producing dilatation of the small bowel on plain film radiographs is discussed in Table 26.**4**.

Table 26.4   Dilatation of Small Bowel

Disease	Radiographic Findings	Comments
Mechanical obstruction without vascular compromise		
Adhesions and bands	Obstructive pattern with site of obstruction commonly in the ileum (right iliac fossa or pelvis).	Most frequent cause of obstruction, almost always due to postoperative scarring (usually 3 weeks or later after surgery) or previous inflammatory process. Congenital bands are rare.
Neoplasm (extrinsic or intrinsic)	Obstructive pattern without predilection for location.	Most often caused by mesenteric metastases or lymphoma. Less common are benign or malignant tumors arising within the small bowel. Mesenteric cyst and endometrial implants are other rare causes of small bowel obstruction.
Strictures	Obstructive pattern without site predilection.	Neoplastic, inflammatory (e.g. Crohn's disease, tuberculosis), ischemic, posttraumatic, postoperative, and post-radiation therapy.
Hematoma	Obstructive pattern without site predilection.	Intramural hematomas can occur posttraumatically or spontaneously in patients with bleeding diathesis (including anticoagulation therapy).
Parasites (e.g., ascaris)	Occasionally a cluster of linear densities representing a mass of worms outlined by gas can be seen at the site of obstruction.	Usually in children.
Foreign body	Obstruction common in terminal ileum. Foreign body may be recognizable if partially opaque.	In children and mentally disturbed or retarded patients. *Bezoars* are primarily found in mentally retarded or edentulous patients or patients who have undergone (partial) gastric resection.
Gallstone ileus (Fig. 26.24)	Obstruction most common in distal ileum. Gallstone may occasionally contain sufficient calcium to be visible radiographically. Demonstration of gas in shrunken gallbladder and/or biliary system is diagnostic.	Usually in elderly women. Caused by a large gallstone entering the small bowel via a fistula from the gallbladder or from the common bile duct to the duodenum.
Periappendiceal abscess	Extrinsic obstruction of terminal ileum. Abscess might be apparent as a right lower quadrant mass. Appendicolith is occasionally seen.	A similar right lower quadrant mass with distal small bowel obstruction can also be found with Crohn's disease, tuberculosis, actinomycosis, lymphogranuloma venereum and lymphoma.
Hernia (external and internal) (Fig. 26.25)	Demonstration of extraperitoneal bowel containing air and/or fluid at characteristic locations is diagnostic. If the herniated bowel contains only fluid, a mass lesion is simulated and incarceration must be strongly considered (see also under "strangulation" in this table). Whereas the diagnosis of external hernia is easily confirmed clinically, internal herniation should be suspected when bowel loops are crowded in circular arrangement in a local area.	Second most frequent cause of small bowel obstruction. External hernias are 20 times more common than internal hernias. External hernias develop in inguinal, femoral, umbilical, or obturator canals and in weakened surgical incisions. Internal hernias occur in diaphragmatic, gastroepiploic (foramen of Winslow), paraduodenal, and mesenteric defects, which may be congenital or acquired (e.g., surgical defects). The left paraduodenal hernia is the most common internal hernia, accounting for over half of all cases.

(continues on page 612)

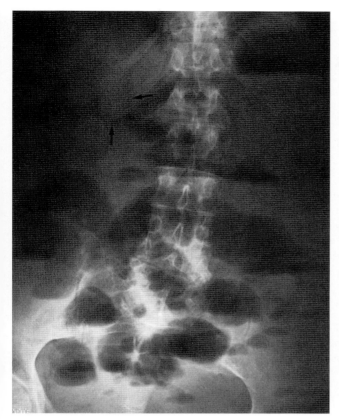

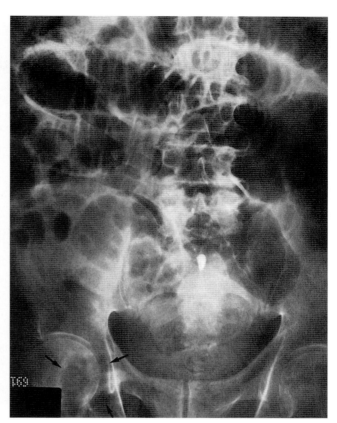

Fig. 26.**24 Gallstone ileus** in upright projection. Small bowel obstruction is caused by a nonradiopaque gallstone lodged in the distal ileum. Distended loops of bowel with inverted U-shape and multiple small air–fluid levels at different heights are seen. The colon is collapsed. The air in the larger bile ducts (arrows) is diagnostic.

Fig. 26.**25   Right inguinal hernia** causing small bowel obstruction in supine projection. Distended loops of small bowel with valvulae conniventes producing a spring-coil appearance are seen. Diagnostic is the herniated, air-containing, small bowel loop projecting into the right inguinal area (arrows).

Table 26.4 (Cont.) Dilatation of Small Bowel

Disease	Radiographic Findings	Comments
Congenital intestinal stenosis or atresia	Triple-bubble sign is seen in infants with proximal jejunal atresia, with the gas being trapped in the stomach, duodenum, and proximal jejunum.	Meconium peritonitis (often calcified) is a common complication of small bowel atresia.
Meconium ileus	Obstruction of the distal ileum in infants by meconium evident as bubbly mass in the right quadrant. Microcolon is also present.	Ileal inspissation with abnormal sticky meconium is commonly associated with cystic fibrosis. May be complicated by stenosis, atresia or volvulus of the small bowel.
Meckel's diverticulum	Obstruction in distal ileum.	Obstruction may be caused by 1) intussusception, 2) internal herniation through congenital band extending from Meckel's diverticulum, and 3) sequelae of chronic inflammation.
Colonic obstruction	Small bowel dilatation occurs with incompetent ileocecal valve. The cecum and to a lesser degree the remaining colon proximal to the obstruction are characteristically distended also.	For differential diagnosis of colonic obstruction, see Table 26.5.
Mechanical obstruction with vascular compromise		
Strangulation	External obstruction of both the afferent and efferent limb of a bowel loop with compromise of mesenteric vessels at the site of obstruction. *Incomplete* strangulation is indistinguishable on plain radiography from simple mechanical obstruction. *Complete* strangulation: Little or no gas but extensive fluid accumulates in the strangulated bowel loop presenting often as mass lesion with characteristically polycyclic outline. Air–fluid levels in prestenotic bowel are initially short and located at different levels, but with rapidly occurring paresis become longer and located at similar levels.	The most common cause of a strangulating obstruction is an *incarcerated hernia*.
Intussusception	Dilated ileum often has beaklike termination at the intussusception site. Intussusception may produce a mass lesion with convex defect in the air column of ascending or transverse colon. On barium examination the classic coiled-spring appearance (barium trapped between the intussusception and the surrounding bowel wall) may be evident.	Common in children between 6 months and 2 years of age ("idiopathic" form). In older children and adults, intussusceptions are much less common and result usually from an associated mass lesion. Ileocolic intussusceptions account for 90% of cases, whereas ileoileal (6%) and colocolic (4%) intussusceptions are rare.
Volvulus	Thickened folds may appear as radiating stripes converging towards the center of the torsion. On upright films, torqued loops may demonstrate long air–fluid levels indicating paresis. The distended small bowel loops often appear disarranged and have a tendency to be located in the right upper quadrant as opposed to a simple mechanical obstruction, where the distended loops are somewhat more often seen in the left upper quadrant.	More common in infants and children than adults. Small bowel volvulus is often associated with anomalies of the mesentery and malrotation. In the latter case, cecum and terminal ileum are usually placed upwards and to the left.

Table 26.4 (Cont.) Dilatation of Small Bowel

Disease	Radiographic Findings	Comments
Nonobstructive dilatation		
Adynamic ileus, localized ("sentinel loop")	Localized dilatation of small and/or large bowel loops adjacent to an acutely inflamed organ, or associated with point tenderness.	Found with acute processes involving the appendix, gallbladder, pancreas, or part of urogenital system.
Adynamic ileus, generalized 1. **Postoperative, posttraumatic** 2. **Shock, sepsis** 3. **Acute disease in abdomen, pelvis, chest (pneumonia, myocardial infarction)** 4. **Electrolyte imbalance (uremia, hypokalemia)** 5. **Drugs (atropine and substitutes, morphines and derivatives, barbiturates, phenothiazines, and hexamethonium)** 6. **Pain (especially colics caused by ureteral or common bile duct stones, torsion of uterine fibroid, or ovarian tumor)** 7. **Neurogenic or neuromuscular disorders (myotonic dystrophy, Parkinsonism, spinal cord lesions, tabes dorsalis)** 8. **Endocrine disorders (diabetes, hypothyroidism, hypoparathyroidism, adrenal insufficiency)**	Dilatation of entire gastrointestinal tract without mucosal or intestinal wall abnormalities is characteristic. Small bowel distension is caused predominantly by air and less by fluid.	Causes of adynamic ileus that clinically mimic small bowel obstruction by frequently being associated with colicky abdominal pain include: *1 Pelvic surgery* *2 Urinary retention* *3 Biliary and ureteral colics* *4 Lead poisoning* *5 Acute porphyria* *6 Idiopathic intestinal pseudo-obstruction* *7 Neonatal adynamic ileus* Conditions simulating adynamic ileus, with gastric dilatation being usually the most prominent finding, are: *1 Aerophagia* *2 Assisted ventilation*
Peritonitis	Findings similar to adynamic ileus, although colonic distension is often very prominent. Restricted diaphragmatic movements, pleural effusions and particularly ascites are associated. *Ascites* may be evident as increased density in pelvis with "dog ears" on urinary bladder, obliteration of hepatic and splenic angles, medial displacement of the liver, spleen, ascending and descending colon from radiolucent (fat) flank stripes which may become thinned, and separation and central location of small bowel loops.	Primary peritonitis (without underlying cause such as perforation or surgery and without evidence of infection elsewhere) is essentially limited to young children and adults with liver cirrhosis. With conventional techniques, usually 200 ml or more of intraperitoneal fluid is required for a diagnosis. Smaller amounts can however, easily be demonstrated with ultrasonography, CT and MRI.
Scleroderma	Dilatation is most prominent in duodenum and jejunum. Air in the esophagus and/or colonic outpouchings (pseudodiverticula) is virtually diagnostic when present.	Disease of middle age with female sex predominance of 3 : 1. Honeycombing in the lung bases may be observed.

(continues on page 614)

Table 26.4   (Cont.) Dilatation of Small Bowel

Disease	Radiographic Findings	Comments
Sprue, tropical and nontropical	Predominantly small bowel dilatation. Pneumatosis and intussusception occur with increased frequency.	Tropical sprue is limited to the Far East, India, and Puerto Rico. Nontropical sprue (adult celiac disease) is an important dietary-related cause of chronic malabsorption in response to the ingestion of gluten found in temperate climates.
Ischemic bowel disease (Fig. 26.26)	Localized or generalized "adynamic ileus" pattern. Submucosal edema or hemorrhage may be evident as "thumb prints." Gas may be seen in bowel wall (streaky appearance as opposed to the bubbly appearance of pneumatosis), portal vein system including intrahepatic branches, and/or peritoneum (poor prognostic sign).	Mesenteric infarction can result from an embolus or thrombus in the superior or inferior mesenteric artery and less commonly from venous thrombosis. Nonocclusive mesenteric ischemia is five times more common in the bowel supplied by the inferior mesenteric artery (descending colon and sigmoid) than superior mesenteric artery. *Neonatal necrotizing enterocolitis* in premature or dehydrated infants is the counterpart of the mesenteric infarction in the elderly.
Acute gastroenteritis and food poisoning	Increased motor activity characteristically causes numerous small air–fluid levels at different heights throughout small and large bowel.	Caused by bacterial, viral, and toxic agents.

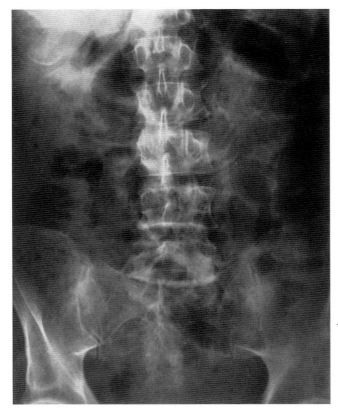

◁ Fig. 26.**26**   **Mesenteric infarction** (supine projection). A generalized adynamic ileus pattern with dilatation of both small and large bowel is seen. In addition, streaky and to a lesser degree mottled radiolucencies are seen scattered throughout small bowel loops indicating intramural gas. Gas is also seen in the portal system of the liver as irregular peripheral radiolucencies. A close-up view of the liver in this patient is shown in Fig. 32.**2**.

Dilatation of the Colon (Megacolon)

A dilated colon (megacolon) can be diagnosed when the colonic diameter exceeds 8 cm. This may be the result of obstruction with prestenotic dilatation, paralysis, or disintegration of the bowel wall. The most important complication of a megacolon is perforation regardless of the etiology of colonic distension (obstruction versus nonobstruction). Colonic rupture can occur when the diameter of the colon exceeds 10 cm. Since the cecum is generally the widest segment of the colon, perforation takes place most often at this site.

Differential diagnosis of a local or generalized dilatation of the colon is discussed in Table 26.**5**.

Table 26.5 Dilatation of the Colon

Disease	Radiographic Findings	Comments
Obstruction		
Fecal impaction (Fig. 26.27)	Large masses of mottled-appearing stool in rectosigmoid area and other colon segments with distension of proximal large and small bowel.	Usually in elderly or bedridden patients. Other rare causes of colonic obturation include foreign bodies, gallstones, and parasites.
Tumor (intrinsic or extrinsic) (Fig. 26.28)	Chronic rather than acute colonic obstruction. Large quantities of fecal material, fluid, and gas distend the colon proximal to the obstruction.	Carcinoma of the colon is by far the most common intrinsic tumor. Extrinsic colonic obstruction may be caused by the invasion of malignant pelvic tumors or metastases (e.g., from carcinomas of stomach or pancreas).
Diverticulitis	Virtually limited to lower descending and sigmoid colon. Obstruction may result from an intramural or intraperitoneal abscess and is usually incomplete and chronic in nature. Abscess may present radiographically as mass that sometimes contains gas within the lesion. Fistulas between sigmoid and bladder (pneumaturia), vagina, flank, or thigh occur. Gas-filled diverticula are occasionally seen but not diagnostic.	*Granulomatous colitis* (Crohn's disease) rarely results in colonic obstruction.
Periappendiceal abscess	Mass in ileocecal area producing small bowel obstruction is characteristic. Rarely, obstruction of the sigmoid colon might occur. Appendicolith may be seen.	
Pelvic abscess	Most often originating from the female genital system. Developing within tubes or pelvic recesses. May obstruct rectum by extrinsic compression.	Commonly gonococcal infection, less often streptococcus, staphylococcus, and tuberculosis.

(continues on page 616)

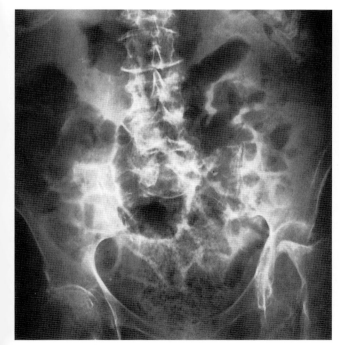

Fig. 26.27 Fecal impaction (supine projection). Large amounts of fecal material is seen in the rectosigmoid area. Distension of the colon and to a lesser degree the small bowel is evident in this immobilized patient with advanced rheumatoid arthritis causing destruction of the left hip.

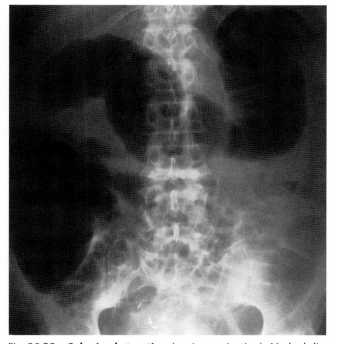

Fig. 26.28 Colonic obstruction (supine projection). Marked distension of the entire colon, with the exception of the rectosigmoid area, was caused by a metastatic ovarian carcinoma invading the sigmoid.

Table 26.5   (Cont.) Dilatation of the Colon

Disease	Radiographic Findings	Comments
Pancreatitis	Strictures occur rarely in the transverse or proximal descending colon, which may simulate primary or metastatic carcinoma, but are usually reversible.	Such a stricture has to be differentiated from an adynamic ileus of the transverse colon in pancreatitis producing the "colon cut-off sign." See under localized adynamic ileus of the colon in this table.
Lymphogranuloma venereum	Rectal strictures are late sequelae of the disease causing chronic obstruction.	In women and homosexual men following an evanescent primary genital lesion with subsequent enlargement of inguinal lymph nodes and fistula formation.
Volvulus (Figs. 26.29, 26.30)	Marked dilatation of twisted colonic segment with only mild to moderate dilatation of prestenotic bowel. Barium column from enema terminates characteristically as beak at point of obstruction. *Sigmoid:* Walls of dilated segment converge in three separate lines toward twisted mesenteric root, evident as soft-tissue density. Adjacent medial walls form a thicker central line, while each lateral wall forms a thinner peripheral line ("coffee bean" sign). Massively dilated, closed loop tends to project into the right upper abdomen. *Cecum:* Depending on torsion axis, markedly dilated cecum presents as single sac preferentially located in the midabdomen ("bag" type), or may have the shape of a kidney located in the left mid to upper quadrant, with the twisted mesentery simulating a dense renal hilum. *Transverse colon:* Twisted loop characteristically to the left of midline. A distended redundant and ptotic transverse colon ("*pseudovolvulus*") must be differentiated by the fact that the walls do not converge towards a twisted mesentery.	Involves colon with mobile mesentery, most commonly the sigmoid, less frequently the cecum, and rarely the transverse colon. Usually in elderly patients, often from nursing homes or mental institutions. Characteristic is acute onset, but may be intermittent or occasionally even chronic. Compromised blood supply leads to bowel necrosis and subsequent perforation when not promptly treated.
Hernias (external and internal)	Similar to small bowel hernias (see Table 26.4) but less common, since only sigmoid and transverse colon have sufficient mobility to herniate.	Interposition of colon (or occasionally small bowel) between liver and diaphragm occurs in asymptomatic patients, but may rarely cause abdominal pain (*Chilaiditi syndrome*).

(continues on page 618)

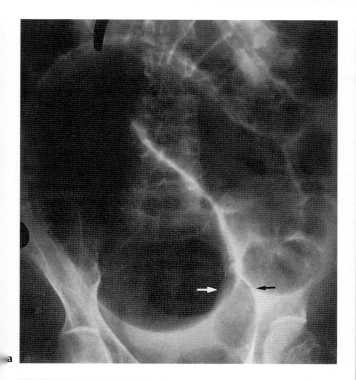

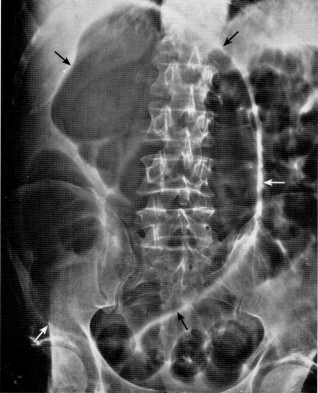

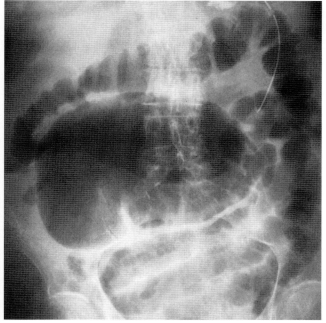

Fig. 26.**29 a–c   Volvulus of the colon** (supine projections). **a** Sigmoid volvulus resembling a "coffee bean". The twisted mesenteric root is indicated by two arrows. **b** Cecal volvulus assuming the shape of a kidney (arrows). **c** Cecal volvulus ("bag" type).

Fig. 26.**30 a–c   Volvulus of the colon. a** Sigmoid volvulus. Walls of dilated segment converge in three separate lines towards twisted mesenteric root (arrows). The adjacent medial walls form a thicker central line while each lateral wall forms a thinner peripheral line. The overall appearance resembles a coffee bean. Note also the moderate prestenotic colon dilatation and the absence of gas and fecal material in the distal sigmoid and rectum. **b** Cecal volvulus. The appearance resembles a kidney with the twisted mesentery simulating a dense renal hilum. Note also the collapsed poststenotic colon. **c** Cecal volvulus ("bag" type). The dilated cecum presents as a saclike lesion in the midabdomen. Note also the collapsed poststenotic colon.
▽

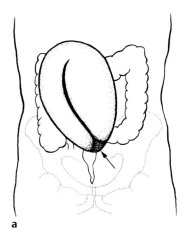

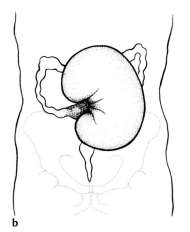

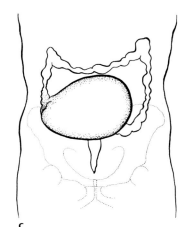

a

b

c

Table 26.5   (Cont.) Dilatation of the Colon

Disease	Radiographic Findings	Comments
Strictures (postoperative, post-irradiation, posttraumatic, postinflammatory, postischemic) (Fig. 26.31)	Obstruction of involved segments, of varying length, is caused by circumferential narrowing (edema, hematoma, or fibrosis).	Postoperative obstruction at a stoma site (colostomy, iliostomy) can be difficult to differentiate on plain films from postoperative adynamic ileus, since dilatation of the bowel down to the stoma is present in both conditions.
Adhesions	Extrinsic or circumferential narrowing of a short segment.	Usually postoperative or postinflammatory, rarely developmental.
Nonobstructive		
Adynamic ileus, localized ("sentinel loop")	Localized colonic distension adjacent to acutely inflammed organ.	For example, terminal ileum and cecum in appendicitis, hepatic flexure in cholecystitis, transverse colon in pancreatitis, and descending colon in diverticulitis. The term "colon cut-off sign" was originally associated with the absence of gas in the spastic transverse colon in pancreatitis, but was later used to describe the adynamic gaseous distension of part or the entire transverse colon with abrupt collapse ("cut-off") of its distal part or the splenic flexure.
Adynamic ileus, generalized	Colonic dilatation is part of generalized gastrointestinal tract dilatation.	See Table 26.**4** for various causes.
Peritonitis	Findings similar to adynamic ileus, but colonic dilatation usually prominent. Signs of ascites.	See Table 26.**4**.
Toxic megacolon (Fig. 26.32)	Dilatation of entire colon occurs, but transverse colon is usually the most affected segment, demonstrating marked distension, thinning of the wall, and loss of haustral markings. In less involved segments, haustra may even appear thickened producing a "thumb print" appearance. A few long air-fluid levels in the colon are usually found on upright or decubitus films. Pseudopolyps recognizable in the air-distended segments are virtually diagnostic for ulcerative colitis.	Characterized clinically by abdominal pain, fever, leukocytosis, and shock. Relatively common (5%) and life-threatening complication of *ulcerative colitis* and rare in other forms of enterocolitis (e.g., *amebiasis, cholera, typhoid fever, bacillary dysentery* and *Crohn's colitis*). Ischemic colitis can also present with identical clinical and radiographic findings.
Ischemic colitis (Fig. 26.33)	Most common presentation is a localized or generalized adynamic ileus. Haustra may be edematous and appear thickened. Intraluminal gas may outline multiple rounded soft tissue densities representing submucosal edema and hemorrhage ("thumb prints"). Presence of streaky gas in bowel wall and portal system is a very ominous sign (see Fig. 26.**26**). Rapidly progressive ischemia may progress to "toxic megacolon" syndrome and perforation. Healing may occur with formation of a stricture and sacculations (pseudodiverticula).	Splenic flexure (at junction of superior and inferior mesenteric artery) is the most common location, followed by descending and sigmoid colon (supplied by inferior mesenteric artery), but every segment can be involved. Similar radiographic findings (adynamic ileus and "thumb printing") may occasionally be seen in a variety of bleeding disorders (e.g., *purpura Henoch-Schönlein, idiopathic thrombocytopenic purpura, anticoagulation therapy*) and *hereditary angioneurotic edema.*
Jejunoileal bypass	Chronic dilatation of entire colon. Cause unknown.	For example, for morbid obesity. Abdominal distension and pain developing 1–3 years following bypass surgery.
Colonic pseudo-obstruction (Ogilvie's syndrome or colonic ileus) (Fig. 26.34)	Disproportionate gaseous distension of the colon without organic obstruction. Massive cecal dilatation is often the dominating feature.	Usually associated with major systemic diseases or following abdominal or pelvic surgery. Cecostomy may be necessary to prevent perforation.

(continues on page 620)

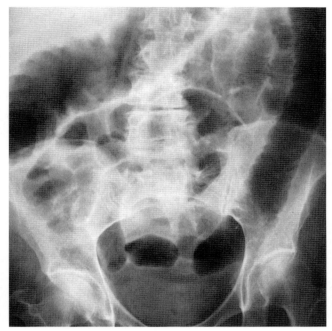

Fig. 26.**31** **Inflammatory stricture of the sigmoid colon** (supine projection). A markedly dilated colon down to the sigmoid area is seen, whereas the rectum appears empty (virtually complete absence of gas and fecal material in this area).

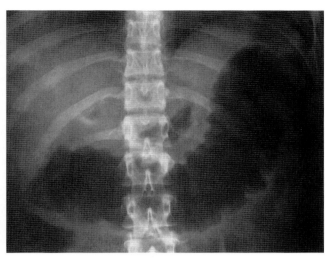

Fig. 26.**32** **Toxic megacolon in ulcerative colitis** (supine projection). Marked dilatation of the transverse colon, loss of haustral markings and "a combination of thumb prints" and pseudopolyps outlined by air are seen.

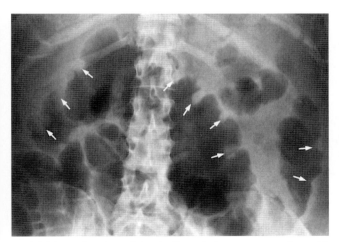

Fig. 26.**33** **Ischemic colitis.** A distended transverse colon with thickened haustra and "thumb printing" (arrows) caused by submucosal edema and hemorrhage is seen.

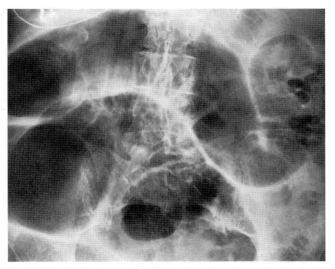

Fig. 26.**34** **Colonic pseudo-obstruction** (supine projection). Dilatation of the entire colon is seen, but is most pronounced in the cecum followed by the transverse colon.

Table 26.5   (Cont.) Dilatation of the Colon

Disease	Radiographic Findings	Comments
Hirschsprung's disease (aganglionosis) (Fig. 26.35)	Chronic dilatation of proximal colon with normal- or narrowed-appearing rectum and/or sigmoid representing the aganglionic segment.	Although characteristically a disease of childhood, it can be seen in adults, presenting with chronic constipation and progressive abdominal distension
Chagas' disease	Besides megaesophagus, megacolon is most common manifestation.	Caused by *Trypanosoma cruzi*, which damages the ganglion cells in the myenteric plexus. Limited to South America.
Scleroderma	Findings usually more pronounced in esophagus and small bowel. Colonic dilatation and loss of haustra occur. Sacculations (pseudodiverticula) on antimesenteric border (as in ischemic colitis) are quite characteristic.	Middle-aged women most commonly affected (male-female ratio, 1:3).
Amyloidosis	Colonic dilatation occurs only in rare cases.	Radiographic findings simulate more often ulcerative colitis (narrowing and thickening of bowel wall, absent haustral markings, and multiple polypoid mass lesions).
Muscular dystrophies	Colonic dilatation may be segmental or complete.	Extracolonic findings are much more conspicuous.
Hypothyroidism	Although entire gastrointestinal tract may be affected, atony and dilatation (acute or chronic) is most striking in the colon.	Nonspecific symptoms of bloating, flatulence, and constipation are frequently present.
Idiopathic ("psychogenic constipation," or "functional constipation")	Chronic dilatation of entire colon and rectum not associated with any disease.	May result from faulty bowel habits or may be the "functional" sequela of a completely healed disease.

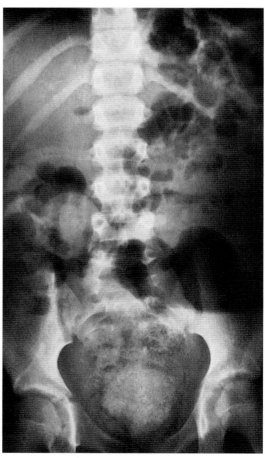

Fig. 26.**35** **Hirschsprung's disease** (upright projection). Chronic dilatation of the colon with a few air–fluid levels and a large amount of fecal material in the rectosigmoid area is seen. The aganglionic segment was limited in this case to the distal rectum.

Extraluminal Gas

Gas collections outside the bowel lumen (e. g. in the bowel wall, peritoneal cavity, extraperitoneal space, and within parenchymal organs) has to be differentiated from both gas within the gastrointestinal tract and peritoneum. Gas in the peritoneal space moves according to body position, whereas intramural or retroperitoneal gas is fixed and often presents as small bubbles that do not coalesce. Compared to plain film, radiography CT, however, is far superior for both localization and characterization of a pathologic abdominal gas collection and nowadays the imaging modality of choice for such an endeavor.

A localized air–fluid level outside the bowel lumen is indicative of an *abscess*. On plain films, the intraabdominal abscess may be radiologically manifested by demonstrating (1) a soft-tissue mass, (2) a collection or pattern of extraluminal gas, (3) viscus displacement, (4) loss of normally visualized structures, and (5) fixation of a normally mobile organ. Secondary signs include scoliosis, elevation or splinting of a diaphragm, localized or generalized ileus, and pulmonary basilar changes.

Extraperitoneal gas following perforation has a mottled appearance and the gas bubbles do not move according to posture. The extraperitoneal collection of gaseous lucencies is often oriented with a general vertical axis, sometimes as linear lucencies, tracking along the fascial planes.

The anterior pararenal space located between the posterior parietal peritoneum and the anterior renal fascia is the most common site of extraperitoneal infection. Most abscesses arise from primary lesions of the alimentary tract, especially the colon, extraperitoneal appendix, pancreas, and duodenum. They originate from perforating malignancies, inflammatory conditions, penetrating peptic ulcers, and accidental or iatrogenic trauma (including endoscopy). The differential diagnosis of extraluminal gas collections is discussed in Table 26.**6**).

Table 26.6 Extraluminal Gas Collections in the Abdomen or Pelvis

Disease	Radiographic Findings	Comments
A. Gas in the Peritoneal Cavity		
Postoperative (laparotomy, abdominal drainage tubes, peritoneal dialysis)	Gas in the uppermost part of the peritoneal cavity without air–fluid level. Best visualized under the right hemidiaphragm in upright position and in the right-side-up decubitus position between the liver and the right lateral peritoneum. Gas may be present up to 24 days after operation; it usually disappears within 3 to 6 days.	Radiograph should be taken 5 to 10 minutes after placing the patient in the appropriate position. Postoperative gas is present more often in asthenic patients than in obese ones, and in greater quantities after upper abdominal or pelvic surgery. Peritonitis has no influence on the disappearance of the gas. A leak should be suspected if gas is not continuously resorbed on subsequent postoperative radiographs or persists after 1 week (earlier in obese patients and children). Colonic interposition between the liver and the diaphragm (Chilaiditi syndrome) may be mistaken for intraperitoneal gas.
Perforated viscus (Figs. 26.36, 26.37)	Free intraperitoneal gas usually with clinical and radiographic signs (peritoneal fluid, paralytic ileus, pain-induced scoliosis) of peritonitis. Gas may also appear as a triangular subhepatic collection overlying the right kidney.	The most common causes are: *perforated peptic ulcer* and *perforated colonic diverticulum*, especially in renal transplant patients, rarely abdominal *trauma, perforated appendicitis* or ruptured *Pneumatosis cystoides intestinalis*. Free intraperitoneal gas is present in two-thirds of perforated ulcers. Gastric and colonic perforation tend to produce larger gas collections than small bowel and appendiceal perforations.
Resuscitation, anesthesia or endoscopic instrumentation	Small amount of intraperitoneal gas with or without gastric dilatation or pneumomediastinum.	Gas leaks from the mediastinum or thinned dilated segment of the intestine without perforation and peritonitis.
Spontaneous pneumoperitoneum without peritonitis (idiopathic)	Free intraperitoneal gas in the absence of disease, or symptoms.	The most common cause is suction of air through the female genital tract. A small amount of free intraperitoneal air after intercourse is a rare but normal finding in females. A *forme fruste* perforation of a peptic ulcer should be considered.

(continues on page 622)

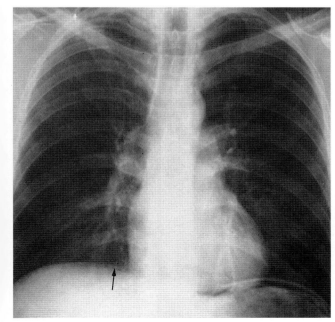

Fig. 26.**36** **Free intraperitoneal gas** under both hemidiaphragms. Perforated duodenal ulcer.

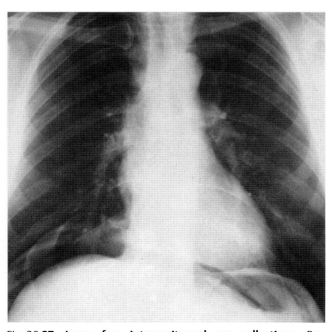

Fig. 26.**37** **Large free intraperitoneal gas collections.** Perforated colon, a complication secondary to ulcerative colitis.

Table 26.6   (Cont.) Extraluminal Gas Collections in the Abdomen or Pelvis

Disease	Radiographic Findings	Comments
B. Gas in the Bowel Wall		
Pneumatosis cystoides intestinalis (Fig. 26.38)	Round extrinsic and intrinsic gas containing cysts in the bowel wall, usually best seen in the colon.	Caused by air spread from the mediastinum or associated with ulcerative disease, acute or chronic distension, or ischemic necrosis of the bowel mucosa. May be postoperative or idiopathic.
Necrosis of the intestine	A lucent line of gas in the diseased segment of intestine.	Necrosis of the intestinal wall may be a complication of vascular occlusion, toxic megacolon, necrotizing enterocolitis or an adjacent abscess.
Intramural leakage after Injury (Fig. 26.39)	Small intramural gas collections adjacent to an intramural perforation of a peptic ulcer or surgical injury (anastomosis).	A rare complication of localized mucosal injury resulting in transmural gas leakage. Very rarely such an incident is secondary to *diabetic infection* or *cystic fibrosis.*
C. Gas in the Biliary Tree		
Abnormal communication (postoperative reflux, cholecystoenteric fistula) (Fig. 26.40)	Lucent lines of gas density overlying the liver with or without gaseous lucency of the gallbladder. The gas is usually near the porta hepatis and in extrahepatic bile ducts. DD: Gas in the portal veins.	The most common cause of intrabiliary gas is a surgical procedure (choledochoduodenostomy, cholecystoenterostomy, sphincterotomy). Without previous surgery, perforation of a gallstone into the intestine is the usual cause, sometimes complicated by a gallstone ileus. Carcinoma is a rare cause of a fistula.
Emphysematous cholecystitis (Fig. 26.41)	Gas in the lumen and/or wall of an enlarged gallbladder with a possible air–bile level. Gas may be present in the bile ducts. DD: Subhepatic or liver abscess, gas in the duodenal bulb.	Blockage of the cystic duct and subsequent overgrowth of gas producing organisms, usually *Clostridium welchii* and *Escherichia coli.* Occurs usually in elderly men with *diabetes.*
D. Gas in the Portal Veins		
Bowel necrosis	Linear streaks of intrahepatic portal venous gas extending toward the periphery of the liver in a severely ill patient. DD; Gas in the biliary tree.	Usually associated with *mesenteric infarction* or *necrotizing enterocolitis.* Gas may be seen in the bowel wall. Rarely it may be seen in severe bowel dilatation or inflammatory bowel disease and emphysematous or corrosive gastritis.
Umbilical vein catheterization	As above.	Accidental, secondary to diagnostic or therapeutic catheterization of a neonate.

(continues on page 624)

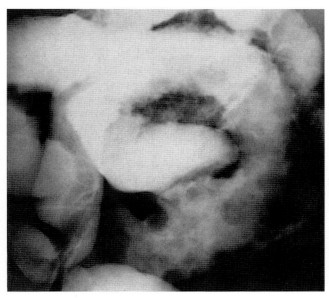

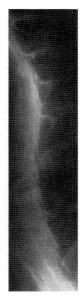

Fig. 26.**38** **Pneumatosis cystoides intestinalis.** Gas-containing cysts in the wall of the colon.

Fig. 26.**39** **Intramural gas** in the colonic wall is seen as a thin stripe, which follows the haustral pattern. A postoperative condition.

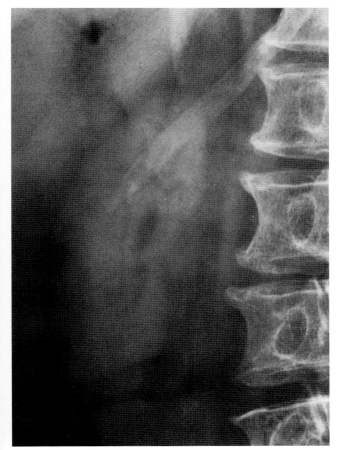

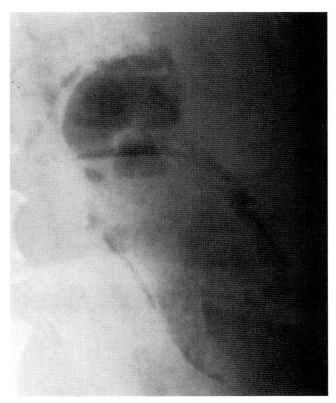

Fig. 26.**40** **Gas in the biliary tree** in a patient with a cholecystoenteric fistula (perforation of a gallstone into the duodenum).

Fig. 26.**41** **Emphysematous cholecystitis.** Gas is seen both in the wall and in the lumen of an enlarged gallbladder. An air–bile level is also present. Thin stripes of gas extend to the bile ducts.

Table 26.6 (Cont.) Extraluminal Gas Collections in the Abdomen or Pelvis

Disease	Radiographic Findings	Comments
E. Diffuse Retroperitoneal Gas		
Rupture or perforation of the descending duodenum (Fig. 26.42)	Gas extends medially beyond the lateral border of the right psoas muscle toward the spine in the anterior pararenal space.	Perforation of duodenum into the extraperitoneal space is usually caused by blunt trauma. The appearance of symptoms may be delayed. There may be accompanying traumatic pancreatitis. Penetrating postbulbar ulcer is a rare cause. Right perirenal gas occurs in only one-third of cases of retroperitoneal duodenal rupture.
Extraperitoneal perforation of the colon or appendix (Fig. 26.43)	Mottled gaseous lucencies overlap the psoas muscle on the right, approach the spine, and do not obscure the flank stripe laterally.	In children, a relatively common cause is extraperitoneal appendicitis associated with an abscess. In adults, it may be a complication of colonoscopy, perforated carcinoma, diverticulitis of the right colon, or secondary to granulomatous ileocolitis. Abscess formation is common in these conditions.
Retroperitoneal sigmoid perforation	Extraperitoneal gas progresses up the left side, extending medially over the psoas muscle. Extension into the posterior pararenal compartment dominates the radiologic findings.	If the sigmoid perforation occurs between the leaves of the mesocolon, the extraperitoneal gas may rise bilaterally within the anterior pararenal spaces. Perforation may be due to diverticulosis or endoscopy.
Rectal perforation	Bilateral spread of extraperitoneal gas parallel to the lateral contour of the psoas muscles outlining the suprarenal and subdiaphragmatic structures.	Usually due to trauma or iatrogenic (leakage of a postoperative anastomosis or after endoscopy and biopsy).
Retroperitoneal gas from pneumomediastinum (Fig. 26.44)	Gaseous lucencies extend preferentially within the flank fat into the posterior pararenal space.	Extraperitoneal gas within the posterior pararenal space may dissect into the immediate subdiaphragmatic tissue planes. It can be differentiated from free peritoneal air, since it parallels a lower plane of the diaphragmatic curvature with a crescenting outline, may be medial or lateral to the apex of the peritoneal cavity, and appears to increase on expiration and decrease on inspiration.
External penetrating trauma	The localization of mottled gaseous lucencies depends on the site of trauma.	

(continues on page 626)

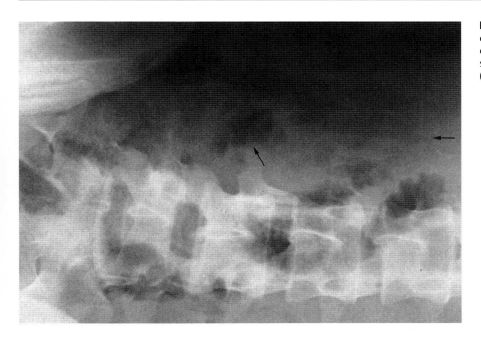

Fig. 26.**42 Traumatic rupture of the duodenum.** Mottled gaseous lucencies are seen in the retroperitoneal space (arrows). They do not coalesce. (A left lateral decubitus projection).

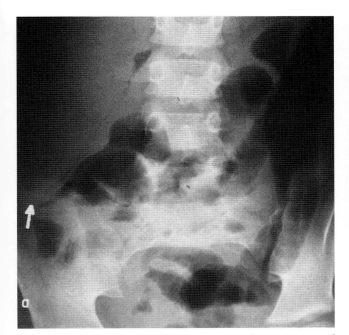

Fig. 26.**43 Perforation of retrocecal appendix.** A "string of pearls" collection of gas rises along the lateral border of the psoas muscle indicating retroperitoneal location of the gas (arrow).

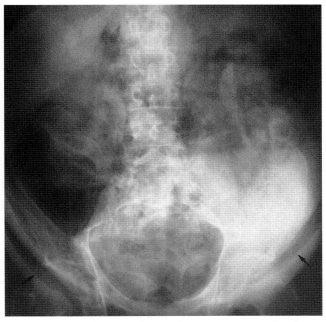

Fig. 26.**44 Retroperitoneal gas from pneumomediastinum.** The pneumomediastinum resulted from respirator treatment for an asthmatic attack. Gaseous lucencies extend within the flank fat (arrows).

Table 26.6   (Cont.) Extraluminal Gas Collections in the Abdomen or Pelvis

Disease	Radiographic Findings	Comments
F. Extraluminal Pelvic Gas Collection(s)		
Pelvic abscess	Extraluminal gas and/or air–fluid level. Extrinsic distortion of the dome of the urinary bladder. Displacement of the sigmoid colon, usually posteriorly or superiorly.	Usually associated with peritonitis, after pelvic surgery, genital infection, or colonic diverticulitis.
Pneumatosis cystoides intestinalis	Gas within the wall of the colon.	See section B of this Table.
Emphysematous cystitis (Fig. 26.45)	Gas bubbles in the wall of the urinary bladder with or without gas in the lumen. DD: Large fecal impaction with multiple trapped gas bubbles.	Usually associated with diabetes, urinary stasis, or bladder outlet obstruction with urinary infection.
Vesicocolic fistula	Gas in the urinary bladder without gas in the bladder wall.	May be congenital or secondary to colonic diverticulitis or malignancy.
Primary pneumaturia	Gas within the urinary bladder in the absence of fistula, instrumentation or other predisposing factors (e.g., fungus ball).	
Emphysematous vaginitis	Focal collection of gas bubbles, varying in diameter from a few millimeters up to 3 cm, confined to the upper two-thirds of the vagina and/or cervix. DD: Normal rectal gas, gas gangrene of the uterus, emphysematous cystitis.	A self-limited, benign condition, most common in pregnant women. Usually asymptomatic except for vaginal discharge. Associated with *Trichomonas vaginalis* or *Hemophilus vaginalis* infection.
Uterine gas gangrene	A large mass (uterus) in the pelvis containing mottled radiolucencies. Gas is present in the uterine wall and often in the cavity and in the fetus if present. Paralytic ileus and retroperitoneal abdominal gas may be present.	A *Clostridium perfringens* infection which is usually secondary to abortive manipulation of a pregnant uterus. An *infected uterine fibroid* is a rare cause of gaseous lucencies in the uterus. Gas in the abdominal wall (postoperatively) may mimic uterine gas collection.
G. Gas within an Abscess (Intraperitoneal or Extraperitoneal Localized Gas Collection with or without Air–fluid Level)		
Subphrenic abscess (Fig. 26.46)	Air–fluid level or mottled gas lucencies intermixed with necrotic material. Elevation and restricted motion of the hemidiaphragm. Pleural effusion (sympathetic). If left-sided, may separate the fundus of the stomach from the diaphragm.	Usually a complication of intra-abdominal surgery. May be secondary to *perforated appendix, peptic ulcer, diverticulitis,* or *cholecystitis.* Left-sided subphrenic abscess usually complicates splenectomy, gastric surgery, left colonic surgery, or hiatal hernia repair. Right-sided subphrenic abscess may follow biliary, gastric, duodenal, or right colonic surgery.
Perirenal abscess (Fig. 26.47)	Extraluminal gas around a kidney and in the retroperitoneal space. Loss of definition of the lower renal outline. Displacement and sometimes axial rotation of the kidney. The lower pole is displaced medially, upward and anteriorly. Margin of the upper segment of the psoas muscle may be invisible. Fixation of the kidney. Restriction of the diaphragmatic motility and scoliosis may be present.	Usually secondary to renal infection (*pyelonephritis, tuberculosis, carbuncle*) and *perforation* of the renal capsule. Often associated with diabetes. Pus collection may displace adjacent bowel. *Osteomyelitis* of the spine may rarely create an abscess in the posterior pararenal space. A *urinoma* does not contain gas. It pushes the lower pole of the kidney up and laterally. It is associated with hydronephrosis and obscures the lower psoas muscle.

(continues on page 628)

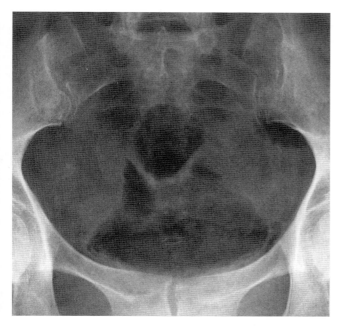

Fig. 26.**45** **Emphysematous cystitis** in a diabetic. Gas is seen both in the wall and in the lumen of the urinary bladder.

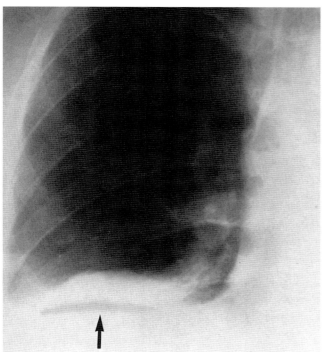

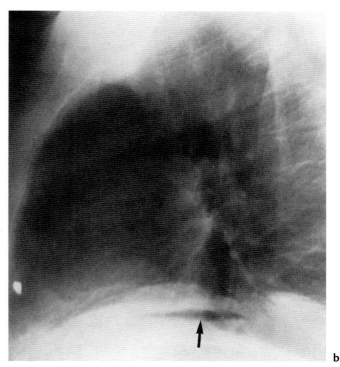

b

Fig. 26.**46 a, b** **Right subphrenic abscess.** An air–fluid level below the right hemidiaphragm (arrow) that projects further away from the lung than free air. Elevation of the hemidiaphragm is associated.

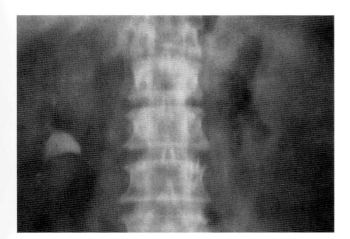

Fig. 26.**47** **Left perirenal abscess.** Extraluminal gas on the medial side of the laterally displaced left kidney.

Table 26.6 (Cont.) Extraluminal Gas Collections in the Abdomen or Pelvis

Disease	Radiographic Findings	Comments
Renal abscess (sub-capsular)	Visualization of the displaced renal capsule or fascia. Flattening or compression of the kidney.	In the absence of gas, a subcapsular hematoma may look identical.
Liver abscess	Gas may occasionally be present in a liver abscess either due to a gas-forming organism or due to connection to the biliary tree. The liver may be enlarged and ascites or pleural effusion may be present.	Can be caused by pyogenic organisms or amebic infestation in severely ill patients, Plain film findings are nonspecific in the absence of gas.
Pancreatic abscess	Peritoneal fat necrosis produces a pathognomonic mottled pattern of normal fat intermingled with areas of water density, best appreciated on CT scans. True gas lucencies may be seen, too. Spread from the head of the pancreas tends to be downward and to the right.	Pancreatic abscess may dissect within fascial planes to the posterior pararenal space, push the kidney and colon forward, and obliterate psoas muscle and flank stripe.
Lesser sac abscess (Fig. 26.48)	A gas–fluid level in the left upper abdomen extending slightly over the midline but not reaching the diaphragm. The stomach is displaced anteriorly and the colon interiorly.	Gas collection in the lesser sac may be due to bowel perforation or a hernia through the foramen of Winslow. A necrotic tumor containing an air-fluid level may mimic an abscess.
Intraperitoneal abscess (Fig. 26.49)	Depending on location: *Right paracolic abscess*: Gas shadow and a mass effect lateral to the ascending colon below the hepatic flexure. *Subhepatic abscess*: Displacement of the proximal transverse colon, lateral wall of the duodenum; loss of visualization of the hepatic angle and of the right kidney, depending on anteroposterior position of the abscess. *Gastrohepatic recess abscess*: Posterior and left displacement of the stomach. *Gastrosplenic recess abscess*: Medial and posterior displacement of the stomach. *Renosplenic recess abscess*: Medial and anterior displacement of the stomach.	A supramesocolic abscess may appear similar to a lesser sac abscess on upright films, but is situated in the midline beneath the central tendon of the diaphragm. As in all abdominal abscesses CT is the primary tool for abscess characterization.
Periappendicular abscess	Appendicolith may be visible (Fig. 27.**8**). Rarely an extrinsic defect of the cecum, with possible displacement of the terminal ileum and multiple gas densities overlying the psoas muscle.	

(continues on page 630)

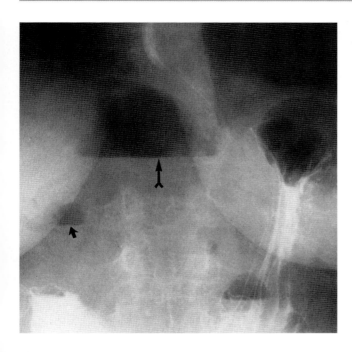

Fig. 26.**48** **Lesser sac abscess** (arrow) and *cholecystoduodenal fistula* (short arrow) in the same patient. A large gas–fluid level is seen in the midline, just below the level of the diaphragm, representing the lesser sac abscess. The smaller gas–fluid level is located in the gallbladder.

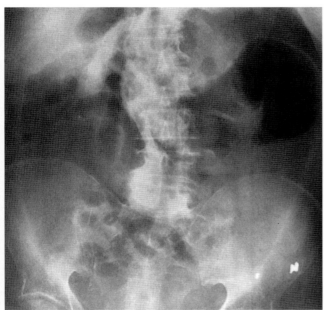

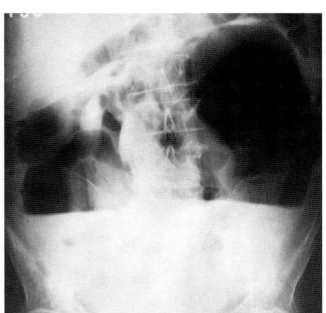

b

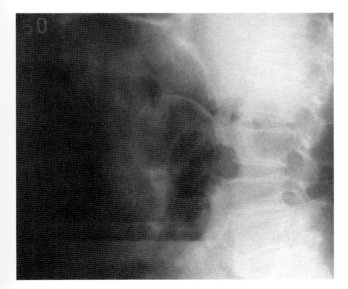

Fig. 26.**49 a–c**   **a** Supine, **b** upright AP, and **c** upright lateral. **A large inframesocolic. intraperitoneal abscess.** A huge gas-containing cavity, which displaces the transverse colon upward. The sigmoid loop is situated within the abscess and its walls are delineated by gas (there is an air–fluid level in the sigmoid colon). The air–fluid level within the abscess does not extend throughout the entire abscess because of loculations within the abscess.

Table 26.6   (Cont.) Extraluminal Gas Collections in the Abdomen or Pelvis

Disease	Radiographic Findings	Comments
H. Gas in Necrotic Tumor		
Gastrointestinal stromal tumor (GIST) (Fig. 26.50)	Large ulcerating necrotic tumors may depict an air–fluid level.	Occurs in both benign and malignant GISTs formerly referred to as leyomyoma and leyomyosarcoma, respectively. Rarely found in neurogenic and lipomatous neoplasms.

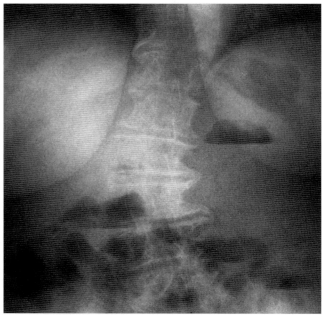

a

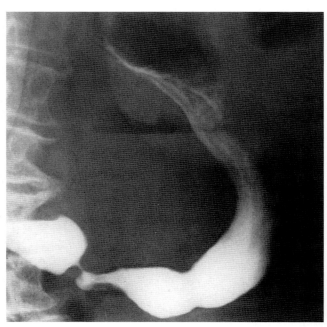

Fig. 26.**50** **Malignant gastrointestinal stromal tumor of the stomach wall** with an air–fluid level. A barium study demonstrates its close proximity to the stomach instead of the lesser sac, which is more posterior in this projection.

27 Abdominal Calcifications

As elsewhere in the body, abdominal calcifications may be *dystrophic*, resulting from precipitation of calcium salts in necrotic tissue (e.g., pancreatitis, granulomas) or may result from *chemical interaction* (e.g., hypercalcemia). Some calcifications develop without known underlying pathology (e.g., prostatic calculi).

The majority of calcifications on the abdominal films are of little clinical significance, but some indicate areas of pathology or allow even a precise diagnosis. Some calcifications can be classified on the basis of their radiographic appearance (location, number, size, shape, distribution, or density). The following calcifications may be of significance in the assessment of an acute abdomen:
– Calcifications of the biliary tract
– Calcified aneurysm of the abdominal aorta or of the hepatic or splenic artery
– Appendicoliths—indicative of appendicitis
– Calcification of an appendiceal mucocele, ringlike or amorphous
– Ribbon-like calcifications in Meckel's diverticulum
– Pancreatic calculi
– Renal, ureteral and vesical calculi
– Calcium deposits in a dermoid cyst

Oblique or lateral projections are of value in differentiating abdominal wall calcifications from calcifications within the intraperitoneal or retroperitoneal space. Calculi less than 1 mm in diameter are not recognizable on plain films but may be obvious on CT.

Intramuscular injections of quinine, calcium gluconate, or calcium penicillin can result in calcifications, usually in the gluteal region. Bismuth injections have a higher density (Fig. 27.1). Injection sites are usually bilateral. They are easy to differentiate from intra-abdominal calcifications.

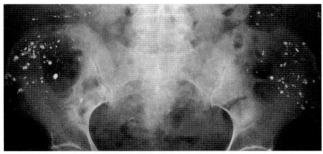

Fig. 27.**1** **Bilateral metal (bismuth) deposits** in needle tracks, a residue of injections given for the treatment of lues. Note the high density of the deposits in comparison with bone.

Table 27.1 Differential Diagnosis of Abdominal Calcifications

Site and Pattern of Calcification	Common Causes	Radiographic Findings and Comments
Calcification in the liver		
A. Disseminated	Histoplasmosis, tuberculosis	Small (up to 3 cm), multiple, dense, scattered throughout the liver. If calcifications of the spleen and lung are associated, the pattern is virtually diagnostic of histoplasmosis.
	Brucellosis	Snowflake, fluffy calcifications. Similar lesions may be seen in the spleen.
	Tongue worm (*Armillifer armillatus*)	Typical comma-shaped or semilunar calcifications occur in the liver, lungs, pleura, peritoneum, and spleen.
	Metastatic mutinous carcinoma (of the colon or rectum, less frequently ovary, breast, stomach).	Finely granular calcifications have a diameter of 2 to 4 mm and a poppy-seed appearance.
	Metastases from other primary tumors (adrenal, bronchogenic, melanoma, mesothelioma, neuroblastoma, osteogenic sarcoma, pancreatic, renal, testicular, thyroid).	Calcification of metastases in these tumors is much rarer than in mucinous carcinomas. They also tend to be larger and denser. Growth indicates malignancy.
B. Cystic	Hydatid cysts (*Echinococcus granulosus*) (Fig. 27.**2a**)	Oval or circular calcifications are characteristic. Arclike daughter cyst calcifications within the mother cyst may occur also. Usually asymptomatic.
	Alveolar hydatid disease (*Echinococcus multilocularis*)	Multiple small (2 to 4 mm) cysts with calcified walls lie within large areas of amorphous calcification; are seen in 70% of cases. Symptomatic, may be fulminant, even fatal.
	Liver cyst (nonparasitic) (Fig. 27.**2b**)	Calcification of the cyst wall is rare.
C. Solitary	Healed liver abscess (pyogenic or amebic)	Dense, mottled calcification, usually solitary. Calcification of an amebic abscess is often associated with secondary infection.
	Coccidioidomycosis Gumma (tertiary syphilis)	These are rare causes of hepatic parenchymal calcification.
	Guinea worm (*Dracunculus medinensis*)	Calcified large worms are more commonly seen in extremities, rarely in the liver.
	Filariasis	Coiled calcified densities are rarely seen in the liver, more commonly in soft tissues.

(continues on page 633)

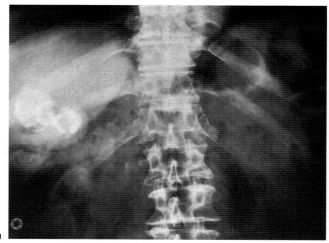

a

Fig. 27.**2a** **Calcified hydatid cysts in the liver.**

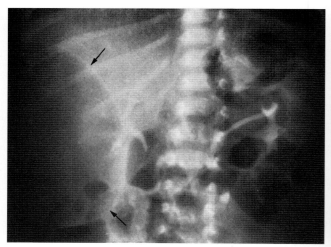

Fig. 27.**2b** **Calcified cystic hematoma in the liver.** A faintly calcified rim (arrows) is seen in this infant.

Table 27.1   (Cont.) Differential Diagnosis of Abdominal Calcifications

Site and Pattern of Calcification	Common Causes	Radiographic Findings and Comments
	Toxoplasmosis Cysticercosis Ascariasis Clonorchiasis	Liver calcifications in these conditions are unusual.
	Cavernous hemangioma	A sunburst pattern of calcified spicules may be seen. Most hemangiomas are not calcified. Unlike hemangiomas of soft tissue elsewhere, calcified phleboliths are uncommon in hepatic hemangiomas.
	Primary carcinoma of the liver	Dystrophic calcification of necrotic tumor tissue may occur, especially in children; seen as flecks or spherical calculi resembling cholelithiasis.
	Hematoma	Traumatic liver hematoma may later calcify.
D. Vascular	Calcified thrombus of the portal vein	A linear density crossing the vertebral column. Rare, usually associated with cirrhosis and portal hypertension.
	Hepatic artery aneurysm	A cracked eggshell appearance typical of aneurysm is rare in the hepatic artery, much more common in the splenic artery. May mimic a calcified cyst.
E. Gallstones	(See biliary calcification in this table)	
F. Capsular	May occur in alcoholic cirrhosis, pyogenic infection, meconium peritonitis, or pseudomyxoma peritonei.	
G. Generalized increase of liver density	May be secondary to hemochromatosis, hemosiderosis, cirrhotic contraction, Thorotrast injection or lipiodol (Ethiodol) embolisation of the liver after lymphography.	

(continues on page 634)

Table 27.1 (Cont.) Differential Diagnosis of Abdominal Calcifications

Site and Pattern of Calcification	Common Causes	Radiographic Findings and Comments
Calcification in the spleen		
A. Disseminated	Phleboliths	Multiple small, round calcific nodules throughout the spleen.
	Granulomatous disease (histoplasmosis, tuberculosis, brucellosis) (Fig. 27.**3**)	Histoplasmosis is the most common cause in endemic areas. Similar lesions are often present throughout the lungs, occasionally in the liver. Calcifications in brucellosis are larger than in histoplasmosis or tuberculosis, about 1 to 3 cm in diameter. They consist of flocculent central calcifications and a surrounding calcific rim. Brucellosis may still be active when calcifications occur.
B. Cystic	Echinococcal cysts (Fig. 27.**4**)	Hydatid cysts are often multiple and heavily calcified in contrast to other cysts.
	Hematoma	A splenic hematoma may occasionally become cystic and calcify.
	Congenital cyst Dermoid Epidermoid	These lesions very rarely calcify in the spleen.
C. Capsular and/or parenchymal calcification	Splenic infarct (Fig. 27.**5**)	Single or, rarely, multiple. Infrequently calcifies as a triangular density, with apex toward the center of the organ.
	Hematoma Abscess (pyogenic or tuberculous)	Plaques of calcification of the splenic capsule may occur secondary to an abscess, although calcification of splenic abscesses is rare.
D. Vascular	Calcified splenic artery (Fig. 27.**3**)	A common finding without clinical importance. Tortuous, corkscrew appearance of the linear calcification is characteristic.
	Splenic artery aneurysm	Circular or bizarre calcification with diameter larger than the normal artery.
E. Generalized increase of splenic density	Sickle-cell anemia	Produced by fine miliary calcifications and iron deposits.
	Hemochromatosis	Iron deposition. May also occur in excessive dietary intake of iron or in thalassemia, Fanconi's anemia, or rarely after multiple transfusions.
	Thorotrast deposits	Thorium dioxide particles are stored in the reticuloendothelial system. A history of thorotrast angiography may be obtained. This contrast medium has not been used since the early 1950s.
Calcification in the pancreas		
A. Disseminated	Alcoholic pancreatitis Gallstone pancreatitis (Fig. 27.**6**)	Alcoholic pancreatitis is the most common cause of pancreatic lithiasis. Numerous irregular, small concretions are widely scattered within the pancreatic ducts throughout the gland. Present in 20–40% of patients with chronic alcoholic pancreatitis. The incidence of calcification in gallstone pancreatitis is only 2%, but the radiographic appearance is similar.
	Hyperparathyroidism	Due to pancreatitis, which develops in up to 20% of patients with hyperparathyroidism. Often associated with renal calcifications.
	Hereditary pancreatitis	Rounded, often relatively large pancreatic calcifications which are already present in childhood.

(continues on page 636)

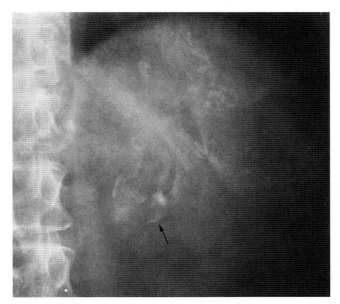

Fig. 27.**3** **Tuberculosis.** Disseminated granulomatous calcifications in the spleen. Calcification of the tortuous splenic artery is associated (arrow).

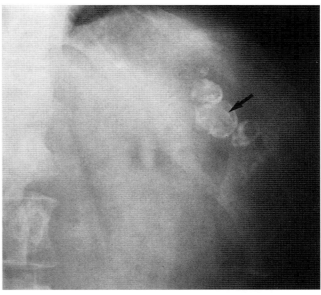

Fig. 27.**4** **Echinococcal cysts of the spleen.** Arclike calcifications (arrow) within the calcified mother cysts represent calcified daughter cysts.

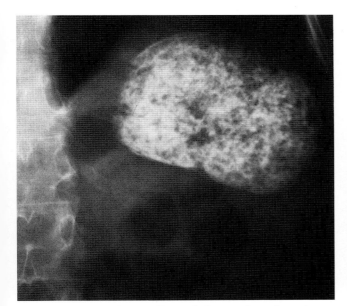

Fig. 27.**5** **Splenic infarct.** Diffuse calcification throughout the entire spleen after infarction.

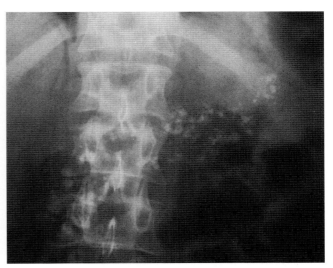

Fig. 27.**6** Pancreatic calcifications secondary to **chronic pancreatitis.** (Courtesy of Dr. Leena Kivisaari, Helsinki University Central Hospital.)

Table 27.1   (Cont.) Differential Diagnosis of Abdominal Calcifications

Site and Pattern of Calcification	Common Causes	Radiographic Findings and Comments
	Cystic fibrosis	Fine granular calcifications of the pancreas in a pediatric patient
	Kwashiorkor (protein malnutrition)	Typical calcifications of chronic pancreatitis in a young patient.
	Hemangioma or lymphangioma	May contain multiple phleboliths.
B. Cystic 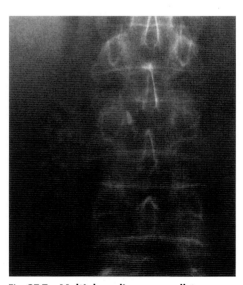	Pancreatic pseudocyst	A rim of calcification occasionally outlines the wall of the pseudocyst. Pancreatic lithiasis is usually associated.
C. Solitary	Cystadenoma Cystadenocarcinoma	10 % of these tumors contain radiographic calcification. Sunburst pattern of calcification is pathognomonic if present. Adenocarcinomas do not calcify.
	Hematoma	Intraparenchymal hemorrhage due to trauma, infarction, or a bleeding intraparenchymal aneurysm.
Calcifications in the biliary tract		
A. Calculous	Gallstone(s) (Fig. 27.**7**)	20 % of gallstones are radiopaque. They tend to have a dense outer rim of calcium salts. Renal calculus or an appendicolith in a long retrocecal appendix may project into the right upper quadrant, but can be differentiated on oblique films. Calculi in the bile duct may be difficult to appreciate and to differentiate from renal stones.
B. Cystic	Porcelain gallbladder	Extensive mural calcification of the gallbladder in chronic cholecystitis. There is a high incidence of gallbladder carcinoma, requiring prophylactic cholecystectomy.
C. Homogenous	Milk of calcium bile	High biliary concentrations of calcium carbonate secondary to chronic cholecystitis and obstruction of the cystic duct. Simulates a contrast-filled normal gallbladder.
D. Punctate	Mucinous adenocarcinoma of the gallbladder	A rare cause of localized fine granular calcification in the gallbladder.

(continues on page 637)

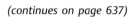

Fig. 27.**7**   **Multiple radiopaque gallstones.**

Table 27.1 (Cont.) Differential Diagnosis of Abdominal Calcifications

Site and Pattern of Calcification	Common Causes	Radiographic Findings and Comments
Calcification in the alimentary tract		
A. Calculous	Appendicoliths (Fig. 27.**8**)	A round, laminated enterolith, usually located in the right lower quadrant. Demonstration of an appendicolith in a patient with fever, leukocytosis and right lower quadrant pain is highly suggestive of acute appendicitis, likely a gangrenous one. May mimic gallstone or ureteral stone.
	Meckel's stone	An occasionally faceted enterolith is seen in Meckel's diverticulum, located low midline or in the right lower quadrant. May be complicated by inflammation, hemorrhage, or perforation.
	Rectal stone	Low midline enterolith with possible rectal symptoms or even fecal impaction.
	Diverticular stone	An enterolith within a colonic diverticulum
B. Cystic	Calcified mucocele of the appendix	A large crescent-shaped or circular calcification in the right lower quadrant. May displace the cecum.
	Calcified appendix epiploica	An infarcted appendix epiploica is seen as a cystic calcification adjacent to the gas-filled colon, most commonly in the ascending portion. May become detached and mobile.
	Mesenteric or peritoneal cysts	Especially chylous and hydatid cysts of the mesentery tend to have calcific walls.
C. Parenchymal	Mucinous adenocarcinoma of the stomach or colon	Small, mottled, or punctate calcifications of mucinous carcinoma occur predominantly in patients under 40.
	Gastrointestinal stromal tumor (GIST)	Calcium deposits occur in 4% of GISTs of the stomach, and even less commonly in the remaining gastrointestinal tract. A large lesion suggests malignancy.
	Mesenteric lipoma Omental fat necrosis	Rare causes of calcification in the alimentary tract.
D. Ingested material	Trapped nonopaque foreign bodies	They tend to have a ring-like appearance due to peripheral deposition of calcium.

(continues on page 638)

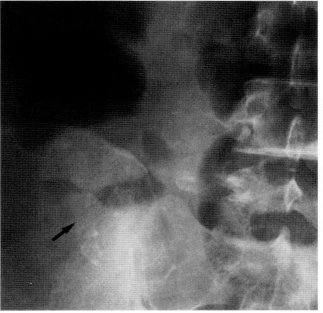

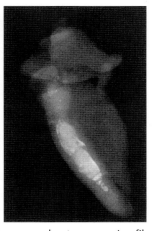

Fig. 27.**8 a, b** **Appendicolith. a** A tubular calcification of the right lower quadrant on a supine film (arrow). **b** Roentgenogram of the surgical specimen.

Table 27.1 (Cont.) Differential Diagnosis of Abdominal Calcifications

Site and Pattern of Calcification	Common Causes	Radiographic Findings and Comments

Calcification in the kidney
 	
A. **Nephrolithiasis** (Figs. 27.9, 27.10)
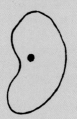
	Often idiopathic but commonly associated with:
	Chronic urinary infection
	Hyperparathyroidism
	Loss of calcium from bones due to immobilization, menopause, senility, or metabolic reasons
	Stasis of urine due to obstruction or neurogenic bladder
	Calcium phosphate stones are uniformly dense. They occur commonly in:
	  – Idiopathic hypercalciuria
	  – Idiopathic hyperuricosuria
	  – Hypercalcemic conditions
	  – Distal renal tubular acidosis
	Calcium oxalate stones are very dense. They occur in:
	  – Intestinal malabsorption, bypass
	  – Crohn's disease
	  – Primary hyperoxaluria
	Struvite (magnesium ammonium phosphate) stones are moderately opaque, often staghorn stones and occur often in:
	  – Persistent urinary tract infection
	  – Neurogenic bladder
	Cystine stones (slightly opaque) occur in:
	  – Cystinuria, seen in children and young adults, may form staghorns
	Uric acid stones are nonopaque. They occur often in:
	  – Gout
	  – Diet high in purines
	  – Rapid cell destruction (e.g., treatment of lymphoma)
		90 % of urinary calculi are sufficiently opaque to be seen on the plain film. Expiration and inspiration films help in correct localization of the calcification. Urate and matrix stones are radiolucent. Staghorn calculi form a cast of the pelvocaliceal system and tend to be relatively radiolucent.

(continues on page 639)

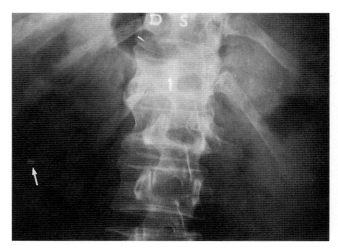

Fig. 27.**9 Caliceal stone.** The intrarenal location is shown with oblique projection.

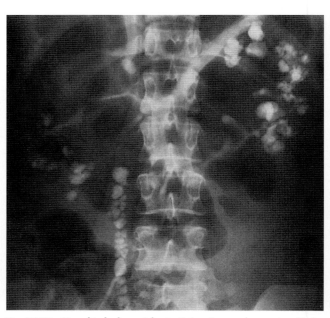

Fig. 27.**10 Renal tubular acidosis.** Extensive nephroureterolithiasis and renal parenchymal calcifications are seen.

Table 27.1 (Cont.) Differential Diagnosis of Abdominal Calcifications

Site and Pattern of Calcification	Common Causes	Radiographic Findings and Comments
B. Predominantly pyramidal nephrocalcinosis	Medullary sponge kidney (Fig. 27.**11**)	Small calcifications within cystic dilatations of the distal collecting tubules, bilateral in 75%, may involve a single pyramid only.
	Hyperparathyroidism (Fig. 27.**12**)	Small nodular or streaky calcifications in renal pyramids are seen in about 25%. Often associated with stones and bone abnormalities.
	Renal tubular acidosis: Primary (idiopathic) or associated with systemic diseases: Ehlers–Danlos syndrome, sickle-cell anemia, thyroiditis, primary hyperparathyroidism, vitamin D intoxication, idiopathic hypercalciuria, medullary sponge kidneys, toxic nephropathy, chronic pyelonephritis secondary to urolithiasis, and hyperoxaluria. (Figs. 27.**10**, 27.**13**)	Inability of the distal portion of the nephron to effectively secrete hydrogen ions to lower urinary pH. Nephrolithiasis and nephrocalcinosis occur in the majority of cases of primary renal tubular acidosis. Staghorn calculi are common.

(continues on page 640)

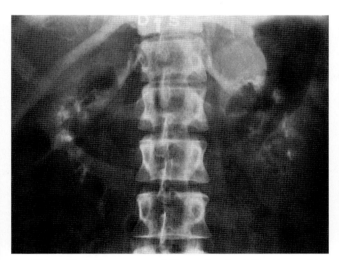

Fig. 27.**11** **Medullary sponge kidney.** Small calcifications within cystic dilatations of the distal collecting tubules are seen bilaterally.

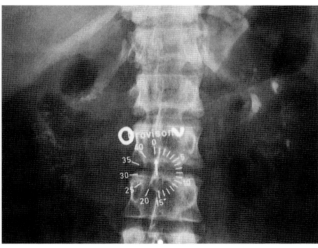

Fig. 27.**12** **Hyperparathyroidism.** Small nodular calcifications are seen throughout the renal pyramids bilaterally.

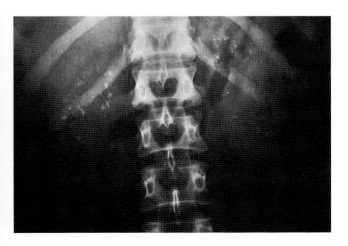

Fig. 27.**13** **Renal tubular acidosis.** Multiple small calcifications throughout the medullary portion of the renal parenchyma are seen.

Table 27.1   (Cont.) Differential Diagnosis of Abdominal Calcifications

Site and Pattern of Calcification	Common Causes	Radiographic Findings and Comments
	Skeletal demineralization secondary to: - Carcinoma metastatic to bone - Paraneoplastic hypercalcemia - Severe osteoporosis - Cushing's disease - Steroid therapy - Paget's disease	Metastatic bone destruction is common, but rarely causes nephrocalcinosis. Paraneoplastic hypercalcemia occurs especially in lung and kidney carcinomas. Immobilization may cause acute demineralization with hypercalcemia and nephrocalcinosis.
	Increased intestinal absorption of calcium in: - Sarcoidosis - Hypervitaminosis D - Milk-alkali syndrome	There is increased intestinal sensitivity to vitamin D in sarcoidosis resulting in increased absorption of calcium. Increased tubular load of calcium and phosphate causes nephrocalcinosis.
	Hyperoxaluria (Fig. 27.**14**): - Primary - Secondary to inflammatory bowel disease, intestinal bypass, or pancreatic insufficiency	Primary hyperoxaluria is a rare congenital disease in which urinary calculi and nephrocalcinosis occur early in childhood. Secondary hyperoxaluria results from increased intestinal absorption of oxalate, most commonly seen in Crohn's disease.
	Renal papillary necrosis secondary to: - Analgesic abuse (e.g., phenacetin) - Diabetes mellitus - Obstructive uropathy - Pyelonephritis - Sickle-cell anemia	A triangular radiolucency surrounded by a dense ring shadow is a characteristic radiographic finding. The pattern may vary and mimic renal tuberculosis or medullary sponge kidney. A detached papilla may form a renal stone. Uroepithelial carcinoma occurs with an increased incidence in analgesic nephropathy.
	DD: Persistent or increasingly dense nephrogram after contrast medium administration (Figs. 27.**15**–27.**17**)	In acute obstructive uropathy, acute tubular blockage (e.g., multiple myeloma, hemoglobinuria, myoglobulinuria, amyloidosis, proteinuria, hyperuricemia and drug-induced), shock (most often as adverse reaction to intravenous contrast material administration), acute tubular necrosis, acute pyelonephritis, early stage of *medullary cystic disease* (rare, usually familial disorder, presenting in adolescents and young adults, and eventually resulting in chronic renal failure) and *infantile (autosomal recessive) polycystic kidney disease* (bilateral glass renal enlargement with slowly increasingly dense striated nephrogram and poor visualization of the collecting system).
C. Predominantly Medullary	Renal tuberculosis (Fig. 27.**18**)	May produce single or multiple flecks of nephrocalcinosis, gross amorphous and irregular calcifications, or massive calcification of the whole kidney (autonephrectomy). There is a history of pulmonary tuberculosis years earlier in most cases.
	Chronic pyelonephritis	Radiographically demonstrable calcifications are rare unless associated with papillary necrosis.
D. Disseminated cortical calcification of kidneys	Acute cortical necrosis secondary to: - Shock - Toxic substances - Acute tubular necrosis - Acute pyelonephritis	Punctate or linear calcifications of the cortex occur within one month of the onset.
	Hyperoxaluria	Calcifications may involve predominantly cortex. See above.
	Hereditary nephritis (Alport's syndrome)	Recurrent microscopic hematuria, slowly progressive renal failure, and later often deafness. May be a disorder of basement membrane synthesis. Fully expressed only in males (X-linked penetrance) who usually die before the fifth decade.
	Chronic glomerulonephritis Dialysis therapy Polycystic disease Sickle-cell disease Fabry's disease Nail-patella syndrome (osteo-onychodysplasia)	These are rare causes of renal cortical calcification. *Fabry's disease*, or *angiokeratoma corporis diffusum universale* (accumulation of ceramide hexoside), is radiologically characterized by cardiomegaly with congestive heart failure and poor renal function.
	Calcified subcapsular hematoma	Linear calcification around the kidney, often associated with hypertension.

(continues on page 642)

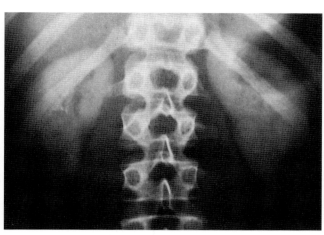

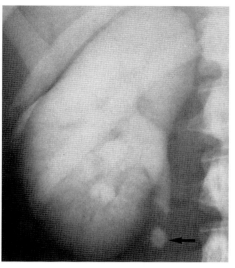

Fig. 27.14 Hyperoxaluria. Both kidneys are abnormally dense. The renal cortices are homogeneously dense and the pyramids contain dense calcific flecks.

Fig. 27.15 Acute obstructive uropathy. An increasingly dense nephrogram is seen 15 hours after contrast injection. Note the acutely obstructing calculus in the proximal ureter (arrow).

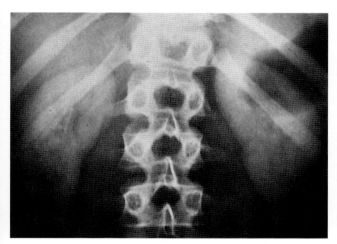

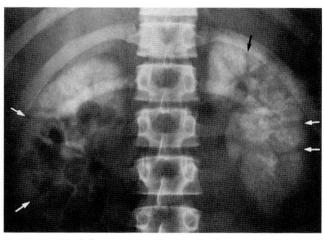

Fig. 27.16 Arterial hypotension secondary to severe contrast reaction. An increasingly dense nephrogram is seen 15 minutes after contrast injection in both kidneys, which had decreased in size when compared with the scout film. Note also the absence of contrast excretion.

Fig. 27.17 Medullary cystic disease (early stage). A striated nephrogram caused by contrast accumulation in dilated tubuli is seen 120 minutes after contrast injection. Note also that the striated nephrogram spares both the outer cortex and columns of Bertin, evident as radiolucent bands (arrows). The poorly opacified collecting system is not dilated.

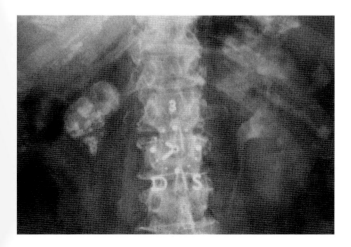

Fig. 27.18 Renal tuberculosis with massive parenchymal calcification of the shrunken right kidney. No excretion of contrast medium on the right side.

Table 27.1   (Cont.) Differential Diagnosis of Abdominal Calcifications

Site and Pattern of Calcification	Common Causes	Radiographic Findings and Comments
E. Focal parenchymal calcification of the kidney	Tuberculosis (Fig. 27.**19**)	May appear as a single nodular or irregular calcification (see above).
	Adenocarcinoma (Fig. 27.**20**)	About 10 % of renal adenocarcinomas calcify. If a renal mass contains calcium in a nonperipheral location, it is very likely malignant. Even a curvilinear cystic peripheral calcification of a mass does not exclude malignancy.
	Nephroblastoma (Wilms' tumor) (Fig. 27.**21**)	Cystic, streaky, or amorphous calcification of the tumor is uncommon, but may occur in older children and adults with nephroblastoma.
	Xanthogranulomatous pyelonephritis (Fig. 27.**22**)	Simulates carcinoma, but inflammatory masses may be multiple and diffusely calcified. A large pelvic calculus is present in the majority of cases, causing pelvocaliceal obstruction.

(continues on page 643)

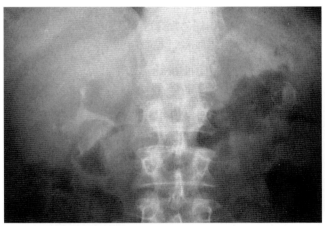

Fig. 27.**19   Renal tuberculosis** of the left kidney with focal calcification. The calcification appears cystic but internal calcifications are also present.

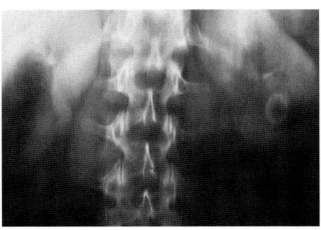

Fig. 27.**20   Adenocarcinoma** of the left kidney with calcification—a thick-walled, somewhat cystic calcification with irregular internal calcific deposits.

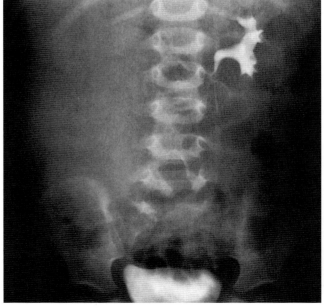

Fig. 27.**21   A large Wilms' tumor** in the right kidney of a three-year-old boy, seen as an enlarged, nonexcreting kidney containing tiny flecks of calcification.

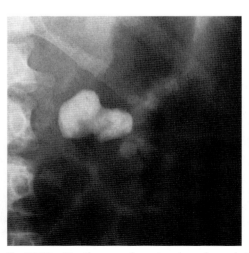

Fig. 27.**22   Xanthogranulomatous pyelonephritis.** Scout film shows pelvic stones and parenchymal calcifications.

Table 27.1 (Cont.) Differential Diagnosis of Abdominal Calcifications

Site and Pattern of Calcification	Common Causes	Radiographic Findings and Comments
F. Cystic (curvilinear) renal calcification	Simple renal cyst (Fig. 27.**23**)	A thin curvilinear calcification can be demonstrated in 3%.
	Adenocarcinoma (Fig. 27.**24**)	20% of thin curvilinear calcifications are due to a calcified fibrous pseudocapsule of a renal adenocarcinoma.
	Polycystic or multicystic disease (Fig. 27.**25**)	Curvilinear calcifications similar to that of a simple cyst may occur.
	Echinococcal cyst	The majority are calcified. Complete circumferential ring of calcium is characteristic but not always present.
	Organized perirenal hematoma (Fig. 27.**26**)	May appear as large cystlike calcification.
	Old perirenal abscess	
	Nephroblastoma (Wilms' tumor)	May appear cystic due to peripheral calcification.

(continues on page 644)

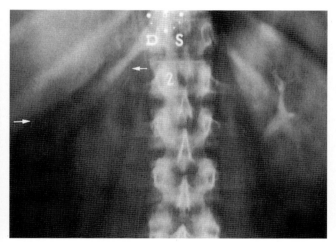

Fig. 27.**23** **Two calcified simple renal cysts** in the right kidney (arrows) are seen.

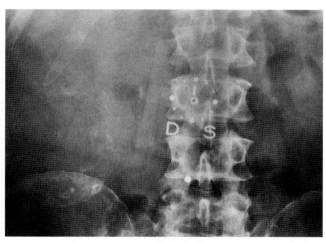

Fig. 27.**24** **Adenocarcinoma of the kidney.** Curvilinear calcification (with possible internal calcifications) in a large tumor of the lower pole of the right kidney.

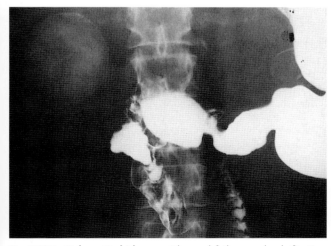

Fig. 27.**25** **Polycystic kidneys** with renal failure and calcification of the cyst walls bilaterally.

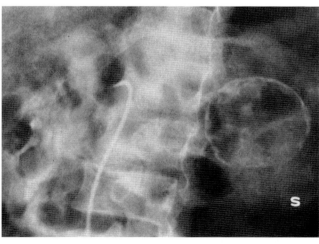

Fig. 27.**26** **Calcification of an organized perirenal hematoma** on the left.

Table 27.1   (Cont.) Differential Diagnosis of Abdominal Calcifications

Site and Pattern of Calcification	Common Causes	Radiographic Findings and Comments
	Renal artery aneurysm	A cracked eggshell-like circular calcification at the renal hilus is seen in about one third of renal artery aneurysms.
	Renal milk of calcium DD: Residual Pantopaque from prior cyst puncture and Pantopaque injection	Calcium-containing sediment in a cyst, caliceal diverticulum, or obstructed renal pelvis. Mimics calculus in supine films. In upright position calcific material gravitates to the bottom of the cyst.
Ureteral calcification	Ureteral calculus: Mostly idiopathic but the following conditions predispose: – Decreased mobility – Pre-existing ureteral obstruction – Metabolic diseases (see nephrocalcinosis) – Pre-existing infection – Postoperative ureteral stump DD: Phleboliths (round, located laterally, and commonly below the interspinous line)	Characteristically irregular, often oval, lodged at three levels: Ureteropelvic junction (large calculi) Pelvic brim Ureterovesical junction (small calculi) Stones less than 4 mm will eventually pass spontaneously in over 80%. 4–6 mm stones will be passed spontaneously in 50%, but often cause renal obstruction. Stones larger than 6 mm rarely pass spontaneously and have a high incidence of serious complications.
	Schistosomiasis	Tubular calcification of the distal ureter occurs in about 15% of patients.
	Tuberculosis (Fig. 27.**27**)	Ureter calcifies less frequently than the kidney and its appearance is variable. Ipsilateral renal calcification is often present.
Adrenal and retroperitoneal calcification **A. Triangular**	Neonatal adrenal hemorrhage	Occurs in infants born to mothers with diabetes and/or with an abnormal obstetric history. The periphery of the adrenal calcifies a few weeks after hemorrhage. Can be an incidental finding.
	Adrenal tuberculosis (Addison's disease)	In about a quarter of patients discrete, stippled densities outline the entire adrenal. Calcification can also be confluent and dense.
B. Cystic (curvilinear)	Adrenal cyst: – Lymphatic – Necrotic pseudocyst (Fig. 27.**28**) – Cystic adenoma – Echinococcal – Old hemorrhage (Fig. 27.**29**)	A thin rim of curvilinear calcification above the kidney.
C. Mottled mass calcification	Adrenal cortical carcinoma Pheochromocytoma (rare) Adrenal cortical adenoma (rare) Adrenal myelolipoma (a small mass of bone marrow and fat) (very rare)	Scattered flecks of calcification throughout the mass.
	Neuroblastoma	Calcification that is fine granular or stippled, rarely massive, occurs in about 50% of neuroblastomas. It is the second most common malignancy in children (after Wilms' tumor).
	Retroperitoneal teratoma	Calcified spicules of cartilage or bone are seen near the midline of the upper abdomen. Teeth inclusions may be identifiable.
	Retroperitoneal cavernous hemangioma (Fig. 27.**30**)	A large mass with multiple phleboliths.

(continues on page 646)

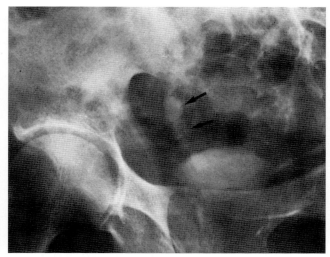

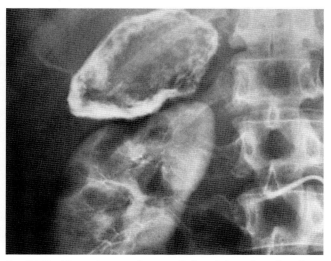

Fig. 27.**27 Tuberculosis of the right distal ureter** with characteristic ribbon-like calcifications (arrows).

Fig. 27.**28 Necrotic pseudocyst of the right adrenal.** A large cystic calcified mass, separate from the kidney, is seen.

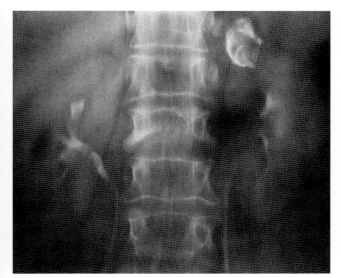

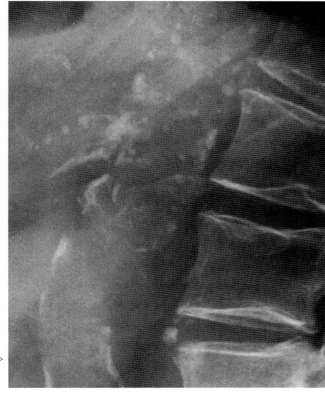

Fig. 27.**29 Calcified old adrenal hemorrhage** above the left kidney.

Fig. 27.**30 Retroperitoneal cavernous hemangioma.** Multiple ▷ phleboliths superimposed on the calcified and ectatic abdominal aorta and anterior to it are seen.

Table 27.1 (Cont.) Differential Diagnosis of Abdominal Calcifications

Site and Pattern of Calcification	Common Causes	Radiographic Findings and Comments
	Other retroperitoneal tumors (Fig. 27.**31**)	Calcification is extremely rare.
	Calcified lymph node(s)	One or more 1 to 1.5 cm dense, often coarse calcifications.
	Retroperitoneal hematoma Tuberculous psoas abscess	May present as a large calcification.
D. Longitudinal tubular calcification	Atherosclerosis	Sclerotic plaques of the aortic wall are common in the elderly. The aorta characteristically narrows toward the bifurcation. It may be curved and simulate an aneurysm.
	Abdominal aortic aneurysm (Fig. 27.**32**)	The walls of the aneurysm tend to calcify more than the normal aorta. Calcified plaques outline the aneurysm that most commonly occurs below the renal arteries, Oblique films can be used to avoid superimposition of the spine.

(continues on page 647)

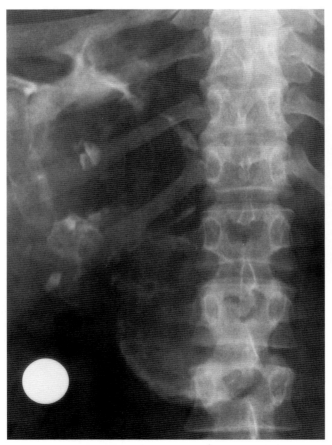

Fig. 27.**31** **Retroperitoneal teratoma.** A large calcified mass originating in the right retroperitoneum with extension into the subhepatic space is seen.

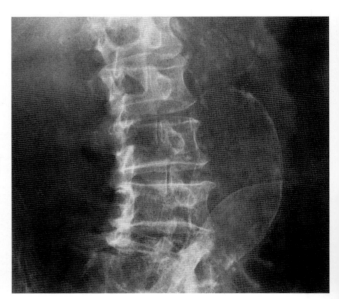

Fig. 27.**32** **Calcified abdominal aortic aneurysm.**

Table 27.1   (Cont.) Differential Diagnosis of Abdominal Calcifications

Site and Pattern of Calcification	Common Causes	Radiographic Findings and Comments
Pelvic calcification		
A. Tubular calcification	Arteriosclerosis	The aorta and the iliac arteries are frequently calcified and seen as irregular plaque-like densities. May be seen in young persons with diabetes.
	Vas deferens Associated conditions: Diabetes mellitus Tuberculosis Degenerative change (Fig. 27.**33**)	Bilaterally symmetric tubular densities that run medially and caudally to enter the base of the prostate, somewhat mimicking a medium-sized arteriosclerotic artery. Vas deferens calcification due to chronic inflammation (tuberculosis, syphilis) is intraluminal and has an irregular pattern.
B. Calcified bladder wall	Schistosomiasis (Fig. 27.**34**)	About 50 % of patients with schistosomiasis of the bladder have visible calcifications of the bladder, most apparent at the base. A linear opaque shadow may surround a relatively normal-sized bladder. A disruption in the continuity of the homogenous line of calcification is suggestive of a squamous cell carcinoma of the bladder, a common complication.
	Tuberculous cystitis	A rare cause of bladder wall calcification. Usually a faint calcified rim is seen in a contracted bladder, associated with calcifications in a kidney and ureter.
	Encrusted cystitis: nonspecific infection post-irradiation	A very rare cause of calcification of the bladder wall.

(continues on page 648)

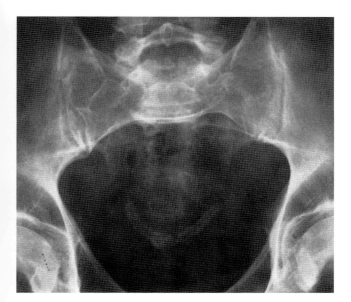

Fig. 27.**33** **Calcified vas deferens** in a 65-year-old patient, an incidental finding.

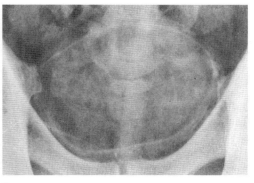

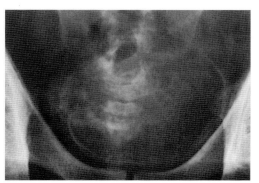

Fig. 27.**34 a, b** **a Schistosomiasis** of the urinary bladder. A linear calcified ring represents the bladder wall. **b** The same patient, two years later. The disruption of the right bladder wall calcification is virtually diagnostic for a complicating squamous carcinoma.

a

b

Table 27.1   (Cont.) Differential Diagnosis of Abdominal Calcifications

Site and Pattern of Calcification	Common Causes	Radiographic Findings and Comments
C. Calculi	Bladder calculi (Fig. 27.**35**) – migrated down the ureter – formed in the bladder secondary to obstruction or infection of the lower urinary tract or formed around a foreign body nidus	Usually circular or oval with variable internal structure. Small calculi may be confused with phleboliths in the vicinity of the bladder.
	Urethral calculi (Fig. 27.**36**) – migrant or primary	Midline stones usually in the subpubic angle. In males they are associated with urethral stricture, in females with diverticula and infection.
	Urachal calculus	An oval or dumbbell-shaped opacity is located anteriorly in the midline and superimposed on the sacrum. On cystograms, the upper portion of the bladder is pear-shaped and points toward the stone.
	Phleboliths	Phleboliths are calcified thrombi within a vein, present in most adults. Round, homogeneous or ringlike, most frequent in the lateral aspect of the pelvis. When seen in great quantity in a localized area, they are suggestive of a *hemangioma*.

(continues on page 649)

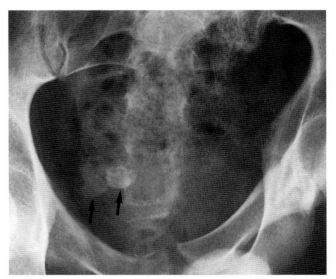

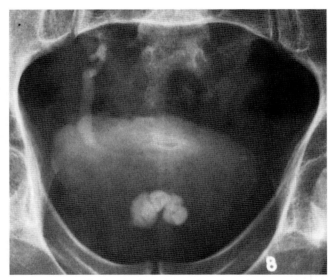

Fig. 27.**35**   **Bladder calculi** (arrows) in a young male (age 22) with trauma, prolonged immobilization and urinary tract infection.

Fig. 27.**36**   **Urethral calculi** in the proximal urethra. A male with gonorrheal urethral stricture.

Table 27.1　(Cont.) Differential Diagnosis of Abdominal Calcifications

Site and Pattern of Calcification	Common Causes	Radiographic Findings and Comments
D. Mass calcifications (stippled or conglomerate) in a female 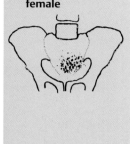	Uterine fibroid (leiomyoma) (Fig. 27.**37**)	The most common calcified lesion of the female genital tract. A mottled or "mulberry" type of calcification is characteristic.
	Ovarian dermoid cyst (Fig. 27.**38**)	About half of them contain calcification, either partial or complete teeth, or the cyst wall is calcified.
	Papillary cystadenoma or papillary cystadenocarcinoma of the ovary (Fig. 27.**39**)	Psammomatous calcifications of these tumors are scattered, and amorphous. They are easily missed on plain films. Implants in the peritoneal cavity may show similar calcifications, but may be mistaken for feces.
	Gonadoblastoma	Circumscribed mottled calcifications in the pelvis are frequent but the tumor is rare.
	Spontaneous amputation of the ovary	Probably the result of torsion and infarction of the adnexa. A small, coarsely stippled calcified mass in the pelvis that moves with changing positions.

(continues on page 650)

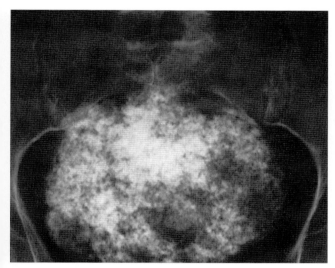

Fig. 27.**37**　**A large calcified uterine fibroid.**

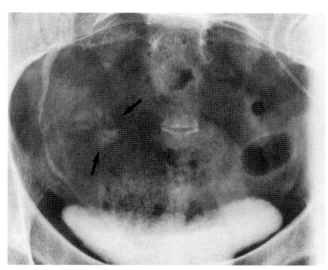

Fig. 27.**39**　**Papillary cystadenocarcinoma** of the right ovary detected as an incidental finding by observing the fine amorphous psammomatous calcifications (arrows).

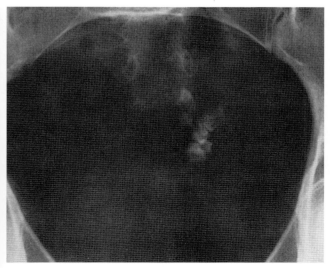

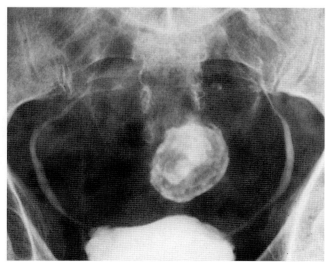

b

Fig. 27.**38 a, b**　**a Ovarian dermoid cyst** containing several teeth. **b** Ovarian dermoid with layered calcification.

Table 27.1   (Cont.) Differential Diagnosis of Abdominal Calcifications

Site and Pattern of Calcification	Common Causes	Radiographic Findings and Comments
	Pregnancy (Fig. 27.**40**)	Fetal bones may be seen
	Placental calcification	Occurs after the 32nd week of fetal life, has an average diameter of 15–20 cm and thickness of 3 cm. Calcification is greatest in the periphery.
	Lithopedion	Fetal skeletal parts are mixed with calcification. Can be intrauterine (old missed abortion) or extrauterine (previous ectopic pregnancy).
Mass calcifications (stippled or conglomerate) in a male 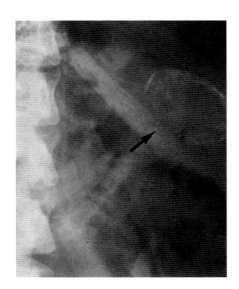	Prostatic calculi: – Primary (idiopathic) – Secondary to obstruction, stasis, or infection – Postoperative (in prostatic fossa, rare)	Frequent in men over 40. Discrete 2 to 4 mm calcifications may be present throughout the prostate or have a horseshoe or ring arrangement. Depending on the size of the prostate they may be seen above, behind, or rarely beneath the symphysis pubis. The most common cause of secondary prostatic calculi is a urethral stricture. *Prostatic tuberculosis* may cause an identical pattern. Postoperative stones are usually large and most common after an open prostatectomy.
	Seminal vesicle calculi	Very rare, variable in diameter, single or multiple.
E. Mass calcifications (stippled or conglomerate) in both sexes	Bladder neoplasm: – Transitional cell carcinoma – Squamous cell carcinoma (usually in schistosomiasis) – Mesenchymal tumors (rarely)	Calcification associated with a mass in the bladder usually indicates the presence of a bladder neoplasm. Tumor calcification can be punctate, coarse, or linear, and is often located on the surface of the tumor.
	Calcified lymph node	Represents old granulomatous infection and has a diameter of 1 to 1.5 cm. Calcification is usually coarser than in phleboliths or in calculi.
"String of pearls" calcification	Tuberculous salpingitis	May be bilateral in the female pelvis.
	Tuberculosis of vas deferens	Intraluminal calcifications may produce an irregular string of densities with a typical course.

(continues on page 651)

Fig. 27.**40** **Normal pregnancy** showing fetal bones. A calcified uterine fibroid, displaced into the left upper quadrant (arrow) is seen as an incidental finding.

Table 27.1 (Cont.) Differential Diagnosis of Abdominal Calcifications

Site and Pattern of Calcification	Common Causes	Radiographic Findings and Comments
Widespread abdominal calcification	Ovarian cystadenocarcinoma with abdominal metastases (Fig. 27.**41**)	Granular or sandlike psammomatous calcifications adjacent to the peritoneal fat stripe are characteristic.
	Pseudomyxoma peritonei (ruptured pseudomucinous cystadenoma of the ovary or mucocele of appendix)	Annular curvilinear calcifications may appear secondary to a foreign body reaction in the peritoneum.
	Undifferentiated abdominal malignancy	Variable forms of calcification may occur rarely.
	Tuberculous peritonitis (Fig. 27.**42**)	Mottled, widespread calcifications may simulate residual barium.
	Meconium peritonitis (Fig. 27.**43**)	Multiple small calcifications secondary to intrauterine perforation of the bowel.

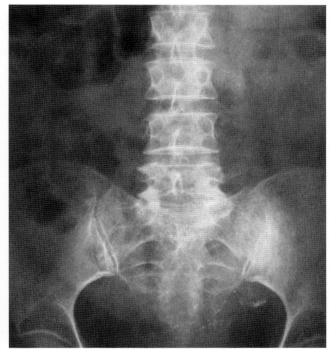

Fig. 27.**41** **Ovarian cystadenocarcinoma** with abdominal metastases. Faint granular psammomatous calcifications as demonstrated in the pelvis are seen throughout the peritoneal cavity.

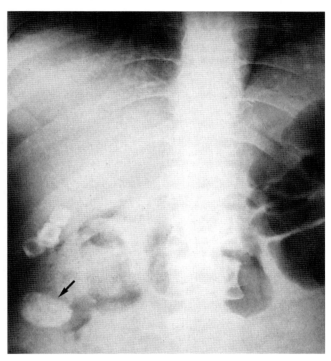

Fig. 27.**42** **Tuberculous peritonitis** (healed) with calcification (arrow). Gallstones are also seen on this film above the peritoneal calcification

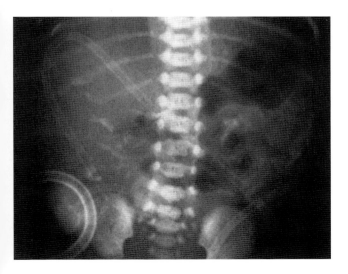

Fig. 27.**43** **Meconium peritonitis** with calcification secondary to ileal atresia. Widespread peritoneal calcifications are seen.

28 Abnormal Mucosal Pattern in the Gastrointestinal Tract

The mucosal pattern of the gastrointestinal tract is best evaluated with a double-contrast examination, i.e., gaseous distension and mucosal coating with a thin layer of high density barium.

The fully distended normal *esophagus* has a smooth mucosal surface (Fig. 28.1). As the esophagus collapses, the mucosal folds become visible as longitudinal, straight, and narrow folds (Fig. 28.2). Rarely, delicate transverse folds appear in the mid-esophagus. They may represent contraction of the muscularis mucosae. Abnormal mucosal patterns include nodularity, superficial ulcerations, and abnormal mucosal folds. They usually represent esophagitis or varices, rarely a superficially spreading carcinoma.

In a fully distended *stomach* with good mucosal coating, the areae gastricae (the faint reticular surface pattern [Fig. 28.3]) are often visible. The areae gastricae are most frequently seen in the antrum, and in some patients also in the proximal body and fundus. The normal diameter of the areae gastricae is about 2 to 3 mm in the antrum, somewhat larger in the body and fundus. The lack of visualization of the areae gastricae may be due to technical factors and is not necessarily indicative of disease (Fig. 28.4). An unusually coarse surface pattern may represent nonspecific inflammation (gastritis), intestinal metaplasia, or rarely, lymphoid hyperplasia of the gastric antrum. The coarse surface pattern is therefore indicative of a benign form of mucosal inflammation with questionable histologic specificity (Fig. 28.5).

In an incompletely distended stomach (Fig. 28.6) and in conventional barium examination, the rugal folds of the stomach are well demonstrated, but they will flatten after proper gaseous distension. Persistence of the antral folds despite adequate distension is almost always due to antral gastritis. Large normal rugal folds in the body and fundus may be difficult to distinguish from those infiltrated by tumor or those caused by dilated veins of the gastric wall. Abnormal folds tend to be stiffer than normal and therefore resist effacement or gaseous distension. Localized abnormalities of the mucosal pattern are usually due to erosions, ulcers, polyps, carcinoma, or lymphoma.

The surface of the *duodenal bulb* is smoother than that of the areae gastricae, representing the fine villous pattern of the duodenal mucosa. Nodularity in the mucosa of the duodenal bulb represents hyperplasia of Brunner's glands, duodenitis, or lymphoid nodular hyperplasia. Radial folds usually represent duodenal ulcer scars.

The major landmarks of the *duodenal loop* are the circular valvulae conniventes and the papilla (ampulla of Vater) with its associated longitudinal folds (Fig. 28.7). Deformation of valvulae conniventes should raise a suspicion of a postbulbar duodenal ulcer, Crohn's disease, or pancreatic disease, especially carcinoma. Thickened or nodular folds point toward duodenitis.

Flocculation of contrast agent may create problems in the interpretation of the *small bowel* mucosal pattern, especially in a single-contrast examination. A double-contrast examination with duodenal intubation enables the examiner to distend the whole small bowel. Combined with compression, this method makes it possible to study fold shapes

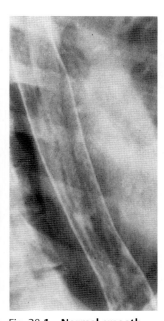

Fig. 28.**1 Normal smooth mucosal surface of the well-distended esophagus.**

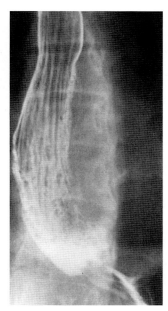

Fig. 28.**2 Longitudinal mucosal folds in the normal esophagus** appear when gaseous distension decreases.

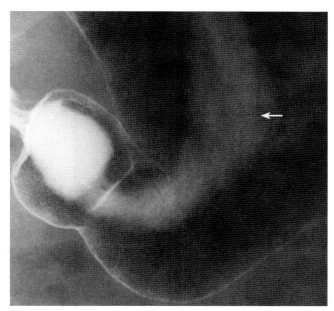

Fig. 28.**3 Normal surface pattern of a well-distended stomach** in double-contrast examination. The areae gastricae have a diameter of 2 to 3 mm in the antrum (arrow).

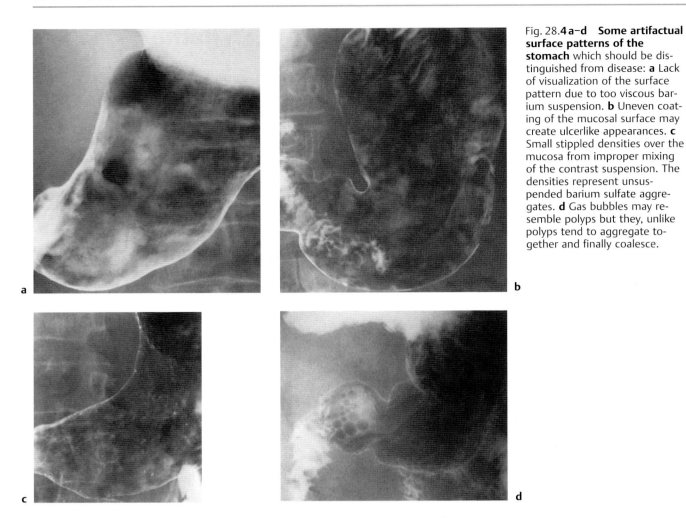

Fig. 28.**4 a–d** **Some artifactual surface patterns of the stomach** which should be distinguished from disease: **a** Lack of visualization of the surface pattern due to too viscous barium suspension. **b** Uneven coating of the mucosal surface may create ulcerlike appearances. **c** Small stippled densities over the mucosa from improper mixing of the contrast suspension. The densities represent unsuspended barium sulfate aggregates. **d** Gas bubbles may resemble polyps but they, unlike polyps tend to aggregate together and finally coalesce.

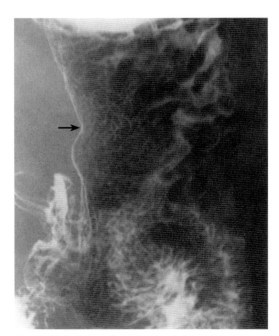

Fig. 28.**5** **Enlarged areae gastricae** (coarse surface pattern [arrow]), a sign of benign mucosal inflammation without histologic specificity.

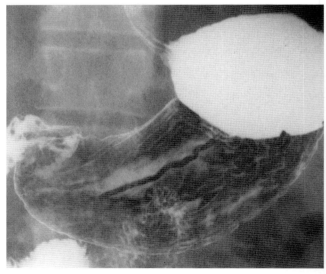

Fig. 28.**6** **Rugal folds** in a normal incompletely distended stomach.

more closely (Fig. 28.**8**). Valvulae conniventes are fewer and less pronounced in the ileum than in the jejunum. With the bowel distended, they run relatively straight across the long axis. Sometimes they may crowd together to create a triangular pattern, which has no diagnostic significance. Normal jejunal folds are about 2 mm thick, ileal folds about 1.5 mm thick. Fold thickness exceeding 2.5 mm in the jejunum and 2 mm in the ileum is considered to be pathological. Usually two to three folds are seen per centimeter in the jejunum and one to three folds in the ileum, depending on the degree of distension. The height of folds has little diagnostic significance. Numerous 2–3 mm rounded elevations, representing lymph follicles, may normally be present in the terminal ileum of children and adolescents (Fig. 28.**9**).

Abnormalities of the mucosal pattern of the small intestine include thickening of folds, with or without nodular appearances. These patterns can be combined with variable degrees of dilatation of the bowel and increase of intestinal fluid. The latter is often considered an unreliable sign, since technical factors may cause poor coating and flocculation of barium, mimicking increased fluid content. The diameter of an undistended, barium-filled small bowel is not more than 2.5 to 3 cm. In a duodenal intubation study, the diameter of the small bowel exceeding 4.5 cm in the upper jejunum, 4 cm in the mid-small bowel, and 3 cm in the distal ileum is considered abnormal.

Inflammatory bowel disease (e.g., Crohn's disease) and malignant tumors (with the exception of small bowel lymphoma) generally produce localized lesions (stenosis, dilatation, or ulceration) rather than diffuse mucosal abnormality.

In the *colon*, the mucosal pattern is best evaluated with double-contrast examination. The normal colonic mucosa is thin, smooth, and straight, essentially featureless except for the haustral markings (Fig. 28.**10**). A series of tightly spaced circular folds may be seen as a transient phenomenon in some patients, most frequently in children. The colonic mucosa may be studded with tiny nodules, 1 to 2 mm in diameter. They represent lymph follicles, and are usually unrelated to disease. Large, umbilicated lymph follicles may represent a response to infection, allergy, or an immunologic deficiency state. Such changes are rare in adults. Abnormal mucosal patterns are encountered in colonic polyposis, diverticulosis, ulcerative colitis, Crohn's disease, and other less common forms of colitis. Granular mucosa, ulceration and inflammatory polyps alone or in combination, and possibly associated with strictures and fistulas may be seen. Flocculation and cracking of the barium sulfate layer on the colonic mucosa represents drying of the suspension on the mucosa and the effect of peristalsis and should be distinguished from a true mucosal abnormality (Fig. 28.**11**).

In the *rectum* there are usually three prominent folds, called the valves of Houston. In a partially collapsed rectum, the columns of Morgagni may be seen in the distal portion. The surface pattern of the rectal mucosa is smooth, similar to that of the colon. Mucosal abnormalities of the rectum are seen in the same diseases which affect the colon. In addition, hemorrhoids may appear as tortuous or polypoid filling defects similar to esophageal varices.

Conditions associated with abnormal mucosal pattern in the gastrointestinal tract are presented in Tables 28.1 through 28.**5**.

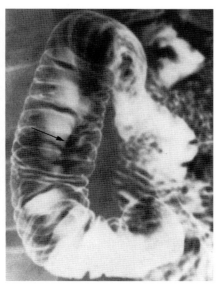

Fig. 28.**7** **Normal mucosal fold pattern of the duodenum.** The longitudinal fold in the posteromedial wall (arrow) is associated with the duodenal papilla.

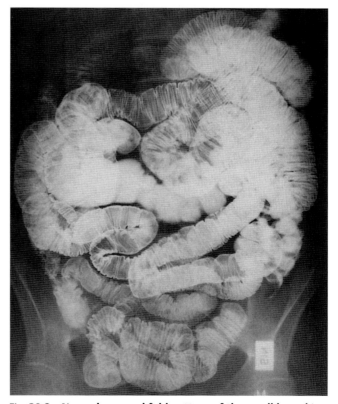

Fig. 28.**8** **Normal mucosal fold pattern of the small bowel** in a double-contrast study. The diameter of small bowel, fold thickness, and the number of folds all decrease from proximal jejunum to distal ileum.

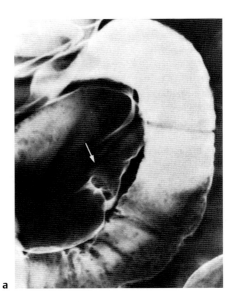

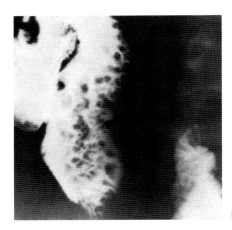

a

b

Fig. 28.**9 a, b   Nodular lymphoid hyperplasia. a** Lymph follicles. 2–3-mm-wide rounded elevations are seen in the distal ileum. The film also demonstrates a typical postappendicectomy deformity in the distal end of the cecum (white arrow). **b** Enlarged lymph follicles. Age 17.

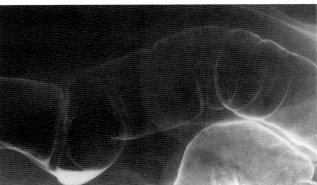

Fig. 28.**10   Normal mucosa of the colon.** Only haustral markings are recognizable.

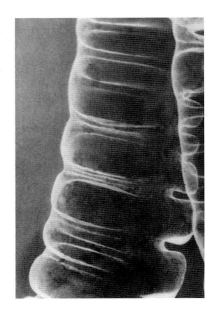

Fig. 28.**11   Flocculation and cracking of the barium sulfate layer** covering the large bowel mucosa. It should not be confused with a mucosal abnormality. This phenomenon increases with time as water is resorbed from the barium suspension.

Table 28.1   Abnormal Mucosal Pattern in the Esophagus

Disease	Radiographic Findings	Comments
Reflux esophagitis (Figs. 28.12–28.13)	Mild forms are radiographically negative. Earliest findings in double-contrast studies consist of streaks or dots of barium in superficial mucosal erosions, or of a diffuse granular or cobblestone pattern. In a single-contrast study, the mucosa is hazy or serrated, possibly with erosions or widened, edematous longitudinal folds.	Reflux may not be demonstrated during the examination. Predisposing conditions include hiatal hernia, prolonged or repeated vomiting, chalasia of infancy, pregnancy, scleroderma, drugs (such as anticholinergics, nitrites, beta-adrenergic agents, and tranquilizers), and esophageal or gastric surgery. Ulcer or stricture may be seen in more severe disease.
Infectious esophagitis (Figs. 28.14–28.16)	Small marginal filling defects with fine serrations may progress to an irregular cobblestone pattern, deep ulcerations, and sloughing of mucosa. Usually the whole esophagus is involved.	The most common cause is *candidiasis* affecting patients with malignancy (especially leukemia, lymphoma, or AIDS) or as a complication of radiation therapy, chemotherapy, corticosteroids, or other immunosuppressive agents. Diabetes mellitus, systemic lupus erythematosus, primary hyperparathyroidism, and renal failure are other predisposing conditions. *Herpetic* esophagitis usually produces an identical radiographic pattern. Rarely, *tuberculous esophagitis* or esophageal *Crohn's disease* may be the cause of a cobblestone pattern.

(continues on page 658)

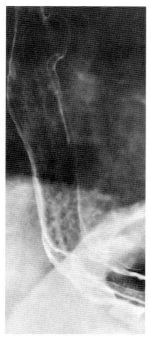

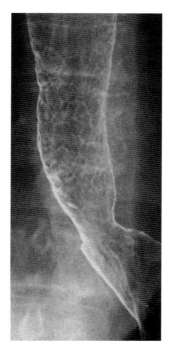

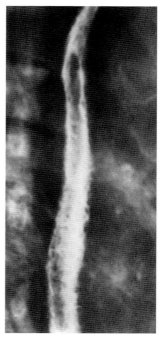

Fig. 28.**12** **Reflux esophagitis.** Thickened folds with irregular barium coating of the mucosa represent surface erosions. A traction diverticulum is demonstrated in the mid-esophagus.

Fig. 28.**13** **Reflux esophagitis** with a flat cobblestone pattern.

Fig. 28.**14** **Esophageal candidiasis.** In a patient receiving cancer chemotherapy. Multiple marginal filling defects and fine serrations are seen.

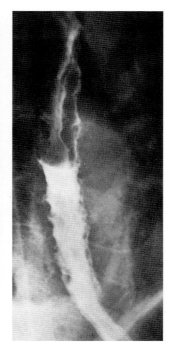

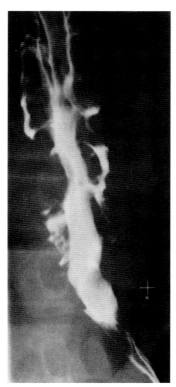

Fig. 28.**15** **Esophageal candidiasis.** Large filling defects and ulcerations as well as sloughing of the mucosa are seen.

Fig. 28.**16** **Esophageal candidiasis** in an AIDS patient. Severe mucosal edema with deep longitudinal ulcerations.

Table 28.1 (Cont.) Abnormal Mucosal Pattern in the Esophagus

Disease	Radiographic Findings	Comments
Esophageal carcinoma (with superficial spread) (Fig. 28.17)	Multiple nodular filling defects associated with impaired distensibility of the wall of the esophagus.	Nodular, submucosal spread is a rare manifestation of esophageal carcinoma. A mass lesion, ulcer, or local stenosis are more common manifestations.
Corrosive esophagitis	Mucosal edema and/or a diffusely granular pattern may be present in early phase.	Alkali tends to produce more severe esophageal injuries than acid. Mucosal ulceration is followed by gradual narrowing of the esophagus within a few weeks.
Radiation esophagitis	Serrations, small marginal filling defects, or a cobblestone pattern; identical to esophageal candidiasis.	Doses greater than 45 Gy frequently lead to severe esophagitis and stricturation. Even doses less than 20 Gy can cause esophagitis if combined with chemotherapy (especially adriamycin or actinomycin D therapy).
Leukoplakia	Small, superficial filling defects with somewhat poorly defined borders, usually in the middle esophagus. Peristalsis is not impaired.	Small round foci of epithelial hyperplasia. Usually found only in esophagoscopy, radiographic presentation is rare.
Acanthosis nigricans	Multiple verrucous proliferations throughout the mucosa, similar to skin changes. May produce a radiographic appearance of finely nodular filling defects.	A premalignant skin disorder characterized by papillomatosis, pigmentation, and hyperkeratosis, which may involve the esophagus.
Intramural esophageal pseudodiverticulosis	Numerous 1–3 mm outpouchings, mimicking multiple ulcers, but appear as a chain of beads. May be associated with a smooth stricture in the upper esophagus and/or candidiasis.	An extremely rare disorder of unknown origin with dilated ducts of the submucosal esophageal glands.
Esophageal varices (Fig. 28.18)	Initially mild thickening of folds and irregularity of esophageal outline, easily hidden behind complete filling with barium. Later tortuous, ribbonlike defects involve the distal esophagus. Early varices are generally situated in the right anterolateral wall of the distal esophagus.	Associated with portal hypertension including liver cirrhosis, superior vena cava obstruction and rarely with noncirrhotic diffuse liver disease or congestive heart failure. Small varices may mimic mild chronic esophagitis (thick folds). Pliability of the wall and the varices differentiates the condition from varicoid esophageal carcinoma.

(continues on page 659)

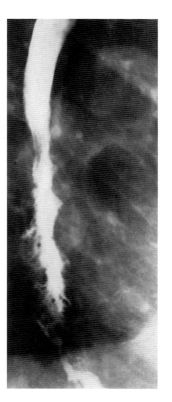

Fig. 28.**17 Esophageal carcinoma.** Filling defects and ulcerations in the narrow esophagus resemble severe esophagitis. The lesion is localized whereas esophagitis usually involves the whole esophagus.

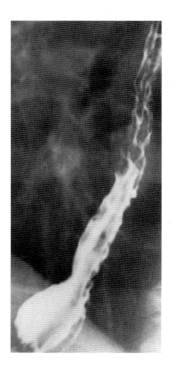

Fig. 28.**18 Esophageal varices.** Tortuous, smooth filling defects are pliable and involve the distal esophagus only.

Table 28.2   Abnormal Mucosal Pattern in the Stomach

Disease	Radiographic Findings	Comments
Normal variant **Hypertrophic gastritis** **Alcoholic gastritis**	Apparent thickening of the mucosal folds, which may be over 5 mm wide in the fundus and proximal body. The folds stretch evenly and appear thinned when the stomach is distended.	Thickening of folds is more common in association with gastritis than in normal population but transient gastritis (e.g., alcoholic) or so-called hypertrophic gastritis cannot be differentiated from normal variant radiographically. Histological evidence of gastritis is often present without radiographic abnormality.
Viral gastritis **(Fig. 28.19)**	Occurs in association with viral gastroenteritis, and is seen as a nonspecific thickening of mucosal folds.	Cytomegalovirus gastroenteritis may complicate AIDS and immunosuppressive therapy.
Antral gastritis	Thickening of mucosal folds is localized to the antrum. Often associated with lack of normal antral distension, asymmetric peristaltic waves, or mucosal wrinkling.	A controversial entity most likely representing one end of the spectrum of peptic ulcer disease.
Corrosive gastritis	Thickened gastric folds, mucosal ulcerations, atony and rigidity of the antrum and lower body.	Usually results from ingestion of acids or highly concentrated alkali.
Infectious gastritis	Thickened gastric folds, possibly gas in the wall of the stomach (if gas-forming organism).	May be associated with botulism, diphtheria, dysentery, typhoid fever, or anisakiasis.
Radiation gastritis	Thickened gastric folds followed by rigidity or luminal narrowing.	A diagnostic possibility if the patient has received more than 45 Gy to the upper abdomen.
Peptic ulcer disease	Thickening of gastric folds, increased gastric fluids despite fasting, and a peptic ulcer may be present.	The degree of enlargement of gastric folds in the body and fundus have a positive correlation to the level of acid secretion. Very prominent folds are characteristic of *Zollinger–Ellison syndrome*, in which ulcers of the distal duodenum are common.
Gastric scarring **(Fig. 28.20)**	Abnormal course of gastric folds, with or without fold enlargement. DD: Gastric carcinoma.	May be secondary to peptic ulcer disease, corrosive gastritis or trauma (surgery).

(continues on page 660)

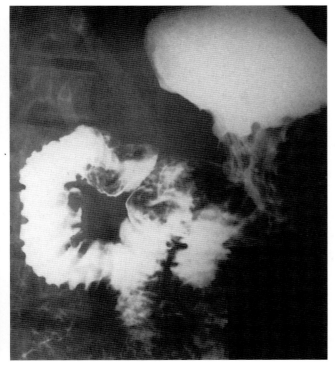

Fig. 28.19   Cytomegalovirus gastroenteritis in an AIDS patient. Gastric and small bowel folds are thick and irregular.

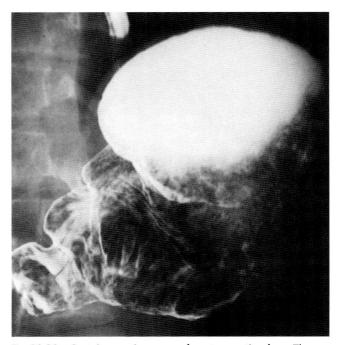

Fig. 28.20   Gastric scarring secondary to peptic ulcer. The gastric folds take an abnormal course and the involved area appears rigid, mimicking carcinoma.

Table 28.2   (Cont.) Abnormal Mucosal Pattern in the Stomach

Disease	Radiographic Findings	Comments
Ménétrier's disease	Massive enlargement of irregular rugal folds, particularly in the greater curvature. Folds may mimic polyps. Excessive mucus may produce mottled mucosal surface.	Hyperplasia and hypertrophy of the gastric glands. May be the cause of a protein-losing enteropathy. Increased incidence of adenocarcinoma of the stomach.
Uremia (Fig. 28.21)	Enlarged rugal folds.	Uremia is often associated with enlargement of gastric and duodenal folds, although not as extensive as in Ménétrier's disease.
Gastric lymphoma (Fig. 28.22)	Thickening, distortion, or nodularity of gastric rugal folds. Often associated with a polypoid and ulcerated lesions, a retrogastric mass, or an enlarged spleen.	May mimic Ménétrier's disease, but often involves also the distal portion of the stomach, the lesser curvature, and even duodenum.
Pseudolymphoma	Enlarged gastric rugal folds, often associated with a large gastric ulcer.	A benign proliferation of lymphoid tissue that can be mistaken histologically for malignant lymphoma.
Gastric carcinoma	Enlarged, tortuous, and coarse gastric folds simulating lymphoma are an unusual presentation of gastric carcinoma. Colloid carcinoma and mucinous adenocarcinoma may contain punctate calcifications (psammoma bodies). A polypoid gastric cancer may have a surface pattern comparable to surrounding areae gastricae, if only the submucosa is involved.	Due to variable radiographic patterns of gastric carcinoma, all mucosal abnormalities require endoscopic verification.
Gastric varices (Fig. 28.23)	Multiple, pliable, smooth, lobulated filling defects in the fundus projecting between curvilinear, crescenting collections of barium. Concomitant esophageal varices are common. May involve the lesser curvature, unlike Ménétrier's disease. Varices do not cause wall rigidity as does malignancy.	Associated with *portal hypertension*. Gastric varices without esophageal varices indicate isolated splenic vein occlusion (e.g., *pancreatitis* or *pancreatic carcinoma*).
Eosinophilic gastritis	Thickening of folds usually in the distal half of the stomach.	A rare diffuse infiltration of the rugal folds by eosinophilic leukocytes associated with blood eosinophilia.
Granulomatous disease, amyloidosis	Rugal enlargement may precede antral narrowing and rigidity.	A rare presentation of *Crohn's disease, sarcoidosis, tuberculosis, syphilis,* or amyloidosis.
Pancreatitis	Selective prominence of the mucosal folds of the posterior wall and the lesser curvature.	Becomes evident a few days after clinical onset of pancreatitis and returns to normal when clinical symptoms improve. Not present in mild pancreatitis.
Pancreatic carcinoma	Enlarged folds predominantly in the greater curvature may be seen.	Caused by direct metastatic invasion.
Gastric polyposis (hyperplastic polyposis, familial adenomatous polyposis, Gardner's syndrome, Peutz–Jeghers syndrome, Canada–Cronkhite syndrome, Cowden's disease) (Fig. 28.24)	Multiple polypoid filling defects in the gastric mucosa, often associated with polyposis in the colon. Hyperplastic polyps are small (less than 1 cm) and uniform in size. Adenomatous polyps tend to be larger (over 2 cm).	Multiple hyperplastic polyps may result from excessive regeneration of the epithelium in chronic gastritis. Numerous small polyps of the stomach are found in patients with familial adenomatous polyposis of the colon and in Gardner's syndrome (polyposis and osteomas), Peutz–Jeghers syndrome (hamartomatous polyposis of small bowel and mucocutaneous pigmentation), Canada–Cronkhite syndrome (diarrhea, alopecia, atrophy of the nails, skin pigmentation, and diffuse gastrointestinal polyposis). Cowden's disease is characterized by multiple hamartomatous polyps, circumoral papillomatosis, and nodular gingival hyperplasia. Filiform gastric polyposis is a rare presentation of *Crohn's disease*.

(continues on page 662)

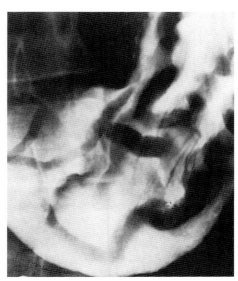

Fig. 28.**21**   **Uremia.** Hypertrophic, irregular gastric folds are seen.

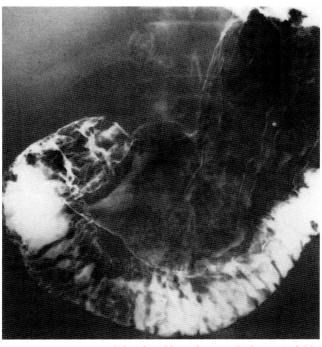

Fig. 28.**22**   **Gastric and duodenal lymphoma.** Thick gastric folds, do not efface even with good gaseous distension. The surface pattern is coarse and irregular.

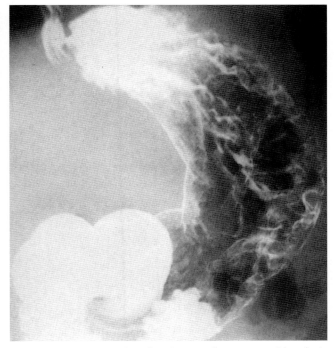

Fig. 28.**23**   **Gastric varices** (carcinoma of pancreas with splenic vein thrombosis). Smooth, enlarged gastric folds in the body and fundus of the stomach are seen. The gastric wall is not rigid. There is no evidence of esophageal varices.

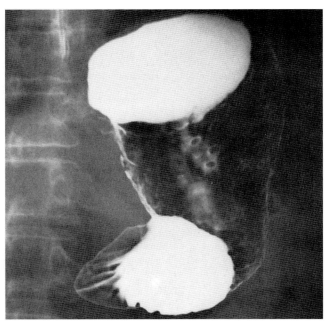

Fig. 28.**24**   **Gastric polyposis.** Multiple polypoid filling defects in the gastric mucosa.

Table 28.2 (Cont.) Abnormal Mucosal Pattern in the Stomach

Disease	Radiographic Findings	Comments
Enlarged areae gastricae (Fig. 28.25, Fig. 28.5)	A coarse surface pattern caused by prominent areae gastricae.	Associated with nonspecific inflammation, intestinal metaplasia, or benign lymphoid hyperplasia.
Erosive gastritis (Fig. 28.25)	Tiny flecks of barium representing erosion, surrounded by a radiolucent halo representing a mound of edematous mucosa. May not be seen in single-contrast examination. Incomplete erosions may not have surrounding reaction and tend to remain undetected.	May be "idiopathic" or associated with predisposing conditions (e.g., alcohol, anti-inflammatory drugs, analgesics, emotional stress). Aphthoid ulcers of Crohn's disease or candidiasis may have an identical appearance.

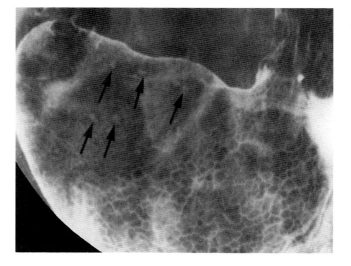

Fig. 28.**25** **Erosive gastritis.** The erosions are seen as tiny flecks of barium surrounded by a radiolucent halo. The surface pattern is coarse (enlarged areae gastricae).

Table 28.3   Abnormal Mucosal Pattern in the Duodenum

Disease	Radiographic Findings	Comments
Brunner's gland hyperplasia	Multiple nodular filling defects or nodular thickening of folds in the duodenal bulb and in the proximal half of the second segment of the duodenum.	Probably represents a response of the duodenal mucosa to peptic ulcer disease.
Benign lymphoid hyperplasia (see Fig. 28.9)	Innumerable tiny nodular defects evenly scattered throughout the duodenum without wall rigidity.	Proliferation of lymphoid aggregates without known cause or associated with hypogammaglobulinemia.
Peptic ulcer disease	Duodenal fold thickening may represent mucosal edema or diffuse hyperplasia of Brunner's glands (nodular thickening).	If associated with enlarged gastric rugal folds and distal ulcerations of the duodenum, one should consider *Zollinger–Ellison syndrome* (non-beta islet cell tumor of pancreas with elevated gastric secretion).
Pancreatitis	Edematous thickened folds in the periampullary region and proximal descending duodenum.	Similar changes can be associated with other types of adjacent periduodenal inflammation, e.g., *cholecystitis*.
Uremia	Irregular, swollen, and stiffened folds in the duodenal bulb and second portion of the duodenum. High incidence of hyperplastic polyps in the same area.	Fold thickening may simulate changes caused by pancreatitis, a frequent complication of uremia.
Crohn's disease	The early lesions consist of superficial erosions, aphthoid ulcers and fold thickening, usually in the bulb and proximal second segment. Later findings consist of narrowing and scarring.	Duodenal involvement has been reported in 1 % to over 20 % of patients with Crohn's disease. Similar changes occur rarely in duodenal *tuberculosis* and *strongyloidiasis*.
Giardiasis (Fig. 28.26)	Nodular thickening and edema of duodenal and jejunal folds. Increased secretions.	A bizarre pattern of nodular fold thickening in the duodenum may represent an early stage of *nontropical sprue*.
Lymphoma (Fig. 28.27)	Coarse, nodular, irregular folds, with or without mass lesions.	A mass lesion is a more common presentation.
Pancreatic carcinoma	May cause localized nodular impressions and thick folds due to impaired lymph drainage.	*Metastases to peripancreatic lymph nodes* can produce a similar appearance.

(continues on page 664)

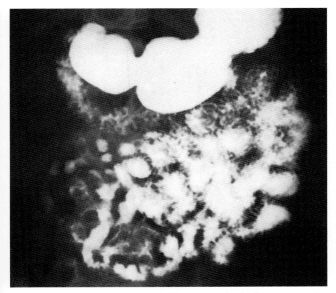

Fig. 28.**26** **Giardiasis** in a child. Mucosal thickening in the duodenum and proximal jejunum with increased secretions seen as poor coating of the mucosa.

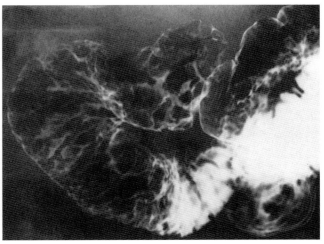

Fig. 28.**27** **Lymphoma.** Coarse, nodular, irregular folds of the duodenal sweep and large, smooth nodular filling defects in the duodenal bulb.

Table 28.3 (Cont.) Abnormal Mucosal Pattern in the Duodenum

Disease	Radiographic Findings	Comments
Whipple's disease Amyloidosis Mastocytosis Eosinophilic enteritis Intestinal lymphangiectasia	Thickening of duodenal folds in association with diffuse small bowel disease.	See Table 28.**4**.
Vascular impressions (duodenal varices, mesenteric arterial collaterals)	Small varices or enlarged arteries may cause a diffuse polypoid or serpiginous mucosal pattern, mimicking fold thickening or Brunner's gland hyperplasia.	Varices are secondary to portal hypertension. Esophageal varices are usually present. True mucosal fold thickening may be present due to venous congestion. Collateral circulation through the gastroduodenal and pancreaticoduodenal arteries is caused by mesenteric arteriosclerotic occlusive disease.
Duodenal hemorrhage	"Stacked coins" appearance of mucosal fold thickening, associated with an intramural mass.	May be a complication of trauma to the upper abdomen or caused by anticoagulant therapy.
Cystic fibrosis	Thickened, coarse, proximal duodenal folds, often associated with nodular indentations and distorted contour of the duodenal sweep.	The cause of these changes is not known.
Erosive duodenitis	Central collections of barium surrounded by a radiolucent halo, most frequently seen in the duodenal bulb.	Erosive changes are only demonstrated by double contrast technique. Erosive, hemorrhagic duodenitis may be associated with a *duodenal ulcer* or be a complication of *myocardial infarction* or *congestive heart failure*.
Duodenal polyposis	Multiple polypoid filling defects in the duodenal mucosa associated with polyps elsewhere in the intestine.	Duodenal polyposis may occur in association with gastrointestinal polyposis syndromes (see Table 28.**5**). Polypoid mucosal hyperplasia in the proximal duodenum occurs frequently in association with uremia.

Table 28.4   Abnormal Mucosal Pattern in the Small Bowel

Disease	Radiographic Findings	Comments
A. Thickened Folds and Small Bowel Dilatation		
Ischemic bowel disease	Dilated bowel with thickening of the mucosal folds due to edema and/or hemorrhage. A plain film may show an ileus pattern.	May be caused by venous insufficiency, thromboembolic disease, or hypoperfusion due to atherosclerosis or low cardiac output. Bowel dilatation without thickening of mucosal folds is a less common presentation.
Metastases Crohn's disease Tuberculosis Radiation enteritis	Dilatation of small bowel that shows thickened folds and edema (secondary lymphangiectasia). May lead to bowel obstruction.	Involvement of the mesentery results in this pattern.
Zollinger–Ellison syndrome	Proximal jejunal dilatation, fold thickening, and increased fluid content with large gastric folds and ulcers in atypical locations. Distal jejunum and ileum are normal.	Acid secretions produce chemical enteritis. 50% of gastrin-secreting tumors are malignant. May be associated with *multiple endocrine adenomatosis*.
B. Thickened Folds and Gastric Involvement		
Lymphoma	Thick, irregular, or distorted folds in the small bowel with or without separation of small bowel loops. Large gastric folds with intraluminal masses, ulceration, or nodular lesions.	Small bowel dilatation may occur in advanced disease.
Ménétrier's disease with hypoproteinemia	Thickened, regular small bowel folds associated with massively enlarged gastric folds. Increased intestinal fluid content.	Extensive protein loss from the stomach may create hypoproteinemia and small bowel changes similar to those seen in cirrhosis and ascites.
Eosinophilic gastroenteritis	Thick, regular, distorted, or nodular folds in the proximal small bowel associated with thickened antral folds, antral narrowing, and occasionally ulcers. Rigidity of the wall may mimick carcinoma or Crohn's disease.	Diffuse small bowel involvement alone occurs as well. Eosinophilia is common. Symptoms and signs follow the ingestion of specific foods.
Zollinger–Ellison syndrome	Enlarged gastric folds and ulcers. Thickened small bowel folds. Increased fluid content.	Proximal small bowel dilatation is often present.
Crohn's disease	A broad spectrum of small bowel abnormalities (ulceration, fold thickening, cobblestoning, strictures, fistulas) may be associated with antral rigidity and deformity mimicking gastric carcinoma	Crohn's disease in the distal ileum is almost always present.
Cirrhosis	Prominent gastric rugae or nodular fundal masses in association with regular thickening of small bowel folds.	Seen in patients with severe liver disease and hypoproteinemia. Esophageal varices are usually present.
Intestinal amyloidosis Whipple's disease	Thickened folds both in the stomach and small bowel, possibly with antral narrowing.	Intestinal amyloidosis may be associated with nonspecific immunoglobulin abnormalities. Both are rare causes of combined gastric and small bowel involvement.
C. Thickened Irregular Folds		
Hemorrhagic bowel disease	Usually localized, regular thickening of small bowel folds with sharply delineated margins ("stack of coins" appearance). Scalloping and thumb printing may be present. The radiographic pattern varies according to the clinical course.	Associated with several conditions including: *Ischemic bowel disease* (atherosclerosis, infarction, trauma, radiation endarteritis) *Vasculitis* (connective tissue diseases, thromboangiitis obliterans, Henoch–Schönlein purpura) *Hemophilia* *Idiopathic thrombocytopenic purpura* (acute in children) *Trauma* *Secondary coagulation defects* (liver disease, leukemia, lymphoma, multiple myeloma, metastatic carcinoma, anticoagulant therapy)

(continues on page 666)

Table 28.4   (Cont.) Abnormal Mucosal Pattern in the Small Bowel

Disease	Radiographic Findings	Comments
Intestinal edema (Fig. 28.28)	Regular thickening of several or all small bowel folds with increased intestinal fluid (flocculation, dilution, poor coating).	The most common cause is *hypoproteinemia* with the albumin level below 2 g/100 ml. Causes of hypoproteinemia include liver cirrhosis, nephrotic syndrome, protein-losing enteropathies (such as Ménétrier's disease, Crohn's disease, Whipple's disease, lymphoma, carcinoma, ulcerative colitis or intestinal lymphangiectasia, constrictive pericarditis, burns, and allergic reactions). *Lymphatic blockage* by tumor or radiation and *angioneurotic edema* are other causes of intestinal edema. Angioneurotic edema tends to cause more localized changes, which rapidly revert to normal.
Intestinal lymphangiectasia (Fig. 28.28)	Regular thickening of mucosal folds due to intestinal edema (see above) and lymphatic dilatation.	*Primary*: Congenital lymphatic blockage; usually a young patient with no evidence of liver, kidney, or heart disease. *Secondary*: A complication of inflammatory or neoplastic lymphadenopathy.
Abetalipoproteinemia	Mucosal fold thickening is most marked in the duodenum and jejunum. Small bowel dilatation, irregularity of folds or even nodular folds may occur.	A rare recessively inherited disease manifested by malabsorption of fat, progressive neurologic deterioration and retinitis pigmentosa. Jejunal biopsy is diagnostic.
Eosinophilic enteritis Amyloidosis Pneumatosis intestinalis	True or apparent regular thickening of mucosal folds may be a feature in these conditions.	Irregular, distorted folds are a more common presentation of eosinophilic enteritis. Radiolucent gas cysts are diagnostic of pneumatosis intestinalis.
D. Irregular Folds without Small Bowel Dilatation		
Whipple's disease (Fig. 28.29)	Extensive thickening and distortion of folds is seen predominantly in the duodenum and jejunum.	Infiltration of the lamina propria by large periodic acid–Schiff stain positive macrophages and Gram-positive bacilli. Diarrhea, arthritis, fever, and lymphadenopathy are common. Jejunal biopsy is diagnostic.
Giardiasis (see Fig. 28.26)	Irregular, distorted, thickened mucosal folds in the duodenum and jejunum. Hypersecretion and hypermotility of the bowel is common. Associated nodular lymphoid hyperplasia points towards an underlying immunodeficiency state.	Symptomatic (gastroenteritis, cramping, malabsorption) usually found in children, post-gastrectomy patients, travelers to endemic areas, and patients with gastrointestinal immunodeficiency. Cysts in the stool or a jejunal smear demonstrating *Giardia lamblia* are diagnostic.
Lymphoma	Thickening or obliteration of mucosal folds. Segmental constrictions, ulcers, or polypoid masses may occur. May be localized to one or several segments or diffusely involve most of the small bowel. Most frequent in the ileum.	May represent *primary* intestinal lymphoma or be a manifestation of a disseminated lymphomatous process that affects many organs (*secondary*). Primary intestinal lymphoma may be a complication of sprue.
Amyloidosis (Fig. 28.30)	Sharply demarcated thickening of folds throughout the small bowel have either regular or irregular appearance. Jejunization of the ileum is characteristic. Nodularity and tumor-like defects may occur. Ulceration, intestinal infarction, or impaired peristalsis may also be evident.	Small bowel involvement occurs in at least 70% of cases of generalized amyloidosis, which can be either primary or secondary to a chronic disease (tuberculosis, osteomyelitis, ulcerative colitis, rheumatoid arthritis, multiple myeloma and other malignant diseases, familial Mediterranean fever). Rectal or jejunal biopsy are diagnostic.
Eosinophilic enteritis	Thickened, initially regular folds, which are most prominent in the jejunum, become irregular with more extensive disease. Bowel wall may have a saw-toothed contour and become rigid.	May simulate Crohn's disease radiographically, but peripheral eosinophilia and gastrointestinal symptoms related to ingestion of specific foods are characteristic.

(continues on page 668)

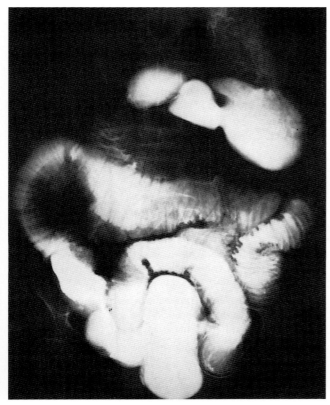

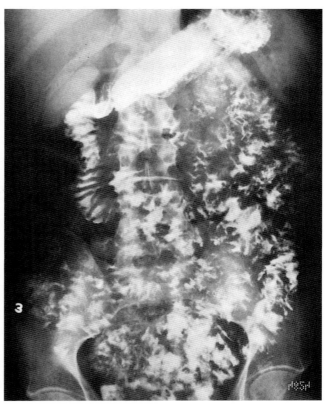

Fig. 28.28 Intestinal edema secondary intestinal lymphangiectasia. Regular thickening of mucosal folds, dilatation of small bowel loops, and increased fluid content of the small bowel are seen.

Fig. 28.29 Whipple's disease. Extensive thickening and distortion of the mucosal folds in the whole small bowel are evident.

Fig. 28.30 Amyloidosis. Sharply demarcated, thick small bowel folds and a few small nodules are seen, but the diameter of the small bowel is normal.

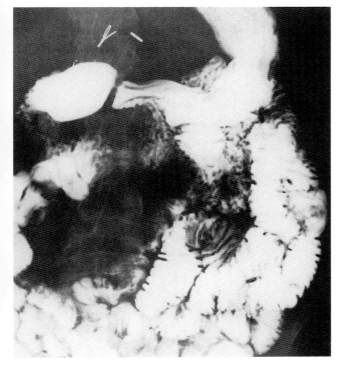

Table 28.4   (Cont.) Abnormal Mucosal Pattern in the Small Bowel

Disease	Radiographic Findings	Comments
Crohn's disease (Fig. 28.31)	The radiographic mucosal changes in their usual sequence of appearance are: - Irregular thickening and distortion of the valvulae conniventes. - Rough cobblestone appearance of the ulcerated, thick mucosa. - Rigid thickening of the bowel wall with narrowing of lumen and loss of mucosal pattern (string sign). The terminal ileum is most commonly involved, but diseased segments are commonly found also in other locations.	Other common radiographic findings include intramural tracking, separation of bowel loops, and fistulas. *Tuberculosis* may produce an indistinguishable pattern, but is usually localized in the ileocecal region only.
Mastocytosis (urticaria pigmentosa) (Fig. 28.32)	Generalized irregular, distorted, and thickened folds. Sometimes a diffuse pattern of sand-like nodules is present.	Mast cell proliferation in the reticuloendothelial system and skin. Lymphadenopathy, hepatosplenomegaly, peptic ulcer, and sclerotic bone lesions may be associated.
Strongyloidiasis (Fig. 28.33)	Irritability of bowel and irregular thickening of the duodenal and proximal jejunal folds, eventually the whole intestinal tract.	May be asymptomatic or mimic acute tropical sprue. Worms or larvae are detected in duodenal secretions.
Yersinia enterocolitis	Coarse, irregular thickening of small bowel mucosal folds is the most common finding, but nodular filling defects and ulceration producing a cobblestone appearance as in Crohn's disease may occur. The changes are usually localized in a short segment of the terminal ileum.	In children, Yersinia infection usually causes acute enteritis, in adolescents and adults an acute terminal ileitis or mesenteric adenitis is the usual presentation.
Typhoid fever	Irregular thickening and nodularity of the terminal ileum. The involvement is symmetric. Skip areas and fistulas do not occur.	An acute illness caused by *Salmonella typhosa* can be distinguished radiographically from Crohn's disease of the terminal ileum. Splenomegaly is common.
Alpha chain disease	Coarsely thickened irregular mucosal folds, possibly with nodules throughout the small bowel.	A disorder of immunoglobulin peptide synthesis causes in defective secretory IgA production, and results in diarrhea and malabsorption.

(continues on page 670)

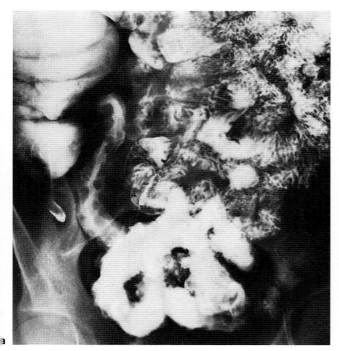

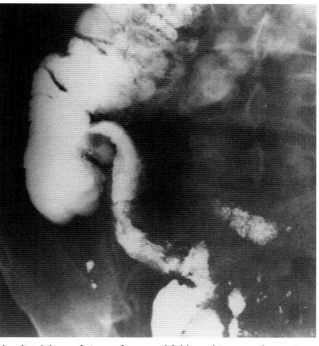

Fig. 28.**31 a, b   Crohn's disease. a** Irregular thickening, distortion and disappearance of valvulae conniventes. The distal small bowel wall appears rigid and thickened. Cobblestone pattern is seen in the distal ileum. **b** Loss of mucosal folds and increased secretions in the distal ileum of another patient.

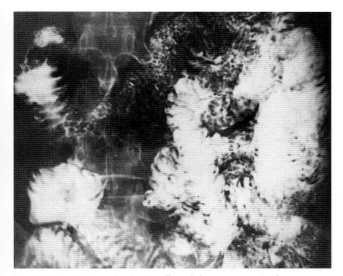

Fig. 28.**32   Mastocytosis.** Small nodules are seen in the mucosa. Mucosal folds are slightly irregular, and the duodenal folds are thick.

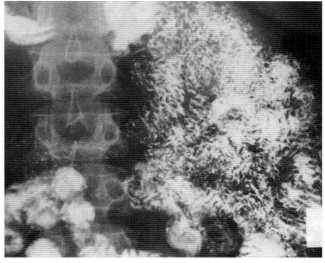

Fig. 28.**33   Strongyloidiasis.** Irregular, thickened mucosal folds are present in the jejunum.

Table 28.4   (Cont.) Abnormal Mucosal Pattern in the Small Bowel

Disease	Radiographic Findings	Comments
Radiation enteritis (Fig. 28.34)	Thickened and/or irregular folds, loss of mucosal pattern, separation of bowel loops, spasticity. Ulcerations and fistulas may occur.	Changes occur at the site of radiation therapy. They may mimic Crohn's disease.
E. Small Bowel Poly-posis		
Peutz–Jeghers syndrome	Multiple polyps (hamartomas) are seen throughout the small bowel and may occur elsewhere in the gastrointestinal tract.	This is the most common small bowel polyposis syndrome. Multiple gastrointestinal polyps are associated with mucocutaneous pigmentation. Hyperpigmentation of the buccal mucosa is characteristic. Increased incidence of adenocarcinoma of duodenum or jejunum and of ovarian cysts and tumors.
Gardner's syndrome	Multiple adenomatous polyps are occasionally seen in the small bowel, predominantly in the distal portion.	Diffuse colonic polyposis associated with osteomas, soft-tissue tumors (desmoids) and eventual colorectal carcinoma.
Familial polyposis	Multiple adenomatous polyps may be seen throughout the gastrointestinal tract.	Extraintestinal lesions of Peutz–Jeghers or Gardner's syndrome are absent. A very rare condition with a high risk of gastrointestinal carcinoma.
Juvenile gastrointestinal polyposis	Polyps (hamartomas) are present throughout the gastrointestinal tract.	If associated with alopecia, nail dystrophy, hyperpigmentation, and malabsorption, it is called the *Canada–Cronkhite* syndrome. The latter disorder presents in later life, unlike other juvenile polyposis syndromes.
Multiple hemangiomas	The combination of phleboliths and multiple filling defects in the small bowel is pathognomonic.	*Benign gastrointestinal stromal tumors (GISTs)* and *carcinoids* are very rarely multiple enough to produce a polyposis pattern.
Neurofibromatosis (Fig. 28.35)	Multiple small bowel neurofibromas have an eccentric distribution. They may mimic sessile or pedunculated polyps.	Café-au-lait pigmentation and cutaneous fibromas are characteristic.
Metastases	Multiple intraluminal or intramural filling defects characteristically have a target or bull's eye appearance.	The most frequent primary neoplasms are melanoma and carcinomas of the breast and lung. Other carcinomas and lymphoma may produce a similar pattern.
F. "Granularity" of the Small Bowel Mucosa		
Macroglobulinemia (Waldenström)	A sandlike radiographic pattern in the small bowel mucosa represents enlarged intestinal villi. The folds are not thickened.	A plasma cell dyscrasia with large amounts of IgM in the serum, anemia, bleeding, lymphadenopathy, and hepatosplenomegaly.
Nodular lymphoid hyperplasia	The bowel mucosa is studded with innumerable tiny polypoid masses uniformly distributed throughout the involved segment, usually jejunum. Enlarged and distorted fold pattern suggests associated giardiasis.	In children and young adults, lymphoid hyperplasia of the terminal ileum is a normal finding. Elsewhere in adults, it is almost invariably associated with a late-onset *immunoglobulin deficiency*. *Giardiasis* is common.
Histoplasmosis	A sandlike covering superimposed on irregular distorted folds.	The lamina propria is infiltrated by histoplasma-laden macrophages creating the appearance of granularity.
Intestinal lymphangiectasia Whipple's disease Yersinia enterocolitis (healing) Eosinophilic enteritis Mastocytosis	Sandlike pattern may occasionally be present in these conditions, but other radiographic features are more characteristic.	See above in this Table.

(continues on page 672)

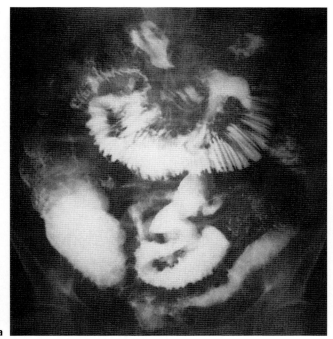

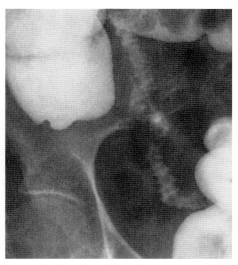

a

b

Fig. 28.**34 a, b**   **Radiation enteritis,** secondary to the therapy of a gynecologic tumor. **a** Thickening and irregularity of both small and large bowel mucosa; loss of normal mucosal patterns is most extensive close to the area of highest radiation dose. Thumb printing is seen in the sigmoid and cecum too. A fistulous tract is seen higher in the midabdomen from one loop of small bowel to another. **b** Smooth but thickened mucosal folds in the distal ileum in another patient with a similar history.

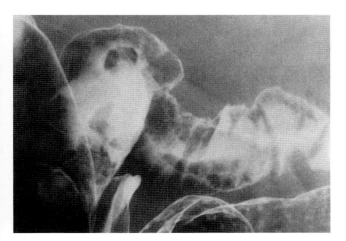

Fig. 28.**35**   Multiple polypoid filling defects in the distal ileum in a patient with **neurofibromatosis**.

Table 28.4 (Cont.) Abnormal Mucosal Pattern in the Small Bowel

Disease	Radiographic Findings	Comments
Mechanical obstruction **Adynamic ileus** **(Fig. 28.36)**	Increased caliber of the small bowel above the obstruction (or throughout in ileus). Increased fluid causes haziness, poor coating, and flocculation of barium suspension, but valvulae conniventes are normal.	For more detailed discussion of bowel obstructions, see Chapter **26**. In *chronic idiopathic intestinal pseudo-obstruction*, radiographic and clinical signs of mechanical obstruction are intermittently present without an organic lesion.
Vagotomy **Drugs**	Prolonged transit time and dilatation of the small bowel with normal folds.	Drugs that cause decreased smooth muscle activity include atropine, morphine, L-dopa and barbiturates.
Sprue **Celiac disease** **(Figs. 28.37, 28.38)**	The barium in the dilated small bowel has a coarse, granular, or hazy appearance due to increased bowel fluid. The contours of the jejunum are smooth, unindented due to atrophy and effacement of mucosal folds ("moulage sign"). Segmentation or flocculation of barium are unreliable signs of malabsorption.	Adult nontropical sprue (celiac disease), tropical sprue (infectious), and celiac disease of children are clinically and radiographically similar. The degree of bowel dilatation is related to the severity of the disease. Diffuse intestinal lymphoma may complicate longstanding sprue and cause thickening and distortion of mucosal folds.
Scleroderma **Dermatomyositis** **(Fig. 28.39)**	Dilated small bowel with normal-sized folds that are closely packed together. Extremely prolonged transit time. Dilatation is most prominent in the duodenum. Large broad-necked pseudosacculations (pseudodiverticula) in the antimesenteric border of the bowel are also characteristic. They are caused by mesenteric fibrosis which also pulls folds asymmetrically together.	Skin changes, joint symptoms, or the appearance of Raynaud's phenomenon usually precede changes in the small bowel. Scleroderma and dermatomyositis produce identical small bowel changes. These two entities can be differentiated from sprue by the absence of hypersecretion, and by the presence of pronounced duodenal dilatation and markedly delayed barium transit time.
Lactase deficiency	A conventional small bowel examination is normal but the addition of lactose into the barium suspension results in dilatation of the small-bowel, increased bowel secretions, and rapid transit.	A common enzyme defect resulting in watery diarrhea and abdominal discomfort soon after ingestion of milk products.
Ischemic bowel disease	Delayed intestinal transit and dilatation of bowel with increased intraluminal fluid.	Thickening of mucosal folds is commonly seen in acute conditions, but in chronic conditions (arteriosclerosis, connective tissue diseases, massive amyloidosis) the fold pattern may remain normal despite bowel dilatation.
Chagas' disease	Small bowel dilatation with normal folds.	Damage to visceral neurons may be the underlying cause. *Diabetes complicated by hypokalemia* may rarely be associated with small bowel dilatation.

(continues on page 674)

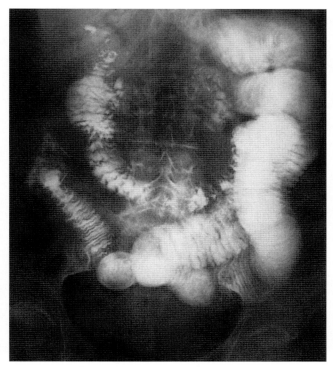

Fig. 28.**36** **Gallstone ileus.** Increased caliber of the small bowel above the impacted stone, and increased secretions, but the valvulae conniventes are normal.

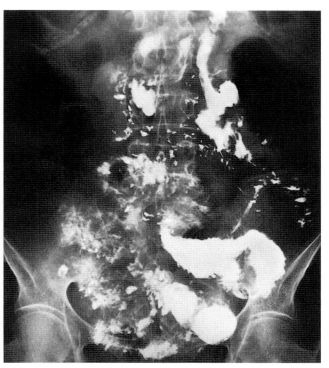

Fig. 28.**37** **Sprue.** Tubular appearance of several bowel segments with effaced mucosal folds is seen (moulage sign). Fragmentation and flocculation of the barium, and an increased amount of fluid in the bowel lumen are also present.

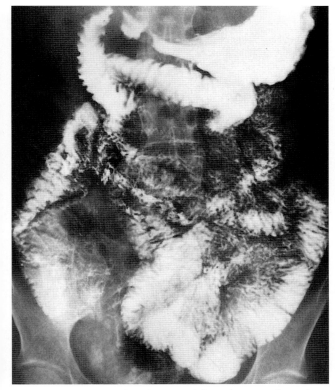

Fig. 28.**38** **Sprue.** In the absence of flocculation and moulage, with the modern barium suspensions, the small bowel loops appear dilated, have slightly thickened folds, and the increased fluid content causes dilution of the barium.

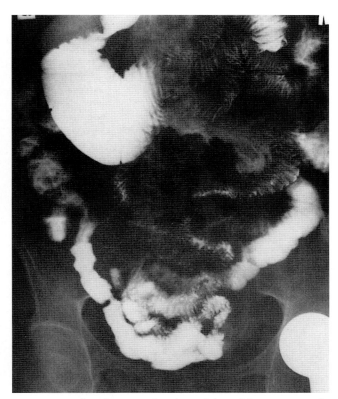

Fig. 28.**39** **Scleroderma.** Dilated small bowel loops, especially the duodenum. Normal-sized folds. Prolonged transit time.

Table 28.5   Abnormal Mucosal Pattern in the Colon and Rectum

Disease	Radiographic Findings	Comments
Ulcerative colitis **(Fig. 28.40)**	The appearance and sequence of mucosal changes depend on duration and severity: - Fine granularity of the mucosa in double contrast or haziness in single contrast (hyperemia and edema). - Stippled mucosal pattern in double contrast, serration or speculation in single contrast (superficial ulcers), which should be differentiated from transient pseudospicules (innominate lines). - Larger marginal ulcerations symmetrically around the circumference of the bowel wall ("collar button" ulcers). - Denuded flat mucosa, possibly with pseudopolyps. Filiform polyposis may occur, seen as thin, straight filling defects. - Shortening and rigidity of the colon ("lead pipe" configuration) combined with mucosal atrophy. - Loss of haustral markings alone is an unreliable sign. Involvement of rectosigmoid is characteristic. Inflammatory changes may occur in the terminal ileum ("*backwash ileitis*").	A majority of patients have mild disease with only distal colonic involvement. Acute fulminating disease is often complicated by perforation or *toxic megacolon* (see Chapter **26**), chronic disease by carcinoma of the colon. Extracolonic manifestations include *arthritis, spondylitis, pericholangitis, liver disease*, and *thrombotic complications*. Even biopsy is not fully diagnostic in some cases, since features of Crohn's disease or nonspecific ulcerating colonic disease may coexist.
Crohn's colitis **(Figs. 28.41, 28.42)**	Mucosal alterations usually appear in the following sequence: - Punctate collections of barium with a halo of edema (aphthoid ulcers) surrounded by normal mucosa or small, irregular nodules. - Deeper, irregular ulcers surrounding mounds of edematous mucosa (cobblestone appearance). - Penetrating asymmetric ulcers form long tracts parallel to the longitudinal axis of the colon or fistulas to adjacent organs. - Stricture formation. - Segmental involvement of the colon with extensive inflammatory changes in the terminal ileum, asymmetric ulceration, fistulas, sinus tracts, and mesenterial thickening are characteristic. Filiform polyposis may occur.	Symptoms such as diarrhea, pain, and weight loss are often more severe than in ulcerative colitis. Extraintestinal complications similar to ulcerative colitis are less frequent. Increased incidence of biliary and renal stones results from ileal disease. Aphthoid ulcers can also occur in other forms of colonic inflammation, e.g., amebic colitis, tuberculosis, yersinia colitis, and Behçet's syndrome.

(continues on page 676)

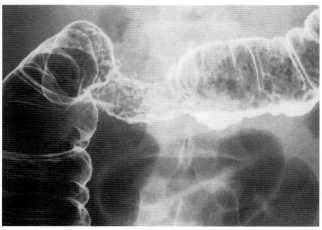

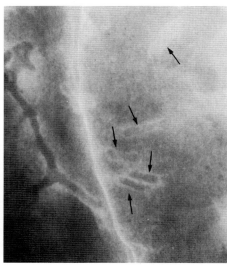

Fig. 28.**41**   **Crohn's colitis.** Segmental narrowing of the proximal transverse colon, with irregular nodules and ulcers.

Fig. 28.**42**   Multiple **filiform polyps** (arrows) in a patient with **Crohn's colitis**.

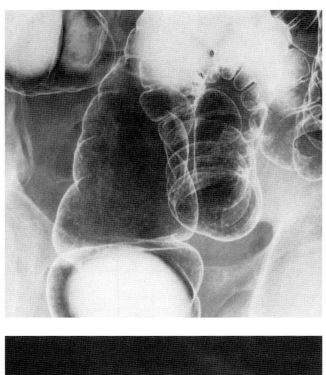
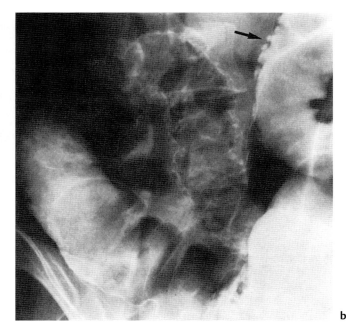

a

b

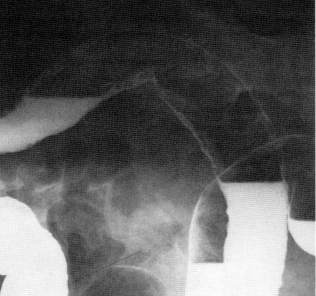
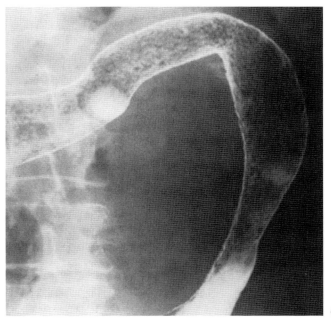

c

d

Fig. 28.**40 a–d   Mucosal changes in ulcerative colitis: a** Stippled mucosa! pattern representing superficial ulcers. **b** Larger marginal ulcerations, including collar button ulcers (arrow). **c** Denuded flat mucosa with numerous pseudopolyps. **d** Short, rigid colon with a mottled surface pattern.

Table 28.5   (Cont.) Abnormal Mucosal Pattern in the Colon and Rectum

Disease	Radiographic Findings	Comments
Ischemic colitis (Fig. 28.43)	Mucosal changes depend on the phase of the disease: – Serrated margin and fine superficial ulcerations are the earliest findings and may simulate ulcerative colitis. – "Thumb printing", pseudopolyposis, and deep ulcers occur later in most cases. – Eventually the changes may disappear, develop into a stricture or proceed into infarction that may be evident by the presence of gas in the bowel wall and in the portal system. The splenic flexure and the sigmoid area are common locations.	Abrupt onset of abdominal pain and rectal bleeding with diarrhea is a common presentation. A history of prior cardiovascular disease is frequent. Mucosal findings may be indistinguishable from ulcerative or Crohn's colitis, but typical history, short clinical course, and the location of changes are helpful. Ulcerating nodularity with pseudopolyps may occur proximal to colonic obstruction. It may be caused by *ischemia secondary to distension of the bowel wall.*
Amebiasis (Fig. 28.44)	Colonic mucosal changes are similar to ulcerative or Crohn's colitis. Segmental involvement of the colon as in Crohn's colitis is common. The cecum is affected in 90% of cases and may have a cone-shaped appearance.	Clinical symptoms have a wide spectrum. Hepatic abscess develops in about one-third of cases of amebic dysentery. Concomitant ileal disease favors Crohn's colitis rather than amebiasis. Stool specimens are usually diagnostic.
Schistosomiasis	The colonic mucosa is edematous and spiculated simulating ulcerative colitis. Small ulcers, spasm, disturbed motility, and loss of haustral pattern are common. Later, characteristic multiple 1–2 cm filling defects develop representing granulomas. The descending and sigmoid colon are most frequently involved.	The parasite penetrates the colonic wall and causes an inflammatory reaction. Detection of ova in freshly passed stools is diagnostic. Very rarely *strongyloidiasis* causes severe ulcerating colitis.
Trichuriasis	Granular mucosal pattern throughout the colon with flocculation of barium and multiple small filling defects.	The pattern is similar to cystic fibrosis. Only found in the tropics and subtropics.
Shigellosis (basillary dysentery)	Shallow, ragged ulcers encircle the colon, which shows mucosal edema and exudation. Barium enema cannot usually be tolerated, but if successful, it shows deep "collar button" ulcerations and intense spasm. The changes may be segmental or generalized.	Incubation period after ingestion of the organisms is usually 2–3 days or more, after which profuse diarrhea begins. The radiographic patterns of salmonellosis and shigellosis may be similar, but involvement of the ileum favors salmonellosis.
Salmonellosis (typhoid fever)	Barium enema is rarely performed due to short course. Small ulcerations and edematous thickening of folds may be seen. Unlike in shigellosis, terminal ileum is usually involved.	Incubation period is often as short as 12 hours, recovery takes place within 4–5 days.
Tuberculous colitis (Fig. 28.45)	Radiographic findings closely simulate Crohn's disease. Cecum and distal ileum are most commonly affected.	If caused by *Mycobacterium tuberculosis,* coexistent pulmonary tuberculosis is often demonstrated radiographically. In tuberculous colitis caused by *Mycobacterium bovis,* pulmonary tuberculosis is usually absent.
Gonorrheal proctitis	Barium enema is usually normal. Mucosal edema or ulceration of the rectum occurs rarely.	Most patients with rectal gonorrhea are asymptomatic and diagnosed by staining and culture of purulent exudates.
Staphylococcal enterocolitis	Radiographic features of generalized ulcerating colitis may be seen in severe cases.	Usually secondary to administration of broad spectrum antibiotics.
Yersinia enterocolitis	Multiple small colonic ulcerations similar to those seen in Crohn's colitis, associated with thick mucosal folds, nodular filling defects, or ulceration of the distal small bowel.	A relatively common cause of ileitis and colitis in children, which causes fever, diarrhea, or symptoms simulating appendicitis.
Campylobacter colitis	Similar to acute or early changes of ulcerative colitis, e.g., mucosal edema and superficial ulcerations.	An acute colitis simulating ulcerative colitis but has a self-limited course.

(continues on page 678)

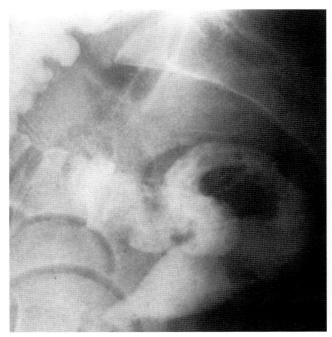

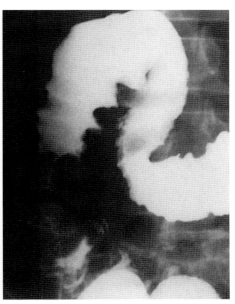

Fig. 28.**43** **Ischemic colitis** (occlusion of the inferior mesenteric artery). Mucosal irregularities with early pseudopolyposis are seen in the sigmoid colon.

Fig. 28.**44** **Amebic colitis.** A mass (ameboma) is present in the cecum. Ulcerations and thumb printing are seen in the proximal colon.

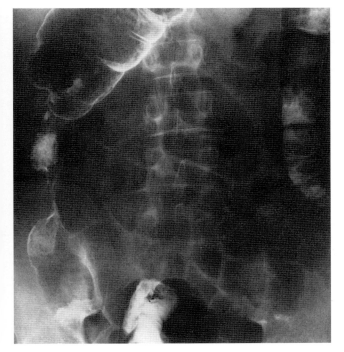

Fig. 28.**45** **Tuberculous colitis.** A long stricture is present in the cecum and ascending colon. Superficial mucosal changes are seen in a small area above the strictured segment. These changes are similar to Crohn's colitis.

Table 28.5 (Cont.) Abnormal Mucosal Pattern in the Colon and Rectum

Disease	Radiographic Findings	Comments
Fungal colitis (candidiasis, histoplasmosis, mucormycosis)	Irritable spastic colon with thick irregular mucosal folds, and occasionally ulcers.	These are rare causes of colitis in chronically ill patients. The fungal infection may be primary or spread from another site in the body. *Actinomycosis* producer a similar radiographic and clinical picture.
Lymphogranuloma venereum	Spasm, irritability, mucosal edema, ulcers, fistulas, or sinus tracts are seen in the rectum. The rest of the colon is not involved.	Rectal involvement is common (25%), especially in women and homosexual men. As the disease progresses, rectal stricture develops.
Herpes zoster	Small ulcerations in a narrowed segment of colon. A pattern of raised polygonal "urticaria" plaques may also occur.	Herpes zoster is a rare cause of colonic ulcerations. Typical clinical history and skin lesions suggest the correct diagnosis.
Cytomegalovirus colitis	Mucosal ulceration, luminal narrowing, "thumb printing," or even tumorlike defects in the cecum.	The most important cause of severe lower gastrointestinal tract bleeding in renal transplant recipients on immunosuppressive therapy and in AIDS patients.
Pseudomembranous colitis (Clostridium difficile disease) (Fig. 28.46)	Barium enema is contraindicated in severe cases. In mild or healing cases thickened colonic wall and haustral markings, irregular bowel wall due to pseudomembranes, and mucosal ulcerations simulating other ulcerating conditions are seen.	A spectrum of colonic inflammatory states usually complicating antibiotic therapy, sometimes surgery, uremia or large bowel obstruction. In the latter cases the course may be fulminant and fatal.
Radiation-induced colitis (Fig. 28.34)	Spasticity and ulceration of the colonic wall are most severe in the segments adjacent the irradiated organs. The anterior rectal wall is most commonly involved. Strictures and fistulas may develop.	Usually secondary to pelvic irradiation for carcinoma of the cervix, endometrium, ovary, bladder, or prostate. The course is usually benign and self-limited.
Caustic colitis	3 to 5 days after exposure, ulcerations and mucosal sloughing similar to other ulcerating lesions may be observed.	A rare complication of a cleansing enema that contains detergents when the fluid is trapped in the proximal colon. Subsides within 3 to 4 weeks.
Pancreatitis	Irregularity or ulcerations and pseudopolyps in the transverse colon and splenic flexure.	Due to spread of pancreatitis along the transverse mesocolon.
Amyloidosis	May occasionally present as ulcerating colitis indistinguishable from other causes.	May occur both in primary or secondary (connective tissue disorders, chronic infection) amyloidosis. Rectal biopsy is diagnostic.
Inorganic mercury poisoning	Ulcerating lesions in the colon are associated with acute renal damage.	
Behçet's syndrome	Diffuse mucosal thickening and ulceration or multiple discrete ulcers in otherwise normal colon may occur. Rectum is spared but terminal ileum may be involved. Ulcers tend to be larger than in Crohn's colitis and easily perforate.	Characterized by ulcerations in the buccal and genital mucosa and skin lesions.
Diverticulosis	Saclike outpouchings with short necks often associated with a sawtooth pattern must be differentiated from ulcers and polyps.	Most common in the sigmoid colon. Ulcerative colitis or Crohn's disease may coexist and simulate diverticulitis.
Solitary rectal ulcer syndrome	Nodularity of rectal mucosa may be followed by ulcerations on the anterior or anterolateral rectum within 15 cm of the anal verge and near a valve of Houston.	Usually occurs in young patients with rectal bleeding. May be associated with rectal mucosal prolapse or pelvic muscle discoordination during defecation. May lead to rectal stricture and simulate inflammatory bowel disease or carcinoma.
Nonspecific benign ulceration of the colon	Usually single, in up to 20% multiple ulcerative lesions usually in the cecum or ascending colon. Most occur in the antimesenteric border, in contrast to diverticula. A masslike effect simulating carcinoma is frequent.	A diagnosis of exclusion, rarely made before operation. No precise cause can be identified. Lesions in the ascending colon may mimic appendicitis, those of descending colon simulate diverticulitis or carcinoma.
Nodular lymphoid hyperplasia	Nodular tiny (~2 mm) filling defects are evenly distributed throughout the colon simulating familial polyposis, pseudopolyposis of bowel inflammation, or nodular lymphoma. A fleck of barium in the center of the nodules (umbilication at the apex of the enlarged lymph follicles) is characteristic.	The filling defects in nodular lymphoid hyperplasia are sessile and uniform in size, whereas polyps in familiar polyposis vary in size and are often pedunculated. They are evenly distributed, and are smaller than the nodules of lymphoma.

Table 28.5   (Cont.) Abnormal Mucosal Pattern in the Colon and Rectum

Disease	Radiographic Findings	Comments
Cystic fibrosis	Multiple poorly defined filling defects give the colonic mucosa a hyperplastic appearance simulating polyposis.	Caused by adherent collections of viscid mucus that are not removed by cleansing enema. *Trichuriasis* causes a similar appearance due to adherent whipworms and associated mucus.
Colonic urticaria (Fig. 28.47)	Large, round or polygonal, raised plaques in a grossly dilated (usually right) colon, representing submucosal edema.	An allergic reaction of the colonic mucosa to medication, with or without concomitant cutaneous lesions. The lesions regress once medication is withdrawn. Similar lesions may occur in *herpes zoster*.
Artifacts Foreign bodies	*Fecal material* adhered to the colonic mucosa is usually irregular and unevenly coated; barium tends to infiltrate into the mass and interpose between the mass and mucosa. *Radiolucent air bubbles* tend to appear as clusters of small bubbles adhered to a larger one. *Mucus strands* are seen as irregular branching defects and occasionally simulate filiform polyposis.	*Foreign bodies*, especially kernels of corn can simulate multiple polyps. Similar to other artifacts, they are usually freely movable and disappear in a repeat examination. *Sharp angulation* of the bowel may result in a long filling defect resembling the stalk of a polyp.
Lymphoma	Multiple irregular filling defects are a rare manifestation and usually associated with ileal changes.	A more common presentation of colonic lymphoma is a single, relatively large lesion, which may occasionally infiltrate over a long segment of the colon.
Leukemia	In lymphocytic leukemia diffuse mucosal or submucosal interlacing filling defects of the colon may occur. In myelogenous leukemia diffuse plaques, nodules, or masses are sometimes seen.	Usually asymptomatic but may cause necrotizing enterocolitis, hemorrhage, or perforation.
Metastases	Spiculations of the bowel contour as in ulcerative colitis. Mucosal thickening, nodular masses, or multiple eccentric strictures can simulate Crohn's disease.	Hematogenous metastases from breast, lung, stomach, ovary, pancreas, uterus, or melanoma may cause this pattern, which clinically usually manifests as bloody diarrhea. Multiple primary carcinomas of the colon occur in 1%.

(continues on page 680)

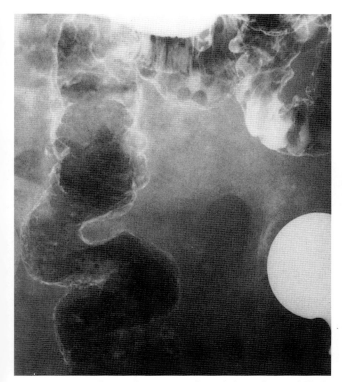

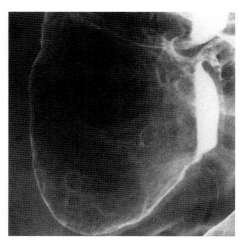

Fig. 28.**46 Pseudomembranous colitis (Clostridium difficile disease).** Pseudomembranes are most obvious in the sigmoid colon, seen as multiple filling defects. Ulcerations are present in the rectal mucosa.

Fig. 28.**47** Raised plaques in the mucosa of the cecum which rapidly vanished and were considered to represent **colonic urticaria**.

Table 28.5 (Cont.) Abnormal Mucosal Pattern in the Colon and Rectum

Disease	Radiographic Findings	Comments
Familial polyposis (Fig. 28.48)	Myriad of small (less than 1 cm) polyps (adenomas) may blanket the whole colon or spare the right colon. May look like a poorly cleansed colon. Other parts of the gastrointestinal tract are usually spared.	An inherited autosomal dominant condition arising around puberty and clinically manifesting usually in the third or fourth decade. Virtually all develop carcinoma of the colon or rectum. *Disseminated gastrointestinal polyposis* may be a variant of familial polyposis. *Turcot syndrome* refers to multiple adenomatous polyps of the colon associated with gliomas which occur in the second decade.
Gardner's syndrome	The colonic lesions are indistinguishable from the pattern of familial polyposis.	Associated with bony overgrowth or osteomas of the skull, keloid formation, soft tissue tumor, sebaceous cysts, and a 100% risk of colorectal carcinoma.
Peutz–Jeghers syndrome	Polyps (hamartomas) are primarily present in the small bowel, but multiple polyps occur in colon and rectum.	An inherited autosomal dominant disorder which manifests during childhood or adolescence. Excessive melanin deposits on the lips and buccal mucosa are characteristic. A slightly increased risk of intestinal carcinoma or ovarian tumor exists.
Multiple hamartoma syndrome (Cowden's disease)	Single or multiple polyps may be present in the colon.	Circumoral papillomatosis and nodular gingival hyperplasia are characteristic.

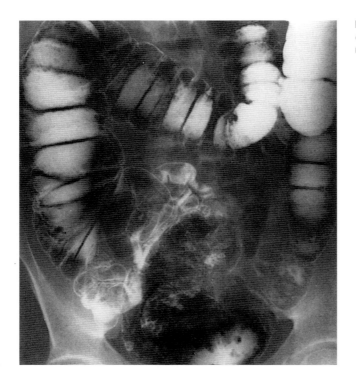

Fig. 28.**48** **Familial polyposis.** A great number of small polyps cover the colonic mucosa. The distal ileum is normal. The pattern mimics a poorly cleansed colon.

Table 28.5 (Cont.) Abnormal Mucosal Pattern in the Colon and Rectum

Disease	Radiographic Findings	Comments
Juvenile polyposis syndromes (juvenile polyposis coli, generalized gastrointestinal juvenile polyposis)	Multiple hamartomatous polyps of the colon usually found in childhood. Polyps may be present also in the stomach and small bowel.	*Canada–Cronkhite syndrome* presents in later life with multiple hamartomatous polyps and malabsorption. The syndrome is characterized by alopecia, nail dystrophy, and hyperpigmentation, and may be lethal soon after being diagnosed.
Neurofibromatosis of the colon	Multiple diffuse intraluminal or intramural nodules tend to be larger than in the hereditary polyposis syndromes, and have a characteristic eccentric distribution, the nodules being located entirely on the mesenteric side.	Characteristic skin lesions (café-au-lait spots and cutaneous fibromas) are diagnostic.
Colonic lipomatosis	Multiple filling defects are seen usually in the right colon without mucosal ulcerations.	Histologic verification is required.
Multiple colonic hemangiomas	Intraluminal or intramural filling defects in the colon.	Can be diagnosed radiographically only if phleboliths are associated with the lesions.
Hemorrhoids	Rectal filling defects may simulate polyps or are seen as linear shadows of enlarged veins.	Hemorrhoids often remain undetected in the barium enema examination. They should be differentiated from the normal rectal columns of Morgagni.
Pneumatosis intestinalis (Fig. 28.49)	Intramural gas collections may simulate broad-based polyps but are more radiolucent.	
Colitis cystica profunda	Multiple irregular filling defects simulate adenomatous polyps. They occur usually in the pelvic colon and rectum.	Mucous subepithelial cysts are frequently associated with proctitis or colitis. A rare condition called *colitis cystica superficialis* is associated with pellagra. Minute cysts are diffusely distributed throughout the colon.

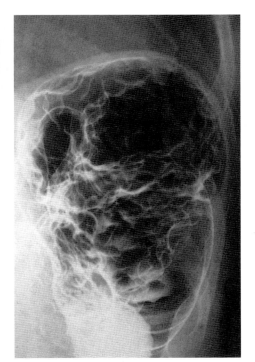

Fig. 28.**49** **Pneumatosis intestinalis.** Intramural gas collections in the splenic flexure simulate broad-based polyps but are radiolucent.

29 Narrowing in the Gastrointestinal Tract

An acquired circumferential narrowing in the gastrointestinal tract is generally caused either by *edema, inflammation* or *hemorrhage* with eventual *scar formation*, or by *tumor encasement*. Other conditions that may occasionally produce a stenosis include *congenital lesions* (e.g., webs or congenital strictures), *localized spasm* or *hypertrophy*, especially of a sphincter (e.g., esophageal sphincter or pylorus), or the *torsion* or *kinking of a freely mobile bowel segment* (e.g., volvulus or herniation).

Radiologic differential diagnosis between benign and malignant stenosis is usually difficult and in the majority of

cases requires a biopsy for an unequivocal diagnosis. A discrete, irregular, and asymmetric narrowing with associated ulcerations or a well-demarcated filling defect with overhanging edges strongly suggest a malignant lesion. A smooth concentric stenosis with tapering margins generally favors a benign condition, but many malignancies can present radiographically in similar fashion.

The differential diagnosis of stenotic lesions in the gastrointestinal tract is discussed in Tables 29.1 to 29.5.

Table 29.1   Narrowing of the Esophagus

Disease	Radiographic Findings	Comments
Web (congenital or acquired) (Fig. 29.1)	Single or less commonly multiple, bandlike concentric or eccentric narrowing, preferentially located in the cervical esophagus. Congenital webs always originate from the anterior wall.	Usually incidental finding without clinical symptoms. *Plummer–Vinson syndrome:* Iron deficiency anemia and acquired esophageal webs that may cause dysphagia. Certain skin diseases (e.g., *epidermolysis bullosa* and *benign mucous membrane pemphigoid*) may also be associated with esophageal webs.
Cartilaginous ring (tracheobronchial rest)	Short stricture-like narrowing in the distal esophagus. Characteristic are tiny fistulas that extend from the narrowed segment and may fill with barium.	Usually diagnosed in infancy, but occasionally in adults with long history of dysphagia. Other *congenital strictures* cannot be differentiated from acquired lesions.
Schatzki's ring (lower esophageal ring) (Fig. 29.2)	Smooth concentric narrowing at the junction between esophageal and gastric mucosa. Only seen in conjunction with a sliding hiatal hernia when the ring is located above the diaphragm.	Symptoms related to the ring (intermittent dysphagia or occasionally total obstruction) are only found when the ring diameter is less than 12 mm.
Carcinoma (primary) (Fig. 29.3)	Annular constriction often with overhanging margins, irregular lumen, and destroyed or ulcerated mucosa. These findings indicate an advanced stage of the disease. Preferred location is middle and lower esophagus in this order. More than one carcinoma might occasionally be present.	Usually in patients over 40 years of age with much higher incidence in men than women, often with both heavy smoking and drinking history.
Metastases (Fig. 29.4)	By direct invasion from carcinoma in adjacent organs or lymph nodes. Narrowing may be relatively smooth and often symmetric (especially from mediastinal metastases of a bronchogenic or breast carcinoma) or irregular and often ulcerated simulating a primary lesion (e.g., by direct extension of a cardia carcinoma into the distal esophagus or by invasion of a larynx, pharynx, or thyroid carcinoma into the cervical esophagus).	
Lymphoma (Fig. 29.5)	Involvement occurs by direct extension of gastric lymphoma, presenting often as a nodular, nonobstructive narrowing that may be difficult to differentiate from a gastric carcinoma progressing to the distal esophagus, or by enlarged, lymphomatous nodes encircling the esophagus and causing a relatively smooth narrowing.	Lymphomatous rather than metastatic carcinomatous involvement is likely in patients below 40 years of age.

(continues on page 686)

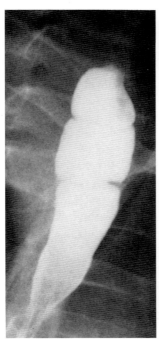
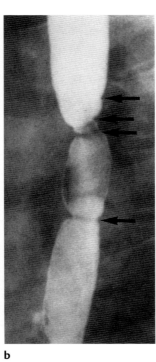

Fig. 29.**1 a, b   Esophageal webs. a** Two webs are seen in Plummer–Vinson syndrome in the upper esophagus. **b** Four concentric webs of unknown etiology are seen in the mid-esophagus (arrows).

a   b

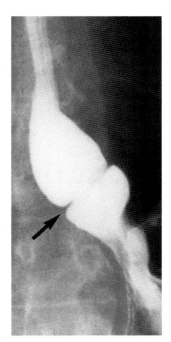

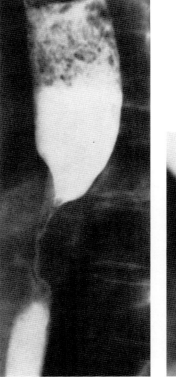

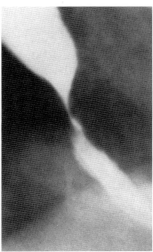

a

b

Fig. 29.2 Schatzki's ring in hiatal hernia. A smooth concentric and symptomatic narrowing with a diameter of 1 cm is seen in a small sliding hiatal hernia (arrow).

Fig. 29.3 a, b Esophageal carcinomas. a A slightly irregular and eccentric stricture is seen in the middle esophagus. **b** A smooth concentric stenosis is seen in the lower esophagus that is indistinguishable from a benign structure.

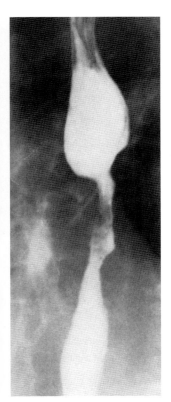

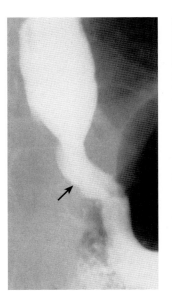

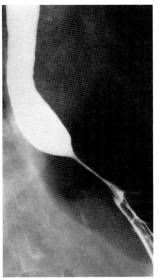

a

b

Fig. 29.4 Metastasis from bronchogenic carcinoma. Extrinsic narrowing of the midthoracic esophagus without apparent mucosal abnormalities is seen. Although the described findings suggest extrinsic metastatic involvement, a primary esophageal carcinoma may present in similar fashion.

Fig. 29.5 a, b Lymphoma (two cases). Moderate concentric narrowing of the distal esophagus (arrow) is seen in **a** and a stricture-like stenosis caused by an encircling lymphomatous mass in **b**.

Table 29.1 (Cont.) Narrowing of the Esophagus

Disease	Radiographic Findings	Comments
Infectious esophagitis (Fig. 29.6)	Smooth, usually symmetric and often long strictures with tapering at both ends are characteristic and develop in the healing phase.	Candida and herpes simplex or zoster esophagitis develop usually in compromised hosts or AIDS patients. Tuberculosis, histoplasmosis, and syphilis are rare.
Crohn's disease and eosinophilic gastroenteritis	Rare causes of an esophageal stricture.	Esophageal involvement invariably associated in both conditions with manifestation of the disease in other parts of the gastrointestinal tract.
Reflux esophagitis (Fig. 29.7)	Often somewhat asymmetric and slightly irregular narrowing of the distal esophagus with funnel-shaped proximal end and absent mucosal pattern. A hiatal hernia is usually associated. A marginal ulcer at the gastroesophageal junction (peptic esophagitis) may be present and cause severe spasm and inflammation.	Changes caused by spasm and inflammation often cannot be differentiated from fibrotic healing, except that the two former are reversible, whereas the latter is not.
Barrett's esophagus (Fig. 29.8)	Smooth but often asymmetric stricture in the mid-esophagus resulting from a healed (Barrett's) ulcer.	Barrett's esophagus consists of islets of gastric mucosa in the esophagus away from the cardia with tendency to produce a peptic ulcer.
Intramural pseudo-diverticulosis	Multiple cystic pouches of 1–3 mm are found in a short segment, or occasionally the entire length, of the esophagus. A stricture, usually of the mid-esophagus, is associated in about two-thirds of patients.	Dysphagia of long duration is often present
Corrosive (caustic) esophagitis (Fig. 29.9)	Long smooth strictures involving the lower and often middle esophagus.	Strictures may appear as early as 2 weeks after ingestion of a caustic liquid.
Mediastinitis (infectious, abscess-forming, or sclerosing)	Concentric or eccentric, usually smooth narrowing of various lengths at different locations of the intrathoracic esophagus.	May be the sequela of a perforated or ruptured esophagus (e.g., post-instrumentation, trauma, or severe vomiting – *Boerhaave's syndrome:* complete tear of all layers of the esophageal wall above the gastroesophageal junction).
Hematoma	Both intramural or paraesophageal bleeding and subsequent fibrosis may produce a smooth narrowing at various levels.	In bleeding disorders, posttraumatic, postinstrumentation, and rarely in the *Mallory–Weiss syndrome* (hematemesis secondary to repeated vomiting caused by mucosal tear usually originating just below the gastroesophageal junction that may extend into the esophagus).
Iatrogenic strictures	Smooth, benign-appearing strictures may develop after repair of hiatal hernia or gastric surgery that permits bile to reflux into the esophagus, after prolonged nasogastric intubation and irradiation.	*Prolonged nasogastric intubation* predisposes to both gastroesophageal reflux (by preventing hiatal closure) and mucosal ischemia (by tube compression). Strictures may also develop after endoscopic obliteration of esophageal varices.
Motility disorders	Achalasia and prolonged lumen-obliterating contractions may simulate smooth organic strictures.	*Secondary contractions* spread simultaneously upwards and downwards from the middle and lower esophagus and produce radiographically a temporary hourglass deformity. See also Chapter 26.

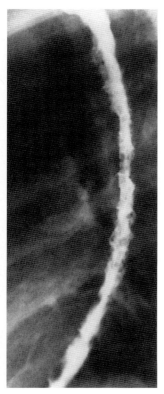

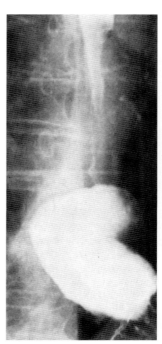

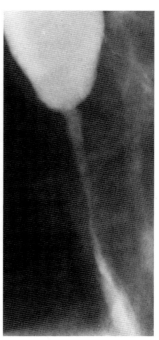

a

b

Fig. 29.6 Infectious esophagitis caused by candida. Narrowing of the entire esophagus with mucosal abnormalities is seen. In this case the disease is still active and has not yet progressed to stricture formation.

Fig. 29.7 a, b Reflux or peptic esophagitis. a A slightly asymmetric and somewhat irregular narrowing of the distal esophagus is seen in conjunction with a hiatal hernia. **b** A stricture in the distal esophagus has formed secondary to peptic esophagitis. The ulcer in the gastroesophageal junction is no longer seen.

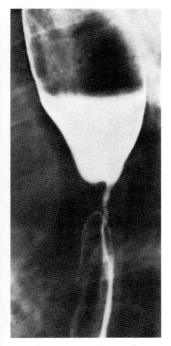

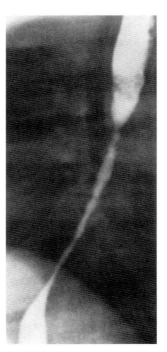

Fig. 29.8 Barrett's esophagus. A short and smooth but eccentric stricture is seen in the mid-esophagus after healing of a Barrett's ulcer.

Fig. 29.9 Corrosive esophagitis. A long and relatively smooth stricture has formed in the distal esophagus several weeks after ingestion of a caustic agent.

Table 29.2   Narrowing of the Stomach (Linitis Plastica Appearance)

Disease	Radiographic Findings	Comments
Carcinoma (scirrhous) (Fig. 29.10)	Part or entire stomach is shrunken into a rigid tubular stricture without peristaltic contractions. Rugal folds are generally flattened or totally obliterated and the mucosal pattern is often effaced. Involvement originates usually near pylorus and progresses slowly upwards, the fundus being least involved.	*Linitis plastica* ("water bottle stomach") refers to all conditions in which the stomach appears as a narrowed rigid tube. By far the most common cause is scirrhous carcinoma of the stomach. The condition is caused by a desmoplastic response stimulated by tumor invasion.
Metastases Fig. 29.11)	Circumferential stenosis to complete linitis plastica appearance may be caused by direct invasion from pancreatic and less common transverse colon carcinoma. Hematogenous metastases (e.g., from carcinoma of breast or lung) can also diffusely infiltrate the stomach wall and produce a similar radiographic appearance.	Tumor invasion from transverse colon carcinoma occurs via gastrocolic ligament.
Lymphoma (Fig. 29.12)	Irregular narrowing usually beginning in the antrum. Abnormal but usually not effaced mucosal pattern, often with small ulcerations. Contrary to carcinoma some flexibility of the stomach wall and residual peristalsis are usually maintained.	Besides the ileum, primary lymphoma affects most often the stomach and is of the non-Hodgkin variety. Secondary gastric involvement is more common and occurs with both Hodgkin's and non-Hodgkin's lymphoma. *Pseudolymphoma* may present also as constricting gastric lesion often associated with a large ulcer crater.

(continues on page 690)

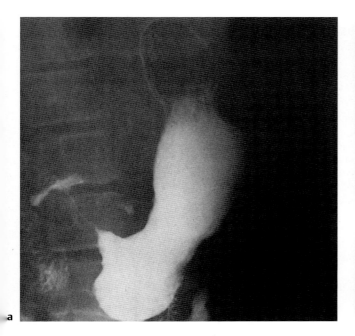

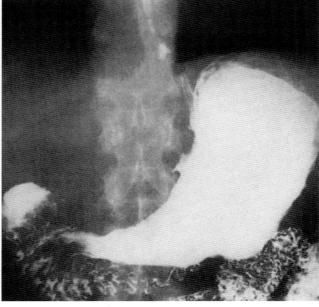

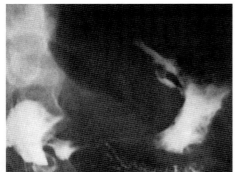

Fig. 29.10 a–c Gastric carcinoma (scirrhous) producing a linitis plastica appearance. In all three cases the carcinoma originated near the pylorus and progressed to a varying degree upward. The involved part of the stomach presents as a rigid tubular stricture without peristaltic contractions and with completely effaced mucosal pattern. **a** Antrum and lower part of the body are involved. **b** Entire stomach is involved and has water bottle appearance. Note also the malignant-appearing flat ulcer on the lesser curvature. **c** Shrinkage of the entire stomach is seen in this most advanced case.

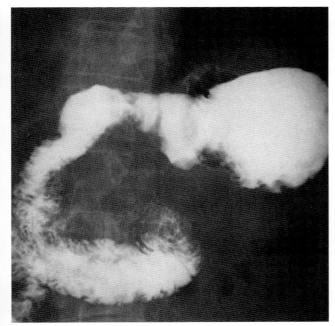

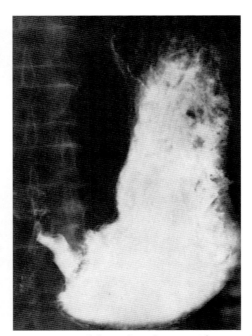

Fig. 29.11 Pancreatic carcinoma invading the stomach. Circumferential involvement of the antrum is seen but the greater curvature is much more severely affected than the lesser curvature. Note also the widening and infiltration of the duodenal sweep.

Fig. 29.12 Hodgkin's lymphoma with secondary gastric involvement. Irregular narrowing of the antrum with destroyed mucosal pattern is seen. Note also the lymphomatous involvement of the greater curvature with nodular lesions, some of which demonstrate central ulcerations.

Table 29.2   (Cont.) Narrowing of the Stomach (Linitis Plastica Appearance)

Disease	Radiographic Findings	Comments
Exogastric mass (Fig. 29.13)	Extrinsic compression of the lesser curvature may produce a markedly narrowed stomach that is otherwise normal.	For example, with severe hepatomegaly or large pancreatic pseudocyst.
Peptic ulcer disease (Fig. 29.14)	Antral rigidity and narrowing can be seen with a distal gastric ulcer and is caused by either intense spasm and edema in the acute stage or fibrosis in the chronic stage. An ulcer may radiographically not be demonstrable in either condition. Fibrotic healing of an ulcer in the body of the stomach may result in characteristic hourglass deformity.	An inflammatory antral process leading to submucosal fibrosis is occasionally termed *"stenosing antral gastritis"* and indistinguishable from healed ulcer disease.
Phlegmonous gastritis	Irregular narrowing in the antrum extending to the body, often with both effaced mucosal folds in one area and thickened in another. Gas-producing organisms may produce intramural air bubbles, that are diagnostic.	Rare bacterial infection of the stomach with high mortality rate. Presents clinically with severe, acute abdominal symptoms (pain, nausea, and vomiting). Purulent emesis is rare but diagnostic when present.
Granulomatous gastritis (tuberculosis, sarcoidosis, syphilis)	Concentric narrowing, preferentially of the antrum, often with erosions and ulcerations.	Rare manifestations of these diseases.
Crohn's disease	Smooth, concentrically narrowed and relatively rigid antrum flaring into a normal gastric body and fundus (ram's horn sign). Duodenal involvement is almost always associated. Ulcerations and fissures are often present. Gastric outlet obstruction is a relatively common complication.	Concomitant involvement of gastric antrum, duodenal bulb and proximal sweep may simulate partial gastrectomy and Billroth I anastomosis ("pseudo-Billroth I").
Eosinophilic gastritis (Fig. 29.15)	Irregular narrowing of the antrum often associated with contiguous spread of the disease into duodenum and small bowel (eosinophilic gastroenteritis).	Benign self-limited condition that is often clinically and radiographically confused with Crohn's disease.
Corrosive (caustic) gastritis (Fig. 29.16)	Rigid and smooth stricture of the stomach with predilection for the antrum and pylorus.	Develops within a few weeks after ingestion of corrosive agent (e.g., alkalis, acids, formaldehyde).
Radiation gastritis	Rigid narrowing of the gastric lumen in the field of previous irradiation may develop in the healing phase.	A fractionated therapeutic dose in excess of 45 Gy is usually required.
Hepatic arterial chemotherapy	Narrowing of the antrum and proximal duodenum, often associated with ulcerations. Involvement corresponds to blood supply of gastroduodenal artery.	Caused by inadequate catheter placement with a high blood concentration of chemotherapeutic agent reaching gastroduodenal artery. May resolve after discontinuation of hepatic artery perfusion.
Gastroplasty (gastric stapling)	Narrowing of an otherwise normal stomach and presence of metallic suture material are characteristic.	This surgical procedure is performed for weight reduction in morbid obesity.
Amyloidosis	Rare cause of rigid narrowing particularly of the antrum.	In systemic primary and secondary amyloidosis with manifestations of the disease in other organs.
Volvulus (Fig. 29.17)	Organoaxial volvulus: Stomach rotates upward around its long axis (line connecting cardia with pylorus). Mesenteroaxial volvulus: Stomach rotates around a line connecting the middle of the lesser curvature with the middle of the greater curvature. Characteristic findings include inversion of the stomach with greater curvature above lesser curvature, cardia and pylorus at the same level, and downward pointing of pylorus and duodenum.	Usually associated with diaphragmatic hernias, eventration or paralysis of the diaphragm. May be asymptomatic when neither vascular compromise nor outlet obstruction is present.

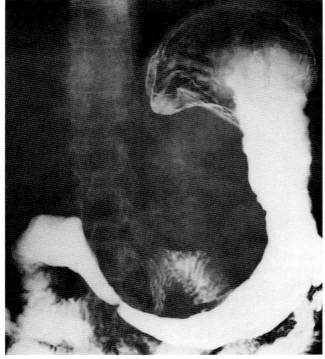

Fig. 29.**13** **Metastatic ovarian carcinoma.** A large and diffusely, faintly calcified mass involving both the left liver lobe and the lesser omentum causes extensive narrowing and elongation of the stomach.

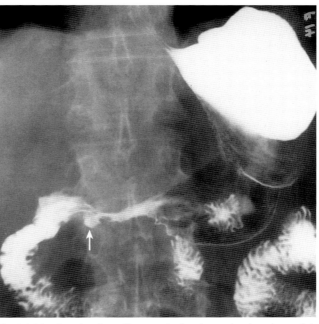

Fig. 29.**14** **Peptic ulcer disease.** A distal gastric ulcer (arrow) is associated with marked narrowing of the antrum due to spasm and edema.

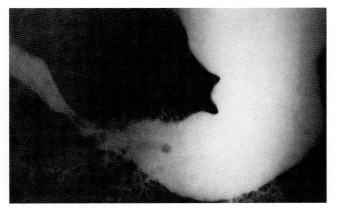

Fig. 29.**15** **Eosinophilic gastritis.** An irregular narrowing of the antrum with mucosal abnormalities and small polypoid filling defects is seen.

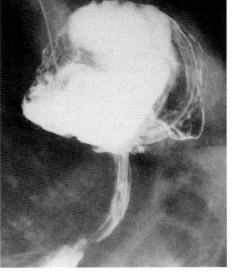

Fig. 29.**17** **Gastric volvulus.** An organoaxial volvulus of the stomach that is partially herniated through the diaphragm is seen.

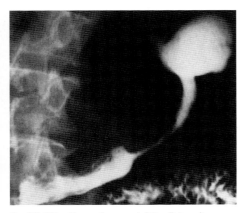

Fig. 29.**16** **Corrosive gastritis.** Extensive narrowing of the body and antrum with relative sparing of the fundus is seen.

Table 29.3 Narrowing of the Duodenum

Disease	Radiographic Findings	Comments
Duodenal atresia/stenosis	Double-bubble sign in infants with complete or high-grade duodenal obliteration.	Presence of gas in the small and large bowel indicates that the duodenal obstruction is incomplete.
Webs (duodenal diaphragms)	Membrane-like structures, preferentially located in the second portion of duodenum, which may cause varying degrees of obstruction.	These diaphragms are congenital and usually diagnosed in infancy and childhood.
Annular pancreas (Fig. 29.18)	Extrinsic narrowing of the second portion of the duodenum from the lateral side and above the level of the ampulla. The mucosa is intact unless duodenal ulceration develops, which is not uncommon in adults with symptomatic annular pancreas.	Annular pancreas may first be diagnosed in adulthood. Obstruction, even in infancy, is almost always incomplete.
Midgut volvulus (Fig. 29.19)	Duodenal obstruction associated with spiraling of small bowel and both inferiorly and to the right displaced duodenojejunal junction (ligament of Treitz) is diagnostic. Cecum is located in midabdomen or on the left side, indicating incomplete rotation of the gut.	Only found with incomplete rotation of the gut, resulting in a narrow mesenteric attachment of the small bowel. Usually diagnosed in childhood.
Ladd's bands (congenital duodenal or peritoneal bands)	Extrinsic duodenal narrowing of anterior wall of the second or third portion of the duodenum.	May cause partial or intermittent obstruction. Symptoms often increase in upright and decrease in supine position.
Duodenal duplication cyst	Intramural or extrinsic fluid-containing mass of spherical or tubular shape that may encroach on the duodenum.	Usually asymptomatic, but may rarely cause a high-grade duodenal obstruction.
Choledochal cyst (Fig. 29.20)	Extrinsic narrowing and widening of the duodenal sweep, when the choledochal cyst occurs near the ampulla of Vater.	Represents a localized dilatation of the common bile duct.
Carcinoma of the duodenum (primary) (Fig. 29.21)	Constricting and narrowing with nodular mucosal destruction, ulcerations, and often overhanging edges. Preferentially located at or distally to the ampulla of Vater.	Clinical symptoms include obstruction and bleeding. Obstructive jaundice is present with periampullary location.
Pancreatic carcinoma (Fig. 29.22)	Narrowing of usually the second portion and rarely the third and fourth portions of the duodenum occurs in advanced stages. Mucosal destruction usually but not always present.	Two-thirds of pancreatic carcinomas originate in the head, the rest in the body and tail, in this order.
Metastases and lymphoma (Fig. 29.23)	Narrowing preferentially located in the distal half of the second portion and third portion of the duodenum. An abnormal mucosal pattern with nodular lesions and ulcerations may be associated.	Caused by neoplastic aortic and pancreaticoduodenal lymph node involvement. A *retroperitoneal sarcoma* can rarely produce similar changes.

(continues on page 694)

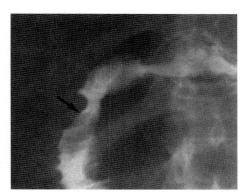

Fig. 29.**18   Annular pancreas.** Extrinsic narrowing of the second portion of the duodenum from the lateral side is seen (arrow).

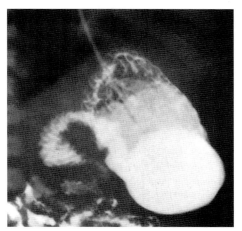

Fig. 29.**19   Midgut volvulus.** Duodenal obstruction and spiraling of the jejunum are characteristic.

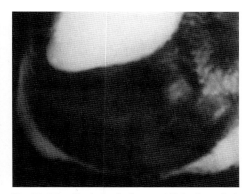

Fig. 29.**20   Choledochal cyst.** Widening of the duodenal sweep with marked extrinsic compression of the duodenum is seen.

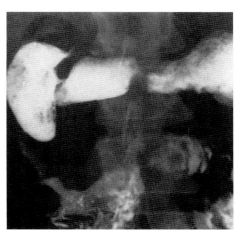

Fig. 29.**21   Duodenal carcinoma.** Irregular narrowing of the duodenal sweep that is not widened is associated with complete mucosal destruction.

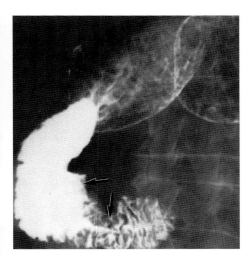

Fig. 29.**22   Pancreatic carcinoma.** Complete obstruction of the third portion of the duodenum with an extrinsic mass defect on the second and third portions of the duodenum (arrows) is seen. Note also the marked prestenotic dilatation.

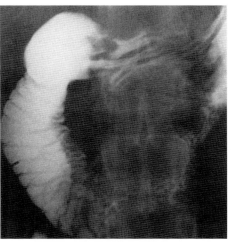

Fig. 29.**23   Non-Hodgkin's lymphoma.** Extrinsic defects on the medial aspect of the distal half of the second portion of the duodenum and narrowing with partial obstruction of the third portion of the duodenum are caused by enlarged aortic and parapancreatic lymph nodes.

Table 29.3   (Cont.) Narrowing of the Duodenum

Disease	Radiographic Findings	Comments
Postbulbar ulcer disease (Fig. 29.24)	Postbulbar ulcers, usually located on the medial wall of the second portion of the duodenum may cause concentric narrowing and obstruction of the duodenum. Abnormal mucosa and demonstration of an ulcer differentiate this condition from an annular pancreas.	Duodenal narrowing and obstruction is caused in the acute stage by spasm and in the chronic stage by a fibrotic stricture.
Crohn's disease (Fig. 29.25)	One or several areas of usually concentric narrowing associated with mucosal effacement, nodularity, and ulcerations. Stomach is almost always involved, also.	Similar findings are seen in *tuberculosis, strongyloidiasis, nontropical sprue* (healing phase after ulceration) and *eosinophilic gastroenteritis*. All these conditions are, similar to Crohn's disease, also associated with manifestations of the disease in other parts of the gastrointestinal tract.
Pancreatitis or pancreatic pseudocyst (Fig. 29.26)	Spasm in the acute stage and fibrosis in the chronic stage may cause narrowing of the second or occasionally, when the mesenteric root is mostly involved, the third portion of the duodenum. Mucosal thickening and spiculation can be seen, but there is no mucosal destruction as in pancreatic cancer. Duodenal narrowing may also result from extensive compression by a pancreatic pseudocyst.	Similar radiographic findings can occasionally be found with *cholecystitis,* but are usually located in the proximal half of the second portion of the duodenum.
Superior mesenteric artery syndrome	Extrinsic anterior narrowing and obstruction of the third portion of the duodenum where it crosses the spine. The duodenal mucosa is intact. Characteristically, the finding is more pronounced in supine position and partially to completely relieved in prone or lateral decubitus position.	Associated with thin patients, hyperlordosis lumbalis, prolonged immobilization, decreased peristalsis, thickened mesenteric root (e.g., by inflammation or tumor), and abdominal aortic aneurysm.
Hematoma (Fig. 29.27)	Compression of second and third portion of the duodenum by hematoma or subsequent fibrosis.	Hematoma might be intramural or retroperitoneal secondary to trauma, anticoagulation therapy, bleeding diathesis, or bleeding aortic aneurysm.
Iatrogenic strictures	Relatively smooth narrowing of the second or third portion of the duodenum.	Following retroperitoneal surgery (e.g., repair of aortic aneurysm, insertion of prosthetic aortic graft) or pancreaticoduodenal surgery and radiation therapy.

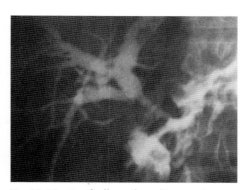

Fig. 29.24 Postbulbar ulcer disease. A concentric narrowing of the upper descending duodenum is seen. Note also the barium reflux into the biliary system that may be caused by either ulcer perforation into a bile duct or incompetence of Oddi's sphincter secondary to scarring.

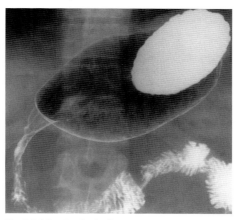

Fig. 29.25 Crohn's disease. Concentric narrowing of the second portion of the duodenum is associated with mucosal irregularities and partial effacement.

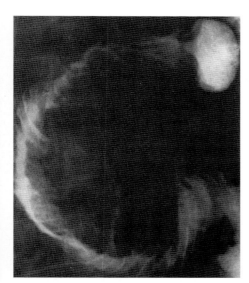

Fig. 29.26 Pancreatitis with pancreatic pseudocyst. Marked widening of the duodenal sweep with extrinsic narrowing is seen. Note also the mucosal spiculation.

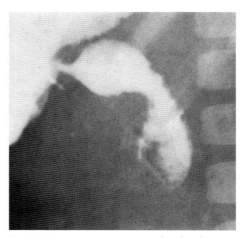

Fig. 29.27 Hematoma. Duodenal obstruction between the second and third portion of the duodenum is seen.

Table 29.4   Narrowing of the Jejunum or Ileum

Disease	Radiographic Findings	Comments
Congenital atresia and stenosis	Minimal to complete obstruction of jejunum or ileum.	Usually diagnosed in infancy or childhood. Atresia is a more severe variant in the newborn, associated with *meconium ileus* (evident as scattered abdominal calcifications). The associated microcolon (thin and ribbon-like) is most pronounced in low ileal atresia and progressively less so with a more proximal location. Meconium ileus is also found in *cystic fibrosis*.
Carcinoid (Figs. 29.28 and 29.29)	Narrowing and angulation of adjacent, preferentially ileal loops, which are fixed and separated from each other. The mucosa of the involved segments is irregularly thickened and transversely elongated producing a spiculated or tethered appearance or is destroyed. One or several small filling defects may be seen but are usually not conspicuous.	This presentation is caused by either the carcinoid itself that has locally infiltrated the mesentery and lymph nodes, or a desmoplastic reaction induced by the tumor.
Carcinoma (Fig. 29.30)	Localized narrowing preferentially of the jejunum with destroyed and ulcerated mucosa.	Obstruction and pain are the most common clinical presentations.
Metastases (Fig. 29.31)	Usually multiple areas of narrowed and fixed loops. Tethering of the mucosa and transverse stretching of mucosal folds often combined with extrinsic or less commonly intrinsic mass lesions, which may undergo ulcerations. May resemble carcinoids or primary carcinoma, but multiple sites of involvement with varying presentations suggest metastases.	Common primary tumors that metastasize to the mesentery and small bowel include carcinomas originating in the gastrointestinal tract, pancreas, urogenital tract, lung, breast, and skin (melanoma).

(continues on page 698)

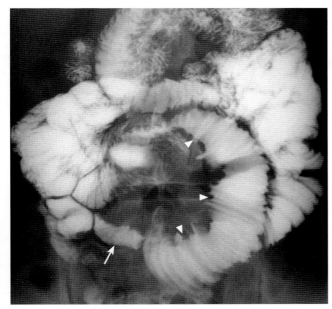

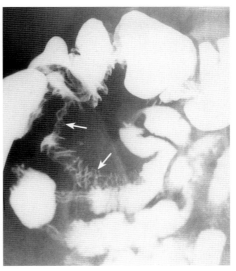

Fig. 29.**28**   **Carcinoid.** A large mass separating the dilated small bowel loops associated with a stenotic segment (arrow) is seen. The prestenotic dilated loops depict characteristic mucosal tethering (arrowheads).

Fig. 29.**29**   **Carcinoid.** A mass separating the ileal loops and encircling the terminal ileum (arrows) with spiculated mucosal folds is seen.

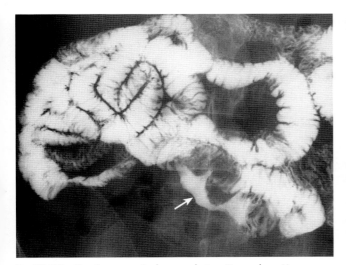

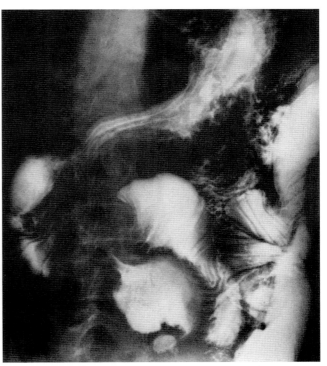

Fig. 29.**30**   **Carcinoma.** A large obstructing ulcerating mass (arrow) with completely destroyed mucosa is seen.

Fig. 29.**31**   **Metastases from colon carcinoma.** Extensive metastatic disease is present involving the greater curvature of the stomach, duodenum, and small bowel loops that are fixed and narrowed at many locations by either extrinsic tumor infiltration or concentric constriction with prestenotic dilatation. Note also the mucosal tethering and destruction in many areas.

Table 29.4   (Cont.) Narrowing of the Jejunum or Ileum

Disease	Radiographic Findings	Comments
Lymphoma (Fig. 29.32)	Narrowing of usually multiple small bowel segments by either extrinsic compression or infiltration of the bowel wall. Irregular, thickened folds with small nodular defects and ulcerations are often present. Loops draped around mesenteric masses are fixed and demonstrate mucosal tethering. Obstruction occurs only in advanced disease. Differentiation from metastases is often impossible.	Primary and secondary involvement of the small bowel is much more common with non-Hodgkin's lymphoma than Hodgkin's disease.
Inflammation of adjacent structures	Localized narrowing of neighboring small bowel that may demonstrate a normal or edematous mucosal pattern, by spasm in the acute and stricture formation in the chronic stage.	For example, in pancreatitis, appendicitis, diverticulitis, and intraperitoneal abscess formation.
Tuberculosis (Fig. 29.33)	Findings similar to Crohn's disease, but are often more localized in the terminal ileum and have a greater tendency for stricture formation and higher incidence of associated cecal and ascending colon involvement.	Rare. Not necessarily associated with pulmonary tuberculosis.
Parasitic infections (giardiasis, strongyloidiasis)	Limited to duodenum and jejunum where the lumen is often narrowed by severe spasm and the mucosa thickened and irregular.	Clinical symptoms of malabsorption are only found with severe infestations.
Crohn's disease (Fig. 29.34)	Development of one or several stenotic segments with obstruction is common and most frequently seen in the terminal ileum but can involve any part of the gastrointestinal tract. In the acute stage, marked ulceration with severe spasm produces the "string" sign evident as narrowed, poorly delineated bowel segment with effaced mucosal pattern resembling a frayed cotton string. In a more chronic stage, pipelike narrowing of varying lengths often separated by normal segments ("skip" lesions) are seen, caused by thickening and fibrosis of the bowel wall. Irregular strictures can be seen in advanced fibrotic stage. Thickened mucosa with ulcerations ("cobblestone" pattern), perforation, fistula, and abscess formations are commonly associated features.	Small bowel obstruction is a common complication in severe Crohn's disease.
Retractile mesenteritis	Narrowing, separation, and angulation of small bowel loops by an apparent mesenteric mass.	A poorly understood, rare condition characterized by fibrosis, inflammation, and fatty infiltration of the mesentery. Related entities include *isolated lipodystrophy* and *lipogranuloma* of the mesentery, *nodular panniculitis* and *Weber–Christian disease*.
Adhesions (Fig. 29.35)	Extrinsic or concentric narrowing of a short segment with obstruction, which may be intermittent by kinking or compression of bowel loops at the site of previous surgery or inflammation.	Most common cause of small bowel obstruction. Usually caused by previous surgery or peritonitis.
Anastomotic stricture	Localized, relatively smooth narrowing at anastomotic site caused initially by edema and hematoma and later by fibrotic stricture formation.	Must be differentiated from local recurrence, which is often irregular and may be associated with a growing mass lesion.

(continues on page 700)

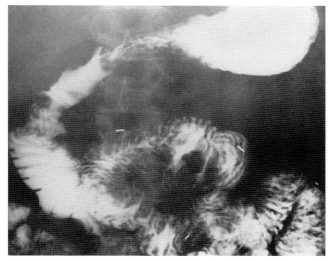

Fig. 29.**32** **Non-Hodgkin's lymphoma.** A jejunal loop draped around a mesenteric mass with mucosal tethering is seen. Note also the circumferential narrowing of the duodenum with destroyed mucosal pattern and nodular defects.

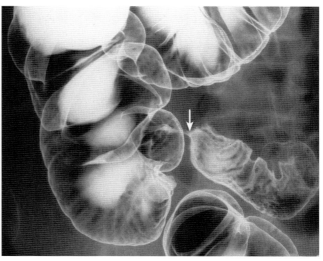

Fig. 29.**33** **Tuberculosis.** A stricture (arrow) is seen in the terminal ileum with abrupt transition from the normal bowel.

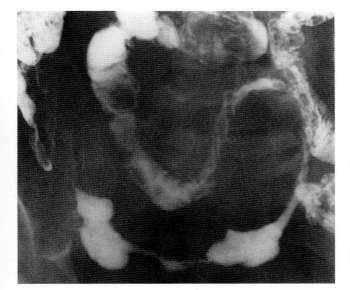

Fig. 29.**34** **Crohn's disease.** Several strictures separated by normally distended bowel segments ("skip" lesions) are seen.

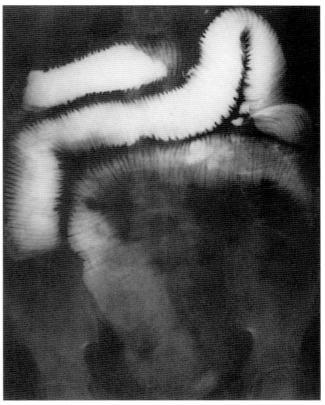

Fig. 29.**35** **Adhesions.** Small bowel obstruction is caused by postoperative adhesions in the pelvis. Note the markedly dilated, prestenotic small bowel loops with circular but not thickened folds.

Table 29.4   (Cont.) Narrowing of the Jejunum or Ileum

Disease	Radiographic Findings	Comments
Radiation therapy (Fig. 29.36)	One or several stenotic segments of varying lengths in the field of irradiation.	Narrowing may be caused by submucosal edema and spasm in the acute stage, where mucosal thickening and shallow ulcerations might be associated, followed by fibrosis in the chronic stage.
Ischemic bowel disease	Narrowing of the involved segment by edema and spasm in the acute stage, with thickened folds and marginal filling defects ("scalloping" or "thumb printing"). With incipient healing, the mesenteric border becomes flattened and rigid and the antimesenteric border plicated forming multiple sacculations or pseudodiverticula. With progressive fibrosis the involved segment becomes tubular with smooth surface and finally forms a stricture up to 10 cm in length.	Usually in elderly patients with cardiac failure. Similar radiographic findings are seen in *connective tissue disorders* (especially *scleroderma*), *thromboangiitis obliterans,* and *Henoch–Schönlein syndrome.*
Graft-versus-host disease (Fig. 29.37)	Narrowing of the bowel lumen is caused by edema and spasm. Folds are either thickened and shaggy or effaced ("ribbon bowel"). The transit time is markedly decreased, but barium coating of abnormal bowel loops may last for hours or even days producing the "small bowel cast" sign.	Occurs in 50% of patients with allogeneic (donor genetically different from host) bone marrow transplant. T-lymphocytes from donor cause selected epithelial damage in gastrointestinal tract, liver, and skin of the transplant recipient.
Hernias (external and internal) (Figs. 29.38 and 29.39)	Narrowing of the herniated bowel loops at characteristic locations with or without vascular compromise that may be evident as mucosal edema. In internal hernias, the trapped bowel loops are packed together into a small confined space and are clearly separated from the remaining small bowel.	External hernias (inguinal, femoral, umbilical, incisional) are the second most common cause of small bowel obstruction after adhesions. Internal hernias result from congenital abnormalities or surgical defects within the mesentery. In left paraduodenal hernias (most common internal hernia) and herniation through the foramen of Winslow, the trapped bowel loops are located in the left upper quadrant.
Volvulus	Twisted small bowel segment with obstruction and vascular compromise.	Rare cause of obstruction in the adult. Associated with defective fixation of the mesentery permitting abnormal rotation or adhesions acting as pivot for small bowel segments to rotate about.

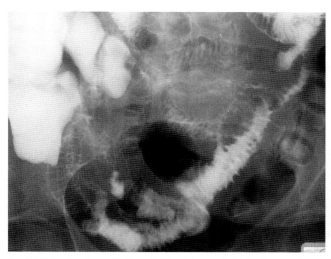

Fig. 29.**36** **Acute radiation ileitis.** Mucosal thickening and narrowing of the ileum is limited to the field of irradiation.

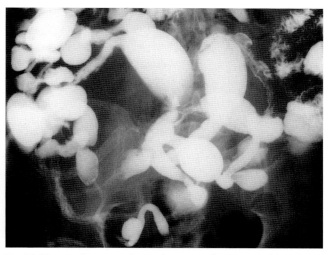

Fig. 29.**37** **Graft-versus-host disease.** Alternating dilated and stenotic small bowel segments with completely effaced mucosal pattern are seen.

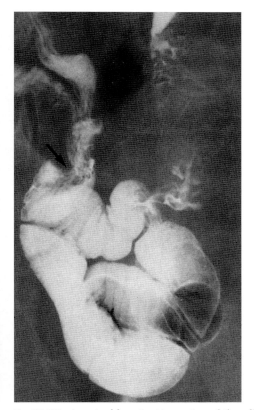

Fig. 29.**38** **Inguinal hernia.** Narrowing of the afferent and efferent ileal loop at the entry into the hernial sac (arrow) while the herniated ileal loops are distended, indicating partial obstruction.

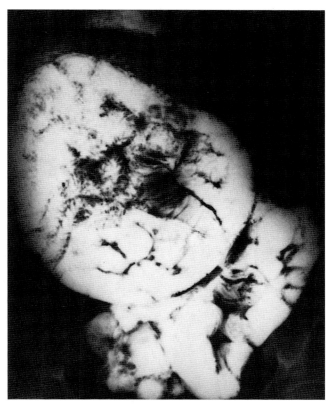

Fig. 29.**39** **Right paraduodenal hernia.** Jejunal loops are bunched together on the right side of the abdomen. Right paraduodenal hernias are associated with incomplete intestinal rotation with the duodenojejunal junction being located in a low right paramedian position.

Table 29.5   Narrowing of the Colon and Rectum

Disease	Radiographic Findings	Comments
Microcolon in neonates	Thin, unused colon associated with complete low small bowel or proximal colonic obstruction. In both distal colonic and rectal atresia and imperforate anus, the colon proximal to the point of obstruction is dilated.	In meconium ileus (e.g., in cystic fibrosis), ileal and colonic atresia. If the obstruction is higher in the jejunum or duodenum, then the colon is normal in size.
Hirschsprung's disease (aganglionosis) (Fig. 29.40)	Segmental narrowing of the rectum and/or distal sigmoid with abrupt transition to grossly dilated prestenotic colon.	Occasionally first diagnosed in late childhood and early adulthood. The narrowed, relatively normal-appearing distal segment is the pathologic part with absence of ganglion cells in the myenteric plexus. Hirschsprung's disease rarely involves other segments of the colon or even the entire colon. *Meconium plug syndrome* (local inspissation of meconium) and *imperforate anus* also produce low colonic obstruction and have to be differentiated in the neonatal period from Hirschsprung's disease.
Transient localized spasm (Fig. 29.41)	Concentric transient localized narrowing with normal mucosal pattern. Spasm is usually relieved with intravenous glucagon.	Occurs anywhere in the colon, but particularly common in the transverse, descending, and sigmoid colon, where the so-called *colonic sphincters* are located.
Endometriosis (Fig. 29.42)	Constricting narrowing with intact mucosa measuring up to several centimeters in length, usually involving the rectosigmoid. Irregular or pleated folds and polypoid filling defects can occasionally be associated.	Limited to women of child-bearing age. This form is seen when the endometrial implant induces a desmoplastic reaction and hyperplasia of the smooth muscle.
Carcinoid	Rarely presents in cecum and ascending colon as circumferential colonic narrowing with destroyed but usually not ulcerated mucosal pattern, simulating adenocarcinoma.	Carcinoids of the colon often occur at a younger age than primary adenocarcinomas.
Carcinoma (Fig. 29.43)	Concentric narrowing is a common presentation of primary adenocarcinoma producing "apple-core" or "napkin-ring" lesions. The abrupt transition from normal bowel to the annular tumor with destroyed and often ulcerated mucosa and the production of a "tumor shelf" with "overhanging edges" are characteristic. Longer stenotic segments (up to 12 cm) with tapered ends and gradual transition to normal colon are seen in the relatively rare scirrhous carcinoma.	Annular carcinomas originate from flat tumor plaques (saddle lesions) that involve originally only part of the circumference of the colonic wall. Approximately 75 % of colon carcinomas occur in the rectosigmoid area. Clinical symptoms are often late and nonspecific (change in bowel habits, anemia, rectal bleeding). Scirrhous carcinomas have a very poor prognosis. The luminal narrowing is caused by an intense desmoplastic reaction in the bowel wall.
Metastases (Fig. 29.44)	Besides extrinsic compression and fungating, often ulcerating intraluminal masses, a smooth or irregular stenosis, and an annular constricture are also common presentations. In contrast to primary carcinoma, however, the ends are often more tapered without a pronounced "tumor shelf" and "overhanging edges" appearance.	By direct invasion from neighboring organs (prostate, uterus, ovary, kidney, pancreas, stomach), intraperitoneal seeding, and hematogenous (e.g., from carcinoma of breast, lung, and melanoma) or lymphangitic spread.

(continues on page 704)

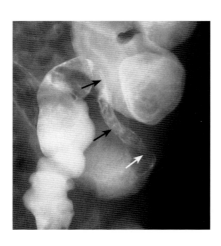

Fig. 29.**40** **Hirschsprung's disease.** Segmental narrowing of the sigmoid (arrows) is seen with abrupt transition to markedly dilated prestenotic colon.

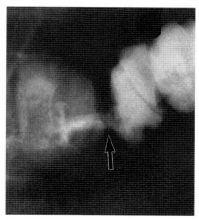

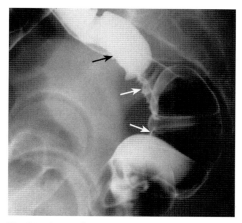

Fig. 29.41 Transient localized spasm of the colon. An area of localized concentric narrowing with intact mucosa is seen in the transverse colon.

Fig. 29.42 Endometriosis. Extrinsic narrowing of the rectosigmoid (arrows) with spiculated adjacent bowel wall but intact mucosal pattern is seen.

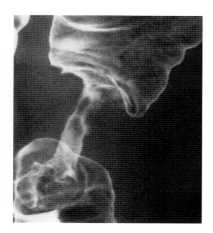

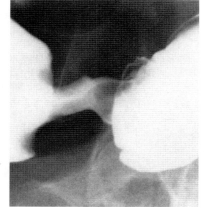

Fig. 29.43 a, b Colon carcinoma. A localized narrowing producing an "apple-core" or "napkin-ring" lesion is seen **a** in the descending colon and **b** in the sigmoid colon. Note the abrupt transition from normal bowel to the annular tumor with destroyed mucosa producing a "tumor shelf" with "overhanging edges."

a   **b**

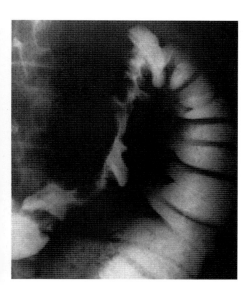

Fig. 29.44 Colonic metastasis from carcinoma of the stomach. An irregular narrowing of the transverse colon with destroyed mucosa and ulceration is seen. Although there is no pronounced "tumor shelf" production with "overhanging edges," this lesion cannot be differentiated from a primary colon carcinoma on the basis of its radiographic appearance alone.

Table 29.5   (Cont.) Narrowing of the Colon and Rectum

Disease	Radiographic Findings	Comments
Lymphoma	Localized narrowing of the colon (especially the cecum) by constricting and infiltrating lesion with mucosal destruction is a rare presentation. Extrinsic compression and narrowing by large mesenteric lymph node masses may also occur.	This manifestation is virtually limited to non-Hodgkin's lymphomas. *Kaposi's sarcoma* (Fig. 29.**45**) may present in a male homosexual AIDS patient anywhere in the gastrointestinal tract as an infiltrating lesion, polypoid mass or multiple submucosal nodules often with central umbilication.
Diverticulitis (Fig. 29.46)	Narrowing of the involved segment (usually the sigmoid) by spasm in the acute and fibrosis in the chronic stage. An extrinsic filling defect caused by paracolic abscess secondary to a perforated diverticulum may be seen. Contrast extravasation from a diverticulum, evident as a tiny collection at the tip of a diverticulum or rarely as the filling of an abscess, is diagnostic. Diverticula adjacent to an abscess are spastic and often draped around it.	Incidence of colonic *diverticulosis* increases with age. In this condition large numbers of diverticula may shorten the involved segment and produce a "saw-tooth" appearance by the thickened circular muscle. This condition is occasionally referred to as *"spastic diverticulosis"*, but its clinical relevancy is controversial. Diverticulitis is a relatively rare complication of diverticulosis in which the diverticular perforations result in the development of peridiverticular abscesses.
Extracolonic inflammatory process (Fig. 29.47)	Localized narrowing by spasm and edema or less commonly, at a later stage, by adhesions and stricture formation.	Caused by adjacent abscess or inflammation (e.g., pancreatitis: narrowing of the distal transverse colon and splenic flexure; cholecystitis: narrowing of the hepatic flexure; appendicitis: narrowing of the cecum). These conditions may also present as a localized ileus instead of a localized spasm in the adjacent colon (see Table 26.**5**).
Bacillary dysentery (shigellosis)	Narrowing of the colon by spasm associated with mucosal edema and superficial ulcerations. May progress to rigid, tubular stenosis with loss of haustration. Preferential location is the rectosigmoid area.	Acute or chronic (with periodic episodes of exacerbation and remission) inflammatory disease of the colon. May resemble clinically and radiographically ulcerative colitis. *Typhoid fever* and *Yersinia enterocolica* infection can produce inflammatory changes in the terminal ileum with narrowing and irregularity of the cecum.
Tuberculosis (Fig. 29.48)	Shortening and narrowing of the cecum ("cone-shaped") is most common manifestation. Involvement of terminal ileum is usually associated with cecal involvement. Segmental narrowing with irregular contours and ulcerations can occur in the remaining colon.	Pulmonary tuberculosis is not invariably associated.

(continues on page 706)

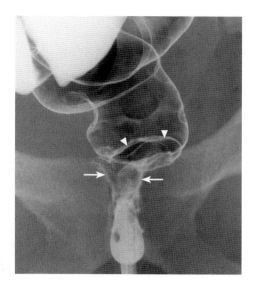

Fig. 29.**45 Kaposi's sarcoma.** A constricting lesion (arrows) associated with a polypoid mass (arrowheads) is seen in the rectum.

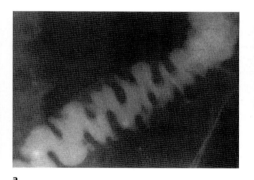

a

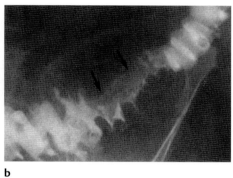

b

Fig. 29.**46 a, b Diverticulosis progressing to diverticulitis** in a two-year interval. **a** A shortened sigmoid colon with "sawtooth" appearance is seen that is caused by thickened and spastic circular muscle in the presence of numerous diverticula. This appearance is occasionally also referred to as "spastic diverticulosis." **b** Two years later, diverticulitis has developed. Narrowing of the involved segment by spasm and abscess formation (arrows) is now seen, besides thin mucosal spiculations.

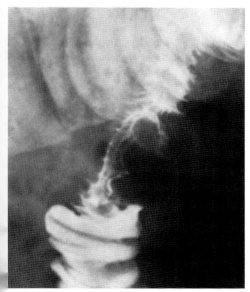

Fig. 29.**47 Pancreatitis with secondary involvement of the descending colon.** Concentric narrowing of the inflamed part of the descending colon by spasm and edema is seen. Note that in contrast to a carcinoma the mucosal pattern in the narrowed segment is intact but edematous. Together with the fine mucosal spiculations, this suggests an inflammatory rather than neoplastic nature of the abnormality.

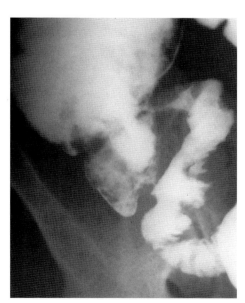

Fig. 29.**48 Tuberculosis.** A narrowed ("cone-shaped") cecum with small polypoid filling defects is associated with a stenotic terminal ileum with a destroyed mucosal pattern and ulcerations.

Table 29.5 (Cont.) Narrowing of the Colon and Rectum

Disease	Radiographic Findings	Comments
Amebiasis (Fig. 29.49)	Cecum is concentrically narrowed and appears cone-shaped, whereas the terminal ileum is usually normal, in contrast to Crohn's disease or tuberculosis. Ileocecal valve is usually thickened and fixed in open position, permitting free reflux into the terminal ileum. Segmental lesions with superficial ulcerations and localized spasm may progress to fibrotic, rather long strictures, which are often multiple and most commonly located in the transverse and sigmoid colon and both flexures. Amebomas may present occasionally as annular constricting mass lesions.	The cecum is involved in 90% of chronic amebiasis. The diagnosis is made by the demonstration of *Entamoeba histolytica* in stool or rectal biopsy.
Fungal disease	Narrowing of the cecum or less commonly the colon, associated with inflammatory mass, often simulates primary adenocarcinoma.	*South American blastomycosis* involving terminal ileum and cecum may be mistaken for Crohn's disease. *Actinomycosis* (a fungus-like bacterial infection) may mimic an appendiceal abscess.
Schistosomiasis	Narrowing of the sigmoid colon or, less commonly, any other segment by progressive fibrosis occurs, especially when the disease originally presented as granulomatous process with extensive pericolonic infiltration. An initial presentation with multiple 1–2 cm polypoid granulomas, however, progresses only rarely to stricture formation.	Chronic debilitating disease that may involve multiple organs and affects over 200 million people in the tropics and subtropics. *Strongyloides stercoralis* can occasionally produce colonic strictures following ulcerating colitis. *Anisakiasis* (ascaris-like nematode) can produce severely inflamed and narrowed terminal ileum, cecum, and ascending colon in people eating raw fish.
Lymphogranuloma venereum (Fig. 29.50)	Short or long tubular rectal stricture of varying length, beginning just above the anus and extending in some cases to the sigmoid, which may be involved also. Ulcerations, fistulas, and perirectal abscesses are commonly associated.	Viral venereal disease particularly common in sexually promiscuous individuals and in the tropics. Presents initially as herpetiform lesion on the external genitalia 2 weeks after infection. *Herpes zoster* may produce short segments of colonic narrowing with small ulcerations. *Cytomegalovirus* infection may produce colonic ulcers, edema and narrowing, especially in immunosuppressed renal transplant recipients.
Nonspecific benign ulcer disease	Stricture formation can be a late sequela, especially in the cecum and rectum.	In the rectum the entity is termed *solitary rectal ulcer syndrome* and must be differentiated from lymphogranuloma venereum.
Ulcerative colitis (Fig. 29.51)	Foreshortening of the colon with depression of flexures, narrowing of the lumen, and absent haustral pattern with relatively smooth surface are characteristic for chronic stage ("lead-pipe" colon). Localized concentric strictures of varying length with relatively smooth contours and tapering margins are seen in different stages of the disease and rarely cause obstruction. Carcinomas complicating ulcerative colitis develop preferentially in the distal half of the colon, may be multicentric in 20% of cases, and are often very difficult to differentiate from a benign stricture, since they present often as a narrowed 2–6 cm segment with tapered ends, but the narrowed lumen is usually somewhat eccentric and the contours tend to be irregular.	Incidence of colon carcinoma is approximately 20 times higher in ulcerative colitis than normal population. Risk of developing carcinoma is particularly high with universal colitis and increases with duration of the disease. Rarely a carcinoma develops during the first 10 years after onset of the disease.

(continues on page 708)

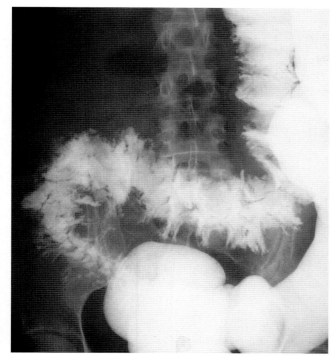

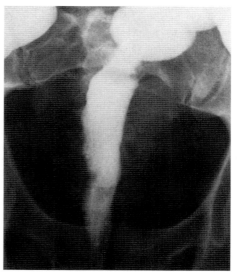

Fig. 29.**49 Acute amebiasis.** Narrowed proximal colon and particularly cecum by edema is associated with extensive mucosal destruction and ulcerations.

Fig. 29.**50 Lymphogranuloma venereum.** Narrowing of the entire rectum beginning just above the anus is seen.

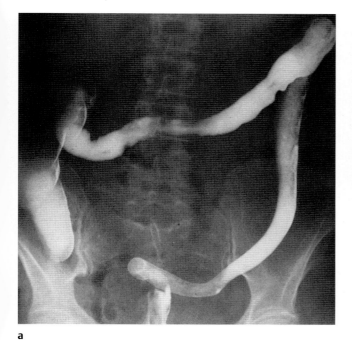

a

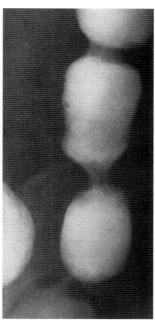

b

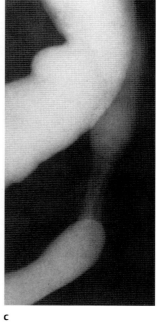

c

Fig. 29.**51 a–c Ulcerative colitis in three different patients. a** "Lead-pipe" colon. Foreshortening and narrowing of the entire colon with more severe involvement of the left side, absent haustral markings, and depression of the flexures is characteristic for the chronic stage. **b** Three areas of benign concentric narrowing are seen in the descending colon of this patient with chronic ulcerative colitis. **c** Carcinoma in chronic ulcerative colitis, presenting as benign-appearing stricture of the descending colon, although the lumen stricture is slightly eccentric.

Table 29.5   (Cont.) Narrowing of the Colon and Rectum

Disease	Radiographic Findings	Comments
Crohn's colitis (Fig. 29.52)	Solitary or multiple stenotic segments are often already encountered in an early stage of the disease when other more characteristic findings are also present ("cobblestone" pattern, skip lesions and fistulas). In the chronic stage, a "lead-pipe" colon identical to ulcerative colitis and localized benign strictures, which occasionally may be eccentric and difficult to differentiate from a carcinoma, are often seen.	The incidence of colon carcinomas in Crohn's colitis is higher than in the normal population, but this association is less striking than in ulcerative colitis. Carcinomas complicating Crohn's colitis present usually as fungating mass lesions in the proximal colon and are therefore relatively easily recognized.
Ischemic colitis (Fig. 29.53)	Besides "thumb printing," annular constricting lesions simulating carcinoma may be seen in the acute phase. During healing, flattening of the mesenteric border combined with pleating of the antimesenteric margin may produce multiple sacculations or pseudodiverticula. Progressive fibrosis may finally result in tubular narrowing and smooth stricture formation. Preferentially located in the splenic flexure, descending and sigmoid colon.	Usually in elderly patients with cardiac failure. A similar sequence of events (from "thumb printing," to smooth stricture formation) may occasionally also be seen with intramural bleeding of different etiologies. Acute ischemic colitis reverts to normal radiographic appearance when adequate collateral circulation is established. This occurs invariably in the rare so-called *"evanescent ischemic colitis"* of adolescents and young adults, in which no apparent underlying cause is found.
Graft-versus-host disease	Spasm, loss of haustration, edema, and a granular mucosal pattern or ulcerations are common findings.	Occurs in 50% of patients with allogeneic bone marrow transplants.
Cathartic colon	Foreshortened tubular colon with loss of haustration similar to burned-out ulcerative colitis. In contrast to the latter, the right side is usually more severely involved and often shows constant areas of concentric narrowing, whereas the rectum and sigmoid appear often normal.	In patients with history of lifelong constipation and habitual use of irritant cathartics for 15 years and longer.
Caustic colitis	Tubular narrowing to severe stricture formation begin within one month after enemas with caustic agents.	For example, following detergent enema.
Pseudomembranous colitis (clostridium difficile disease)	Healing may occasionally result in a tubular colon without haustral markings. Strictures can develop very rarely.	Complete healing without any radiographic sequelae occurs usually after discontinuation of the offending antibiotic (especially clandamycin) or chemotherapeutic agent, respectively.
Radiation therapy (Fig. 29.54)	Segmental narrowing of varying lengths in the field of previous irradiation, most commonly found in the sigmoid and rectum. Narrowing is caused by spasm in the acute stage and associated with mucosal edema, serrations, and ulcerations, whereas a smooth tubular stricture is found in the chronic fibrotic stage.	Fibrotic tubular strictures develop 6 to 24 months after irradiation with a dose in excess of 40 Gy.
Anastomotic stricture	Localized, smooth narrowing with at least limited distensibility at anastomotic site is caused by edema and hematoma in the immediate postoperative period and may progress to a fibrotic stricture.	Must be differentiated from a local recurrency where the stricture is often irregular, nondistensible, and progressively worsening.
Adhesions	Short smooth stenotic areas with intact mucosa.	Secondary to abdominal surgery or inflammation.

(continues on page 710)

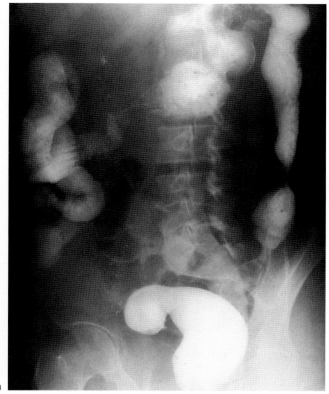

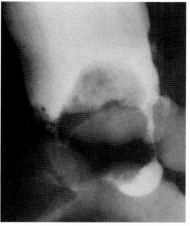

Fig. 29.**52 a, b Crohn's colitis** in a patient with ileocolostomy performed four years earlier for colon carcinoma. **a** Several benign stenotic segments are seen in the remaining distal half of the colon with the two most severe strictures being located at the anastomotic side between ileum and transverse colon and in the descending colon. Note also the abnormal mucosal pattern in both ileum and colon with relative sparing of the rectosigmoid. **b** The carcinoma had originally presented as a fungating mass in the ascending colon in this patient with a long history of Crohn's disease.

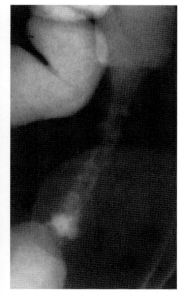

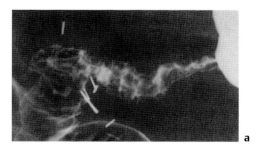

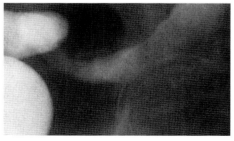

Fig. 29.**53 Ischemic colitis.** A constricting lesion with "thumb printing" is seen in the descending colon.

Fig. 29.**54 a, b Radiation colitis, a** in the acute and **b** in the chronic phase. A localized narrowing of the sigmoid colon is seen in both phases. Mucosal abnormalities including ulcerations are associated in the acute stage, whereas a tubular stricture is seen in the chronic stage.

Table 29.5 (Cont.) Narrowing of the Colon and Rectum

Disease	Radiographic Findings	Comments
Pelvic lipomatosis (Fig. 29.55)	Narrowing and vertical elongation of the rectum and sigmoid with intact mucosa and distensible wall. The increased pelvic radiolucency caused by the excessive fat deposition may already be appreciated by conventional radiography; otherwise CT is diagnostic.	Benign condition with increased deposition of normal adipose tissue in the pelvis. A similar narrowing of the rectosigmoid may occasionally be seen with *retractile mesenteritis,* which more commonly involves the small bowel.
Pelvic fibrosis	Narrowing of the rectum and/or sigmoid.	After pelvic surgery, trauma, inflammation, irradiation, and edema (e.g., chronic obstruction of the inferior vena cava).
Pelvic carcinomatosis and lymphoma	Narrowing of the rectum and/or sigmoid with or without tumor infiltration.	Metastases from urogenital or intestinal malignancies.
Pelvic mass	Extrinsic narrowing and often elongation of the rectum and/or sigmoid.	Ovarian cyst, enlarged uterus, neurogenic and sacral lesions (retrorectal), hematoma (pelvic fractures), abscess, urinoma, and lymphocele.
Amyloidosis	Rare cause of rigid narrowing with effacement of haustral markings preferentially in the rectosigmoid area.	May mimic chronic ulcerative colitis.
Volvulus (cecal and sigmoid) (Figs. 29.56 and 29.57)	The tapered contrast column at the level of obstruction has characteristically the appearance of a "bird's beak."	Plain film findings may already be diagnostic. See Chapter **26** (Figs. 26.**29** and 26.**30**).
Hernias (Fig. 29.58)	Localized narrowing and obstruction of displaced transverse or sigmoid colon, often complicated by strangulation.	Inguinal, femoral, umbilical, diaphragmatic, incisional as well as internal hernias (e.g., through the foramen of Winslow) occur.

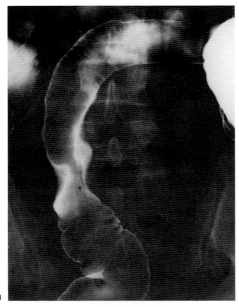
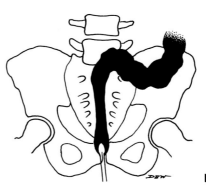

a   b

Fig. 29.**55 a, b** **Pelvic lipomatosis.** Narrowing and vertical elongation of the rectum and distal sigmoid with intact mucosa and distensible wall is characteristic.

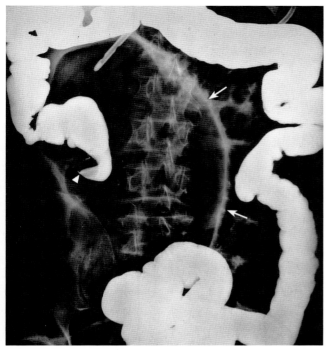

Fig. 29.**56** **Cecal volvulus.** A markedly dilated cecum (arrows) is associated with a smooth tapered obstruction of the ascending colon (arrowhead).

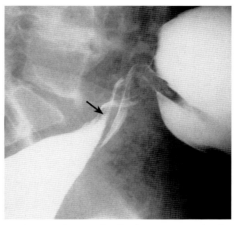

Fig. 29.**57** **Sigmoid volvulus.** A tapered edge of the obstructed contrast column ("bird's beak") pointing toward the site of torsion is characteristic (arrow).

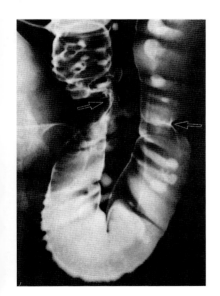

Fig. 29.**58** **Inguinal hernia.** Localized extrinsic compression of the afferent and efferent loop of the sigmoid colon at the site of entry into the hernial sac is seen (arrows). Note also the multiple diverticula.

30 Filling Defects in the Gastrointestinal Tract

In the gastrointestinal tract, space-occupying lesions are visualized during barium examinations as filling defects. A variety of normal and pathologic structures can produce a filling defect in the gastrointestinal tract, although neoplasms are the most common cause. They may originate from the mucosa, the remaining bowel wall, or an adjacent organ. Depending on the site of origin, intrinsic and extrinsic mass lesions can be differentiated radiographically.

An *intrinsic lesion* is characterized by the fact that the larger portion of the mass projects into the lumen of the bowel. Using this definition, any lesion with a stalk obviously falls into this category. Lesions in which the barium column forms an acute angle between the mass and bowel wall, when viewed in profile, are also intrinsic (Fig. 30.1). If such a lesion involves the entire circumference of the bowel, acute angles ("shouldering") may be seen on both sides of the lumen. Most intrinsic lesions originate from the mucosa, but occasionally an intramural lesion (e.g., a gastrointestinal stromal tumor [GIST] of the bowel wall) may produce radiographic features characteristic of an intrinsic or polypoid mass.

When the barium column forms an obtuse angle between the lesion and bowel wall in profile projection, the tumor can be either intrinsic or extrinsic. An infiltrating carcinoma presenting as a plaque would be an example of an intrinsic lesion that can present radiographically in this way. A similar filling defect can be produced by an *extrinsic mass,* but in this case only a small segment of the mass protrudes into the lumen, while the larger portion of it is located outside the bowel lumen (Fig. 30.1). Assuming the extrinsic mass has a more or less globular shape, the radiographically visualized tumor segment is always smaller than the part of the lesion projecting outside the lumen. Assessment of the size of the extraluminal component may be the only clue to help differentiate between an intrinsic and extrinsic lesion when both form an obtuse angle with the bowel wall.

Extrinsic filling defects in the gastrointestinal tract can be caused by normal, or more commonly by pathologically altered organs in the immediate vicinity. In the esophagus, this includes the spine, thyroid, trachea, left main bronchus, aorta, heart, lymph nodes, and other tissue structures of the posterior mediastinum (Fig. 30.2). Displacement of an esophageal

segment, however, is not only caused by *extrinsic compression,* but may at times also result from *retraction* produced by a scarring process. This occurs, for example, in apical pleuropulmonary fibrosis.

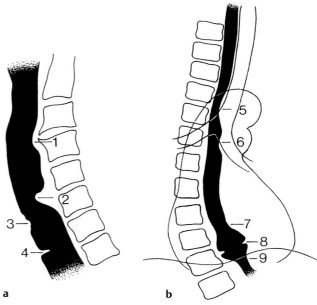

a   b

Fig. 30.**2 Normal and pathologic filling defects in the esophagus. a** Lateral cervical esophagus. **b** Left posterior oblique thoracic esophagus.
1 Posterior defect caused by osteophytes.
2 Intermittent posterior defect at the C5/C6 disk level by cricopharyngeus muscle.
3 Anterior impression at the C6 level caused by pharyngeal venous plexus.
4 Esophageal web arising characteristically from the anterior wall.
5 Left anterior impression caused by aortic arch.
6 Anterior impression caused by left main bronchus.
7 Junction between tubular esophagus and phrenic ampulla (vestibule).
8 Lower esophageal or Schatzki's ring.
9 Narrowing caused by diaphragmatic hiatus.

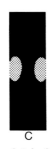
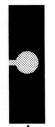
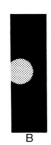
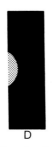
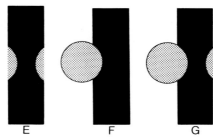

A   B   C   D   E   F   G

Fig. 30.**1 Differentiation between intrinsic** (A to E) **and extrinsic** (F and G) **lesions**. Radiographic signs of an intrinsic lesion include the demonstration of a pedicle (A) or the demonstration of an acute angle between lesion and bowel wall (B and C). An obtuse angle between lesion and bowel is not diagnostic, since it can be

found with both intrinsic (D and E) and extrinsic (F and G) lesions, both producing the same radiographic profile. However, with extrinsic lesions a larger extraluminal component is invariably present, as shown in F and G.

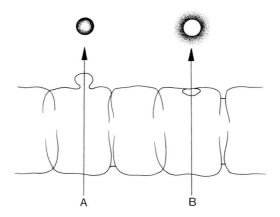

Fig. 30.**3**   **Differentiation between diverticulum** (A) **and polyp** (B) when viewed face-on in double-contrast examinations. A diverticulum has a sharp outer border and a fuzzy inner border (A), whereas a polyp has a sharp inner border and a fuzzy outer border (B).

Differentiation between *benign* and *malignant* mass lesions can be difficult. Rigidity of the involved bowel segment, a destroyed mucosal pattern, and ulcerations associated with a mass strongly suggest a malignancy. A soft and pliable or pedunculated mass lesion with a normal mucosal pattern favors a benign process. Tumor size is an unreliable criterion for differentiating between benign and malignant lesions, although polypoid lesions measuring less than 10 mm in diameter are likely to be benign. On the other hand, an increase in the size of a mass on follow-up examination is very likely to indicate a malignant process. The growth rate of gastrointestinal malignancies can occasionally be very slow, with tumor-doubling times exceeding three years. One has to keep in mind that an increase in diameter of only 26% is required to double the volume of a spherical lesion.

In air contrast studies, differentiation between a *polypoid lesion* and a *diverticulum* may be difficult when the lesion is seen face-on in a double-contrast examination. In these conditions, a sharp inner border of barium around the lesions is characteristic for a polypoid lesion, whereas in a diverticulum the outer border is sharply defined (Fig. 30.3).

The differential diagnosis of filling defects in the gastrointestinal tract is discussed in Tables 30.1 to 30.5.

Table 30.1 Filling Defect in the Esophagus

Disease	Radiographic Findings	Comments
Normal structures: Cricopharyngeal muscle (Fig. 30.2)	Intermittent posterior filling defect at the pharyngoesophageal junction (at the C5/C6 disk level).	*Cricopharyngeal achalasia:* Functional disturbance with dysphagia caused by failure of this muscle to relax. Produces a persistent filling defect radiographically. Idiopathic, or associated with a variety of neuromuscular disorders or partial pharyngectomy. Hypertrophy of the cricopharyngeus may also occur after laryngectomy with the development of esophageal speech.
Pharyngeal venous plexus	Occasional shallow anterior impression at the level of C6.	
Left main bronchus (Fig. 30.2)	Anterior impression below aortic arch.	
Vascular structures: **Aortic arch (Fig. 30.2)**	Left anterior impression best demonstrated in right anterior oblique projection.	Extrinsic filling defect much more pronounced with anteriosclerotic or aneurysmatic aortic arch.
Arteriosclerosis or aneurysm of descending aorta	Displacement of esophagus varies, but is often anterior.	
Right aortic arch	Type 1: Characteristic right anterior impression. Type 2: Characteristic large posterior defect in esophagus.	Type 1: Mirror-image branching, commonly associated with congenital heart disease. Type 2: Posterior right aortic arch. Most common type, not associated with congenital heart disease. Associated aberrant left subclavian artery and left ligamentum arteriosum may form complete vascular ring.
Double aortic arch	Large posterior defect caused by the junction of both arches and small and higher anterior defect produced by trachea pressed against esophagus. Right and left lateral impression corresponds to each arch.	May cause dysphagia and dyspnea by compression.
Aberrant right subclavian artery	Posterior defect with characteristic appearance. In frontal projection the esophageal defect is oblique, begins at the upper border of the aortic arch, and ascends from left to right at an angle of 70 degrees.	Usually an incidental finding, but may occasionally cause dysphagia.
Aberrant left pulmonary artery	Anterior indentation of esophagus at level of carina by left pulmonary artery arising from right pulmonary artery.	Signs of respiratory obstruction and infection may be present.
Left atrial enlargement	Localized compression and displacement of esophagus posteriorly and to the right below carina.	Mitral valve disease is by far the most common cause of isolated left atrial enlargement. When the left ventricle is also enlarged, the esophagus is displaced posteriorly along the entire length of its contact with the heart.

(continues on page 716)

Table 30.1 (Cont.) Filling Defect in the Esophagus

Disease	Radiographic Findings	Comments
Cysts (intramural and mediastinal) (Fig. 30.4)	Smooth round extrinsic or, less commonly, intrinsic filling defects.	Rare. Besides congenital or duplication cysts, retention cysts originating in the esophageal glands occur.
Benign esophageal tumors (Figs. 30.5, 30.6)	Smoothly outlined intramural lesions that bulge into the esophageal lumen or may be pedunculated. *Leiomyomas* are usually found in the lower third of the esophagus and may occasionally ulcerate.	Rare and usually asymptomatic. Besides leiomyomas (most common), *lipomas, angiomas, neurogenic tumors, granular cell myoblastomas, polyps* (fibromuscular or inflammatory), *papillomas,* and *villous adenomas* are found.
Thyroid enlargement or tumor	Significant extrinsic displacement of both the trachea and the cervical or paratracheal esophagus occurs even with a relatively small goiter including in the substernal location. Thyroid carcinomas may invade the esophagus, causing an abnormal mucosal pattern.	All thyroid mass lesions, which do not infiltrate into the surrounding structures, move up and down with the larynx during swallowing. Fluoroscopy is virtually diagnostic.
Carcinoma of the esophagus (Fig. 30.7)	An irregular circumferential lesion with destroyed or ulcerated mucosa, overhanging edges and abrupt transition to normal tissue is the most common presentation. A fungating mass with superficial ulceration is less frequently found. Early spread into mediastinal tissue occurs, possibly because of lack of serosal membrane on the esophagus.	The majority are squamous cell carcinomas. Adenocarcinomas, verrucous carcinomas (exophytic or warty tumors that rarely metastasize), primary melanomas, and metastases are rare intrinsic esophageal malignancies of epithelial origin.
Carcinoma of the stomach (Fig. 30.8)	Irregular mass in the distal esophagus.	Caused by gastric carcinoma of the cardia extending upward.
Leiomyosarcoma (Fig. 30.9)	Extrinsic or intrinsic bulky mass lesions with a smooth or irregular outline. Ulcerations occur frequently.	*Malignant gastrointestinal stromal tumors (GISTs)* are uncommon in the esophagus. *Carcinosarcomas* and *pseudosarcomas* are other rare tumors that present as large intrinsic mass lesions with irregular outline.

(continues on page 718)

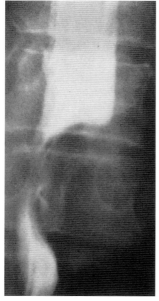

Fig. 30.**4** **Intramural esophageal cyst.** A smooth filling defect is seen.

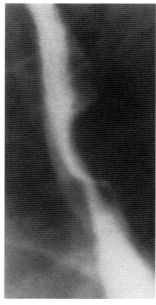

Fig. 30.**5** **Leiomyoma.** A smooth semicircular defect is seen.

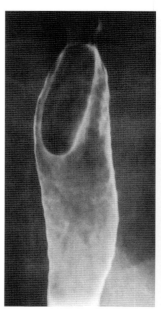

Fig. 30.**6** **Lipoma.** A smooth, oval deformable mass is seen in the upper esophagus.

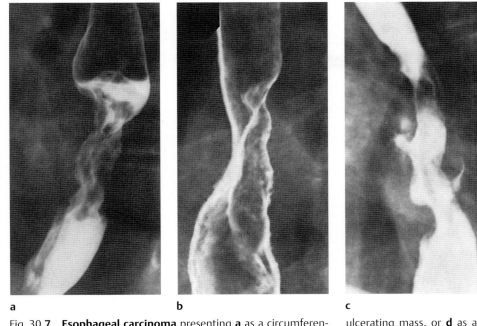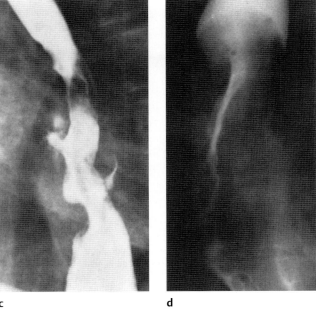

a   b   c   d

Fig. 30.**7** **Esophageal carcinoma** presenting **a** as a circumferential lesion with destroyed mucosa, **b** as a plaque-like lesion, **c** as an ulcerating mass, or **d** as an intraluminal mass with overhanging edges.

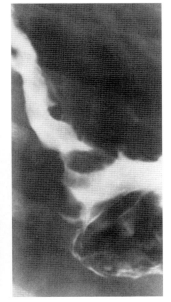

Fig. 30.**8** **Carcinoma of the stomach** invading the distal esophagus. An irregular mass is seen in the distal esophagus.

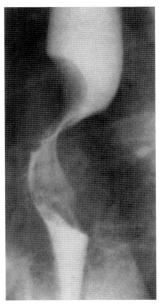

Fig. 30.**9** **Leiomyosarcoma.** A large spiraling mass with mainly extrinsic tumor component is seen.

Table 30.1   (Cont.) Filling Defect in the Esophagus

Disease	Radiographic Findings	Comments
Lymphoma	One or several extrinsic filling defects caused by mediastinal lymphadenopathy are the most common presentation. Infiltration of the esophagus from mediastinal lymph nodes or stomach producing irregular filling defects can occur. Primary lymphoma of the esophagus is extremely rare.	Occurs with Hodgkin's and non-Hodgkin's lymphoma.
Mediastinal tumors	Extrinsic filling defects caused by tumors or lymphadenopathy of the posterior mediastinum.	Common. *Metastases* (e.g., from bronchogenic carcinoma) and lymphoma may cause dysphagia at a relatively early stage. Primary mediastinal tumors are much less common and may cause considerable displacement without causing dysphagia. For further differentiation see Table 17.**3**.
Infectious esophagitis	Multiple small round or oval filling defects are occasionally seen, and are usually associated with a shaggy mucosa and fine ulcerations.	Usually caused by candidiasis and rarely by herpes in compromised hosts and AIDS patients.
Mediastinal abscess (see Fig. 30.24 b)	Localized extrinsic mass that may contain air.	Usually due to esophageal rupture, which is diagnosed by extravasation of ingested contrast material.
Granulomatous mediastinitis	Anterior esophageal compression by enlarged paratracheal lymph nodes, which may be calcified.	Patient usually asymptomatic. *Tuberculosis, histoplasmosis,* and *sarcoidosis* are the most common etiologies. *Sclerosing mediastinitis* may rarely produce a filling defect similar to a carcinoma.
Mediastinal hematoma	Extrinsic compression of the esophagus, usually in the upper mediastinum.	Trauma, surgery, aortic dissection.
Varices (Fig. 30.10)	Round or oval filling defects predominantly in the distal esophagus, often resembling beads of a rosary. Normal peristalsis and change in appearance between esophageal dilatation and contraction, where they usually disappear, are diagnostic.	In *portal hypertension* caused by liver cirrhosis or Budd–Chiari syndrome (both associated with ascites and abnormal liver functions) or splenoportal vein occlusion (usually no ascites and normal liver functions).
Food or foreign body (Fig. 30.11)	May simulate intraluminal mass, particularly when located in prestenotic segment (organic stenosis or persistent spasm).	*Air bubbles* coated with barium cause only transitory changes and can easily be differentiated.
Spondylosis and spondylitis (see Fig. 30.2 a)	Osteophytes of the cervical spine may produce one or more smooth extrinsic defects in the posterior wall of the esophagus. Infectious spondylitis can present as a posterior fusiform mass with vertebral destruction, It usually originates from the cervical or lower thoracic spine.	Tuberculous and nontuberculous spondylitis.

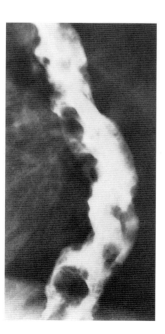

Fig. 30.**10** **Varices.** Large round and oval filling defects are seen in the distal esophagus. The absence of obstruction, normal peristalsis, and change in appearance between esophageal dilatation and contraction are characteristic.

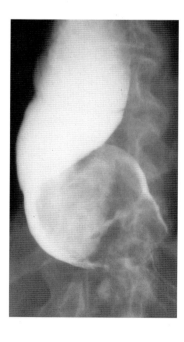

Fig. 30.**11** **Bezoar.** A large intraluminal mass is seen in the dilated distal esophagus just proximal to the gastroesophageal junction.

Table 30.2   Filling Defects in the Stomach

Disease	Radiographic Findings	Comments
Web (Fig. 30.12)	Circular membrane-like defect, usually located in antrum.	Rare congenital lesion.
Ectopic pancreas (aberrant) (Fig. 30.13)	Nodule measuring 1–4 cm in diameter and preferentially located in the antropyloric region. A central depression (umbilication) is characteristically present and can simulate an ulcer.	Heterotopic pancreatic tissue may occur anywhere in the gastrointestinal tract, but is most common in the stomach. Patient is normally asymptomatic.
Duplication cyst	Usually solitary 3–12 cm intramural lesion, preferentially on greater curvature. Alteration in configuration under external compression may indicate cystic nature of lesion.	Majority of duplication cysts are diagnosed in childhood.
Polyps and benign tumors (Figs. 30.14 and 30.15)	Usually present as solitary and small submucosal nodules with intact mucosa. Ulcerations occur in *gastrointestinal stromal tumors (GISTs), neurogenic tumors,* and *lipomas.* Polyps, lipomas, and GISTs may be pedunculated. *Hyperplastic polyps* present as small (1 cm or less) and often multiple filling defects that are caused by excessive regenerative hyperplasia in an area of chronic gastritis, and must be differentiated from adenomatous polyps that are potentially malignant.	Any polypoid lesion larger than 2 cm should be suspected of being malignant and should therefore be removed. Even histologically, it is often difficult to differentiate between benign and malignant gastrointestinal stromal tumors (GISTs) and adenomatous polyps, respectively. The latter have a high incidence of malignancy and are often found in chronic atrophic gastritis. Multiple gastric polyps may also be seen in *familial polyposis* of the colon and in the *Gardner's syndrome* (see Table 30.**5**). Multiple hamartomas presenting as small polypoid lesions are found in *Peutz–Jeghers, Canada–Cronkhite* and *Cowden's syndrome.* In all three conditions they are associated with hamartomas in other parts of the gastrointestinal tract (see Table 30.**5**).

(continues on page 720)

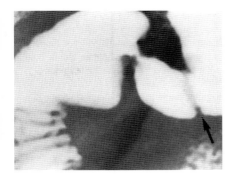

Fig. 30.**12   Congenital antral web.** A circumferential membrane-like defect is seen in the antrum (arrow).

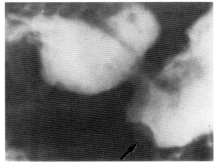

Fig. 30.**13   Ectopic (aberrant) pancreas.** A small nodule with central umbilication (arrow) is seen in the greater curvature of the prepyloric region.

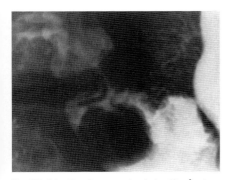

Fig. 30.**14   Benign gastrointestinal stromal tumor (GIST).** A nodular lesion is seen in the antrum.

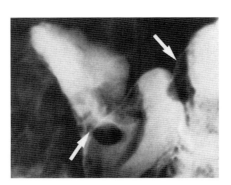

Fig. 30.**15   Adenomatous polyps.** Two round-to-ovoid filling defects with pedicles (arrows) are seen in the antrum.

Table 30.2   (Cont.) Filling Defects in the Stomach

Disease	Radiographic Findings	Comments
Villous adenoma (Fig. 30.16)	Usually a solitary, sessile mass of varying size. Because of the softness of the tumor, change in shape occurs with peristaltic contractions or external compression. Barium trapped between strands may produce a frondlike appearance.	Rare gastric tumor with relatively high incidence of malignancy.
Carcinoma (Fig. 30.17)	Ranging from polypoid lesions to large fungating masses with destroyed mucosal pattern (amputation of folds), ulcerations, and rigidity of the adjacent stomach wall are often present. May occur at any location, but slight preference for lesser curvature, especially near gastric incisura. Mucus-producing carcinomas may occasionally contain calcifications.	Other radiologic presentations of gastric carcinoma are the ulcerating form and the infiltrative (scirrhous) type.
Sarcoma (Fig. 30.18)	Intramural lesions with intraluminal component that varies greatly in size. Ranges from small circumscribed nodules to large exophytic masses, often with deep central ulceration. Calcifications are rarely present.	A *malignant gastrointestinal stromal tumor (GIST)* is the most common gastric sarcoma. *Neurogenic sarcomas, liposarcomas,* and *fibrosarcomas* are rare.
Lymphoma (Fig. 30.19)	Ranges from thickened folds with nodular lesions to large intrinsic or extrinsic masses. Ulcerations are relatively common.	Primary gastric lymphoma is usually of the non-Hodgkin's variety. When it presents as a localized gastric mass, it is radiographically indistinguishable from a *pseudolymphoma*. Secondary involvement of the stomach occurs with both Hodgkin's and non-Hodgkin's lymphoma.
Kaposi's sarcoma	Focal or diffuse, sharply defined submucosal nodules (5–20 mm) with or without central umbilication are characteristic.	In homosexual males with AIDS.
Metastases (hematogenous) (Fig. 30.20)	Rare. Usually multiple, sharply delineated filling defects, often with central ulcerations ("target lesions").	Metastases from melanoma are most common, followed by breast and lung carcinomas and rarely other malignancies.
Extrinsic mass (Fig. 30.21)	Extrinsic defects may be caused by normal or enlarged adjacent organs and inflammatory or neoplastic lesions. Gastric mucosa is characteristically normal unless infiltrated by a malignant lesion (e.g., carcinoma of pancreas infiltrating greater curvature and posterior wall of the stomach and simulating gastric carcinoma).	Extrinsic impression on anterior wall and lesser curvature is often caused by a normal or more often by an enlarged *liver*. In the distal antrum and pyloric region, an extrinsic defect may be caused by a *hypertrophic pylorus*. Extrinsic impression on the posterior wall and greater curvature can be caused by the *spleen*, *colon*, an enlarged retroperitoneal organ (especially *pancreas*, including pancreatic pseudocysts, *left kidney*, and *left adrenal*), or a pathologic process in the *lesser sac*. *Intraperitoneal metastases* may involve all surfaces of the stomach.

(continues on page 722)

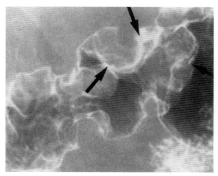

a

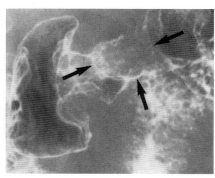

b

Fig. 30.**16 a, b**   **Villous adenoma** (histologically with early carcinomatous transformation). A sessile, soft mass (arrows) that changes shape with peristaltic contractions (note the difference between **a** and **b**) is seen in the antrum, but there is only minimal barium trapping between its villous strands.

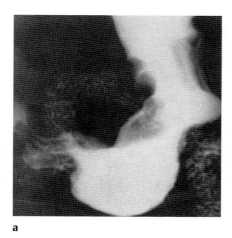

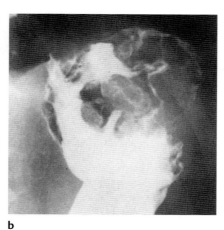

a

b

Fig. 30.**17 a, b   Gastric carcinoma** in two different patients. **a** A mass originating from the lesser curvature that is completely rigid in this area, is seen. **b** A fungating mass with destroyed mucosal pattern and ulcerations is seen in the fundus.

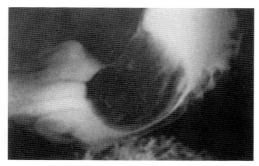

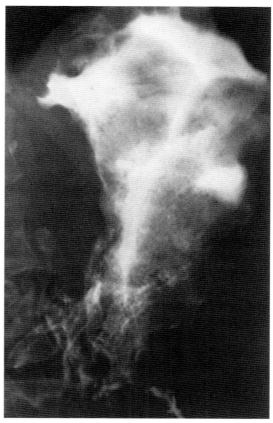

Fig. 30.**18   Malignant gastrointestinal stromal tumor (GIST).** A large mass lesion is present in the body of the stomach.

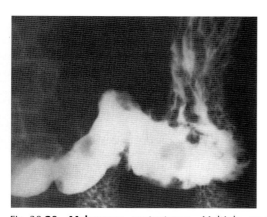

Fig. 30.**20   Melanoma metastases.** Multiple nodular lesions some of which with central ulcerations ("target lesions") are seen in the body and antrum of the stomach.

Fig. 30.**19   Non-Hodgkin's lymphoma.** A large mass lesion involving the fundus and body of the stomach is seen.

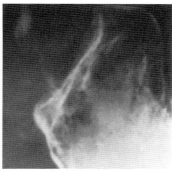

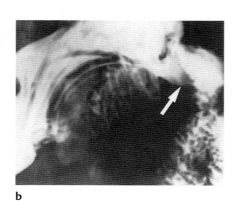

a

b

Fig. 30.**21 a, b   Extrinsic mass lesions.** Extrinsic defects without mucosal involvement are seen **a** in the fundus, caused by an *accessory spleen,* and **b** on the greater curvature, caused by *non-Hodgkin's lymphoma.* Note also the abnormal mucosal pattern in the distal duodenum and the ulceration in the duodeno-jejunal junction (arrow), which is caused by lymphomatous infiltration.

Table 30.2 (Cont.) Filling Defects in the Stomach

Disease	Radiographic Findings	Comments
Eosinophilic granuloma (inflammatory fibroelastic polyp) (Fig. 30.22)	Polypoid mass lesion measuring up to 9 cm in diameter. May be pedunculated. Almost always located in the gastric antrum. Ulceration is very rare.	This lesion is neither associated with peripheral eosinophilia nor food allergy and has nothing to do with the eosinophilic granuloma of the Langerhans cell histiocytosis complex.
Ménétrier's disease (giant hypertrophic gastritis) (Fig. 30.23)	Multiple nodular filling defects caused by markedly enlarged gastric folds are seen, preferentially located in the fundus and along the greater curvature.	Ménétrier's disease is a protein-losing enteropathy. Similar nodular defects caused by enlarged gastric folds are occasionally seen in *Crohn's disease, eosinophilic gastritis, tuberculosis,* and *sarcoidosis.*
Peptic ulcer	Mucosal edema around the ulcer may occasionally simulate an ulcerating tumor. A large indentation on the greater curvature opposite an ulcer on the lesser curvature should not be mistaken for a mass ("ulcer finger").	A *double pylorus* (short fistula connecting the prepyloric lesser curvature with the duodenal bulb secondary to peptic ulcer disease) may produce the appearance of an intraluminal prebulbar defect that is caused by the two pyloric channels surrounding the scar tissue in between.
Hematoma	Rare. Intramural mass of varying size.	Usually history of trauma or bleeding disorder is present.
Postoperative defect (Fig. 30.24)	Postoperative defects can measure up to 5 cm in areas of suturing. They may become less prominent or even disappear with time. *Fundoplication* deformities after hiatal hernia repair produce masslike defects in the gastric fundus, caused by the invaginated esophagus.	A postoperative defect that increases in size on follow-up studies indicates complication (hematoma, abscess, etc.) or tumor recurrence.

(continues on page 723)

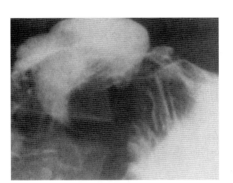

Fig. 30.**22** **Eosinophilic granuloma.** A large round mass lesion is seen in the antrum.

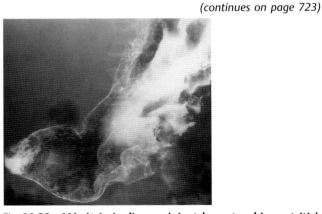

Fig. 30.**23** **Ménétrier's disease (giant hypertrophic gastritis).** Multiple nodular filling defects caused by markedly enlarged gastric folds are seen in the fundus and along the greater curvature.

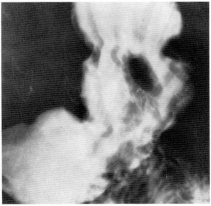

a

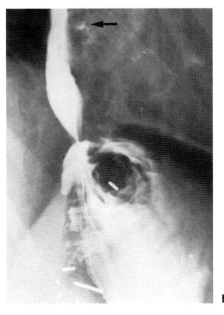

b

Fig. 30.**24 a, b** **Postoperative defects. a** An oval filling defect is seen in the body of the stomach. Note also the postoperative indentation on both the lesser and greater curvature at the same level. **b** Nissen fundoplication: a characteristic filling defect is seen in the cardia. Note also the small iatrogenic perforation (arrow) with abscess formation causing a gentle extrinsic compression in the lower esophagus.

Table 30.2 (Cont.) Filling Defects in the Stomach

Disease	Radiographic Findings	Comments
Amyloidosis	Solitary or more commonly multiple, often ulcerated filling defects.	Usually associated with involvement of other parts of the gastrointestinal tract.
Varices (Fig. 30.25)	Multiple smooth lobulated filling defects preferentially located in the fundus. Occasionally, a single filling defect is caused by a large varix. Change in size and shape is characteristic. Usually associated with esophageal varices and splenomegaly.	Gastric varices not associated with esophageal varices occur in splenic vein occlusion (e.g., in pancreatitis or carcinoma of pancreas). The collateral flow passes in these cases from the short gastric veins via the left and right gastric veins to the portal vein.
Intussusception (Fig. 30.26)	Intraluminal, often polycyclic defect with characteristic circular and semicircular springlike folds.	Occurs in resected stomach, or is caused by a pedunculated lesion.
Bezoar (Fig. 30.27)	Freely mobile, intraluminal mass with often characteristic mottled appearance, conforming to the shape of the stomach. May cause gastric dilatation and fill the entire lumen.	Phytobezoars are composed of plant products and trichobezoars of hair.
Foreign body, ingested food, blood clots (Fig. 30.28)	Single or multiple freely mobile filling defects of varying shape and size.	A *gallstone* passing either retrograde from the duodenum or through a cholecystogastric fistula can rarely produce an intraluminal filling defect.

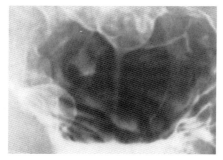

Fig. 30.**25** **Gastric varices.** Smoothly lobulated nodular lesions are seen in the fundus.

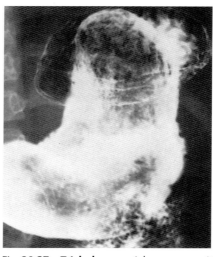

Fig. 30.**27** **Trichobezoar.** A large mass with mottled appearance is seen in the stomach.

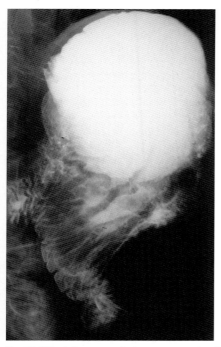

Fig. 30.**26** **Jejunogastric intussusception in Billroth II.** Invagination of small bowel loops through the gastrojejunal anastomosis into the partially resected stomach produces the characteristic lesion with "coiled spring" appearance.

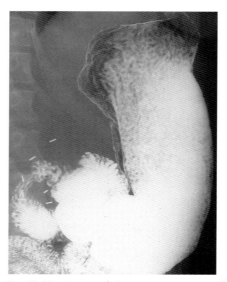

Fig. 30.**28** **Ingested rice.** Large amounts of ingested rice mimics a granular mucosal pattern in the stomach.

Table 30.3   Filling Defects in the Duodenum

Disease	Radiographic Findings	Comments
Web	Circumferential membrane-like filling defect usually located in the second portion of the duodenum. May cause varying degrees of obstruction.	Congenital abnormality.
Ectopic (aberrant) pancreas	Usually submucosal nodules, measuring 1 to 2 cm (rarely up to 4 cm). Central umbilication is characteristic and should not be confused with an ulcerating mass.	Aberrant pancreatic tissue in the gastrointestinal tract is found in 2% of all routine postmortems, most commonly located in stomach and duodenum.
Annular pancreas	Extrinsic ringlike or predominantly lateral defect on the superior part of the descending duodenum.	Often only diagnosed in adulthood, since no significant obstruction occurs in majority of cases.
Hypertrophy of Brunner's glands (Fig. 30.29)	Multiple diffuse or circumscribed small polypoid filling defects, measuring from a few millimeters ("cobblestone" pattern) to 1 cm in diameter. Preferential location is first portion of duodenum.	Often associated with peptic ulcer disease. Small *glandular adenomas* of *Brunner's glands* have also been described, but probably represent localized areas of hypertrophy rather than true neoplasms.
Nodular lymphoid hyperplasia (benign)	Innumerable tiny, 1–5 mm filling defects evenly distributed throughout the entire duodenum.	Usually an incidental finding but may be associated with hypogammaglobulinemia.
Heterotopic gastric mucosa	Multiple filling defects similar to benign lymphoid hyperplasia but more irregular and limited to the duodenal bulb.	Incidental finding. Compared to Brunner's gland hypertrophy, the filling defects are smaller and less uniform.
Duplication cyst	Intrinsic or extrinsic mass in first or second portion of duodenum. May become tubular in shape when communication with normal lumen occurs.	Very rare in the adult. May cause duodenal obstruction in infancy.
Choledochal cyst (Fig. 30.30)	Extrinsic mass on the inner aspect of the duodenal sweep, which might be widened and compressed, when the lesion is large enough.	Usually in girls under the age of 10, presenting with jaundice, right upper quadrant mass, and abdominal pain.
Intraluminal diverticulum (Fig. 30.31)	Rare form of duodenal diverticulum originating in the descending portion of the duodenum The wall of the diverticulum may be seen as a radiolucent line ("halo sign"). May be confused with communicating duplication cyst that is filled with barium.	
Polyps and benign tumors (Fig. 30.32)	Solitary or rarely multiple nodules that may be pedunculated. Central ulcerations can occur. Nodular lesions located in the bulb are usually benign.	May mimic ulcer symptoms and bleed. Histologically, *adenomas, gastrointestinal stromal tumors (GISTs), lipomas, neurinomas,* and others are found, but radiologic differentiation is usually not possible. Multiple hamartomatous polyps may be present in *Peutz–Jeghers syndrome.* *Villous adenomas, carcinoids,* and *islet cell tumors* are potentially malignant lesions located preferentially in the first or second portion of the duodenum. Severe peptic ulcer disease or diarrhea is usually associated with carcinoids and islet cell tumors.
Duodenal carcinoma (Fig. 30.33)	Circumferential constricting lesion with mucosal destruction or polypoid mass, often with ulceration. Usually located distal to the papilla.	Most of the primary duodenal malignancies are adenocarcinomas, the rest sarcomas and lymphomas.

(continues on page 726)

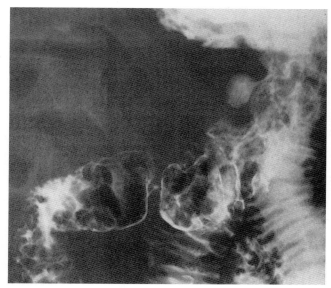

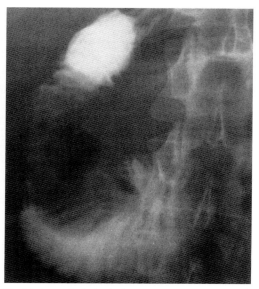

Fig. 30.29 Hypertrophy of Brunner's glands. Multiple polypoid lesions measuring up to 1 cm are seen in the proximal duodenum, and are associated with a large peptic ulcer in the lesser curvature of the stomach.

Fig. 30.30 Choledochal cyst. An extrinsic filling defect is seen on the medial aspect of the second portion of the duodenum.

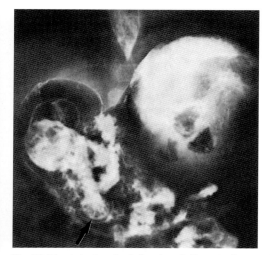

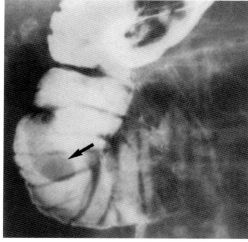

Fig. 30.31 Intraluminal duodenal diverticulum. A barium-filled fingerlike sac is seen in the second portion of the duodenum. Note the characteristic radiolucent band around its distal end (arrow) representing the wall of the diverticulum ("halo sign").

Fig. 30.32 Duodenal polyp. A smooth ovoid filling defect with a large pedicle is seen in the second portion of the duodenum (arrow).

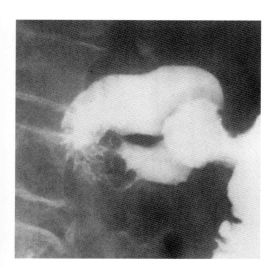

Fig. 30.33 Duodenal carcinoma. An irregular filling defect with small ulcerations is seen in the duodenum.

Table 30.3   (Cont.) Filling Defects in the Duodenum

Disease	Radiographic Findings	Comments
Metastases (Fig. 30.34)	Extrinsic compression with or without invasion of the duodenum by malignancy from an adjacent organ. Invasive metastases are associated with mucosal destruction, ulceration and mass formation. Intracanalicular and hematogenous metastases presenting as solitary or multiple nodular lesions are rare. Central ulceration in these metastases is quite characteristic (target lesions).	Found with carcinomas from neighboring organs such as the pancreas and biliary system, retroperitoneal malignancies, or by direct extension from the stomach (e.g., in lymphoma). Metastases presenting as target lesions originate usually from breast and lung carcinomas, melanoma or Kaposi's sarcoma.
Enlargement of the papilla of Vater (ampullary carcinoma, impacted gallstone) (Figs. 30.35 and 30.36)	Extrinsic or intrinsic defect at medial border of second portion of duodenum.	Filling defects smaller than 1.5 cm are within normal limits. Somewhat larger filling defects are seen with inflammation (e.g., papillitis, pancreatitis, cholangitis) or edema (e.g., post iatrogenic manipulation or stone passage). Ampullary carcinomas and impacted gallstones are usually associated with obstructive jaundice.
Choledochocele (intraduodenal choledochal cyst)	Filling defect at the medial border of the second portion of the duodenum caused by the prolapse of the cystic dilated portion of the terminal common bile duct.	Congenital or acquired. It is usually only associated with obstructive jaundice when complicated by an impacted gallstone or secondary inflammatory changes.
Blood clots, food, foreign bodies, gallstones	Rare intraluminal, fully mobile filling defects of various sizes and shapes. A gallstone eroded into the duodenum may rarely cause obstruction.	Reflux of barium through a fistulous tract into the biliary system supports the diagnosis of gallstone erosion into the duodenum.
Prolapsed gastric mucosa	Lobulated, mushroom-shaped filling defect at the base of the duodenal bulb with varying appearance during peristalsis.	Prolapse of redundant antral mucosa with peristaltic wave is usually an incidental finding of no clinical significance.
Prolapsed antral polyp (Fig. 30.37)	Usually a solitary round or oval filling defect at the base of the duodenal bulb.	Any polypoid gastric tumor may be the lead for a *gastric intussusception into the duodenum* (Fig. 30.**38**) causing symptoms of acute or chronic obstruction.
Peptic ulcer	Surrounding edema and swelling may be prominent, simulating an intraluminal mass with central ulceration.	Inflammatory swelling most pronounced in fresh ulcers and in children.
Superior mesenteric artery syndrome	Characteristic extrinsic anterior impression of the third portion of the duodenum in supine position. Partial-to-complete relief in prone position.	In young, thin, asthenic or hyperlordotic individuals, in prolonged immobilization (e.g., body cast and after severe burns) and in persons with reduced duodenal peristaltic activity (e.g., scleroderma).
Varices	One or more filling defects, often simulating enlarged mucosal folds.	Varicose dilatation of pancreaticoduodenal veins is rare in portal hypertension,

(continues on page 728)

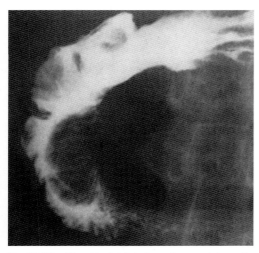

Fig. 30.**34** **Non-Hodgkin's lymphoma.** A large irregular mass indistinguishable from an ampullary carcinoma is seen in the medial aspect of the second portion of the duodenum. However, the correct diagnosis can be suggested by the nodular and ulcerative involvement of the proximal duodenum.

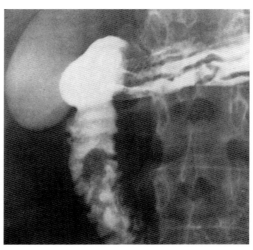

Fig. 30.**35** **Normal papilla of Vater.** An unusually large smooth filling defect is seen in the second portion of the duodenum. The gallbladder was opacified by an unrelated previous radiographic examination.

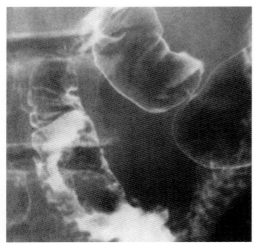

Fig. 30.**36** **Ampullary carcinoma.** An irregular filling defect is seen on the medial aspect of the second portion of the duodenum.

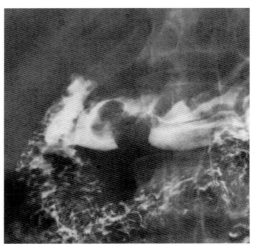

Fig. 30.**37** **Prolapsed antral polyp.** A smooth ovoid filling defect is seen in the duodenal bulb.

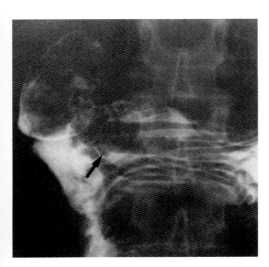

Fig. 30.**38** **Gastric intussusception** into the duodenum caused by antral mass (non-Hodgkin's lymphoma). The intussuscepted antrum occupies the entire duodenal bulb, whereas the antral polypoid lymphomatous lesion is no longer recognizable. Note also the coiled-spring appearance in the prepyloric part of the antrum caused by the intussusception (arrow). There is also an extrinsic defect on the greater curvature of the antrum caused by enlarged lymph nodes.

Table 30.3   (Cont.) Filling Defects in the Duodenum

Disease	Radiographic Findings	Comments
Hematoma (intramural or retroperitoneal) (Fig. 30.39)	Extrinsic filling defects commonly in the posterolateral aspect of the second and third portion of duodenum.	In bleeding disorders, posttraumatic or rarely spontaneous.
Postoperative defect	Extrinsic- or intrinsic-appearing defect in area of suturing.	A *stitch abscess* may produce a similar finding.
Pancreatic head enlargement (carcinoma, inflammation) (Fig. 30.40)	Widened duodenal loop with extrinsic impression on its inner border. Second portion may assume shape of inverted figure 3 ("inverted 3 sign"). Mucosal destruction, tumor invasion, and ulcerations suggest carcinoma; mucosal edema, calcifications, and pseudocysts (large extrinsic mass lesions in stomach or bowel) favor pancreatitis.	Elevated amylase levels are the most important clinical finding in *acute pancreatitis,* whereas *carcinoma of the head of the pancreas* is associated with jaundice in the great majority of cases. *Macrocystic adenomas* and *adenocarcinomas* may occasionally widen the duodenal sweep (Fig. 30.**41**), although the majority of these tumors originate in the body and tail of the pancreas.
Gallbladder and dilated common bile duct (Fig. 30.41)	A physiologically distended gallbladder may cause an extrinsic defect on the anterolateral aspect of the junction between the first and second portions of the duodenum. An extrinsic impression of tubular shape on the posterior wall of the duodenal bulb may be caused by an abnormally dilated common bile duct.	Although an extrinsic duodenal impression is already seen with a normal gallbladder, larger defects can be found with pathologically altered gallbladders (e.g., hydrops, pericholecystic abscess, carcinoma).
Hepatic mass	Extrinsic posterolateral filling defect on the first and second portions of the duodenum.	Hepatic cyst, abscess, benign and malignant tumors, or focal hypertrophy (e.g., of the caudate lobe) may cause extrinsic duodenal filling defects.
Subhepatic abscess	Extrinsic lateral filling defect on the second portion of the duodenum.	For example, postsurgical or secondary to ruptured gallbladder in acute cholecystitis.
Colon	Anterolateral filling defect in the fourth portion of the duodenum.	May be caused by fecal material or a mass in the transverse colon.
Retroperitoneal mass (Figs. 30.42 and 30.43)	Extrinsic defects in the second and adjacent third portions of the duodenum, either on the posterolateral wall (e.g., enlarged right kidney or adrenal) or on the posteromedial wall (e.g., retroperitoneal lymphadenopathy, sarcoma, abscess, and aortic aneurysm).	Retroperitoneal mass lesions causing filling defects on the posteromedial wall of the second portion of the duodenum are radiographically similar to the findings in pancreatic head enlargement.

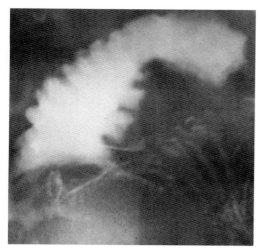

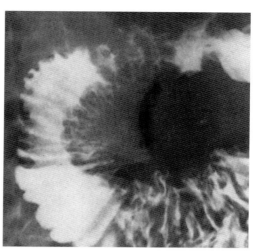

Fig. 30.**39** **Posttraumatic hematoma.** A large filling defect is seen at the junction between the second and third portion of the duodenum with almost complete obstruction and significant prestenotic dilatation.

Fig. 30.**40** **Pancreatic carcinoma.** An extrinsic impression on the inner border of the second portion of the duodenum with rnucosal destruction is seen.

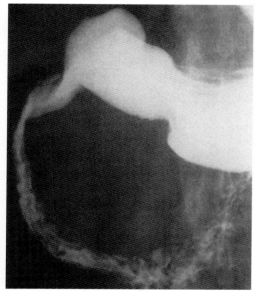

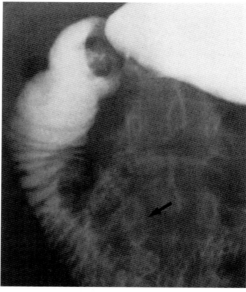

Fig. 30.**41** **Extrinsic defects caused by distended gallbladder and macrocystic adenoma of the pancreas.** The extrinsic impression on the anterolateral aspect of the junction between the first and second portions of the duodenum is caused by a distended gallbladder, whereas the widening of the duodenal loop is caused by a large macrocystic adenoma in the head of the pancreas.

Fig. 30.**42** **Non-Hodgkin's lymphoma** involving aortic lymph nodes. An extrinsic filling defect is seen in the inner aspect of the second and third portions of the duodenum. A markedly enlarged aortic lymph node is still faintly opacified from previous lymphography (arrow).

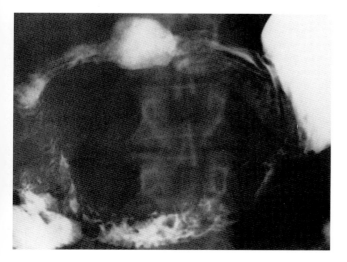

Fig. 30.**43** **Retroperitoneal hemangiosarcoma.** A marked widening of the duodenal loop by an extrinsic mass is seen. Mucosal destruction and nodular defects in the duodenum are caused by tumor invasion.

Table 30.4 Filling Defects in the Small Bowel (Jejunum and Ileum)

Disease	Radiographic Findings	Comments
Ectopic pancreas	Small submucosal nodule. Central umbilication is characteristic, but not always present.	Rare in small bowel (common in stomach and duodenum).
Duplication cyst	Intrinsic or extrinsic filling defect of varying size, usually in distal ileum.	Rare. May sometimes communicate with bowel lumen producing saclike structure.
Meckel's diverticulum (inverted) (Fig. 30.44 a, b)	Intraluminal filling defect in the middle or distal portion of ileum.	May progress to intussusception and cause small bowel obstruction.
Endometrioma (Fig. 30.45)	Small, usually solitary extrinsic or intrinsic mass, preferentially located in the ileum.	Rare. Clinical symptoms related to menstrual cycle.
Nodular lymphoid hyperplasia (benign) (Fig. 30.46)	Multiple nodular filling defects with predilection for the terminal ileum, but may be found throughout small bowel and colon.	Usually in children and adolescents. May be associated with dysgammaglobulinemia.
Benign tumors and polyps (Fig. 30.47 a, b)	Single or multiple filling defects. May be pedunculated. Central ulceration secondary to necrosis occurs. _Benign gastrointestinal stromal tumor (GIST)_: Extrinsic or intrinsic filling defect, almost always single, often ulcerated, and occasionally pedunculated. Preferentially located in the jejunum. True leiomyomas are much less common, but present in similar fashion. _Polyps_ (adenomatous and hamartomatous): Single or multiple, commonly pedunculated lesions, usually less than 5 cm in diameter. Preferentially located in the ileum. _Lipoma_: Solitary relatively small filling defect that may be pedunculated. Characteristically changes shape when compressed. Preferentially located in the distal ileum and ileocecal valve area. _Hemangiomas_: Commonly multiple and measuring less than 1 cm in diameter. Phleboliths are occasionally associated. _Neurofibromas_: Single or multiple, sessile or pedunculated, with or without ulcerations.	A benign GIST is the most common nonmalignant neoplasm of the small bowel measuring usually less than 5 cm. _Peutz–Jeghers_ syndrome: multiple (hamartomatous) polyps in the small bowel often associated with colonic and gastric polyps and characteristic pigmentation of skin and mucous membranes. _Rendu–Osler–Weber_ syndrome: familial disorder with multiple telangiectatic lesions. Spider telangiectasia or multiple nodular angiomas occur in the small bowel. Multiple polypoid lesions in the small bowel are also found with _Cowden's_ syndrome, _Canada–Cronkhite_ syndrome, _Gardner's_ syndrome, and _familial polyposis_. These conditions, however, are more common in the colon and therefore discussed in more detail in Table 30.**5**.
Carcinoid	One or, rarely, several small intraluminal masses, virtually always located in ileum (particularly the terminal portion) and characteristically associated with a fixed, kinked loop of bowel causing obstruction.	Most common neoplasm of the small bowel. Besides the primary lesion, mesenteric lymph node metastases may also cause small bowel obstruction. The carcinoid syndrome, characterized by skin flushing, diarrhea, and involvement of the right heart valves, is caused by extensive serotonin release into the blood. The syndrome is usually only found in the presence of extensive liver metastases.
Adenocarcinoma	A sharply demarcated nodular or annular filling defect with abnormal mucosal pattern is characteristic. Flat ulcerations are occasionally found. Most tumors are located in the jejunum. Presentation as a broad-based polyp occurs, but is relatively uncommon, whereas presentation as a pedunculated polyp is very unusual. Obstruction is a common complication.	Patients present commonly with small bowel obstruction or, less frequently, with chronic gastrointestinal blood loss.

(continues on page 732)

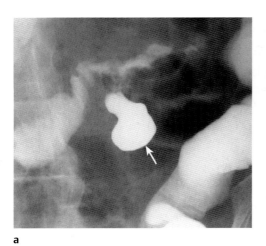

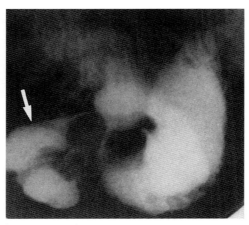

Fig. 30.**44 a, b** **Meckel's diverticulum** (two cases). A large, irregularly shaped outpouching (arrow) of the distal ileum is seen in **a**. Partial inversion of the Meckel's diverticulum (arrow) is seen in **b** causing a lobulated intraluminal filling defect in the distal ileum with partial obstruction.

a
b

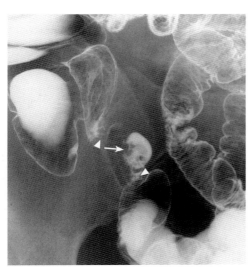

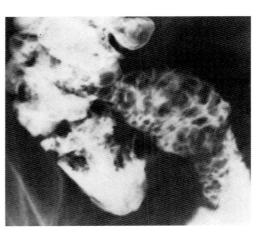

Fig. 30.**45** **Endometrioma.** A small irregular intraluminal mass (arrow) in the terminal ileum is associated with two short stenotic areas (arrowheads).

Fig. 30.**46** **Nodular lymphoid hyperplasia.** Multiple small nodular defects are seen in the terminal ileum and to a lesser degree in the cecum.

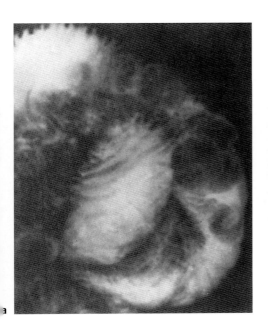

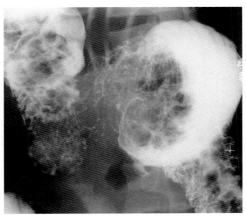

Fig. 30.**47 a, b** **Peutz–Jeghers syndrome** (two cases). **a** Several polypoid lesions are seen in the jejunum with early obstruction caused by intussusception. **b** A large, obstructing, intraluminal mass caused by a jejunojejunal intussusception with characteristic "coiled spring" appearance is seen associated with multiple polypoid lesions in both the afferent and efferent loop.

a
b

Table 30.4   (Cont.) Filling Defects in the Small Bowel (Jejunum and Ileum)

Disease	Radiographic Findings	Comments
Malignant gastrointestinal stromal tumor (GIST) (Fig. 30.48)	Extrinsic or intrinsic (broad-based or rarely pedunculated) filling defect without site predilection. Deep central ulcerations occur in approximately half of cases. Benign and malignant GISTs cannot be reliably differentiated.	Approximately half of the GISTs in the small bowel are malignant, the other half benign. The vast majority of formerly diagnosed leiomyomas and leiomyosarcomas are now considered to represent GISTs. Other sarcomatous tumors, including true *leiomyosarcomas*, are very rare.
Lymphoma (Fig. 30.49)	Single or multiple nodular extrinsic (secondary lymphoma) or intrinsic (polypoid to annular) masses without site predilection. Thickened folds, often with corrugated or tethered appearance, may be associated. Complete effacement of mucosal pattern and large ulcerations are commonly seen.	Primary and secondary small bowel involvement occurs quite commonly with non-Hodgkin's lymphomas, whereas in Hodgkin's disease small bowel manifestations are rare and almost always secondary.
Metastases (hematogenous and mesenteric) (Fig. 30.50)	Single or multiple extrinsic or intrinsic masses without site predilection. Central ulcerations ("bull's eyes" or "target lesions") are particularly common in melanomas. A fixed loop of bowel associated with an extrinsic mass invading the bowel wall and causing an annular or eccentric defect is characteristic for mesenteric metastases. Mucosal tethering of the involved loop that is fixed by mesenteric metastases is a common finding.	Hematogenous metastases originate most commonly from melanoma, breast, and bronchogenic carcinomas. Mesenteric metastases (lymphatic spread or per continuitatem) are often found with carcinomas originating from the gastrointestinal or urogenital tract. Direct invasion of small bowel from a carcinoma in an adjacent organ (e.g., pancreas or colon) is also possible.
Kaposi's sarcoma	Multiple extrinsic or intrinsic nodules throughout the entire intestinal tract, often with central ulcerations.	Characteristic skin lesions (ulcerated hemorrhagic dermatitis).
Inflammatory pseudotumor	Localized submucosal filling defect or polypoid lesion.	May occasionally lead to an intussusception.
Intussusception (Fig. 30.51)	Intraluminal, often lobulated mass, characteristically with "coiled spring" appearance.	Idiopathic only in infants and young children. In adults virtually always secondary to intraluminal mass (benign or malignant), an inverted Meckel's diverticulum or sprue.

(continues on page 734)

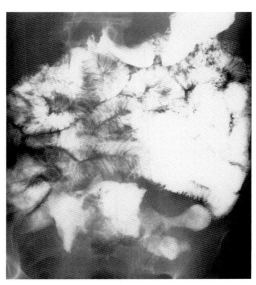

Fig. 30.**48 Malignant gastrointestinal stromal tumor (GIST).** A very large ulcerating mass is seen in the distal ileum on the bottom of the radiograph.

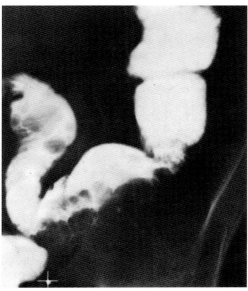

Fig. 30.**49 Non-Hodgkin's lymphoma.** Extrinsic invasion of the ileum is seen producing nodular defects and mucosal tethering.

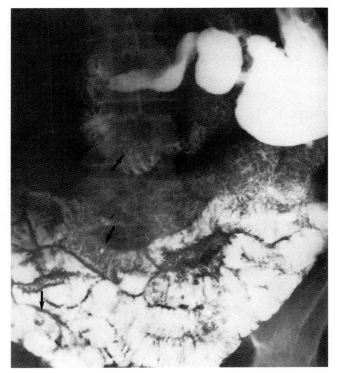

Fig. 30.**50 Melanoma metastases.** Multiple small nodules with central ulcerations are seen throughout the small bowel (arrows).

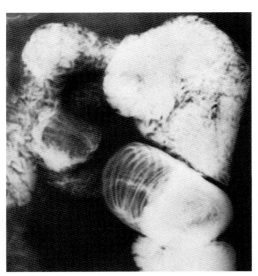

Fig. 30.**51 Intussusception in Hodgkin's lymphoma.** An intraluminal mass with characteristic "coiled spring" appearance is seen in the jejunum.

Table 30.4 (Cont.) Filling Defects in the Small Bowel (Jejunum and Ileum)

Disease	Radiographic Findings	Comments
Hematoma	Extrinsic mass may be caused by mesenteric hematoma. Often associated with intramural bleeding evident as "stacked-coin" appearance.	Usually with anticoagulation therapy or hemophilia. "Stacked-coin" appearance is more striking in jejunum than ileum because of better developed jejunal folds.
Gallstone	Usually solitary intraluminal mass (radiolucent or opaque), most often seen in the distal ileum (narrowest portion) where the stone can become impacted and cause mechanical obstruction. Air or contrast reflux into the biliary system is diagnostic.	Elderly women are most often affected. In more than 50% of cases, gallstone perforation into the gut does not cause obstruction.
Food, foreign bodies, pills	Solitary or multiple freely mobile intraluminal filling defects of varying shapes and sizes.	Fruit pits trapped in a blind loop or area of narrowing can become calcified (enterolith). Air bubbles may temporarily mimic round intraluminal masses.
Worm infestations (Ascaris, Strongyloides, hookworm or tapeworm) (Fig. 30.52)	Elongated radiolucent filling defects that can be coiled up and produce an intraluminal mass. Barium in the gastrointestinal tract of the worm is often seen presenting as a thin longitudinal line along the length of the worm.	No symptoms are found with mild infections, but large numbers of worms may produce abdominal pain and obstruction. A mass of coiled Ascaris contrasted by intestinal gas can occasionally be diagnosed without barium.
Pneumatosis intestinalis (primary or idiopathic) (Fig. 30.53)	Radiolucent cystic lesions along the contour of the bowel wall are diagnostic. A symptomless pneumoperitoneum that does not require surgical intervention is sometimes associated.	Secondary pneumatosis intestinalis is found with bowel necrosis (e.g., ischemic bowel disease and necrotizing enterocolitis in infants), peptic ulcer disease, inflammatory bowel disease, post gastrointestinal surgery, and in obstructive pulmonary disease. In these conditions, the air in the bowel wall tends to have a more streaky or crescent, linear appearance.

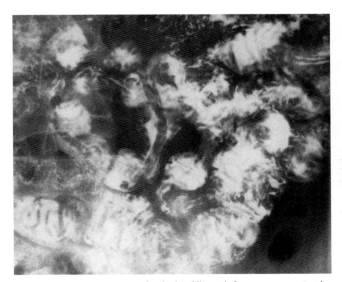

Fig. 30.**52** **Ascaris.** Several tubular filling defects are seen in the small bowel.

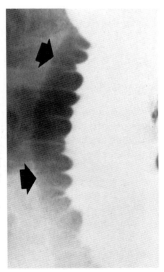

Fig. 30.**53** **Pneumatosis intestinalis.** A radiolucent band consisting of numerous confluent radiolucent cystic lesions is seen.

Table 30.5   Filling Defects in the Colon and Rectum

Disease	Radiographic Findings	Comments
Ileocecal valve (Fig. 30.54)	*Normal*: Intrinsic round-to-oval filling defect not exceeding 4 cm in diameter and arising from the medioposterior wall of the colon at the junction of the cecum and ascending colon. *Lipomatous infiltration* or *hypertrophy*: Enlarged, often slightly lobulated ileocecal valve with smooth surface and intact mucosa. *Ileal mucosal prolapse*: Radial folds in the form of a star are seen in a normal or slightly enlarged ileocecal valve viewed face-on.	Histologically, lipomatous infiltration is characterized by submucosal fatty infiltration and lack of a capsule. Enlargement of the ileocecal valve may also be caused by benign or malignant neoplastic and inflammatory diseases (e.g., *Crohn's disease, tuberculosis, amebiasis*). In these conditions, the mucosal surface may no longer be smooth. A *neoplasm* may furthermore cause an asymmetric or polypoid enlargement. Rarely, an *intramural hematoma* or *impacted gallstone* or foreign body may cause or simulate an enlarged ileocecal valve.
Appendix (intussusception or inverted stump) (Fig. 30.55)	Oval, round, or less commonly finger-like intrinsic filling defect arising from the medial wall of the cecum without visualization of the appendix. DD: Extrinsic cecal filling defect caused by appendiceal abscess. An appendicolith is occasionally present.	Postoperative defects secondary to inversion of the appendiceal stump or incomplete resection of the appendix may measure up to 3 cm in diameter. Intussusception of the appendix usually occurs in the presence of an *appendiceal tumor* or *mucocele* (obstructed appendix filled with sterile mucus) that may present with peripheral calcifications.
Duplication cyst	Rare extrinsic spherical or tubular mass with intact mucosa anywhere in the colon, producing often partial to complete obstruction.	Occasionally, duplication may communicate with the colonic lumen, producing a double-barrel appearance.
Lipoma (Fig. 30.56)	Smooth, relatively sharply outlined, deformable, and somewhat radiolucent intrinsic filling defect, preferentially located in the right half of the colon. A pedicle that appears to be wider than the thin stalk of an adenomatous polyp may develop in larger lipomas.	*Gastrointestinal stromal tumors (GISTs)* and other benign mesenchymal neoplasms are relatively rare in the colon.
Endometrioma	Usually solitary extrinsic or intrinsic, broad-based filling defect, preferentially located in the sigmoid. May cause tethering of the adjacent mucosa due to secondary fibrosis, or produce an annular constricting lesion that simulates a carcinoma.	Usually diagnosed between ages 20 and 40, rarely in postmenopausal females.

(continues on page 736)

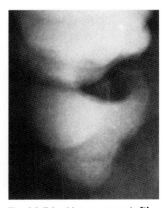

Fig. 30.**54** **Lipomatous infiltration of the ileocecal valve.** A slightly lobulated, smooth filling defect is seen originating from the medioposterior wall of the junction between the cecum and ascending colon.

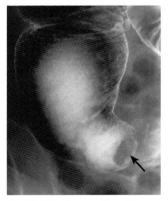

Fig. 30.**55** **Appendiceal intussusception.** An oval filling defect (arrow) is seen in the cecum without visualization of the appendix.

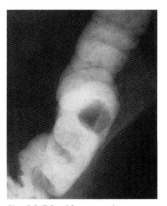

Fig. 30.**56** **Lipoma.** A smooth and relatively sharply outlined filling defect is seen in the descending colon.

Table 30.5 (Cont.) Filling Defects in the Colon and Rectum

Disease	Radiographic Findings	Comments
Polyp (adenomatous) (Fig. 30.57)	Solitary or multiple spherical filling defects with smooth surface, often measuring less than 1.5 cm in diameter. May be lobulated when larger. Pedicles are common and may occasionally measure several centimeters in length. A barium-coated, air-filled *diverticulum* must be differentiated (see Fig. 30.**3**).	Premalignant condition: Incidence of malignancy correlates with size of lesion. Sessile and broad-based polyps measuring more than 2 cm in diameter are malignant in almost half of cases. *Hyperplastic polyps* are smooth sessile mucosal elevations of less than 5 mm in diameter without malignant potential. They are found at autopsy in up to 50 % of colons of asymptomatic adults. Radiographically, they cannot be differentiated from tiny adenomatous polyps.
Polyposis (Figs. 30.58–30.62)	*Familial polyposis*: Innumerable, sessile polyps ranging from 1 to 2 mm to 1 to 2 cm in diameter. Small pedicles can occasionally be identified in some lesions. Usually the entire colon is involved, though left colon and rectum involvement is often more pronounced. Segmental colonic involvement is unusual. In less than 5 % of cases, polyps are also found in the stomach and small bowel (Fig. 30.**58**).	Autosomal dominant inheritance. Sporadic cases without traceable family history occur rarely. Usually diagnosed in young adults. Carcinoma of the colon will develop in virtually all patients when untreated (approximately 15 years after the appearance of colonic polyps).

(continues on page 738)

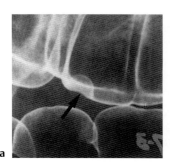
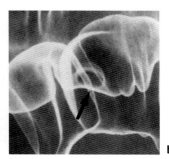

Fig. 30.**57 a, b** **Polyp. a** in profile and **b** in oblique projection. A small polyp (arrows) with the appearance of a bowler hat is seen in **b**.

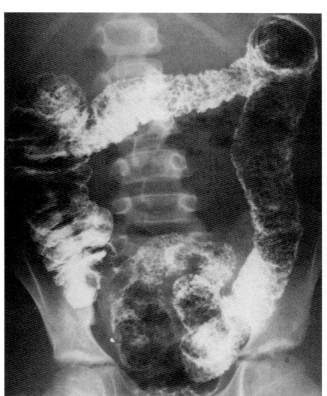

Fig. 30.**58** **Familial polyposis.** Innumerable small polyps throughout the colon and rectum are seen.

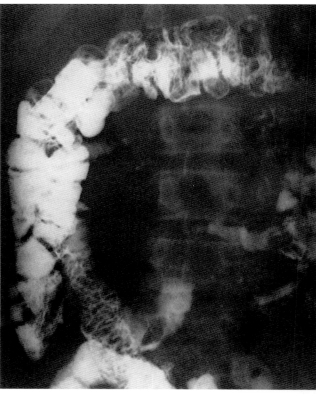

Fig. 30.**59** **Nodular lymphoid hyperplasia.** Multiple tiny polyps are seen in this small bowel follow-up examination in the colon. Note that the greatest number of lesions is characteristically seen in the terminal ileum.

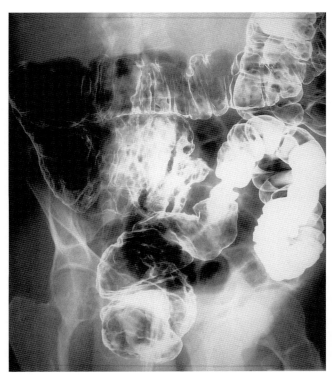

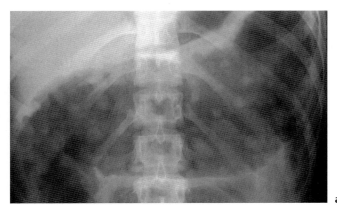

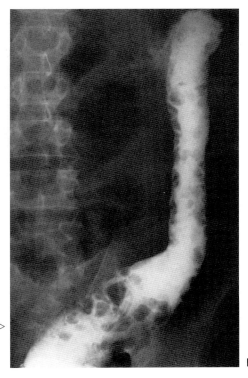

Fig. 30.**60** **Lymphoma.** Multiple polypoid lesions are seen in the terminal ileum and scattered throughout the entire colon.

Fig. 30.**61 a, b** **Pseudopolyposis in ulcerative colitis** (two ▷ cases). **a** A markedly dilated transverse colon (toxic megacolon) with multiple polypoid lesions is seen (plain film). **b** Numerous polypoid lesions are seen in the descending and sigmoid colon.

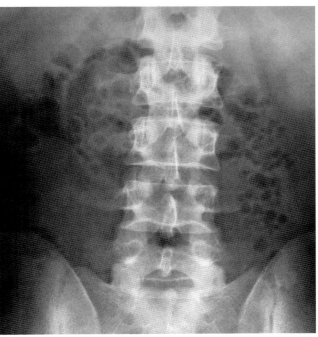

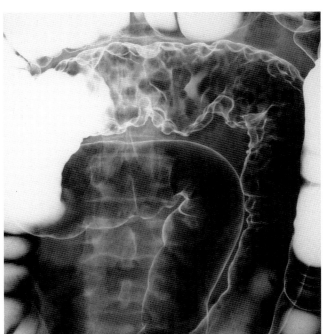

Fig. 30.**62 a, b** **Pneumatosis cystoides coli.** Multiple gas-containing polypoid lesions are seen in the sigmoid colon. **a** (plain film), **b** (double contrast enema).

Table 30.5 (Cont.) Filling Defects in the Colon and Rectum

Disease	Radiographic Findings	Comments
	Gardner's syndrome: Colonic polyps (rarely stomach and small bowel) radiographically indistinguishable from familial polyposis. Osteomas and soft-tissue lesions (e.g., a desmoid of the mesentery presenting as a large extrinsic mass) may be seen.	Autosomal dominant syndrome consisting of colonic polyposis predisposing to carcinoma, osteomatosis, and cutaneous soft tissue lesions (mesenchymal tumors and cysts). Tendency for excessive scar formation (keloids).
	Turcot syndrome: Colonic polyposis with potential for malignancy associated with brain tumors (astrocytomas).	Autosomal recessive inherited.
	Canada–Cronkhite syndrome: Polyps in colon, small bowel, and stomach.	Gastrointestinal hamartomatous polyposis and ectodermal abnormalities (alopecia, hyperpigmentation, and nail atrophy). Develops in the elderly and has no familial or sexual predilection. Presents with malabsorption and severe diarrhea.
	Juvenile polyposis: Multiple hamartomatous colonic polyps, usually in children under 10 years of age, rarely in adults.	DD: *Multiple juvenile polyps*: One or a few polypoid lesions containing multiple mucin-filled cysts and abundant connective stroma are found in young children, presenting often with diarrhea and rectal bleeding. Polyps have a tendency to autoamputate or regress spontaneously.
	Cowden's syndrome (multiple hamartoma syndrome): Multiple polyps (rarely solitary lesions) may be found in the entire gastrointestinal tract.	Rare hereditary disorders associated with multiple tumors and malformations in different organs. Circumoral papillomatosis and nodular gingival hyperplasia are characteristic clinical features.
	Peutz–Jeghers syndrome: Only a few colonic polyps can be seen at best, since the disease primarily involves the small bowel.	See Table 30.**4**.
	Colonic neurofibromatosis: Multiple filling defects varying in diameter from one to several centimeters. Characteristic is the eccentric location of the lesions which are all located on the mesenteric side.	Associated with type I neurofibromatosis (von Recklinghausen's disease) presenting with (cutaneous neurofibromas and "café-au-lait" pigmented skin lesions.
	Nodular lymphoid hyperplasia of the colon: Innumerable, tiny filling defects of uniform size, measuring only a few millimeters in diameter (Fig. 30.**59**).	Usually in children and rare in adults. DD: Polypoid lesions in lymphoma tend to be larger, vary in size, and are associated with thickened folds.
	Lymphoma: Multiple polypoid lesions are not an unusual presentation (Fig. 30.**60**).	Metastases from melanoma and carcinomas of breast and lung rarely may also present as polypoid colonic lesions.
	Inflammatory pseudopolyps: Associated with radiographic evidence of an inflammatory process (Fig. 30.**61**).	For example, ulcerative colitis, granulomatous colitis, amebiasis, and schistosomiasis.
	Pneumatosis cystoides coli: Round extrinsic and intrinsic filling defects with increased radiolucency (gas-containing cysts) that can already be seen on plain film radiograph (Fig. 30.**62**).	May be idiopathic or caused by air spread from the mediastinum (e.g., in chronic obstructive pulmonary diseases) or associated with peptic ulcer disease or secondary to surgery.
Villous adenoma (Fig. 30.63 a–c)	Solitary, broad-based, often lobulated intrinsic filling defect that is commonly located in rectum or sigmoid. Tumor is often walnut-sized, but may range from 0.5 to 15 cm in diameter. Its appearance is characteristic when barium is trapped between villous strands, producing an irregular reticulated surface. Since the tumor is soft, it changes shape and may even be effaced by compression.	Usually diagnosed in the middle-aged and elderly, who may present with mucous diarrhea. Incidence of adenocarcinoma is high and increases with the size of the tumor.

Table 30.5   (Cont.) Filling Defects in the Colon and Rectum

Disease	Radiographic Findings	Comments
Carcinoid	Two different clinicopathologic entities: 1 Benign, small sessile, polypoid lesion, measuring less than 2 cm in diameter and preferentially located in appendix or rectum. 2 Broad-based bulky intraluminal filling defect measuring several centimeters at the time of diagnosis and commonly associated with lymph node and liver metastases. Usually located in cecum or right colon.	The benign variety located in appendix and rectum occurs usually in the younger and middle-aged patient, and is much more common than the malignant colonic form, which is usually seen in the elderly patient.
Carcinoma (Fig. 30.64)	Usually, solitary polypoid or annular filling defects varying greatly in size. The surface may be smooth, ragged, or ulcerated. Fungating polypoid carcinomas are preferentially located in the cecum, ascending colon, or rectum, whereas annular ulcerating lesions, characteristically with "overhanging edges", are more commonly seen in the transverse, descending, and sigmoid colon. Abrupt transition from tumor to healthy mucosa is typical. Rarely curvilinear and/or mottled calcifications are seen in the primary and metastatic lesions (lymph nodes and liver).	Colon cancers present with occult blood in the stool, but are otherwise asymptomatic until late in their course, when complications develop. These include obstruction, perforation (peritonitis or, when sealed off, abscess formation), and invagination. Calcifications are seen in mucus-producing adenocarcinomas.

(continues on page 740)

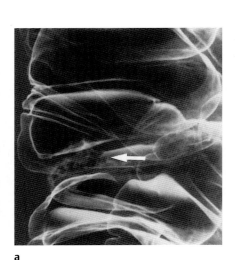
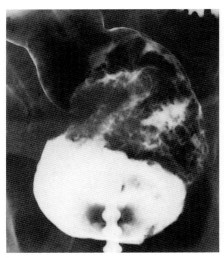
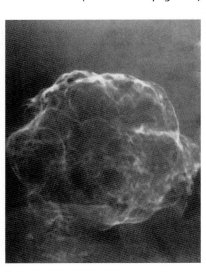

a   b   c

Fig. 30.**63**   **Villous adenoma** (two cases). **a** The small spongelike lesion (arrow) in the ascending colon was histologically completely benign. **b** The bulky mass in the rectum, with an irregular reticulated surface, revealed a malignant transformation at its base histologically. **c** The post evacuation film often best demonstrates the 6characteristic spongelike pattern caused by barium trapped between villous strands.

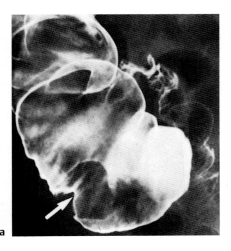
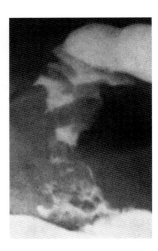

a   b

Fig. 30.**64 a, b**   **Colonic adenocarcinomas** in two different patients. **a** An irregularly outlined polypoid mass is seen in the cecum. Retraction of the colonic wall at the site of origin of the lesion strongly suggests malignant nature of the polypoid mass (arrow). **b** A circumferential, ulcerating mass lesion is seen in the sigmoid colon in the second case.

Table 30.5   (Cont.) Filling Defects in the Colon and Rectum

Disease	Radiographic Findings	Comments
Lymphoma and sarcoma (Fig. 30.65)	Localized form may present as a polypoid or annular, often ulcerated mass, preferentially located in the cecum and less commonly in the rectum. Extrinsic filling defects can occur from lymphoma involving adjacent organs or lymph nodes.	Diffuse colonic involvement by lymphoma presenting with thickened folds, nodules and ulcerations is a more common presentation. Involvement of the colon by non-Hodgkin's lymphoma is much more common than by Hodgkin's disease. Colonic sarcomas (e.g., *Kaposi's sarcoma* with localized or multicentric involvement) and *malignant gastrointestinal stromal tumor (GIST)* with only localized involvement may present radiographically similar to lymphoma.
Metastases (Figs. 30.66 and 30.67)	Present as solitary or multiple extrinsic filling defects with intact mucosa, or as an intrinsic mass lesion mimicking a primary colon carcinoma. In the pelvis, extrinsic metastases may simulate pelvic lipomatosis (vertical elongation, elevation, and narrowing of the rectum and urinary bladder).	Pathways of involvement: 1 Direct invasion from carcinomas in adjacent organs (e.g., gastrointestinal and urogenital systems). 2 Hematogenous (e.g., from breast carcinoma and rarely from bronchogenic carcinoma and melanoma). 3 Intraperitoneal seeding (transported by ascites).
Appendiceal abscess (Fig. 30.68)	Extrinsic filling defect, usually in the cecum and terminal ileum, but it may develop anywhere in the abdomen with an abnormally located or unusually long appendix. Extrinsic mass may have mottled appearance simulating fecal material or an air–fluid level on upright and decubitus films. An appendicolith (oval-shaped with laminated calcifications) within the lesion is diagnostic but is found only in a small minority of cases.	Perforated appendicitis is the most common cause of intra-abdominal abscess in a patient who has not previously undergone surgery.
Diverticulitis with abscess formation (Fig. 30.69)	Solitary or less commonly multiple, extrinsic filling defects, usually in the sigmoid colon. Barium may occasionally enter abscess cavity. In the acute stage, spasm of the involved colon segment is usually present and the adjacent diverticula may be draped over the abscess ("drape sign"). In the chronic stage, an intramural abscess is often associated with a markedly narrowed bowel lumen, simulating colonic carcinoma.	Predominant clinical symptoms are localized tenderness and fever.

(continues on page 742)

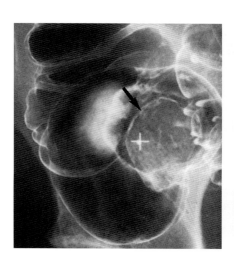
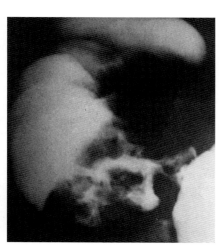

Fig. 30.**65 a, b   Non-Hodgkin's lymphoma** involving the cecum (two cases). In **a** a round intraluminal mass (arrow) is seen, whereas in **b** an ulcerating destructive lesion is present. Radiographically, both cases are indistinguishable from adenocarcinomas at this location.

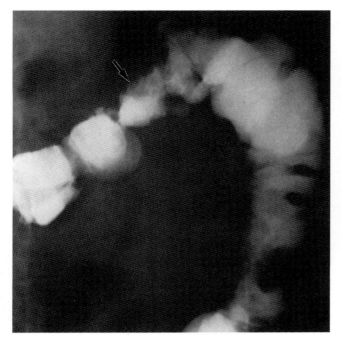

Fig. 30.**66 Metastases from carcinoma of stomach.** Both extrinsic and intrinsic nodular lesions are seen. Note also the irregular marginal spiculation of the superior (mesenteric) border of the transverse colon caused by mesenteric metastases (arrow).

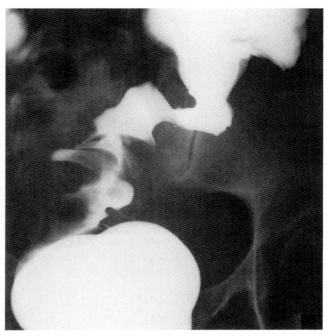

Fig. 30.**67 Metastases from ovarian carcinoma.** Circumferential narrowing of the shortened and fixed sigmoid with large filling defects is seen.

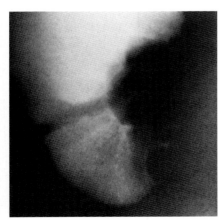

Fig. 30.**68 Appendiceal abscess.** An extrinsic defect is seen on the medial aspect of the cecum. Other inflammatory mass lesions (e.g., Crohn's disease) cannot be differentiated in the absence of an appendicolith.

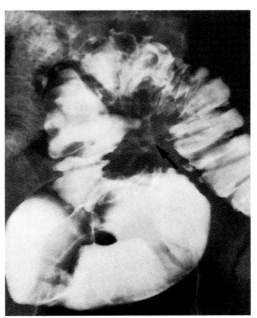

Fig. 30.**69 Diverticulitis with abscess formation,** A mass lesion with barium entering the abscess cavity (arrow) and the edematous sigmoid draped around it is seen.

Table 30.5 (Cont.) Filling Defects in the Colon and Rectum

Disease	Radiographic Findings	Comments
Amebic colitis (Fig. 30.70)	Thumb printing and multiple filling defects caused by pseudopolyposis and amebomas are seen besides ulcerations. The disease may involve any part of the colon, but the cecum is involved in up to 90% of cases. The ileum is not involved. Contrast reflux through a "gaping" ileocecal valve helps to differentiate cecal amebiasis from a carcinoma when present.	An *ameboma* is a hyperplastic granuloma of the large bowel caused by secondary bacterial invasion of an amebic abscess. Radiographically, it usually presents as an annular, constricting mass lesion with apple core appearance that is often indistinguishable from a carcinoma. Demonstration of small ulcers adjacent to the ameboma and the relatively young age of the patients are both helpful in differentiating it from carcinoma.
Tuberculosis	Localized tuberculosis of the colon is usually limited to the cecum, which appears shrunken and retracted. An intraluminal mass is rarely seen. A narrowed and ulcerated terminal ileum is commonly associated, but barium refluxes only infrequently into the terminal ileum because of spasm and thickening of the ileocecal valve.	With the exception of the cecum, localized tuberculous involvement of the colon or rectum is rare.
Actinomycosis	Cecal mass similar to tuberculosis, but greater tendency towards fistulization.	Develops secondary to appendicitis or appendiceal abscess.
Ulcerative colitis (Fig. 30.71 a–c)	Pseudopolyps present usually as numerous small filling defects associated with other signs of the disease (ulceration, absence or irregularities of haustral folds, narrowing and foreshortening of the colon). Rarely, a pseudopolyp may present as large fungating mass. When localized, the rectosigmoid area is preferentially involved.	Can affect all ages, although two peaks occur, the first between 20 and 25 and the second between 50 and 60 years of age. Characteristic clinical presentation consists of intermittent episodes of diarrhea and rectal bleeding. Pseudopolyps can already be seen in the acute stage, where they represent edematous mucosal remnants, but they are usually more prominent in the subacute and chronic stages, when epithelial regeneration has occurred.
Crohn's colitis (Fig. 30.72)	Uniform filling defects ("cobblestone" appearance) may be created by swollen mucosa separated by deep, linear, longitudinal and vertical ulcers. When localized, the right colon, including terminal ileum, is preferentially involved. Skip lesions and presence of fistulas are characteristic.	Occurs primarily in adolescence and young adults, presenting with diarrhea but without gross bleeding.

(continues on page 744)

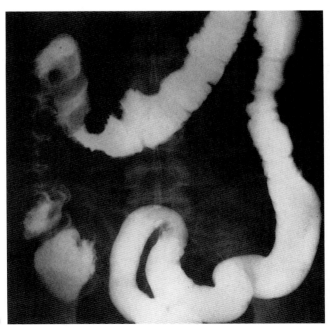

a

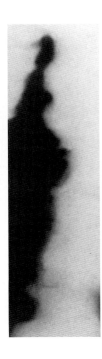

b

Fig. 30.**70 a, b   Amebic colitis. a** Thumb printing and filling defects are limited to the right colon, whereas tiny ulcerations, some of them with a "collar button" appearance, are seen throughout the entire colon with the exception of the sigmoid. The are shown in the magnified view of the descending colon in **b**.

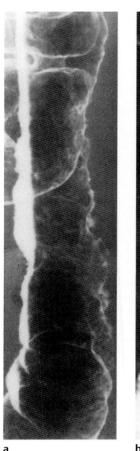
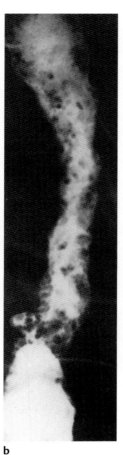
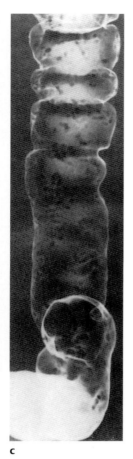

a   b   c

Fig. 30.**71 a–c   Ulcerative colitis. a** Acute stage: marginal ulceration including collar button ulcers are evident. **b** (5 years after a): Multiple pseudopolyps, varying considerably in size, are now present, in addition to mucosal ulcerations and spasm. **c** (10 years after **a**). The pseudopolyps have decreased in size, the ulcers have healed, and a normal haustral pattern has returned.

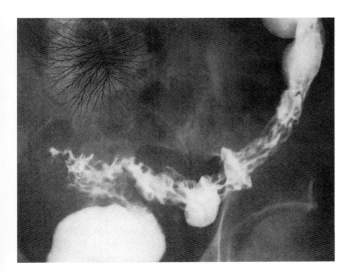

Fig. 30.**72   Crohn's disease.** A combination of ulceration, edematous mucosa and pseudopolyposis produces a cobblestone appearance in the foreshortened sigmoid. Note also that the rectum is not involved.

Table 30.5 (Cont.) Filling Defects in the Colon and Rectum

Disease	Radiographic Findings	Comments
Inflammatory pseudo-tumor (Fig. 30.73)	A localized large intraluminal mass with irregular surface mimicking a carcinoma is occasionally found with ulcerative colitis and Crohn's disease.	The bulky mass is produced by a cluster of pseudopolyps.
Ischemic colitis (Fig. 30.74)	Pseudopolyps and "thumb printing" are seen in addition to ulcerations in a more advanced stage that is often indistinguishable from ulcerative colitis. Preferential involvement of splenic flexure and left colon, but characteristically sparing the rectum.	Presents typically in the elderly as acute episode of abdominal pain and bleeding.
Pseudomembranous colitis (clostridium difficile disease) (Fig. 30.75)	Large polypoid defects and "thumb printing" to wide transverse bands of thickened colonic wall can be seen throughout the entire colon, but are usually most prominent in the transverse colon.	Usually develops after a course of broad-spectrum antibiotics (e.g., clindamycin) or chemotherapy. Severe diarrhea without significant rectal bleeding is the usual clinical presentation.
Colonic urticaria	Large, round or polygonal raised plaques in grossly dilated (usually right) colon, representing submucosal edema.	This condition is most often associated with an allergic reaction secondary to medication in which condition it may be very transient. Less common causes of submucosal edema presenting in this fashion include ischemia, chronic obstruction of various etiologies, and infections such as herpes zoster. "Thumb printing" is, however, a far more common radiographic presentation of submucosal edema.
Schistosomiasis	Usually multiple polypoid filling defects measuring up to 2 cm, preferentially in the sigmoid and rectum. A single larger lesion is less common, and may cause obstruction and simulate carcinoma.	Filling defects are caused by granulomas, which are a late manifestation of the disease after heavy infestation and chronic exposure.
Worm infestations (Ascaris or Trichuris)	Solitary intraluminal filling defect by a bolus of ascaris or numerous irregular defects throughout the colon caused by excessive mucus production induced by trichuris trichiura that are attached to the bowel wall.	*Trichuris trichiura* (whipworm) is a frequent inhabitant of the cecum and appendix of man. Infections (trichuriasis) are common in the subtropics and tropics.
Cystic fibrosis	Multiple poorly defined filling defects caused by viscous mucus adherent to the wall.	In children and young adults.
Colitis cystica profunda	Usually multiple filling defects measuring up to 2 cm in diameter and preferentially limited to the rectosigmoid area.	Filling defects are caused by submucosal cysts, lined with mucus-producing epithelium. Present clinically with bright rectal bleeding, mucus discharge, and diarrhea.

(continues on page 746)

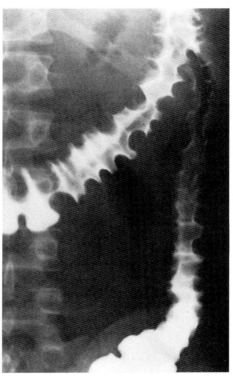

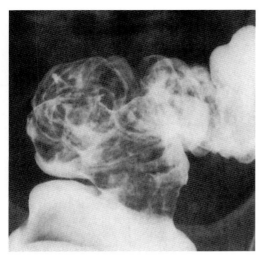

Fig. 30.**73 Inflammatory pseudotumor in Crohn's disease.** A localized fungating mass is produced in the foreshortened sigmoid by a cluster of pseudopolyps. (Same case as in Fig. 30.**72**, 1 year later).

Fig. 30.**74 Ischemic colitis.** Large marginal filling defects ("thumb printing") are seen in the distal transverse and descending colon.

Fig. 30.**75 Pseudomembranous colitis (Clostridium difficile disease).** In addition to ulcerations, extensive submucosal edema is evident throughout the entire colon causing markedly thickened haustra and "thumb printing."

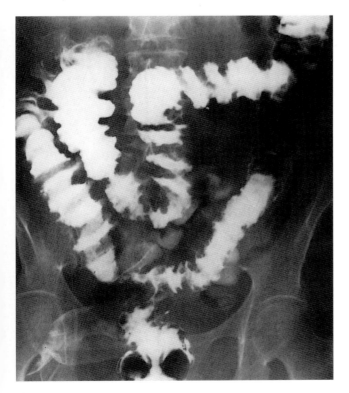

Table 30.5   (Cont.) Filling Defects in the Colon and Rectum

Disease	Radiographic Findings	Comments
Pneumatosis cystoides coli (Fig. 30.76)	Multiple deformable round filling defects with increased radiolucency.	See also under "polyposis" in this table.
Suture granuloma	Filling defect at anastomotic site that characteristically decreases in size with time.	Patient's history is important.
Intussusception (ileocolic or rarely colocolic) (Fig. 30.77)	Solitary filling defect, usually in the right colon. Obstruction and vascular compromise are often associated. "Coiled spring" appearance is characteristic.	In adults, the leading points of intussusceptions are commonly an inverted Meckel's diverticulum, lymphoma, mesenteric nodes, or polyps.
Hemorrhoids (internal)	Multiple polypoid filling defects in the rectum, usually associated with tubular filling defects caused by the veins from which the hemorrhoids arise.	May cause intermittent bleeding that is characteristically found on the outside of the stool.
Amyloidosis	Rare cause of single or multiple filling defects in the rectum and colon.	Since histologic involvement of rectal submucosa in both primary and secondary amyloidosis is common, rectal biopsies are often diagnostic even with a normal-appearing rectum.
Adhesions and fibrous bands	May produce extrinsic filling defects simulating a tumor.	Usually secondary to previous abdominal surgery. *Enlarged appendices epiploicae* may rarely produce similar filling defects.
Feces, artifacts, undigested food particles, air bubbles	Solitary ("fecaloma") or multiple intraluminal filling defects, which may be freely mobile or adherent to the wall and confused with polypoid lesions.	Undigested food particles caught in a diverticulum may calcify and produce *enteroliths*. Rarely, a *gallstone* trapped in the sigmoid may present as an intraluminal filling defect.

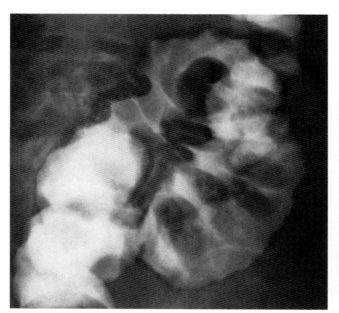

Fig. 30.**76   Pneumatosis cystoides coli.** Multiple round filling defects with increased radiolucency are seen in the descending and sigmoid colon. In some areas, the cystic lesions have become confluent and form a broad radiolucent band along the barium column.

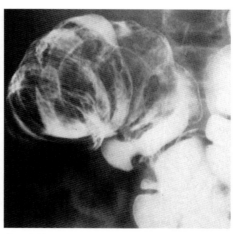

Fig. 30.**77   Intussusception in non-Hodgkin's lymphoma.** Complete obstruction by an intraluminal mass with "coiled spring" appearance is seen in the hepatic flexure.

31 Ulcers, Diverticula, and Fistulas in the Gastrointestinal Tract

Ulcers

An *ulcer* in the gastrointestinal tract is defined as a loss of mucous surface, causing gradual disintegration and necrosis of the tissues. Partial or complete loss of the mucosa only, without penetration into the submucosa, is generally called an *erosion*. In this chapter, solitary ulcerations, either single or multiple, will be discussed. Erosions and ulcers may be widespread and therefore create a generalized abnormality of the mucosal surface. Such conditions are discussed in Chapter **28**. Single ulcers also cause abnormalities of the surrounding mucosa, either due to inflammatory changes or scarring.

Although deformity of the mucosal surface may be helpful in locating an ulcer, an ulcer crater should be demonstrated, preferably both in profile and en face, to make a definitive diagnosis. An ulcer crater on the dependent wall in the double-contrast examination and in the single-contrast examination may collect a pool of barium. An ulcer crater filled by a blood clot and viewed en face will be seen as a ring shadow. Artifacts such as the stalactite phenomenon (a hanging drop of barium), patchy coating, precipitation, and flaking of barium or insufficient separation of the anterior and posterior walls ("kissing" artifact) may create shadows that simulate an ulcer or other mucosal abnormalities. Colonic or small bowel diverticula may mimic the ring shadow of an ulcer.

Malignant versus Benign Ulcers

It is a common practice to obtain an endoscopic and histologic verification as soon as an ulcer in the gastrointestinal tract has been demonstrated radiographically. Certain features are helpful in the differential diagnosis of benign and malignant ulcers (Figs. 31.**1** and 31.**2**). This applies especially to the stomach, where both malignant and benign ulcerations occur frequently, whereas in the duodenum, the most common site of ulcers, the vast majority are benign. If a lesion is highly suggestive of malignancy on radiologic grounds, negative endoscopic or cytologic findings should not be taken as definitive evidence of its benign nature. Such lesions require follow-up studies.

Diverticula

A *diverticulum* is a circumscribed pouch created by herniation of the lining mucous membrane through a defect in the muscular coat of the wall. *True diverticula* are herniations of the mucous membrane and the submucous layers, whereas intestinal *false diverticula* are formed by protrusion of the mucous membrane alone through a tear in the muscular coat. Protrusions as a result of pressure from within are called *pulsion diverticula*. *Traction diverticula* are bulgings of the full thickness of the wall of the esophagus caused by adhesions resulting from some external lesion. If a diverticulum is shown by double contrast en face, the appearance may simulate the ring shadow around a polyp. The meniscus of barium in a diverticulum fades centrally, whereas around a polyp it fades peripherally. Criteria for differentiating are presented in Figure 31.**3**. When seen in profile, they are easily differentiated. The mucosal lining and a narrow and long neck relative to the pouch itself help to differentiate a diverticulum from an ulcer.

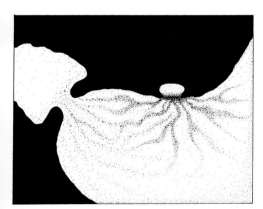

Fig. 31.**1 Radiologic features of a benign gastric ulcer:** (1) Penetration beyond the normal contour of the stomach, (2) mucosal folds radiate into the orifice of the crater, (3) a smooth mound of edema surrounding a sharply defined crater, (4) signs of undermining of the mucosa (Hampton's line, ulcer collar).

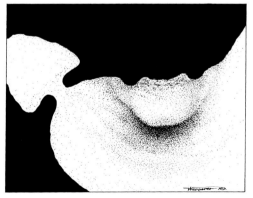

Fig. 31.**2 Radiologic features of a malignant gastric ulcer:** (1) Nodularity of the tissue surrounding the ulcer crater and in the orifice and floor of the crater, (2) tumor rim, (Carman's meniscus sign), (3) the crater fails to project beyond the normal gastric lumen, (4) radiating mucosal folds do not reach the orifice of the ulcer, (5) the crater is wider than it is deep.

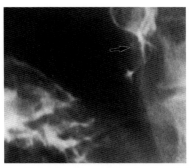

Fig. 31.**3**   An **ulcer niche in the distal esophagus** (arrow) surrounded by an ulcer collar and spasm.

Fistulas

A *fistula* refers to an abnormal communication from the gastrointestinal tract into another part of the bowel (enteric-enteric), to another organ (internal), or to the surface of the body (external). A fistula permitting the escape of pus is often called a *sinus tract*. The demonstration of fistulas in the barium examination of the gastrointestinal tract depends on the patency of the channel at the given moment. Fistulas may be better demonstrated by thin barium alone than in a double-contrast examination. Fistulas that open to the surface of the body may be cannulated and filled with contrast (fistulography). Fistulas may be congenital or secondary to an ulcer, chronic inflammation, malignancy, or trauma.

Table 31.1   Ulcers, Diverticula, and Fistulas in the Esophagus

Disease	Radiographic Findings	Comments
Reflux esophagitis (Fig. 31.3)	Penetrating marginal ulcer in the region of the junction between the esophagus and stomach or hiatal hernia. The ulcer is a nichelike projection surrounded by ulcer collar and esophageal spasm.	Gastroesophageal reflux is often demonstrated. May be complicated by penetration into adjacent structures. Healing may result in stricture. For earlier signs of reflux esophagitis, see Chapter 28.
Barrett's esophagus (Fig. 31.4)	Esophageal ulceration usually at a distance from the cardia. Usually deep, penetrating, and identical to other peptic ulcerations. Often associated with a narrowed segment (spasm or stricture).	An ulcer in an islet of gastric mucosa in the esophagus complicating reflux esophagitis. A sliding hiatal hernia with gastroesophageal reflux is commonly demonstrated. In contrast to marginal ulceration of reflux esophagitis, Barrett's ulcer is separated by a variable length of normal-appearing esophagus from the hiatal hernia or cardia. Bears a high risk of malignant transformation.
Granulomatous esophagitis	Single or multiple ulcers, narrowing of the lumen, and numerous nodular filling defects. Fistulous tracts are common.	*Tuberculosis* of the esophagus is rare and usually associated with advanced disease in the lungs. *Crohn's disease*, *syphilis*, and *histoplasmosis* of the esophagus are likewise rare. Crohn's disease is suggested by concomitant Crohn's disease elsewhere. *Actinomycosis* of the adjacent tissues may also cause fistulization.
Carcinoma of the esophagus (Figs. 31.5–31.8)	The ulcer crater is surrounded by a bulging mass which projects into the esophageal lumen. The ulcerated surface is rigid. Purely ulcerating appearance with a flat meniscoid mass is rare. Broncho-esophageal or tracheoesophageal fistulas occur.	Esophageal carcinomas often present signs of ulceration but other radiographic features like narrowing or mass are more prominent. *Lymphomas* or *metastases* with "bull's eye" ulcerating lesions, (e.g., melanoma), are rare in the esophagus. 50 % of acquired esophageal fistulas are due to malignancy in the mediastinum.

(continues on page 750)

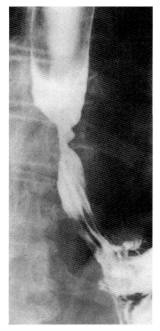

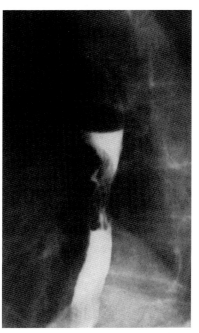

Fig. 31.**4** **Barrett's esophagus.** An ulcer and stricture is present about 10 cm above the esophagogastric junction. Esophageal folds below the ulcer are slightly thickened.

Fig. 31.**5** **Carcinoma of the esophagus.** A crater surrounded by a mass.

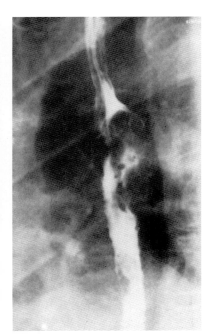

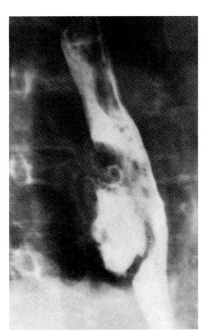

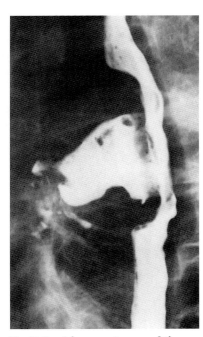

Fig. 31.**6** **Bull's eye ulcer of the esophagus.** Primary melanoma of the esophagus, a rare entity.

Fig. 31.**7** **Carcinoma of the esophagus.** A large ulceration with Carman's meniscus sign is seen.

Fig. 31.**8** **Adenocarcinoma of the esophagus.** A large ulceration and an esophagobronchial fistula are seen.

Table 31.1 (Cont.) Ulcers, Diverticula, and Fistulas in the Esophagus

Disease	Radiographic Findings	Comments
Leiomyoma (Fig. 31.9)	A large mass with central ulceration, no concentric narrowing of the lumen.	Carcinoma may have an identical appearance.
Corrosive esophagitis	Ulceration associated with sloughing of destroyed mucosa, eventually associated with gradual narrowing of the esophagus. A fistula may follow esophageal perforation.	Ulceration always occurs following ingestion of corrosive materials. Alkali tends to produce more extensive changes in the esophagus than acid.
Drug-induced ulcer	Solitary esophageal ulceration complicating drug treatment. The ulcer itself has no distinctive features.	Associated with delayed esophageal transit time (supine position, hiatal hernia, reflux, abnormal peristalsis, stricture, left atrial enlargement). Most common caused by potassium chloride tablets.
Intramural esophageal pseudodiverticulosis	Innumerable pinhead-sized outpouchings project from the lumen. A proximal esophageal stricture is common.	Dilated esophageal glands probably secondary to an inflammatory process.
Zenker's diverticulum (Figs. 31.10, 31.11)	A saccular outpouching protrudes posteriorly in the upper esophagus (C5–6 level). It may extend downward and posteriorly, displace the cervical esophagus anteriorly, and cause narrowing of the lumen.	A pulsion diverticulum at a point of weakness between the oblique and circular fibers of the cricopharyngeal muscle. May be seen as a retroesophageal air–fluid level on plain films.
Diverticula of the thoracic esophagus (Fig. 31.12)	Most are seen in the middle third opposite the bifurcation of the trachea. May have a funnel, cone, tent, or fusiform shape and usually best visualized in the left anterior oblique projection. Perforation of a diverticulum may rarely cause mediastinitis and a fistulous tract.	Most are traction diverticula that develop in response to the pull of fibrous adhesions following infection of the mediastinal lymph nodes and often seen adjacent to a calcified lymph node. Pulsion diverticula of the mid-esophagus or traction diverticula of the cervical esophagus are rarely seen.
Epiphrenic diverticula	A broad, short-necked outpouching in the distal 10 cm of the esophagus with normal mucosal appearance and an absence of spasm.	A pulsion-type diverticulum, usually associated with motor abnormalities of the esophagus, which may simulate an esophageal ulcer.
Congenital tracheoesophageal fistula (Fig. 31.13)	Type III: Most common (85 to 90%); the upper segment of esophagus ends in a blind pouch at the level of the bifurcation or slightly above. The lower segment is connected to the trachea. Air in the stomach. Type I: The next most common type; both the upper and lower segments of the esophagus are blind pouches, no air below the diaphragm. Type II: The upper esophageal segment communicates with the trachea, no air below the diaphragm. Type IV: Either both segments of the esophagus are connected with the trachea or there is a single fistulous tract (H-fistula).	Results from failure of complete separation of the trachea and upper alimentary tract. An H-fistula may not be detected in infancy and may cause only occasional symptoms, whereas the others are symptomatic immediately after birth. Associated anomalies include: – Vertebral or rib abnormalities. – Atrial or ventricular septal defects. – Tetralogy of Fallot. – Duodenal or anal atresia.
Traumatic laceration or perforation of the esophagus	Pneumomediastinum is a common initial finding in esophageal perforation, followed by development of mediastinitis and a fistulous tract. Laceration may be seen as a persistent linear collection of contrast material.	Perforation is usually a complication of esophagoscopy, dilatation of the esophagus, crush injury, or rarely due to severe vomiting (*Boerhaave's syndrome*). The mucosal–submucosal laceration and hemorrhage of the esophagus following severe vomiting, called *Mallory–Weiss syndrome*, is always located at the esophagogastric junction, and is rarely detected radiographically.

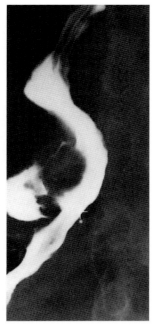

Fig. 31.**9** **Leiomyoma of the esophagus.** A large ulcerated mass mimics esophageal carcinoma, but luminal narrowing is not present.

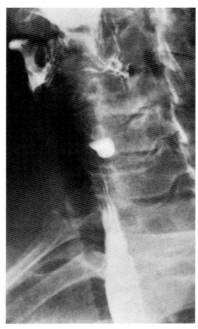

Fig. 31.**10** **Zenker's diverticulum.** Barium remains in the posterior saccular outpouching at the pharyngoesophageal junction after swallowing.

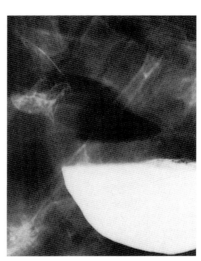

Fig. 31.**11** A large **Zenker's diverticulum** presents as a retroesophageal air-fluid level and barium collection.

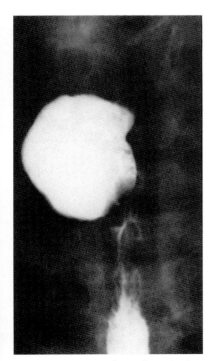

Fig. 31.**12** **Giant pulsion diverticulum** of the upper esophagus.

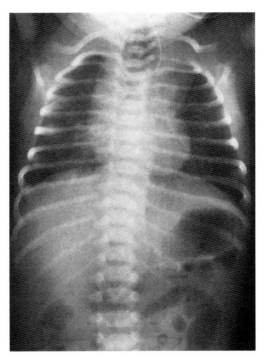

Fig. 31.**13** **Congenital tracheoesophageal fistula.** The nasopharyngeal tube makes a loop in the blind, air-containing pouch of the upper esophagus. Air in the bowel indicates a connection between the lower esophagus and the trachea.

Table 31.2   Gastric Ulcers, Diverticula, and Fistulas

Disease	Radiographic Findings	Comments
Peptic ulcer disease (Figs. 31.14–31.16)	Signs of benign gastric ulcer: Ulcer projects outside the normal gastric lumen. Undermining of mucosa with minimal edema, a lucent line (Hampton line) parallels the base of the crater. Edema may create an ulcer collar, an ulcer mound, or trapping of barium in the ulcer. Smooth, slender mucosal folds extend into the edge of the crater or, in the absence of folds, the surrounding tissue has a smooth contour. Decreases to one half or even more within 3 weeks and often disappears completely in 6 weeks, but residual deformity may remain.	A large ulcer mound can simulate a neoplasm by extending beyond the limits of the ulcer. The size or shape of the ulcer has no practical value as far as malignancy is concerned. Benign ulcers of the greater curvature may demonstrate features that suggest malignancy (intraluminal location, nodular surroundings). Practically all ulcers above the level of the cardia are malignant.
Gastritis	A crater with signs of a benign ulcer may be seen in the absence of peptic ulcer disease.	Other radiographic features (e.g., thickening of mucosal folds, enlargement of areae gastricae or hypersecretion) are more characteristic.
Granulomatous infiltration of the stomach (Fig. 31.17)	Ulcer associated with mucosal abnormalities and usually disease elsewhere in the gastrointestinal tract (Crohn's disease) or lungs (tuberculosis).	Involvement of the terminal ileum suggests Crohn's disease.
Gastrointestinal stromal tumor (GIST) (Fig. 31.18)	Usually a large mass with central ulceration, often in the gastric fundus.	Benign and malignant GISTs are radiographically indistinguishable.
Radiation injury	Peptic ulcerlike radiographic findings without a history of relationship to meals. A high incidence of perforation and hemorrhage.	A complication of a dose more than 45 Gy to the high para-aortic or upper abdominal area, which occurs from 1 month to 6 years (average 5 months) after treatment.

(continues on page 754)

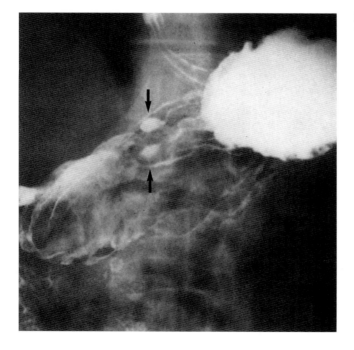

Fig. 31.**14**   **Two superficial gastric ulcers** (arrows) seen as collections of barium surrounded by mucosal edema.

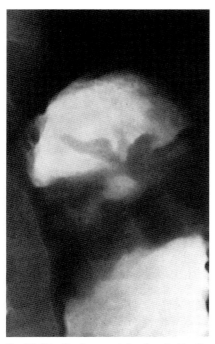

Fig. 31.**15** **Benign gastric ulcer** in the fundus—a rare location for a benign ulcer. Mucosal folds here tend to be thick. The folds extend into the edge of the crater.

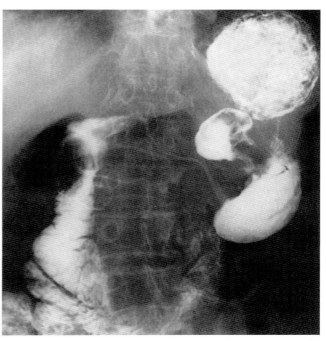

Fig. 31.**16** **Giant benign gastric ulcer** with the appearance of a diverticulum.

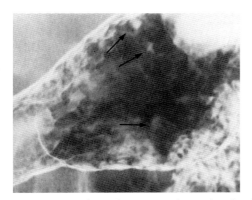

Fig. 31.**17** **Crohn's disease** involving the distal stomach. Tiny aphthoid ulcers and mucosal irregularity are seen in the antrum (arrows).

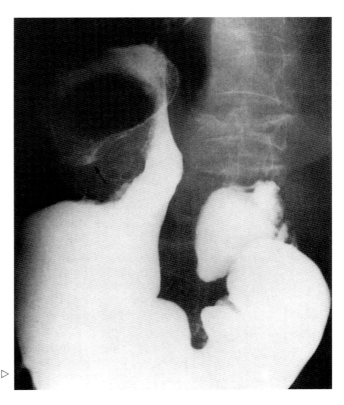

Fig. 31.**18** **Malignant gastrointestinal stromal tumor (GIST).** ▷ A large intramural mass in the fundus with a central ulceration (arrow) is seen.

Table 31.2 (Cont.) Gastric Ulcers, Diverticula, and Fistulas

Disease	Radiographic Findings	Comments
Pseudolymphoma	A large ulcer surrounded by a mass and associated with enlarged rugal folds.	A benign proliferation of lymphoid tissue that can simulate malignant lymphoma. May represent a reaction to chronic peptic ulcer disease. May not be distinguishable from malignant lymphoma in frozen sections or biopsy.
Gastric carcinoma (Figs. 31.19, 31.20)	Signs of a malignant gastric ulcer: – The ulcer projects inside the normal lumen. – Radiating folds merge into a mound of polypoid tissue around the crater or may be clubbed. – Gastric mucosa surrounding the ulcer is abnormal. A rim of tumor may be seen (Carman's meniscus sign). Practically all ulcers above the level of the cardia are malignant.	The radiographic appearance is extremely variable. Most gastric carcinomas can ulcerate.
Lymphoma (Fig. 31.21)	A large ulcerated mass, usually indistinguishable from other malignancies. A single huge ulcer or multiple ulcers suggest lymphoma.	About 2% of all gastric neoplasms are lymphomas, usually associated with diffuse disease. Enlargement of the spleen and retrogastric lymph nodes are often observed.
Metastatic lesion	Bull's eye lesion(s) with central, relatively large ulceration.	Most commonly seen in malignant melanoma but can occur in carcinoma of the breast and lung. Direct extension from neighboring organs can cause gastric ulceration.
Eosinophilic granuloma	A discrete polypoid mass (unlike eosinophilic gastroenteritis) that may demonstrate central ulceration.	Gastrointestinal eosinophilic granuloma is most frequent in the stomach, but may rarely occur elsewhere in the bowel. This entity is neither related to eosinophilic gastroenteritis nor to the Langerhans cell histiocytosis complex.
Marginal ulceration post partial gastrectomy (Fig. 31.22)	A benign ulcer is usually situated in the jejunal side, within the first few centimeters of the anastomosis. It usually has a tent-shaped or conical configuration, but it may be superficial and undetectable. Secondary signs such as edema, flattening, or rigidity of the jejunum are helpful.	A postoperative complication of gastric surgery for the treatment of duodenal peptic ulcer disease, usually within 2–4 years of partial gastrectomy. May be difficult to detect radiographically due to postoperative distortion.
Gastric stump carcinoma	Gastric stump carcinoma may present as an ulcer on the gastric side.	Any ulcer on the gastric side of the anastomosis should be considered malignant unless proven otherwise, since carcinoma in gastric remnant occurs frequently (up to 20% in 20 years).
Erosive gastritis (superficial gastric erosions) (see Fig. 28.25)	Tiny flecks of barium (erosion) surrounded by a radiolucent halo (edema). Defects in the epithelium do not penetrate beyond the muscularis mucosae and are rarely detected on conventional barium examination.	May be the cause of gastrointestinal bleeding. Usually an incidental finding, but may be associated with gastric irritation (alcohol, drugs), Crohn's disease, or candidiasis.
Ectopic pancreas (Fig. 31.23)	A smooth submucosal mass, usually 2 cm or less in diameter, that has a central dimple. This represents the orifice of the duct from the pancreatic tissue and may mimic an ulcerated lesion.	Most common on the distal greater curvature of the gastric antrum within 3–6 cm of the pylorus.
Double pylorus	An accessory channel connects the lesser curvature of the prepyloric antrum with the duodenal bulb (gastroduodenal fistula). An ulcer is usually seen within or adjacent to the accessory channel.	Associated with peptic ulcer disease.

(continues on page 756)

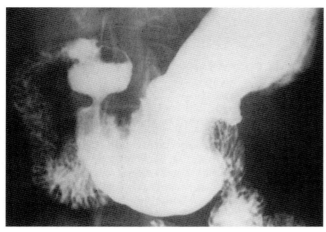

Fig. 31.**19** **Gastric carcinoma** with characteristic features of a malignant ulcer. The ulcer projects inside the lumen. Its margins are irregular.

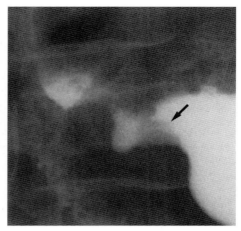

Fig. 31.**20** **Gastric carcinoma** with Carman's meniscus sign (arrow).

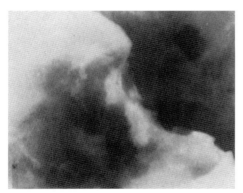

Fig. 31.**21** **Lymphoma.** A large mass with multiple ulcerations is typical for lymphoma.

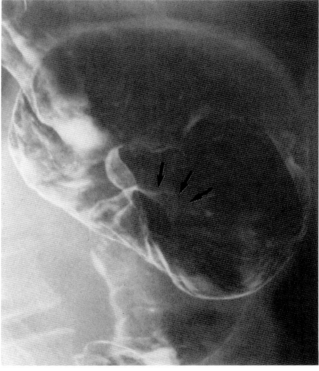

Fig. 31.**22** **Superficial marginal ulceration** (arrows) of the gastric stump. The marginal mucosal ulceration is difficult to detect radiographically.

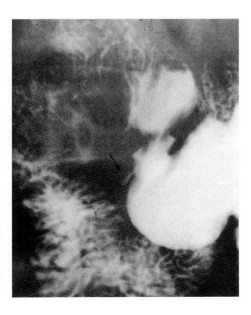

◁ Fig. 31.**23** **Ectopic pancreas** in the distal greater curvature. The duct (arrow) mimics a penetrating narrow ulcer crater. An indentation is seen in greater curvature.

Table 31.2   (Cont.) Gastric Ulcers, Diverticula, and Fistulas

Disease	Radiographic Findings	Comments
Hypertrophic pyloric stenosis (Fig. 31.24)	A small triangular outpouching from the greater curvature side of the long, narrowed pyloric canal is pathognomonic (Twining recess) and may mimic an ulcer.	Radiographically, adult and infantile forms are identical. Gastric ulcer is a common complication in adults but it does not involve the hypertrophied pyloric canal.
Gastric diverticulum (Fig. 31.25)	An outpouching of the gastric wall in the region of the fundus or cardioesophageal junction. A narrow neck and gastric folds running into it allow it to be differentiated from a large ulcer.	Most gastric diverticula are congenital. A small congenital intramural gastric diverticulum may simulate a dilated pancreatic duct of an ectopic pancreatic rest. Acquired diverticula may occur at the stoma after gastroenterostomy, or following healing of a perforated peptic ulcer. *Pseudodiverticulum* of the greater curvature may result from fibrosis and shortening of the lesser curvature (e.g., in severe peptic ulcer disease).
Gastrojejunal fistula (gastrojejunostomy) (Fig. 31.26)	Some or all of the contrast medium bypasses the duodenum.	Gastrojejunostomy is usually created surgically for the therapy of gastric retention.
Gastrocolic fistula	May not be detected on upper gastrointestinal series but frequently during barium enema.	Usually a complication of gastric or colonic carcinoma, more rarely pancreatic carcinoma. Benign ulcer of the greater curvature or posterior wall of the antrum in patients receiving steroids, chronic ulcerating bowel disease, or marginal ulceration following gastric surgery are rare causes.
Internal fistula involving the stomach	Passage of barium into an irregular cavity through a fistulous tract. Extraluminal gas (in pseudocyst, abscess, or biliary tree) may be seen.	The most common cause is spontaneous (or surgical) communication into a pancreatic pseudocyst. Cholecystogastric fistulas are rare.
External fistula involving the stomach	May not be completely visualized on the upper abdominal series if not adequately drained and associated with abscesses.	Usually a complication of surgery on the pancreas, failing gastrointestinal anastomosis or postoperative abscess.

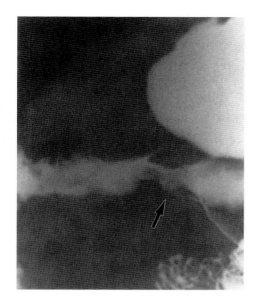

Fig. 31.**24** **Hypertrophic pyloric stenosis.** The pyloric canal is long. An outpouching on its greater curvature side (arrow) is pathognomonic and mimics an ulcer.

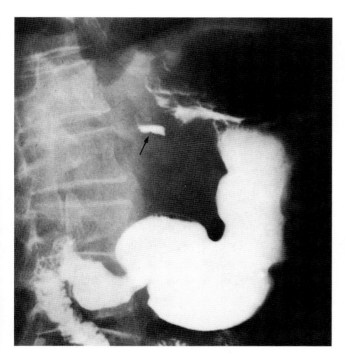

Fig. 31.**25** **Gastric diverticulum** near the cardioesophageal junction (arrow). The patient also has gastric carcinoma of the greater curvature.

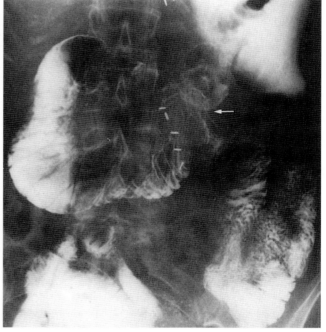

Fig. 31.**26** **Spontaneous fistula between the stomach and the duodenojejunal junction** (arrow) following radiotherapy of left renal carcinoma. Usually this kind of bypass is surgically performed (gastrojejunostomy).

Table 31.3   Ulcers, Diverticula, and Fistulas in the Duodenum

Disease	Radiographic Findings	Comments
Peptic ulcer of the duodenal bulb (Fig. 31.27)	Demonstration of the ulcer crater both in supine air contrast and compression radiographs is necessary. Thickened folds radiating toward the crater help in the localization. Only a minority of patients have deformity of the duodenal cap, spasm, or tenderness. Spasm, edema, or scarring may cause gastric outlet obstruction and nonvisualization of the bulb without hypotonization.	85% of ulcer craters are round, 15% are linear. Multiple ulcers occur in 10 to 15% of cases. Ulcers occur with equal frequency in anterior and posterior walls of the bulb. A *giant duodenal bulb ulcer* may appear like a normal bulb in shape but is fixed and rigid and has irregular margins (ulcer within an ulcer).
Postbulbar peptic ulcer (Fig. 31.28)	A shallow, flattened niche on the medial aspect of the upper second portion of the duodenum, associated with eccentric local spasm or later with ring stricture. Penetration into the pancreas may cause pancreatitis and widening of the duodenal sweep.	One quarter of duodenal ulcers in *Zollinger–Ellison syndrome* are postbulbar or even more distal. Postbulbar ulceration may occur also in benign peptic ulcer disease, but multiple distal ulcers and thickened gastric folds suggest the presence of an islet cell tumor of the pancreas and Zollinger–Ellison syndrome.
Gastrointestinal stromal tumor (GIST) (Fig. 31.29)	An intramural ulcerated mass lesion. May mimic a mound of edema surrounding a peptic postbulbar ulcer.	Differentiation between benign and malignant variety is radiographically impossible.
Adenocarcinoma	Narrowing of the duodenum and ulceration may occur at any point along the sweep.	Gardner's syndrome and Peutz–Jeghers syndrome have an increased risk of developing an otherwise rare duodenal adenocarcinoma.
Spread of carcinoma from adjacent organs	Tumor may invade duodenum and cause ulceration and deformity at any point.	Pancreatic carcinoma tends to involve the inner wall of the sweep, other carcinomas (colon, right kidney, gallbladder) the outer aspects of the sweep or bulb.
Metastases	Hematogenous metastases may ulcerate and create a target lesion appearance.	
Lymphoma	Solitary involvement of the duodenum is rare and has variable appearances, including ulcerations.	Lymphoma may mimic all common duodenal deformities (ulcer, pancreatitis, Crohn's disease, hyperplasia of Brunner's glands).
Crohn's disease Tuberculosis	Granulomatous disease is characterized by duodenal nodularity and postbulbar ulceration.	Crohn's disease is almost invariably associated with the same process elsewhere in the gastrointestinal tract. Duodenum is involved in approximately 1%.
Ectopic pancreas	May simulate a postbulbar small ulceration surrounded by edema, but characteristic spastic incisure is absent.	
Duodenal diverticulum (Figs. 31.30, 31.31)	Most common in the medial side of the sweep and in the periampullary region. Diverticula have a smooth, rounded shape. They are often multiple. They may contain inspissated food particles. A large gas-filled diverticulum may mimic an abscess, dilated cecum, or a pancreatic pseudocyst on plain films.	An incidental finding in up to 5% of barium examinations and usually asymptomatic. Duodenal diverticulitis may mimic cholecystitis, peptic ulcer disease, or pancreatitis, and may be complicated by hemorrhage, retroperitoneal perforation, abscess, or fistulas. Opening of bile and pancreatic ducts into a diverticulum (3%) may predispose to obstructive biliary or pancreatic disease.
Duodenal pseudo-diverticula	Exaggerated outpouchings of the inferior and superior recess of the duodenal bulb secondary to a peptic ulcer ("clover leaf deformity").	
Duodenocolic fistula	A communication between abnormal duodenum and colon is better demonstrated on barium enema than on upper gastrointestinal series.	May be associated with Crohn's disease involving the duodenum or carcinoma of the colon infiltrating into the duodenum. Other enteroenteric fistulas, e.g., *duodenojejunal*, may be present in Crohn's disease.

(continues on page 760)

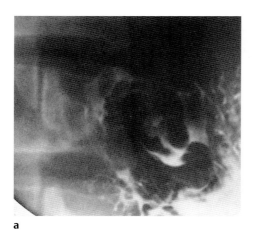

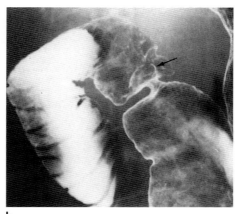

Fig. 31.**27** **Peptic ulcer** of the duodenal bulb. **a** Ulcer crater between thickened folds as demonstrated with single-contrast technique. **b** Another case, demonstrated with double-contrast technique. An arrow points to the round ulcer crater.

a   **b**

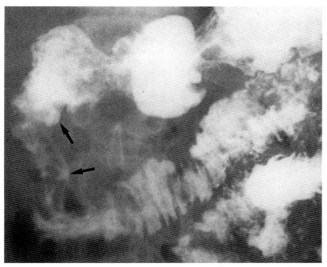

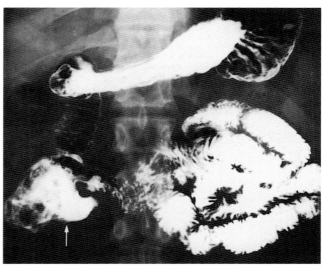

Fig. 31.**28** **Zollinger–Ellison** syndrome. Postbulbar ulcers (arrows) on the medial side of the descending duodenum. Irregular duodenal folds and increased secretions.

Fig. 31.**29** **Benign gastrointestinal stromal tumor (GIST) of the duodenum.** A large ulcerated mass lesion (arrow) is seen at the junction between the second and third portions of the duodenum.

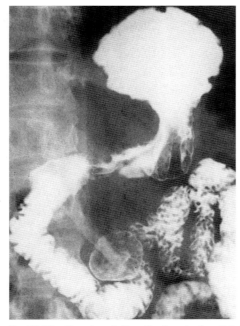

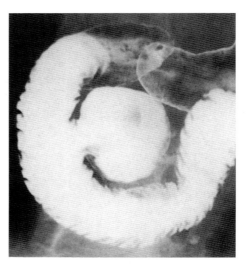

Fig. 31.**30** **Duodenal diverticulum** in the distal duodenum, filled with food.

Fig. 31.**31** A large **duodenal diverticulum** on the medial side of the descending duodenum. A food particle causes a filling defect.

Table 31.3   (Cont.) Ulcers, Diverticula, and Fistulas in the Duodenum

Disease	Radiographic Findings	Comments
Cholecystoduodenal fistula (Fig. 31.32)	Plain films demonstrate gas in the gallbladder or biliary tree, and on upper gastrointestinal series barium usually refluxes into the fistula. (The fistula may occasionally extend to the stomach, hepatic flexure, or jejunum, but most commonly into the duodenum.)	Most (90%) are secondary to acute cholecystitis, usually complicating a gallstone disease. Penetrating duodenal or gastric ulcer, trauma, or tumor are rare causes. The fistula may be surgical (cholecystoduodenostomy, choledochoduodenostomy).
Duodenorenal fistula (Fig. 31.33)	A communication to the right perirenal space may be demonstrated on upper gastrointestinal series. A communication to the renal pelvis is best demonstrated on retrograde pyelography.	Secondary to a rupture of a right perirenal abscess into the duodenum (often in renal tuberculosis) or rarely due to a penetrating duodenal ulcer.

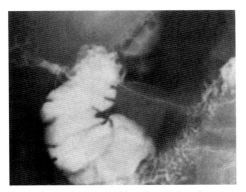

Fig. 31.**32** **Cholecystoduodenal fistula** in a patient with gallstone ileus.

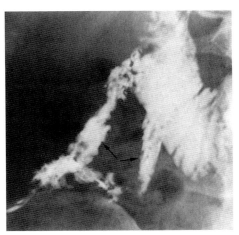

Fig. 31.**33** **Duodenorenal fistula** secondary to rupture of a perirenal abscess into the duodenum. The abscess contains mottled gaseous lucencies. Two fistulous tracts (arrows) are demonstrated with water-soluble contrast medium.

Table 31.4 Ulcers, Diverticula, and Fistulas in the Small Bowel

Disease	Radiographic Findings	Comments
Zollinger–Ellison syndrome (peptic ulcer disease)	Peptic ulcer of the proximal jejunum may occur. Association with multiple duodenal ulcers and enlarged gastric rugae is characteristic.	See also Fig. 31.**27**.
Partial gastrectomy (peptic ulcer disease)	Benign ulcer in the jejunum may occur near the gastrojejunostomy stoma.	An ulcer on the gastric side of the stoma has to be considered malignant unless proven otherwise.
Carcinoid tumor	Most small-bowel carcinoids present as one or more filling defects or as small bowel obstruction. An intramural or intraluminal mass with gross ulceration (bull's eye lesion) is a less common manifestation.	The most common tumor in the small intestine. Most are located in the distal ileum. *Carcinoid syndrome* refers to systemic effects of circulating serotonin. Most symptomatic patients have extensive metastases. Urinary excretion of 5-hydroxyindole acetic acid is elevated.
Gastrointestinal stromal tumors (GISTs)	A pedunculated or intramural mass with a deep, pitlike ulcer crater is characteristic. May cause small bowel obstruction.	GISTs are the most common benign neoplasm of the small intestine (most frequent in the duodenum). About one-sixth of them are malignant, but benign and malignant GISTs are radiographically indistinguishable.
Adenocarcinoma	A plaquelike ulcerated mass is an infrequent presentation. An annular short constrictive process and/or bowel obstruction is a typical presentation.	Most occur in the duodenum or jejunum. May rarely present as a bull's eye lesion.
Lymphoma	A relatively long lesion involving the entire circumference of the bowel wall with extensive ulceration is a typical presentation of a solitary small bowel lymphoma.	Primary lymphoma of the small intestine occurs usually in the jejunum or ileum, very rarely in the duodenum. Separation of bowel loops due to a mesenteric mass is common.
Metastatic melanoma	Round or oval nodules with sharply demarcated borders and a relatively large ulcer (bull's eye lesion).	Gastrointestinal metastases can be the first clinical presentation of metastatic melanoma. Ulcerated metastases to the jejunum or ileum from other, more common carcinomas are rare.
Kaposi's sarcoma	Metastases to the small bowel are relatively common and they characteristically appear as multiple bull's eye lesions.	A systemic disease with multiple soft bluish nodules of the skin with hemorrhages, similar to infectious granulomas but has a neoplastic character. Common in AIDS and in elderly men in parts of Africa, eastern Europe, and northern Italy.
Jejunal diverticula	Thin-walled, atonic outpouchings with narrow necks on the mesenteric side of the small bowel. Leakage of gas through diverticula may cause pneumoperitoneum without peritonitis.	Jejunal diverticulosis may cause malabsorption secondary to overgrowth of bacteria. Jejunal diverticulitis is a rare complication, which may cause a mesenteric abscess or mass displacement of the jejunal loops.
Pseudodiverticula	Large sacs with squared, broad bases involving the antimesenteric side of the small bowel.	Pseudodiverticula result from smooth muscle atrophy and fibrosis. They are characteristic of *scleroderma*. In *Crohn's disease* they are associated with strictures. They may also occur in *lymphoma*.
Meckel's diverticulum (see Fig. 30.44)	Rarely demonstrated radiographically as a wide-necked outpouching that arises from the antimesenteric side of the distal ileum.	Rudimentary omphalomesenteric duct, usually within 100 cm from the ileocecal valve. It has an incidence of 1 to 4% in autopsies. Usually asymptomatic, but may cause bleeding, intestinal obstruction, or inflammation (simulates appendicitis clinically).
Ileal diverticula	Small outpouchings near the ileocecal valve, which resemble those commonly seen in the sigmoid colon.	Usually asymptomatic and rarely cause complications. If infected, they simulate late appendicitis clinically.

(continues on page 762)

Table 31.4   (Cont.) Ulcers, Diverticula, and Fistulas in the Small Bowel

Disease	Radiographic Findings	Comments
Enteric–enteric fistulas (Fig. 31.34)	Fistula formation associated with abnormal bowel mucosa, stricturation, and mesenteric thickening of the involved segments. The distal ileum is almost invariably affected.	Fistulas are a hallmark of chronic *Crohn's disease* (seen in 50%), whereas they are rare in *ulcerative colitis* (0.5%). Enteric-enteric fistulas are most common, but fistulas extending to bladder, vagina, abscesses, or perianal skin also occur. Enteric–enteric fistulas involving the small bowel may occur also secondary to *primary* or *metastatic malignancy*, *radiation therapy*, ulcerative colitis, and infections (*tuberculosis, pelvic inflammation, actinomycosis, amebiasis, shigellosis*).
Diverticulitis	Single or multiple fistulous communications between the colon and small bowel occur in 10% of patients with diverticulitis.	
Postoperative gastro-jejunocolic fistula	In barium enema examination, contrast extends directly from the transverse colon into the stomach.	A grave complication of marginal ulceration after gastric surgery. Associated with diarrhea, weight loss, and/or bleeding.

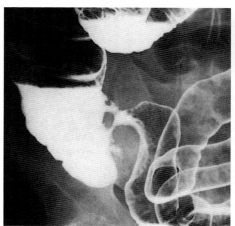

a

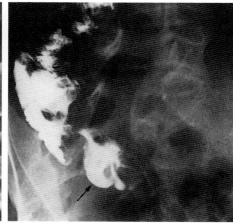

b

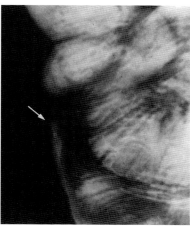

c

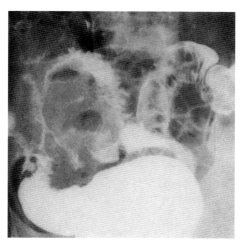

d

Fig. 31.**34 a–d**   **Crohn's disease. a** Ileocolic fistulas through a mass between the distal ileum and cecum. **b** Pseudodiverticulum (arrow) of the distal ileum, narrowing of the ileal lumen. **c** External fistula (arrow) originating from the jejunum and descending towards the pelvis. **d** Numerous fistulous tracts through a mass in the right iliac fossa.

Table 31.5 Ulcers, Diverticula, and Fistulas in the Colon and Rectum

Disease	Radiographic Findings	Comments
Ulcerative colitis (Fig. 31.35)	Discrete and widely separated marginal ulcers are unusual. Monotonous symmetric ulceration of the mucosa is more characteristic. Enteric–enteric fistulas are rare (about 0.5%).	See Fig. 28.**40**, for the patterns of mucosal changes. Generalized ulceration occurs also in *shigella, salmonella,* and *staphylococcus* infections, in *pseudomembranous colitis, (clostridium difficile disease),* and in severe *strongyloidiasis.*
Crohn's disease	Aphthoid ulcers surrounded by normal mucosa. Deeper irregular ulcers may penetrate beyond the contour of the bowel and coalesce to form long (over 10 cm) tracts parallel to the longitudinal axis of the colon. Fistulous tracts to adjacent bowel, bladder, vagina, perineum, or abdominal wall are common.	Similar deep ulcers and fistulas involving primarily cecum may occur in *tuberculosis* and *amebiasis.* Cecal ulceration may also be a manifestation of *cytomegalovirus* infection. Aphthoid ulcers may occur in *amebiasis, tuberculosis,* and *yersinia* infections and in *Behçet's syndrome.*
Ischemic colitis	Single or multiple ulcers surrounded by pseudo-polyposis and "thumb printing" mucosal edema.	Most common in the splenic flexure and sigmoid. The disease may resolve rapidly or progress to stricture formation.
Radiation-induced colitis	Spasm, fine serrations of the bowel wall, and superficial to penetrating ulcerations can be found in the field of irradiation. Fistulas and strictures develop often.	The most common site of localized injury is the anterior rectal wall, since it often receives the highest radiation dose during the treatment of gynecologic, prostatic, and bladder carcinomas.
Lymphogranuloma venereum	Multiple shaggy ulcers of the rectum associated with fistulas and sinus tracts of varying length, sometimes progressing to tubular rectal stricture.	Sinus tracts can be short and blind or connected to a perianal abscess. Involvement of the whole rectum (rarely distal colon) and barium spicules projecting into the lumen distinguish this condition from other causes of rectal ulceration.
Solitary rectal ulcer syndrome	Pre-ulcerative nodulation is followed by ulcer formation within 15 cm of the anal verge and near the valve of Houston. Longstanding ulceration leads to fibrosis and rectal stricture.	A rare condition that may be difficult to differentiate from inflammatory bowel disease or malignancy. Manifests mainly in young patients as rectal bleeding. Probably associated with pelvic muscle discoordination during defecation.

(continues on page 764)

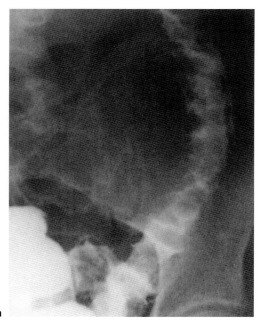
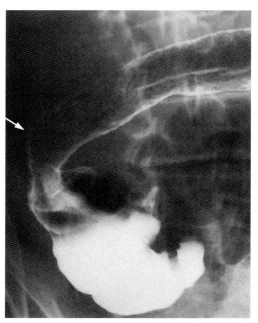

a

b

Fig. 31.**35 a, b Ulcerative colitis. a** Pseudopolyps originating from the ulcerated mucosa create the appearance of double track-ing in the descending colon. **b** Discrete ulcerations (arrow) are seen at the hepatic flexure.

Table 31.5 (Cont.) Ulcers, Diverticula, and Fistulas in the Colon and Rectum

Disease	Radiographic Findings	Comments
Nonspecific benign ulceration of the colon	Usually single (in 20% multiple) colonic ulcer arising usually from the antimesenteric wall. Radiographically, a carcinoma of the colon is usually suspected due to the masslike effect of the inflammatory reaction.	A diagnosis of exclusion only. Most frequent in the cecum and ascending colon where it can clinically mimic appendicitis. May perforate.
Carcinoma of the colon	Early saddle cancer may be seen as a flat, plaque-like lesion, which shows central ulceration. Double tracking of the sigmoid colon, representing pericolic sinus tracts or fistulas, may occur.	A more common pattern in left colon is an annular "apple-core" tumor with eventual mucosal destruction or a large fungating mass in the right colon. *Rectal carcinoids* may also ulcerate.
Metastatic carcinoma	May rarely present as bull's eye lesions or enteric–enteric fistulas.	*Lymphomas* and *leukemias* may also rarely present as mucosal ulcerations or ulcerating mass lesions in the colon.
Diverticulosis (Figs. 31.36, 31.37)	Round outpouchings beyond the confines of the lumen, usually less than 2 cm in diameter. They commonly occur in the sigmoid colon, but may also involve other segments of the colon. They are very rare in the rectum.	A huge sigmoid diverticulum probably represents a slowly progressing *diverticular abscess*. Diverticula appear around the mesenteric tenia. The distensibility of the colon is retained in the absence of inflammation.
Diverticulitis (Fig. 31.38)	A complication of diverticulosis in which perforation of a diverticulum leads to the development of a peridiverticular abscess. Extravasation of barium beyond the diverticulum, either as a tiny projection of contrast from the tip of the diverticulum or as obvious filling of a pericolic abscess, is diagnostic. A more common but less specific sign is the demonstration of a pericolic soft-tissue mass (abscess). Colonic obstruction, short (3 to 6 cm) parasigmoid tracts (double tracking), and fistulas may be associated.	Clinically, the most common presentation is "left-sided appendicitis." Colonic cancer associated with diverticular disease can be difficult to differentiate from diverticulitis, although the latter usually involves a longer segment. Fistulas into the small bowel (10%) and adjacent organs may occur, mimicking Crohn's disease. Colocutaneous fistulas may complicate surgical treatment.
Pseudodiverticula (Fig. 31.39)	Sacculations with squared, broad basis on the antimesenteric border at the colon, Characteristic of *scleroderma* and *healing ischemic colitis*.	Pseudodiverticula are produced by fibrosis involving primarily the mesenteric border of the colon.

(continues on page 766)

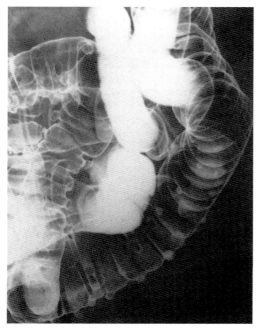

Fig. 31.**36** **Sigmoid diverticulosis.** Several diverticula are seen in profile and end-on.

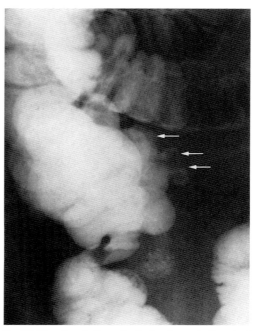

Fig. 31.**37** **Cecal diverticulosis.** Several diverticula contain fecal material or gas (arrows).

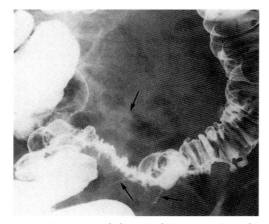

Fig. 31.**38** **Sigmoid diverticulitis.** Narrowing of a segment with short fistulous tracts (lower arrows) and perisigmoid soft tissue mass (upper arrow) is seen.

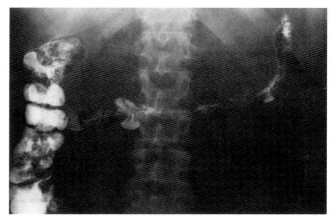

Fig. 31.**39** **Two pseudodiverticula** of the inferior (anti-mesenteric) margin of the transverse colon in scleroderma are seen.

Table 31.5 (Cont.) Ulcers, Diverticula, and Fistulas in the Colon and Rectum

Disease	Radiographic Findings	Comments
Fistulas involving the colon or rectum (Figs. 31.40–31.42)	Fistulous tracts are not always demonstrated by barium enema despite passage of feces or gas through the fistula. Urinary fistulas are best demonstrated by voiding cystourethrography.	*Acquired fistulas* are usually associated with Crohn's disease or radiation necrosis, less commonly with other inflammatory disease or malignancy. *Congenital fistulas* (rectovesical, rectovaginal, rectourethral, rectoperineal and rectolabial fistulas) may be associated with an imperforate anus.

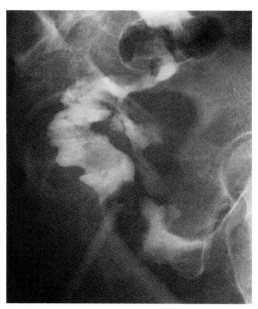

Fig. 31.**40 Rectouterine fistula** as a complication of radiotherapy of carcinoma of the cervix. Contrast medium leaks from the anterior wall of the rectum into the uterine cavity and further into the vagina.

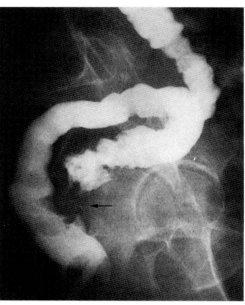

Fig. 31.**41 Rectosigmoid fistula** (arrow), a complication of radiotherapy of carcinoma of the cervix.

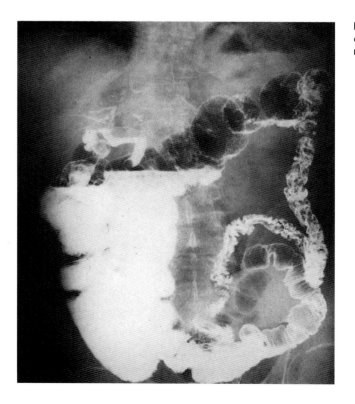

Fig. 31.**42 Choledochocolic fistula.** Filling of the biliary tree during barium enema is seen. A complication of carcinoma of the right kidney.

32 Gallbladder and Bile Duct Abnormalities

Plain Radiography

The normal gallbladder and the biliary ducts are not seen on plain radiography with the possible exception of thin patients, in whom a very faint density caused by the gallbladder is occasionally recognizable. Therefore, the presence of gas or calcification is required in the biliary system before it becomes visible on plain radiography.

Gas in the biliary system is virtually limited to two conditions: (1) an abnormal communication between the gastrointestinal and biliary tracts allowing the reflux of air (and also barium) from the bowel into the biliary system and (2) the presence of gas-producing organisms within the biliary system (Fig. 32.1). Biliary gas has to be differentiated from other gas collections in the right upper quadrant. Both the duodenal bulb and a large duodenal diverticulum can be confused with an air-filled gallbladder, but an upper gastrointestinal barium examination or CT will clearly identify these structures. Hepatic and subhepatic abscesses may be more difficult to differentiate because of their anatomic proximity to the gallbladder and a symptomatology similar to that of emphysematous cholecystitis. In these cases, ultrasonography appears most useful to locate the abnormal gas collection. Other pathologic gas collections (e.g., retroperitoneal and abdominal wall abscesses) are easily differentiated from air in the gallbladder with conventional radiography in two projections, since they will project outside the expected gallbladder area in at least one view.

Differentiation between *gas in the biliary ducts* and *gas in the portal system* can at times be difficult. As a general rule, gas in the biliary system tends to be located in the larger ducts near the hilum of the liver, whereas portal vein gas is preferentially seen in the liver periphery. The most common cause of gas in the portal system is bowel infarction, that may also be evident radiographically (adynamic ileus with thickened folds and/or haustra, "thumb prints," and streaky or linear crescent gas in the bowel wall), thus supporting the diagnosis of intraportal gas (Fig. 32.2). Small mottled gas collections within the liver parenchyma can also be seen with *liver abscesses,* which are often multiple, but with only a small minority containing gas.

In *emphysematous cholecystitis,* gas is seen in either the lumen or the wall of the gallbladder, or in both (Fig. 32.3). The gallbladder usually has a generous size. Although cystic duct obstruction is almost always associated, cholelithiasis may not be present. Upright or decubitus films may disclose an air–bile level.

The incidence of emphysematous cholecystitis is approximately five times greater in males than females, and is associated with diabetes in a majority of cases. Gallbladder perforation is an extremely serious but not unusual complication. Gas-forming organisms of the *Clostridium* group are the most common germs, but *Escherichia coli, anaerobic Streptococci,* and others have also been implicated. Ascending cholangitis caused by these organisms generally does not

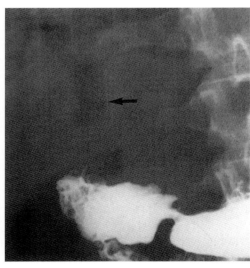

Fig. 32.1 Biliary gas secondary to choledochoduodenostomy. The dilated extrahepatic bile ducts (arrow) are contrasted by gas, whereas the barium has not yet refluxed into the biliary system.

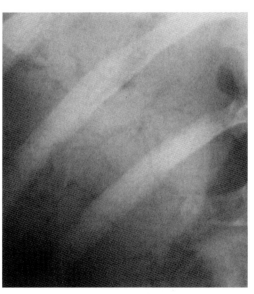

Fig. 32.2 Portal gas secondary to mesenteric infarction. Irregular tubular radiolucencies are seen in the liver periphery. The supine abdominal film of this patient is shown in Fig. 26.**26**.

produce enough gas in the bile ducts to be detectable by conventional radiography.

Spontaneous or postoperative *cholecystoenteric fistulas* are the most common cause of gallbladder air. However, in these cases the gallbladder is small to normal in size and air is never seen in the gallbladder wall, but commonly in the lumen of bile ducts. *Gallstone perforation* into the duodenum or less commonly into the colon is the most common cause of a spontaneous cholecystoenteric fistula. Rarely, a *carcinoma* of the gastrointestinal tract, pancreas, or biliary system may produce an enterocholic fistula that is radiographically evident by intraluminal air in the bile ducts and/or gallbladder. Perforation of a peptic ulcer into the biliary system is even more unusual. By far the most common cause of intrabiliary air results from *surgical procedures* such as choledochoduodenostomy, cholecystoenterostomy, and sphincterotomy. On upper gastrointestinal examination, barium refluxes freely into the biliary system in these cases. Small amounts of gas in the common bile duct are occasionally seen with an *incompetent Oddi's sphincter*. This may be drug-induced (cholecystokinin, anticholinergica), caused by local inflammation and scarring (e.g., postbulbar ulcer disease), or a carcinoma originating in the region of the ampulla of Vater. The sphincter incompetence is rarely idiopathic. Similarly, gas or contrast material reflux into the pancreatic duct can occasionally also be seen in these conditions.

Gallstones are by far the most common cause of calcification in the biliary system, despite the fact that only approximately 20% contain sufficient calcium to be radiopaque. Ultrasonography is, therefore, the procedure of choice to diagnose cholelithiasis, since both calcified and noncalcified gallstones are readily demonstrated by this technique. There is a great variation in the radiographic appearance and size of gallstones. They are present as homogeneous or ringlike densities, which is unfortunately also the radiographic manifestation of many other calcified right upper quadrant lesions (Fig. 32.**4**). Calcifications in the right kidney, retroperitoneum, and costal cartilage may all project into the gallbladder area on an anteroposterior film, but can easily be differentiated from gallstones in an oblique or lateral view. Ultrasonography or computed tomography may, however, be required to differentiate gallstones from vascular, hepatic, and lymph node calcifications located in the proximity of the biliary system. Faceted gallstones or the demonstration of stellate radiolucencies representing gas within the gallstones ("Mercedes-Benz" sign) are relatively rare but diagnostic findings for cholelithiasis (Fig. 32.**5**).

Opacification of the gallbladder on plain radiography (without the administration of any contrast medium) is caused by innumerable sandlike calcified particles dispersed in a thick, pastelike bile. It is termed *milk of calcium* or *limy bile syndrome* (Fig. 32.**6**). In this condition, the gallbladder is chronically inflamed and the cystic duct obstructed by a stone that is often calcified. The visualization of a cystic duct stone and the often slightly granular appearance of the milk of calcium bile may help to differentiate this condition from a gallbladder opacified by contrast medium. One has to be aware that the gallbladder may occasionally remain opacified for up to two weeks after oral cholecystography and that vicarious biliary excretion of a urographic contrast agent resulting in gallbladder opacification occurs with poor renal function, with acute unilateral ureteral obstruction and a normally functioning contralateral kidney, or when large urographic contrast material dosages are used.

Porcelain gallbladder refers to calcifications in the gallbladder wall that can occur in chronic cholecystitis (Fig.

32.**7**). Gallstones are almost always present with one usually obstructing the cystic duct. Malignant degeneration of the porcelain gallbladder develops with a high enough frequency to warrant prophylactic cholecystectomy even in asymptomatic patients. Rarely, a *mucinous adenocarcinoma* of the gallbladder can disclose fine punctate calcifications.

Contrast Examination

Visualization of the gallbladder and/or bile ducts can be achieved by oral administration of biliary contrast agents or by direct injection of contrast into the biliary system. The latter is attained by transhepatic, transjugular or endoscopic retrograde cholangiography and postoperative T-tube cholangiography.

Diagnostic visualization of the biliary system by oral cholecystography is virtually limited to nonjaundiced patients. In the presence of normal liver function, failure to visualize the gallbladder with oral cholecystography is highly suggestive of gallbladder disease (e.g., *cholecystitis* or *cystic duct obstruction*. Rare causes of *nonvisualization* that are related neither to the liver nor to the biliary system include diseases and abnormalities of the gastrointestinal tract, malabsorption syndromes, and interference by a variety of drugs with the cholecystographic agents in the resorption from the gut or the biliary excretion. The diameter of the common bile duct ranges from 1 to 7 mm in healthy individuals. After cholecystectomy, the average bile duct diameter tends to be slightly larger than in the noncholecystectomized patient. A diameter in excess of 15 mm strongly suggests bile duct obstruction in any patient.

The differential diagnosis of filling defects in the opacified gallbladder and bile ducts is discussed in Tables 32.1-32.**3**. *Mucosal outpouchings* (diverticula) from the gallbladder are usually multiple and present radiographically as small oval collections of contrast material adjacent to the gallbladder wall. They are referred to as *Rokitansky–Aschoff sinuses* (Fig. 32.**8**), are best seen after gallbladder contraction (e.g., after a fatty meal), and represent one of several manifestations of gallbladder adenomyomatosis (see also Tables 32.**1** and 32.**2**). The differential diagnosis of saccular lesions originating from bile ducts is the subject of Table 32.**4**. It has to be remembered that in a jaundiced patient, gallbladder and bile duct lesions are only visualized with direct (e.g., transhepatic or endoscopic retrograde) cholangiography, whereas oral cholecystography results in nonvisualization of the biliary system in these cases. However, ultrasound is nowadays the imaging method of choice to investigate gallbladder and biliary diseases and to differentiate between hepatic and obstructive jaundice.

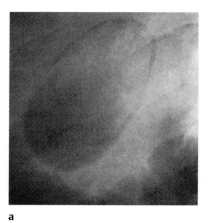
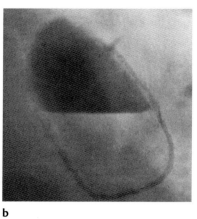

a   b

Fig. 32.**3 a, b   Emphysematous cholecystitis** in a diabetic patient **a** in supine and **b** in right lateral decubitus projections. Both intramural and intraluminal gas are seen in the gallbladder. On the lateral decubitus film, an air–bile level is seen.

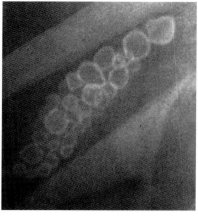

Fig. 32.**4   Gallstones.** Multiple gallstones are evident as ringlike densities with a radiolucent center.

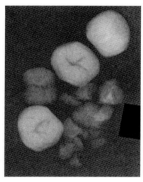

Fig. 32.**5   Gallstones** with "Mercedes-Benz" sign. Gas within the gallstones is evident as stellate radiolucencies.

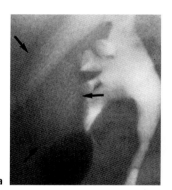
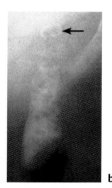

a   b

Fig. 32.**6 a, b   Milk of calcium bile** or **lime bile syndrome** (two cases). **a** Innumerable sandlike calcific densities are coincidentally seen in the gallbladder (arrows) during intravenous urography. **b** A radiopaque shrunken gallbladder containing numerous small nonopaque gallstones is associated with a larger ovoid cyst duct calculus with faint rim calcification (arrow).

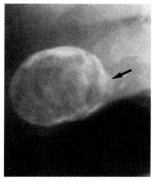

Fig. 32.**7   Porcelain gallbladder.** Calcification of the gallbladder wall is seen. Note the additional density next to the gallbladder neck representing the obstructing cystic duct stone (arrow).

Fig. 32.**8   Rokitansky–Aschoff sinuses.** Multiple punctate collec- ▷ tions of contrast medium along both sides of the markedly contracted gallbladder neck after a fatty meal are seen (arrows). The apparent filling defects in the gallbladder fundus are caused by superimposed gas in the colon.

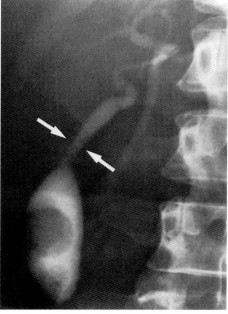
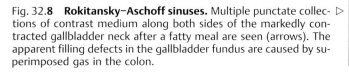

Table 32.1   Linear of Bandlike Filling Defects in the Opacified Gallbladder

Disease	Radiographic Findings	Comments
Septate gallbladder	Septa of variable length and number in a normal-sized gallbladder.	Rare. Stasis in different gallbladder compartment predisposes to infection and gallstone formation.
Phrygian cap (Fig. 32.9)	A radiolucent line, caused by an incomplete circumferential septum of varying thickness, partially separates the fundus from the body.	Developmental anomaly without clinical significance.
Gallstones (Fig. 32.10)	A layer of innumerable tiny calculi may form a thin-to-thick radiolucent band on upright or lateral decubitus films, but cannot be seen on supine examination.	
Cystic fibrosis	Multiple weblike trabeculations in a small gallbladder with marginal irregularities.	Opacification of the gallbladder with oral cholecystography is usually poor.
Adenomyomatosis (Fig. 32.11)	Localized adenomyomatosis of the "circumferential" type may cause compartmentalization of the gallbladder ("hourglass gallbladder"). Gallstones are often present in distal compartment.	Adenomatosis consists of mucosal proliferation, increased thickness of the muscularis, and mucosal outpouchings. Disease may be localized or diffuse. In the latter case, mucosal outpouchings may present as multiple oval contrast collections of varying size round to adjacent to the gallbladder wall.

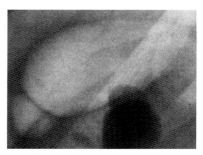

Fig. 32.**9 Phrygian cap.** The radiolucent line between the fundus and the body of the gallbladder is caused by an incomplete circumferential septum.

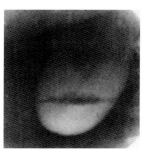

Fig. 32.**10 Gallstones.** A layer of numerous small cholesterol stones forms a radiolucent band on this film taken with horizontal beam in upright position.

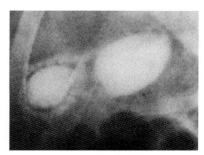

Fig. 32.**11 Adenomyomatosis.** Compartmentalization of the gallbladder producing an "hourglass" deformity is seen. Note also the multiple Rokitansky–Aschoff sinuses presenting as a string of beads around the circumference of the distal compartment.

Table 32.2 Round or Masslike Filling Defects in the Opacified Gallbladder

Disease	Radiographic Findings	Comments
Gallstones (Fig. 32.12)	Single or multiple filling defects, varying greatly in shape and size, ranging from 1 mm to 5 cm. Characteristically, gallstones are freely movable, thus changing the location within the gallbladder in different positions. Rarely, a stone may become adherent to the wall and simulate a mural lesion.	80% are composed predominantly of non-radiopaque cholesterol. Two-thirds of the patients are asymptomatic. Peak age is the fifth and sixth decades with a 3:1 female predominance. A higher incidence of gallstones is also found with cirrhosis, diabetes, pancreatitis, Crohn's disease, and hyperparathyroidism. Bilirubin stones are associated with excessive red blood cell destruction (hemolytic anemias).
Cholesterolosis Cholesterol polyp (Fig. 32.13)	Single, or more commonly several, round-to-oval filling defects of varying size, but usually measuring less than 1 cm. They can be differentiated from gallstones by their fixed location in the gallbladder.	Abnormal deposits of cholesterol esters in fat-laden macrophages in the lamina propria ("strawberry gallbladder").
Adenomyoma (Fig. 32.14)	Solitary filling defect characteristically located in the fundus of the gallbladder. An "ulcer niche" is occasionally seen in the center of the lesion representing a solitary Rokitansky–Aschoff sinus.	Localized manifestation of adenomyomatosis caused by focal hyperplasia of the gallbladder wall.
Adenomyomatosis (Fig. 32.15)	Multiple small filling defects often associated with other manifestations of the disorder such as compartmentalization or narrowing of the fundus and Rokitansky–Aschoff sinuses.	May be associated with symptoms of chronic gallbladder disease.
Benign tumors, intramural cyst, or ectopic tissue	Extremely rare causes of one or more small mural filling defects in the gallbladder.	Benign tumors include adenomas, papillomas, carcinoids, and different mesenchymal tumors. Intramural cysts include epithelial and mucus retention cysts. Ectopic tissue implanted into the gallbladder wall may originate from the pancreas or stomach.
Carcinoma (Fig. 32.16)	Nonvisualization of gallbladder is the common presentation in oral cholecystography. Irregular filling defect may be found in an opacified gallbladder.	May originate in gallbladder or represent a local extension of a biliary or hepatic carcinoma. Other less common malignancies include *hematogenous metastases* (e.g., from melanoma) and *sarcomas* (e.g., leiomyosarcoma).
Inflammatory pseudo-tumors	Solitary or multiple filling defects developing during the course of chronic cholecystitis.	*Xanthogranulomatous cholecystitis* is a rare form of chronic cholecystitis that presents with nodular lesions and is usually associated with cholelithiasis. *Parasitic granulomas* can occasionally be found with ascariasis and paragonimiasis.
Extrinsic mass	Extrinsic filling defects measure usually several centimeters and tend to be semicircular or may cause an hourglass deformity. Normal anatomical structures (e.g., dilated duodenum or colon) and mass lesions originating from liver, porta hepatis, and pancreas may produce extrinsic filling defects.	*Postoperative defects* may present in similar fashion. Small extrinsic defects may occasionally be caused by *vascular structures*.
Air in bowel (see Fig. 32.8)	Superimposed bowel air may simulate one or more true filling defects. Projection of the air outside the opacified gallbladder on one film allows correct diagnosis.	

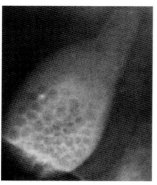

Fig. 32.**12** **Gallstones.** Multiple small filling defects caused by nonradiopaque cholesterol stones are seen.

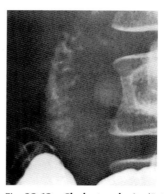

Fig. 32.**13** **Cholesterolosis** ("strawberry gallbladder"). Multiple small polypoid filling defects are seen in the contracted gallbladder.

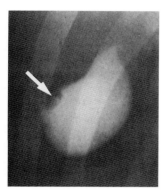

Fig. 32.**14** **Adenomyoma.** A solitary small defect is seen in the contracted gallbladder with a Rokitansky–Aschoff sinus presenting as central contrast collection (arrow).

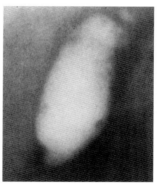

Fig. 32.**15** **Adenomyomatosis.** Several small filling defects and a constricting narrowing of the gallbladder fundus are seen.

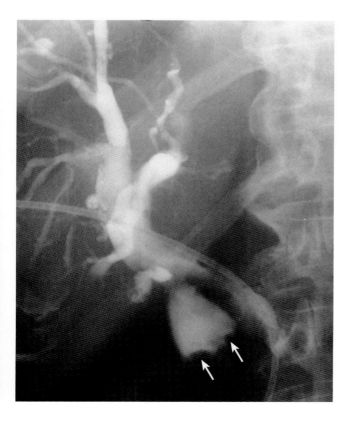

Fig. 32.**16** **Gallbladder carcinoma.** A relatively large, irregular filling defect (arrows) is seen in the gallbladder fundus. Dilatation of the biliary system is caused by tumor extension into the common bile duct.

Table 32.3 Filling Defects and/or Localized Stenosis of Opacified Bile Ducts

Disease	Radiographic Findings	Comments
Congenital membrane	Rare cause of partial obstruction of common hepatic duct by membranous diaphragm.	Usually diagnosed in young adults. Recurrent jaundice for many years characteristic. DD: *Biliary atresia* of the neonate is the result of a progressive inflammatory obliterative process during fetal life.
Calculi (Fig. 32.17)	Bile ducts usually dilated by partial or complete obstruction. Stones may be freely mobile. Impacted stones characteristically produce a convex filling defect with smooth border.	*Mirizzi syndrome*: Gallstone impacted in the cystic duct, causing partial common hepatic duct obstruction (Fig. 32.**18**)
Cholangiocarcinoma and metastatic extrinsic or intrinsic carcinoma (Figs. 32.19–32.22)	Configuration of the biliary duct at point of obstruction is similar for extrinsic and intrinsic tumors. It may be blunt, rounded, jagged, tapered or show a "rat tail" deformity. *Pancreatic carcinoma* (Fig. 32.**19**): Obstruction usually associated with large mass and located at superior margin of pancreas (the level at which the common bile duct changes from a medial and slightly caudal course to a lateral and steeper caudal direction) or more distally. *Metastases* (Fig. 32.**20**): Obstruction of common hepatic duct often in porta hepatis. *Gallbladder carcinoma* (Fig. 32.**20**): Mass in gallbladder area usually associated with cystic duct obstruction and often combined with common hepatic duct obstruction when the latter is invaded. *Bile duct carcinoma* (Fig. 32.**21**): Originate in 95 % anywhere in the extrahepatic biliary system. May produce intraluminal masses of varying sizes or more commonly infiltrating stenotic lesions of varying length. *Ampullary carcinoma* (Fig. 32.**22**): Obstruction of the distal common bile duct, often without traceable tumor. Occasionally an irregular or polypoid mass measuring less than 2 cm is found.	Middle-aged and elderly patients with unremittant progressive jaundice and pruritus. *Lymphoma* involving the nodes in the porta hepatis presents like metastases. *Klatskin tumors* are cholangiocarcinomas that originate from the junction between the right and left hepatic duct. They tend to grow slower and metastasize later than the usual cholangiocarcinomas.

(continues on page 776)

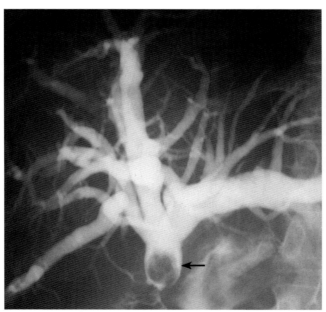

Fig. 32.**17   Biliary calculus.** An impacted stone (arrow), evident as a around filling defect completely surrounded by contrast medium is seen in the common hepatic duct causing marked dilatation of all hepatic ducts proximal to this calculus.

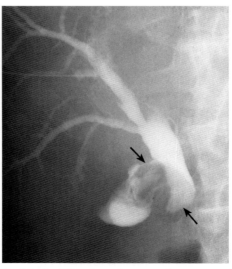

Fig. 32.**18   Mirizzi syndrome.** A large, nonradiopaque gallstone (arrows) impacted in the cystic duct protrudes into the common hepatic duct causing obstruction of the latter.

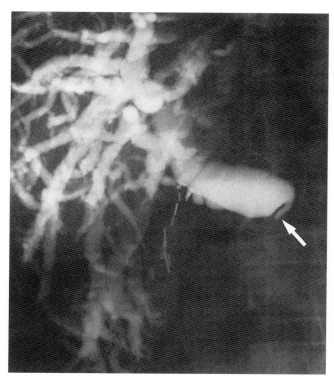

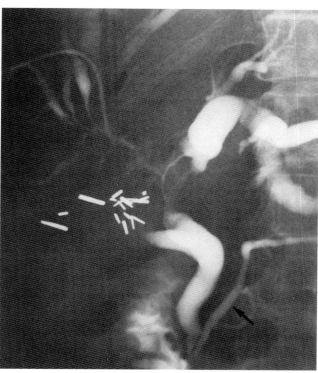

Fig. 32.**19 Pancreatic carcinoma.** Obstruction of the common bile duct in characteristic location (level at which it changes from a medial and slightly caudal course to a lateral and steeper caudal direction) is present. The beaklike termination of the occluded duct is often seen in this condition (arrow). Cholecystectomy was performed in the past.

Fig. 32.**20 Metastatic gallbladder carcinoma.** A large metastasis in the porta hepatis causes obstruction of the relatively smoothly tapered right hepatic ducts and a marked prestenotic dilatation of the left hepatic duct. Note also the contrast reflux into the pancreatic duct (arrow).

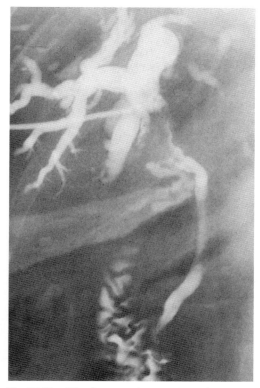

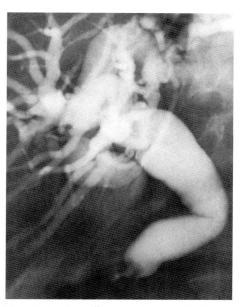

Fig. 32.**21 Bile duct carcinoma.** Irregular stenosis of the common hepatic duct and, to a lesser extent, of the common bile duct is seen.

Fig. 32.**22 Ampullary carcinoma.** An irregular stenosis of the ampullary portion of the bile duct combined with a polypoid lesion, producing an irregular filling defect in the obstructed distal common bile duct, is virtually diagnostic.

Table 32.3   (Cont.) Filling Defects and/or Localized Stenosis of Opacified Bile Ducts

Disease	Radiographic Findings	Comments
Benign tumors and inflammatory pseudotumors	Rare cause of a sessile polypoid filling defect that may or may not cause obstruction.	*Adenomas* and a wide variety of other benign neoplasms are encountered. *Papillomas* may be multiple, and the combination of intraluminal nodules and thick mucous production may cause biliary obstruction. *Tuberculosis, sarcoidosis,* and other granulomatous diseases involving the lymph nodes in the porta hepatis rarely cause extrinsic compression and obstruction of the biliary system.
Pancreatitis, chronic (Fig. 32.23)	Smooth stricture of distal common bile duct is characteristic. Complete obstruction is rare. Pancreatic pseudocyst may cause displacement of bile ducts. Pancreatic calcifications are occasionally seen.	May present with recurrent cholangitis and obstructive jaundice. *Acute pancreatitis*: A reversible smooth narrowing of the distal common bile duct by the enlarged and edematous pancreas head is occasionally seen.
Inflammation/fibrosis of papilla of Vater	Incomplete distal common bile duct obstruction with or without contracted (spastic) Oddi's sphincter may simulate a polypoid lesion. DD: calculus or ampullary carcinoma.	Causes: Acute or chronic inflammatory disease (e.g., bile ducts, pancreas). Postoperative or post instrumentation. Idiopathic (hypertrophy of Oddi's sphincter).
Cholangitis		
Acute cholangitis	Narrowing of the ducts by edema and spasm	Ascending nonsuppurative and suppurative cholangitis are differentiated.
Recurrent pyogenic cholangitis (intrahepatic pigment stone disease)	Marked dilatation of proximal intrahepatic and extrahepatic ducts, cholelithiasis and strictures may be seen.	Endemic in Asia (Hong Kong disease). Often associated with *Clonorchis sinensis* or *Ascaris* infestation.
Primary sclerosing cholangitis (Fig. 32.24)	Multiple extrahepatic and intrahepatic bile duct strictures resulting in alternating segments of normal or slightly dilated and circumferentially stenotic ducts ("beaded appearance") and small saccular outpouchings (pseudodiverticula). Diffuse obstruction of the peripheral intrahepatic bile duct radicles results in a "pruned tree" appearance.	Associated with inflammatory bowel disease (especially ulcerative colitis), cirrhosis, pancreatitis, and retroperitoneal fibrosis. *Secondary sclerosing cholangitis* is associated with chronic bacterial cholangitis from bile duct stricture or cholelithiasis and ischemic bile duct damage (e.g., *post liver transplant*). DD: 1. *Sclerosing cholangiocarcinoma*: Marked ductal dilatation upstream from a dominant stricture or intraductal mass > 1 cm is characteristic. 2. *Primary biliary cirrhosis*: Disease is limited to the intrahepatic ducts
AIDS cholangitis (Fig. 32.25)	Irregular mild dilatation of intra- and extrahepatic bile ducts similar to sclerosing cholangitis and/or papillary stenosis of the common bile duct.	Caused by cytomegalovirus and cryptosporidium.
Worm infestation (ascaris, liver flukes, echinococcus) (Fig. 32.26)	Characteristic filling defects by an ascaris (up to 20 cm in length) that may extend into the duodenum or be coiled in the bile duct, causing partial obstruction.	Ascaris and liver flukes ascend from the duodenum into bile ducts. Liver flukes (*Clonorchis sinensis* and *Fasciola hepatica*) are nematodes, measuring 1 to 2 cm in length. They inhabit the smaller bile ducts and produce oval-to-linear filling defects. *Echinococcus*: Round or irregular filling defects caused by cyst membranes, daughter cysts or scolices discharged from a communicating hepatic cyst.
Postoperative and posttraumatic (e.g., hematomas and strictures)	Filling defects or smooth localized narrowing.	Following bile duct surgery or interventional radiologic procedures.
Blood clots	Mobile filling defects of varying shape, simulating radiolucent calculi or worms.	Usually postoperative, rarely with bleeding disorders.
Air bubble (Fig. 32.27)	Round, mobile, nonobstructive filling defects.	

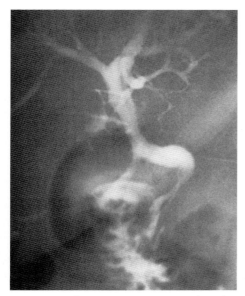

Fig. 32.**23   Chronic pancreatitis.** A relatively smooth stricture of the distal common bile duct is seen that begins at the superior margin of the pancreas (the level at which the common bile duct changes from a medial course to a lateral and steep caudal direction).

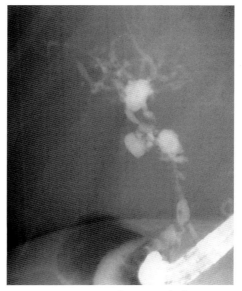

Fig. 32.**24   Primary sclerosing cholangitis in ulcerative colitis.** Alternating stenotic and nonstenotic segments in the extrahepatic and major intrahepatic bile ducts ("beaded appearance") are associated with saccular and cystic outpouchings (pseudodiverticula) of varying sizes. Note also the diffuse obstruction of the peripheral intrahepatic bile ducts producing a "pruned tree" appearance.

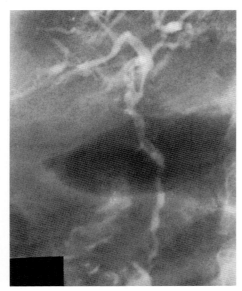

Fig. 32.**25   AIDS cholangitis.** Alternating stenotic and nonstenotic segments in the extrahepatic and major intrahepatic bile ducts are seen.

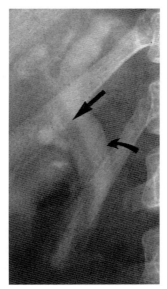

Fig. 32.**26   Ascaris.** A tubular filling defect caused by an ascaris (straight arrow) ascending into the common bile duct (curved arrow) is seen producing partial obstruction.

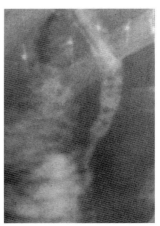

Fig. 32.**27   Air bubbles simulating biliary calculi.** Multiple small round radiolucencies are seen in a normal-sized and nonobstructed common bile duct in this postoperative T-tube cholangiogram.

Table 32.4 Saccular and Diverticular Lesions of the bile Ducts

Disease	Radiographic Findings	Comments
Congenital hepatic fibrosis	Irregular cystic spaces of varying sizes communicating with intrahepatic bile ducts ("lollipop-tree" appearance).	Rare disorder that radiographically simulates Caroli's disease. Associated with periportal fibrosis and portal hypertension.
Choledochal cyst (Figs. 32.28 and 32.29)	Segmental dilatation of the common bile duct and adjacent portions of common hepatic duct and cystic duct. Separate segmental dilatation of intrahepatic and extrahepatic ducts represents a rare variant of the disease. Diverticulum-like extrahepatic and intrahepatic lesions ("congenital hepatic diverticulum") are also included in this entity and comprise about 1%.	Most common congenital bile duct lesion, with male:female ratio of 1:4. Present classically with jaundice, right upper quadrant mass, and/or abdominal pain in children or adults. Congenital biliary cysts may be classified as 1) choledochal cyst, 2) diverticulum of extrahepatic duct, 3) choledochocele, 4) multiple segmental cysts (4a intrahepatic and extrahepatic, 4b extrahepatic only), 5) intrahepatic cysts only (Caroli disease).
Choledochocele (Fig. 32.30)	Cystic dilatation of intramural portion of the common bile duct in the duodenal wall with pancreatic duct entering it.	Insertion of the common bile duct into a duodenal diverticulum must be differentiated.
Caroli's disease (Fig. 32.31)	Segmental saccular dilatation of intrahepatic bile ducts.	Congenital malformation, but usually first diagnosed in adulthood, when the following complications occur: intrahepatic stone formation, cholangitis, liver abscess, and septicemia. There is a high incidence of associated medullary sponge kidneys.
Hepatic abscesses (Fig. 32.32)	Multiple small intrahepatic contrast collections are characteristically found with direct cholangiography in severe suppurative cholangitis and are diagnostic for complicating abscesses.	Hematogenous hepatic abscesses rarely communicate with the biliary system.
Sclerosing cholangitis (Fig. 32.33)	Prestenotic dilatation with small saccular outpouchings can be seen in addition to localized areas of narrowing and may be the dominating radiographic feature. Involvement occurs in extrahepatic and major intrahepatic ducts.	Usually secondary to longstanding partial biliary obstruction. A primary form tends to occur with inflammatory bowel disease, especially ulcerative colitis.
Echinococcal cyst	Irregular intrahepatic cavity with or without marginal calcification and often sharply defined round filling defects (daughter cysts). Detached daughter cysts may produce filling defects in the extrahepatic ducts and lead to total obstruction.	Communication with the biliary tree is the most common complication of hepatic echinococcal disease. Intermittent pain and jaundice may be caused by periodic discharge of fragments of the cyst membrane or its contents.
Fistula	Irregular cavity communicating with the extrahepatic biliary system.	Usually postoperative.
Cystic duct remnant	Tubular structure in characteristic location in patients who have undergone cholecystectomy.	No clinical significance unless associated with stones or inflammation.

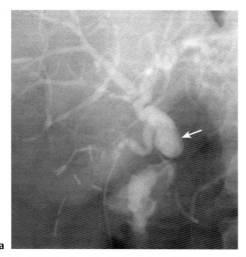

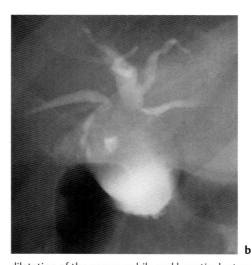

a

b

Fig. 32.**28 a, b** **Choledochal cysts** (two cases). **a** Segmental dilatation of the common bile duct (arrow) and adjacent portions of the common hepatic duct and cystic duct is seen. **b** Marked ovoid dilatation of the common bile and hepatic duct causes obstruction of the intrahepatic biliary system.

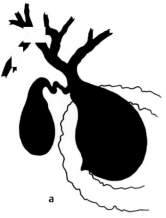

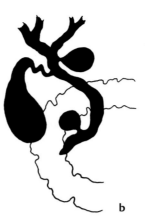

Fig. 32.**29 a, b**   Choledochal cysts. **a** A segmental dilatation of the common bile duct, which may reach such proportions that widening and extrinsic compression of the duodenal sweep occur, is the most common presentation. **b** Diverticulum-like outpouchings from the extrahepatic bile ducts and rarely the intrahepatic ducts are an unusual manifestation of the choledochal cyst entity.

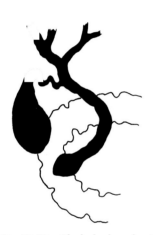

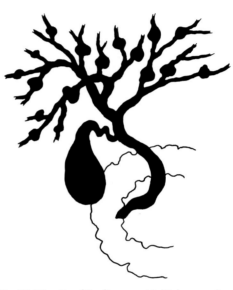

Fig. 32.**30   Choledochocele.** Cystic dilatation of the intramural portion of the common bile duct. Produces a smooth filling defect in the second portion of the duodenum on an upper gastrointestinal examination.

Fig. 32.**31   Caroli's disease.** Multiple saccular dilatations of the intrahepatic ducts are characteristic.

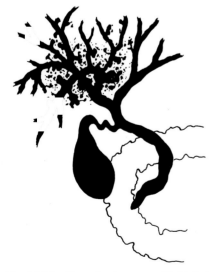

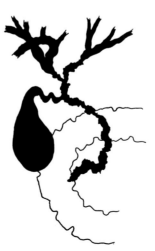

Fig. 32.**32   Hepatic abscesses.** Multiple intrahepatic contrast collections can be found in severe suppurative cholangitis.

Fig. 32.**33   Sclerosing cholangitis.** Prestenotic duct ectasia with small saccular outpouchings may be interspersed with areas of localized narrowing.

33 Abnormal Renal Papillae and Calices

Many renal diseases manifest themselves originally in an alteration of the papilla, the calix, or the relationship between them. Some abnormalities are entirely confined to this area. Most of these conditions are briefly mentioned in other chapters of the abdominal section, but they will be summarized and discussed here in greater detail.

The calix is the peripheral end of the collecting system, capping usually one, and rarely multiple, papillae. Therefore, the number of calices relates directly to the number of pyramids, which average about 10 per kidney but may be as many as 18. Larger calices with somewhat irregular appearance are occasionally seen in the polar areas and may receive more than one papilla *(compound papillae)*. This should not be confused with caliceal destruction or caliectasis. There is a tendency toward symmetry in the configuration and number of calices between the right and left side. Any asymmetry between the two sides should raise suspicion of an abnormality, although this may occasionally represent a normal variation.

In the anteroposterior projection, the majority of calices are seen more or less in profile and project laterally, superiorly, and inferiorly but never medially. If the majority of calices are not viewed in profile on an anteroposterior projection, and particularly if calices project medially, a *malrotation* or *nonrotation* of the kidney should be diagnosed.

With large intravenous contrast material dosages, a blush may be seen extending from the papilla to the rest of the pyramid in a fanlike fashion, but no distinct contrast accumulation should occur. Fine linear and parallel lines of contrast converging from the renal pyramid may be seen with ureteral obstruction caused by external compression or when an obstructive lesion is present.

The normal calix is characterized by sharp forniceal angles. The loss of this sharp angle is usually the first radiographic sign of a caliceal abnormality before any destructive process can be identified. The fornices are also very vulnerable to an increased pressure in the urinary tract, so that contrast extravasation occurs almost invariably first at this location. A pathologic process involving the papilla and calix may progress to *"clubbing"* where the normally concave caliceal cup has become a straight or slightly convex border (Fig. 33.1). "Clubbing" is seen as end result of chronic pyelonephritis, refluxing nephropathy, tuberculosis, papillary necrosis, and hydronephrosis. "Clubbing" of a single calix in an otherwise normal kidney is usually caused by chronic obstruction of the corresponding infundibulum caused by a transitional cell carcinoma, tuberculosis or, rarely, another inflammatory stricture, by calculus, or by an anomalous vessel.

Diffuse renal parenchymal calcifications *(nephrocalcinosis)* occur most often in the renal medulla and are usually most evident in the papilla, where the largest urine concentration is attained (Table 33.1 and Fig. 33.2). *Cortical nephrocalcinosis* is rare and limited to diseases primarily involving the renal cortex (e.g., acute cortical necrosis and occasionally chronic glomerulonephritis, Alport syndrome [hereditary nephritis and deafness], primary oxalosis, chronic paraneoplastic hypercalcemia, and rejected renal transplants).

The differential diagnosis of processes involving primarily the renal papilla and calix are summarized in Table 33.2.

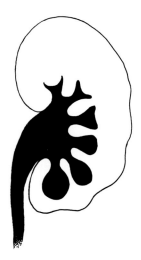

Fig. 33.**1** **Normal calix progressing to "clubbing."** A normal calix with sharp forniceal angles is seen on the top. Loss of the sharp forniceal angles and flattening of the papillary indentation in the caliceal cup are the next stages before "clubbing" finally occurs. Note also the loss of cortical tissue that is normally associated. "Clubbing" may be seen as the end result of *chronic pyelonephritis, refluxing nephropathy, tuberculosis, papillary necrosis,* and *hydronephrosis.*

Table 33.1 Medullary Nephrocalcinosis (commonly associated with nephrolithiasis) (Fig. 33.2)

Medullary sponge kidney
Oxalosis (primary and secondary [enteric hyperoxaluria])
With hypercalcemia and/or hypercalciuria:
　Hyperparathyroidism (primary, less commonly secondary)
　Renal tubular acidosis (primary and secondary)
　Bartter's syndrome (tubular disorder with potassium and sodium wasting, hyperaldosteronism and hypokalemic
　　acidosis)
　Milk–alkali syndrome
　Cushing's syndrome (endogenous, exogenous)
　Paraneoplastic syndrome (ectopic parathormone production in lung and kidney carcinoma)
　Hypervitaminosis D and E
　Sarcoidosis
　Bone metastases
　Multiple myeloma
　Senile osteoporosis
　Paget's disease
　Immobilization (prolonged)
　Hyperthyroidism
　Drug therapy (furosemide in infants and ACTH therapy)
　Idiopathic hypercalcemia
　Idiopathic hypercalciuria

Table 33.2 Abnormalities in the Renal Papillae and Calices

Disease	Radiographic Findings	Comments
Pyelorenal backflow (Fig. 33.3)	*Pyelosinus backflow*: Contrast medium extravasates from the fornices along the infundibula, renal pelvis, and proximal ureter. Repeated episodes may result in urinomas or peripelvic and retroperitoneal fibrosis at a later stage. Most common form of backflow (Fig. 33.**3a**). *Pyelotubular backflow*: Wedge-shaped area of increased density extending from the calix into corresponding papilla. Individual tubules can occasionally by appreciated as fine and uniform lines radiating in a brushlike fashion from the calix toward the periphery (Fig. 33.**3b**). Rarely, the contrast extends beyond the pyramid up to the subcapsular space (*interstitial backflow*). *Pyelolymphatic backflow*: Visualization of a few small lymphatics draining medially. Usually associated with other types of backflow or chyluria (e.g., in filariasis bancrofti) (Fig. 33.**3a**). *Pyelovenous backflow*: Forniceal rupture into venae interlobares or venae arcuatae. Extremely rarely seen radiographically because of the rapid clearance of the contrast medium from the vein (Fig. 33.**3a**).	Secondary to increased pressure in the collecting system (e.g., retrograde pyelography, intravenous urography with large contrast dosages, ureteral obstruction, or external compression).
Medullary sponge kidney (tubular ectasia) (Fig. 33.4)	Mild but irregular dilatation to small cyst formation of the collecting ducts in one or several papillae. May be bilateral. Numerous tiny calculi may form in ectatic tubuli indistinguishable from medullary nephrocalcinosis. (For differential diagnosis, see Table 33.**1**).	Developmental defect in collecting ducts that only becomes manifest in young to middle-aged adults, who may be asymptomatic or present with nephrolithiasis, hematuria, or recurrent urinary tract infections. May be associated with *Ehlers–Danlos syndrome, parathyroid adenoma*, and *Caroli's disease*. Bilateral tubular ectasia seen in the first decade of life is suspect for *childhood polycystic kidney disease* or *medullary cystic disease*, since medullary sponge kidney is very uncommon at that age.

(continues on page 784)

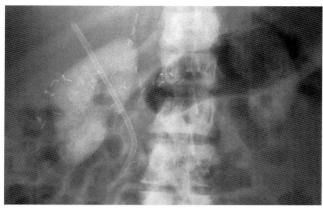

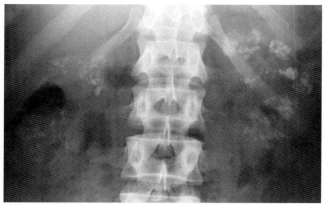

Fig. 33.**2 a, b Nephrocalcinosis. a Cortical (diffuse) nephrocalcinosis** in **oxalosis.** Bilateral small and universally dense kidneys are seen. Note also the markedly increased bone density with woolly appearance in the spine. **b Medullary nephrocalcinosis** in **primary hyperparathyroidism.** Punctate calcifications are seen in the renal medulla with sparing of the cortex.

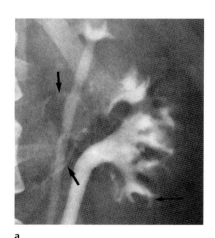

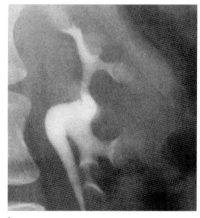

Fig. 33.**3 a, b Pyelorenal backflow, a** with retrograde urography and **b** with intravenous urography performed with external compression.
a *Pyelosinus backflow* is evident as contrast extravasation from the caliceal fornices causing irregular contrast puddles around the calices and infundibula. *Pyelolymphatic backflow* is evident from the opacification of small lymphatics (short arrows). *Pyelovenous backflow* is seen by the visualization of an interlobar vein (long arrow). **b** *Pyelotubular backflow* is evident as an area of increased density composed of fine radiating lines extending from the calices into the corresponding papillae.

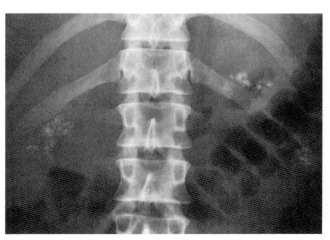

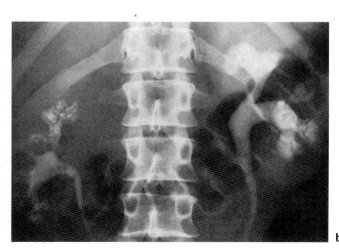

Fig. 33.**4 a, b Medullary sponge kidney, a** before and **b** after contrast injection. Numerous tiny calculi indistinguishable from nephrocalcinosis are seen in **a. b** After contrast injection, it is evident that the calculi are located in irregularly dilated collecting tubules of enlarged papillae.

Table 33.2   (Cont.) Abnormalities in the Renal Papillae and Calices

Disease	Radiographic Findings	Comments
Papillary necrosis (necrotizing papillitis) (Figs. 33.5–33.8)	Papillary swelling is the earliest radiographic abnormality but usually very difficult to differentiate from a normal variant. Tract formation extending from the calix (especially the fornix) may present the first conclusive radiologic finding. In a more advanced stage, two types of papillary necrosis are distinguished: 1. The *medullary type* (or partial papillary slough) presents as a single, irregular cavity located concentric or eccentric in the papilla and varies in shape from round to oblong, with the long axis of the cavity paralleling the long axis of the papilla. 2. The *papillary type* (or total papillary slough) presents as a line of contrast running across the base of the papilla. This line progressively widens until complete separation of the ultimately sloughed papilla occurs, which may be evident as a radiolucent triangular filling defect in the now saccular calix ("clubbing"). Occasionally a necrotic papilla does not slough and the silhouette of the papilla remains preserved, although it may shrink slightly with time *("necrosis in situ")*. Calcification of the necrotic papillary tissue is not unusual and is seen just outside the cup of an involved calix. It may be circular or triangular, conforming to the shape of the necrotic papilla. Demonstration of such calcifications is often the only reliable way to diagnose a papillary necrosis in situ.	Papillary necrosis if found with the following diseases: 1 *Analgesic nephropathy*: Usually in middle-aged to elderly women with a long history of analgesic drug abuse (especially phenacetin). 2 *Diabetes mellitus*: Usually but not invariably associated with chronic or recurrent urinary tract infections. 3 *Sickle-cell anemia*: Changes in homozygous S-hemoglobinopathy are much more severe than in heterozygous S-hemoglobinopathy. 4 *Urinary tract obstruction* and *infection.* 5 *Renal transplants.* 6 Rare in *renal vein thrombosis, liver cirrhosis,* and *posttraumatic.*
Tuberculosis (Fig. 33.9)	Irregularities at the surface of one or several papillae or calices is the earliest radiographic abnormality ("smudged" papilla). May progress to irregular tract formations from the calix into the papilla or small cavity formations within the papilla and finally result in extensive destruction of papillae and calices, producing large irregular cavities. End stage is an autonephrectomized kidney with dense calcifications. Other characteristic radiographic findings in advanced tuberculosis include stricture formation in the collecting system and ureters, shrunken bladder, and focal amorphous calcifications (tuberculomas) in the renal parenchyma.	Renal tuberculosis is usually a late manifestation of the disease occurring in patients with history of tuberculosis at another site (e.g., lung or bone). On the other hand, tuberculosis of the urogenital system originates almost always in the kidney. Early recognition of the disease is essential to initiate prompt treatment so that severe and irreparable damage can be prevented.

(continues on page 786)

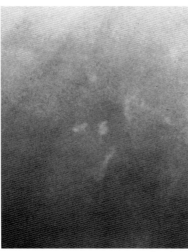

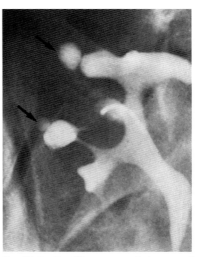

Fig. 33.**5 Papillary necrosis in situ** in diabetes. Bilateral shrunken kidneys with small calcifications in the area of the papillae were seen, but are only shown for the right side.

Fig. 33.**6 Papillary necrosis** in a renal transplant. Abnormal calices with two round cavities (arrows) are seen.

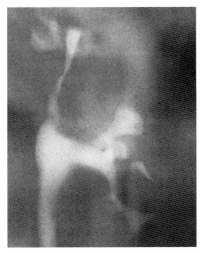

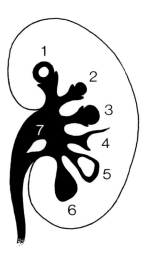

Fig. 33.**7** **Papillary necrosis** in sickle-cell anemia. Abnormal calices with tracts extending from the fornices, irregular cavities, and "clubbing" are seen. Similar findings were present in the right kidney.

Fig. 33.**8** **Papillary necrosis.** Different presentations of papillary necrosis are summarized. 1 to 3: Medullary type or partial papillary slough. 4: Tract extending from a fornix. 5 and 6: Papillary type or total papillary slough. 7: Filling defect caused by sloughed papilla.

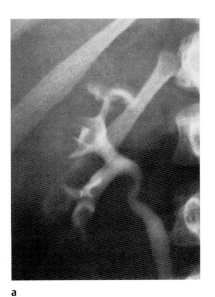

a

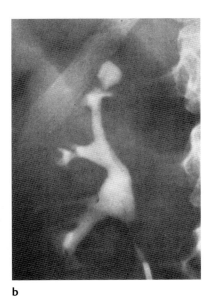

b

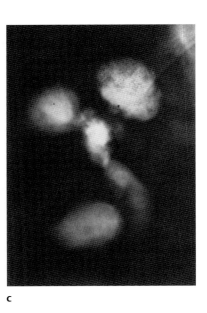

c

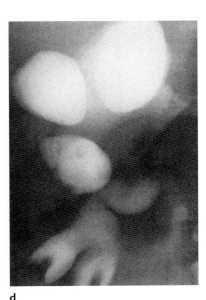

d

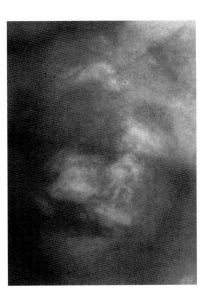

e

Fig. 33.**9 a–e** **Renal tuberculosis** in five different cases. **a** Poor definition of calices with fuzzy appearance and early destructive lesions in the papillae, evident as irregular contrast accumulations, are seen. **b** The cup of the most superior calix has an indistinct and irregular border and is connected with a small cavity in the corresponding papilla. **c** The major calices are completely destroyed and incorporated in large irregular cavities. **d** Involvement of the renal pelvis has caused strictures of the infundibula resulting in hydrocalices of varying degrees. **e** The end stage of renal tuberculosis is a small heavily calcified kidney that no longer excretes any contrast medium (autonephrectomy).

Table 33.2   (Cont.) Abnormalities in the Renal Papillae and Calices

Disease	Radiographic Findings	Comments
Chronic atrophic pyelonephritis (refluxing nephropathy) (Fig. 33.10)	Clubbed dilated calices caused by retraction of the papillae combined with localized depressed cortical scars over the involved calices are the hallmark of the disease. It may be unifocal or multifocal with preferential involvement of the poles, whereas the midportion is usually only involved in combination with at least one pole. The disease may be unilateral or bilateral. In the latter case, one kidney is usually much more severely affected, resulting in a significantly smaller kidney when compared with the contralateral site.	In young adults (especially women) presenting often with chronic urinary tract infection, hypertension, or chronic renal failure. The disease is the end stage of vesicoureteral reflux and recurrent urinary tract infections (usually *escherichia coli*) in infancy and early childhood, although the disease is often asymptomatic and consequently not recognized at that age. Predilection of the disease for the renal poles results from the fact that intrarenal (pyelotubular) reflux occurs primarily in compound papillae, the majority being located in the polar regions of the kidney.
Postobstructive renal atrophy (Fig. 33.11)	Generalized uniform caliectasis that may have clubbed appearance and diffuse smooth loss of cortical thickness in a normal to moderately shrunken kidney. Renal pelvis and infundibula can be normal.	Result of prolonged or several intermittent episodes of previous obstruction.
Congenital megacalices (megacalicosis) (Fig. 33.12)	Dilated calices have frequently a polygonal or faceted appearance. Renal cortex and kidney size are both normal. Bilateral in 20 % of cases.	Congenital nonobstructive enlargement of calices due to malformation of renal papillae (possibly secondary to temporary intrauterine obstruction).
Ureteropelvic junction (UPJ) obstruction	Persistent or intermittent hydronephrosis that may progress to a hydronephrotic sac, with the remaining renal parenchyma reduced to a thin surrounding rim.	Usually caused by intrinsic or extrinsic compression from a band or vessel, or by poor conduction of urine through the junction secondary to abnormal muscle development, injury, or inflammation.
Obstructive uropathy (Fig. 33.13)	Dilatation of the collecting system (calices, infundibula, and renal pelvis) and ureter down to the point of obstruction in normal or enlarged kidney with markedly delayed opacification after intravenous contrast material administration.	At a late stage, the kidney can become small.
Nonobstructive hydronephrosis	Dilatation of collecting system always associated with dilated ureter (hydroureter).	May be caused by different entities: *Reflux* (incompetent ureterovesical valve). *Functional obstruction* in the *juxtavesical ureter segment* with vigorous prestenotic peristaltic waves. Megacalices are rarely seen in this condition. *Endotoxic paralysis* of smooth muscle of urinary tract (e.g., bacterial endotoxins released during acute pyelonephritis). Physiologic relaxation of ureteral muscle during *pregnancy* and *postpartum*, both associated with extrinsic pressure from the enlarged uterus. *Nephrogenic diabetes insipidus* (rarely in pituitary diabetes insipidus).

(continues on page 788)

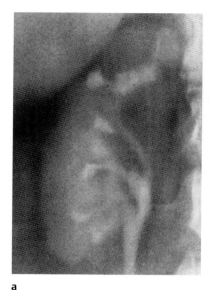

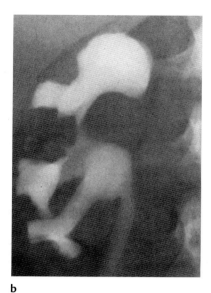

a

b

Fig. 33.**10 a, b Chronic atrophic pyelo-nephritis** in two different cases. **a** A small scarred kidney with abnormal calices ranging from flattening of the papillae to "clubbing" is seen. Note that the upper and lower pole calices are the ones most severely involved and associated with the greatest loss of cortical tissue in both poles. **b** Clubbed calices with complete loss of cortical tissue are seen in this retrograde urogram.

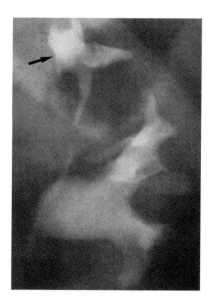

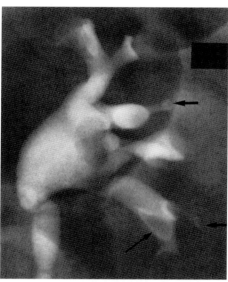

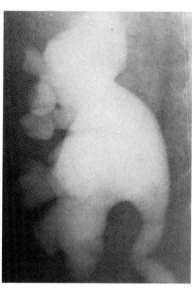

Fig. 33.**11 Postobstructive renal atrophy.** A dilated double collecting system with calicectasis, flattened papillae, and clubbing in some areas is associated with a generalized smooth loss of cortical tissue. A calculus in the upper collecting system is concealed by the contrast (arrow).

Fig. 33.**12 Congenital megacalices and microcalices** (normal variant). Large calices, some of them with faceted appearance (long arrow) and two microcalices (short arrows) are seen.

Fig. 33.**13 Obstructive uropathy** caused by pelvic metastases (cervix carcinoma). Dilatation of the entire collecting system and ureter is seen.

Table 33.2   (Cont.) Abnormalities in the Renal Papillae and Calices

Disease	Radiographic Findings	Comments
Localized caliectasis (Fig. 33.14)	*Compound calix*: Multiple calices without discrete infundibula and often somewhat irregular appearance preferentially in the upper pole producing a hammerhead or T-shaped appearance (normal variant). *Megacalix (congenital)*: Dilated calix without evidence of obstruction (see megacalices). *Postobstructive caliectasis (localized)*: Dilated calix secondary to previous infundibular obstruction. *Hydrocalix*: Dilated calix with delayed opacification secondary to infundibular obstruction (e.g., by calculus, stricture, anomalous vessel, or tumor). *Papillary necrosis* (localized). *Tuberculosis* (localized).	A *microcalix* consists of a minified infundibulum and calix, that is present at birth and does not change in size with growth (see Fig. 33.**12**).
Amputated calix	Nonvisualization of an isolated calix due to complete infundibular obstruction or calix destruction.	Caused by transitional cell carcinoma, renal carcinoma, tuberculosis, inflammatory stricture, calculus, or blood clot.
Caliceal diverticulum (pyelogenic cyst) (Figs. 33.15, 33.16)	Solitary, sharply delineated, often spherical cystic space, measuring up to 3 cm in diameter. Delayed opacification during intravenous urography occurs by retrograde filling through a narrow channel that originates characteristically, but not always, from a caliceal fornix.	Suggested etiologies include parenchymal cyst draining into a calix, ruptured cortical abscess, and dilatation of either a renal tubule or a blind end of a branching Wolffian duct.

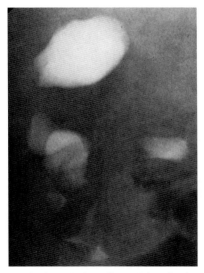

Fig. 33.**14**   **Hydrocalices.** Dilated calices caused by infundibular obstruction secondary to lymphoma are seen in the upper and middle calices, whereas the lower calices are not obstructed.

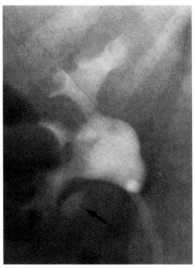

Fig. 33.**15**   **Caliceal diverticulum.** An oblong diverticulum (arrow) is seen in the lower pole connected to and filled retrogradely from the adjacent caliceal fornix.

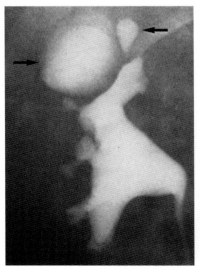

Fig. 33.**16**   **Caliceal diverticula** secondary to renal abscess. Two smoothly outlined cystic lesions (arrows) are seen in the upper pole in this patient with a long history of renal abscess. It appears likely that these lesions represent burned-out abscess cavities connecting with the collecting system. The patient was completely asymptomatic at this stage.

34 Filling Defects in the Urinary Tract

Filling defects in the urinary tract may be caused by (1) intraluminal lesions, (2) masses originating from the mucosa or wall of the urinary tract, and (3) extrinsic normal and pathologic structures impressing on the urinary tract. *Intraluminal lesions* are by far the most common cause of filling defects, of which the overwhelming majority are *calculi*. They are radiopaque in approximately 90% of cases. Nonopaque calculi and other intraluminal defects such as blood clots or air bubbles can, however, only be differentiated from a polypoid mucosal lesion when they can be separated from the adjacent wall in their entire circumference; that is, when they are always completely outlined by contrast in multiple projections covering a 180° range. However, this is usually only possible in the bladder, whereas the lumen of both collecting system and ureter are so narrow that nonattached intraluminal lesions are at least, in some projections, in contact with the adjacent wall. Proof of free mobility of filling defects within the urinary tract is another more useful sign to diagnose a nonattached lesion. Calculi can, however, also become impacted and may therefore not change their location.

The differentiation between a *mucosal (intrinsic)* and *extrinsic mass* is similar to a mass in the gastrointestinal tract (see Fig. 34.1). A mucosal (or occasionally intramural) lesion can be diagnosed when it is attached to the wall by a stalk or when an acute angle is present between lesion and adjacent wall. The latter occurs also, however, with intraluminal lesions such as calculi. Extrinsic lesions almost always form an obtuse angle between the lesion and adjacent wall, but this is by itself not a useful radiographic criterion to differentiate them from intramural or mucosal lesions, since the latter may have the same appearance when they are broad-based. Both extrinsic and intrinsic lesions may produce complete or incomplete urinary tract obstruction, which will be dealt with in Chapter 35.

Filling defects in the collecting system and ureter are discussed in Table 34.1 and defects in the urinary bladder are the subject of Table 34.2. Filling defects in the urethra are relatively rare and will be included in Table 35.5.

Table 34.1   Solitary or Multiple Filling Defects in the Collecting System and Ureter

Disease	Radiographic Findings	Comments
Aberrant papilla	Oval or round defect in a major infundibulum without obstruction. Broad-based attachment may be seen when viewed in profile. Rarely multiple.	Papilla without calix. A normal calix seen end-on in one projection may have a similar appearance, but can clearly be differentiated by its normal appearance in another projection when viewed in profile.
Pseudotumor (Fig. 34.1)	Smooth extrinsic defects in collecting system.	Normal renal tissue mimicking an abnormal mass. May be congenital (thick *column of Bertin* and *suprahilar* or *infrahilar bulges*) or acquired (*focal hypertrophy of renal parenchyma* in area of destruction). Renal scan, contrast-enhanced computed tomography, or magnetic resonance imaging demonstrate normal functioning renal tissue.
Cysts (Figs. 34.2–34.4)	Solitary or multiple sharply defined extrinsic defects in collecting system. A small intrinsic-appearing filling defect in the renal pelvis may be caused by an epithelial cyst. Multiple bilateral cysts in grossly enlarged kidneys are characteristic for *adult (autosomal dominant) polycystic kidney disease.*	Any etiology (cortical cysts, medullary cysts, peripelvic cysts, echinococcal cyst etc.). *Epithelial cysts* of the renal pelvis are rare small solitary lesions within the transitional cell epithelium measuring less than 1 cm in diameter.
Diverticulum (Fig. 34.5)	Localized extrinsic compression on the collecting system or rarely the ureter by a slightly delayed opacified cystic lesion is characteristic.	*Ureteral diverticula* are rare congenital, or less commonly acquired, solitary or occasionally multiple outpouchings along the course of the ureter without clinical significance. They are round or tubular in shape; the latter may represent small blind-ending ureters. If they enlarge because of infection, stone formation or obstruction, they may cause an extrinsic defect or narrowing of the adjacent ureter and no longer opacify with contrast.
Valves	Transverse filling defects often resulting in obstruction with a sharp linear cut-off, especially in the distal ureter.	Rare. True congenital valves consisting of mucosa and smooth muscle must be distinguished from pseudovalves, which may be acquired (e.g., chronic inflammation) and consist only of redundant mucosa.
Lipomatosis of renal sinus (Fig. 34.6)	Extrinsic compression of the collecting system with elongated infundibula and trumpetlike calices.	Bilateral in obesity and in senile renal atrophy. Unilateral and often simulating a mass when composed of both granulation tissue and fat in an area of parenchymal destruction.
Endometriosis	Intraluminal defect or stricture formation in the distal ureter below pelvic rim.	Intrinsic ureteral endometriosis is four times less common than the extrinsic form that causes ureteral deviation and compression. In women in the later childbearing years with characteristic cyclic symptoms, including pain and hematuria. History of previous gynecologic or abdominal surgery is often present.
Cholesteatoma	Irregular defect in the renal pelvis, occasionally with onion-peel appearance when contrast material penetrates between laminated layers. Often causing obstruction and irregular dilatation of the pelvis and calices with mucosal striation.	Rare benign lesion representing sloughed keratinized epithelium after squamous metaplasia of uroepithelium in middle-aged persons, often associated with chronic infection and impaired urinary drainage. Renal calculi coexist in about half of the patients.

(continues on page 792)

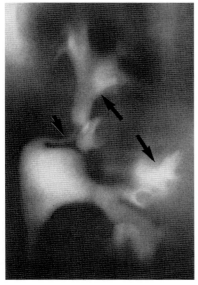

Fig. 34.**1** **Pseudotumors.** A hypertrophic column of Bertin simulates an extrinsic mass between upper and middle caliceal group, causing an extrinsic defect on these structures (long arrows) and a suprahilar bulge displaces the major infundibulum of the upper caliceal group downward (short arrow).

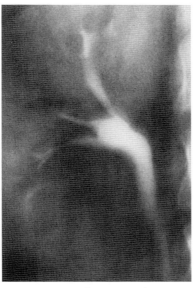

Fig. 34.**2** **Peripelvic cyst.** A large cyst located below the renal pelvis causes displacement and extrinsic compression of the renal pelvis and lower calices.

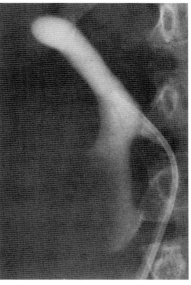

Fig. 34.**3** **Echinococcal cyst.** Splaying and extrinsic compression of the abnormal collecting system is caused by a huge echinococcal cyst involving most of the kidney.

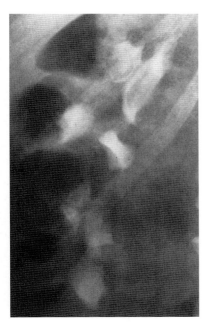

Fig. 34.**4** **Adult polycystic kidney disease.** An enlarged kidney with splayed collecting system and multiple extrinsic defects is seen. Similar changes were also present in the left kidney.

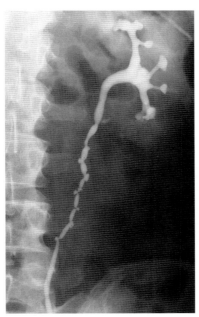

Fig. 34.**5** **Ureteral diverticula.** Multiple small outpouchings are seen in the proximal ureter.

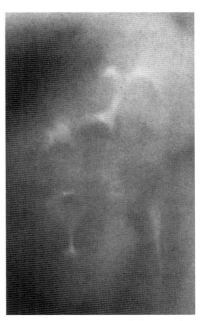

Fig. 34.**6** **Lipomatosis of the renal sinus.** Extrinsic compression of the renal pelvis and infundibula without obstruction is caused by an irregular radiolucent mass in the renal hilum.

Table 34.1 (Cont.) Solitary or Multiple Filling Defects in the Collecting System and Ureter

Disease	Radiographic Findings	Comments
Leukoplakia (Fig. 34.7)	Small defect or local mucosal irregularity often with striation in the collecting system. Occasionally causing caliceal or infundibular obstruction. May rarely be bilateral.	Squamous metaplasia of transitional cells in patients with history of chronic infection and calculi (in approximately 50%). Leukoplakia and cholesteatoma are often considered to represent the same entity, but leukoplakia differs from the latter by its smaller size and the frequent association with carcinoma.
Mesenchymal tumor (Fig. 34.8)	Usually small and smooth defect, preferentially located in the renal pelvis and calices. May have mottled appearance when larger.	Rare. *Hemangioma* (bleeding tendency), *lipoma*, and *leiomyoma* are found. *Fibroepithelial polyps* (fibrous polyps) are frequently multiple (renal pelvis and proximal ureter) and occasionally bilateral and occur in children and young adults with an increased male incidence.
Ureteral polyp (Fig. 34.9)	Elongated filling defect with smooth margin and rarely causing obstruction. Preferentially located in proximal ureter.	Usually in patients between 20 and 40 years of age with intermittent pain. Hematuria is rare.
Papilloma (papillomatosis) (Fig. 34.10)	Round, irregular defect, preferentially located in lower ureter, but is also found in proximal ureter and renal pelvis. Frequently causes obstruction. Often multiple. Urinary bladder involvement may be associated.	Although histologically benign, papillomas are considered for all practical purposes as low grade malignant tumors. Present usually in patients older than 50 with hematuria.
Transitional cell carcinoma (Figs. 34.11–34.14)	Irregular shaggy or smooth filling defect anywhere in the urinary tract causing early obstruction. Contrast material may be trapped between the interstices of the papillary tumor fronds, producing a characteristic stippled appearance. In the ureter, the wall is often infiltrated and stiff, producing a fixed local ureteral dilatation with abnormal mucosal pattern above and below the lesion (in contrast to the collapsed ureter below a benign intraluminal obstruction). A predominantly infiltrating lesion may present as a short or long stricture. There is sometimes evidence of a mass extending beyond the urogenital tract, especially in the kidney. Multicentric locations or metastatic seeding along the urogenital tract, with a second lesion more distally in the ureter or bladder, is not uncommon.	Transitional carcinomas occur usually in the 50–70 age group. Hematuria, pain, and palpable mass (hydronephrosis) are common presenting symptoms. Primary squamous cell carcinomas, adenocarcinomas, and sarcomas are very rare.

(continues on page 794)

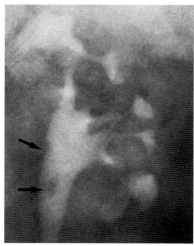

Fig. 34.**7** **Leukoplakia.** Two small irregular defects (arrows) are seen in this case with chronic atrophic pyelonephritis.

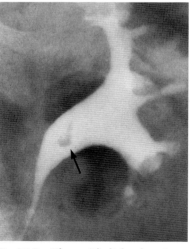

Fig. 34.**8** **Fibroepithelial polyp.** A small smooth defect is seen in the renal pelvis (arrow).

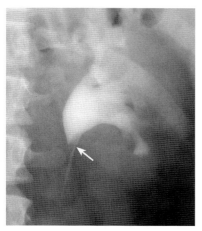

Fig. 34.**9 Ureteral polyp.** An elongated filling defect with smooth margin is seen in the proximal ureter just below the ureteropelvic junction (arrow).

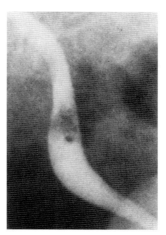

Fig. 34.**10 Papilloma.** A small irregular defect is seen in the distal ureter.

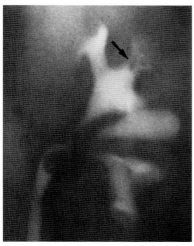

Fig. 34.**11 Transitional cell carcinoma.** A smooth oval filling defect is seen at the ureteropelvic junction that is associated with infiltration and obstruction of the renal pelvis. Note also the small defect in major infundibulum (arrow) that proved to be an aberrant papilla.

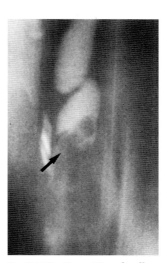

Fig. 34.**12 Transitional cell carcinoma.** An irregular defect causing severe obstruction is seen in the distal ureter (arrow). The more proximal bandlike defect running obliquely across the dilated ureter is caused by a postoperative adhesion.

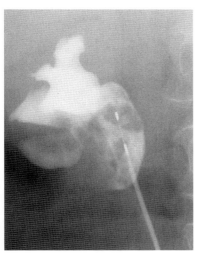

Fig. 34.**13 Transitional cell carcinoma.** A large irregular filling defect is seen in the renal pelvis causing obstruction of the deformed and dilated calices.

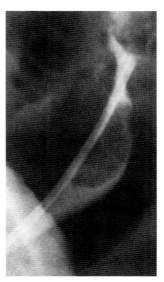

Fig. 34.**14 Transitional cell carcinoma.** A slightly irregular ovoid filling defect is seen in the distal ureter. Note also the mucosal irregularities above the lesion and a constant dilatation of the ureter below the lesion indicating wall stiffness caused by tumor infiltration.

Table 34.1 (Cont.) Solitary or Multiple Filling Defects in the Collecting System and Ureter

Disease	Radiographic Findings	Comments
Renal carcinoma (Fig. 34.15)	An irregular intrinsic filling defect in the renal pelvis is rare, whereas extrinsic compression distortion and local obstruction of the collecting system is a common presentation.	Extrinsic defects on the collecting system can also be produced by other malignant tumors (e.g., *lymphoma, metastasis*) or by benign tumors (e.g., *angiomyolipoma*) and *inflammatory mass lesions* located in the renal parenchyma.
Metastases	Irregular defects most commonly in the distal ureter from intracanalicular seeding, direct invasion, or rarely hematogenous spread. However, encasing stricture-like lesions are a more common presentation with the latter two patterns of metastatic spread.	Intracanalicular seeding with metastases in the distal ureter is common from a transitional cell carcinoma in the renal pelvis or proximal ureter and rarely from a renal cell carcinoma. Direct invasion occurs most often from carcinoma of the urinary bladder and the cervix, or occasionally the rectosigmoid, and rarely from retroperitoneal malignancies including Hodgkin's disease and non-Hodgkin's lymphoma. Hematogenous metastases to the urogenital tract are extremely unusual (e.g., carcinoma of the prostate, breast, or lung).
Pyeloureteritis cystica (Fig. 34.16)	Numerous round sharply defined and usually only measuring a few millimeters filling defects predominantly in the collecting system and proximal ureter. Occasionally the bladder may be involved also. Frequently unilateral.	Usually in association with chronic urinary infection. Rarely an *allergic urticaria* or *submucosal hemorrhage* (e.g., with anticoagulation therapy) may mimic ureteritis cystica. Air bubbles have also to be differentiated during antegrade or retrograde pyelography.
Pyeloureteritis (nonspecific) (Fig. 34.17)	Fine linear striations in renal pelvis and proximal ureter caused by redundant mucosal folds.	More common in children than adults. Found with reflux and infection. Mucosal striations due to leukoplakia are more coarse and irregular.
Tuberculosis	Dilatation and fuzzy or moth-eaten appearance of mucosa in collecting system and ureter due to mucosal ulceration and edema in the early stage. Multiple stricture formation giving the ureter a "beaded" appearance is the hallmark of the disease in the advanced stage. Involvement of the entire ureteral length produces a shortened ureter with thickened walls ("pipe-stem" appearance). Ureteral calcifications are rare, whereas the renal parenchyma (including papillae), seminal vesicles and epididymis are often calcified in tuberculosis.	Urogenital tuberculosis is a hematogenous infection, usually originating from a focus in the lung. Earliest urographic findings usually involve papillae and calices showing irregularities and early destructive lesions.
Schistosomiasis	Round defects in the distal, usually dilated ureter which are almost always associated with defects in the bladder. Progresses to stricture formation with obstruction. Linear, semicircular, or rarely punctate wall calcifications are often associated.	Almost always due to schistosoma hematobium, with a much higher incidence in males than females.
Malakoplakia	Small, single or multiple round filling defects, preferentially located in the distal ureter. May spread to the proximal ureter and renal pelvis or rarely involve the latter primarily. Can cause obstruction.	Rare granulomatous plaques of unknown etiology, most commonly seen in the bladder, from which they may extend into the ureters. Four times more common in females than males, with the highest incidence in the fifth decade. Usually associated with chronic urinary tract infection.

(continues on page 796)

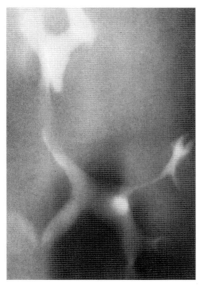

Fig. 34.**15   Renal carcinoma.** A large mass lesion between the upper and middle caliceal group with splaying and partial obstruction of the upper calices is seen.

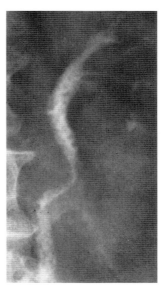

Fig. 34.**16   Pyeloureteritis cystica.** Numerous small round filling defects are seen in the renal pelvis and proximal ureter.

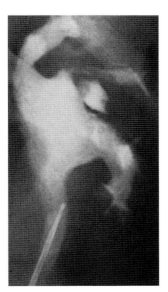

Fig. 34.**17   Pyeloureteritis.** Fine mucosal striations are seen in the collecting system and proximal ureter in this patient with chronic urinary tract infection.

Table 34.1   (Cont.) Solitary or Multiple Filling Defects in the Collecting System and Ureter

Disease	Radiographic Findings	Comments
Calculi (Figs. 34.18–34.21)	Round-to-oval, often mobile filling defects, usually less than 1 cm in diameter when located in the ureter. May be concealed by the contrast when the latter is of similar density as the calculus. Tend to become impacted in areas of normal anatomic narrowing, namely at the ureteropelvic junction, at the ureteral crossing with sacrum and iliac vessels, and at the ureterovesical junction. Obstruction with prestenotic dilatation is the main complication. Larger calculi are seen in the collecting system, where they may form a cast of the pelvis and calices (staghorn calculi). Renal parenchymal calcifications must be differentiated from renal calculi. The former may be localized (e.g., in cortical abscesses, tumors, and cysts) or diffuse in nephrocalcinosis. Medullary nephrocalcinosis (e.g., in primary hyperparathyroidism, medullary sponge kidney, tubular acidosis, and hypercalcemia) is, however, frequently associated with urolithiasis. Multiple stone fragments found in a ureter after lithotripsy are referred to as *"steinstrasse"*.	Over 90 % of calculi are opaque, the majority containing calcium as oxalate or phosphate, or as a mixture of both. They are seen in the following conditions: 1. Hypercalcemia and/or hypercalciuria 2. Renal tubular acidosis 3. Hyperoxaluria 4. Medullary sponge kidney 5. Idiopathic Magnesium ammonium phosphate calculi are also opaque and found with recurrent urinary tract infections and xanthogranulomatous pyelonephritis. Cystine and xanthine calculi are usually faintly opaque (seen in cystinuria and xanthinuria, respectively, which are two rare hereditary disorders), as are matrix calculi found with poorly functioning infected kidneys. Uric acid calculi are nonradiopaque and found in exogenous (dietary) or endogenous hyperuricemia (e.g., gout, hematologic and myeloproliferative diseases, chronic renal diseases, and certain drugs, especially chemotherapeutic agents).
Gas (Fig. 34.22)	Gas bubbles present as round, freely mobile intraluminal defects, not associated with any signs of obstruction. They must be differentiated from superimposed intestinal gas that projects at least partially outside the urinary tract in different projections or in subsequent films.	Intraluminal gas is found with: *Preceding instrumentation, trauma,* or *surgery.* *Emphysematous pyelonephritis, ureteritis,* or *cystitis,* where it is associated with gas in the soft tissues. It is a rare disease, usually found in patients with diabetes. *Surgical anastomosis or spontaneous fistulas* between gastrointestinal and urinary tract (e.g., secondary to Crohn's disease or carcinoma).
Blood clots (Fig. 34.23)	Irregular defects of varying size or shape (e.g., produce a cast of surrounding structure). May change shape and disappear with time. May cause temporary obstruction.	Gross hematuria is characteristically present. Tumor, trauma, instrumentation, vascular malformations, nephritis, bleeding disorders, and anticoagulation therapy are common causes.
Sloughed papilla, necrotic tissue debris, inspissated pus, or fungus ball	Rare cause of irregular defects.	In papillary necrosis and severe necrotizing pyelonephritis (e.g., in diabetes) or pyonephrosis.

(continues on page 798)

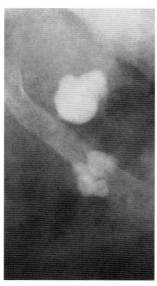

Fig. 34.**18** **Caliceal calculi** in chronic atrophic pyelonephritis (scout film). Two irregular calcific densities are seen that were located in dilated calices.

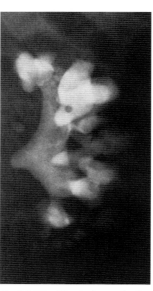

Fig. 34.**19** **Staghorn calculus** (scout film). The calculus has formed a cast of the collecting system.

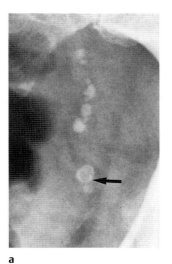
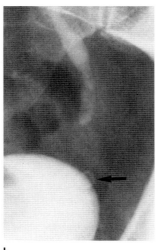

a   b

Fig. 34.**20 a, b** **Multiple ureteral calculi** in a patient with medullary sponge kidney **a** before and **b** after contrast medium injection. **a** Several small calculi are seen aligned in a string-like fashion just below the sacroiliac joint. Note the two phleboliths located more distally, one of which has a characteristic radiolucent center (arrow). **b** After contrast administration, the ureteral calculi are largely concealed by the contrast, but partial obstruction is evident at this level. Note also that the two phleboliths (arrow) are located outside the distal nonobstructed ureter.

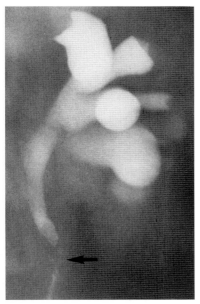

Fig. 34.**21** **Impacted calculus.** An oval radiolucent calculus is impacted above a stricture (arrow) causing partial obstruction and hydronephrosis.

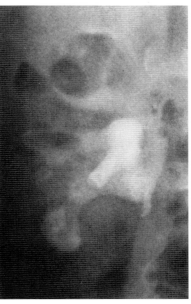

Fig. 34.**22** **Emphysematous pyelonephritis in diabetes.** Poor contrast excretion occurs into an abnormal collecting system with clubbed calices, some of which are outlined by air and already visible on the scout film.

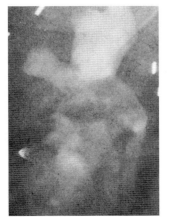

Fig. 34.**23** **Blood clot.** A large irregular radiolucent filling defect is seen in the renal pelvis post pyelolithotomy.

Table 34.1 (Cont.) Solitary or Multiple Filling Defects in the Collecting System and Ureter

Disease	Radiographic Findings	Comments
Blood vessels (Fig. 34.24)	Solitary, extrinsic, often bandlike defect with mild obstruction at the crossing of normal arteries or less commonly veins.	Caused by the renal artery or one of its major branches in the collecting system, or accessory renal artery, iliac artery, or gonadal vein in the ureter. *Congenital bands* and *postoperative adhesions* are rare and can produce imprints on the urogenital tract that are radiographically indistinguishable from aberrant vessels (see Fig. 34.12).
Arterial collaterals (Fig. 34.25)	Multiple small marginal defects (vascular notching), most often in the proximal ureter.	Usually in renal artery stenosis or occlusion. Occasionally in occlusion of the distal abdominal aorta or iliac artery, in renal arteriovenous malformations, and renal carcinomas. Ureteral notching is occasionally seen also in *polyarteritis nodosa*.
Aneurysm or arteriovenous fistula of renal artery	Localized filling defect in the renal pelvis.	Congenital, mycotic, posttraumatic, or postoperative.
Renal vein thrombosis	Extrinsic filling defects in the renal pelvis by distended renal veins or collaterals. Small nodular defects in the renal pelvis and proximal ureter by mural edema or hemorrhage. Vascular notching by venous collaterals.	Defects in renal pelvis and proximal ureter are only seen with retrograde pyelography; opacification with intravenous urography is usually insufficient.
Venous collaterals	Vascular notching of the ureter and renal pelvis is radiographically indistinguishable from arterial collaterals.	In renal vein thrombosis, occlusion of the inferior vena cava, or ureteral vein varicosity (congenital or after pregnancy).
Ovarian vein syndrome	Extrinsic compression, usually of the right ureter at the level of the first sacral segment, causing mild to moderate obstruction.	Caused by a markedly dilated ovarian vein or possibly by a locally induced periureteral fibrosis after several pregnancies.
Stricture (Fig. 34.26)	Usually conical narrowing, but when eccentric and short may occasionally simulate an extrinsic defect.	Benign strictures are congenital or acquired. Congenital strictures are most often located in the ureteropelvic and ureterovesical junctions. Benign acquired strictures may be the sequelae of inflammation, stone passage, trauma, surgery, or instrumentation. Malignant strictures are commonly caused by transitional cell carcinoma and metastases.
Ureteral spasm and peristalsis	May simulate a localized filling defect or "vascular notching," but is not persistent.	

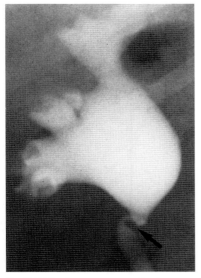

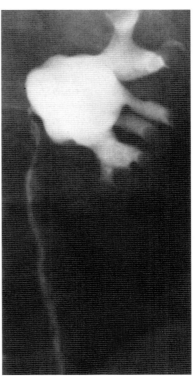

Fig. 34.**24** **Accessory renal artery** causing ureteropelvic junction obstruction. Dilatation and obstruction of the collecting system is caused by an accessory renal artery causing an extrinsic filling defect at the ureteropelvic junction (arrow).

Fig. 34.**25** **Vascular notchings.** Small marginal defects are seen ▷ in the proximal ureter of this patient with renal artery stenosis.

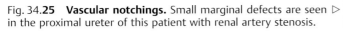

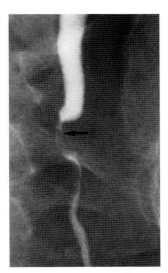

Fig. 34.**26** **Postsurgical stricture.** A short eccentric stricture is seen simulating an extrinsic mass lesion (arrow).

Table 34.2   Solitary or Multiple Filling Defects in the Urinary Bladder

Disease	Radiographic Findings	Comments
Congenital septa	Bandlike intravesical defects dividing the bladder completely or incompletely into two (bladder reduplication) or several (multilocular bladder) compartments.	Usually associated with other anomalies.
Simple ureterocele (Fig. 34.27)	Unilateral or bilateral dilated distal segment of ureter within bladder separated from the opacified urine by a 2–3 mm wide radiolucent line representing the prolapsed ureter wall and bladder mucosa ("cobra head" appearance).	Prolapse of the dilated distal ureteral orifice into the bladder lumen. Congenital or acquired. May predispose to obstruction, infection, and stone formation, but is often discovered incidentally. A ureterocele or ectopic ureter should not be confused with a *"jet" of contrast* that traverses the bladder obliquely from the ureteral orifice and represents a normal transitory peristaltic phenomenon (Fig. 34.**28**).
Ectopic ureterocele (Fig. 34.29)	Smooth defect of varying size and shape at the base of the bladder associated with a duplicated system. The ureterocele is arising from the ureter draining the upper segment, which is nonfunctioning or hydronephrotic.	Congenital and in 90% of cases unilateral lesion, usually diagnosed in children and young adults presenting with dysuria, pyuria, and flank pain. Much more common in females.
Endometriosis	Smooth extrinsic or intrinsic, round to lobulated filling defect, usually located in the posterior wall.	Presents usually with pain or cyclic urinary symptoms, including hematuria. History of previous gynecologic or abdominal surgery common.
Amyloidosis	Irregular, lobulated defect in the bladder with slight preference for the lateral wall and rarely involving the trigone.	In primary amyloidosis with systemic involvement, or limited to the bladder, or as part of secondary amyloidosis.
Mesenchymal tumors	Small polypoid to large often fungating mass lesions. Benign and malignant varieties cannot be differentiated unless there is evidence of wall infiltration. A stalk is occasionally present and favors benign lesion (e.g., *fibro-epithelial polyp*).	*Leiomyomas* and *rhabdomyomas* (or myosarcomas), *neurofibromas* (or sarcomas), pheochromocytomas (benign or malignant), *hemangiomas,* and *fibromas* or *fibrosarcomas* occur. Bladder *pheochromocytoma* presents characteristically with sudden episodic hypertension, tachycardia, and flushing during micturition. *Rhabdomyosarcoma* is the most common bladder tumor in children, often referred to as *"sarcoma botryoides."*
Papilloma (papillomatosis) (Fig. 34.30)	Solitary or multiple (25%) polypoid defects with smooth or serrated margins. Lesions may be pedunculated, No signs of bladder wall infiltration.	Histologically benign, but multiple recurrences occur. Tumors are therefore considered as low-grade malignancies and sometimes classified as grade I transitional cell carcinomas.

(continues on page 802)

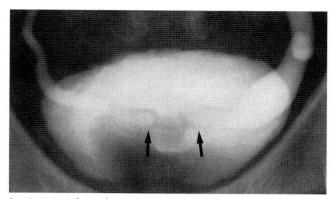

Fig. 34.**27** **Bilateral simple ureteroceles.** The bilateral distal ureter segments that are prolapsed into the bladder produce the characteristic "cobra head" appearance (arrows). On the left side the ureterocele causes partial obstruction, evident from the markedly dilated distal ureter.

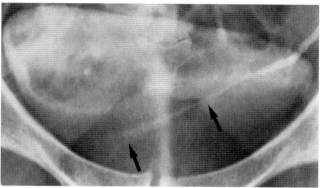

Fig. 34.**28** **"Jet" of contrast.** A jet of contrast originates from the left ureteral orifice and traverses the bladder obliquely across the midline. It represents a normal peristaltic phenomenon and should not be confused with a simple ureterocele which does not cross midline.

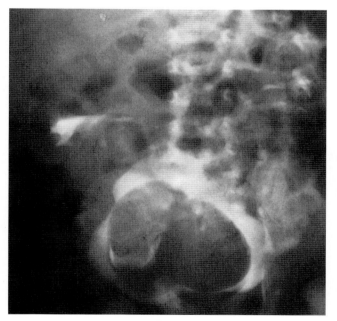

Fig. 34.**29** **Ectopic ureterocele.** A large smooth filling defect is seen in the bladder associated with a duplicated right system, of which the nonfunctioning upper system displaces characteristically the functioning lower collecting system downwards.

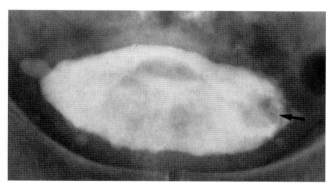

Fig. 34.**30** **Papilloma.** A polypoid irregular defect with serrated margin is seen originating from the left lateral bladder wall (arrow). Note also the prostatic hypertrophy causing a large midline extrinsic defect originating from the bladder floor and trabeculation of the bladder wall.

Table 34.2 (Cont.) Solitary or Multiple Filling Defects in the Urinary Bladder

Disease	Radiographic Findings	Comments
Transitional cell carcinoma (Figs. 34.31–34.33)	Irregular defect of varying size, fixed in position. (DD: blood clot or stone). Rigidity of thickened bladder wall sloping towards the tumor and asymmetry of the bladder are signs of bladder wall infiltration. Extrinsic defects occur with perivesical lymph node metastases. Early ureter obstruction results from tumors originating near the ureteral orifices (about 70%). Calcifications are rare but may be punctate or nodular. Tumors are frequently multicentric (e.g., associated with lesions in collecting system, ureter, or other locations in the bladder).	Usually in patients over 50 years of age, with higher incidence in males. Hematuria, frequency, or dysuria are the most common presenting symptoms. Tumors may also originate in diverticula or very uncommonly in the remnants of the urachus (adenocarcinomas). Squamous cell carcinomas (a complication of schistosomiasis) and adenocarcinomas are otherwise rare.
Metastases (Fig. 34.34)	Extrinsic defect with irregular surface when bladder is invaded by tumor originating from a neighboring organ. Solitary or multiple, usually intrinsic filling defects with smooth or irregular margins can be seen with canalicular or hematogenous metastases. Extrinsic impression on the bladder from enlarged but noninvading lymph nodes or mass are the most common presentations.	Direct extension from primary carcinomas of prostate, cervix, uterus, ovary, or rectosigmoid. Canalicular metastases from kidney and ureter. Hematogenous metastases are rare (e.g., from lung or breast carcinoma and melanoma).
Lymphoma	Irregular defect caused by direct invasion from perivesical lymphoma. Solitary (e.g., primary lymphoma) and multiple smooth filling defects are rare. Extrinsic impression on the bladder from enlarged but noninvading lymph nodes is the most common presentation.	Primary lymphoma of the bladder is exceedingly rare. Secondary involvement occurs with advanced lymphoma. Diffuse infiltration or localized bladder masses are occasionally seen in *leukemia*.
Cystitis	Thickened irregular wall, often associated with vesicoureteral reflux or occasionally ureter obstruction.	Reliable radiographic diagnosis is usually not possible.
Hemorrhagic cystitis (Fig. 34.35)	Irregular wall, occasionally with blood clots in the bladder lumen.	Acute cystitis affecting all ages. May be seen with frequent sexual intercourse ("honeymoon cystitis").
Abacterial (acute interstitial) cystitis	Similar to hemorrhagic cystitis.	Usually seen in young males presenting with abacterial pyuria, often associated with gross hematuria.

(continues on page 804)

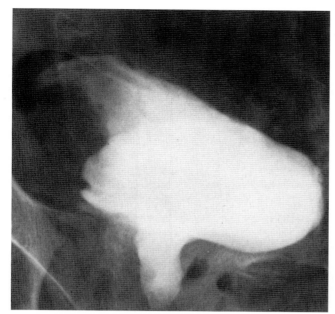

Fig. 34.**31** **Bladder carcinoma (transitional cell carcinoma).** A large irregular defect is seen in the anterolateral wall of the bladder. Note also the fingerlike cavity extending downwards from the bladder floor secondary to transurethral prostatectomy.

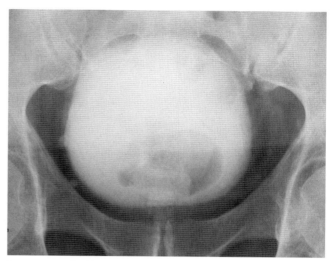

Fig. 34.**32** **Bladder carcinoma (transitional cell carcinoma).** A relatively smooth filling defect is seen in the bladder floor causing complete obstruction of the right ureterovesical junction (nonfunctioning right kidney).

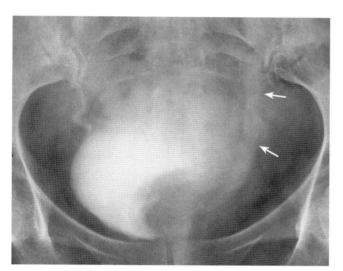

Fig. 34.**33** **Bladder carcinoma (transitional cell carcinoma).** An irregular poorly demarcated filling defect is seen in the bladder floor with partial obstruction of the left ureterovesical junction evident by the dilated distal left ureter (arrows).

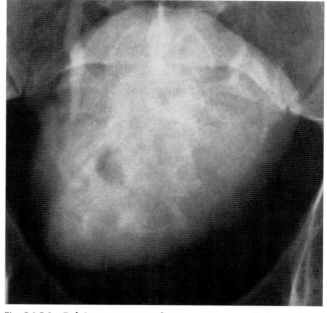

Fig. 34.**34** **Pelvic metastases from carcinoma of the rectum.** Asymmetric elevation of the bladder floor with extrinsic compression of the left lateral side is caused by extensive pelvic metastases.

Fig. 34.**35** **Hemorrhagic cystitis.** Mucosal irregularities are seen throughout the bladder.

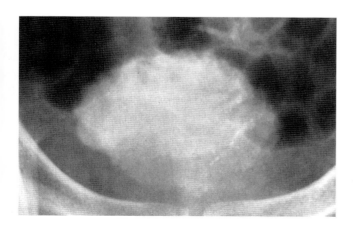

Table 34.2   (Cont.) Solitary or Multiple Filling Defects in the Urinary Bladder

Disease	Radiographic Findings	Comments
Bullous edematous cystitis (Fig. 34.36)	Irregular wall with smooth extrinsic or intrinsic defects measuring up to 2 cm.	Acute cystitis often secondary to indwelling catheters.
Interstitial cystitis (chronic)	Thickened irregular wall in small bladder.	Chronic disease of unknown etiology.
Eosinophilic cystitis	Irregular often greatly thickened wall with indentations or multiple polypoid defects of grape size.	Acute, possibly allergic, cystitis that may progress to chronic stage.
Granulomatous cystitis	Thickened irregular wall with nodular defects or larger mass.	Chronic primary disease of the bladder or secondary to an extension of granulomatous disease of the bowel or prostate.
Emphysematous cystitis (Fig. 34.37)	Small intramural gas-filled vesicles protruding into the lumen, or intramural gas streaks. Free intraluminal gas is often present.	Usually in diabetes. Postoperative intramural gas may produce similar findings.
Cystitis cystica	Multiple cysts of varying size projecting into lumen especially in trigone and bladder base.	Chronic. May be associated with pyeloureteritis cystica.
Cystitis glandularis	Multiple smooth defects or a larger irregular lesion, preferentially located at the dome of the bladder.	Chronic proliferative disorder of unknown etiology with proliferation of glandular elements.
Cyclophosphamide cystitis	Nodular defects in acute stage. May progress to bladder contracture.	Acute stage 24–48 hours after large intravenous cyclophosphamide dosages.
Tuberculosis	Mucosal irregularities with progressive shrinkage of the bladder. Calcification of the bladder wall is rare.	Usually associated with renal tuberculosis.
Fungus ball	Single large or multiple small intraluminal mobile filling defects, often containing gas that produces a mottled appearance in the defects. Contrast may impregnate the fungus ball and enhance its visibility.	Most often caused by *Candida albicans* in debilitating diseases, immunosuppressed patients, prolonged antibiotic or steroid therapy, and diabetes.
Schistosomiasis	Multiple polypoid filling defects, associated with bladder wall calcifications.	Usually caused by *Schistosoma hematobium*. With male predominance.
Malakoplakia	Single or multiple, smooth, round-to-oval intrinsic defects, preferentially located on the floor of the bladder and rarely larger than 1 cm. Occasionally the distal ureter is also involved with nodular lesions.	Rare inflammatory condition, predominantly found in women and usually associated with chronic coliform urinary tract infection.

(continues on page 806)

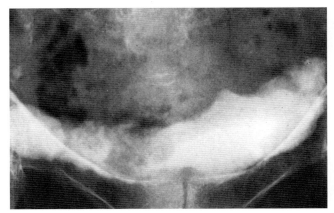

Fig. 34.**36 Bullous edematous cystitis.** An irregular wall with predominantly extrinsic defects is seen.

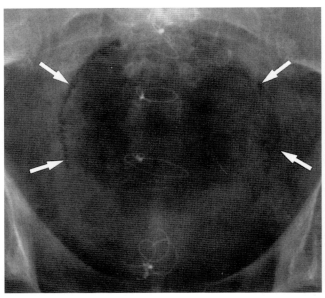

Fig. 34.**37 Emphysematous cystitis in diabetes.** Intramural gas (arrows) is evident as radiolucent streaks or small vesicles. Note also the free intraluminal gas seen as a large radiolucent area within the bladder in this supine film.

Table 34.2 (Cont.) Solitary or Multiple Filling Defects in the Urinary Bladder

Disease	Radiographic Findings	Comments
Calculi (Figs. 34.38 and 34.39)	Single or multiple smooth calcifications of varying size and shape (round, laminated, faceted, or star-shaped). Characteristically change intravesical location with different positions. (DD: calcified tumor [Fig. 34.40], bladder wall calcification, prostatic calculi, phleboliths). Nonopaque calculi are more common in the bladder than in the collecting systems and ureters, and are only seen after bladder opacification. Calculi occur frequently in bladder diverticula.	May originate from the kidneys or form in the bladder (or diverticulum) secondary to stasis, infection, immobilization, foreign bodies, bladder surgery, and trauma. Most often found in elderly men with prostatism. May also complicate a neurogenic bladder.

(continues on page ■■)

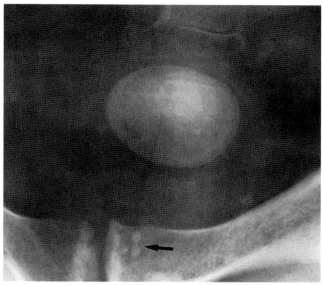
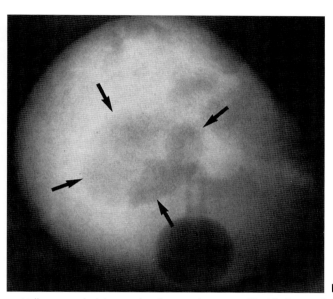

Fig. 34.**38 a, b Bladder calculus. a** before and **b** after contrast injection. **a** A solitary oval bladder stone is seen in the scout film. Note also the small prostatic calcifications projecting over the symphysis (arrow). **b** After bladder opacification, the calculus is partially concealed (arrows), whereas the water-filled balloon of the Foley catheter at the bladder floor is now well visualized. Note also the vague radiolucent areas projecting into the superior part of the bladder, caused by superimposed bowel gas.

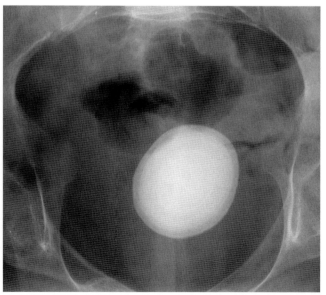
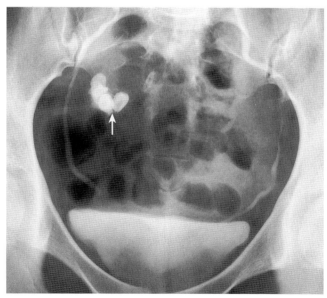

Fig. 34.**39 Bladder calculus.** A large, very dense, laminated bladder calculus is seen that was completely obliterated by the contrast medium after intravenous contrast medium administration (not shown).

Fig. 34.**40 Dermoid.** A small lesion containing four rudimentary teeth (arrow) located outside the right ureter and bladder is seen.

Table 34.2   (Cont.) Solitary or Multiple Filling Defects in the Urinary Bladder

Disease	Radiographic Findings	Comments
Air	Smooth, round, freely mobile intraluminal defect producing an air–fluid level with horizontal roentgen beam. Intraluminal gas (pneumaturia) is often associated with intramural gas evident as linear streaks or small round lucencies, and gas outside the bladder wall. Both intraluminal and intramural gas must be differentiated from superimposed gas in the lower gastrointestinal tract.	Pneumaturia (intraluminal gas) is found with: 1 instrumentation, 2 post surgery, 3 penetrating trauma, 4 fistula to gas-containing hollow organs, and 5 emphysematous cystitis (usually in diabetic patients).
Blood clots (Fig. 34.41)	Irregular intraluminal filling defects of varying sizes. Small filling defects are mobile. Large filling defects that occupy almost the entire lumen are still completely surrounded by contrast, thus allowing differentiation from tumors. Blood clots often change in size and shape or disappear over a period of several days.	Hematuria is usually present. Blood may originate from the kidney or the bladder itself. Common causes of bleeding include tumor, trauma, instrumentation, vascular malformations, hemorrhagic cystitis, bleeding disorders, and anticoagulation therapy.
Intramural hematoma or edema (Fig. 34.42)	Irregular or smooth intramural filling defects that may be associated with intraluminal blood clots.	Post surgery, instrumentation, and trauma. May resolve or proceed to granulation tissue formation with subsequent fibrosis.
Trauma (Fig. 34.43)	Intraluminal (blood clots) and intramural (hematoma) filling defects occur. Extravesical hemorrhage (with or without bladder rupture) produces elongation and elevation of the bladder (inverted "teardrop" appearance). Pelvic fractures are commonly associated.	*Intraperitoneal rupture:* Contrast extravasation around dome of bladder with smooth often band-like appearance. *Extraperitoneal rupture:* Contrast overlies lower half of bladder and has irregular, often streaky or feathery appearance.
Foreign body (including Foley catheter)	Opaque or nonopaque filling defects. Most common intraluminal defect is caused by the inflated balloon of a Foley catheter.	If any foreign material is present for a prolonged period of time, it often forms a nidus for calculus formation.
Pelvic organs (normal or enlarged) (Fig. 34.44)	Extrinsic defect, often associated with bladder displacement.	*Uterus* (including fibroid uterus and pregnancy), distended *rectosigmoid* (fecal impaction), *prostate*, and *ectopic kidney*. A *contracted levator* ani may produce slight and symmetrical elevation of the bladder floor. Impressions may also be caused by the *sacrospinous ligaments* producing symmetrical outpouchings of the lateroinferior aspect of the bladder.

(continues on page 808)

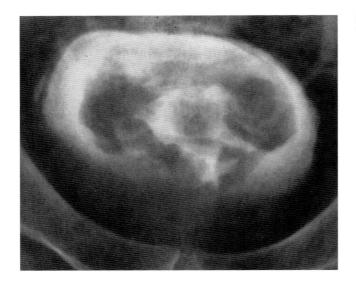

Fig. 34.**41**   **Blood clot.** A large intraluminal filling defect is seen in the bladder.

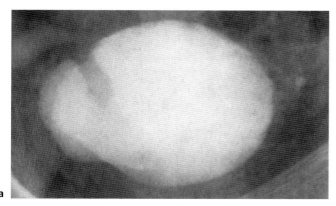
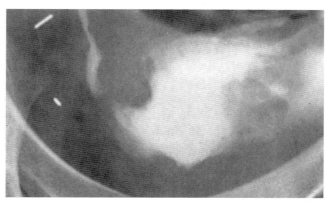

a   b

Fig. 34.**42 a, b   Postoperative edema and hematoma** in two renal transplant recipients. **a** A smooth filling defect caused by edema is seen at the site of the ureter implantation. **b** An irregular larger defect caused by a hematoma is seen at the site of the ureter implantation. Note also the irregular intraluminal filling defects in the left half of the bladder caused by blood clots.

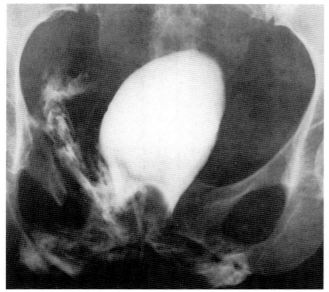
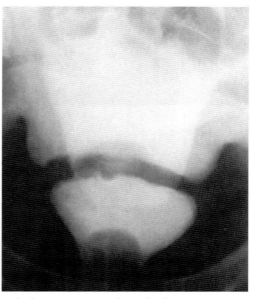

a   b

Fig. 34.**43 a, b   Bladder rupture. a** Extraperitoneal rupture of the bladder. Multiple pelvic and sacral fractures are seen, with pelvic hematoma causing extensive narrowing, elongation, and elevation of the bladder. Extraperitoneal contrast medium extravasation with characteristic streaky or feathery appearance is also present. **b Intraperitoneal rupture of the bladder**. A large amount of homogeneous intraperitoneal contrast medium projects above the dome of the collapsed bladder.

Fig. 34.**44   Fibroid uterus.** An extrinsic filling defect on the bladder dome by a markedly enlarged uterus and bilateral distal ureter obstruction are seen.

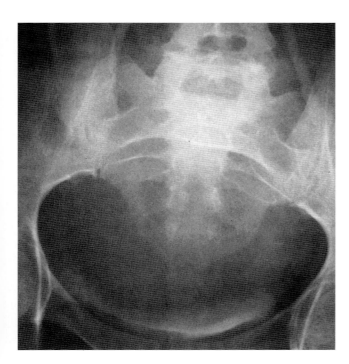

Table 34.2 (Cont.) Solitary or Multiple Filling Defects in the Urinary Bladder

Disease	Radiographic Findings	Comments
Prostatic enlargement (Figs. 34.45 and 34.46)	Extrinsic smooth or irregular filling defect of varying size at the base of the bladder. Distal ureters often demonstrate a "fish-hook deformity" or a "right angle turn." In chronic enlargement of the prostate, trabeculation of the bladder, diverticula, bilateral dilatation of the collecting systems and ureters secondary to bladder outlet obstruction, or occasionally by direct compression of the ureteral orifice are found. Multiple prostatic calculi may be seen, but are of little differential diagnostic value.	Prostatic hypertrophy and carcinoma are by far the most common causes and usually cannot be differentiated unless tumor invasion into neighboring organs or distant metastases are evident.
Extrinsic pelvic mass (Fig. 34.47)	*Lateral displacement* or *lateral defect* are caused by: 1 uterine tumor (especially fibroid, which is often densely calcified), 2 lymphadenopathy, 3 tuboovarian mass lesion, 4 osseous tumor, 5 rectosigmoid mass, 6 abscess, 7 aneurysm, 8 hematoma, and 9 hip arthroplasty. *Anterior displacement* or *posterior defect* are caused by 1 uterine tumor (most commonly fibroid), 2 neurogenic (presacral) tumor or meningocele, 3 rectal mass, and 4 osseous tumors originating from sacrum or coccyx.	*Dermoids* (see Fig. 34.**40**) have a characteristic appearance and can often reliably be diagnosed by demonstrating a radiolucent mass or a mass surrounded by radiolucent fat containing dense calcifications (e.g., tooth fragments).
Vesical fistula (Fig. 34.48)	Perivesical mass (abscess or tumor) causing a crescent-shaped defect or, in a more advanced stage, an irregular intrinsic mass that is often associated with gas in the bladder. Opacification of an irregular tract within the mass is diagnostic.	*Vesicointestinal fistulas* occur secondary to diverticulitis (51 %), colorectal carcinomas (16 %), Crohn's disease (12 %), bladder carcinoma (5 %), and rarely after surgical injury (e.g., prostatectomy), irradiation, foreign bodies, and abscesses (prostatic, pelvic, or appendiceal, the latter may occasionally result in a vesicoappendiceal fistula). *Vesicovaginal fistulas* are most commonly secondary to hysterectomy, but are also found with radiation therapy, malignant tumors of bladder, cervix, uterus, and rarely vagina, penetrating or obstetric injuries, and pelvic fractures. *Vesicouterine fistulas* are rare and usually secondary to cesarean section. *Vesicocutaneous sinuses* are almost always secondary to surgery, whereas *vesicoretroperitoneal sinuses* may result from operations, inflammations, and malignancies.

(continues on page 810)

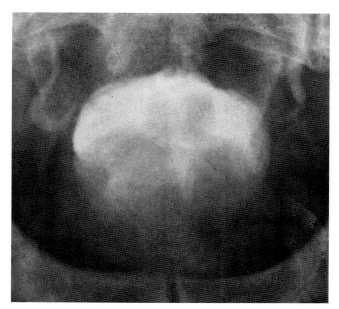

Fig. 34.**45** **Prostatic hypertrophy.** A symmetrical semicircular filling defect originating from the bladder floor is seen. The distal right ureter demonstrates a "fishhook deformity," whereas the left ureter makes a "right angle turn" at its distal end, both of which are quite characteristic for prostatic enlargement. The round radiolucency on top of the defect caused by the enlarged prostate is produced by the inflated balloon of a Foley catheter.

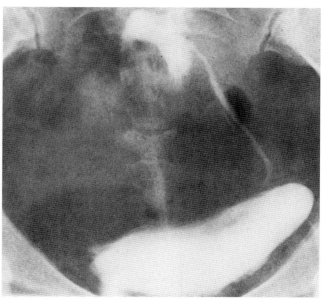

Fig. 34.**46** **Prostatic carcinoma.** A large and irregular defect is seen in a slightly trabeculated bladder. Note also the thickened and irregular right lateral wall of the bladder secondary to tumor infiltration.

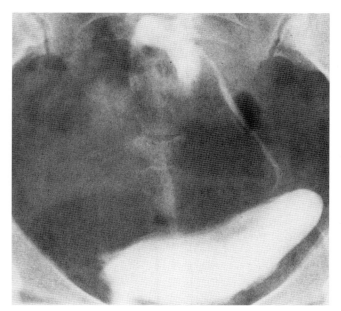

Fig. 34.**47** **Ovarian cystadenoma and pelvic kidney.** Lateral displacement of the bladder and a slight impression on the bladder dome are caused by these two conditions.

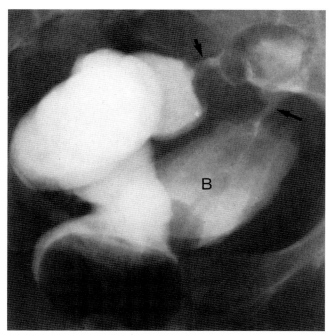

Fig. 34.**48** **Vesicocolonic fistula** secondary to carcinoma of the sigmoid. A fistulous track (long arrow) is seen between the sigmoid colon and the bladder (B). Note also the constricting sigmoid carcinoma (short arrow).

Table 34.2   (Cont.) Solitary or Multiple Filling Defects in the Urinary Bladder

Disease	Radiographic Findings	Comments
Pelvic lipomatosis (Fig. 34.49)	Elevation, narrowing, and vertical elongation of the bladder, often with inverted "teardrop" or "pear-shaped" appearance, by a relatively radiolucent pelvic mass (fat). Medial displacement of the distal ureters may occasionally be associated with some ureteral obstruction. Straightening, elongation, and elevation of the rectosigmoid with or without extrinsic compression are characteristically also present.	Strong male predominance. Similar radiographic appearances except for the increased radiolucency are seen in the following conditions that can also present as a more localized extrinsic defect on the bladder when the involvement is not so extensive. *Pelvic carcinomatosis* and *lymphoma.* Rarely in benign lymphadenopathy with considerable node enlargement (e.g., *lipoplastic lymphadenopathy*). *Perivesical hemorrhage* especially after trauma (see Fig. 34.**43**). *Obstruction of inferior vena cava* causing pelvic edema, usually associated with edema in the lower extremities. *Lymphoceles,* usually after lymphadenectomy or extensive pelvic surgery. *Urinoma* associated with bladder fistula of various etiologies. *Pelvic fibrosis* resulting from treated pelvic malignancies (e.g., radiation therapy) or secondary to perivesical hemorrhage, pelvic inflammation, obstruction of the inferior vena cava, lymphoceles, and urinoma. Rarely, the pelvis is also involved in retractile mesenteritis caused by an idiopathic fibro-adipose tissue proliferation.
Pelvic cysts and cyst-like lesions	Extrinsic defect or bladder displacement by soft, deformable mass.	Cysts originating from urachus, Müllerian duct, Gartner's duct, prostate, seminal vesicle, vas deferens, ovary, and vagina. Other cystic lesions include nonopacified bladder diverticula, hydrocolpos, hydrosalpinx, and anterior meningoceles. Urinomas and lymphoceles are usually posttraumatic or postoperative. Echinococcal cysts may show calcifications.

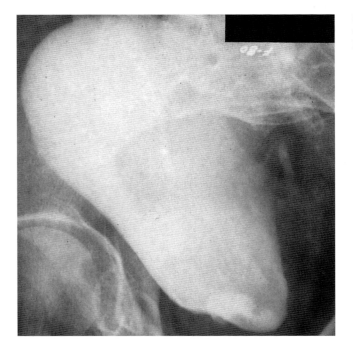

Fig. 34.**49**   **Pelvic lipomatosis.** Elevation, narrowing and vertical elongation of the bladder is seen, producing a "pear shape" appearance.

35 Urinary Tract Obstruction and Dilatation

Obstruction in the urinary tract commonly occurs at sites where a normal anatomic narrowing exists. These include, from top to bottom, the infundibula (branches of major or minor calices), ureter, bladder outlet, and urethra. In the ureter both the ureteropelvic and ureterovesical junctions are particularly prone to obstruction. The hallmark of any obstructive lesion, regardless of etiology and degree of obstruction, is the prestenotic dilatation. Segmental dilatation of the urinary tract is not, however, always secondary to a more distally located obstruction, but may also be caused by nonobstructive diseases. The various causes of caliceal dilatation have been discussed in Chapter **33**. The different etiologies of a dilated ureter and bladder are summarized in Tables 35.**1** and 35.**2**, respectively.

A ureter that is obstructed at its lower end becomes redundant with time and produces characteristic deviations. The proximal ureter is laterally displaced just below the ureteropelvic junction, whereas the ureter over the sacrum is often slightly medially deviated. Many causes of extrinsic ureter obstruction at various levels can be diagnosed from ureter displacement rather than from the contour changes produced by the extrinsic lesion on the ureter itself (Fig. 35.**1**).

An abnormal ureteral course may also be associated with renal displacement caused by a mass lesion or resulting from a congenital anomaly. A *pelvic kidney* frequently represents a *renal transplant*, but an *ectopic kidney* is another consideration. The latter may be located on the opposite side of its ureteral orifice (*crossed ectopica*). In both the *horseshoe kidney* (both kidneys joined at poles by parenchymal or fibrous isthmus) and the *discoid (pancake) kidney* (bilateral fused pelvic kidneys) the renal pelvis and ureters are situated anteriorly.

The differential diagnosis of an obstructed ureter is the subject of Table 35.**3**, and the various etiologies of a contracted urinary bladder are summarized in Table 35.**4**. Abnormalities of the urethra with or without obstruction are discussed in Table 35.**5**.

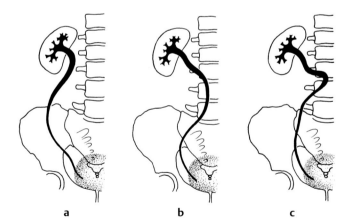
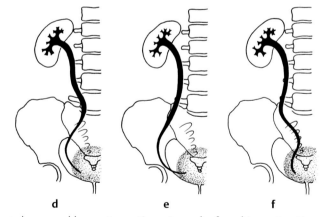

Fig. 35.**1 a–f   Ureter deviations. a** Lateral displacement of the proximal ureter is commonly caused by metastases or lymphoma in aortic lymph nodes, retroperitoneal sarcoma, abscess, or hematoma and aortic aneurysm. **b** Medial displacement of the proximal ureter is commonly caused by a large tumor or cyst originating from the lower pole of the kidney and may occasionally be seen with any condition that more commonly causes lateral displacement of the proximal ureter (see **a**). **c** Localized medial displacement of the right ureter at L3 is characteristic for a retrocaval ureter. A similar displacement of the left ureter is extremely rare and may be caused by a retroaortic ureter or be found in conjunction with a left-sided or double inferior vena cava. **d** Medial displacement of the ureter in the lumbosacral area is seen with retroperitoneal fibrosis where it is usually bilateral. **e** Lateral displacement of the distal ureter is seen with a central pelvic mass (enlarged uterus, ovary, or rectosigmoid). **f** Medial deviation of the distal ureter is often caused by pelvic carcinomatosis and lymphoma or an aneurysm of the iliac arteries. It is also seen following abdominoperineal surgery.

Table 35.1   Dilated Ureter (Megaureter)

Disease	Radiographic Findings	Comments
Obstruction of ureter (Fig. 35.2)	Unilateral prestenotic dilatation of ureter and collecting system (hydronephrosis and hydroureter).	Mechanical obstruction most commonly caused by calculus, tumor or stricture. For further differentiation, see Table 35.**3**.
Obstruction of bladder outlet or urethra (Fig. 35.3)	Dilated bladder. Abnormal trabeculation and diverticula formation in the bladder wall are found with chronic obstruction. Bilateral dilatation of ureters and collecting systems are associated.	For further differentiation, see Table 35.**5**.
Postobstructive hydronephrosis and hydroureter (Fig. 35.4)	Dilatation of the collecting system (particularly calices) and ureter without evidence of obstruction. Unilateral or bilateral.	Results from one prolonged or several intermittent episodes of previous obstruction.
Nonobstructive hydroureter (congenital ureterectasis)	Usually unilateral dilatation of ureter with normal pelvis and calices and without demonstrable abnormality in the ureter.	Congenital malformation of ureteral wall that is nonprogressive.
Megaloureter (congenital)	Functional, smoothly tapered narrowing of the juxtavesical ureter segment with minimal to extensive (up to 5 cm in diameter) dilatation of the pelvic ureter. Vigorous, non-propulsive peristaltic waves occur, similar to achalasia in the esophagus. May occasionally progress to dilatation of entire ureter and collecting system. Bilateral in 20 to 40% of cases.	Usually diagnosed in young adults, either coincidentally or with vague lower quadrant pain. May remain unchanged for years unless infection or decompensation (progressive dilatation) occurs.

(continues on page 814)

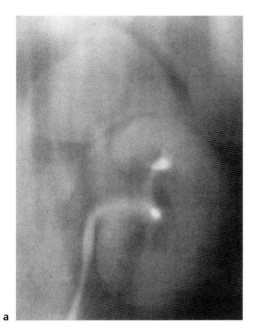

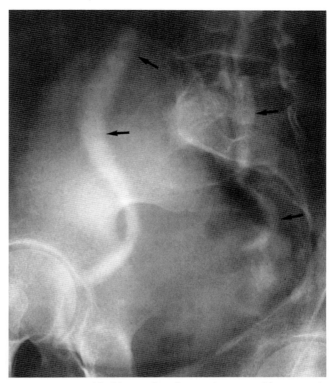

Fig. 35.**3** **Acute bladder outlet obstruction** caused by prostatic carcinoma. A markedly dilated bladder with bilateral hydroureters (arrows) is seen.

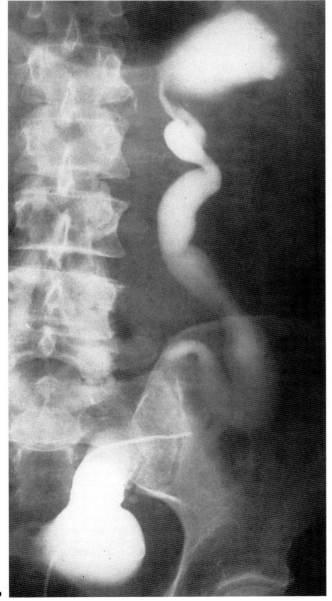

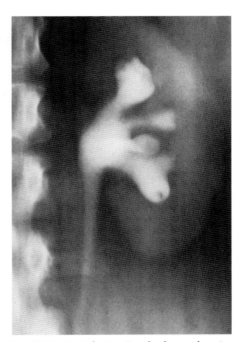

Fig. 35.**4** **Postobstructive hydronephrosis and hydroureter.** A dilated collecting system with partially clubbed calices and hydroureter is seen without delay in contrast excretion.

◁ Fig. 35.**2 a, b** **Duplication with obstruction of the upper segment** during **a** intravenous and **b** retrograde urography. **a** A nonfunctioning mass is seen on the upper pole of a small left kidney. **b** Retrograde urography reveals a duplicated system with marked hydronephrosis and hydroureter of the upper segment caused by obstruction at the ureterovesical junction.

Table 35.1 (Cont.) Dilated Ureter (Megaureter)

Disease	Radiographic Findings	Comments
Vesicoureteral reflux (Fig. 35.5)	Unilateral or bilateral. Ranges from retrograde opacification of a normal distal ureter to marked dilatation of entire ureter and collecting system with caliceal clubbing. Demonstration of actual contrast reflux from the bladder into ureter is not always possible (may be present in one examination and absent in the next).	More common in children than adults. May be congenital or acquired. *Congenital causes:* 1 Abnormalities in ureterovesical junction. 2 Complete duplication of ureters, with reflux usually occurring into the ureter draining the lower renal segment. 3 Ectopic ureter to bladder neck or urethra. Also in duplication when the ectopic ureter draining the upper renal segment is not obstructed. 4 Megacystis syndrome (see Table 35.2). 5 Congenital diverticula. 6 Congenital syndromes: e.g., "prune belly" (absent musculature of the abdominal wall, renal hypoplasia, dilated and tortuous ureters and cryptorchism) and exstrophy of the bladder. *Acquired causes:* 1 Cystitis 2 Neurogenic bladder 3 Previous ureterovesical surgery 4 Obstruction of bladder outlet or urethra
Pyelonephritis (acute)	Mild to moderate dilatation of the collecting system and ureter. Usually unilateral.	Paralysis of the smooth muscles in the urinary tract, caused by bacterial endotoxins.
Cystitis	Mild dilatation of the lower third of the ureters may be associated, especially with recurrent infections.	Probably caused by a combination of urinary reflux and smooth-muscle paralysis.
Chagas' disease	Dilatation of both ureters, usually with bladder dilatation.	In chronic *Trypanosoma cruzi* infection, causing destruction of the myenteric plexus. Endemic in South and Central America,
Pregnancy and postpartum (Fig. 35.6)	Dilatation of collecting system and ureter, usually more pronounced on the right side.	Combination of physiologic relaxation of ureteral wall and extrinsic compression by enlarged uterus.
Diabetes insipidus (Fig. 35.7)	Bilateral dilatation of ureters and collecting systems is often associated with an overdistended bladder.	Young adults with polydipsia and polyuria. Usually in nephrogenic diabetes insipidus (no tubular response to endogenous or exogenous antidiuretic hormones), but only rarely in pituitary diabetes insipidus.
Neurogenic bladder (Fig. 35.8)	Unilateral or bilateral dilatation of ureter and collecting system, associated with a characteristic neurogenic bladder (large and flaccid, or contracted with mural trabeculation and diverticula formation).	Caused by reflux (incompetent ureteral orifices) and/or bladder outlet obstruction (spastic external sphincter or pseudosphincter formation between the internal and external sphincter).
Absence of abdominal musculature (prune belly syndrome)	Renal dysplasia with dilated and markedly redundant ureters and enlarged smooth bladder.	Characteristic triad of absent musculature of the abdominal wall, causing a wrinkled (prunelike) appearance of the abdomen, urinary tract malformations, and cryptorchism.

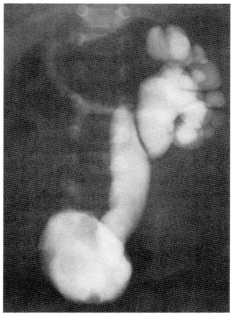

Fig. 35.**5** **Unilateral vesicoureteral reflux.** Contrast reflux from the bladder into a markedly dilated ureter and collecting system with clubbed calices is seen.

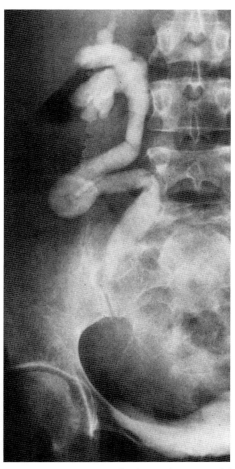

Fig. 35.**6** **Postpartum hydronephrosis and hydroureter.** A dilated right ureter caused by both physiologic atony and extrinsic compression of the enlarged uterus is seen.

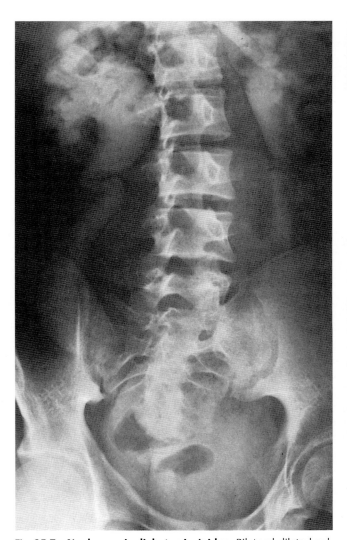

Fig. 35.**7** **Nephrogenic diabetes insipidus.** Bilateral dilated collecting systems and ureters are seen with a smooth, overdistended bladder.

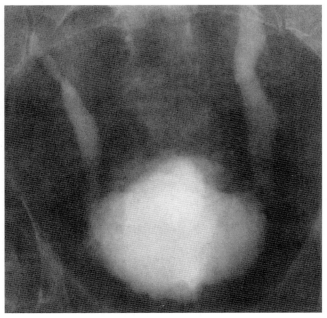

Fig. 35.**8** **Neurogenic bladder.** Bilateral dilated ureters are seen with a hypertonic neurogenic bladder showing increased trabeculations and multiple cellules.

Table 35.2   Dilatation of the Urinary Bladder (Commonly Associated with Bilateral Dilated Ureters)

Disease	Radiographic Findings	Comments
Obstruction of bladder outlet or urethra (Fig. 35.9)	Dilated bladder with increased trabeculation and one or multiple diverticulum formation, which may become larger than the bladder itself. With prolonged obstruction the bladder may become thin-walled and atonic.	Most common cause is prostatic hypertrophy or carcinoma. Acquired and congenital urethral strictures and urethral valves are other causes. The latter two conditions are usually diagnosed in children. For further differentiation see Table 35.5.
Bladder neck obstruction (primary) (Fig. 35.10)	Dilated bladder with posterior or anterior indentation or collar formation around the bladder neck. It may also demonstrate incomplete funneling or failure of relaxation during voiding.	In children assumed to be caused by muscular hypertrophy, local fibrosis, or bladder neck dysfunction. Existence of this entity as a true disorder of organic or functional etiology is still debated.
Bladder prolapse (Fig. 35.11)	Dilatation of the bladder may be caused by outlet obstruction. Base of bladder projects below the inferior margin of the symphysis, but this might sometimes only be evident in upright position.	*Cystocele* is a prolapse of the bladder and the anterior vaginal wall into the vaginal cavity usually following childbirth. May be associated with *stress incontinence* (Fig. 35.12).
Chagas' disease	Dilatation of the bladder often associated with ureteral dilatation.	Rare complication of *Trypanosoma cruzi* infection. Endemic in South and Central America.
Neurogenic bladder (Fig. 35.13)	Markedly dilated bladder presents in atonic or hypertonic form: 1 Atonic: smooth, thin-walled and commonly oval-shaped. 2 Hypertonic: heavily trabeculated, often with multiple cellules or saccules, but rarely with larger diverticula. A "pine tree" shape of the bladder is characteristic, but only present in a minority of cases.	Neurogenic bladder can also be significantly contracted (see Table 35.4). Large hypertonic bladders are usually associated with outlet obstruction (e.g., spastic external sphincter or pseudosphincter formation).

(continues on page 818)

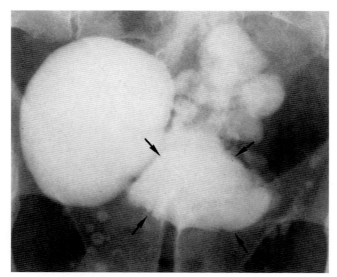

Fig. 35.**9** **Chronic bladder outlet obstruction** caused by prostatic hypertrophy. Multiple diverticula with characteristic smooth walls are seen. The largest diverticulum on the right side has become considerably larger than the trabeculated bladder (arrows).

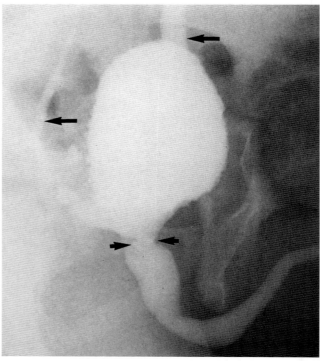

Fig. 35.**10** **Primary bladder neck obstruction.** A collar formation (short arrows) is seen around the bladder neck during voiding. Note also the contrast reflux into both ureters (long arrows).

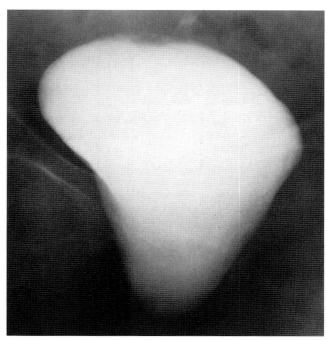

Fig. 35.**11** **Bladder prolapse.** Base of the bladder projects below the symphysis. DD: Cystocele where the bladder and anterior wall of the vagina prolapse into the vaginal cavity.

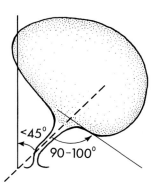

Fig. 35.**12** **Evaluation of stress incontinence** in the female bladder. The normal posterior urethrovesical angle (the angle between the axis of the upper urethra and the posterior bladder floor) ranges between 90° and 100°. The normal urethra inclination angle (the angle between the axis of the upper urethra and the vertical axis of the patient) is smaller than 45°. Stress incontinence type I: The posterior urethrovesical angle is smaller than 90° during straining or voiding, whereas the urethra inclination angle remains normal. Stress incontinence type II: The posterior urethrovesical angle is larger than 100° and the urethra inclination angle is larger than 45°.

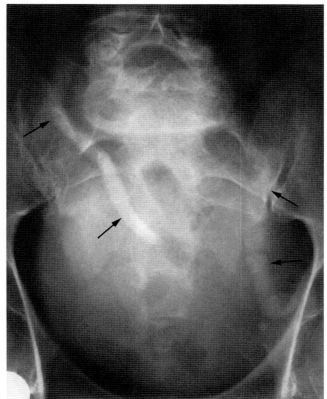

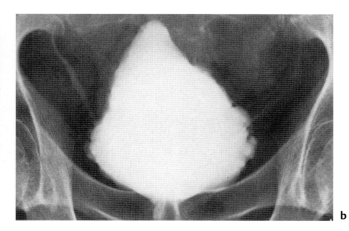

Fig. 35.**13 a, b** **Neurogenic bladders.** **a** atonic form and **b** hypertonic form. **a** A markedly dilated bladder with a smooth, thin wall is seen. Note also the dilated ureters (arrows). **b** A heavily trabeculated bladder with numerous small saccules is seen. Note also the "pine tree" shape of the bladder.

Table 35.2 (Cont.) Dilatation of the Urinary Bladder (Commonly Associated with Bilateral Dilated Ureters)

Disease	Radiographic Findings	Comments
Diabetes	Radiographic manifestation is similar to large atonic neurogenic bladder.	Neurogenic bladder dysfunction occurs in about 1–2% of cases.
Diabetes insipidus (see Fig. 35.7)	Dilated smooth or trabeculated bladder, usually associated with dilated ureters and collecting systems.	Usually in young adults. Much more common in nephrogenic than pituitary diabetes insipidus.
Megacystis syndrome	Large, smooth-walled, or slightly trabeculated bladder with vesicoureteral reflux during voiding. Bladder neck often fails to funnel and distend during voiding.	Usually seen in childhood, more frequently in girls than boys. Bladder voiding is usually complete, without a significant urinary residue remaining on postvoid films.
Absence of abdominal musculature (prune belly syndrome) (Fig. 35.14)	Renal dysplasia with dilated and markedly redundant ureters and enlarged smooth bladder.	Characteristic triad includes absent musculature of abdominal wall causing a wrinkled (prunelike) appearance of the anterior abdominal wall, urinary tract malformations, and cryptorchism. Poor prognosis, with about half of the children dying within the first few years of life.
Miscellaneous (hysteria, infrequent voider, drugs, idiopathic)	Smooth, markedly distended bladder with normal function.	Drugs include tranquilizers and muscle relaxants.

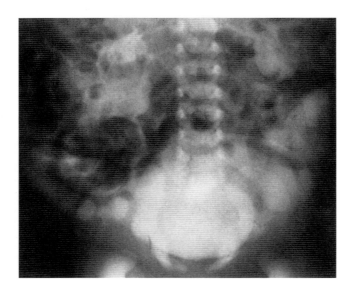

Fig. 35.**14 Prune belly syndrome.** A large, smooth bladder, with bilateral dilated and markedly redundant ureters, is seen.

Table 35.3 Obstruction of the Ureter

Disease	Radiographic Findings	Comments
Ureteropelvic junction (UPJ) obstruction (Fig. 35.15)	Persistent or intermittent hydronephrosis. Ureter occasionally appears to leave the markedly dilated pelvis not at its most dependent portion but at a point higher on the anterior or medial surface, because the pelvis may enlarge behind the relatively fixed junction. If the obstruction is not relieved, progressive loss of renal parenchyma may eventually result in a hydronephrotic sac, with the renal parenchyma reduced to a thin rim surrounding it.	Most often congenital. Caused by intrinsic stenosis or extrinsic compression from a band or vessel, or by poor conduction of urine through the junction secondary to abnormal muscle development, injury or inflammation. Ureteropelvic junction obstruction may also be associated with vesicoureteral reflux and may be secondary to the reflux. Ureteropelvic junction obstruction is especially common in horseshoe and incompletely rotated kidneys.
Ureteral valves	Linear cut-off with obstruction, preferentially located in the distal ureter.	Valves are transverse folds of redundant ureteral mucosa. Either congenital (valves consisting of both mucosa and smooth muscle) or acquired (secondary to chronic inflammation).
Simple ureterocele (Fig. 35.16)	Unilateral or bilateral oval or round filling defects caused by the dilated distal ureter prolapsed into the bladder. Separation of the opacified urine in the cystic, dilated and prolapsed ureter from the opacified urine in the bladder by the ureteral wall and bladder mucosa produces the characteristic cobra head appearance. The cause is presumed to be a congenital or acquired stenosis of the ureteral orifice. Both infection and calculus formation may aggravate the obstruction in the ureterocele.	Congenital or acquired ureteroceles often disappear spontaneously when the cause of obstruction is eliminated (e.g., after passage of calculus trapped in a ureterocele). Voiding cystoureterogram (VCUG): The dilated distal ureter may evert during voiding, producing a temporary ureterocele-like appearance. DD: *Pseudoureterocele*: Obstruction of an otherwise normal intramural ureter mimicking ureterocele caused by bladder tumor or edema (e.g., impacted ureteral calculus or following ureteral instrumentation).
Ectopic ureterocele	Stenotic ectopic ureteral orifice associated with hydronephrosis or nonvisualization of the involved ureter and collecting system. Almost always associated with a duplicated system, the ureterocele arising from the ureter draining the upper segment. A smooth and often lobulated defect at the base of the bladder, or occasionally in the proximal urethra, represents the dilated submucosal portion of the ectopic ureter.	A congenital, and in 90% unilateral, lesion. Usually diagnosed in children and young adults presenting with dysuria, pyuria and flank pain. Much more common in females.

(continues on page 820)

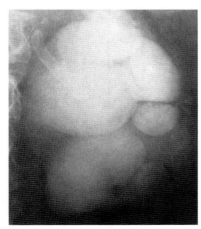

Fig. 35.**15** **Ureteropelvic junction (UPJ) obstruction.** A markedly hydronephrotic collecting system is seen.

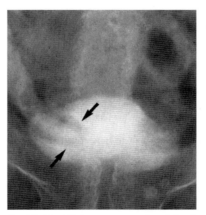

Fig. 35.**16** **Right ureterocele with obstruction.** A characteristic "cobra head" appearance (arrows) with dilatation of the right ureter is seen. The ureteral obstruction was caused by an opaque calculus in the ureterocele now concealed by contrast medium.

Table 35.3 (Cont.) Obstruction of the Ureter

Disease	Radiographic Findings	Comments
Endometriosis	Intrinsic (rare) or extrinsic obstruction of the distal ureter, usually below the pelvic rim.	Usually in women of late childbearing age. Hematuria in association with menstrual period characteristic, but only present in a minority of cases. History of previous gynecologic or abdominal surgery is common.
Amyloidosis	Narrowed and somewhat rigid, occasionally constricted ureter with proximal hydronephrosis.	Primary, secondary, or focal (localized) amyloidosis may involve any ureter segment.
Benign ureteral tumors	Rare cause of ureteral obstruction.	See Table 34.1, for further differentiation.
Ureter carcinoma (Figs. 35.17, 35.18)	One (occasionally two or more) often irregular filling defects, without site predilection, causing usually mild to complete obstruction. Infiltrating carcinomas may also present as an irregular stricture with overhanging margins or as smooth, short or long stenotic segments simulating a benign process.	See Table 34.1, for further differentiation of ureteral malignancies.
Bladder carcinoma (Fig. 35.18)	Unilateral or bilateral obstruction of the ureterovesical junctions is particularly common with infiltrating tumors, especially when they originate in the trigone. Distal ureters may also be obstructed by encasement or direct invasion from lymph node metastases.	See Table 34.2, for further differentiation of bladder malignancies.
Cystitis acute or chronic	*Acute*: Compression of intramural ureters by edema and inflammation. *Chronic*: Obstruction of the ureterovesical junction by fibrosis or inflammatory mass lesions.	See Table 34.2, for further differentiation of acute and chronic cystitis.
Tuberculosis (Fig. 35.19)	Multiple strictures are common. If the strictures are short and follow in close sequence, a "beaded" or "corkscrew" appearance may result. Total ureteral involvement may produce a short, narrowed ureter with thickened wall and absent peristalsis ("pipe-stem" appearance).	Late manifestation. Almost always associated with renal tuberculosis (see Table 33.2). A shrunken bladder is often present also.

(continues on page 822)

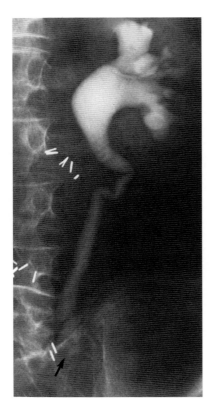

Fig. 35.**17** **Transitional cell carcinoma** of the ureter. An irregular filling defect (arrow) is seen in the ureter with prestenotic dilatation.

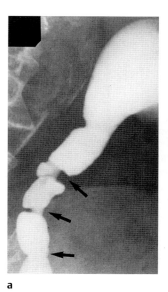
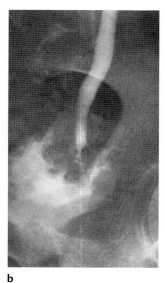
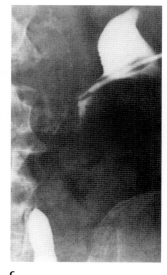
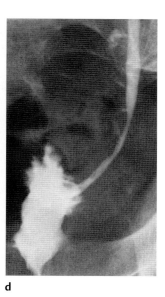

a **b** **c** **d**

Fig. 35.**18 a–d** **Multicentric transitional cell carcinoma** involving the proximal and distal ureter and bladder. **a** Three areas of localized eccentric narrowing are seen in the proximal ureter (arrows). **b** An irregular filling defect caused by carcinoma is seen in the bladder with extension and obstruction of the distal ureter. Note also the calcified aortic aneurysm displacing the hydronephrotic renal pelvis and most proximal part of the ureter laterally (**a, c**).

c, d Six months after **a** and **b**. **c** The three areas of localized narrowing in the proximal ureter have progressed to a long stricture with almost complete obstruction. **d** Involvement of the distal ureter presents now as another long stricture. The bladder involvement has also markedly progressed and is now evident as a small shrunken bladder with irregularly thickened wall.

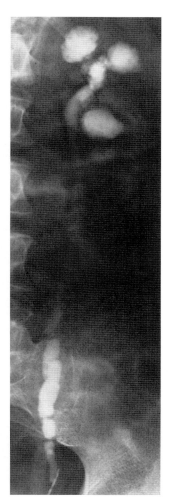

Fig. 35.**19** **Tuberculosis.** Multiple short strictures in close sequence are seen in the distal ureter producing a characteristic "beaded" appearance. Note also the destruction of the collecting system.

Table 35.3 (Cont.) Obstruction of the Ureter

Disease	Radiographic Findings	Comments
Schistosomiasis (Fig. 35.20)	Strictures, aperistalsis, and calcifications (usually linear or occasionally punctate) in the distal ureter are characteristic.	End stage of the disease, almost always associated with bladder wall calcification.
Radiation therapy	Gradual ureteral stricture and obstruction developing several months to years after treatment. With pelvic irradiation (e.g., for uterine carcinoma), the stricture develops usually 1–2 cm above the ureterovesical junction.	Stricture formation more common when the ureter was originally involved with carcinoma. Tumor recurrence is often impossible to differentiate from a radiation-induced fibrosis, even when the time factor is considered.
Post surgery and instrumentation (Fig. 35.21)	Localized narrowing of the ureter (e.g., with accidental ureter ligation, edema of ureter wall, or stricture formation) or diffuse narrowing by extrinsic compression. Displacement of the ureter by abscess, hematoma, or urinoma, all of which might progress to retroperitoneal fibrosis, is often associated.	Instrumental perforation usually heals rapidly and without sequelae when less than 50% of the ureter circumference is involved and no distal obstruction is present. Inadvertent disrupture of the blood supply to the ureter may cause necrosis of the ureteral wall several weeks later leading to fistulization. Ligation of both ureters results in anuria 8–10 hours after major pelvic surgery.
Stricture (Figs. 35.21, 35.22)	*Congenital*: Commonly located at the ureteropelvic and ureterovesical junctions (see also under ureteropelvic junction obstruction in this table). *Acquired*: Smooth ureteral narrowing without site predilection. May be very short or involve a longer segment. Secondary to inflammatory disease (ureteritis), extrinsic inflammation, surgical or instrumental injury, radiotherapy, or neoplasm. In the latter case, the stricture is often irregular.	In retrograde studies, narrowing of the ureteral lumen that is often indistinguishable from a stricture may be caused by *ureteral spasm* secondary to catheter manipulation.

(continues on page 824)

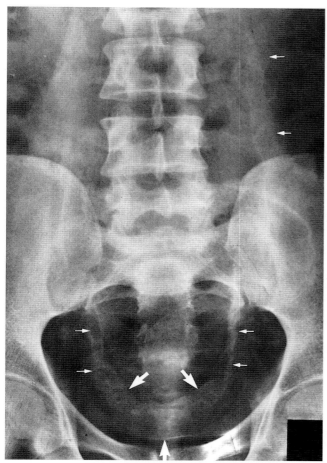

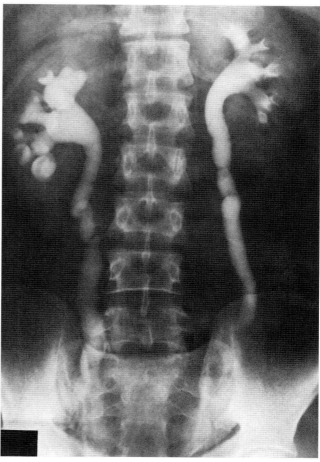

Fig. 35.**20**   **Schistosomiasis. a** Scout film. Linear calcifications of the bladder wall (long arrows), both distal ureters (short arrows) and the left mid-ureter (short arrows) are characteristic. **b** After in-travenous contrast medium administration bilateral symmetric dilatation of both collecting systems and ureters caused by a combination of aperistalsis and mild distal ureteral obstruction is seen.

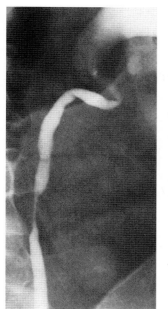

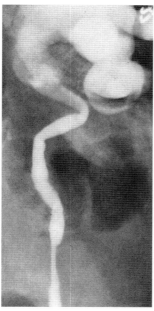

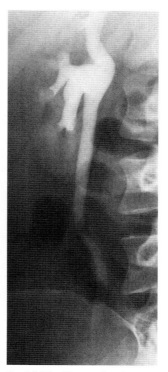

Fig. 35.**21 a, b   Benign ureteral stricture, a** before and **b** four months after resection and reanastomosis. **a** A short and slightly irregular stricture is seen in the proximal ureter with prestenotic dilatation (idiopathic periureteral fibrosis or secondary to chronic urinary tract infection). **b** After resection and reanastomosis a similar, but this time perfectly smooth, stricture reoccurred at the same location.

Fig. 35.**22**   **Ureteral stricture** in Crohn's disease. A smooth tapering of the ureter with prestenotic dilatation is seen.

Table 35.3   (Cont.) Obstruction of the Ureter

Disease	Radiographic Findings	Comments
Calculus (Fig. 35.23)	About 90% of calculi are radiopaque enough to be visualized on plain films. May be partially or completely obstructing, especially when located at physiologically narrowed sites (e.g., ureteropelvic or ureterovesical junctions). Positions of calculi and sites of obstruction may change between examinations. While nonopaque calculi are evident as lucent filling defects after proper opacification of the ureters, radiopaque calculi may be concealed by the contrast medium if both have a similar radiodensity.	Obstructing nonopaque calculi can reliably be diagnosed with ultrasonography because, like all stones, they produce a characteristic posterior shadowing. Computerized tomography may also be useful to differentiate nonopaque calculi from intraluminal tumors on the basis of the higher attenuation values of the calculi.
Blood clots	Irregular radiolucent filling defects that may produce temporary and usually incomplete obstruction.	Usually secondary to renal trauma, bleeding disorders, anticoagulation therapy, surgery or tumors. Ureteral injury secondary to trauma is rare, since the ureters are not fixed and are well protected in their entire course.
Sloughed papilla	Ureteral obstruction by an irregular filling defect in patients with evidence of papillary necrosis.	See Table 33.2, for radiographic findings in papillary necrosis.
Inspissated pus or necrotic tumor debris	Irregular filling defect occasionally causing ureteral obstruction.	In patients with severe inflammatory process or necrotic tumor in the kidney.
Vascular compression (Figs. 35.24, 35.25)	Crossing vessel may cause extrinsic imprints on the ureter at various levels with usually mild dilatation of the more proximal ureter but rarely significant obstruction. *Proximal ureter*: Normal and aberrant renal arteries. *Middle ureter*: Iliac vessels at L5/S1. Occasionally the ureter is retroiliac. In this condition a marked vascular impression, slight medial displacement, and a more pronounced obstruction are usually present. An extrinsic impression on the right ureter at the SI level with mild to moderate obstruction is also seen in the *ovarian vein syndrome* (see Table 34.1). *Pelvic ureter*: Aneurysmatic dilatation of internal iliac artery may cause a localized medial displacement of the ureter below the pelvic brim, but rarely obstruction.	Ureteral obstruction by a crossing vessel is more severe when the involved artery is arteriosclerotic or aneurysmatically dilated. Similar changes can be seen with *congenital* or *acquired* bands.
Aneurysm of abdominal aorta or common iliac artery	Extrinsic compression with localized or diffuse lateral displacement of the ureter above the pelvic brim. Calcifications of the aneurysm are diagnostic when present.	Most commonly with an arteriosclerotic aneurysm, but also with dissecting and mycotic aneurysms.
Retrocaval ureter (Fig. 35.26)	Mild obstruction of the right ureter with characteristic "hook like" medial displacement at the level of L3.	The right ureter is located posteriorly and medially to the inferior vena cava. A similar displacement of the left ureter is extremely rare and may be caused by a retroaortic ureter or associated with a left-sided or double inferior vena cava.
Herniation of ureter (Fig. 35.27)	Abnormal course of a redundant ureter, often associated with obstruction. *Femoral* or *inguinal hernia*: Ureter loop in femoral or inguinal canal, may occasionally extend into the scrotum. *Sciatic hernia*: Lateral angulation of pelvic ureter. Obstruction is rare. *Internal hernia*: Ureter trapped under peritoneal folds or iliac fascia or between iliac vessels.	Ureter hernias are rare and represent either congenital anomalies or are seen following pelvic surgery.

(continues on page 826)

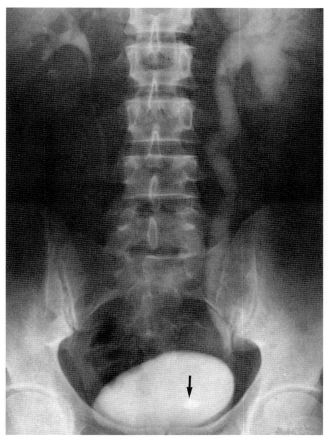

Fig. 35.**23** **Calculus at the ureterovesical junction.** Hydrone-phrosis and hydroureter is caused by an opaque calculus (arrow) impacted in the left ureterovesical junction.

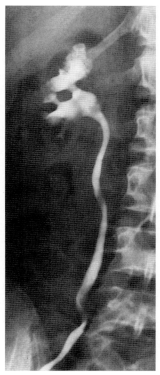

Fig. 35.**24** **Retroiliac ureter.** An extrinsic impression on the ureter with slight medial displacement is seen at the L5/S1 level. Note also the changes caused by medullary sponge kidney in the upper calices.

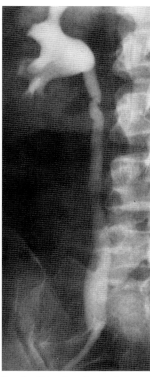

Fig. 35.**25** **Ovarian vein syndrome.** Narrowing of the right ureter with prestenotic dilatation is seen at S1.

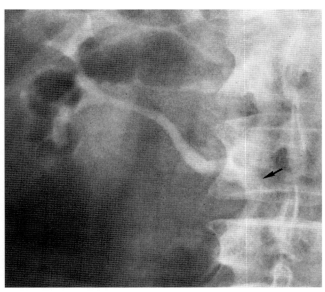

Fig. 35.**26** **Retrocaval ureter.** Characteristic "hooklike" medial displacement of the right ureter without significant obstruction is seen (arrow).

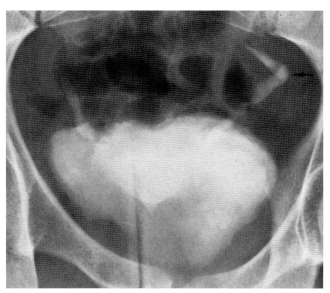

Fig. 35.**27** **Sciatic ureter hernia.** Lateral angulation of the pelvic ureter without obstruction is seen (arrow). Bladder wall thickening and irregularities were caused by abacterial pyuria.

Table 35.3 (Cont.) Obstruction of the Ureter

Disease	Radiographic Findings	Comments
Bladder diverticulum (Fig. 35.28)	Congenital diverticula are usually solitary and located near the ureteral orifice, and may occasionally obstruct the distal ureter by extrinsic compression.	Congenital bladder diverticula usually occur in children. Urinary infection and vesicoureteral reflux are much more common complications than ureteral obstruction. A diverticulum above and lateral to the ureteral orifice, often producing an obstructed ureter just above the bladder ("notch sign") and primarily found in paraplegics, has been termed *Hutch diverticulum*. Acquired diverticula occur later in life, are often multiple, have no site predilection, and result usually from bladder outlet or urethral obstruction.
Retroperitoneal fibrosis (Fig. 35.29)	Unilateral or more commonly bilateral narrowing and frequently medial deviation of both urethras in the area of the lower lumbar and upper sacral segments with prestenotic dilatation.	Most common between 40 and 60 years of age, with male predominance. The etiology is unknown. History of prolonged drug ingestion (e.g., ergot derivatives, phenacetin, methyldopa) is occasionally available. A similar process involves occasionally the proximal ureter and kidney *(Gerota's fasciitis)* or the distal ureters and bladder *(pelvic fibrolipomatosis)*. A similar fibrotic process may coexist at other sites (e.g., fibrosing mediastinitis, sclerosing cholangitis, retractile mesenteritis, Riedel's thyroiditis, retro-orbital pseudotumor).
Retroperitoneal abscess (Fig. 35.30)	Lateral displacement of kidney and ureter with extrinsic compression. Retroperitoneal gas collections are rarely seen but diagnostic when present. Calcifications occur, especially with a tuberculous psoas abscess.	May originate from spondylitis (particularly tuberculous), perinephric abscess, urinary tract infection, pancreatitis, perforated duodenum, or develop following retro-peritoneal surgery.
Retroperitoneal hematoma	Smooth lateral displacement of ureter and kidney (unilateral or bilateral) with extrinsic compression of the ureter, The psoas margin is usually preserved, but appears widened and more dense.	In trauma (usually with laceration of the kidneys, fractured lumbar vertebral bodies, or transverse processes, respectively), ruptured aortic aneurysm, postoperative, bleeding disorders, and anticoagulation therapy. May progress to retroperitoneal fibrosis.

(continues on page 828)

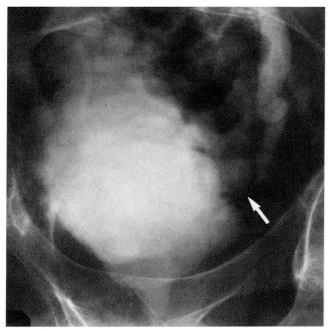

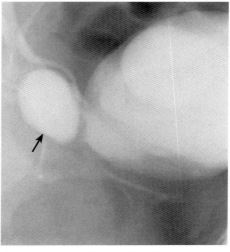

a

b

Fig. 35.**28 a, b Bladder diverticula** including **Hutch diverticulum. a** Neurogenic bladder. **b** Bladder outlet obstruction (urethral stricture). Multiple bladder diverticula including a Hutch diverticulum (arrow) is seen in both patients. Note also the extrinsic narrowing ("notch sign") of the adjacent ureters by the Hutch diverticula. A funnel-shaped dilatation of the prostatic urethra caused by spasm of the external sphincter is seen in **a**.

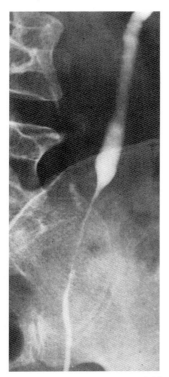

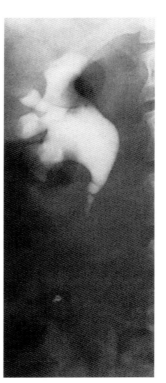

Fig. 35.**29 Retroperitoneal fibrosis.** A long, smooth narrowing of the slightly medial deviated left ureter is seen in the lumbosacral area. A similar stricture was present in the right ureter also.

Fig. 35.**30 Retroperitoneal abscess.** Lateral displacement of the proximal ureter with extrinsic obstruction is seen.

Table 35.3   (Cont.) Obstruction of the Ureter

Disease	Radiographic Findings	Comments
Retroperitoneal tumor (Fig. 35.31)	Lateral or rarely medial displacement of proximal ureter with obstruction, caused by extrinsic compression, encasement, or invasion.	*Metastatic* (e.g., from carcinoma of the urogenital system, pancreas, melanoma of lower extremities, or rarely from carcinoma of the rectosigmoid or descending colon) or *lymphomatous involvement of the retroperitoneal lymph nodes* is by far the most common cause. Primary retroperitoneal tumors are much less common (e.g., *liposarcomas* and other malignant or rarely benign, mesenchymal tumors). Retroperitoneal *pheochromocytomas* may produce characteristic symptoms (hypertension, tachycardia, and flushing). Tumors originating from the urogenital ridge remnants may have characteristic calcifications (e.g., *teratomas, dermoids*). Rarely, retroperitoneal cysts occur.
Benign pelvic mass (Fig. 35.32)	Lateral deviation of pelvic ureter (unilateral or bilateral) with occasionally mild to moderate extrinsic obstruction by large central mass.	With ovarian cyst, uterine fibroids, enlarged uterus (pregnancy or postpartum), or occasionally markedly distended rectosigmoid.
Pelvic malignancy (extrinsic)	Obstructed distal ureter is characteristically straightened or medially displaced.	In pelvic carcinomatosis or pelvic lymph node metastases (e.g., from carcinoma of rectosigmoid, bladder, cervix, and ureters) and pelvic lymphoma.
Pelvic abscess or inflammatory disease (Fig. 35.33)	Unilateral or bilateral obstructed pelvic ureters, usually in normal location or rarely medially displaced.	In diverticulitis, Crohn's disease, appendiceal abscess, or postoperative.
Pelvic lipomatosis (Fig. 35.34)	Gentle bilateral and symmetrical medial displacement of pelvic ureters, which may be incompletely obstructed. Excessive fat deposition may produce an increased radiolucency that can easily be confirmed with computed tomography or magnetic resonance imaging.	Elevated bladder, often with inverted "teardrop" or "pear-shaped" appearance and straightening and elongation of the rectosigmoid are usually associated (see Table 34.2, for additional information).

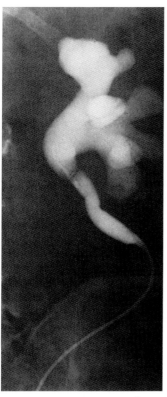

Fig. 35.**31** **Retroperitoneal non-Hodgkin's lymphoma.** Lateral displacement of the proximal ureter with complete obstruction is seen.

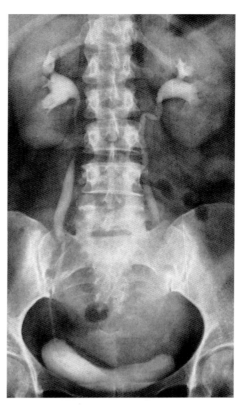

Fig. 35.**32** **Ovarian cyst.** A large pelvic mass is seen causing an extrinsic impression on the bladder dome and lateral deviation of both pelvic ureters with mild obstruction.

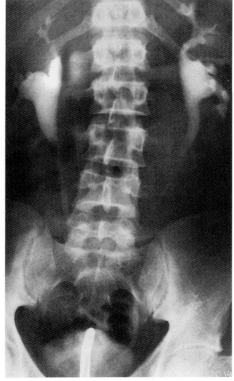

Fig. 35.**33** **Pelvic abscess.** Mild obstruction of both ureters that are slightly medially displaced in the pelvis is seen.

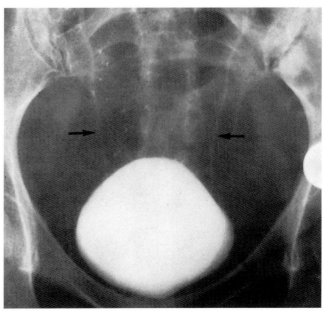

Fig. 35.**34** **Pelvic lipomatosis.** Gentle bilateral and symmetrical medial displacement of the pelvic ureters is seen (arrows). Note also the increased radiolucency in the pelvis caused by the lipomatosis. The bladder depicts the characteristic "pear-shaped" appearance.

Table 35.4   Small Urinary Bladder

Disease	Radiographic Findings	Comments
Transitional cell carcinoma (Fig. 35.35)	Usually somewhat asymmetrically contracted bladder with an irregular and thickened wall and indentations. Markedly deformed bladders occur with localized tumor infiltration. Unilateral or bilateral ureter obstruction is commonly associated. Fine granular calcifications on the tumor surface (encrusted) occur, but are unusual (about 1%).	*Squamous cell carcinomas* are rare in the bladder but present often in a primarily infiltrating form and have an extremely poor prognosis. This histologic type is associated with schistosomiasis. *Adenocarcinomas* may develop in remnants of the urachus.
Cystitis (acute) (Fig. 35.36)	Severe mucosal and intramural edema may cause a thickened irregular bladder wall. The bladder volume may be markedly decreased due to spasm. Ureteral reflux or less common obstruction may be associated. Changes are reversible.	See Table 34.2, for further differentiation.
Cystitis (chronic) Fig. 35.37)	Small bladder with trabeculation and wall irregularities. Ureteral reflux or obstruction occurs occasionally. Findings change little with time.	*Interstitial cystitis* is a chronic inflammatory disorder characteristically associated with a very small bladder. For further differentiation of chronic cystitis see Table 34.2. A small bladder with linear wall calcifications is occasionally seen in *chronic cyclophosphamide cystitis* and *alkaline-encrusted cystitis* (e.g., drug-induced).
Tuberculosis (Fig. 35.38)	Thickened and trabeculated bladder wall (early stage) with progressive decrease in capacity and becoming more smooth-walled. In the late stages, the bladder may disappear nearly completely with the ureters practically entering the urethra directly. Short ureters with multiple strictures and reflux are commonly associated. Calcification in the bladder wall is rare, but common in seminal vesicles and vas deferens.	Almost invariably associated with renal tuberculosis, where the disease originates and spreads via the ureters into the bladder.

(continues on page 831)

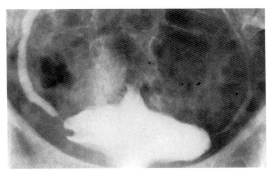

35.35

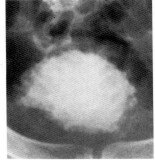

35.36

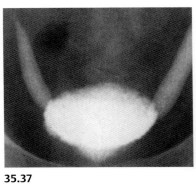

35.37

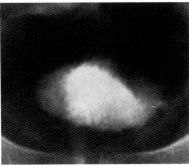

35.38

Fig. 35.**35**   **Transitional cell carcinoma of the bladder.** A shrunken and irregularly deformed bladder with thickened wall and partial obstruction of the right ureterovesical junction is seen.

Fig. 35.**36**   **Acute cystitis.** A small spastic bladder with severe mucosal and interstitial edema causing a thickened irregular wall is seen.

Fig. 35.**37**   **Chronic cystitis.** A small bladder with thickened and slightly trabeculated wall is seen. Dilatation of both ureters is caused by vesicoureteral reflux.

Fig. 35.**38**   **Tuberculous cystitis.** A markedly shrunken bladder with a slightly irregular wall is seen.

Table 35.4   (Cont.) Small Urinary Bladder

Disease	Radiographic Findings	Comments
Schistosomiasis (Fig. 35.39)	In advanced disease the capacity of the fibrotic bladder is often somewhat decreased and commonly associated with wall calcifications. Nodular, often calcified lesions may also be seen. Dilated distal ureters (obstruction or reflux) with calcifications and round filling defects are often associated.	Calcification may surround bladder completely in a 1 to 3 mm wide, dense line located in the lamina propria or muscularis. The uncommon squamous cell carcinoma of the bladder develops in this condition with a much higher frequency than in the general population.
Radiation cystitis (Fig. 35.40)	Contracted bladder with smooth or irregular surface. May rarely calcify.	Develops several months to several years after completion of irradiation.
Postoperative bladder	Decreased bladder capacity.	Post partial resection.
Neurogenic bladder (Fig. 35.41)	Contracted bladder with markedly reduced capacity and irregular thickened wall, trabeculations, sacculations, and cellules. Besides a round or oval shape, the bladder may also present with an "hourglass" or "pine tree" appearance. The latter configuration is also seen with enlarged neurogenic bladders.	Neurogenic bladder can also present with significant dilatation (see Table 35.2).
Defunctionalized bladder	Small, usually smooth-walled bladder. Reflux into ureters or ureteral stumps may occur. If infected ("empyema cystis"), bladder wall is usually irregular.	Bladder may be either completely defunctionalized after urinary diversion or partially in end-stage kidney disease, in which there is little or no urine production.

(continues on page 832)

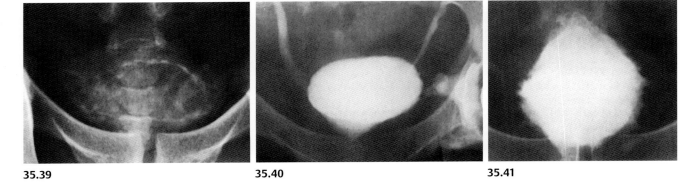

35.39   **35.40**   **35.41**

Fig. 35.**39 Schistosomiasis.** Complete ringlike calcification of the entire bladder wall is present.

Fig. 35.**40 Radiation cystitis.** A small bladder with a relatively smooth surface is seen, four years after irradiation of an endometrial carcinoma.

Fig. 35.**41 Neurogenic bladder.** A contracted bladder with thickened wall and "pine tree" appearance is seen.

Table 35.4   (Cont.) Small Urinary Bladder

Disease	Radiographic Findings	Comments
Bladder hernia (Fig. 35.42)	Small, often asymmetric bladder with displacement of both ureters and trigone toward the side of herniation. The herniated part of the bladder is not always opacified during intravenous urography.	Inguinal bladder hernias are more common in males, whereas femoral hernias are predominant in females.
Total bladder incontinence	Small capacity bladder because of inadequate filling.	For example, following total prostatectomy.
Extrinsic perivesical bladder compression (Figs. 35.43, 35.44)	Elevation of a narrowed bladder often with characteristic inverted "teardrop" or "pear-shaped" appearance.	In pelvic lipomatosis (extrinsic mass has increased radiolucency), pelvic hematoma (associated with pelvic fractures), pelvic edema (e.g., obstruction of inferior vena cava), and pelvic neoplastic or inflammatory disease.

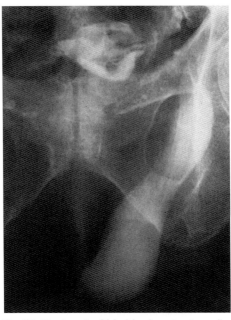

Fig. 35.**42   Inguinal bladder hernia.** A small asymmetric bladder that is displaced toward the side of herniation is seen in the pelvis, whereas the larger part of the bladder has herniated into the scrotum.

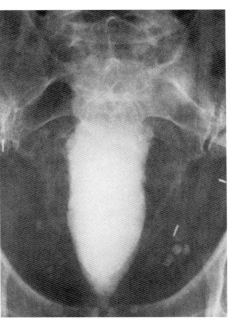

Fig. 35.**43   Pelvic carcinomatosis** secondary to prostatic carcinoma. Extrinsic compression and elongation of the bladder is caused by extensive pelvic metastases and secondary edema.

Fig. 35.**44   Pelvic hematoma.** Elevation and elongation of the narrowed bladder by a large hematoma, resulting from multiple pelvic and sacral fractures, are seen.

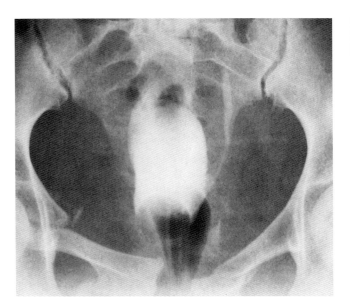

Table 35.5   Abnormal Urethra

Disease	Radiographic Findings	Comments
Posterior urethral valves (males) (Fig. 35.45)	Dilatation of the posterior urethra down to the level of the urogenital membrane.	Majority diagnosed in newborn period. In less severe forms it may become manifest in childhood or adolescence with urinary tract infection, hematuria, enuresis, or incontinence. Anterior urethral valves in males and valves in females are rare.
Enlarged verumontanum	Round to oval filling defect in prostatic urethra, but rarely causes obstruction.	Congenital or acquired (benign hypertrophy or secondary to infection: verumontanitis).
Ureterocele (ectopic)	May occasionally prolapse through the bladder neck into posterior urethra, producing a filling defect with some degree of obstruction.	Ectopic ureteroceles are almost always associated with a duplicated system, the ureterocele arising from the ureter draining the upper segment. Prolapse of the ureterocele occurs during voiding, either intermittently or chronically.
Bladder neck obstruction (Fig. 35.46)	Small, narrowed bladder neck, occasionally with anterior or posterior indentation, diaphragm, or collar formation at the bladder neck opening and failure of funneling during voiding.	Controversial entity that may be congenital or acquired. Postulated causes include: 1 muscle hypertrophy, 2 fibrous ring, 3 chronic inflammation, 4 bladder neck dyskinesia.
Spasm of external sphincter (neurogenic bladder) (Fig. 35.47)	Saccular or funnel-shaped dilatation of the prostatic urethra, with the widest portion at the bladder neck.	Associated with hypertonic neurogenic bladder. *Pseudosphincter* formation between the internal and external sphincters may have a radiographically similar appearance.

(continues on page 834)

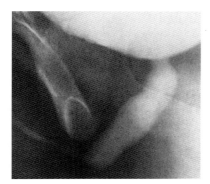

Fig. 35.**45**   **Posterior urethral valve.** Marked dilatation of the posterior urethra is seen.

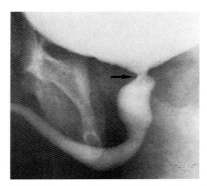

Fig. 35.**46**   **Bladder neck obstruction.** A dilated bladder with collar formation around the bladder neck is seen (arrow).

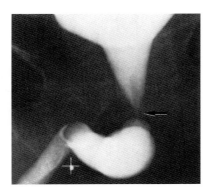

Fig. 35.**47**   **Spasm of external sphincter in neurogenic bladder.** Localized circumferential narrowing in the posterior urethra is caused by spastic external sphincter (arrow). Note also the characteristic funnel-shaped prestenotic dilatation of the urethra.

Table 35.5 (Cont.) Abnormal Urethra

Disease	Radiographic Findings	Comments
Incompetence of external sphincter (neurogenic bladder) (Fig. 35.48)	Smooth widening of prostatic and membranous urethra associated with incontinent neurogenic bladder.	*External sphincterotomy* produces a similar radiographic appearance.
Prostatectomy (Fig. 35.49)	Irregular cavitary widening of prostatic urethra.	Bladder incontinence is present when external sphincter is also involved.
Prostatic utricle (Müllerian duct remnant)	Normally not visualized, or seen as a small pit at the center of the verumontanum or as a narrow outpouching posterior to prostatic urethra extending toward the bladder. Enlargement may be congenital or secondary to distal urethral obstruction (Müllerian duct cyst).	The utricle is a rudiment of the Müllerian ducts in the male, corresponding to the upper vagina and uterus in the female.
Prostatic hypertrophy (Fig. 35.50)	Elongated prostatic urethra. Anterior tilting of proximal urethra with middle lobe enlargement, often associated with a filling defect (enlarged subcervical prostate) causing the contrast to flow around it (Y-effect). Lateral lobe enlargement compresses the urethra from the side, producing a slitlike appearance in the frontal and a widened, saberlike appearance in the lateral projection.	Benign prostatic hypertrophy is the most common cause of urethral obstruction in elderly males.
Prostatic carcinoma	Prostatic urethra irregularly narrowed in all projections without angulation and elongation.	Carcinoma and benign prostatic hypertrophy are frequently associated. In these cases, the radiographic findings are often more characteristic of the latter condition.
Acute prostatitis	Narrowed, elongated, and straightened prostatic urethra, often with tread-like appearance.	Acute inflammation of the prostate is caused most often by *Escherichia coli* or *Staphylococcus*.
Prostatic abscess	Prostatic cavity varying from several millimeters to several centimeters with usually fairly smooth walls.	If the abscess does not communicate with the urethra, radiographic findings are indistinguishable from benign prostatic hypertrophy.
Chronic prostatitis (Fig. 35.51)	Narrowing and straightening of the prostatic urethra. Opacification of dilated prostatic ducts is characteristic, but only present in a minority of cases.	A common clinical entity, affecting 35% of men over 35 years of age. Symptoms are nonspecific and include low backache, frequency, burning on urination, hematospermia, and decreased potentia. Prostate is normal or small.
Tuberculous prostatitis (Fig. 35.52)	Filling of greatly dilated prostatic ducts and cavity formations in a more advanced stage are characteristic. Calcifications are common but indistinguishable from ordinary prostatic calculi.	Usually associated with tuberculosis elsewhere in the urogenital tract.
Polyps and benign tumors (Fig. 35.53)	Round or oval filling defects, preferentially in posterior urethra. May change position when pedunculated. Stalk can occasionally be identified	*Condylomata acuminata* may present as multiple sessile filling defects, which may spread to the bladder and are almost always associated with cutaneous condylomata.
Carcinoma	Irregular narrowing or urethra, often with contrast extravasation into the tumor.	Rare. Majority are epidermoid carcinomas, but transitional cell carcinomas and adenocarcinomas occur also.
Metastases	*Direct invasion* from bladder, prostate, or rectum. Posterior urethra is involved. *Canalicular spread*: carcinoma of bladder or prostate. *Hematogenous spread*: to corpora cavernosa penis (often multiple) with secondary invasion of the anterior urethra (from kidney, lung, testis, and colon).	Metastases are more common in the urethra than primary carcinomas.

(continues on page 836)

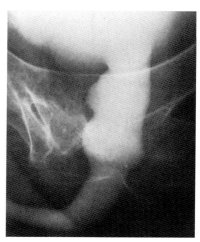

Fig. 35.**48** **Incompetence of external sphincter in neurogenic bladder.** An incontinent bladder with dilated urethra is seen. The same radiographic finding can also be found after external sphincterotomy.

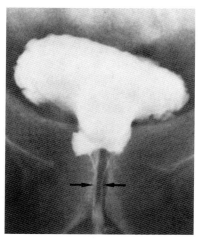

Fig. 35.**49** **Transurethral prostatectomy.** Irregular widening of the proximal prostatic urethra is seen. Prostatic regeneration again causes obstruction of the distal prostatic urethra, where the contrast outlines in two thin lines a filling defect caused by regenerating prostatic tissue (arrows).

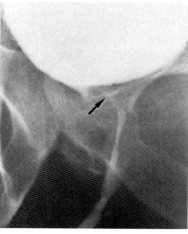

Fig. 35.**50** **Benign prostatic hypertrophy.** Elongation and narrowing of the prostatic urethra in this oblique projection is caused by lateral lobe enlargement, whereas the anterior tilting at the bladder neck (arrow) suggests median lobe hypertrophy.

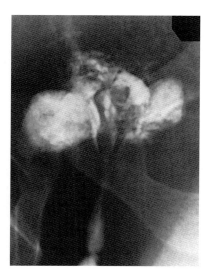

Fig. 35.**51** **Chronic prostatitis.** Narrowing of the prostatic urethra with extensive contrast material reflux into the dilated prostatic ducts is seen.

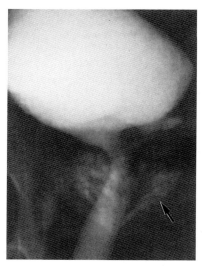

Fig. 35.**52** **Tuberculous prostatitis.** Contrast reflux into irregularly dilated prostatic ducts is seen. Note also the opacification of a Cowper's gland (arrow).

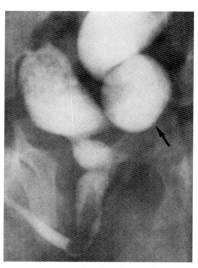

Fig. 35.**53** **Urethral polyp.** A long filling defect is seen in the posterior urethra. Note also the contrast reflux into the massively dilated left ureter (arrow).

Table 35.5   (Cont.) Abnormal Urethra

Disease	Radiographic Findings	Comments
Urethritis (Fig. 35.54)	No radiologic abnormalities in acute episode. Secondary changes in chronic urethritis include irregularities of urethral lumen and stricture formations. Littre's glands (tiny, often slightly irregular dots on the dorsal aspect of the penile urethra), Cowper's glands and ducts which originate from the bulbous urethra, extend parallel to it on its posterior side and terminate in a pair of round or oval shaped glands (see Figs. 35.52 and 35.55), prostatic ducts, ejaculatory ducts, and seminal vesicles may all retrogradely opacify with contrast medium in chronic urethritis. Occasionally periurethral abscesses with smooth or serrated margins can be visualized, located usually in the bulbous or membranous urethra.	Caused by gonococcus, or a variety of nonspecific bacterial, viral, fungal, or protozoan infections. Usually symptomatic in males, but often asymptomatic in females. *Reiter's syndrome* consists of nonspecific urethritis, conjunctivitis, mucocutaneous manifestations, and arthritis and is usually seen in young males. *Urethritis cystica.* Rare. Tiny round filling defects in urethra. *Tuberculosis* of the urethra is rare and may present with stricture, abscess, and fistula formation, and is usually associated with a more characteristic involvement of the prostate.
Stricture (Fig. 35.55)	Usually smooth narrowing of urethral lumen of varying length (valvelike, circumferential indentation, or tubular). Multiple strictures occur in about 10%. Preferential location is the bulbomembranous urethra.	Strictures may be congenital (commonly at the external urethral meatus and often associated with hypospadias), inflammatory (gonorrhea, tuberculosis, syphilis, or nonspecific infections), traumatic, postoperative or neoplastic (primary urethral carcinoma or secondary from carcinoma of bladder or prostate). *Amyloidosis* (primary or secondary) may rarely cause a urethral stricture also.
Fistula (Fig. 35.56)	Urethrorectal, urethrocutaneous, urethrovesical (rare), and urethrovaginal fistulas occur. Abnormal communication and luminal opacification of neighboring organs are usually best demonstrated with urethrocystography, but this is not always successful.	Congenital or acquired (secondary to trauma, surgery, inflammatory disease, neoplasm, and radiation therapy).
Perforation and rupture (Figs. 35.57, 35.58)	Contrast extravasation at the site of laceration is diagnostic. In the male, the posterior urethra (prostatic, membranous, or bulbous urethra) is usually involved. Traumatic urethral ruptures are commonly associated with pelvic fractures and bladder injuries. False passages secondary to instrumentation present commonly as irregular tracts with varying lumen diameters, usually located in the bulbous and membranous urethra.	Secondary to instrumentation, foreign bodies, external trauma (including saddle falls), penetrating injuries, or spontaneous in urethral obstruction.

(continues on page 838)

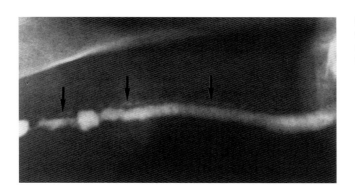

Fig. 35.54   Chronic gonococcal urethritis. Irregularities of the urethral lumen, strictures, and opacification of Littre's glands evident as tiny irregular dots on the dorsal aspect of the penile urethra (arrows) are seen.

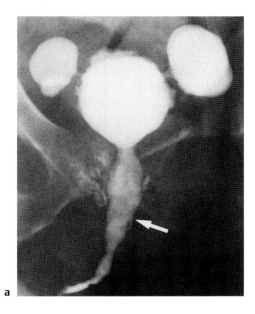

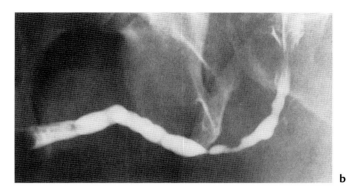

Fig. 35.**55** **Gonorrheal strictures. a** Voiding cystogram. A trabeculated bladder with two bladder diverticula, dilated prostatic urethra, and contrast medium reflux into the prostatic ducts and the duct of a Cowper's gland (arrow) is seen. **b** Retrograde urethrogram: multiple strictures are seen in the anterior urethra, with the most severe involvement found in the bulbous part.

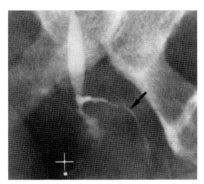

Fig. 35.**56** **Urethral fistula.** An atretic urethra, with a fistulous tract (arrow) connecting the posterior urethra with the rectum, is seen.

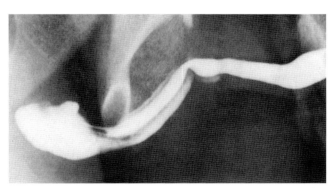

Fig. 35.**57** **Traumatic urethral rupture.** Contrast medium extravasation from the bulbous urethra, tracking along both sides of the urethra, is seen.

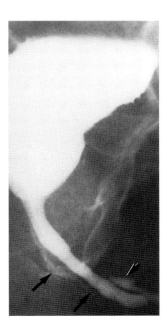

Fig. 35.**58** **False passage secondary to instrumentation.** An irregular contrast-filled cavity (short arrow) is seen in the bulbous urethra just proximal to a short stricture. Note also the opacification of an irregular Cowper's duct and gland (long arrows), which should not be confused with a fistulous tract. The marked dilatation of the bladder neck and prostatic urethra is secondary to prostatectomy.

Table 35.5   (Cont.) Abnormal Urethra

Disease	Radiographic Findings	Comments
Urethrocavernous reflux (Fig. 35.59)	Extravasation of contrast, most commonly in the pendulous and bulbous urethra, is evident as narrow, diffuse dense lines spreading distally and without apparent urethral connection or as extensive, diffuse spreading of contrast on either side of the urethra. Opacification of veins is diagnostic but not always seen.	Occurs during retrograde urethrography or by voiding against obstruction.
Diverticula (Fig. 35.60)	Tubular, round or oval, smooth outpouchings that communicate with the urethra.	Congenital (e.g., Gartner's duct, Wolffian duct) or acquired (secondary to trauma, instrumentation, urethral stones, infection, and stricture). Acquired diverticula are much more common in females.
Calculi and foreign bodies (Fig. 35.61)	Solitary or less common multiple, usually radiopaque filling defects.	Primary calculi are formed in the urethra (usually obstructed and infected), diverticulum, or prostate. A foreign body may be the nidus for encrustation and calculus formation. Secondary calculi are passed from the bladder.
Blood clots and air bubbles	Solitary or multiple, mobile radiolucent filling defects.	Air bubbles are usually iatrogenic and rarely due to pneumaturia.

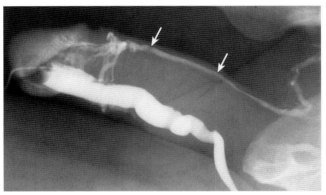

Fig. 35.59 Urethrocavernous reflux. Contrast medium extravasation occurs during retrograde urography with immediate opacification of the dorsal vein of the penis because of spasm of the external urethral sphincter. The finding has no clinical relevancy and should not be confused with a traumatic urethral rupture (see Fig. 35.57).

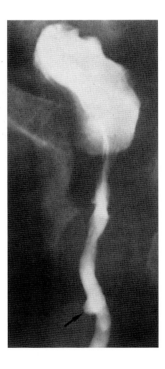

Fig. 35.**60 Posttraumatic diverticulum.** A smooth, round outpouching is seen (arrow). The irregularities in the small bladder and posterior urethra are also secondary to trauma and subsequent surgical repair.

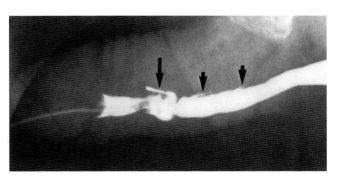

Fig. 35.61 Foreign body. A metallic pen cap (long arrow) is seen in the penile urethra, causing localized irregularities and some narrowing. Note also the two small fistulous tracts more proximally in the urethra (short arrows).

References

General

Burgener FA, Kormano M. Differential Diagnosis in Computed Tomography. Stuttgart: Thieme; 1996.

Burgener FA, Meyers SP, Tan RK, Zaunbauer W. Differential Diagnosis in Magnetic Resonance Imaging. Stuttgart: Thieme; 2002.

Dähnert W. Radiology Review Manual. 5th ed. Baltimore: Williams and Wilkins; 2003.

Damjanow I, ed. Anderson's Pathology. 8th ed. St Louis: Mosby; 1996.

Ebel K-D, Blickmann H. Differential Diagnosis in Pediatric Radiology. Stuttgart: Thieme; 1999.

Federle MP, Megibow AJ, Naidich DP. Radiology of AIDS. New York: Raven Press; 1988.

Goldman L. Cecil's Textbook of Medicine. Philadelphia: Saunders; 2007.

Gray HL, Bannister LH, Williams PL. Gray's Anatomy. Edinburgh: Churchill Livingstone; 2004.

Kasper D. Harrison's Principles of Internal Medicine. New York: McGraw-Hill Co; 2005.

Keats TE, Lusted LB. Atlas of Roentgenographic Measurement. Chicago: Year Book Medical; 2001.

Keats TE. Atlas of Normal Roentgen Variants that May Simulate Disease. St Louis: Mosby; 2001.

Kreel L. Outline of Radiology. London: Heinemann Medical; 1992.

Kuhn J. Caffey's Pediatric Diagnostic Imaging. Chicago: Year Book Medical; 2003.

Kumar V, Cotran RS, Collins SL. Robbins Pathologic Basis of Disease. Philadelphia: Saunders; 2005.

Meschan I. Analysis of Roentgen Signs in General Radiology. Philadelphia: Saunders; 1973.

Mims C. Medical Microbiology. London: Elsevier Science; 2004.

Reeder MM. Reeder and Felson's Gamuts in Radiology. New York: Springer; 2003.

Reeders JW, Mathieson JR. Imaging in AIDS. Philadelphia: Saunders; 1974.

Sutton D. A Textbook of Radiology and Imaging. Edinburgh: Churchill Livingstone; 2002.

Swischuk LE. Imaging of the Newborn, Infant and Young Child. Baltimore: Williams and Wilkins; 2003.

Taybi H, Lachman RS. Radiology of Syndromes, Metabolic Disorders. Chicago: Mosby; 1997.

Townsend C. Sabiston Textbook of Surgery: The Biological Basis of Modern Surgical Practice. Philadelphia: Saunders; 2004.

Bone

Browner B. Skeletal Trauma. Philadelphia: Elsevier Science; 2003.

Freyschmidt J, et al. Borderlands of Normal and Early Pathological Findings in Skeletal Radiography. Stuttgart: Thieme; 2003.

Greenspan A, Duprey L. Orthopedic Imaging: A Practical Approach. Philadelphia: Lippincott; 2004.

Resnick D. Diagnosis of Bone and Joint Disorders. Philadelphia: Saunders; 2002.

Resnick D, Kransdorf MJ. Bone and Joint Imaging. Philadelphia: Saunders; 2005.

Stoller DW, Tirman PFJ, Bredella M. Diagnostic Imaging Orthopaedics. Salt Lake City: Amirsys; 2004.

Chest

Felson B. Chest Roentgenology. Philadelphia: Saunders; 1999.

Fraser RS, Müller NL, Coleman NC, Paré PD. Fraser and Paré's Diagnosis of Diseases of the Chest. Philadelphia: Saunders; 1999.

Müller NL, Fraser RS, Coleman NC, Paré PD. Radiologic Diagnosis of Diseases of the Chest. Philadelphia: Saunders; 2001.

Reed JC. Chest Radiology: Patterns and Differential Diagnosis. Chicago: Year Book Medical; 2003.

Singleton EB, Wagner ML, Dutton RV. Radiologic Alas of Pulmonary Abnormalities in Children. Philadelphia: Saunders; 1988.

Webb WR, Müller NL, Naidich DF. High Resolution CT of the Lung. Philadelphia: Lippincott; 2000.

Abdomen

Davidson AJ, Hartman DS, Choyke PL, Wagner BJ. Davidson's Radiology of the Kidney and Genitourinary Tract. Philadelphia: Saunders; 1998.

Eisenberg RL. Gastrointestinal Radiology: A Pattern Approach. Philadelphia: Lippincott; 2003.

Frimann-Dahl J. Roentgen Examination in Acute Abdominal Diseases. 3rd ed. Springfield, IL: Thomas; 1974.

Levine MS, Rubesin SE, Laufer I. Double Contrast Intestinal Radiology. Philadelphia: Saunders; 1999.

Margulis AR, Burhenne HJ. Alimentary Tract Radiology. 4th ed. St. Louis: Mosby; 1989.

Marshak RH, Lindner AE. Radiology of the Small Intestine. 2nd ed. Philadelphia: Saunders; 1976.

Marshak RH, Lindner AE, Maklansky D. Radiology of the Colon. Philadelphia: Saunders; 1980.

Marshak RH, Lindner AE, Maklansky D. Radiology of the Stomach. Philadelphia: Saunders; 1983.

McCort JJ, Mindelzun RE, Filpi RG, Rennell C. Abdominal Radiology. Baltimore: Williams and Wilkins; 1981.

Meyers MA. Dynamic Radiology of the Abdomen: Normal and Pathologic Anatomy. Heidelberg: Springer; 2000.

Ney C, Friedenberg RM. Radiographic Atlas of the Genitourinary System. Philadelphia: Lippincott; 1981.

Pollack HM, Mc Clennan BL, Dyer RB, Kenney PJ. Clinical Urography. Philadelphia: Saunders; 2001.

Singleton EB, Wagner ML, Dutton RV. Radiology of the Alimentary Tract in Infants and Children. Philadelphia: Saunders; 1997.

Skucas J. Advanced Imaging of the Abdomen. Heidelberg: Springer; 2006.

Index

Page numbers in **italics** refer to illustrations